Self-Medication

Reference for Health Professionals

Volume One

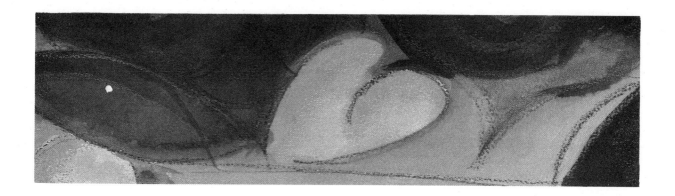

FOURTH EDITION

CANADIAN PHARMACEUTICAL ASSOCIATION

Self-Medication

Reference for Health Professionals

Volume One

FOURTH EDITION

Published By
Canadian Pharmaceutical Association
Ottawa, Ontario, Canada

Director of Publication and Professional Services
Carmen M.E. Krogh, B.Sc.Pharm.

Editorial Division
Patricia Carruthers-Czyzewski, BScPhm, MSc (Pharmacology), *Editor*
Louise Travill, B.S.P., *Associate Editor*
Robin McIntosh, B.A., *Assistant Editor*
Dianne Letwin, Med.Sec., *Administrative Assistant*

Production Division
Dick Logan, *Design and Production Director*
Kathleen Cullis, *Typesetting Supervisor*
Andrew Webber, *Typesetter/Programmer*
Elizabeth Iles, Lucienne Prévost, Brian Proulx and Marilyn Birtwistle, *Typesetters*

Information Service
Monique Holmes, *Manager*
Kathleen Kearns, *Coordinator*
Darquise Leblanc, *Assistant*

The editors gratefully acknowledge the assistance of Roxanne Bisson, Claire Gillis, Angèle Gobeil, Suzanne Krogh, Angèle Leroux, Debbie Mallette, Rita Tremblay and Louise Welbanks in the production of this edition.

For information on electronic applications, contact the Canadian Pharmaceutical Association.

Copyright, 1992
by the Canadian Pharmaceutical Association/
Association pharmaceutique canadienne
ISBN: 0-919115-33-0 Set
ISBN: 0-919115-38-1 Volume 1

First Edition 1980
Reprinted 1981, 1983
Second Edition 1985
Third Edition 1988

Published by Canadian Pharmaceutical Association
1785 Alta Vista Drive
Ottawa, Ontario, Canada
K1G 3Y6

Tel. (613) 523-7877
Fax (613) 523-9445

Illustrations by Mary Trafford
Index by Editor's Ink
Printed in Canada by CK Productions, Toronto

Canadian Cataloguing in Publication Data

Main entry under title:
Self-medication: reference for health professionals
4th ed.
First-2nd eds. published under title: Canadian self-medication; 3rd ed., under title:
Self-medication: a reference for health professionals
Includes index.
Includes bibliographical references.
Contents: v. 1. Reference for health professionals.—v. 2. Product information.
ISBN 0-919115-33-0 (Set)—ISBN 0-919115-38-1 (v. 1)—ISBN 0-919115-39-X (v. 2).
ISSN 1188-9284 (applicable to vol. 2 only which will be updated annually)

1. Self-medication. 2. Drugs, Nonprescription. I. Carruthers-Czyzewski, Patricia A., date. II. Travill, Louise, date.
III. McIntosh, Robin, date. IV. Canadian Pharmaceutical Association

RM671.5.C3C35 1992   616.02'4   C92-090401-7

Contents

Chapters

Appendices

Authors

Lesia M. Babiak, B.Sc.Pharm., Pharm.D.
Head, Clinical Research, Therapeutic Areas
Glaxo Canada Inc.
Toronto, Ontario

Marie Berry, B.Sc.(Pharm.), B.A., LL.B.
Vimy Park Pharmacy
Winnipeg, Manitoba

Arthur G. Blouin, Ph.D., C.Psych.
Director of Research
Department of Psychiatry, Ottawa Civic Hospital
Assistant Professor, Faculty of Medicine
University of Ottawa
Ottawa, Ontario

Jane Blouin, Ph.D., C.Psych.
Psychologist, Eating Disorders Clinic
Ottawa Civic Hospital
Assistant Professor, Department of Psychiatry
Faculty of Medicine, University of Ottawa
Ottawa, Ontario

Paul Brisson, M.D., C.S.P.Q., F.R.C.P.C.
Staff, Ottawa General Hospital
Clinical Assistant Professor
Faculty of Medicine, University of Ottawa
Ottawa, Ontario

Glen R. Brown, B.S.P., Pharm.D.
Assistant Director, Clinical
St. Paul's Hospital
Vancouver, British Columbia

R. Frank Chandler, B.Sc.Pharm., M.Sc., Ph.D
Professor of Pharmacy
College of Pharmacy
Dalhousie University
Halifax, Nova Scotia

William R. Cornish, B.Sc.Phm.
Drug Use Evaluation
Department of Pharmacy
Sunnybrook Health Science Centre
North York, Ontario

Patrick S. Farmer, B.S.P., M.Sc., Ph.D.
Associate Professor, College of Pharmacy
Dalhousie University
Halifax, Nova Scotia

Dawn M. Frail, B.Sc.(Pharm.), M.Sc.
Vice President of Pharmacy
Lawtons Drugs
Dartmouth, Nova Scotia

Kathleen F. Gesy, B.S.P.
Pharmacist
Royal University Hospital
Saskatoon, Saskatchewan

Linda R. Hensman, B.Sc.(Pharm.), Pharm.D.
Director of Pharmacy
St. Clare's Mercy Hospital
St. John's, Newfoundland

**Shirley A. Heschuk, B.Sc.(Pharm.),
  M.Sc.(Pharmacology)**
Sessional Lecturer
Professional Practice Coordinator
Faculty of Pharmacy and Pharmaceutical Sciences
University of Alberta
Edmonton, Alberta

Debra A. Kent, Pharm.D.
Program Supervisor, Education
B.C. Drug and Poison Information Centre
Clinical Assistant Professor
Faculty of Pharmaceutical Sciences
University of British Columbia
Vancouver, British Columbia

Robert A. Locock, B.Sc., M.Sc., Ph.D.
Associate Professor
Faculty of Pharmacy and Pharmaceutical Sciences
University of Alberta
Edmonton, Alberta

Lily Lum, B.Sc.Pharm.
Drug Information Pharmacist
Ontario College of Pharmacists
Drug Information Centre
Toronto, Ontario

Brenda J. McBean Cochran, B.Sc.Pharm., M.Sc.Pharm.
Consumer Health Education Consultant—BMC Health
  Associates
Sessional Lecturer—College of Pharmacy
Dalhousie University
Halifax, Nova Scotia

Betsy Miller, BScPharm
Regulatory Affairs Associate
Ortho-McNeil, Inc.
Don Mills, Ontario

Penny F. Miller, B.Sc.(Pharm.), M.A.
Senior Instructor, Faculty of Pharmaceutical Sciences
Clinical Pharmacist, Department of Family Practice
University of British Columbia
Vancouver, British Columbia

Louis A. Pagliaro, M.S., Pharm.D., Ph.D., F.A.B.M.P.
Professor, Department of Educational Psychology
University of Alberta
Edmonton, Alberta

William A. Parker, B.Sc.Pharm., Pharm.D., M.B.A.
Associate, Shoppers Drug Mart
Sessional Lecturer, Dalhousie University
Halifax, Nova Scotia

Sanna G. Pellatt, B.Sc.(Pharm.)
Pharmacist, B.C. Cancer Agency, Vancouver Clinic
Clinical Instructor, Faculty of Pharmaceutical Sciences
University of British Columbia
Vancouver, British Columbia

Laura-Lynn Pollock, B.Sc.(Pharm.)
Clinical Pharmacist Consultant
Victoria, British Columbia

Michel Quesnel, B.Sc., B.Sc.Pharm., L.Ph.
Associate, Jean Coutu
Hull, Québec

Debra J. Ricciatti-Sibbald, B.Sc.Phm.
President, Debary Dermatologicals
Mississauga, Ontario
Tutor, Faculty of Pharmacy, University of Toronto
Toronto, Ontario

Glenwood H. Schoepp, B.S.P
Manager, St. Anthony's Clinic Pharmacy
Victoria, British Columbia

Yvonne M. Shevchuk, B.S.P., Pharm.D.
Associate Professor of Pharmacy
College of Pharmacy
University of Saskatchewan
Saskatoon, Saskatchewan

Keith Simons, B.Sc.(Pharm.), M.Sc., Ph.D.
Professor
Faculty of Pharmacy
University of Manitoba
Winnipeg, Manitoba

Linda G. Suveges, B.S.P., M.Sc., Ph.D.
Associate Professor
College of Pharmacy
University of Saskatchewan
Saskatoon, Saskatchewan

Jeffrey G. Taylor, M.Sc.
Assistant Professor
College of Pharmacy
University of Saskatchewan
Saskatoon, Saskatchewan

Michael G. Tierney, M.Sc.
Assistant Director, Drug Consultation Services
Pharmacy Department
Ottawa General Hospital
Ottawa, Ontario

Lynn Torsher, BSc.Pharm.
Drug Information/Staff Pharmacist
Children's Hospital of Eastern Ontario
Ottawa, Ontario

Lynn R. Trottier, B.Sc.(Pharm.)
Acting Assistant Director, Patient Care, Education &
  Research
University Hospital, UBC Site
Clinical Assistant Professor, Part-time
Faculty of Pharmaceutical Sciences
University of British Columbia
Adjunct Professor, Gerontology Program
Simon Fraser University
Vancouver, British Columbia

David S. Wing, B.S.P., M.S.
Coordinator of Outpatient Pharmacy and Research
Foothills Hospital
Calgary, Alberta

Irene Worthington, B.Sc.Phm.
Drug Information Pharmacist
Ontario College of Pharmacists
Drug Information Centre
Toronto, Ontario

Dale E. Wright, B.S.P., M.Sc.(Pharmacol.)
Consultant Pharmacist
Calgary, Alberta

Foreword

Patricia Carruthers-Czyzewski, BScPhm, MSc (Pharmacology)
Editor

While this edition of *Self-Medication* builds largely upon the 3rd edition, it also introduces a whole new concept for the publication. The reference is now presented in two volumes to allow for easy retrieval of the information. *Volume 1* summarizes the scientific and technical information which provides the rationale for treatment of specific self-limiting ailments. *Volume 2* focuses on product information thereby complementing the scientific information contained in *Volume 1*.

The information in *Volume 1* has been updated by original authors wherever possible. The algorithms depicted in many of the chapters provide an overview of the individual topic and serve as a therapeutic guide for the professional.

The major change for this edition is *Volume 2*. It is designed as an easy-to-use reference, to be updated annually. As new products are introduced on the Canadian market, this annual supplement will allow us to bring you the most up-to-date product information. I wish to acknowledge the Nonprescription Drug Manufacturers Association of Canada for their support of this concept. We particularly wish to recognize the manufacturers who have committed resources and time to the development of this volume by highlighting their specific products. Their participation in this new venture recognizes the need for an up-to-date, centralized source of information on products for self-medication. Furthermore, this sharing of information encourages the safe and effective use of consumer products.

The extensive product tables which are included in *Volume 2* provide an overview of products available for the treatment of a specific problem. The cooperation of the Bureau of Pharmaceutical Surveillance of the Drugs Directorate, Health and Welfare Canada, in adapting their publication, *Canadian Drug Identification Code,* made it possible to collate the product table information. Their assistance is gratefully acknowledged. A tremendous amount of work by professional and technical staff at CPhA was required to bring these tables together.

I am grateful to have worked on this project with Robin McIntosh and Louise Travill who literally "picked up where I left off". Their hard work and perseverance ensured the successful completion of the book. The efforts of other CPhA publication staff members who contributed their time, when the help was needed, is very much appreciated. It was certainly a team effort.

And team work is exactly what is needed to contribute positively to the health practices of consumers. Professionals, consumers and manufacturers need to work together to achieve maximum benefits from self-medicating products. The sharing of information ensures professionals are better prepared to meet the needs of a more increasingly sophisticated consumer. This edition is one of many significant tools required for this challenge.

1

Consumer Counselling

Brenda J. McBean Cochran

A step-by-step counselling guide describes the art of questioning, assessing symptoms and medical history, selecting a suitable product, counselling on products and non-pharmacologic approaches, and encouraging appropriate follow-up. Discussions of non-verbal communication and special counselling situations—such as dealing with potentially embarrassing subjects, talkative consumers or the hearing-impaired consumer—complete the chapter.

Advising on self-medication can be a complex process, especially when one considers the amount of information that needs to be exchanged between a pharmacist and consumer. In most cases, pharmacists need a thorough description of the problem before advice can be given. And when self-medication is indicated, consumers need information about the safe and effective use of nonprescription products. Considering the workload in most pharmacies, the pharmacist must be able to perform these activities in a reasonable amount of time.

During the past several decades, scientists studying communication and learning behavior have contributed much knowledge that applies to self-care counselling. An understanding of information-gathering skills, adult education principles and the influence of non-verbal behavior can help the pharmacist make the most productive use of time available for counselling. Some situations, such as potentially embarrassing discussions, require special communication awareness and skills so both the pharmacist and consumer are comfortable discussing a health problem.

The Pharmacist and Self-Care

Self-care may be broadly defined as "all the things that people do to protect, maintain or improve their own health." Within this context, self-treatment refers to the process of selecting suitable drug and nondrug measures for the prevention and treatment of diseases or symptoms. About 85 per cent of symptoms are self-treated, and of all "ill" people, about 30 per cent are known to use nonprescription drugs. Although valid reasons exist for self-medication, unwise reliance on this form of treatment may result in inaccurate or delayed diagnosis of significant disease, adverse drug-drug or drug-disease interactions, unnecessary adverse reactions and risks, and/or delayed treatment with more effective measures.

Pharmacists are given sole jurisdiction over many nonprescription drugs on the basis that they will provide responsible advice and control over their use. For each request, the pharmacist must help the consumer decide the best course of action. Recommendation choices include: referral for medical opinion; self-treatment with nonprescription drugs, nonpharmacologic measures or both; or reassurance that no intervention is necessary. This decision-making process should not be confused with diagnosis. Although pharmacists are trained extensively in pharmacology, they are not expected to have the knowledge or skills to medically diagnose a problem. They must, however, be able to screen individual symptoms and exclude certain diagnoses before recommending self-treatment.

There are guidelines to help pharmacists fulfil this responsibility. Following the initial work of an ad hoc committee of the Canadian Pharmaceutical Association (CPhA), a task force of the association was formed in 1983 to help pharmacists respond to questions from consumers and to establish criteria for referring consumers for medical attention. A number of broad guidelines were developed by this committee, many based on a comprehensive report by the Pharmaceutical Society of Great Britain. Figure 1 summarizes the task force recommendation. These guidelines, along with the right communication and interviewing skills, should help the pharmacist meet the needs of individual consumers in an effective, efficient and comfortable manner.

Information-Gathering Communication Skills

Most, if not all, self-care counselling requires assessment of an individual's problem. The importance of effective information-gathering skills cannot be overemphasized, especially when one considers that consumers' self-reports are often the sole basis for recommending a course of action.

Pharmacist inquiries can range from simple questions, such as determining someone's age, to more involved problems such as defining what is meant by "stomach upset." Although this process may seem straightforward, experience and research show the quality of information received from consumers is not always the best. The way a pharmacist asks a question influences the accuracy, breadth and depth of this information. For example, to the question "Do you use any other drugs?" people may respond with an emphatic "no!" if they think the pharmacist is referring to street drugs, or if they do not consider nonprescription items to be drugs.

The effective use of information-gathering skills can improve the questioning process. Often called "probes," information-gathering skills may be defined as "virtually any behavior that elicits a response from the other person." For the purpose of this discussion, these skills

Consumer Counselling

Figure 1 *Pharmacists' Responses to the Self-Medicating Consumer*

A	B	C

I General principles

The standard of care
When responding to the self-medicating consumer, a pharmacist is able to assess those presenting symptoms to determine the most appropriate action:
• refer for medical opinion
• recommend nonprescription drug and/or nonpharmacologic treatment
• reassure the consumer that no treatment is necessary at that time.

Regarding a medical diagnosis
A pharmacist does not have the knowledge, skills nor training to make a medical diagnosis. However, he or she should be able to differentiate between those symptoms indicative of a serious condition and those treatable by obtaining symptomatic relief.

Consumer/Pharmacist communications
To achieve effective communication with consumers, a pharmacist must consider:
• developing a systematic approach when responding to a request for advice
• establishing an appropriate degree of privacy
• eliminating physical barriers
• phrasing the technical information in nontechnical terms.
• establishing good eye contact and understanding the meaning of body language.

II Screening
A pharmacist is able to review a variety of factors and symptoms to judge when to refer consumers to a practitioner or when to suggest self-treatment.

General factors
The following are to be considered whenever a pharmacist is determining how to respond to a request for advice:
• age
• sex
• allergies
• general health of the individual and the clustering of several symptoms
• other medication being taken
• pregnancy
• lactation
• previous medical diagnosis for these symptoms
• duration of symptoms.

Referral for medical advice
Consumers with the following symptoms or conditions should be immediately referred for medical advice as these symptoms are strongly associated with a serious health condition.
CAUTION: This list is not exhaustive. Other symptoms should be evaluated especially when associated with a General Factor.
• anorexia
• loss of blood from any orifice
• yellowing of the skin
• increasing breathlessness
• any discharge from the penis or vagina
• increased urinary frequency
• pain upon urination
• swelling and/or lumps of any size, including those around the joints
• persistent or recurrent fever, cough and/or hoarseness
• skin or mouth conditions that fail to heal or change in size
• loss of weight
• spontaneous bruising
• ankle swelling
• unusual changes in the sputum, particularly if it is yellow or green
• discoloration of urine
• menstrual abnormalities
• difficulty in swallowing
• severe pain in the chest, abdomen, head or ears
• diarrhea, particularly with infants
• reduced ability to see, hear or taste.

Responding to symptoms
The following symptoms are often associated with minor or self-limiting conditions and frequently respond to a specific regimen of self-treatment by the consumer. When recommending self-medication, a pharmacist is able to give advice on the dosage, storage, administration, adverse effects and precautions associated with the particular medications recommended.
CAUTION: These symptoms may be part of a more serious condition and pharmacists must vigilantly assess them in light of "General Factors".
• insomnia
• fever
• common cold
• diarrhea
• foot problems, warts, corns
• symptoms of the eye, ear or mouth
• burns
• headache
• sinus congestion
• constipation
• pain
• rash, itching of skin
• allergic symptoms
• fatigue.

III Evaluating results
When medications are recommended, a pharmacist is able to suggest a time period within which the suggested treatment should be effective along with a reassessment or referral at that time.
Special considerations: A pharmacist is to emphasize the following points:

Symptomatic treatment should never be continued for more than a few days.

Repeated use of symptomatic medications may mask serious conditions.

Any adverse change in the original symptoms could indicate a more serious underlying condition that should be reported to the physician.

Adapted from: "Pharmacists' responses to the self-medicating patient," (Draft). Ottawa: Canadian Pharmaceutical Association, 1985.

are addressed under the general headings of questioning techniques and facilitation.

Questioning Techniques
Closed-Ended Questions

Also referred to as direct or specific questions, closed-ended questions are those which ask for a specific piece of information and which limit the answer options of the patient. Although it may not be the questioner's intention, closed-ended questions often restrict answers to "yes" or "no". For example, "Have you had the pain long?" and "Are you nauseated?" are two closed-ended questions that might be used to assess the need for medical referral.

Although there are times when closed-ended questions are helpful, their routine use is discouraged for several reasons.

First, because closed-ended questions seek specific information, a series of such questions may be needed to get the necessary information, adding to the time it takes to assess an individual's symptoms.

Second, the pharmacist is more likely to miss potentially significant information about the complaint. The restrictive or rapid-fire nature of these questions can create an air of interrogation, which causes many people to become passive or "closed" in their communication. If the pharmacist neglects to ask about a particular aspect of a condition, the subsequent decision may be based on incomplete data.

Third, many closed-ended questions leave the pharmacist unsure of what the response means. For example, a "yes" to the question "Do you know how to use this product?" does not tell the pharmacist what the consumer knows. The pharmacist must then rephrase or ask additional questions to ensure the individual has appropriate information.

Fourth, people can respond to some closed-ended questions without really knowing the answer. For example, an individual may answer "no" to the question "Do you have any allergies?" simply to avoid having to say "I don't know." Similarly, closed questions allow people to give an answer they think the pharmacist wants to hear, or to avoid discussing a potentially uncomfortable topic. "Do you drink much alcohol?" elicits a "no" from many people, a response that may or may not be accurate.

Open-Ended Questions

The best information is usually obtained with open-ended questions. In contrast to the closed format, these questions cannot be answered "yes" or "no" and usually require a response of more than a few words. Open-ended questions are often built around the words "what" or "how", and the topic is normally specified in broad terms. "What symptoms are you experiencing?" and "How do you normally use this product?" are examples of two open-ended questions used in self-care counselling.

Initially, open-ended questions may be more difficult to formulate, and a certain skill is required to minimize repetitive, confused or unimportant responses. With practice, however, these questions can provide a significant amount of information with minimal effort. Their use is encouraged for several reasons.

First, because open-ended questions are nonrestrictive, consumers may spontaneously provide all information the pharmacist needs to make an appropriate recommendation.

Second, the open format increases the possibility of obtaining unsolicited information about a condition. For example, an individual may reveal details that the pharmacist would not have addressed with the closed format, or a response may provide clues to other questions that should be asked.

Third, open-ended questions encourage people to talk with minimum guidance and input from the pharmacist, allowing the practitioner more time to listen and observe. This is especially important in self-care counselling where observation may reveal important details about an individual's condition.

Fourth, because the open format allows people to express symptoms in their own words, the pharmacist will be able to use similar terminology and avoid words that might alarm or antagonize someone. The pharmacist can also assess the consumer's current level of knowledge and focus counselling efforts on gaps or misconceptions in that person's understanding.

Finally, open-ended questions are easier to answer because respondents can do so from their own point of reference. This consideration is particularly helpful with nontalkative people, although some studies suggest that for all people, the more an individual is allowed to speak, the more successful the interview. Similarly, the open format conveys a willingness to listen, a factor likely to promote a positive and ongoing relationship with the consumer.

Despite these advantages, open-ended questions should not be used exclusively. As described later, most successful interviews use a combination of open-ended and closed-ended questions.

Follow-up Questions

An initial question may not provide the specific information being sought. Follow-up or secondary questions are then needed. These questions seek more detail in a specific area and indicate a larger perspective is required. For example, questions such as "In what way do you feel worse?" or "Can you tell me more about how the medication affected you?" are helpful when the response to an initial question—whether open or closed—is incomplete, vague or suggests a problem area. As these examples illustrate, follow-up questions are usually asked in relatively general terms. Even though some can be answered "yes" or "no", they imply the need for more than a one-word answer.

Multiple Questions   Avoid

A common pitfall in assessment is the multiple question. These are questions with more than one point of inquiry ("How long have you been taking this, and has it helped?") or that ask for more than one item of information ("Do you have any vision changes, stomach upset or dizziness?"). Multiple questions should always be avoided. They are confusing, as people do not know how, or to which portion, they should respond. Similarly, when answered, the pharmacist may not be sure to which part the respondent is referring, and the efficiency of the interview decreases. In addition, people often answer only one part of the question, and important information may be lost as other parts are forgotten.

Leading Questions   Avoid

Another pitfall is leading the consumer. Leading questions are a form of the closed question that strongly imply a desired answer. Questions such as "You take your blood pressure pills all the time, don't you?" and "The pain isn't worse after meals, is it?" can be threatening, and leave little room for disagreement by the respondent. Leading questions should always be avoided.

Why Questions

Questions beginning with "why" should also be avoided. Although the intention is usually to get additional information, questions like "Why didn't you tell your doctor about this?" and "Why didn't you follow the directions?" can put respondents on the defensive by implying that they must justify their behavior. "Why" questions are almost impossible to answer completely and can result in a response that becomes complicated even for a highly trained psychologist. Because the pharmacist has little control over a person's answer, the efficiency of the discussion is reduced. Alternatives to "why" questions are those using "what", "how" or "was there a special reason" in place of "why".

Facilitation

Other approaches for obtaining information fall under the broad heading of facilitation. Defined as "the purposeful encouragement to continue talking," facilitation techniques are nondirective and can include any manner, gesture or word that encourages people to say more about a particular topic. Reflection and attentive silence are particularly helpful for guiding a discussion without biasing an individual's response.

Reflection

As the name implies, reflection is the technique of "mirroring" or repeating back the last few words of a person's sentence. The words usually take on the inflection of a question, and may simply repeat the area in which a questioner wishes more information. For example, a person may say "I've had this stomach ache for the last few days." Reflection with "stomach ache?" encourages description of that symptom in greater detail.

Reflection is especially useful for nontalkative people, although everyone responds favorably to hearing their own words. As with all facilitation techniques, reflection should not be overused. As a general rule, no more than one or two reflective statements about the same topic are appropriate.

Attentive Silence

Silence is one of the most powerful tools available for obtaining information. Although practitioners—particularly those new to counselling—may be uncomfortable with periods of silence, people often need time to organize their thoughts. Interrupting this silence may destroy the opportunity to get valuable information.

During periods of silence, it is important to "attend" to the other person, as nothing will end a discussion faster than if it appears the pharmacist is not listening. This is usually conveyed nonverbally, with gestures like a nod of the head or leaning forward with an interested, expectant facial expression. Equally effective is the use of encouraging comments such as "hmmm-mmm," or the interjection of "yes" or " I see". These comments are useful alternatives to head-nodding, which tends to be overused. If a person stops talking about a subject on which more information is needed, a simple "Tell me more about that" will encourage further description.

As with reflection, silence must not be used excessively. Too much silence, especially when someone expresses feelings of anxiety or depression, may be interpreted as cold or distant. Similarly, pauses may occur when the listener does not understand a question or comment; the pharmacist must be aware of faulty communication as a cause of silence.

Other communication skills, such as empathy and assertiveness, can help the pharmacist obtain information from a consumer. A description of these skills is beyond the scope of this chapter; the reader is referred to other written material for a comprehensive discussion of these subjects.

Systematic Approach to Self-Care Counselling

According to Dr. Lawrence Weed, father of the problem-oriented medical record, a basic criterion for problem-solving is ". . . how well a clinician can identify patients' problems and organize them for solution". An important interviewing principle can help the pharmacist achieve this goal; counselling will be more successful if the pharmacist uses a pre-planned, structured approach during discussions with consumers. In other words, counselling will be more effective and efficient if the pharmacist has developed a *logical sequence* for questioning and educating patients, and has a *mental image* of the order in which this information ideally is exchanged.

Figure 2 illustrates one such approach for self-care counselling. As with all "structured" interviews, the Systematic Approach is divided into two phases—the information-gathering phase and the recommendation phase. The main purpose of the information-gathering phase is to determine the advisability of self-treatment. Step 1 defines the person's problem. If nonprescription therapy seems appropriate, Step II identifies factors in the medical history that might influence the choice of product. At any point during the information-gathering phase, the pharmacist may also recommend referral to another health professional, or simply provide reassurance

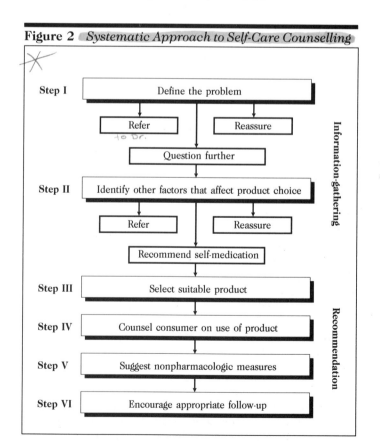

Figure 2 *Systematic Approach to Self-Care Counselling*

Step I — Define the problem

Refer (to Dr.) | Reassure

Question further

Step II — Identify other factors that affect product choice

Refer | Reassure

Recommend self-medication

Information-gathering

Step III — Select suitable product

Step IV — Counsel consumer on use of product

Step V — Suggest nonpharmacologic measures

Step VI — Encourage appropriate follow-up

Recommendation

that treatment is not necessary. When self-treatment is indicated, the pharmacist proceeds to the recommendation phase to select a suitable product (Step III), provide relevant information about that product (Step IV), suggest nonpharmacologic measures (Step V), and/or encourage appropriate follow-up and monitoring of symptoms (Step VI).

Both the broad and specific steps in the Systematic Approach are based on principles of medical interviewing, therapeutic drug monitoring and adult education. At least four reasons can be identified why this type of approach increases productivity of pharmacists' self-care counselling.

First, although the pharmacist may be aware in principle of the questions needed to define a problem, without a predetermined course of action it is easy to become sidetracked and miss potentially significant information. A mental image of the order of information exchange increases the likelihood that all factors are considered before a recommendation is made.

Second, the pharmacist has better control over the flow of information. People seldom articulate their history in a concise, logical manner. Pharmacists who have a clear idea of the information they need at each step are better able to guide the discussion in an orderly fashion.

Third, and equally important, asking questions in a logical order can prevent unnecessary questions. For instance, if the pharmacist determines near the beginning that a backache has persisted more than a few days, or is accompanied by pain on urination, the consumer should be immediately referred to a physician, and the counselling encounter thus ends.

Finally, because information required by consumers is organized into stages in the pharmacist's mind, he or she will be better able to transmit these ideas one at a time. In turn, the educational process will be more effective.

The following sections describe the systematic approach in detail. Examples of questions for assessing symptoms are provided, along with suggestions for wording with which consumers are more familiar. As with any counselling tool, pharmacists must use their own judgment when applying this approach in practice. Although the broad headings are a helpful memory aid, all steps may not apply to each consumer. Based on information in Step 1, for example, the pharmacist may choose simply to reassure a consumer and, skipping Steps II through V, provide advice about appropriate follow-up if the symptoms change in any way (Step VI).

Step I: Define the Problem *may be done by Technician*

The initial task with any request for self-medication is to find out more about the person's problem. Step I has two objectives. First and foremost is the need to rule out more serious health conditions; if the pharmacist cannot be reasonably certain symptoms are self-treatable, individuals should be encouraged to see a doctor. Second, when self-treatment seems appropriate, details in Step I will identify ingredients most likely to help a person's symptoms.

Before symptom-specific questions are asked, 3 introductory steps need to be considered: identity of the person with the complaint; previous recommendations about that complaint; and, in some cases, an explanation of why questions need to be asked.

Check Identity

People often ask for a product on behalf of others. Since the pharmacist's recommendation may depend on who has the symptoms,

missing this step can have time-consuming, if not serious, consequences. For example, a 9 month old infant with diarrhea should be seen by a doctor and knowing the age early in a discussion may eliminate the need for more specific questions.

Identify Previous Recommendations

It is worthwhile near the beginning of a discussion to determine whether other health professionals have been consulted about the symptoms in question. For example, finding out about a second opinion in the early stages may prevent having to explain why the pharmacist suggests a different product than, say, the physician.

Identifying other recommendations also may eliminate the need for additional information. If a physician has recommended a specific product, Steps I through III can likely be omitted and the pharmacist can concentrate on details for the safe and effective use of that product.

At the same time, one must be cautious about automatically attributing symptoms to an alleged previous diagnosis, since other pathological factors might have developed. Additionally, the pharmacist must establish whether other instructions were given at the time of the original diagnosis. For example, some people may have been advised to return to their doctor if symptoms recur or worsen. Closely related people often self-diagnose their ailments and request specific medications based on these self-assessments. The pharmacist must be careful about accepting these assessments at face value and encourage referral if there is any question about the advisability of self-treatment.

Explain Purpose of Further Questions

In some cases, explaining why questions need to be asked may be helpful. People may not have had a pharmacist question them in detail and, if uneasy with this process, are unlikely to give accurate or complete responses.

The explanation should be brief, but may include the amount of time or number of questions to be asked, subjects to be covered, and benefits to the consumer. For example, the statement "To help you find the best treatment for your symptoms, I'll need to ask you a few questions about . . ." is a succinct way of indicating that questions are asked not out of superficial curiosity, but out of a genuine desire to help.

Clarify Symptoms

Although identifying a problem in general terms is straightforward (a "cold" or "stomach upset"), obtaining a thorough description of that problem may be more complex. For example, Table I illustrates 8 categories of questions used in medical history-taking, and Part II of the CPhA guidelines shows other factors that need to be considered when assessing the advisability of self-treatment with nonprescription drugs (see Figure 1).

The best approach for obtaining this information is to gradually restrict the open-endedness of a series of questions. This key principle for any information-gathering situation is especially important when the pharmacist attempts to identify the nature of a medical problem. In practice, this approach can be broken into three distinct stages to help the pharmacist achieve a smooth and efficient flow of information: ask the broadest possible question first; identify all general symptoms; and ask specific questions to fill in gaps.

Ask the broadest question first: For example, when someone asks

Duration or recurring symptoms

for a cold remedy, an appropriate first question might be "What symptoms do you have?" This approach allows people to respond in their own words. In some cases, the pharmacist may be able to make an immediate recommendation on the basis of this information.

Identify all general symptoms: The efficiency of many information-gathering situations can be improved if the next set of questions identifies all general symptoms. For the person with a "cold", the presence or absence of nasal involvement, cough, sore throat, fever, aches or pains should be determined before detailed questions are asked about each symptom. A nonspecific question, such as "Do you have any other symptoms?", is appropriate. Alternatively, the pharmacist may ask directly about symptoms commonly associated with the presenting complaint, or that might suggest the person has something other than a minor, self-limiting condition.

There are four reasons why identifying all symptoms at this stage can decrease counselling time. First, finding out about certain symptoms early in the discussion may eliminate the need for more detail. For example, symptoms listed in Part IIB of the CPhA guidelines strongly suggest more serious health problems, and people describing any of these should be referred for medical advice.

Equally important is clustering of symptoms. As a general rule, the presence of related symptoms is a criterion for referral; again, the pharmacist may save time by obtaining this information near the beginning of a discussion.

Identifying symptoms in a general way also allows the pharmacist to focus next on those more likely to need medical attention. For example, a sore throat is potentially more serious than a stuffy nose and investigating that symptom first may eliminate the need for details about the nasal symptoms.

Finally, identifying all general symptoms allows the pharmacist to begin thinking about ingredients. Although products are not chosen at this stage, the pharmacist can at least forget about those with unnecessary ingredients. For instance, if a cold is confined to the head, products containing expectorants and antitussives can mentally be eliminated from the list of possibilities.

Ask specific questions to fill in gaps: The pharmacist should now have a fairly clear picture of an individual's problem. Some symptoms may however require further elaboration. This stage of assessment is perhaps the most difficult, particularly when complaints are vague or when a substantial amount of information is still needed. Since a goal at this stage is to rule out the need for referral, the most productive questions will be those that help the pharmacist differentiate between serious conditions and ones that are minor or self-limiting.

Of the 8 dimensions in Table I, chronology is the most important. The time required to make a decision about referral can be substantially reduced if the pharmacist asks about the duration of symptoms early in the line of questioning. For example, a headache that has lasted 3 days may indicate serious disease; one that has lasted 2 hours probably does not require immediate medical assessment. Information about recurring symptoms may be equally important. Symptoms that return frequently may indicate a major pathologic condition and should be referred, particularly since the repeated use of symptomatic medications can mask the condition and delay appropriate diagnosis.

The relative importance of the remaining categories in Table I varies with individual symptoms. As with all assessment questions, the ability to elicit this information efficiently requires an understanding of disease states and their presentation. Each chapter in this

Table I *Dimensions of Present Illness*

Chronology	How long has the consumer had the symptom? Has the consumer had this symptom before?
Related symptoms	What other symptoms does the individual have? Is there any clustering of symptoms? What is their chronological relationship to each other?
Bodily location	Where does the symptom occur? Specific questions related to depth, radiation and areas(s) may be needed to localize the symptom.
Quality	How is the symptom described? If pain, is it sharp, dull, constant, throbbing, etc.? Descriptions will range from mild to severe and need to be evaluated in light of temperament.
Quantity	Specific questions about frequency (how often?), size (how big?) and volume (how much?) may be necessary.
Setting	Under what circumstances does the symptom occur? Is it worse (or better) at a particular time of day? Can it be related to factors in environment or lifestyle?
Aggravation or alleviation	Is there anything that makes the symptom worse or that relieves the symptom? What medication has been tried? What were the results?
Possible health-related causes	Does the individual have other health conditions that might explain the current symptoms? Is it a side effect of other medication being taken?

Note: Some diseases do not manifest in all dimensions and others have symptoms not fully covered by these categories. By and large, however, their use in history-taking is reliable and can serve as a guide to the clinician in organizing a description of an illness.

text provides a list of formulated questions to ask about specific conditions. The reader is referred to these as well as basic therapeutic textbooks to develop priorities for the order of questions at this stage.

Referring a Consumer

Although there are no hard and fast rules, the above discussion identifies three guidelines for referral: the presence of symptoms strongly suggesting serious disease; clustering of symptoms; and long-lasting or recurring symptoms. Another consideration is general appearance. If the person with a 2 hour history of headache looks ill, the possibility of a potentially serious condition cannot be excluded and medical assessment should be advised.

These guidelines are not meant to be exhaustive. During discussions with consumers, other considerations of a more general nature may emerge. Some people simply may be seeking encouragement to see a physician; an individual's perception of symptoms must always be taken into account. In other cases, as with acne, referral may be in order when symptoms might respond better to prescribed medication. Finally, a cardinal rule of assessment is to discourage

Consumer Counselling

self-treatment if any uncertainty exists about the cause of the symptom. If the pharmacist cannot reasonably exclude the possibility of a more serious underlying condition, the person must be referred for medical opinion.

A proper referral reflects consideration of three factors: whom the person should see; when the person should be seen; and why referral is recommended. The pharmacist should use both tact and firmness, so the person understands the importance of follow-up without becoming unduly alarmed. Wording similar to the following can be effective in most situations: "From what you have told me, I think it is a good idea (or important) to see your doctor. It may be a simple case of . . . , but it is better to be safe, and I'm sure your doctor would want to see you about this."

People are more likely to follow pharmacists' advice for referral if they understand why they have been referred. If a consumer appears reluctant to bother a doctor for seemingly minor complaints, the importance of having symptoms medically evaluated may need to be stressed. Questions such as "Do you have a regular doctor?", "Can you reach your doctor today (or within an appropriate time frame)?" and "Do you want me to call and explain your symptoms?" may provide needed encouragement.

Step II: Identify Other Factors That Affect Product Choice   *Only by Pharmacist* *step II-VI*

When self-medication seems advisable, the next step is to evaluate other factors in the consumer's history that may affect the choice of product. Depending on the situation, it may be necessary to find out about some or all of the following areas.

Health of the consumer: Are there any other illnesses or health conditions that affect the choice of product? For example, when considering a sympathomimetic, the pharmacist must know if there is a history of diseases like high blood pressure or diabetes. Since conditions such as pregnancy and lactation may affect the choice of product, questions about health should not be restricted to illness or disease.

Other drugs: Is the person taking any other drugs, including nonprescription drugs or home remedies, that may interact with the ingredients being considered? Classic examples include tetracycline for people requesting an antacid and warfarin when acetylsalicylic acid (ASA) is considered.

Allergies and previous adverse effects: Does the person have an allergy to specific ingredients? Has the person had adverse reactions to the product or product category under consideration? For example, people react differently to different antihistamines. Past drowsiness from one may make another choice in this category more appropriate.

Some of this information may have been obtained in Step I. If not, direct or closed-ended questions are usually the most efficient at this stage. These questions may follow an initial broad question, and a technique known as bridging may be useful. For example, when considering an analgesic, the statement "You mentioned you take...Are you taking any other prescription or nonprescription medicines?" can be followed with questions about blood thinners, medicines for gout and other classes of drugs that interact with the product the pharmacist has in mind.

Step III: Select Suitable Product

In the absence of drug or disease interactions, the next step in the systematic approach is to select a suitable product. This process is guided primarily by information obtained in Steps I and II. Another important consideration is the safety and efficacy of products. Many pharmacists evaluate products within a category and have 2 or 3 in mind for each set of symptoms.

Other drug variables, such as dosage form and side effects, should be matched with consumer variables, such as lifestyle or work conditions. A topical decongestant may be more appropriate than an oral antihistamine combination for someone who needs to be alert. Or, children's dosage forms may be better for certain age groups. Because elderly people sometimes have difficulty swallowing, liquid preparations or coated tablets might be more suitable for them.

A person's past experience with a product is also important. By finding out which products have been used, the pharmacist can avoid recommending those found unsuitable in the past. Conversely, if a product gave excellent results in the past, the pharmacist can accept and encourage that choice, as long as other criteria for selection have been met.

Finally, although not a sole criterion, the pharmacist should consider the relative cost of products. Different dosage forms may represent a cost saving, and people will appreciate receiving a less expensive remedy.

Step IV: Counsel Consumer on Use of Product

Although consumers today are relatively well informed, a number of studies suggest errors occur with nonprescription drugs. Often these errors are due to lack of knowledge. Once a product is chosen, the pharmacist must ensure the consumer has sufficient information to use that product in the most beneficial and least toxic manner. Although the type and amount of information varies with each person, five general categories need to be considered: intended benefits; administration instructions; potential side effects; potential interactions; and storage instructions.

For each category the pharmacist's goal is to provide accurate, understandable and practical information. One principle of adult education states that people are more likely to remember and follow advice if they understand the reason for doing so. Therefore the pharmacist should explain the rationale for instructions whenever possible. This explanation not only helps ensure proper use of nonprescription products, but reinforces that these items are drugs and must be used carefully. The time spent educating consumers can be more productive if the pharmacist begins by finding out what is known about a product. This approach allows the pharmacist to identify and correct any misconceptions, and in many cases to avoid unnecessary duplication of information. In accordance with another principle of adult education, new information will have more meaning, because it can be related to what an individual already knows. As well, the pharmacist will be able to use more appropriate terminology, taking cues from words the individual uses.

Intended Benefits

An integral part of nonprescription drug counselling is an explanation of the intended benefits of a product. This usually is as simple as explaining why that product was chosen and, in the case of multiple-ingredient preparations, describing the purpose of each ingredient.

Explanations should be brief, specific to the consumer's problem and in understandable terms. A pharmacist might recommend a combination cold product for nasal congestion and nonproductive cough,

Consumer Counselling

but a person told it contains a sympathomimetic and antitussive seldom learns the benefits of the product. A more meaningful explanation might be as follows: "This ingredient (referring to the package) will help relieve nasal stuffiness, and this one (the antitussive) helps stop coughing so there is less irritation to the throat."

When explaining the choice of product, the pharmacist should also bear in mind the power of the placebo effect. Statements such as "This medicine is often helpful for conditions such as yours" or "This is an excellent product for . . ." go a long way toward relieving symptoms. This approach is particularly important with products that have become so common the public tends to underestimate their efficacy, and with conditions such as pain that have a large psychological component. For similar reasons, the pharmacist should avoid appearing hesitant about a product. Statements like "Well, I guess this might help" do little to inspire confidence in the value of the product.

Consumers should also be told when benefits are likely to appear. Symptom relief may be almost immediate, but products such as bulk-forming laxatives, acne remedies or dandruff treatments do take longer to work. People who expect immediate relief may become prematurely discouraged unless they know what to expect. Also, certain people may need to be cautioned about benefits. For example, masking muscular pain with an analgesic may lead to overactivity of the injured muscle.

Administration Instructions

Nonprescription drugs may be ineffective simply because they are administered improperly. Although most labels give complete instructions, studies show that some people do not read, let alone correctly interpret, this information. In some cases, the print may be too small for the visually impaired, and several studies show that some information is written at a level higher than the average consumer can comprehend. An estimated 5 per cent of Canadians and 18 per cent of those over age 65 are considered functionally illiterate, and these people in particular are unable to interpret written directions.

For these reasons, it is important for the pharmacist to verbally review or supplement package information in some or all of the following areas: the amount per single dose; the number of doses per day; the times of administration; the specific method of administration; and the suggested length of treatment.

The amount per single dose: A review of manufacturers' single-dose recommendations is important. Since consumers tend to view nonprescription drugs as safe and may believe "if one is good, two are better," it is especially important to outline the consequences of exceeding these recommendations. On the other hand, individuals who are sensitive to drugs may be well advised to reduce initial doses when trying new preparations.

Number of doses per day: For similar reasons, the maximum amount of medication that may be taken in a 24-hour period, as well as the suggested interval between doses, needs to be pointed out. Undercompliance, on the other hand, is seldom a problem, as most people are motivated by symptoms to use a nonprescription product. However, the pharmacist may encounter people who take a nonprescription drug for a chronic problem on the advice of their physician. In these cases, the importance of using the medication regularly needs to be stressed. It is best to be extremely specific in this explanation. The following example, which can be adapted for most medical conditions, illustrates a succinct way of conveying information to a person with arthritis: "Some people take ASA only when required for the relief of pain. However, in your case, it is important to take it 4 times a day, even when you feel well, to help prevent the pain and swelling that comes from arthritis."

Times of administration: Depending on the drug, information about specific times of administration may include: when to take the drug in relation to food (for example, with ASA); when to take the drug in relation to other medication (for example, with antacids); or when during a 24 hour period the effects of the medication are least disruptive (for example, with certain laxatives).

Specific method of administration: Many self-care products require special administration. People receiving suppositories, vaginal products, or otic, ophthalmic or nasal preparations should receive detailed explanations on how those products should be used. When products feature diagrams on the package, it may be sufficient to point these out, encouraging consumers to call if they have questions. A less obvious consideration is with drugs with a special coating. Elderly people often have difficulty swallowing products like enteric-coated ASA, and it is not unusual for these people to crush or chew their drugs.

Length of therapy: The appropriate length of therapy usually is discussed in relation to a person's symptoms (see Step VI: Follow-up and Monitoring). However, there may be instances—as with the number of consecutive days for nose drops—when this information is more drug-specific.

As a general rule, symptomatic treatment should not be continued for more than a few days without medical supervision. Although little harm can be done in advising self-treatment if the pharmacist follows this guideline, longer or shorter recommendations are appropriate in some cases. For instance, using an acne or dandruff product beyond a few days is reasonable, but an antinauseant for this length of time may not be advisable.

Side Effects

Common concerns about discussing side effects are that people will experience those effects through the power of suggestion, or be frightened out of taking the drug. Numerous studies indicate that few people react this way. Most people want to know what side effects drugs might cause. Perhaps more importantly, these concerns must be weighed against the potential consequences of an inadequately informed consumer.

A discussion about every adverse drug reaction associated with nonprescription products is seldom necessary. As a rough guideline, people should be advised about those effects they can recognize and for which appropriate precautionary measures can be taken. About 70 to 80 per cent of side effects can be predicted as an extension of pharmacologic action. Within this category, consumers should be informed about the following:

- annoying side effects that can be minimized or eliminated by consumer initiated measures. For example, a dry mouth can be resolved by chewing sugarless gum or taking small, frequent sips of ice water.
- side effects that might otherwise cause undue alarm. For example, drug-induced urine or stool color changes should be discussed before these changes occur.
- bothersome side effects that are transient. For example, some acne treatments cause initial peeling or reddening of the affected area, and people are more likely to tolerate this side effect, and continue with treatment, if they understand the effect's short-term nature.

- side effects that impair ability to perform. Any person receiving a product that causes drowsiness, dizziness, blurred vision or other impairment of physical or mental capacity needs to be forewarned of these effects. Of all side effects, this is perhaps the most important, as failure to inform may result in serious harm to the user.

The remaining 20 to 30 per cent of side effects include more serious, usually unpredictable, toxicities such as allergic reactions and drug-induced diseases. The former may be prevented by questioning the consumer's medical history. The latter as a rule do not require detailed discussion, since people usually do not administer non-prescription products for prolonged periods. On the other hand, advising against long-term use without a physician's advice becomes doubly important for drugs such as antihistamines, which are associated with more serious adverse effects over time.

The potential for alarming consumers or for psychologically inducing side effects can be reduced considerably by following a few general principles.

Avoid definitive statements about the drug's side effects: Comments like "This drug causes stomach problems" or "You'll probably feel drowsy after you take this" not only are more likely to produce a side effect, but the pharmacist does not know whether the user will experience the reaction in question. A less alarming, and more accurate approach, is to avoid the word "you" in favor of general descriptions like: "Some people find this upsets their stomach" and "A few people find they are drowsy after taking this product."

Set the stage, if necessary: If several side effects are to be discussed, it may help to preface information with a general phrase putting these in perspective. For example, "Some people experience unwanted effects with this product. You may not necessarily get these, as the drug affects different people in different ways. However, it is important to be aware of these effects and what to do if they occur."

Gauge the consumer's initial reaction: The pharmacist should be particularly observant at the beginning of a side effects discussion. If a person appears concerned, additional reassurance about the nature and likelihood of the side effect may be needed.

Provide practical advice: Consumers need to be told more than "This drug may cause dizziness, drowsiness, stomach upset ..." They also need to know when a side effect is likely to appear and, more importantly, what to do to minimize its occurrence. For example, if a product causes gastric irritation, the user should be advised to take the drug with food, or crackers and water. It is also helpful to encourage people to call back if a side effect occurs, as another product can often be recommended.

Interactions

Any person taking a product which interacts with alcohol needs to be forewarned of that possibility. The phrasing of this information is important. It is advisable not to leave the impression that alcohol-drug combinations are similar to increased alcohol consumption, as some people see this as a beneficial outcome. Wording to help prevent this interpretation might be: "You may experience an unpleasant feeling, such as extreme drowsiness or disorientation, if you drink alcoholic beverages around the time you take ..."

Counselling about alcohol consumption also requires tact. All pharmacists have heard people react to statements about alcohol with an indignant, "I don't drink!" Often these reactions occur before the pharmacist has a chance to provide relevant information. The following response might be helpful in these situations: "I like to mention this point because a number of people have wine with their meals or the odd beer, and this product should be avoided within ... hours of having a drink." Alternatively, to prevent this reaction, phrases like "social drink" or "wine with meals" are preferable to "alcohol" or "drink(ing)." Another effective approach is to preface any statement about alcohol with "This may not apply to you, but ..."

Depending on the product, other drug interaction advice may be needed. Reviewing all future possibilities at the time of sale, however, is usually an inefficient use of time, as people are unlikely to remember this much detail. The most efficient way to address potential drug interactions is to provide general information, along with encouragement to contact a health professional as situations arise. For example: "This product can affect the way other medicines work [avoiding the word 'interact'] so if you start any new medicines while using this product, be sure to call your doctor or me first so we can tell you whether there is any problem."

Storage

Information about storing nonprescription products may be relevant in some cases—for example, with diabetic testing supplies. Pharmacists should emphasize that the bathroom may not be the best place to store medication since higher temperatures and moisture can cause certain medicines to break down. As well, the statement "Keep out of the reach of children" can be elaborated by suggesting storage in a locked cupboard to prevent accidental poisoning.

Step V: Nonpharmacologic Approaches

Apart from product-specific information, a major component of self-care counselling is advice about nonpharmacologic approaches. Information may be given in conjunction with a product—for example, water with expectorants—or on its own. Nonpharmacologic advice is particularly helpful when contraindications to drug therapy exist and when a physician cannot be seen immediately—for example, in the evening or on weekends.

The pharmacist needs to be aware of nonpharmacologic measures for both prevention and treatment. Such advice may include eating and other lifestyle habits to relieve constipation, the use of a humidifier for cold symptoms and the application of cold compresses for headache. Many excellent pamphlets are available through health agencies, provincial and federal health departments, and pharmaceutical companies. Supplying this information not only adds to consumers' appreciation of the pharmacist, but is an efficient way to educate people about their symptoms.

Suggest humidifier for cold symptoms

Step VI: Follow-up and Monitoring

Consumer counselling should be concluded with encouragement for appropriate follow-up. Since most nonprescription drugs should be used only for minor or self-limiting conditions, the pharmacist needs to ensure the consumer has a clear understanding of what action to take if relief is not obtained.

The foremost consideration for follow-up is an allowable duration of symptoms. Self-treatment, with or without drugs, should be continued only for the time normally required for a particular symptom to resolve on its own. The actual number of days varies with each condition—simple indigestion usually clears within 24 hours, but the common cold typically lasts a week. When advising appropriate follow-up periods, the pharmacist must consider the duration of symptoms before advice was sought at the pharmacy.

Follow-up is also recommended if a nonprescription drug fails to

Consumer Counselling

relieve symptoms within an expected period of time. For example, analgesics usually relieve a headache within a few hours. As well, information about symptoms that may indicate a more serious disease is needed in some instances. The appearance of new symptoms, such as fever with a cold, or a change in original symptoms, such as green sputum, may suggest an underlying pathology and should always be assessed by a physician. Similarly, the repeated use of nonprescription drugs may mask serious problems, and people should be encouraged to see their physicians if symptoms recur frequently.

Encouraging appropriate follow-up requires the same tact and firmness as referral for initial medical advice. In addition, the following phrase may be helpful: "If your symptoms are not relieved by this product or if you are not better in (whatever time scale is appropriate for that condition), contact your doctor. Be sure to explain you have been using this product." This latter statement reinforces that non-prescription items are drugs and of interest to the physician.

As a concluding statement, many pharmacists find it helpful to encourage feedback. A comment such as "Please call and let me know how you manage" indicates an interest consumers appreciate. Equally important, it gives pharmacists an opportunity to evaluate the appropriateness of their advice.

If you see patient again - ask how it worked etc.

Nonverbal Communication

Effective communication depends not only on words, but the nonverbal behavior of the people involved. Consumers are as likely to respond to the way the pharmacist looks, the manner in which words are delivered and accompanying facial expressions, as they are to spoken words.

The importance of nonverbal communication—which encompasses all behavior outside the spoken word—is underlined by findings that up to 90 per cent of meaning in face-to-face discussions can be attributed to nonverbal sources. Unlike verbal communication, nonverbal communication is a continuous process. It begins before the first word is spoken and continues until a particular encounter ends, regardless of how much, or how little, is said.

Nonverbal communication is more spontaneous than verbal communication, and more often reflects the true feelings of a speaker. When verbal and nonverbal messages contradict each other, the nonverbal are more believable. For example, if someone stalks out of the room, slams the door and shouts, "I'm not the least bit angry!", the nonverbal behavior obviously is the most credible.

Nonverbal signs are highly subject to misinterpretation and can be misleading. Without verbal information, a listener can only infer the meaning of a particular behavior and does so in a totally personal manner. A quick look at a wristwatch during a conversation may mean: it is a boring conversation, it is time for coffee or simply that the listener has a new wristwatch. Similarly, the person who appears to be loitering or avoiding the pharmacist's gaze may be preparing to shoplift, or may simply be embarrassed about purchasing a particular product.

The pharmacist's ability to send and receive nonverbal messages influences the quality of relationships with consumers. Though nonverbal behavior is an unconscious process in everyday life, it can be controlled if one is aware of the elements involved. Elements particularly relevant to self-care counselling include the following: kinesics or body language; proxemics or the study of space, position and objects in relation to communication; paralanguage or nonword vocalizations; and the personal style of people engaged in commu-

nication. The application of these elements in counselling is described briefly below. Several excellent references are available for a more complete discussion of nonverbal communication.

Body Language

One of the richest categories of nonverbal communication is body language or kinesics. Often mistakenly equated with the entire process of nonverbal communication, this category refers to the wide range of body movements and facial expressions that accompany the spoken word. Of all nonverbal elements, the use or misuse of body language can have the most dramatic impact on a message.

Within this category, the presence or absence of eye contact is critical. Many pharmacists, without realizing it, do not look at consumers when talking to them. Instead, they tend to look at a product or product section, or to be distracted by other demands such as people waiting at the dispensary. Lack of eye contact is one of the largest barriers to communication. People may interpret it as lack of interest or lack of confidence on the part of the pharmacist. Either of these can inhibit participation in the discussion. Particularly in self-care counselling, not looking at an individual also limits the pharmacist's ability to watch for clues about the severity of a condition, or for people's reactions to product information. At the same time, good eye contact does not mean continually staring at another person. Prolonged eye contact may be interpreted as a sign of arrogance or disrespect. Generally speaking, the best approach is brief eye contact that continues throughout the conversation. *Don't stare*

Closely related, the pharmacist's overall facial expression is important. For instance, mannerisms such as biting the lips, puckering the mouth, or knitting or lowering the eyebrows in response to a question, could be interpreted as suspicion, disapproval or a lack of knowledge. Pharmacists need to be aware of how they unintentionally send messages, especially ones that do not communicate competence as a pharmacist and respect for the consumer.

The pharmacist's willingness to talk to consumers can be detected on the basis of body stance. For example, a "closed posture" occurs when arms are folded across the chest, legs are crossed at the knees and the head faces downward. Although none of these behaviors by itself is necessarily bad, a combination of such nonverbal acts (called "cue clusters") can signal a desire to be doing something other than talking to the consumer.

The best approach for counselling is an "open cue cluster." Communicating openness generally includes the following: brief, consistent eye contact throughout the discussion; a relaxed facial expression that conveys interest and willingness to listen; a relaxed posture with legs uncrossed and arms by the side; a frontal appearance with shoulders square or rotated toward the other person; an erect body position, with head up and shoulders back; a slight lean toward the other person, if sitting; appropriate comfortable gestures, for example, with the hands; and absence of distracting motions.

The open posture contributes to the perception that the pharmacist is willing to devote time to individual consumers. Several studies show a positive relationship between consumer satisfaction and the degree of interest communicated nonverbally by a health professional. In addition, the open posture may influence people's ability to understand and recall information. One study of physicians' nonverbal behavior found that a greater degree of openness, expressed through a forward lean and body orientation, resulted in higher levels of understanding. The authors postulated that the positive interest shown by the practitioner motivated people to listen more closely and, therefore, to retain more information.

Paralinguistics

A second major element of nonverbal communication is the manner in which words are delivered—the tone, rate, pitch and volume of voice and the presence of nonword vocalizations such as "uh," throat clearings or nervous giggles. As much as one-third of nonverbal communication takes place through such vocal cues or "paralanguage."

A varied and interesting voice is ideal, but as long as one's speech is not too extreme, there should be little interference with communication. On the other hand, people can become remarkably upset because an inappropriate tone of voice has been used, often creating an entirely different meaning than the speaker intended. Similarly, a monotone or flat voice is difficult to listen to; adding even modest inflection can help keep the listener's attention. Listening to the inflection, rate and volume of one's voice on tape is a helpful exercise; many people find they sound far different than expected.

Vocal cues can also be used to give and request permission to speak. Four identifiable vocal cues that indicate "turn-taking" have been postulated: turn-yielding cues in the form of silence, or a higher or lower pitch at the end of a comment; turn-requesting cues such as an audible inspiration of breath during pauses; turn-maintaining cues, which include increasing one's volume and rate when the listener indicates a desire to speak; and turn-denying cues, which include silence and slower than normal reinforcement of the other person's comment. Missing any of these cues can contribute to an unintentional message of rudeness or inconsideration. On the other hand, these cues may be helpful during telephone conversations in which nonverbal signals such as facial expression are absent. They can also be effective during discussions with talkative people.

Proxemics

The most familiar example of proxemics (the structure and use of space in communication) is the typical dispensary design. Many prescription counters act as a physical and psychological barrier, and communication is often improved when the pharmacist steps out from behind the counter to talk to a consumer. This gesture is especially important when the dispensary platform is elevated. High-low physical relationships can suggest a superior-inferior relationship, and consumers who perceive themselves to be in the inferior position are less likely to participate in a discussion.

A less familiar component of proxemics is the closeness of body position between the pharmacist and the consumer. There are four identifiable distances in North American culture that reflect the purpose of an interaction as well as the acquaintance level of the participants. Anything less than 45 cm is reserved for those with whom one has an intimate relationship. When a stranger or non-intimate associate enters this space, anxiety or anger at the "invasion of privacy" may result. The next level is 45 to 120 cm (casual-personal distance), which represents the most comfortable distance for conversation between friends and acquaintances. The most accepted distance between two people involved in professional transactions lies between 1 and 4 m (social-consultative distance). Distances over 4 metres are generally reserved for occasions when one speaks to an audience (public distance) and imply that little or no interruption will occur.

Obviously, the pharmacist who counsels from a public distance—shouting advice or directions from a dispensary platform—does little to encourage active participation by the consumer. The distance the pharmacist chooses to counsel a person depends on the relationship with that person as well as the context and topic of discussion. Many pharmacist-consumer exchanges occur at the social-consultative level, but for explanations about products such as vaginal or rectal medication, the pharmacist may choose the outer limits of the casual-personal distance—close enough for privacy, but with enough room for each person to feel comfortable.

The ideal situation is to have a private area near the dispensary for selected consultations. In the absence of this service, the pharmacist can take a number of steps to provide psychological privacy. A particularly helpful arrangement is to form a triangle using the consumer, pharmacist and wall shelf or gondola as the three sides. The positioning signals to others that the consultation is private and not to be interrupted. Even in the most crowded pharmacy, privacy can also be achieved by stepping into a quieter aisle.

The pharmacy itself may project a nonverbal image. Colors used in the pharmacy's decor, lighting, background noise and the use of space (wide or narrow aisles, filled or empty shelves, boxes on the floor) have all been documented as important nonverbal communication channels. The general appearance of the pharmacy can also play an important role in conveying whether the pharmacist is a skilled professional. Dirt, clutter and general untidiness in any business carries a negative nonverbal message, which can be even stronger in those associated with health-care products.

Personal Style

Just as a sloppy, unkempt pharmacy can project a negative image, so too can the appearance of the pharmacy's employees. The style, cleanliness and fit of clothing affect how, or if, consumers respond to the pharmacist. People quickly make assumptions about intelligence, credibility, reliability, breadth of experience and a host of personality characteristics on the basis of physical appearance. If there is any question about the power of personal style, think about how one reacts to people with dirty clothes, dirty hands and fingernails, and greasy hair.

Nonverbal Communication From Consumers

Effective communication requires the detection of nonverbal behavior in others. The elements described above apply equally to consumers, and the pharmacist needs to observe consumers' nonverbal behavior when counselling them about the selection and use of nonprescription drugs.

Awareness of consumers' nonverbal behavior often provides valuable feedback on the effectiveness of counselling efforts. Body language and paralinguistics are particularly relevant. For example, a quizzical look in response to questions or product information should alert the pharmacist that further explanation is required. Similarly, hesitations in speech or a concerned look may suggest that more discussion about a particular topic is needed.

The pharmacist should also be familiar with nonverbal signs indicating anxiety, anger and embarrassment, as these emotions may mean a different style of interaction is needed. Swinging a leg, tapping a foot or drumming fingers may all suggest a state of nervousness. Repeatedly clenching and unclenching one's fist might indicate a certain level of anxiety, or even hostility. People often demonstrate a unique set of body movements for expressing reactions to illness, including self-manipulating movements such as wringing the hands, licking the lips or scratching the nose and face during stressful situations. Since people's emotional state influences how much is gained from counselling, the pharmacist is well advised to address these emotions before providing advice and information about drug therapy.

Finally, nonverbal behavior is influenced by cultural background. For example. although lack of eye contact in American culture is tantamount to denying another person's existence, Oriental people are taught to communicate respect by decreasing eye contact. In the Bulgarian culture, shaking the head from side to side is a sign of agreement. Middle Eastern people may not have the same need to intimate space discussed under proxemics. Pharmacists who provide services to populations of particular racial or cultural origin can find out more about nonverbal behaviors of these groups by reading appropriate texts. However, one must be cautious, as some individuals may have been raised in North America, and their nonverbal behavior will reflect that background.

Special Counselling Situations

Some situations in self-care counselling require additional attention to communication skills. Although it is difficult to generalize, the following sections outline approaches to help the pharmacist in 3 areas: discussing potentially embarrassing subjects; handling overtalkative people; and counselling hearing-impaired geriatric consumers.

Potentially Embarrassing Subjects

In self-care counselling, the pharmacist often encounters subjects that embarrass the consumer. Since pharmacists deal with symptoms and drugs every day, it is easy to forget that some people are acutely distressed by any discussion relating to sex, intimate body parts or bodily functions. Purchasers of laxatives, suppositories, enemas, hemorrhoid preparations or vaginal creams may be reluctant to discuss problems with the pharmacist. The social implications of certain products may also cause embarrassment, as when teenagers buy their first package of condoms or parents purchase a pediculicide for their children.

Most embarrassing situations can be predicted and handled in a smooth, professional manner. With attention to specific communication skills, pharmacists can reduce the likelihood of embarrassing an individual, and can take appropriate steps to set obviously embarrassed people at ease.

As a first step, the pharmacist should anticipate which topics might be embarrassing. In these cases, the discussion should be general at first and questions should be structured from less personal to more personal areas. This gives people time to observe the pharmacist's approach and to see that sensitive issues will be addressed in a professional manner.

When personal questions must be asked, it is best to avoid open-ended ones. People usually find it easier to answer closed-ended questions in embarrassing situations. For example, someone requesting a pediculicide may be uncomfortable responding to the question "Where do you have the problem?" On the other hand, if the pharmacist explains that the area to be treated affects the choice of product, it becomes relatively easy to answer "yes" or "no" to a question such as "Is it in the groin area?" Another approach is to provide relevant information and let the consumer choose the proper

formulation. For instance, with the information "The lotion or shampoo is used for the pubic area, the shampoo for the scalp, and cream or lotion for the skin," most consumers can choose the best product for their symptoms.

In any potentially sensitive situation, the pharmacist should provide as much privacy as possible for the discussion. (See the section on nonverbal communication). Voice level is also important: the pharmacist should keep a low tone so the consumer understands their privacy is respected. At the same time, a hushed voice may suggest there is something to be embarrassed about, and should be avoided.

Pharmacists also need to project a degree of comfort with subjects of a personal nature. Apart from avoiding a subject altogether, one of the worst things a health professional can do is discuss a delicate problem vaguely or euphemistically. For example, if the pharmacist says, "Does it hurt down there where, uh, you know," avoiding words like "vagina" or "groin" may make consumers feel they must also not use these words.

At the other extreme, some pharmacists may attempt to compensate for discomfort by using street language or making light of a situation. Or they may feel they are creating an open and relaxed atmosphere by speaking bluntly. Although important advice may be given, consumers may well be so embarrassed by the brash approach, they tune out anything useful the pharmacist says.

The best terminology for potentially sensitive topics is straightforward, matter-of-fact words. Technical terminology is especially awkward in sensitive situations; if people do not know the meaning of a word, they may be too embarrassed to ask. In these instances, extra effort should be made to use understandable terms, and to rephrase a question or response if the other person seems confused.

Closely related, certain terms may have emotional overtones. Saying "symptoms" rather than naming a particular problem (for example, "lice") and choosing words like "fluid" instead of "pus," "contraception" for "birth control" and "pain medicine" rather than "narcotic" reduce the chance of upsetting an individual. An open-ended approach at the beginning of the interview helps identify words with which the consumer is comfortable. By using a common vocabulary, the pharmacist can help people feel more comfortable discussing sensitive issues.

Despite the pharmacist's best intentions, people may still be embarrassed in sensitive situations. Sometimes the response is obvious—a blush or stammer is relatively easy to read—but often the message is more subtle, and the pharmacist must pay close attention to the consumer's nonverbal behavior. Signals such as indirect or seemingly pointless questions, general evasiveness, or hesitations may point to a consumer who is embarrassed, or who is concerned that the discussion will not be kept in confidence.

A natural tendency in these situations is to tell the person not to be embarrassed. Although some form of reassurance may be in order, judgments about a person's reaction should be avoided. Pharmacists who say, "There's no reason to be embarrassed" have not solved the problem—the person is still embarrassed. Similarly, one should avoid any tendency to laugh or tease. If someone thinks a health professional is intentionally poking fun at a delicate situation, an automatic barrier to effective communication is created. Even lighthearted teasing, such as sometimes accompanies the sale of a laxative or antidiarrheal, should be avoided.

If embarrassment interferes with the transfer of information, two techniques may be appropriate. One is confrontation, in which a comment like "You seem to be having difficulty talking about this" may encourage discussion about the source of embarrassment. Closely related, a statement which recognizes the feelings of the other person (empathy) may be helpful. In embarrassing situations, an empathic statement might be something like, I know it is often difficult to talk about this subject" or, "Many people I talk with are uncomfortable discussing . . ." Again, once people are given an opportunity to verbalize their embarrassment, they may be better able to continue the discussion.

No more than one or two confrontational or empathic statements are appropriate in any given discussion. It is important not to push too far and certainly to avoid backing an individual into a corner with pointed and detailed questions. Despite the pharmacist's attempts to respect a person's privacy, to use appropriate language and to provide opportunities to discuss a problem, some people do not want to open up. The best route in these situations is to provide as much information as possible and leave an opening with something to the effect of, "If you have any questions about these products, I'll be happy to answer them." As well, written information and telephone counselling are effective alternatives for educating consumers in these situations.

Talkative Consumers

A difficult problem for experienced and beginning practitioners alike is the talkative consumer. These people are often seen as barriers to efficiency and may be major sources of irritation. Although complete control is usually impossible, a number of techniques can increase the productivity of discussions with these people.

One type of talkative person is the obsessive individual, who insists on giving an overdetailed account of symptoms. When interviewing such people, pharmacists should be particularly aware of their own nonverbal behavior, avoiding overfacilitation with encouraging nods, gestures or phrases. Instead, pharmacists should limit their show of interest in trivial data, and show greater interest when relevant information is provided. Closed-ended questions can be introduced earlier in the sequence of questioning than they might be otherwise. A courteous interruption when enough information has been obtained about a given point, followed by another specific question, keeps the interview focused and makes it possible to obtain information in a reasonable period of time. A mental image of the order in which questioning is to proceed is particularly helpful in these situations, because it increases the pharmacist's ability to refocus the discussion into areas where information is required.

Another type of overtalkative person is one who rambles or shows similar evidence of confusion and poor organization. A polite interruption is appropriate when these people wander away from the topic at hand. Bridging, or transition, is a particularly useful technique for accomplishing interruption without appearing rude. The following example illustrates how bridging and the use of specific questions might work with a talkative person:

Consumer (with stomach upset): . . . and my husband—he's a teacher you know—he's going to take March break off—he usually doesn't but I insisted this time—and we're going skiing. I think we'll probably go to Lake Louise—maybe not, maybe we'll go to that new place . . . (slight pause).

Pharmacist: It sounds like a wonderful time and I can see you are excited about getting away. Since you'll be travelling, it might be best if I gave you a tablet form of antacid. Are you having any gas with the stomach upset?

Written material also is helpful with these people. Pointing out directions or instructions on a product container or written sheet attracts consumers' attention. Because they are concentrating on the written word, they are less likely to interrupt with unrelated thoughts.

A third type of talkative person is the one who makes every attempt to prolong a discussion. Many of these people simply cannot be hurried. The pharmacist may choose to continue chatting (depending on the time available), or several techniques for closing an interview can help the pharmacist exit these situations gracefully. The first is a summation of important points covered during the interview. Not only does this technique reinforce information, but it subtly indicates that the discussion is coming to a close. Following summation, the pharmacist can use sentences that have concluding words, such as "Well, I think that about covers it. Do you have any questions?" or "If you have any questions, please feel free to call." Certain nonverbal behavior can also be a powerful form of communication; adopting a closed stance is an effective but discreet way to signal that the discussion is finished. Last but not least, pharmacists may indicate they need to terminate the discussion. Most people respect a clinician whose manner suggests strength and self-assurance. They are not offended by an assertive but polite statement, such as "I'd really like to hear more about . . . sometime, but I am busy right now and should get some of these prescriptions filled."

Geriatric Consumers

Counselling seniors often presents a challenge for the pharmacist. In addition to increased pharmacologic and therapeutic considerations, some older people have a degree of sensory loss that makes the exchange of information difficult, if not frustrating, for both parties.

The most common sensory deficit accompanying aging is hearing impairment, a general term used to describe all hearing problems from minute loss to profound deafness. Compared to a rate of about 10 per cent in the total population, an estimated 60 per cent of individuals over age 65 have some degree of impairment. At least 35 per cent of these individuals experience enough hearing loss to interfere with normal conversation.

The older adult is extremely susceptible to drug-use problems and often benefits most from a discussion with the pharmacist. Declining physical function usually requires multiple medications, and although the elderly represent one-tenth of the population, they consume one-quarter of all prescribed medication. In addition, several surveys have identified this group as major consumers of certain nonprescription products. This use of drug products, coupled with the fact that several physicians are likely to be involved in an older person's care, makes screening for drug interactions particularly important. Physiologic changes associated with aging may also alter the presentation of certain illnesses (for example, the elderly do not mount fevers to the same degree as younger people), which complicates the assessment of certain conditions. Similarly, altered response to drugs places the elderly person at greater risk for adverse reactions, a factor that must be taken into account when assessing complaints and recommending products.

The growing number of elderly people makes it increasingly important to understand and respond to their needs. Currently about 10 per cent of the Canadian population, this age group is projected to increase by more than three-quarters by the end of this century and to about 17.6 per cent of the population in the next 50 years. Although many pharmacies now service a large elderly population,

Consumer Counselling

a substantial increase in the older population can be expected in the decades ahead.

Counselling the Hearing-Impaired

The most common form of hearing loss in the elderly is presbycusis, a communication disorder characterized by progressive degenerative breakdown in auditory function. It causes a loss in level as well as clarity of hearing, which makes speech difficult to hear and understand. Specific techniques for communicating with these people are divided into nonverbal, or attending, communication skills and verbal communication skills.

Attending communication skills refer to all nonverbal considerations in communication. Although important in any counselling situation, these are crucial for the hearing-impaired, who are as dependent on nonverbal communication as they are on the spoken word.

The first consideration is to select a quiet environment for the discussion. A common misconception about hearing impairment is that the level at which a person can hear simply declines. However, a major characteristic of hearing impairment (called auditory discrimination difficulty), is a disproportionate and increased sensitivity to sounds. This sensitivity, coupled with distortion of sound within the auditory system, makes it extremely difficult to differentiate between background noise and a speaker's voice.

Testing several locations within the pharmacy will identify which has the least extraneous noise. One should listen for such sounds as peripheral conversations between other people or the sound of a cash register, telephone, computer printer, radio and even pill-counting tray. Many pharmacists are surprised by how much background noise exists in the pharmacy and gain an appreciation for how frustrating it must be to listen for instructions when other sounds are amplified by comparison. Hearing aids generally do not correct auditory discrimination difficulties, so the need for a quiet environment applies equally to these people.

Second, the pharmacy should have good lighting. Many hearing-impaired people rely on lipreading. The counselling area should provide good lighting for the pharmacist's face and upper body so people can take advantage of important visual cues. Similarly, individuals should be positioned so they do not have to look into bright or concentrated sources of light (such as lamps or sunshine) to see the pharmacist. Looking into light makes it extremely difficult to see a speaker's face, and attempts at lipreading will be quickly frustrated. Other distractions that make lipreading difficult include pencil-chewing, smoking, placing hands near or on the lips, and moustaches that cover the mouth.

Third, the pharmacist should face the consumer. It is important to look directly at the individual, as even a slight turn of the head can obscure the lips. In pharmacies with raised platforms, the pharmacist should come to the same level as the consumer. If the consumer is sitting, it may be necessary to bend down so the conversation can take place face-to-face. Good eye contact helps convey a feeling of direct communication.

Finally, the pharmacist should indicate when he or she is ready to speak. A common cue when someone is about to speak is an audible intake of breath immediately before the first word. People with a hearing impairment often miss this cue. To ensure the first parts of a sentence are not missed, pharmacists should use another cue to indicate when they are ready to speak. Attention can be attracted with an upraised hand, a tap on the shoulder or arm, or simply by making eye contact before speaking.

Pathophysiologic changes within the auditory system make attention to **verbal communication skills** equally important.

First, the pharmacist should consider voice level. A natural tendency with the hard-of-hearing is to shout. However, since increased sensitivity and distortion of loud sounds is characteristic of hearing impairment, a shouted message is less likely to be understood. The best results are achieved when one speaks slowly and distinctly, using a well-modulated and firm tone of voice. At the same time, exaggerating or over-emphasizing words makes lipreading difficult. The best rule is to speak clearly and naturally.

Second, the pharmacist should pay attention to voice pitch. Most older people have difficulty hearing high-frequency sounds. Lowering the pitch may help. Female pharmacists, in particular, may need to adjust the pitch of their voices when speaking with the elderly.

Third, pacing needs to be considered. Older adults, particularly those with a hearing impairment, may have difficulty understanding speech as a result of delayed central processing and reaction time. Because these people take longer to process a message, a slow and relaxed pace should be consciously maintained. Particularly during the assessment phase, ample time must be given for responses to the pharmacist's questions. Consumers also should be encouraged to ask for repetitions when a message is not understood.

Periods of silence are common when talking with the hearing-impaired older adult. Silence should not be regarded as a breakdown in communication unless it persists for an extended period of time, for example, more than 20 or 30 seconds. These pauses may simply reflect an attempt to interpret an instruction or recall a fact. As noted earlier, the pharmacist should wait attentively during these silences.

Finally, the pharmacist should pay close attention to vocabulary. Consonant discrimination is often more difficult for the hearing-impaired. Short, simple sentences and a familiar vocabulary consisting of words of as few syllables as possible (for example, drug or pills instead of medication or prescription) are usually easier to comprehend. Re-emphasizing the same point in various ways is also preferable to repeating the same phrase several times. The pharmacist should be careful not to overload the individual with information. Elderly people in particular may be confused by large amounts of information and, confronted with an abundance of facts, may decide to ignore part or all of what is said. As well, sudden changes in subject matter are hard to follow with diminished hearing acuity; explaining when a new subject is about to be discussed helps avoid confusion.

An attitude of respect and consideration is vital to effective communication with the hearing-impaired person. The pharmacist must keep in mind that hearing impairment is not a problem of intelligence, but rather of physical disability. If individuals interpret altered and simplified patterns of speech as condescending, they are likely to dismiss the pharmacist's advice.

Counselling the Deaf Person

Many of the above techniques are equally applicable to deaf people. In addition, some communicate via paper and pencil, in which case the pharmacist should do the same. Others use interpreters who are familiar with their sign language. If an interpreter is present, the pharmacist should continue talking directly to the deaf person, maintaining eye contact throughout the discussion to convey a feeling of direct communication. Questions to the interpreter such as, "Does

Consumer Counselling

he always take it in pill form?" or "Will she remember to mix it with water?" should always be avoided. These can be both degrading and impersonal to a deaf person.

Recognizing the Hearing-Impaired

Many people are reluctant to disclose a hearing problem. They may accept hearing loss as an inevitable part of aging and not feel the need to mention it. Conversely, they may ignore the disability because they are uncomfortable with the idea of getting older. Others are so fed up with having to say "pardon?" they eventually give up all attempt to communicate. With any of these people, the pharmacist needs to be alert to characteristic behaviors of hearing loss so appropriate communication techniques can be implemented.

A common clue to partial hearing impairment is when a person tilts the head so the good ear is directed toward the speaker. Other important nonverbal behaviors include a blank facial expression during conversation, restless limb movements or irregular posture shifts, and noticeable attempts to read lips. Verbal clues include frequent requests for repetition, special difficulty with rapid speech, a loud voice, abnormal spacing or pauses while speaking, and the omission of word endings, especially those with high-frequency sounds such as t, s, sh, f and v.

Although not always receptive to this advice, individuals identified by pharmacists as having a hearing impairment should be encouraged to seek audiology assessment and therapy. Most, if not all, communities have a Canadian Hearing Society office or contact person who can help. Along with a number of excellent programs and services for the hearing-impaired, this group offers a variety of materials for the health professional who deals with these people.

Summary

Often the pharmacist is the only health professional seen about self-medication. Although self-care counselling is almost as old as the profession of pharmacy, it has undergone renewed interest in the past several years. Increasing numbers of people are moving toward self-care as a treatment alternative, and numerous studies show the pharmacist is seen as a valuable source of self-care information. To help meet the growing demand for this service, the pharmacist needs to be aware of how to make the best use of time available for counselling consumers about self-medication.

Traditional emphasis in pharmacy education has been on providing "correct" answers. In practice, however, the pharmacist must be able to elicit and define an individual's problem so the best advice can be given. Interviewing is the principle tool used to accomplish this task. It is a skill that must be mastered if the pharmacist is to be productive. Other communication skills described in this chapter will help improve the effectiveness, efficiency and ease with which self-care counselling is conducted. Just as experience enables the pharmacist to interpret and fill prescriptions with confidence, the ability to apply communication skills with individual consumers will be a direct result of use over time.

References

The Pharmacist and Self-Care

Anonymous. Response to symptoms in general practice pharmacy. Pharm J 1981;226:14–6.

Chiles VK. Self-medication in perspective. In: Chiles VK, ed. Canadian self-medication. Ottawa: Canadian Pharmaceutical Association, 1980:x–xix.

Final report of the task force on responding to the self-medicating patient. Presented to the Canadian Pharmaceutical Association Council of Delegates, 1984.

Guidelines on the sale of nonprescription medications—report of the ad hoc committee to develop guidelines on the sales of nonprescription medication. Presented to the Canadian Pharmaceutical Association Board of Directors and Council of Delegates, 1983.

Haunholter JT. Negligence and the pharmacist: a consideration of some of the aspects. Can Pharm J 1978;111(1):12–6.

Health for all: the role of self-medication. Proceedings of the sixth general assembly. Ottawa: World Federation of Proprietary Medicine Manufacturers, 1981.

Skinner D. Consumer use of nonprescription drugs. Can Pharm J 1985; 118:206–13.

The active health report. Highlights. Ottawa: Health Promotion Directorate, Health and Welfare Canada, 1986:7.

To the year 2000: the changing roles of nonprescription medicines and the practice of pharmacy. Ottawa: The Nonprescription Drug Manufacturers Association of Canada, August 1991.

Information—Gathering Communication Skills

Anonymous. Obtaining additional specific information; direct questioning, system review and physical examination. In: Enelow AJ, Swisher SN. Interviewing and patient care. New York: Oxford University Press, 1979:51–65.

Beardsley RS. The patient interview. In: Tindall WN, Beardsley RS, Curtiss FR, eds. Communication in pharmacy practice: a practical guide for students and practitioners. Philadelphia: Lea & Febiger, 1984:71–81.

Enelow AJ, McKinney, Adler A. Basic interviewing. In: Enelow AJ, Swisher SN. Interviewing and patient care. New York: Oxford University Press, 1979:19–50.

King M, Novik L, Citrenbaum C. Irresistable communication: creative skills for the health professional. Philadelphia: WB Saunders, 1983.

Kitching JB. Communication and the community pharmacist. Pharm J 1986;237(6401):449–54.

Pillow WF. Communicating with the patient. Concepts and skills for interpersonal communication. Eli Lilly and Company, 1985:39–41.

Ray MD, ed. Basic skills in clinical pharmacy practice. Carrboro: American Society of Hospital Pharmacists, 1983.

Reiser DE, Klein Schroder A. The interview process. Patient interviewing—the human dimension. Baltimore: Waverly Press, 1980:111–36.

Reiser DE, Klein Schroder A. Patient interviewing—the human dimension. Baltimore: Waverly Press, 1980.

Russell CG, Wilcox EM, Hicks CI. Interpersonal communication in pharmacy: an interactionist approach. New York: Appleton-Century-Crofts, 1982.

Smith DL. Medication guide for patient counselling. Philadelphia: Lea & Febiger, 1981:3–35.

Stimmell G, Crary W. Techniques for successful patient interaction. California Pharmacist 1980;27:26–8.

The Schering report VII. What's right with pharmacy—the pharmacist's growing influence in the expanding otc market. Kenilworth: Schering Laboratories, 1985.

Tindall WN, Beardsley RS, Curtiss FR, eds. Communication in pharmacy practice: a practical guide for students and practitioners. Philadelphia: Lea & Febiger, 1984.

Systematic Approach to Self-Care Counselling

Ackerman SJ. Doing more harm than good with children's medications. FDA Consumer 1989;23(2):28–31.

Anonymous. Storage and shelf life of drugs: when is it important? Drug Ther Bull 1977;15(21):81–3.

Balon ADJ. Counselling. Pharm J 1986;236(6401):452–4.

Barber ND, Raynor DK. Understanding medicine labels: the effect of plain English. Pharm J 1989;242(6521)(Suppl):R13–17.

Becker MH, Rosenstock IM. Compliance with medical advice. In: Streptoe A, Mathews A, eds. Health care and human behavior. London: Academic Press, 1984;175–203.

Consumer Counselling

Busson M, Dunn APM. Patients' knowledge about prescribed medication. Pharm J 1986;236(6380):624–6.

Chartier MR. Clarity of expression in interpersonal communication. In: Jones JE, Pfeiffer JW, eds. The annual handbook for group facilitators. La Jolla: University Associates, 1976:149–55.

Cluff LE, Caranasos GJ, Stewart MS. Clinical problems with drugs. In: Smith LH, ed. Major problems in internal medicine, Volume V. Philadelphia: WB Saunders, 1975:21.

Decima Research. Attitudes, perceptions and behaviour relating to ethical medicines. A research report to the Department of National Health and Welfare. Drugs Directorate, Health Protection Branch, Department of National Health and Welfare. Ottawa: Minister of Supply and Services Canada, 1990.

Doak C, Doak L, Root J. Teaching patients with low literacy skills. Philadelphia: JB Lippincott Company, 1985.

Doak LG, Doak CC. Patient comprehension profiles; recent findings and strategies. Patient Counselling and Health Education 1980;2(3):101–6.

Edwards C, Stillman P. Minor illness or major disease? Responding to symptoms in the pharmacy. London: The Pharmaceutical Press, 1982:1–2.

Eustace CA, Johnson GJ, Gault MH. Improvements in drug prescription labels for patients with limited education or vision. Can Med Assoc J 1982; 127:301–2.

Holt GA, Hollon JD, Hughes SE, Coyle R. OTC labels: can consumers read and understand them? Amer Pharm 1990;NS30(11):51–4.

Holt GA. How adults learn. Am Pharm 1981;NS21(7):46–7, 70.

Inciardi JA. Over the counter drugs: epidemiology, adverse reactions, overdose deaths and mass media promotion. Addict Dis Int J 1977;3(2):253–72.

Karpinski K. Summary report—national non-prescription drug survey (Draft). For submission to Drugs Directorate of Health Protection Branch by the Bureau of Non-Prescription Drugs, 1981:March.

Kishi DT, Watanabe AS. A systematic approach to drug therapy for the pharmacist. Am J Hosp Pharm 1974;31:494–7.

Klein-Schwartz W, Hoopes JM. Patient assessment and consultation. In: Handbook of nonprescription drugs. Washington: American Pharmaceutical Association, 1982:9–18.

LaPierre G, Mallet L. Readability of materials. Can Pharm J 1987;120:718–28.

Larmour I. My medication, your information. Aust J Hosp Pharm 1985; 15(2):85–91.

Ley P. Communicating with patients. Improving communication, satisfaction and compliance. New York: Croom Helm, 1988.

Liguori S. A quantitative assessment of the readability of ppi's. Drug Intell Clin Pharm 1978;12:712–6.

Lively BT, Baldwin HJ, Carlton BR, et al. The relationship of knowledge to perceived benefits and risks of oral contraceptives. Drug Information J 1981;15:153–9.

Maiman LA, Becker MH, Katlic AW. How mothers treat their children's physical symptoms. J Community Health 1985;10(3):136–55.

Matte DA, McLean WM. Self medication, abuse or misuse? Drug Intell Clin Pharm 1978;12:603–11.

McBean BJ. Blackburn JL. An evaluation of four methods of pharmacist conducted patient education. Can Pharm J 1982;115:167–72.

McKenzie MW. How to conduct a patient medication history interview. In: Ray MD, ed. Basic skills in clinical pharmacy practice. Carrboro: American Society of Hospital Pharmacists, 1983:79–128.

McQueen EG. Pharmacological basis of adverse drug reactions. In: Avery GS, ed. Drug treatment: principles and practice of clinical pharmacology and therapeutics. New York: Adis Press, 1980:202–31.

Meyer LE, Reis JC, Reeder W, Olson DL. Impact of perception on side effects. Drug Intell Clin Pharm 1985;19:213.

Myers ED, Clavert EJ. The effect of forewarning in the occurrence of side effects and discontinaunce of medication in patients on dothiepin. J Int Med Res 1976;4:237–40.

Myers ED, Clavert EJ. The effect of forewarning on the occurrence of side effects and discontinuation of medication in patients on amitriptyline. Br J Psychiat 1973;122:461–4.

Ormand EA, Caulfield C. A practical guide to giving oral medications to young children. Am J Maternal Child Nursing 1976;Sept-Oct:320–5.

Population. School attendance and level of schooling. Canada, provinces, urban and rural. 1981 census of Canada. Statistics catalogue 92–914 (Vol 1 national series). Ottawa: Minister of Supply and Services Canada, 1981.

Reiser DE, Klein Schroder A. Components of the medical history. In: Patient interviewing—the human dimension. Baltimore: Waverly Press, 1980: 163–82.

Rogers A. Teaching adults. Philadelphia: Open University Press, 1986.

Rudd CC. Teaching and counselling patients about drugs. In: Ray MD, ed. Basic skills in clinical pharmacy practice. Carrboro: American Society of Hospital Pharmacists, 1983:153–86.

Russell CG, Wilcox EM, Hicks CI. Language and meaning. In: Interpersonal communication in pharmacy: an interactionist approach. New York: Appleton-Century-Crofts, 1982:107–19.

Smith DS. Patient education—its time has come. Am Pharm 1981; NS21(7):14–9.

Spadari DC, Robinson LA, et al. Assessing readability of patient information materials. Am J Hosp Pharm 1980;37:215–21.

Srnka QM, Self TH. Systematic medication profile review—a self study guide for the pharmacist. Memphis: American College of Apothecaries, 1982.

Sumner ED. Handbook of geriatric drug therapy for health care professionals. Philadelphia: Lea & Febiger, 1983:11.

Tabor M. Minimizing the menace of otc drugs. Occup Health Saf 1982; 51(5):14–9.

Walmsley A. A lowly pill's aspirations. Macleans 1981;Feb 16:53–5.

Woods D. Drug labelling—plainer English needed. Can Med Assoc J 1987; 136:321.

Nonverbal Communication

Anonymous. Professional service areas mandatory in Saskatchewan. Can Pharm J 1986;119:113–4.

Asbell B. What they know about you. Toronto: Random House Inc., 1991.

Barnard D, Barr JT, Schumacher GE. Person to person—"empathy." Bethesda: American Association of Colleges of Pharmacy, 1982:13.

Barnard D, Barr JT, Schumacher GE. Person to person—"nonverbal communication." Bethesda: American Association of Colleges of Pharmacy, 1985.

Brands AJ. The patient's pharmacist. Am J Hosp Pharm 1979;36:311–5.

Condon JC, Yousef FS. An introduction to intercultural communications. Indianapolis: The Bobbs-Merrill Co Inc, 1975.

Cresswell S. Doctor/patient communications: a review of the literature. Ont Med Rev 1983;Nov:559–66.

DiMatteo MR, Taranta A, Friedman HA, Prince LM. Predicting patient satisfaction from physicians' nonverbal communication skills. Med Care 1980;18(4):376–87.

Hall ET. The silent language. New York: Doubleday, 1959:163–4. (Cited in Barnard D, Barr JT, Schumacher GE. Person to person—"nonverbal communication." Bethesda: American Association of Colleges of Pharmacy, 1985:8.)

Hunter RH. Nonverbal communication in pharmacy. In: Tindall WN, Beardsley RS, Curtiss FR, eds, Communications in pharmacy practice: a practical guide for students and practitioners. Philadelphia: Lea & Febiger, 1984: 13–23.

King M, Novik L, Citrenbaum C. Nonverbal communication. In: Irresistable communication. Creative skills for the health professional. Philadelphia: WB Saunders, 1983:63–74.

Knapp ML. Nonverbal communication in human interaction. New York: Holt, Rinehart, Winston, 1978. (Cited in Russell CG, Wilcox EM, Hicks CI. Nonverbal variables. Interpersonal communication in pharmacy: an interactionist approach. New York: Appleton-Century-Crofts, 1982:75–90.)

Larsen KM, Smith KC. Assessment of nonverbal communication in the patient-physician interview. J Fam Pract 1981;12(3):481–8.

Mehrabian A. Silent messages. Belmont: Wadsworth Publishing, 1971. (Cited in Barnard D, Barr JT, Schumacher GE. Person to person—"nonverbal communication." Bethesda: American Association of Colleges of Pharmacy, 1985:3.)

Pillow WF. Communicating with the patient. Concepts and skills for interpersonal communication. Eli Lilly and Company, 1985:26–7.

Ranelli PK. The utility of nonverbal communication in the profession of pharmacy. Soc Sci Med 1979;13A:733–6.

Reinsmith WA. Patient-centered community pharmacy: a mirage. Am Pharm 1985;NS25(1):6–8.

Consumer Counselling

Russell CG, Wilcox EM, Hicks CI. Nonverbal variables. Interpersonal communication in pharmacy—an interactionist aproach. New York: Appleton-Century-Crofts, 1982:75–90.

Samovar LA. Understanding intercultural communictaion. Belmont: Wadsworth, 1981.

Spencer H. The hidden meaning of body language. Am Pharm 1981; NS21(7):48–9,56.

The Dichter Institute for Motivation Research. Communicating the value of comprehensive pharmaceutical services to the consumer. Washington: American Pharmaceutical Association, 1973.

Special Counselling Situations

Anonymous. Courtesy to the hard of hearing (Pamphlet). Toronto: The Canadian Hearing Society, no date.

Anonymous. Emotional and behavioral responses to illness and to the interviewer. In: Enelow AJ, Swisher SN, eds. Interviewing and patient care. New York: Oxford University Press, 1978:102–24.

Anonymous. Focus on aging: communication disorders and aging. Toronto: Programme in Gerontology, 1981:2(2).

Anonymous. Tips on one-one communication with a deaf person (Pamphlet). Toronto: The Canadian Hearing Society, no date.

Ascione FJ, Shimp LA. Effectiveness of four education strategies in the elderly. Drug Intell Clin Pharm 1984;18:926–31.

Barnard D, Barr JT, Schumacher GE. Person to person—"empathy." Bethesda: American Association of Colleges of Pharmacy, 1982.

Burns B, Phillipson C. Drugs, aging and society. Social and pharmacologic perspectives. London: Croom Helm, 1986:1–9.

Chermak G, Jinks M. Counselling the hearing-impaired older adult. Drug Intell Clin Pharm 1981;15:377–82.

Darnell JC, Murray MD, Martz BL, Weinberger M. Medication use by ambulatory elderly—an in-home survey. J Am Geriatr Soc 1986;34(1):1–4.

Denton FT, Spencer BG. Canada's population and labour force, past, present and future. In: Marshall VW, ed. Aging in Canada. Don Mills: Fitzhenry and Whiteside, 1980:21.

Ellor JR, Kurz DJ. Misuse and abuse of prescription and nonprescription drugs by the elderly. Nurs Clin North Am 1982;17(2):319–30.

Health care for the elderly. Today's challenges—tomorrow's options. Ottawa: The Canadian Medical Association, 1987.

Jinks MJ. Geriatric therapy. In: Katcher BS, Young LY, Koda-Kimble MA, eds. Applied therapeutics, the clinical use of drugs. San Francisco: Applied Therapeutics, 1983:1513–29.

Klein LE, German PS, Levine DM, et al. Medication problems among outpatients. A study with emphasis on the elderly. Arch Intern Med 1984; 114:1185.

Lamy PP. Over the counter medication: the drug interactions we overlook. J Am Geriatr Soc 1982;30(Suppl11):69–75.

Lofholm P. Self medication by the elderly. In: Kayne RC, ed. Drugs and the elderly. Los Angeles: Ethel Percy Andrus Gerontology Center, University of Southern California, 1978:8–28.

Oliver CH. Communication awareness: Rx for embarrassing situations. Am Pharm 1982;NS22(10):21–3.

Ostrom JR, Hammarlund ER, Christensen DB, et al. Medication usage in an elderly population. Med Care 1985;23:157.

Reiser DE, Klein Schroder A. Obtaining the medical history. Patient interviewing—the human dimension. Baltimore: Waverly Press, 1980:206.

Smith MC, Sharpe TR. A study of pharmacists' involvement in drug use by the elderly. Drug Intell Clin Pharm 1984;18(6):525–9.

Sumner ED. Handbook of geriatric drug therapy for health care professionals. Philadelphia: Lea & Febiger, 1983.

The Canadian world almanac and book of facts. Toronto: Global Press, 1986:352.

Vestal RE. Drug use in the elderly: a review of problems and special considerations. Drugs 1978;16:358.

Summary

Hetherington M. The self-med megatrend. Drug Merch 1985;66:16,19–20.

Naisbitt J. Megatrends: ten new directions transforming our lives. New York: Warner Books, 1982:133–9.

Popcorn F. The popcorn report. New York: Doubleday, 1991:64–8.

Rachlis M, Kushner C. Second opinion—what's wrong with Canada's health care system and how to fix it. Toronto: Collins Publishers, 1989.

2
Topical First Aid

Marie Berry

Pharmacists should be aware of the types, causes and treatment—both nonpharmacologic and using nonprescription drug products—of minor cuts and wounds, musculoskeletal injuries, burns, frostbite, heat-related injuries, insect bites and stings, and dermatitis. Pharmaceutical products available for first aid include dressings, astringents, antiseptics, topical antibiotics, antipruritics, topical anesthetics and topical anti-inflammatory agents.

Structure of the Skin

The skin is the largest organ of the human body, making up 16 per cent. It covers the body, prevents dehydration and protects the underlying structures.

The skin protects against bacterial infections through three mechanisms: it acts as a physical barrier, minimizing bacterial penetration; the sebaceous glands secrete an oily substance (sebum) that prevents bacterial infestations; and the skin's pH does not support bacterial growth. The skin also acts as a thermoregulator for the body. The rich supply of capillaries in the dermis can contract to retain heat or dilate to transmit and eliminate heat. With its subcutaneous layer of fat, the skin acts as an insulator, and the sweat glands in the skin lower the body temperature through evaporation. The skin provides sensory perception and fluid retention. An injury to the skin can result in fluid loss, sensory perception loss, alteration in body temperature and infection.

Minor Cuts and Wounds

A wound damages the skin, breaking its continuity. Severe bleeding and infection are dangers; even wounds that appear minor may bleed profusely and are susceptible to infection. Penetrating injuries caused by contaminated objects, such as a rusty nail, may require tetanus prophylaxis. Animal bites may require rabies prophylaxis. Alone, the surface appearance of a wound is an unreliable guide to the wound's severity. A careful history of how the injury occurred and a thorough medical profile is required. Hemophiliacs, the elderly and people with diabetes must be especially cautious due to their compromised circulatory system and inadequate healing mechanisms. People with a history of endocarditis face the possibility of systemic infection and damage to cardiac tissue.

Infection commonly complicates injury. The acronym SHARP (swelling, heat, ache, redness and pus) points out the symptoms of an infected wound. Swelling and edema may occur in the tissue and lymph nodes adjacent to the injury. The injury may feel warm to touch and may be accompanied by fever, malaise or headache. Redness may appear around the wound or as streaks extending from the injury. An aching, throbbing wound with local pain indicates infection, as does an accumulation of pus (dead lymphocytes and sloughed tissue wastes).

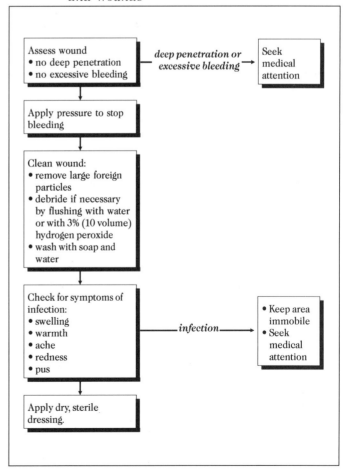

Figure 1 *Suggested Approach for Treating Minor Cuts and Wounds*

Assess wound
• no deep penetration
• no excessive bleeding

deep penetration or excessive bleeding → Seek medical attention

Apply pressure to stop bleeding

Clean wound:
• remove large foreign particles
• debride if necessary by flushing with water or with 3% (10 volume) hydrogen peroxide
• wash with soap and water

Check for symptoms of infection:
• swelling
• warmth
• ache
• redness
• pus

infection → • Keep area immobile
• Seek medical attention

Apply dry, sterile dressing.

Topical First Aid

Table I *Types of Wounds*

	Type	Description
Minimal bleeding	Abrasion	Outer layers scraped, may be contaminated with foreign objects
	Puncture	Foreign object penetrating the skin, e.g., nail, bullet, bee sting
Profuse bleeding	Avulsion	Tissues torn from the body, e.g. an earlobe.
	Incision	Sharp cut to the skin, may penetrate to cause nerve, muscle or tendon damage
	Laceration	Jagged, irregular wound, associated with much tissue damage

Adapted from: Parcel GS, ed. Basic emergency care of the sick and injured. Toronto: CV Mosby, 1982:79–93.

Staphylococcus aureus, a bacteria commonly found on the skin, can infect a wound. The number of organisms present determines the degree of infection with *Staphylococcus aureus*. Once the bacterial count reaches 10^5 the infection is considered serious. *Pseudomonas aeruginosa* and beta-hemolytic streptococci are more invasive; once their presence is evident countermeasures must be taken.

Wounds heal in four stages:

- Cells migrate over the skin defect in a process called epithelization. This process begins about 12 hours after the damage occurs, and continues until the wound is bridged, about 24 to 48 hours. Epithelization requires a sterile environment and is hindered by dry conditions, as moisture is needed for cell movement.
- Inflammation occurs as the required substrates (amines, enzymes, fluids and proteins) accumulate. The inflammation is accompanied by edema, which may occur as late as the second to third day.
- Scar tissue forms with the synthesis of collagen by the fibroblasts. This synthesis begins 4 to 6 days after the injury occurs and can continue for up to 6 weeks.
- The scar begins to mature about 6 weeks after the injury, when the scar is 50 per cent as strong as the normal skin. As the strength of the scar tissue increases, hypervascularity of the scar tissue fades and the scar returns to normal skin color, contracts and flattens.

In open wounds, the formation of granulation tissue produces active contraction and draws the wound edges together. These four stages occur in small as well as large wounds; the scar tissue forms and matures faster in a smaller wound.

The following general first aid measures promote healing and prevent infection.

Table II *Types of Bleeding*

Arterial bleeding	Bright red blood spurting from a wound, most serious
Venous bleeding	Dark red blood flowing from a wound
Capillary bleeding	Blood oozing from a superficial wound

Adapted from: Parcel GS, ed. Basic emergency care of the sick and injured. Toronto: CV Mosby, 1982:79–93.

- Stop the bleeding. If bleeding is severe, seek medical attention.
- Remove any large foreign object from the wound without contaminating the wound further. Debridement (removal of debris) is necessary and can be accomplished with repeated dressing changes. Clean the injury by flushing it with water. Hydrogen peroxide 3 per cent may be used to remove debris. It also possesses a hemostatic property, and a feeble germicide activity. If necessary, clean with soap and water.
- Removal of splinters may be eased by the application, for 12 hours, of a 40 per cent salicylic acid patch covered with a bandage. The salicylic acid hydrates the skin making the splinter easier to remove. Very young children and individuals with impaired circulation are not suitable candidates.
- Apply a dry, preferably sterile dressing. Wet dressings facilitate bacterial growth and should be avoided.
- Observe the injury for any signs of infection (SHARP). If they are present, medical attention is necessary. Keep the infected part immobile, as movement assists the spread of microorganisms. A warm, wet but sterile cloth applied as a compress to the wound, followed by a sterile dry dressing, is sometimes of use (see Figure 1).

Table III *Steps in Wound Treatment*

Primary concern	Control bleeding, using direct pressure and pressure points. Use of tourniquet is discouraged. Prevent or relieve shock. Keep individual warm.
Supportive care	Apply ice, compression bandage, elevation, splints.

Adapted from: Parcel GS, ed. Basic emergency care of the sick and injured. Toronto: CV Mosby, 1982:79–93.

Musculoskeletal Injuries

The musculoskeletal system gives the body support and affords movement. An injury to this system usually does not threaten life, but does impede mobility. Musculoskeletal injuries are classified according to the structure damaged.

A fracture is a break in a bone. Fractures can damage nerves and blood vessels and puncture internal organs. In a closed fracture the skin is not broken; an open fracture has an open wound. The fracture may be complete or incomplete depending on whether the bone breaks completely. At the point of a break there is usually severe pain. Movement increases pain and worsens damage.

The fracture must be immobilized by a splint before moving the injured person. The splint should not be so tight it impairs circulation. Materials such as pillows, newspapers or even the other leg in the case of a leg fracture, serve as suitable splints. If the fracture is open, bleeding must be controlled and care taken not to contaminate the wound.

Medical attention is necessary for all fractures, but especially important for fractures of the skull, clavicle or collarbone, and the vertebral column. Pressure on a skull fracture can result in further internal damage. Spinal cord injury is a concern in a vertebral column fracture. A collarbone fracture is painful and makes it difficult to support the arm.

Figure 2 *Suggested Approach for Treating Musculoskeletal Injuries*

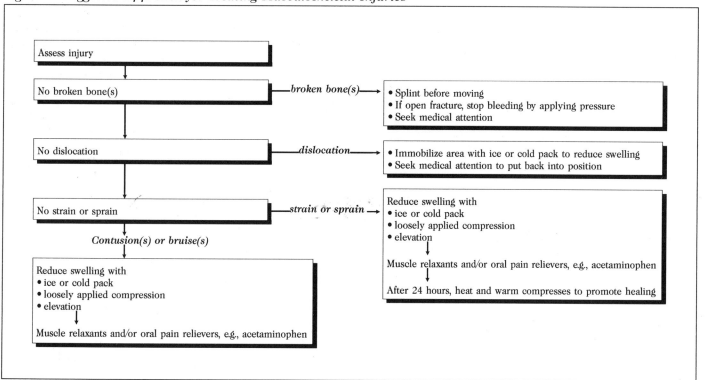

A dislocation is the displacement of a bone from its normal place. Severe pain intensifies if movement is attempted. The dislocated part appears deformed when compared to the uninjured side. Swelling is evident. The joint requires immobilization and ice or cold packs to reduce swelling. The dislocated part should be put back into place with medical supervision.

A subluxation is a partial dislocation in which the bone returns spontaneously to its proper place, possibly damaging surrounding structures.

Stretching or tearing a ligament and soft tissue is a sprain. Depending on whether the damage is a stretch, tear or combination, sprains are classified as mild to severe. Ice or a cold pack controls internal bleeding. A loosely applied compression bandage and elevation of the injured part control swelling and edema. Medical examination may be necessary if the sprain is severe.

Table IV *Questions to Differentiate Among Musculoskeletal Injuries*

1. What happened? How did the injury occur?
2. Where is the pain? Subjective information may help, e.g., muscle vs joint.
3. What is the nature of the pain? Point of extreme sensitivity? Dispersed? Intense? Mild?
4. How does the injured side compare to the normal side? Deformity present or absent?
5. Is there loss of function?

Adapted from: Parcel GS, ed. Basic emergency care of the sick and injured. Toronto: CV Mosby, 1982:127–47.

Strains stretch or tear muscle and tendon fibres. Strains are the most common musculoskeletal injury. They result from overexertion or an uncoordinated movement. A history of what the person was doing and the location of the pain (in a joint or along a muscle) differentiates between strains and other musculoskeletal injuries. The pain of a strain occurs when the affected muscle is used. Pain is not as severe as that of a sprain. Swelling is alleviated with prompt application of ice or cold packs. Compression and elevation of the area further reduce swelling. Chronic problems can result from neglecting strains. After 24 hours, heat and warm compresses are appropriate, increasing circulation. If applied sooner, the heat may increase the interstitial bleeding and consequently the swelling. Heat may be dry, moist or electrical (for example, a heating pad). Liniments are best avoided because they may aggravate already sensitive skin areas. Oral muscle relaxants, such as orphenadrine, chlorzoxazone and methocarbamol, also reduce pain. (See the chapter on internal analgesics.)

A direct blow causing damage produces contusions or bruises. Local pain, stiffness, discoloration and sometimes swelling are symptoms of contusions. Immobilization of the area, cold compresses and elevation help reduce pain and swelling (see Figure 2). Repeated damage can lead to calcification of the damaged tissue mass.

Burns

Burns to the skin are classified as chemical or thermal. The severity of the burn depends on a variety of factors including the type of burn, the temperature produced and the length of time the skin was exposed to the burning agent. Major complications of severe burns include tissue damage, shock, infection, hypoproteinemia, and fluid and electrolyte loss.

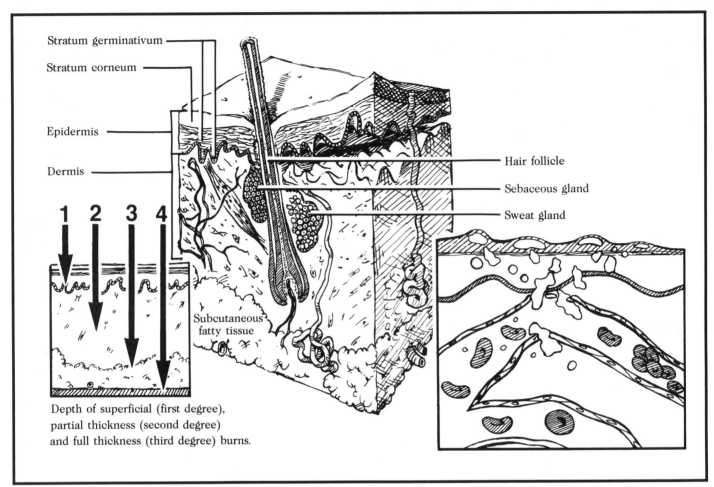

Figure 3 *Severity of Burns*

Thermal (or physical) burns result from exposure to a hot or scalding liquid, a flame or radioactive material, or contact with a hot surface or an electrical current, including lightning. The degree of damage relates to temperature of the burning agent and length of exposure to that agent. An electrical current may involve deeper tissues because of the current's conduction along nerves and blood vessels. Direct current is less dangerous than alternating current, as alternating current causes ventricular fibrillation. With high voltages (over 1,000 volts) respiratory failure may occur. Lightning strikes cause a characteristic "flower-like" electrical burn, along with central nervous system damage. Lightning burns range from superficial, healing spontaneously, to second and third degree burns requiring medical attention.

Chemical burns result from exposure to a corrosive chemical. The degree of damage relates to the nature of substance (for example, alkalies are more corrosive than acids) and the length of exposure time.

Severity of Burns

Traditionally, burns have been classified as first, second, third and fourth degree, depending on the depth of tissue damaged. More recently, the terms superficial, partial thickness and full thickness have been used as classifications (see Figure 3). A first degree or superficial burn involves the outer layers of skin. The skin is red and painful. A common example is a bathwater burn. A second degree or partial thickness burn involves the deeper layers of epidermis. These burns produce blisters and may be complicated by delayed healing and infection. An example of a second degree burn is one produced by a hot iron or a droplet of hot oil. Skin grafting may be needed in an extensive second degree burn. A third degree or full thickness burn involves the full thickness of the skin, including sebaceous glands, sweat glands and hair follicles. A flame can cause third degree burns. Char or fourth degree burns destroy not only the full thickness of the skin, but the underlying subcutaneous structures as well (see Table V).

The severity of burns depends on the percentage of the total body involved as well as the depth of damage. The Rule of Nines divides the body surface into areas of about 9 per cent or multiples of 9 per cent of the total body area (see Figure 4). To compensate for different body proportions, children under age 10 require an adjustment in the Rule of Nines. Generally, a child's head is considered 19 per cent of the surface area at birth and decreases by 1 per cent each year. The difference is added in equal portions to each lower limb. In an adult, a first degree burn involving about one-half a leg means an involvement of 4.5 per cent of body area (0.5 multiplied by nine per cent) and is considered a minor burn. Any second or third degree burn involving more than 20 per cent of the body is considered severe and requires medical attention. A burn that covers 40 per cent of the body surface is severe and requires hospitalization. A burn

Topical First Aid

Table V *Classification of Burns According to Severity*

Burn type	Characteristics	Healing
First-degree (Superficial)	Painful, redness	2–3 days, without treatment
Second-degree (Light partial thickness) (Deep partial thickness)	Painful, blisters are formed	7–30 days, with treatment
Third-degree (Full thickness)	Firm, dry wound, coagulated blood vessels may appear, painless due to loss of sensory receptors	Hospitalization is required
Fourth-degree (Deep thermal necrosis)	Black, charred appearance, dry wound, pain due to damage of underlying structure	Hospitalization is required

Adapted from: Parcel GS, ed. Basic emergency care of the sick and injured. Toronto: CV Mosby, 1982:79–93.

involving both legs and the torso involves 36 per cent of the body area and requires medical attention, if not hospitalization. An exception to this rule is any third degree burn that involves the face, hands, feet or genitalia. These burns always require hospitalization.

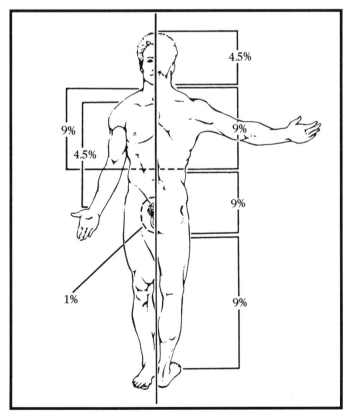

Figure 4 *Rule of Nines*

Determining the depth and severity of the burn wound is necessary for appropriate treatment. Scalds are usually first or second degree burns because the hot liquid touches the skin for a short time, but if the contact is due to immersion, especially of a baby in a bath, or if the clothing is soaked (for example, if a hot liquid is spilled), a scald may be a third degree burn. Flame burns are usually third degree because they involve longer contact with the skin. Electrical currents conduct readily through skin layers; though they may appear to cover a small area, electrical burns may represent a deep necrotic burn.

After a thermal injury, rapid loss of fluid into and around the injury site results in edema. The fluid loss may be significant due to the loss of the protective outer layer of skin. Thermoregulation is lost, and maintaining body temperature may become difficult.

Infection is another major concern when the outer layer of skin is destroyed, as these layers act as a barrier to infection. People especially susceptible to infections are those with debilitating diseases, impaired host defence mechanisms, poor nutritional status and those who are very young or very old. A history of other disease, such as diabetes or endocarditis, may also be a factor. *Staphylococcus aureus*, due to its ubiquitous nature, is a primary infective organism in burn wounds, but *Pseudomonas aeruginosa* and beta-hemolytic streptococci are more invasive when infecting a burn wound.

Treatment

Controversy exists over the use of antibiotics in burn therapy. Burn eschar (thermally damaged skin layers) is dead tissue with no blood supply; systemic antibiotics do not penetrate it. However, sufficient systemic antibiotics may penetrate discharge fluids so that organisms present in burn eschar may develop resistance to these antibiotics. Topical antibiotics may reduce the numbers of infecting organisms, but overgrowth may become a problem. The ointment and cream bases of many topical products provide a moist environment that encourages bacterial growth. In theory, both systemic and topical antibiotics are useful in burn therapy, but in practical terms the burn requires only thorough cleansing. Antibiotic therapy becomes a medical decision made in a hospital setting or by a physician.

The type and severity of the burn must be assessed. Presence of blisters, absence of feeling, severity of pain and remaining vascularity determine the depth of the burn; by using the Rule of Nines, severity can be estimated. Hypovolemic shock is a threat when 20 per cent or more of the body surface is involved. Loss of plasma with a corresponding loss of blood volume and drop in blood pressure occurs in hypovolemic shock. A compensatory vasoconstriction temporarily reduces the size of the vascular bed and may temporarily maintain the blood pressure. The pulse is rapid but weak. The burn wound heals in the same manner as an open wound injury.

Minor Burns

Removing the offending agent and cooling the area are the first lines of therapy. The aim of first aid treatment of minor burns is to relieve pain and reduce risk of infection. Immersion in ice-cold water provides subjective pain relief because the low temperature blocks cutaneous nerve conduction. As well, cold water lowers tissue temperature, reduces vasodilation, promotes vasoconstriction and limits edema. Histamine release from mast cells has a temperature threshold; with the cooling temperatures, histamine release diminishes, decreasing capillary permeability and reducing edema even further. Cooling temperatures also promote protein coagulation; hence, the

Topical First Aid

Figure 5 *Suggested Approach for Treating Burns*

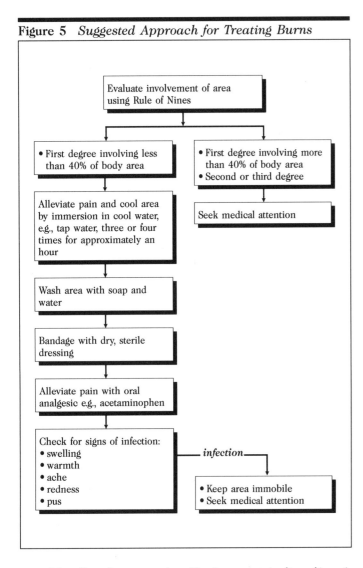

burns. Controversy exists over whether blisters should be broken. Breaking blisters reduces the risk of infection; if the blister is left intact, the serum provides an excellent growth medium for bacteria. If blisters are not broken, epithelization is quicker in the moist environment. Flushing the burn area removes some of the debris. Wrapping the person in a wet towel or sheet may relieve pain. A severe burn is not packed in ice because the cold may damage more exposed tissue. Fluid loss may be apparent, but oral fluids are not given since vomiting may occur. Quick transportation to a hospital is necessary. Skin grafts, either homografts or heterografts, may be needed. Scarring and contracture of joints occur with severe burns. Splinting a joint reduces contracture, and Jobst (compression) garments relieve swelling and reduce scarring (see Table VI).

Table VI *Treatment for Serious Burns*

Chemical	Remove contaminated clothing. Flush with copious amounts of water (injured area held under a tap or a shower is most appropriate). If antidote is available, use as per instructions. Seek medical help.
Electrical	Break electrical contact (turn switch off, knock person away with nonconductive object). If victim is not breathing, clear air passage if needed and begin cardiopulmonary resuscitation. Electrical burns appear simple, but deep muscle necrosis may occur. Treat secondary injuries, fractures. Seek medical attention.
Flame burn	Do not roll (rolling only exposes more area to the flame); smother the flame with a blanket or coat. Wrap individual in clean towel or sheet. Seek medical help.
Hot water burn	Remove hot, wet clothing. Wrap individual in clean towel or sheet. Seek medical help.

size of the affected areas is reduced by decreasing the flow of lymph and its protein concentrations.

Cool water (20 to 25°C) appears to be as effective as cold water. Tap water is about 10°C and is the most available cooling fluid. Cooling should last an hour or more for optimal pain relief and minimized injuries. The burn wound is immersed until the cold temperature causes discomfort, then is removed and reimmersed. Repeating this procedure three or four times is usually sufficient. Overzealous cooling (for example, direct and continued application of ice) must be avoided, as cold injury (such as frostbite) may occur.

After cooling, the burn wound is washed with soap and water and a clean, dry dressing is applied. Specialized burn dressings, for example 2nd Skin, provide a cool barrier protecting the wound. Traditional substances, such as butter, bacon fat and ointments, for example Ozonol, must not be applied to the burn, as they are difficult to remove. However, boiled potato peel dressings, another traditional treatment, have been found successful in wound healing.

Serious Burns

The treatment of serious burns depends on the cause. Hypovolemic shock and the threat of infection are concerns with more serious

Topical anesthetics are best avoided, as they may produce local sensitization and worsen the burn wound. Topical antibiotics are of questionable value when applied by the first aider; these agents should be applied by hospital personnel, and only for the following reasons: to prevent or minimize bacterial invasion of surrounding tissue and the blood stream; to promote early eschar removal and the generation of granulation tissue; to protect newly formed granulation and epithelial tissue; and to establish an early tissue barrier, facilitating wound closure.

Frostbite

Frostbite occurs when tissue is injured or destroyed by freezing. The nose, cheeks, ears, fingers and toes are the areas most commonly affected. High winds may exacerbate damage. When the temperature

Table VII	*Frostbite Injury Classification*
Degree	**Appearance**
First	White hard plaques
Second	Clear fluid, superficial blisters
Third	Purple fluid, deep blisters, discolored skin

Adapted from: McCauley RL, et al. Frostbite injuries: a rational approach based on the pathophysiology. J Trauma 1983;23(2):143–7.

is cold, touching bare skin to cold metal, gasoline or other volatile products can cause severe and immediate frostbite.

Initially, the affected areas become flushed or reddened, turning to a greyish yellow or white. Symptoms associated with frostbite include coldness, numbness and occasionally pain. Usually, other people bring the condition to the attention of the affected person. Frostbite is classified according to the depth of tissue damage (see Table VII).

When the injury begins to thaw, pain, itching, swelling, scabbing and ulceration occur. Hypothermia is a major complication of frostbite. Infection and bruising of the affected area can lead to gangrene.

Two other types of cold injuries are produced by lowering the temperature of tissues rather than by freezing. Local nonfreezing injuries may occur either in wet conditions (for example, trench foot) or in dry conditions (for example, chilblain). Trench foot is not common in civilian populations. It involves the skin and subcutaneous tissue.

Figure 6 *Suggested Approach for Treating Frostbite*

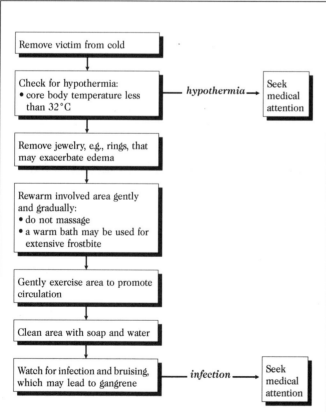

Chilblain produces red, itchy skin lesions, usually on the legs.

Hypothermia is the unintentional lowering of body temperature due to prolonged or extreme exposure. People at risk include the elderly, the inactive, those with cardiovascular disease and mental impairment, and those taking sedative drugs or alcohol.

Treatment

Avoiding cold, wet areas, dressing warmly and avoiding drugs or alcohol that affect judgment and alter peripheral circulation help prevent frostbite. Smoking nicotine-containing cigarettes produces vasoconstriction, which contributes to frostbite. Frostbite wounds heal like burn or open wounds with one exception: the frostbite wound does not contract. Burn and open wounds reduce in size as their edges draw together with the granulation tissue; the frostbite wound does not reduce in size.

Treating frostbite begins by removing the person from the cold environment. Rewarming should be gentle; warm baths are preferred. Once the area is red, it is exercised to promote circulation. To prevent further tissue damage, a frostbitten area is not massaged. Soap and water can be used to clean the injured area as infection is a threat. Although one study reported success with application of topical aloe vera every 6 hours, the benefit of aloe vera is questionable, as other treatment measures were included. Care is needed in treating the delicate areas between the fingers and toes. In anticipation of edema, common after frostbite, jewelry should be removed, especially rings. Hypothermia is evident if the core body temperature falls below 32°C. Under these circumstances, vigorous rewarming is needed, and is best done under full medical supervision (see Figure 6).

Heat-Related Injuries

Heat-related injuries encompass mild to serious conditions ranging from prickly heat to the marathon runner's heat cramps. Heat-related deaths, especially in the very young and very old, occur during heat waves.

The body produces heat when muscles work. The environment contributes to body heat by radiation, convection and conduction. Evaporation of sweat removes excess heat from the body, but depletes the body's volume of water. Dehydration results; once the volume of water is depleted there is no further water for sweating. The resulting increase in body heat with a corresponding decrease in blood volume increases the strain on the cardiac and respiratory systems. Salt (sodium) and other electrolyte depletion may produce muscle cramps. Salt content of the diet is usually enough to satisfy day-to-day body needs. Salt tablets are marketed for prophylactic use in extreme environments. Commercial beverages with a high sodium content are available for athletes' use (for example, Gatorade).

Heat transfers from warmer to cooler objects. When air temperature is lower than body temperature, fans circulate heat away from the body. If the air is warmer, heat transmits to the body, and fans only contribute to this transmission. If the humidity of the surrounding air is too high to allow evaporation, body cooling does not occur.

Prickly heat refers to rashes caused by continuous sweating, especially in areas covered by clothing (for example, waistbands and diaper areas). Recurrences of prickly heat can lead to more serious dermatitis.

Topical First Aid

Table VIII *Symptoms of Heat-Related Injuries*

	Heat exhaustion	Heat stroke
Face	Pale	Red, flushed
Skin	Moist	Hot, dry
Sweating	Profuse	None
Pulse	Weak, rapid	Strong, rapid
Behavior	Subdued	May be erratic at onset
Unconscious	Not usually	Usually

Adapted from: Parcel GS, ed. Basic emergency care of the sick and injured. Toronto: CV Mosby, 1982:184–95.

Heat cramps are painful muscle spasms in the arms and legs. Replacing fluids and electrolytes alleviates heat cramps.

Heat exhaustion occurs in athletes, soldiers, workers in hot climates, infants and incapacitated adults unable to express their need for water. The individual shows progressive weakness and must be moved immediately to the coolest place possible and encouraged to drink cool liquids.

Heat stroke is characterized by an increase in body temperature, salt loss and dehydration. It is usually associated with physical exertion. Drugs such as LSD and amphetamines that increase heat production and drugs such as antihistamines, phenothiazines, propranolol and anticholinergics that decrease sweating can worsen heat exhaustion to the point of heat stroke.

Several measures can prevent heat-related injuries: wearing appropriate clothing that allows for heat loss, acclimatization when working in hot climates, the use of shade and hats, reducing work load, a good intake of fluids and good physical conditioning.

Insect Bites and Stings

Insect bites can be caused by the Diptera class of insects, which includes mosquitos, flies, gnats, bedbugs, ticks and lice. Insect stings may be caused by the Hymenoptera class of insects, including bees, wasps, hornets, yellow jackets and ants. An insect bite involves mandibles and other mouth parts; a sting occurs when the insect injects venom into its victim through a piercing organ or stinger. Hymenoptera stings are more dangerous, because the insect injects venom into the victim by means of a specialized ovipositor or stinger composed of the piercing apparatus, lateral plates and appendages (for movement and attachment), and the venom sac and glands. Only female hymenoptera have stingers.

Certain hymenoptera have a serrated stinger, complete with venom sac, that may remain in the wound (for example, the honeybee). These stingers must be removed since they work their way into the skin. The stingers of other hymenoptera are smooth and less likely to remain in the wound. Stingers deposited near the eye have been reported to work their way into the globe of the eye.

The greatest risk of stings comes from colonized hymenoptera. Ants and bees use their stingers solely as a defence mechanism, whereas the carnivorous hornets and wasps use theirs to kill small insects upon which they prey. African bees introduced into Brazil in 1957, are an aggressive species of Hymenoptera, but their northward advance along with their threat to Canadians is difficult to determine.

Insect venom consists of a complex mixture of proteins, peptides and enzymes that can elicit an immunoglobulin E-mediated allergic reaction. There is sharp pain lasting several minutes, localized swelling, redness and intense itching. Within a few hours the symptoms subside. The venom of the hymenopteran differs among species, but is similar enough to produce cross-sensitivity. Five hundred stings are considered a lethal dose in man, but accounts exist of people surviving more than 4 times as many stings.

The very young, very old and people with debilitating disease or compromised immune systems are more at risk of sensitivity to hymenopteran venom. There are reports that individuals taking beta blockers and/or calcium channel blockers have more severe reactions and, in some instances, relapses to the stings. Beta blockade with its unopposed cholinergic activity and secondary bradycardia may be the reason for this effect.

When the Diptera class insects bite their victims to obtain food, they secrete a small amount of saliva into the wound to assist feeding. The saliva contains proteins that can cause an allergic reaction. The response to a bite is initial pain at the site, then the triple response of wheal formation, erythema (redness) and flare (swelling and heat).

The Diptera class insects also carry disease. The Ixodid tick are vectors responsible for the spread of *Borrelia burgdorferi* or Lyme disease. The Anopheles mosquitoes carry Plasmodium infections or malaria. Equine encephalitis is spread by the Culex and Culiseta mosquitoes. These diseases, along with the many others that these insects carry, are treatable, however prevention of the initial insect bite is preferred.

Hypersensitivity can complicate insect bites and stings. Immunological sensitivity responses are classified in four categories or types. Type I is an immediate reaction (for example, anaphylaxis) and is mediated by immunoglobulin E. Type II occurs when the reaction is between antibodies and tissue antigens (for example, transplant organ rejection). Type III is produced by an antibody and antigen complex (for example, serum sickness). Type IV is a delayed hypersensitivity reaction (for example, contact dermatitis) and is mediated by immunoglobulin M and immunoglobulin G.

A more useful classification of hypersensitivity when considering insect bites and stings is either immediate response (corresponding to Type I reactions) or delayed response (corresponding to Type IV reactions).

The immediate response in a hypersensitive person is an anaphylactic reaction, usually occurring within 5 to 20 minutes of the bite or sting. Urticaria (hives), pruritus (itching), angioedema and gastrointestinal disturbances are seen initially followed by laryngeal edema, bronchospasm, vascular collapse and cardiac arrhythmias. Cardiac arrest occurs thereafter. The delayed reaction occurs some hours after a bite or sting and is manifested by swelling at the site, bruising of the area, and sometimes blistering or necrosis of superficial tissues.

Siphonaptera (fleas), Hemiptera (bedbugs) and Anoplura (lice) also are biting insects. Bites produced by these insects appear similar to those of other insects, but treatment includes eradication of the insect from the affected person and decontamination of personal items. (See the chapter on topical antiparasitics.)

Treatment

General treatment of insect bites and stings includes oral antihistamines, cool compresses, topical antipruritics, beta agonists (for example pseudoephedrine), analgesics for pain relief and elevation of the limb or affected part to discourage venom spread (see Figure 7). Prevention is preferred to treatment.

Figure 7 *Suggested Approach for Treating Insect Bites and Stings*

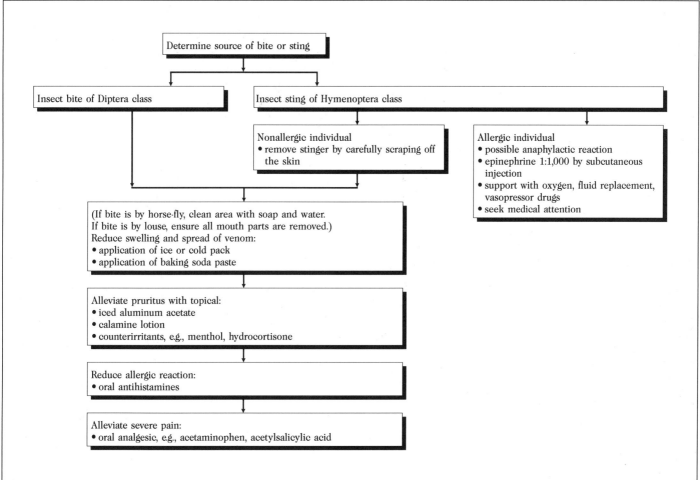

Bites

Symptomatic treatment of insect bites include oral antihistamines, cool compresses and antipruritics. Oral antihistamines are preferred over topical antihistamines with their sensitization potential. They are useful for both urticaria or generalized pruritus. Sedation may be a problem with oral antihistamines; alternatively the sedation may enable the bitten individual to rest overnight. Non sedating oral antihistamines appear to be as effective for relief of urticaria and pruritus.

Chilled aluminum acetate, calamine lotion, counterirritants, hydrocortisone, and even a paste of baking soda are useful topical antipruritics. Topical anesthetics may offer some degree of symptomatic relief despite their sensitizing ability. Colloidal oatmeal baths, for example Aveeno, may alleviate severe itching experienced by an extensively bitten individual. Ammonia-containing bite "neutralizers", for example After Bite, provide a cooling sensation which may be caused by the evaporation of the vehicle.

In treating a horsefly bite, the area of the bite should be cleansed thoroughly with soap and water to remove debris left by this particularly dirty insect. In treating tick bites, the tick's mouth parts must be completely removed, otherwise irritation and infection will result. Tweezers and/or an organic solvent such as a drop of oil will aid removal. Hot objects such as a cigarette should not be used.

Stings

In a nonallergic person, appropriate first aid therapy includes application of an icepack to prevent the spread of venom, application of a paste of baking soda and water, or application of papain, either as a lotion (Stop Itch) or a paste to relieve wheal formation. Papain is found in meat tenderizers (for example, Adolph's) and is able to break down some of the proteins of insect venom and reduces the potential for allergic reaction and wheal formation. Timing is important; if the papain powder is applied too late, the proteins in the insect venom will have elicited the maximum reactions.

If a person is stung by a honeybee, the stinger must be removed. The stinger cannot be grasped and pulled out because the pinching movement squeezes more venom from the still attached venom sac into the person. Instead, the stinger must be scraped off the skin. Chilled aluminum acetate solution or calamine lotion relieves pruritus. Counterirritants (for example, menthol) and hydrocortisone also alleviate pruritus. Oral antihistamines are able to reduce the allergic reaction.

Anaphylactic reactions must be treated immediately with subcutaneous epinephrine (1:1,000), oxygen, fluid replacement and vasopressor drugs. The use of parenteral corticosteroids is controversial, but may be considered for the person with protracted anaphylaxis and delayed reactions. Desensitization may be required if an individual has previously experienced anaphylactic reactions to insect bites. Desensitization involves injecting a minute quantity of the antigenic insect venom, which, in turn, builds the level of venom-specific antibodies. The desensitization program itself may cause anaphylactic reactions. Beekeepers who are frequently stung may develop an immunity. Desensitization protection is only temporary and the person regains sensitivity gradually over 6 to 10 months.

Prevention

To avoid insects and insect bites, individuals should avoid brightly colored clothing, strong and flowery perfume, overripe fruit and clover fields. Covering up with clothing, tucking pant legs into socks and using mosquito netting provide physical barriers to insects.

Individuals allergic to stings should wear identification bracelets. Commercially produced anaphylaxis kits are available for field use. People at risk should always carry preloaded epinephrine syringes, such as EpiPen (0.3 mg epinephrine in an automatic injector), EpiPen Junior (0.15 mg epinephrine in an automatic injector) or AnaKit (two injections of 0.3 mL of 1:1,000 epinephrine in a regular syringe, plus alcohol swabs, a tourniquet and chewable antihistamine tablets). Insect venom extracts are available for diagnosis and for treatment of people prone to anaphylactic reactions from insect bites. These extracts consist of freeze-dried venom from several hymenoptera species and may cause systemic allergic reactions.

The active ingredient in most commercial insect repellents is diethyltolumide (DEET) combined with ethohexadiol or dimethyl phthalate. Repellents are effective against most biting insects, but not those that sting. Once applied insect repellents surround the application site with a vapour which deters insects. Wind, rain, time and perspiration are able to reduce the size of this vapour barrier, and reapplication is necessary. Insect repellents should not be applied near eyes, mucous membranes or broken skin. Application to clothing is an alternative, however a test area should be used to evaluate possible damage to fabric.

Toxicity reactions have been documented. Children who have received repeated and extensive applications of DEET have experienced encephalopathy: slurred speech, staggering gait, agitation, tremors. Accidental ingestion of DEET containing repellents have resulted in toxicities and in one report death. Preparations containing less than 50 per cent DEET are considered free of side effects when applied to the skin of adults, although there have been occasional reports of contact dermatitis. Users should follow directions carefully and be alert to signs of reactions.

Citronella based repellents provide short term protection from mosquitos, but are not effective against other insects. Permethrin, an insecticide, applied as a spray to clothing deters ticks. Other purported repellents include Avon's Skin-So-Soft and oral thiamine (vitamin B1), but data is lacking as to their effectiveness.

Dermatitis

Dermatitis is a general term for various skin disorders involving inflammation with possible damage by chemical or mechanical irritants. Erythema, pruritus, bullae formation (blisters) and urticaria may all be present. The dermatitis may be superficial or there may be deep destruction in the underlying dermal layers. Dermatitis is discussed in depth in its own chapter, but several classifications are

of special interest to the first aider: dermatitis actinica (sunburn), poison ivy contact dermatitis and urticaria (hives).

Dermatitis actinica results from overexposure or hypersensitivity to sunlight or other sources of actinic rays (for example, tanning beds). Some drugs may cause photosensitivity (phenothiazines, sulfones, chlorothiazides, griseofulvin, oral antidiabetic agents, oral contraceptives and some antibiotics). Perfumes and antiseptics can cause contact photosensitivity.

Figure 8 *Suggested Approach for Treating Poison Ivy Dermatitis*

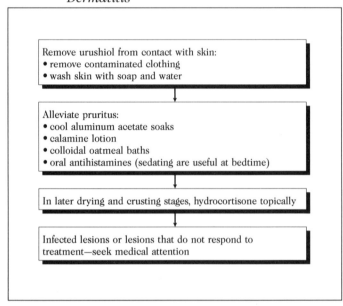

Sunburned skin is red and inflamed. There may be edema and general malaise, exfoliation and pigment changes (tanning). Sunscreens with a sun protection factor (SPF) of 15 are recommended by the Canadian Cancer Society and the Canadian Dermatology Association. A sunscreen that protects against both UVA and UVB and gradual exposure prevents more severe reactions. Treatment includes oral analgesics for pain, cool wet dressings and calamine lotion as an antipruritic. Hydration of the skin must be maintained, but anything applied to the sunburn has to be removed eventually and greasy preparations may be difficult to remove. Topical anesthetics afford temporary relief, but they must be used sparingly to prevent sensitization. (See the chapter on sunscreens.)

Poison ivy contact dermatitis is caused by exposure to urushiol, which is in the resin of poison ivy, oak and sumac. Urushiol is sticky and can be carried on such things as the fur of animals, garden tools, golf balls and clothing. Burning poison ivy liberates vapors that can also cause contact dermatitis. Because it is an allergy, the first exposure may not elicit any skin eruptions, but rather enables antibodies to form and produce dermatitis on subsequent exposures.

Prophylaxis of poison ivy dermatitis includes avoiding the plants and areas where they grow. Ideally a barrier applied in advance of exposure would offer protection. However, the various barriers tested, (organoclay, silicone, bentonite and kaolin) have not been successful. Desensitization therapy (treating the person with Rhus antigens) results in shorter and milder outbreaks of dermatitis. The therapy

Topical First Aid

is a temporary measure and may last only six months. In addition, the person needs desensitization therapy for every season of the plant. Objective relief is the main advantage of desensitization therapy.

Lesions develop within 12 to 48 hours. Redness and swelling are followed by blister formation. Pruritus is evident. The lesions heal rapidly, within 7 to 14 days. The severity of the reaction increases with age. The goal of therapy is to prevent the itching and enable the lesions to heal without secondary complications such as infection. Cool aluminum acetate soaks, tap water compresses, bland lotions such as calamine, and tepid baths with colloidal oatmeal are used. Oral antihistamines help, especially when they produce drowsiness at bedtime. If sedation is not desired, nonsedating antihistamines appear as effective. The use of acetylsalicylic acid in large doses (0.6 g every 4 to 6 hours) provides dramatic relief to some individuals. In the oozing stages of the dermatitis, topical corticosteroids are ineffective, but they benefit in the later drying, crusting stages. (See the chapter on dermatitis.)

Table IX *Causes of Urticaria (Hives)*

Cause	Frequency
Foods, e.g., shellfish, citrus fruits, berries, eggs, nuts, chocolate	Common in all ages
Drugs, e.g., penicillin, sulfonamides	Common in all ages
Pollen	Common in adults
Physical agents, e.g., pressure, cold, heat, sunlight	Less common in adults Least common in children
Infection, e.g., infectious mononucleosis, hepatitis B	Occasional More common in children
Secondary to other disease, e.g., lymphoma, systemic lupus erythematosus, dermatomyositis	Occasional

Adapted from: Mills J, Ho MT, Trunkey DD, eds. Current emergency diagnosis and treatment. Los Altos: Lange, 1983:595–607.

Table X *Checklist for History of Urticarial Reaction (Hives)*

1. Urticaria itself—timing; relation to meals or exercise; pattern of rash itself
2. General health—specific enquiry about each organ system
3. Known allergies—atopic features
4. Detailed dietary history
5. Occupational details
6. Home environment—hobbies, pets
7. Cosmetics
8. Emotional disorders
9. Drug history
10. Dental history
11. Travel history
12. Past history of major and minor illnesses
13. Nature and results of any past treatment for urticaria
14. Family history of urticaria

Urticaria or hives results from an immunological reaction with antigen-antibody complex formation and a subsequent release of chemical mediators. Histamine is the most common biochemical mediator in urticaria, although other kinins and amines may also be released (for example, serotonin). Pruritus and the triple response of wheal, erythema and flare are produced.

Discovering and eliminating the cause resolves urticaria (see Table IX). Symptomatic relief includes oral antihistamines; both sedating and nonsedating appear equally effective. Cimetidine, a prescription drug, has been used successfully in emergency treatment of urticaria. Short-term local treatment includes aluminum acetate soaks and calamine lotion (see Figure 8). Because dry skin perpetuates attacks of chronic hives, hydration of the skin is important.

Pharmaceutical Agents
Dressings

The scab over a wound is nature's dressing. This crust of dried serum is impermeable and keeps the wound clean. It minimizes protein and fluid loss and reduces pain by insulating sensitive tissues. Most important, the scab holds the wound in place. A pharmaceutical dressing attempts to fulfil all these requirements by maintaining the cleanliness of the wound, controlling the wound environment, controlling edema, eliminating the space between tissues when the dressing is held tight against the wound, immobilizing the tissues and reducing scar formation. Table XI outlines the steps involved in applying a dressing.

Table XI *Application of a Dressing*

Wash hands.

Allow the wound to bleed slightly. Do not squeeze a puncture wound to make it bleed. If the puncturing object or part of it remains in the wound, it can be pushed further into the wound.

Use a sterile gauze pad saturated with soap and water to gently wash dirt away from the wound's edges.

Gently flush the wound with large amounts of water; do not apply antiseptics.

Cover the wound with a sterile gauze dressing using commercially available materials whenever possible. Open the package according to directions and handle the dressing only by a corner. Be sure the dressing extends well beyond the edges of the wound.

Cover the gauze dressing with a bandage and secure adhesive tape. Do not impede circulation by bandaging the wound too tightly.

Refer the individual to a physician for the necessary follow-up.

Ointments provide protection, soften skin for greater permeability, provide a moist environment for wound healing and act as a vehicle for other medication (for example, antibacterials). However, anything that goes on a wound eventually has to be removed; in the case of a burn, an ointment may be difficult to remove.

Occlusive dressings keep the healing tissues moist. Their advantages include rapid healing, reduced pain, fewer dressing changes, exclusion of microorganisms and better cosmetic results. Dermatitis, both contact and atopic, blistering diseases and pruritic skin benefit from occlusive dressings. Alternatively, there are disadvantages of occlusive dressings: accumulation of pus, possible hematoma, silent infections, trauma to adjacent skin and adherence of the dressing to the new tissue.

Bandages are occlusive and enhance penetration of medication. Gauze is the primary constituent of bandages and acts as an absorbent and protectant. Gauze is made by weaving bleached cotton into an open-mesh cloth. The natural waxes and impurities are removed from the cotton to increase its absorbing capacity. Gauze is classified either according to its mesh or to the number of threads per inch. Viscous rayon (regenerated cellulose) is also used in bandages, and many dressing pads include both cellulose and cotton. Most dressing pads are packaged in sterile individual packages.

Self adhesive bandages (for example, Band-Aids, Elastoplast) are convenient alternatives to gauze and tape. Butterfly closures are self adhesive bandages intended to pull and hold the edges of small wounds together to encourage healing. Butterfly closures are no substitute for stitches in larger wounds.

Nonadherent gauze is an easily removed dressing that provides the same protection as ordinary gauze. It is preferred as the primary dressing, next to the wound, because the healing process is not disturbed when the dressing is removed and because it provides increased comfort. The gauze can be rendered nonadherent by one of two methods: viscous rayon is impregnated with an oil-in-water emulsion so the resulting gauze dressing remains absorbent; or one side of the gauze is covered with plastic that has numerous holes that allow the gauze to absorb but not to adhere to the wound.

Gauze bandages may be medicated with an ointment. Medicated gauze allows easy removal and provides a delivery system for antibiotics and antiseptics. Petrolatum gauze removes easily and acts as a protectant for the underlying skin. Antiseptic-impregnated gauze contains chlorhexidine or povidone-iodine to prevent infection and to ease removal of the dressing. Antibiotic-impregnated gauze, such as framycetin sulfate is used in the prophylaxis and treatment of infection, but is obtained by prescription only.

Protective dressings may be either mechanical or physical in nature. Collodion is a viscous solution of pyroxylon in an ether and alcohol vehicle; flexible collodion is a collodion containing camphor and castor oil. Traditionally, both have been used to seal small wounds such as mosquito bites. Aerosol polymer sprays, for example Opsite Spray, provide flexible protective films on the skin. They are impermeable to wound exudate and reduce fluid loss. Hydrogels, for example DuoDerm, and hydrocolloids, for example 2nd Skin, Actiderm and OpSite Dressing, are a matrix with a high percentage of water. They are soft and comfortable while providing optimum conditions for wound healing. Hydrocolloids are absorptive and consequently should be changed daily. Siloxane dressings, for example Biobrane, adheres directly to the wound, separating after about 5 to 7 days, to protect. However, petrolatum gauze and other medicated gauzes are currently used more often.

Hydrophilic bead mixtures and matrixes, for example Desibran and DuoDerm Granules, are debridement agents that, applied as a dressing, absorb wound secretions and encourage wound healing.

Astringents

Astringents are locally applied protein precipitants that have low cell permeability, so they act on the skin surface. Astringents decrease cell permeability and contract and wrinkle the skin, protecting the underlying tissue. Edema, inflammation and exudation are reduced

because the endothelium of the capillary hardens, lessening transcapillary movement of proteins. Astringents reduce minor hemorrhaging by coagulating blood. They may cause skin irritation in high concentrations. Most astringents have mild antiseptic properties.

Aluminum salts are the most commonly used astringent agents. Aluminum sulfate is used in solutions of 5 to 10 per cent for foul discharges from mucous membranes and also as a local application for ulcers. A 20 per cent solution of aluminum sulfate (Singose) relieves insect stings and bites. Aluminum acetate (Burow's solution) is used as a wet dressing in oozing areas (for example, poison ivy dermatitis, athlete's foot and acute eczema). Gauze soaked in a 1:10 dilution and applied to the wound promotes a cooling effect. The dressing should not be covered. Aluminum acetate compresses also promote drying of oozing areas and formation of protective crusts. They are usually applied for 30 minutes 3 or 4 times daily. Aluminum chlorhydrate and aluminum chloride can cause irritation and are reserved for use in antiperspirants.

Bismuth salts protect mucosal and raw surfaces. They are weak astringents and antiseptics. At one time bismuth salts were widely used in dusting powders, but they are now considered unsafe for use as an astringent due to their questionable efficacy and potential toxicity. They are found in gastrointestinal products (for example, Pepto Bismol) and hemorrhoid products (for example, Nupercainal suppositories).

Tannic acid once was a widely used antiseptic, but has few, if any, legitimate medical uses today. It is readily absorbed through damaged skin and mucous membranes, causing liver damage. Witch hazel or hamamelis contains tannins, gallic acid, a bitter principle and a trace of volatile oil. Distilled witch hazel was once used for its astringent properties, as a cooling soak for sprains and bruises and in dressings for small superficial wounds and minor skin irritations. Use in recent times is limited to hemorrhoid therapy.

Exsiccated (dried) alum acts as a hemostat for superficial abrasions and cuts. Styptic pencils are molded potassium alum fused with potassium nitrate. They are kept in airtight containers and must be wet before use. Dilute alum solutions have been used for mouthwashes.

Antiseptics

Antiseptics are applied to living tissues to kill or prevent growth of microorganisms. Disinfectants destroy microorganisms and are applied to inanimate objects. Both antiseptics and disinfectants operate by denaturing the cellular proteins of microorganisms. Prophylactic use of both is common, although the development of resistant organisms may occur. In treating wounds, antiseptics do not replace proper mechanical cleaning and the use of a clean dressing. Factors to consider in choosing an antiseptic include: its actions against a broad spectrum of microorganisms; its potency; whether it is bactericidal or bacteriostatic (bactericidal is preferred); its therapeutic index; the incidence of hypersensitivity reactions; whether it has low surface tension to facilitate cell penetration; if it is active in the presence of exudated material; and if it has rapid but sustained action (see Table XII).

Alcohols are antiseptic at a 70 per cent concentration. Isopropyl and ethanol are the two most common antiseptics. Alcohols evaporate quickly and must be rubbed on the skin for about 2 minutes to be effective. Because alcohols cause drying and irritation they are not used on open wounds. Isopropyl alcohol is more effective than ethanol as it has a lower surface tension. As well, it is a common vehicle for many other topical agents. However,

Topical First Aid

Table XII *Comparison of Antiseptics*

Agent	Spectrum	Bactericidal/ Bacteriostatic	Advantage/Disadvantage
Alcohols (ethanol, isopropyl)	All common bacteria	Bactericidal	Used commonly as a vehicle; causes dryness
Boric acid		Bacteriostatic	Unwarranted reputation
Chlorhexidine	Gram positive, gram negative	Bactericidal	Good choice as antiseptic
Chlorine (sodium hypochlorite)	Gram positive, gram negative, some spores and viruses	Bactericidal	Effectiveness decreased by organic matter
Iodine and iodophors (povidone-iodine)	Gram positive, gram negative, fungi, protozoa, yeast	Bactericidal	Povidone-iodine less irritating
Mercurial compounds (merbromin, nitromersol)	Gram positive, gram negative, fungi	Bacteriostatic	Less effective and more toxic than other antiseptics
Silver compounds (silver nitrate)	Gram positive, gram negative	Bactericidal	Nonpresciption use usually as caustic pencils
Oxidizing agents (benzoyl peroxide, hydrogen peroxide, potassium permanganate)	Broad spectrum, especially anerobes	Bactericidal	Benzoyl peroxide used in acne; hydrogen peroxide for debridement
Substituted phenols (hexachlorophene, triclosan)	Gram positive especially staphylococci	Bacteriostatic	Hexachlorophene requires prescription; triclosan found in bar soap.
Quarternary ammonium compounds (benzalkonium chloride, cetrimide)	Gram positive, gram negative, some viruses, fungi and protozoa	Bactericidal	Used as disinfectants as well

isopropyl alcohol causes vasodilation beneath the surface of application, so needle punctures and incisions bleed more than when ethanol is used.

The reputation of *boric acid* as a germicide and astringent is unwarranted. It is no longer used as a therapeutic agent due to the possibility of systemic absorption when applied to abraded skin and accumulative boron toxicity within the central nervous system.

Chlorhexidine, a biguanide, is effective against both gram-positive and gram-negative bacteria, including *Pseudomonas aeruginosa*, although it is less effective against gram-negative organisms. Hibitane is available as both a 4 per cent and a 2 per cent solution of chlorhexidine; the former is used for general asepsis and the latter for maintenance of asepsis. Chlorhexidine is not easily removed from the skin, so it has cumulative effects. It rarely causes contact dermatitis and is widely used as a hand scrub for health care personnel. Little of the active drug is absorbed through the skin, the mucous membranes or the gastrointestinal tract (if swallowed). High germicidal potency, a wide therapeutic index and persistent activity in the presence of body fluids makes chlorhexidine a good choice as an antiseptic.

Chlorine-containing products are bactericidal to both gram-positive and gram-negative bacteria, as well as to some spores and viruses. Common household bleach is one example of a chlorine-containing disinfectant; a sodium hypochlorite solution (Hygeol, Eusol and Dakin's) is an example of a clinical antiseptic. These solutions liberate elemental chlorine, which may irritate. The effectiveness of all chlorine-containing antiseptics is decreased by organic

matter and alkaline pH. Hypochlorite solution is usually used for disinfection, although it may be used do deodorize and cleanse wounds and ulcers when diluted with water. Modified Dakin's lotion (sodium hypochlorite 0.5 per cent) can be prepared with household bleach (sodium hypochlorite 4 per cent): 5 mL in 995 mL boiled water. It may be diluted 1:3.

Table XIII *Relative Chlorine Content*

	Available chlorine	Hygeol/ Water ratio	Hygeol/Water volumes imperial (oz)	metric (ml)
Hygeol	1%	—	—	—
Dakin's (Hygeol ½)	0.5%	1:1	80/80	2200/2200
Eusol (Hygeol ¼)	0.25%	1:3	40/120	1100/3300
Eusol ½ (Hygeol ⅛)	0.125%	1:7	20/140	550/3850
Eusol ¼ (Hygeol 1/16)	0.0625%	1:15	10/150	275/4125
Eusol ⅛ (Hygeol 1/32)	0.031%	1:31	5/155	137.5/4262.5

Prepared by Drug Information Centre, Ottawa General Hospital.

Topical First Aid

Iodines and **iodophors** are bactericidal and are used to treat small wounds and abrasions. Iodines are available as solutions (2.2 per cent in water) and tinctures (2.5 per cent in alcohol). The tincture is widely used as an antiseptic because it is effective, economical and has low toxicity, although there may be pain upon application to raw surfaces. The alcohol base of the tincture has its own antiseptic activity as well as enhancing dispersion and penetration of the iodine. When a wound exudes material, iodine's antiseptic activity rapidly deteriorates, but its action on intact skin persists several hours. Discolored iodine has no efficacy.

Iodine solution (Lugol's solution) and povidone-iodine ointment, an iodophor, are relatively painless when used topically and should be preferred when raw surfaces are involved. Iodine and iodides can cause allergic dermatitis, whereas povidone-iodine is less sensitizing. Iodine tincture is the most effective form of iodine. It may even be used to render contaminated water safe to drink by adding 5 to 10 drops to 1 L of water and allowing the mixture to stand for 15 minutes before using. Absorption of topically applied iodine is marginal, although systemic absorption may occur if topical application is greater than 20 per cent of the body surface.

Iodophors are aqueous complexes of iodines available as ointments and solutions (for example, povidone-iodine). They can release up to 10 per cent of free iodine. The lower their pH, the more effective they are. Iodophors have less bactericidal action, but they irritate less. The spectrum of activity includes both gram-positive and gram-negative bacteria. Iodophors are also active against Candida infections and against some viruses.

Iodine and iodophors should not be applied under occlusive dressings. Reapplication of iodophors is not required, as the iodine slowly releases from the complexes. Both iodine and iodophors stain the skin reddish-brown. The stain can be removed with sodium thiosulfate solution (2 to 8 per cent).

Heavy metals used as antiseptics include mercury and silver. **Mercurial compounds** are bacteriostatic and fungistatic and are affected by the presence of organic matter (for example, serum or wounded skin tissue). In general, they are poor antiseptics. The vehicle of the mercurial compound is sometimes a more effective antiseptic than the compound itself. Mercurial compounds can be absorbed if used extensively or on large areas of abraded skin. As well, the compounds can act as contact photosensitizers and most irritate tissue. They are not recommended.

The main mercurial compound is thimerosal. Used in a concentration of 0.1 per cent, it is more active against fungi than other agents, but less effective than the less toxic ethanol. For this reason, thimerosal is no longer available as a single ingredient product (previously available as Merthiolate), however it can still be found in some contact lens solutions, but even here its use is declining.

Other mercurials include merbromin, nitromersol, phenylmercuric salts and ammoniated mercury. Merbromin is one of the least effective mercurial compounds. It is used preoperatively (2 per cent aqueous) to lessen bacteria. However, serous fluids reduce its effectiveness. Nitromersol, available as a 1:200 diluted tincture, is more effective than other mercurial compounds but less effective than ethanol. Phenylmercuric salts are active against gram-positive and gram-negative bacteria and topical fungi. The activity of these compounds is not reduced by skin and serum. Ammoniated mercury is an inorganic form of mercury that has antiseptic properties. It is used in combination preparations (5 and 10 per cent) for scaling, local irritation and sensitization reactions.

Silver compounds, the second group of heavy metal antiseptics, are bactericidal because they can precipitate protein within the cellular components of microorganisms. Organic silver compounds irritate less than inorganic compounds. Silver compounds are the topical preparations of choice in treating *Pseudomonas aeruginosa* and Proteus infections.

Silver nitrate is strongly bactericidal and astringent, as well as caustic. In aqueous solutions, silver nitrate (0.5 per cent) prevents infection in second and third degree burns. Depletion of chloride ions and subsequent electrolyte imbalance may occur with extensive use of silver nitrate, limiting its therapeutic use. Toughened silver nitrate is available as a caustic pencil used to remove warts.

Oxidizing agents include hydrogen peroxide, benzoyl peroxide and potassium permanganate. Benzoyl peroxide is used in concentrations of up to 20 per cent to treat acne and to manage decubitus ulcers. In concentrations of 20 per cent, benzoyl peroxide may cause contact dermatitis and irritation. Hydrogen peroxide has little effect on intact skin, but is useful in debriding wounds. Its effectiveness lasts only as long as oxygen is released. Hydrogen peroxide is unstable in solution and only freshly prepared solutions should be used. For use as an antiseptic, hydrogen peroxide 3 per cent is recommended. Stronger solutions, such as those in hair bleaches (6 per cent), burn the skin and leave a white eschar.

Potassium permanganate is an oxidizing agent that has disinfectant, deodorant and astringent properties. It is used in a strength of 1 per cent as an astringent to treat poison ivy dermatitis. Solutions are used in a concentration of 1:100 to treat athlete's foot, in a concentration of 1:4,000 as a gargle and in a concentration of 1:1,000 to clean ulcers and abcesses. Solutions must be freshly prepared, and they leave an objectionable purple stain.

Substituted phenols are more commonly used than phenol which is irritant and caustic in solutions greater than 1 per cent. It has local anesthetic and antipruritic effects at concentrations of 0.5 to 1.5 per cent and is often included in topical antipruritic formulations. Substituted phenols (for example, thymol, hexachlorophene, triclosan and resorcinol) irritate less and have a greater lipid solubility, hence a greater ability to penetrate tissue. These substituted phenols are more commonly used as antiseptics for their less irritating nature.

Hexachlorophene (for example, PhisoHex) is active against gram-positive bacteria, but is less active against gram-negative bacteria. In the 1960s, hexachlorophene was used routinely to bath newborns for prophylaxis against Staphylococcus infections. The practice stopped when brain damage was linked directly to the hexachlorophene. Hexachlorophene can only be obtained by prescription.

Triclosan, another substituted phenol, is effective against gram-positive infections and is commonly found in bar soap formulations (for example, Coast, Dial, Zest, Safeguard and Teraseptic). Triclosan in a dilute solution (1:5,000) is bacteriostatic and in a stronger solution (1:500) is bactericidal and fungicidal.

Thymol has both antibacterial and antifungal action. It has little use as a topical antiseptic and is found mainly in vaginal deodorants and mouthwashes as it is water-soluble. Creosols are substituted phenol derivatives used routinely as disinfectants. Resorcinol is known mainly as a keratolytic, with minor antiseptic properties.

Anionic surfactants (for example, soaps) are used for supportive cleansing but are not as effective as other antiseptics. Soaps are composed of metallic salts of fatty acids. They are surface active agents that concentrate at oil-water interfaces and possess emulsifying, hence cleansing, properties. Anionic surfactants dissociate in an

Topical First Aid

aqueous solution to form relatively large and complex anions responsible for the surface activity. Superfatted soaps tend to be slightly alkaline in solution (pH 9.5 to 10.5); synthetic surfactants added to soap solutions produce a neutral pH (about 7.5). Antimicrobial and antiseptic agents are sometimes added as deodorants to soap. Inert aluminum oxide, polyethylene or sodium tetraborate decahydrate particles are added to abrasive soaps.

Quaternary ammonium compounds are cationic surfactants that precipitate and denature proteins and are bactericidal against gram-positive and gram-negative organisms, some viruses, fungi and protozoa. Bacterial spores are resistant. Quaternary ammonium compounds are inactivated by soaps and other anionic cleansers. Before applying them, the skin must be rinsed carefully of any soap residue. The presence of organic matter also reduces the activity of these compounds

Benzalkonium chloride and cetrimide are two common quaternary ammonium compounds. They act rapidly for moderately long duration. They are well tolerated; skin irritation is the most common side effect. They are particularly irritating to the eyes. On broken skin, concentrations of 1:5,000 to 1:20,000 are recommended; a concentration of 1:750 is effective on intact skin. Cationic surfactants are absorbed into cotton, rubber and other porous material.

Topical Antibiotics

Staphylococcus aureus is the most common organism on the surface of the skin. An overgrowth of the organism may result in infection of an injury. Beta-hemolytic streptococci and hemolytic staphylococci are more invasive pathogens. They can be responsible for primary systemic and primary skin infections and for skin infections secondary to other skin damage.

Gram-negative bacteria (for example, *Pseudomonas aeruginosa*) can also be present in secondary pyoderma, especially in warm moist areas.

Considerable controversy surrounds the therapeutic value of antibiotics to treat moderate to severe infections, as they do not eliminate the causative organism nor penetrate to the desired dermal level. As well, systemic absorption and the potential to develop resistant organisms are complications associated with the use of topical antibiotics.

The value of these antibiotics has been proven clinically only in burn wounds, and they are considered useful for only the most superficial pyoderms. The Food and Drug Administration in the United States considers topical antibiotics safe for use only if they do not interfere with wound healing. Most topical antibiotic preparations contain a combination of antibiotics or an antibiotic in combination with other surface active agents.

Table XIV *Bacteria Most Likely to Cause Acute Infections to the Skin and Subcutaneous Tissues*

Skin infections:
Staphylococcus, coagulase positive
Streptococcus pyogenes (Group A)
Dermatophytes and *Candida albicans*
Gram-negative bacilli
Treponema pallidum

Burns:
Staphylococcus, coagulase positive
Streptococcus pyogenes (Group S)
Pseudomonas aeruginosa or other gram-negative bacilli

Decubitus wound infections:
Staphylococcus, coagulase positive
Escherichia coli (or other gram-negative bacilli)
Streptococcus pyogenes (Group A)
Streptococcus anaerobius
Clostridia
Enterococcus
Bacteroides

Traumatic and surgical wounds:
Staphylococcus, coagulase positive
Streptococcus anaerobius
Gram-negative bacilli
Clostridia
Streptococcus pyogenes (Group A)
Enterococcus

Adapted from: Anonymous. Handbook of antimicrobial therapy. New Rochelle: Medical Letter, 1974:8.

Table XV *Factors to Consider When Recommending a Topical Antibiotic*

Age of individual: infant's skin is more permeable than adult's

Blood supply to the area: the greater the blood flow, the greater the chance of systemic absorption

Hydration of the area

If occlusive bandages are being used

Dryness of skin: dry skin is less permeable

Thickness of skin

Concentration and duration of exposure to the proposed drug

Vehicle base and solubility of the drug

Before recommending a topical antibiotic it is necessary to assess the type of injury and any predisposing skin disorders. If proper facilities are available for minimizing contamination and for proper dressing and debridement, topical antibiotics are not necessary.

Bacitracin is a polypeptide antibiotic that inhibits the synthesis of the bacterial cell wall. It is effective against both gram-negative and gram-positive organisms and is especially effective against *Treponema pallidum*. Bacitracin is absorbed systemically and may be nephrotoxic in high doses. This effect is rarely seen, as the quantity of ointment required to reach toxic levels is too irritating to the skin. Resistance to bacitracin is rare, and although hypersensitivity has been reported, it is uncommon. Bacitracin is unstable in aqueous solutions and when exposed to light. It is stable only in a petroleum base.

Gramicidin, a polypeptide antibiotic, alters the cation content of the bacterial cell wall. Gramidicin is too toxic to use systemically, causing hemolysis and kidney and liver damage. Due to its potent hemolytic activity, gramicidin is never applied in any way to allow it access to the blood stream (for example, to nasal or closed body cavities). Gramicidin effectively treats gram-positive infections.

Iodochlorhydroxyquin is antibacterial and antifungal in concentrations of 3 per cent. Systemic preparations have been withdrawn

Topical First Aid

because of its potential to cause subacute myelo-opticneuropathy. Studies indicate that topical absorption, especially through abraded skin, may be significant, so care is required with its use. Irritation at the site of application has been reported.

Polymyxin B acts on the cytoplasm of bacteria, distorting the cell wall and causing leakage of the cytoplasmic components. Polymyxin B effectively treats pyodermas due to gram-negative bacteria (for example, pseudomonas). It is inhibited in the presence of anionic compounds, such as soap and water, because it acts as a cationic agent. Resistance develops slowly and hypersensitization is uncommon.

Mupirocin inhibits bacterial protein and RNA synthesis. It is effective against staphylococci and streptococci, but is less active against other gram-positive and most gram-negative organisms. For individuals with primary or secondary superficial skin infections, a 2 per cent mupirocin ointment is effective applied two or three times daily for 5 to 14 days. Because of its unique chemical structure cross resistance is not seen, however there have been reports of resistance to mupirocin itself after months of use.

Antipruritic Agents

Topical antihistamines, although logical in concept, lack penetration ability and are formulated in concentrations too low to be topically effective (for example, for prophylaxis against dermatitis caused by poison ivy). As well, topical antihistamine usage is associated with a high incidence of contact dermatitis. These agents should never be recommended for urticaria, pruritus or contact dermatitis. Antihistamines, both sedating and non sedating, are more effective if used systemically to curtail the peripheral release of histamine in urticaria and pruritus.

Sensitization to antihistamines may develop, especially in inflamed skin, and cross-sensitivity occurs among all antihistamines. Sensitized individuals may also react to oral administration of substituted ethylamines. Ethanolamines have lower sensitization potential, but because they are common ingredients in nonprescription products, they have been linked to dermatitis reactions. Cross-sensitivity also occurs with phenothiazines.

Zinc salts have mild antiseptic properties due to their ability to precipitate protein. Zinc sulfate, applied topically with sulfurated potash, is used to treat acne, poison ivy and contact dermatitis. Zinc oxide is a mild astringent and antiseptic, but is used more widely as an antipruritic in a variety of skin disorders, such as diaper rash (zinc oxide acts as a medical protective), prickly heat, eczema and ringworm. Zinc oxide is safe and effective for topical use in concentrations of 15 to 25 per cent, and is available in ointments and creams. Zinc oxide is insoluble in water.

Calamine lotion contains zinc oxide (8 per cent) and calamine (8 per cent). It is used as an antipruritic and is safe and effective for nonprescription use.

Crotamiton is used mainly as a scabicide in 10 per cent concentrations. It occasionally causes irritation, especially on inflamed skin. Paradoxically, it has antipruritic and mild anesthetic properties. (See the chapter on topical antiparasitics.)

Topical Anesthetics

Topical anesthetics prevent transmission of nerve impulses along nerve fibres and at nerve endings. Myelinated A fibres are the most affected. The anesthetics inhibit depolarization and potassium and sodium ion exchange at the cell membrane level. The base of the anesthetic must penetrate the lipoprotein nerve sheath before it can act, and its effectiveness depends on concentration at the nerve fibre ends. Effects are reversible.

Topical anesthetics are poorly absorbed through intact skin, but readily absorbed through mucous membranes. They are effective in selected disorders affecting the mucous membranes, mucocutaneous junctions, and abraded and inflamed skin. Most topical anesthetics are antipruritic and anti-inflammatory in nature. Lidocaine has a low sensitizing potential; others, such as benzocaine, are more likely to sensitize especially when applied to inflamed skin.

When recommending a topical anesthetic, pharmacists consider prior sensitization history, the desired duration of anesthetic action and the vehicle for delivery. Very young and very old people have more permeable skin and are more susceptible to topical anesthetic effects. Topical anesthetics should not be used in eyes or when there is a secondary bacterial infection. Spray formulations are applied without rubbing and have the advantage of not irritating sensitive skin further.

Topical anesthetics absorbed systemically through abraded skin can cause central nervous system stimulation (restlessness, excitement, nervousness, blurred vision, nausea and vomiting, muscle twitching and convulsions), central nervous system depression (drowsiness, respiratory failure and coma), and cardiovascular depression (pallor, sweating, arrhythmia and cardiac arrest). Skin sensitization is the most common effect, occurring with repeated use in allergic individuals. Topical anesthetics used most often are amides and esters, with the esters most often causing sensitization. Cross-sensitivity between the amide and ester types is not common. Cocaine is an ester topical anesthetic, but is no longer used as such.

Amides

Dibucaine has a long duration of action (about 2 to 4 hours) and a high lipid solubility. Dibucaine (1 per cent) is used on painful skin and mucous membranes. There is a danger of systemic toxicity when it is applied over debrided areas in large quantities. Dibucaine should be used infrequently.

Lidocaine is used widely in topical preparations, especially for the ear, and begins to act within two to five minutes for 30 to 45 minutes. Lidocaine is usually used in concentrations of 5 per cent and is soluble in both water and alcohol.

Esters

Benzocaine may produce a high degree of sensitivity. Concentrations of less than 10 per cent or acidic preparations are ineffective on intact or mildly sunburned skin. The duration of action is 30 to 45 minutes. Available concentrations range from 5 to 30 per cent and are suitable for use on ulcerated surfaces, burns or wounds. Benzocaine is poorly absorbed and only slightly soluble; therefore it remains in contact with the skin for long periods, lengthening its onset of action.

Butamben picrate is another long-acting topical anesthetic. It is poorly absorbed and only slightly soluble.

Tetracaine is found in ophthalmic preparations. When used topically, its onset is slow and its duration of action relatively short (about 45 minutes).

Others

Dimethisoquin hydrochloride has a long duration of action, lasting 2 to 4 hours. Its sensitization potential is low. It is used at 0.5 per cent in lotions and ointments.

Table XVI *Antihistamines and Other H₁ Receptor Antagonists Used in Topical Preparations*

Agents	Comments
Phenothiazines* Tripelennamine tartrate Promethazine HCl	Worst offenders of allergic dermatitis, contact dermatitis May evoke a photoallergic dermatitis (360nm wave length is involved and sunscreens and window glass offer no protection), which can be activated by incandescent and fluorescent light Once topically sensitized, oral preparations will cause severe dermatitis
Ethanolamines Diphenhydramine Doxylamine succinate Carbinoxamine maleate	Lower sensitization capacity Common ingredients in nonprescription medications Resulting dermatitis, especially in children, clears upon removal of offending agent
Ethylenediamines Antazoline phosphate Tripelennamine citrate Methapyrilene HCl	Active in producing contact dermatitis First reported to cause contact dermatitis Topical and oral administration can both cause dermatitis Sensitized people may also react to aminophylline (theophylline and ethylenediamine)
Alkylamines Brompheniramine maleate Chlorpheniramine maleate Pheniramine maleate Dimethidene maleate Tripolidine HCl	Pheniramine, phenenamine and pyrilamine are capable of causing contact dermatitis
Piperazines Cyclizine HCl Meclizine HCl	Not usually found in topical preparations

*Phenothiazines are not antihistamines but rather are H₁ receptor antagonists.
Adapted from: Drug evaluations annual 1991. Chicago: American Medical Association, 1991:1048.

Pramoxine hydrochloride may be of use for people sensitive to amide and ester topical anesthetics, as it shows little cross-sensitivity. It is used at 1 per cent in creams, ointments and suppositories.

Diperodon hydrochloride is used as an ointment for skin irritations, abrasions, pruritus and hemorrhoids. It is used most often at strengths of one per cent.

Menthol acts as a counterirritant and mild anesthetic, leaving a cooling sensation when applied. In high concentrations (16 per cent), menthol can irritate the skin, causing initial pain. Menthol should not be applied to mucous membranes, because it is slightly caustic.

Camphor, applied vigorously to the skin, acts as a rubefacient, but it can impart a feeling of coolness when not applied vigorously. As well, camphor has mild local anesthetic properties, producing local numbness. If taken orally, camphor is toxic, causing nausea, vomiting and convulsions.

Topical Anti-inflammatory Agents
Corticosteroids

Hydrocortisone and hydrocortisone acetate are safe and effective for nonprescription use. Minor skin irritations respond to topical corticosteroids. Hydrocortisone temporarily relieves contact dermatitis due to poison ivy, oak, sumac, soaps, detergents, cosmetics and jewelry; itching and rashes due to atopic dermatitis (eczema); and insect bites. It is also used to treat ano-genital pruritus. Hydrocortisone is the least potent of the corticosteroids, both topically and systemically. Hydrocortisone 0.5 per cent is generally considered to be effective. In some studies formulations of 0.25 per cent were found to be effective; in other studies they were no better than a placebo.

The mechanism of action of topical corticosteroids is not well understood. Topically, hydrocortisone causes vasoconstriction and thus may reduce swelling and discomfort due to swelling. Hydrocortisone can reduce membrane permeability, thereby preventing the release of chemical mediators and inhibiting pain and pruritus caused by these mediators. Suppression of the immune response and mitotic activity may also account for some of the effectiveness of hydrocortisone.

The therapeutic efficacy of hydrocortisone depends on its release from the vehicle and its solubility and absorption at the skin site. Hydrocortisone is available in gels, creams, lotions, aerosols and ointments. Exudative skin conditions (for example, poison ivy) are best treated with a lotion, dry skin with an ointment and hairy skin areas with a lotion, gel or aerosol. Lotions, gels and aerosols may sting at the site of application. Greasy bases are generally more occlusive and are preferred for dry, scaly lesions.

There are several factors to consider when selecting a product: skin hydration; age of the individual; site of the lesion; severity of the lesion; whether the lesion is wet or dry; and how long the lesion has existed.

The hydration of the skin determines the base chosen and the strength of the product needed. As well, hydrated skin absorbs more of the topical corticosteroid. Children, especially those under two years of age, should be treated with a topical corticosteroid only on the advice of a physician, due to the threat of systemic absorption. Systemic absorption may be a problem with prolonged or exuberant application, in skin areas that are thin (for example, face, armpits and groin) and when the skin is damaged. A more severe, moister and longer existing lesion absorbs more of the active ingredient and systemic effects may be evident.

Systemic absorption can affect fetal development, the growth of children and disease conditions such as diabetes, stomach ulcers and

Topical First Aid

tuberculosis. Occlusion by oleaginous ointments, a film of polyethylene or adhesive tape enhances systemic absorption by promoting increased hydration of the skin.

Paradoxically, hydrocortisone may cause skin eruptions, skin atrophy and sloughing. The skin, especially on the face, may become thin and shiny or may develop strial marks (stretch marks) due to rupture of subcutaneous collagen fibres. Topical hydrocortisone should not be applied in the eye, on the eyelids or near the eyes and should not be used when bacterial, viral or fungal infections are present. These precautions eliminate hydrocortisone's use in tuberculosis of the skin, vaccinia, varicella and herpes simplex (cold sores). Hydrocortisone should not be used in the ear if the ear drum is perforated. When the lesion appears cancerous, hydrocortisone should not be used, because it temporarily suppresses the lesion growth and delays appropriate treatment. Prolonged use in children is discouraged because the larger skin surface area to body weight ratio of children means a greater chance of systemic effects.

Topical hydrocortisone effectively treats minor inflammation and pruritus when used appropriately for short periods of time. Hydrocortisone in concentrations of 1 per cent and less has significantly lower incidence of local adverse effects than fluorinated corticosteroids. Only 0.5 per cent hydrocortisone is available in Canada without a prescription.

Pharmacists can provide the following advice to people using topical hydrocortisone:

• Apply thinly and do not use more than necessary (a maximum of 4 applications daily for no more than 7 days).
• If the lesion does not respond, discontinue use.
• Use occlusive dressings only on the advice of a physician (in the diaper area, tight diapers and rubber pants act like occlusive dressings).
• Take care when using it on children, as children have higher skin permeability than adults.
• Do not use if signs of infection are present (SHARP).
• Do not use if signs of irritation occur or worsen during use (for example, burning, itching, blistering or peeling).
• Do not use if the lesion may be cancerous.

Others

Bufexamac is a nonsteroidal agent possessing anti-inflammatory, analgesic, antipyretic and anti-exudative properties. It exerts its anti-inflammatory effects by stabilizing lysosomal membranes. Applied topically as a 2 per cent cream or ointment, it alleviates pruritus and reduces inflammation. Bufexamac is usually applied two to three times daily and massaged in thoroughly to facilitate dermal penetration.

Vitamin E, an antioxidant, is popularly used to treat inflammatory skin conditions. Topically its base provides hydration and it is this hydration that may be responsible for any success. Aloe vera, used widely in cosmetics, is reported to alleviate inflammation and pruritus and promote healing. Again, it is the vehicle that may be the source of any benefit.

First Aid Kits

Pharmacists are often asked to assist consumers in choosing a first aid kit for car, home, work or school. While commercially available first aid kits, for example the St. John Ambulance First Aid Kit, are

Table XVII *Contents of a First Aid Kit*

Self adhesive bandages, a variety of sizes
Gauze, both rolled and sterile pads
Adhesive tape, sensitive skin type
Scissors
Tweezers
Elastic bandage
Ice bag
Hot water bottle
An antiseptic such as hydrogen peroxide
Thermometer
First aid manual
Telephone number list of emergency numbers

Other items to consider, especially if the first aid kit is intended for travel

Analgesic, antipyretic such as acetaminophen (acetylsalicylic acid and ibuprofen are alternatives and are discussed in Chapter 14)
Antacid with an antiflatulent
Antidiarrheal
Antipruritic such as calamine lotion and/or an oral antihistamine
A sun burn remedy
Foot care products if the trip is going to include walking or hiking
Any prescription drugs, in sufficient quantities, properly labelled and stored

All expiry dates should be checked and all items can be placed in a water proof container.

complete and convenient; packing a personalized first aid kit may be more economical. Table XVII describes the recommended content of a kit.

Summary

To treat an injury it is necessary to determine how and when the injury occurred, and any underlying clinical conditions (for example, diabetes). The nature of the injury should be considered. If the wound is deep or a severe burn, medical attention should be sought. Basic first aid measures (cleansing and bandaging the wound) should be taken.

The use of topically applied antiseptics, antibacterials, antihistamines and anesthetics is questionable. Appropriate systemic treatment (for example, oral antihistamines and oral antibiotics) is preferred for serious injuries. Uncomplicated injuries can be treated effectively by simply cleansing and bandaging the area. Topical corticosteroids are effective for minor skin irritations if used properly. The ad hoc use of these agents should be discouraged due to their narrow therapeutic role in topical first aid.

Ask the Consumer

Q. Describe the injury. How did it happen?

■ Determining the nature of the wound helps in recommending first aid. For example, the recommended treatment for a first degree sunburn covering the entire body is different from treatment for a second degree burn from a droplet of boiling water.

Topical First Aid

Q. When did the injury occur?
■ The time between injury and treatment affects the potential for infection.

Q. What has been done to treat the injury?
■ Prior self-treatment may hinder subsequent therapy. For example, butter applied to a hot water burn is difficult to remove.

Q. Have you any allergies? Are you taking any medication?
■ Before recommending treatment, determine potential drug interactions, underlying disease states such as diabetes, or drug-induced states such as phototoxicity.

Q. Have you used this product before?
■ Correct use of a product is paramount in first aid treatment.

Q. Is there swelling? Is the injury warm to the touch? Does it ache? Is it red? Is there pus at the injury site?
■ Swelling, heat, ache, redness and pus are signs of infection. The extent to which they appear indicates the degree of infection and the need for medical attention.

References

Minor Cuts and Wounds
Copelan R. Chemical removal of splinters without epidermal toxic effects. J Amer Acad of Dermatol 1989;20(4):697–8.

Feingold DS, Hirschmann JV, Leyden JJ. Bacterial infections of the skin. J Amer Acad of Dermatol 1989;20(3):469–75.

Finley JM. Practical wound management. Chicago: Year Book Medical Publishers, 1980:3–10,13–22,25–7.

Hunt TK. Wound management and infection. J Trauma 1979;19(11):890–1.

Rinear CE, Parcel GS. Management of wounds and hemorrhaging. In: Parcel GS, ed. Basic emergency care of the sick and injured. Toronto: CV Mosby, 1982:79–93.

Musculoskeletal Injuries
Bergeron JD, Greene HW. Coaches' guide to sports injuries. Champaign: Human Kinetics Books, 1989:61–73.

Parcel GS. Musculoskeletal injuries. In: Parcel GS, ed. Basic emergency care of the sick and injured. Toronto: CV Mosby, 1982:127–47.

Proctor H, London PS. Principles for first aid for the injured. Toronto: Butterworths, 1977:32–47.

Burns
Davies JWL. Prompt cooling of burned areas: a review of benefits and effector mechanisms. Burns 1982;9(1):1–6.

Demling RH. Burns. N Engl J of Med 1985;313(22):1389–98.

Erskin JF. Electrical accidents. Practitioner 1979;222(1332):777–81.

Frank DH, Fisher JC. Complications of electrical injury-lightning injury. In: Greenfield LJ, ed. Complications in surgery and trauma. Philadelphia: JB Lippincott, 1990:27–8.

Fraser-Darling A. Electrocution, drowning, and burns. Br Med J 1981; 282:530–1.

Ghezzi KT. Lightning injuries. Postgrad Med 1989;85(8):197–208.

Gillespie RW. Emergency care of burn injuries. Occup Health Saf 1982; 51(7):43–7.

Harrison DH, Parkhouse N. Experience with upper extremity burns. Hand Clin 1990;6(2):191–209.

Keswani MH, Vartak AM, Davis JWL. Histological and bacteriological studies of burn wounds treated with boiled potato peel dressings. Burns 1990; 16(2):137–43.

MacMillan BG. Infections following burn injury. Surg Clin of N Amer 1980;60(1):185–96.

Moleski RJ. The burn wound—topical therapy for infection control. Drug Intell Clin Pharm 1978;12(1):28–35.

Molloy HF. Sunburn and other superficial burns. Med J of Aust 1991; 154(4):263.

Munster AM. The early management of thermal burns. Surgery 1980; 87:29–40.

Pegg SP. The role of drugs in the management of burns. Drugs 1982; 24:256–60.

Tolhurst DE. The treatment of burns. Ann R Coll Surg Engl 1980;62(2):120–4.

Frostbite
Anonymous. Treatment of frostbite. Med Lett Drugs Ther 1980;22(26):112–4.

Dexter WW. Hypothermia. Postgrad Med 1990;88(8):55–64.

Li AK, Ehrlich HP, Trelstad RL. Differences in healing of skin wounds caused by burn and freeze injuries. Ann Surg 1980;191(2):244–8.

McCauley RL, et al. Frostbite injuries: a rational approach based on the pathophysiology. J Trauma 1983;23(2):143–7.

McCauley RL, Heggers JP, Robson MC. Frostbite. Postgrad Med 1990; 88(8):67–77.

Zingg W. Cold injury. In: Maddin S, ed. Dermatologic therapy. Philadelphia: WB Saunders, 1982:91–2.

Heat Related Injuries
Anonymous. Treatment of heat injury. Med Lett Drugs Ther 1990;31:66–9.

Cantor RM. Heat illness from mild to malignant. Emerg Med 1991;23(11): 93–100.

Collins KJ. Heat illness: diagnosis, treatment and prevention. Practitioner 1977;219:193–203.

O'Donnell TF Jr. Management of heat stress injuries in the athlete. Orth Clin N Am 1980;11(4):841–55.

Mahan JM. Heat-related illnesses and emergencies. In: Parcel GS, ed. Basic emergency care of the sick and injured. Toronto: CV Mosby, 1982;184–95.

Scott J. Heat-related illness. Postgrad Med 1989;85(8):154–64.

Squire DL. Heat illness. Sports Med 1990;37(5):1085–109.

Insect Bites and Stings
Anonymous. Are insect repellents safe? Lancet 1980;ii(8611):610–1.

Anonymous. Insect repellents. Med Lett Drugs Ther 1989;31:45–7.

Anonymous. Insect venom extracts. Med Lett Drugs Ther 1980; 22(9):37–8.

Anonymous. Treatment of Lyme disease. Med Let Drugs Ther 1989;31:57–9.

Awai LE, Mekori YA. Insect sting anaphylaxis and beta adrenergic blockade: a relative contraindication. Ann Allergy 1984;53(1):48–9.

Elgart GW. Ant, bee, and wasp stings. Dermatol Clin 1990;8(2):229–36.

Graft DF. Stinging insect allergy. Postgrad Med 1989;85(8):173–80.

Harves AD, Millikan LE. Current concepts of therapy and pathophysiology in anthropod bites and stings: part 2. insects. Int J Dermatol 1975; 14(9):621–34.

Holmes HS. Stings and bites. Postgrad Med 1990;88(1):75–8.

Ingall M, Goldman G. Beta blockade in stinging insect anaphylaxis. JAMA 1984;251(11):1432.

Kivity S, Yarchovsky J. Relapsing anaphylaxis to bee sting in a patient treated with beta blocker and Ca blocker. J Allergy Clin Immunol 1990; 85(3):669–70.

Lockey RF, et al. The Hymenoptera venom study III: safety of venom immunotherapy. J Allergy Clin Immunol 1990;86(5):775–80.

Millikan LE. Anthropod bites and stings. In: Maddin S, ed. Dermatologic therapy. Philadelphia: WB Saunders, 1982:43–4.

Nadelman RB, Wormser GP. A clinical approach to Lyme disease. Mt Sinai J Med 1990;57(3):144–56.

Pedersen J, et al. Exaggerated reaction to insect bites in patients with chronic lymphocytic leukemia. Clinical and histological findings. Pathology 1990;22(3):141–3.

Rahn DW. Treatment of Lyme disease. Postgrad Med 1990;87(6):159–64.

Rapoport HG. Disarming insect stings. Drug Ther 1975;125–32.

Riches HR. Insect bites and stings. Practitioner 1977;219:199–203.

Roland EH, Jan JE, Rigg JM. Toxic encephalopathy in a child after brief exposure to insect repellents. Can Med Assoc J 1985;132:155–6.

Topical First Aid

Tenenbein M. Severe toxic reactions and death following the ingestion of diethyltoluamide-containing insect repellents. JAMA 1987;258(11):1509–11.

Toewe CH. Bug bites and stings. Am Fam Physician 1980;1(5):90–5.

Dermatitis

Anonymous. Desensitization to poison ivy. Med Lett Drugs Ther 1981;23(8):40.

Anonymous. Photoplex—a broad spectrum sunscreen. Med Lett Drugs Ther 1989;31:59–60.

Davis SA. Dermatologic emergencies. In: Mills J, Ho MT, Trunkey DD, eds. Current emergency diagnosis and treatment. Los Altos: Lange, 1983; 595–607.

Dromgoole SH, Maibach HI. Sunscreen agent intolerance: contact and photocontact sensitization and contact urticaria. J Amer Acad Dermatol 1990;22:1068–78.

Epstein WL. Topical prevention of poison ivy/oak dermatitis. Arch Dermatol 1989;125:499–501.

Epstein L. Poison ivy dermatitis including poison oak. In: Maddin S, ed. Dermatologic therapy. Philadelphia: WB Saunders, 1982: 368–9.

Mathews KP. The urticarias: current concepts in pathogenesis and treatment. Drugs 1985;30(6):552–60.

Nurse DS. Urticaria: diagnosis and management. Drugs 1975;9:292–8.

Pray WS. Poison ivy: know it, avoid it. US Pharmacist 1991;16(8):16–24.

Sheffer AL. Drug treatment of urticaria and angioedema. Semin Drug Treat 1973;2(4):413–8.

Wooldridge WE. Acute allergic contact dermatitis. Postgrad Med 1990; 87(4):221–4.

Dressings

Eaglstein WH. Experiences with biosynthetic dressings. J Amer Acad Dermatol 1985;12(2):434–40.

Marshall DA, Mertz PM, Eaglstein WH. Occlusive dressings. Arch Surg 1990;125:1136–9.

McKay M. Topical dermatologic therapy. Prim Care 1983;10(3):513–6.

Antiseptics

Anonymous. Topical antiseptics and antibiotics. Med Lett Drugs Ther 1977;9(20):83–4.

Harvey SC. Antiseptics and disinfectants, fungicides, ectoparasiticides. In: Gilman AG, Goodman LS, Rall TW, Murad F, eds. Goodman and Gilman's the pharmacological basis of therapeutics. New York: Macmillan, 1985:964.

Laufman H. Current use of skin and wound cleansers and antiseptics. Amer J Surg 1989;157:359–65.

Rodeheaver G, et al. Bacterial activity and toxicity of iodine-containing solutions in wounds. Arch Surg 1982;117:181–6.

Sheikh W. Comparative antibacterial efficacy of Hibiclens and Betadine in the presence of pus derived from human wounds. Curr Ther Res 1986; 40(6):1096–102.

Topical Antibiotics

Feingold DS, Wagner RF. Antibacterial therapy. J Amer Acad Dermatol 1986;14(4):535–48.

Geronemus RG, Merts PM, Eaglstein WH. Wound healing. The effects of topical antimicrobial agents. Arch Dermatol 1979;115:1311–4.

Hirschmann JV. Topical antibiotics in dermatology. Arch Dermatol 1988; 124:1691–700.

Rahman M, et al. Mupirocin resitant staphylococcus aureus. Lancet 1987; 2:237–8.

Ward A, Campoli-Richards DM. Mupirocin: a review of its antibacterial activity, pharmacokinetic properties and therapeutic use. Drugs 1986;32(5):425–44.

Witkowski JA, Parish LC. Bacterial skin infections. Postgrad Med, 1982; 72(4):166–85.

Antipruritic Agents

Wahlgren C-F, Hagermark O, Bergstrom R. The antipruritic effect of a sedative and a non sedative antihistamine in atopic dermatis. Br J Dermatol 1990;122:545–51.

Yaffe S, et al. Antihistamines in topical preparations. Pediatrics 1973; 51(2):299–301.

Topical Anesthetics

Anonymous. Anesthetic sprays and wipes. Med Lett Drugs Ther 1969; 11(17):70–1.

Bickers DR, Hazen PG, Lynch WS. Clinical pharmacology of skin disease. New York: Churchill Livingstone, 1984:252–69.

Drug Evaluations Annual 1991. Chicago: American Medical Association, 1991:1048.

Topical Anti-inflammatory Agents

Anonymous. Topical hydrocortisone without a prescription. Med Lett Drugs Ther 1980;22(9):38–9.

Drug Evaluations Annual 1991. Chicago: American Medical Association, 1991:1025–9.

3
External Analgesics

Yvonne M. Shevchuk

Pain from various musculoskeletal conditions can be relieved by external analgesics and nonpharmacologic treatment. The most commonly used external analgesics—counterirritants—include allyl isothiocyanate, strong ammonia solution, methyl salicylate, triethanolamine salicylate, turpentine oil, capsicum preparations, camphor, menthol, eucalyptus oil, esters of nicotinic acid and dimethyl sulfoxide. Clinical considerations and dosage forms vary for each agent.

Muscle soreness, strains, sprains, joint inflammation and related musculoskeletal conditions resulting from overexertion and athletic activities are common causes of pain for which consumers seek self-medication products. External analgesics are an important group of nonprescription medications purchased for temporary pain relief. With increasing interest in physical fitness and the growing number of weekend athletes, this market is booming. Consumers also purchase these products to relieve "rheumatism" and arthritic conditions of a chronic nature. Capsaicin products are currently being promoted for chronic pain syndromes such as postherpetic neuralgia and diabetic neuropathy. Pharmacists should be aware of the benefits these products provide as well as limitations of their use.

An external analgesic is a topically applied drug used to relieve pain. It may have analgesic properties resulting from depression of cutaneous sensory receptors (for example, camphor and menthol) or counterirritant properties to stimulate cutaneous sensory receptors (for example, methyl salicylate, allyl isothiocyanate and methyl nicotinate). The desired effect of external analgesics is from local action rather than percutaneous absorption and systemic effects. This chapter concentrates on the drugs that act as counterirritants.

Counterirritants are rubbed into the skin over a painful joint, tendon, ligament or muscle to relieve pain. They may be described as rubefacients, which cause redness; vesicants, which induce blistering; or pustulants, which cause more severe irritation and ulceration. These differences are quantitative rather than qualitative; higher concentrations of rubefacients or applications for prolonged periods produce blistering or severe irritation. A number of nonpharmacologic methods have been used to produce counterirritation for relief of pain. These include radiant heat, hot water bottles, poultices and hot water compresses, application of cold, diathermy and galvanic electrical currents.

Although internal analgesic drugs are currently regarded as the treatment of choice for most pain, the use of counterirritants dates back to primitive cultures. Topical application of any number of substances has always been a part of medical practice. External analgesics, when used appropriately, can provide the desired pain relief in many situations while avoiding the unwanted systemic effects of internal analgesic products.

Uses

External analgesics are used for a variety of ailments. These include acute problems such as sprains, strains and bruises resulting from sports injuries. People may also purchase external analgesics for chronic symptoms associated with rheumatoid arthritis, osteoarthritis, chronic tendinitis or bursitis, or chronic pain syndromes such as postherpetic neuralgia. Although external analgesics do not alter the underlying disease process, local treatment for short periods may provide temporary pain relief.

A sprain refers to partial or complete rupture of a ligament. A strain is an injury to a muscle-tendon unit. A bruise describes the rupture of tissue resulting in a hematoma. Bursitis, tendinitis and traumatic arthritis also cause acute pain. Bursitis and tendinitis are more common in individuals over the age of 50 and may be associated with certain occupations or activities (for example, tennis elbow and housemaid's knee). Bursal sacs are lined with synovial membranes that secrete and absorb liquid providing lubrication between bones, ligaments, tendons, muscles and skin. Inflammation and swelling of a bursae, referred to as bursitis, is a common cause of joint pain and tenderness. Activity and mobility are often limited. Tendinitis refers to strain or injury of tendons. Traumatic arthritis results from a blow or forced abnormal motion of a joint causing acute pain or swelling. The knee is a common site. The inflammatory process can spread from one structure to another and often accompanies degenerative or inflammatory joint disease. Textbooks covering these topics in

Table I *Effects of Counterirritants*

- Local vasodilation
- Dispersal of pain-producing substances secondary to vasodilation
- Lower muscle action potential
- Increase speed of nerve conduction
- Increase muscle capacity to work
- Placebo effect

External Analgesics

sports medicine do not mention the use of external analgesics as a treatment option.

Other causes of skeletal muscle pain include poor posture; prolonged, fixed or stressful conditions producing muscle strain; and stiffness resulting from cold, dampness, temperature changes and air currents. These conditions may be relieved temporarily with counterirritants.

Postherpetic neuralgia may follow acute infection with herpes zoster, particularly in older persons. Burning pain, aching or severe pruritus occurs in the dermatome(s) involved in acute infection. Response to systemic analgesics, tricyclic antidepressants and anticonvulsants is disappointing. The use of capsaicin in this disorder has generated significant interest.

Organic disease, especially in the pelvis, abdomen or spine, may cause referred pain in skeletal muscles. The consumer may misinterpret such pain to be local in origin and attempt to self-medicate with external analgesics. In this case, the use of external analgesics may delay diagnosis.

General Treatment

Several general treatment measures may be beneficial in treating localized acute or chronic pain. Applying heat causes temporary muscle relaxation and relief of pain. In acute injury, applying cold may decrease swelling and reduce pain. Massage results in a number of therapeutic benefits, both physiological and psychological. Other measures such as elevating the limb, firm bandaging, splinting and bracing may be required to reduce swelling and limit movement in the injured area. Controlled exercise programs and physical therapy are used to restore function and regain muscle power.

Pharmaceutical Agents
Mechanism of Action

Few scientific studies deal with the mechanism of action or effects of counterirritants. A 1962 article comments on the scarcity of literature on the topical treatment of rheumatic diseases. Although articles published in the 1940s and 1950s report the effects of counterirritants, the scarcity of current data continues. Possible mechanisms of action and the effects of counterirritants will be discussed despite the lack of scientific evidence (see Table I).

Counterirritants act by producing a transient, mild, local inflammatory reaction at the site of application. Pain relief is desired at another site, usually the underlying structure such as a joint or muscle. The intensity of response depends on the irritant used, its concentration, the solvent in which it is dissolved and the period of contact with the skin.

A phenomenon called the pain paradox can be described simply as one pain inhibiting another. The pain paradox theory assumes the brain can deal with only a limited amount of information at any specific time. When a new stimulus is presented to the central nervous system, the brain is unable to process information about the preexisting pain. Application of counterirritants acts as a new stimulus and distracts the brain, making it less likely to concentrate attention on the original pain.

The most popular pain theory is referred to as the gate control theory. The "gate" is in the dorsal horn of the spinal cord and is called the substantia gelatinosa. The substantia gelatinosa works to increase or decrease transmission of nerve impulses from peripheral input to pain centres in the thalamus and cerebral cortex. Peripheral impulses can be modified by attention, emotion, previous pain experience and other cortical functions. Large A fibres carrying touch, pressure and thermal stimuli, as well as small C fibres carrying cutaneous pain and cold, stimulate a set of neurons referred to as T cells. C fibre activity causes excitation of T cells and inhibition of substantia gelatinosa cells. Inhibition of substantia gelatinosa cells results in opening of the gate and facilitation of pain perception. A fibre activity also causes increased firing of T cells, but with excitation rather than inhibition of substantia gelatinosa cells. This effect results in closing of the gate; T cell activity does not increase and no pain results. Theoretically, applying counterirritants stimulates pain or other sensory receptors, resulting in closure of the gate (see Figure 1).

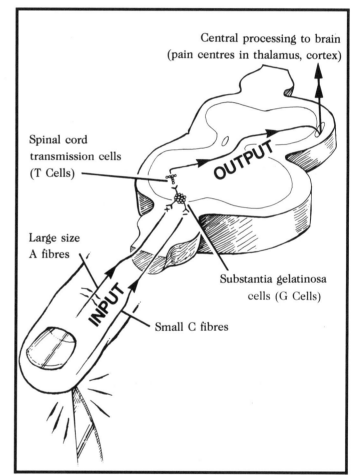

Figure 1 *Gate Control Theory of Pain*

Peripheral afferent fibres with cell bodies in the dorsal root ganglia contain neuropeptides including substance P, cholecystokinin and somatostatin. Substance P is important in transmitting pain stimuli via small fibres. It is also involved in the inflammatory response associated with cutaneous injury and pain. Axon reflex vasodilation may be mediated by substance P. Depletion of substance P from neurons decreases transmission of painful stimuli from the periphery to the spinal cord. Capsaicin is the best studied agent with respect to effects on substance P.

External Analgesics

Counterirritants cause local vasodilation. This vasodilation results in a feeling of warmth and increased comfort. The extent of vasodilation produced by counterirritants is unknown. It may occur only on the skin surface. It is unlikely the effects reach deeper structures such as muscle.

Vasodilation may permit the dispersal of pain producing substances. As postulated in the spasm metabolic waste theory, overworking muscles cause an accumulation of metabolic wastes such as lactic acid. These wastes affect the muscle fibre and irritate nerve endings, resulting in pain, muscle contraction and ischemia. Vasodilation should enhance removal of irritating substances.

Increased blood flow to the area was assumed to result in an increase in local skin temperature. However, spray application of counterirritants resulting in a drop in skin temperature may still relieve pain. Beneficial effects are therefore not solely related to increasing skin temperature.

An increase in skin temperature does not reflect activity in deeper structures such as muscle. Researchers attempted to measure temperature change after applying a preparation containing capsicum, methyl salicylate, oil of camphor, oil of pine, menthol, eucalyptus and turpentine. A significant increase in skin temperature was recorded, but only a slight change could be detected at a depth of 2.5 cm below the surface and no change was recorded at 4 cm.

Blood flow has been measured by other techniques, such as plethysmography or laser-Doppler flowmetry. As measured by plethysmography, applying a counterirritant results in a significant increase in blood flow in the area of erythema with a simultaneous rise in blood flow in nonerythematous distal areas. The increased blood flow was not compared with relief of pain. Local vasodilation is also demonstrated by an increase in oxygen concentration of venous blood after applying a counterirritant. This effect is local and confined to the arm of application. No effect is evident in the opposite arm, suggesting a lack of systemic effect.

Electromyography has been used to measure muscle action potential. Applying a counterirritant lowers muscle action potential; placebo does not. Increased muscle activity in muscles adjacent to painful joints may result from unconscious muscle contraction in an attempt to immobilize the joint. This muscle contraction produces wastes or metabolites that stimulate nerve endings and result in pain. The pain leads to further muscle contraction with further production of metabolites, resulting in a vicious cycle. Improvement of the blood supply by axon reflex stimulated by counterirritants removes metabolites and reduces pain. Axon reflex is the local neural mechanism by which afferent impulses in sensory nerves from the skin cause stimulation of sensory nerves innervating blood vessels. These impulses produce vasodilation.

Applying counterirritants may cause reflex vasodilation of painful tissues under the skin by liberating vasodilatory substances such as histamine, bradykinin and serotonin. No scientific evidence for this theory exists.

Applying counterirritants increases the speed of nerve conduction measured by electromyographic motor nerve conduction velocity testing, as does radiant heat. This increased nerve conduction velocity is maintained in direct proportion to the length of time the medication is in contact with the affected area. The effect is thought to be mediated through the vasomotor system. The study that reported these findings was performed with normal volunteers. Only nerve conduction velocity was studied. No measure of pain relief was performed.

A study using electromyography to detect changes in the amplitude of muscle action potential showed that applying an unnamed counterirritant spray increases a muscle's capacity to work by increasing the time required to fatigue. These results have not been corroborated with subsequent studies, but the findings suggest a possible benefit to using counterirritants. The danger of overworking an already fatigued muscle may also exist.

The placebo effects of counterirritants should not be overlooked. These products have a "medicinal" smell and quickly provide visual and tactile evidence of activity in the form of redness, warmth and a burning sensation. The physical evidence provides the user with a sense of satisfaction. Also, applying the counterirritant may require massage of the affected area, which may provide some relief.

The placebo effect may be particularly important in chronic debilitating conditions such as rheumatoid arthritis, osteoarthritis and postherpetic neuralgia. Treating rheumatoid arthritis sufferers with lactose tablets or subcutaneous saline injections results in placebo responses exceeding 50 per cent. Response to placebo has also been demonstrated in tendinitis, bursitis and other orthopedic problems. Topical application of placebo ointments produces high placebo response in single blind and double blind trials. Placebo response is important for two reasons. First, people with conditions resulting in chronic pain—potential placebo respondents—often purchase external analgesic products. Second, placebo response should be considered when evaluating the effectiveness of external analgesics in treating various conditions. Studies of counterirritant efficacy may provide little valuable information if a placebo control group has not been included.

Although the mechanism of action of these agents is far from clear, the response to counterirritants has been studied and a number of interesting results noted. For example, the number of rubs used to apply a counterirritant ointment does not affect the magnitude of the erythema or the time to achieve it. Redness is not proportional to the concentration used. Mild pains are often permanently relieved by counterirritants, but more severe pain may not be relieved at all. If counterirritation is too great, summation of pain with increased discomfort results; if too weak, there is little effect on the pain. The most effective intensity of counterirritation is slightly less than that which produces discomfort on normal skin. The most effective site of application is directly over the painful stimulus.

Individual Agents

Most commercially available external analgesic products contain more than one active ingredient. The United States Food and Drug Administration (FDA) monograph for external analgesic products states that "any two, three or four counterirritant active ingredients may be combined provided the combination contains no more than one active ingredient from each therapeutic group except that a combination of no more than one redness producing irritant, one vasodilation producing irritant and one irritant that does not produce redness may be combined with both camphor and menthol." Although marketed as combinations, individual active ingredients are discussed in the following section according to the classification in Table II. All doses given are the recommended adult doses. No guidelines are available for the use of these products in children less than 2 years of age. Rarely is the use of counterirritants appropriate for this age group.

External Analgesics

Know

Table II *Counterirritants*   *does*

Irritants that produce redness
> Allyl isothiocyanate
> Strong ammonia solution
> Methyl salicylate
> Turpentine oil

Irritants that do not produce redness
> Capsaicin *for shingles*
> Capsicum
> Capsicum oleoresin

Irritants that produce cooling sensation *in ice products.*
> Camphor
> *mostly* Menthol
> Eucalyptus oil

Irritants that produce vasodilation
> Methyl nicotinate

Adapted from: Food Drug Cosmetic Reporter. Vol I Drugs/Cosmetics. Drug Monograph. Commerce Clearinghouse Inc 1986;Sec:a)72,068.

Allyl Isothiocyanate

Allyl isothiocyanate, also known as volatile mustard oil, is obtained from the seeds of black mustard plant or produced synthetically. Black mustard seed contains the glycoside sinigrin. When the seeds are crushed and exposed to moisture, hydrolysis by myrosin results in the formation of allyl isothiocyanate. White mustard contains sinalbin, which is chemically related to sinigrin and has similar action. Allyl isothiocyanate is an extreme irritant and may produce blistering and severe pain if in contact with the skin too long. In plasters and poultices (mustard plaster), formation of allyl isothiocyanate is slower and therefore less likely to cause blistering. To avoid skin damage, plasters and poultices containing mustard oil should not be left on the skin longer than 15 to 20 minutes. Local effects may last 24 to 48 hours.

Few studies have examined the clinical usefulness of allyl isothiocyanate. Volatile oil of mustard 3 per cent in simple ointment is effective in relieving pain caused by intramuscular injection of hypertonic saline under experimental conditions. The allyl isothiocyanate produces severe irritation, but only mild flushing of the skin.

If ingested, gastrointestinal irritation with vomiting results. Allyl isothiocyanate is usually applied in a concentration of 0.5 to 5 per cent, not more than 3 to 4 times daily in adults and children older than 2 years.

Strong Ammonia Solution

Strong ammonia solution is a counterirritant that produces redness. For use as a counterirritant, it must be diluted to produce a concentration of 1 to 2.5 per cent ammonia. Undiluted, the solution is caustic and vapors are extremely irritating to the respiratory tract and eyes. Ingestion results in severe pain, coughing, vomiting and esophageal or gastrointestinal tract strictures or perforation. Convulsions may also occur.

Ammonia is usually formulated as a liniment. It should be applied no more than 3 to 4 times daily.

Methyl Salicylate — *Oil of Wintergreen (Rub A535 – 18%)*

Methyl salicylate is the most common counterirritant ingredient and is readily identified by its characteristic odor. It is also referred to as sweet birch oil, wintergreen oil, gaultheria oil, betula oil and teaberry oil. It may be obtained from the willow or produced synthetically.

Methyl salicylate is absorbed through intact skin. Initially, it was thought to have the systemic effect of salicylates. Metabolites of salicylates can be detected in the urine after topical application. Only 12 to 20 per cent of the salicylate applied to various areas of the body, with occlusive dressing, is absorbed into the systemic circulation after 10 hours of application. Estimated steady state salicylate plasma concentrations are much lower than levels required for control of rheumatoid arthritis. In some cases, plasma concentrations and antiplatelet effects are detected only in the arm to which the counterirritant is applied. (Salicylates are known to have antiplatelet effects when taken orally.) Although some absorption of methyl salicylate does occur, evidence to suggest a central or systemic effect is lacking.

A combination of 15 per cent methyl salicylate and 10 per cent menthol produces a feeling of warmth within 30 seconds of application and subjective improvement of pain in most people; placebo cream produces no effect. In individuals with rheumatoid arthritis and osteoarthritis, subjective data indicates a combination of 15 per cent methyl salicylate and 10 per cent menthol is more effective than placebo cream in reducing pain. A decrease in resting muscle action potential occurs with the combination product.

In sufferers of rheumatoid arthritis and osteoarthritis using a similar combination product, both the placebo and the counterirritant produce temperature effects in most people. However, the counterirritant produces a significant decrease in the perceived pain as compared to placebo. Both placebo and counterirritant significantly increase range of motion in the joint and improve dexterity, but the effect is greater with the counterirritant product.

Adverse reactions to topical salicylates are uncommon. Local reactions such as redness, itching and dermatitis can occur. The dermatitis may reappear following oral ingestion of salicylate. Considering the widespread use of salicylates, the incidence of topical sensitization is probably low. In a survey of 30,000 users, only two verified cases were identified. People with hypersensitivity reactions to acetylsalicylic acid should use caution since the salicylate moiety is absorbed to some extent through the skin.

Systemic toxicity due to absorption through the skin is uncommon. Toxic levels are achieved only if methyl salicylate has been applied to damaged skin or to large areas of skin with occlusive dressings. Local application of heat should not be used in conjunction with methyl salicylate. The use of topical methyl salicylate and menthol preparation with a heating pad in a 62 year old man produced severe, local skin and muscle necrosis, and renal damage resulting in prolonged hospitalization. These severe effects were attributed to increased percutaneous absorption of the drugs due to local heat application. Levels of salicylate adequate to potentiate the anticoagulant effects of warfarin have been reported in at least twelve cases. There are no prospective studies available examining the potential interaction, however case reports indicate elevated prothrombin times, evidence of bleeding and detectable salicylate blood concentrations in people using topical methyl salicylate and warfarin concurrently. Patients should be instructed to avoid the combination, particularly if increased potential for methyl salicylate absorption

External Analgesics

exists (for example, applications to damaged skin). Methyl salicylate should be used sparingly in children and avoided in people with burns or skin diseases.

The most serious adverse effect is toxicity resulting from oral ingestion, especially by children. The characteristic odor may appeal to small children, especially since some candies have this odor and taste. As little as 4 mL in a child and 6 mL in an adult can be fatal. Intoxication results in gastrointestinal, acid-base, metabolic and coagulation disturbances. The characteristic odor will be present on the breath, in urine and in vomitus. Appropriate toxicology texts should be referred to for details regarding symptoms and management.

Methyl salicylate is used in concentrations ranging from 10 to 60 per cent and may be applied to the affected area no more than 3 to 4 times daily.

Triethanolamine Salicylate

Triethanolamine salicylate (TEA), a salicylate ester, is a topical analgesic agent. The FDA External Analgesic Monograph places TEA in Category III—ingredients for which there is insufficient data and for which further testing is required before classifying into Category I or II. (FDA Category I is a drug product generally recognized as safe and effective and not misbranded. FDA Category II is a drug product not generally recognized as safe and effective or would result in the product being misbranded.) The FDA states that insufficient quantities of ester are absorbed through the skin to provide systemic analgesia. Since this FDA classification, two studies have been undertaken. Oral radiolabelled acetylsalicylic acid was compared to radiolabelled TEA 10 per cent. Serum salicylate levels were much lower with the topical preparation than with the oral salicylate; topical application resulted in synovial fluid concentrations of about 60 per cent of the oral concentration at 1 and 2 hours. Equivalent pain relief was observed with both topical and oral preparations in 4 out of 6 people.

A larger double blind study of 40 people with rheumatic pain compared 10 per cent topical TEA to oral salicylate. Improvement was determined jointly by the physician and the user. Relief of mild to moderate and moderate pain was equivalent with TEA and oral salicylate. TEA was more effective than oral salicylate for severe pain. The response of people with osteoarthritis to both agents was poor. There was a tendency for TEA to provide faster pain relief. A significantly greater number of people experienced adverse effects with oral therapy, and the number of people requiring discontinuation was much higher in the oral salicylate group.

The use of 10 per cent TEA in 25 people with osteoarthritis for 1 week produced the following results: 8 people preferred TEA, 6 people preferred placebo and 11 people had no preference. The results may be questioned because many people had severe arthritis and many received concurrent oral anti-inflammatory agents.

Triethanolamine salicylate is available as a 10 or 15 per cent cream and is massaged into the area of soreness 2 to 3 times daily.

Turpentine Oil

Turpentine oil is used as a counterirritant and is available as turpentine liniment or white liniment. The oil is obtained by distillation and rectification of turpentine from pine trees. No published trials report the efficacy of turpentine oil as a counterirritant for arthritic conditions or muscle soreness. When applied, it produces redness and a sensation of burning. Application may result in hives and blisters. It may sensitize the skin and result in eczema-like conditions.

Vomiting may occur in some individuals due to absorption through the skin.

Toxicity results from ingestion of turpentine oil. As little as 15 mL may be fatal in children. Severe gastroenteritis, irritation of the urinary tract and pre-existing inflammatory processes occur. Petechiae and thrombocytopenia may occur. The person may exhibit central nervous system excitation and seizures or central nervous system depression.

The topical dose is a 6 to 50 per cent concentration applied 3 to 4 times daily.

Capsicum Preparations

Capsicum preparations are counterirritants derived from cayenne pepper and include capsaicin, capsicum and capsicum oleoresin. Small concentrations of capsaicin have been used topically for many years, for short term management of arthralgias and arthritis. Capsicum products are generally available in concentrations of 0.025 to 0.25 per cent capsaicin. Recently, the drug has undergone both open and placebo controlled trials for management of chronic pain syndromes such as postherpetic neuralgia.

Application of capsicum causes erythema and a feeling of warmth. The irritant action is potent, and severe burning can occur on tender skin. With continued use, tachyphylaxis to the burning sensation occurs. Capsaicin does not cause blistering presumably due to a lack of effect on blood vessels. In normal male volunteers, application of capsicum 0.1 per cent cream did not increase forearm blood flow despite local erythema and a sensation of warmth or burning.

Capsaicin is probably the most extensively studied topical analgesic. It exerts its analgesic effect by causing release of substance P from peripheral sensory C nerve fibres. This results in depletion of substance P from the neuron. Substance P is the principal transmitter of nociceptive impulses from the peripheral to the central nervous system and is a potent vasodilator. Capsaicin also inhibits axon reflex vasodilation which is mediated by substance P. Application of capsaicin reduces synthesis of substance P by peripheral nerves.

On initial application capsaicin produces burning and hyperesthesia followed by desensitization to burning and pain. The burning diminishes with repeated use presumably as a result of depletion of substance P. Application 3 to 4 times daily is recommended for maximal effect. Less frequent application prevents total depletion of substance P resulting in decreased efficacy and increased local side effects. One study suggested pretreatment with topical lidocaine 5 per cent for the first 2 weeks to control burning at the site of application. Other adverse effects include stinging or erythema at the site of application, cough and respiratory irritation.

Suggested uses for topical capsaicin include rheumatoid and osteoarthritis, diabetic neuropathy, postherpetic neuralgia (PHN), postmastectomy neuroma, reflex sympathetic dystrophy, vulvar vestibulitis, psoriasis, apocrine chromhidrosis and hemodialysis related itching.

Initial research was in patients with PHN. The results of both open and placebo controlled trials have been reviewed elsewhere, however, in general, pain relief occurred in 60 to 78 per cent of patients. Intolerable burning was the major reason for dropout of study patients. Pain relief requires a minimum of 14 to 28 days of treatment. Maximum response occurs after 4 to 6 weeks of continuous therapy; some patients require therapy indefinitely to prevent return of pain. Both 0.025 and 0.075 per cent cream have been studied.

The length of treatment required before the desired response is achieved and the frequency of application must be stressed to the patient. Noncompliance will result in decreased efficacy and increased local adverse effects. The patient should also be told that burning on application decreases with time.

Camphor

Camphor has weak analgesic and rubefacient action and may have mild local anesthetic action. It produces numbness at the site of application. It has a hot bitter taste; ingestion of small amounts produces a feeling of warmth in the stomach. Flushing of the skin may be minimal unless massage is vigorous. Natural camphor is obtained from the camphor tree, but most commercial camphor is produced synthetically.

The major problem with this external analgesic is accidental ingestion. It is often mistaken for castor oil. As little as 5 mL can result in life threatening illness and may be fatal to a child. Ingestion causes gastrointestinal tract irritation with nausea and vomiting. Shock and severe dehydration due to vomiting may occur. Central nervous system toxicity occurs (excitement, hallucinations, delirium, muscular excitability, tremors and tonic clonic seizures). Other signs and symptoms include urinary retention, albuminuria and transient changes in liver enzymes. In some provinces (for example, British Columbia and New Brunswick) camphorated oil is restricted to "No Public Access" areas of the pharmacy in an attempt to decrease the number of poisonings by this agent.

At concentrations of 0.1 to 3 per cent, camphor exhibits analgesic properties. When used as a counterirritant, 3 to 11 per cent is effective and may be applied 3 to 4 times daily.

Menthol

Menthol is derived from peppermint oil or produced synthetically. It is an irritant that has a cooling effect when applied in low concentrations (0.1 to 1 per cent). At these concentrations it selectively stimulates sensory nerve endings, causing a cooling sensation and analgesia. When used for muscle aches in rubs and liniments, a higher concentration (1.25 to 16 per cent) produces a prickly or burning sensation. Topical application in counterirritant concentrations produces a feeling of coolness followed by a sensation of warmth. It is applied to the affected area 3 to 4 times daily. It may cause sensitization in some people, although this adverse effect is uncommon.

Eucalyptus Oil

Eucalyptus oil is in many counterirritant products. It is placed in FDA category III (lacking sufficient information to permit final classification) and also appears in the FDA list of inactive agents used in external analgesic products. Eucalyptol is the most important constituent of eucalyptus oil. This agent is listed as a flavoring agent and expectorant and as having bacteriostatic properties, but not as a counterirritant. Like camphor and menthol, it produces a cooling sensation when applied topically. The usual concentration in external analgesics is 0.5 to 3 per cent eucalyptus oil. cooling then warms

Esters of Nicotinic Acid

A number of esters of nicotinic acid have been used as counterirritants, including tetrahydrofurfuryl nicotinate, beta-butoxyethyl nicotinate, benzyl nicotinate, ethyl nicotinate, n-hexylester nicotinic acid and methyl nicotinate. Methyl nicotinate is the most commonly used. Application results in vasodilation causing redness and warmth.

Application of a 5 per cent solution results in redness, tingling and heat in 5 to 10 minutes and lasting 0.5 to 1 hour. In some cases a full response is delayed 2 to 4 hours. This may not correlate with pain relief.

The mechanism of nicotinic acid esters is thought to be due to vasodilation. Nicotinic acid ester cream (2.5 per cent) raises forearm blood flow significantly, as measured by venous occlusion plethysmography. A significant increase in blood flow can be shown in the flushed area after application of tetrahydrofurfuryl nicotinic acid ester (5 per cent cream or 20 per cent aqueous glycerin mixture). There is a simultaneous rise in blood flow in the distal part of the treated forearm. This effect is rapid, occurring 4 to 5 minutes after application and lasting at least 30 minutes. Application of 0.025, 0.05 and 0.1 per cent hexyl nicotinate to healthy skin in normal volunteers produces a dose related increase in skin blood flow measured by laser Doppler flow. This occurs even in the absence of significant erythema. Injection of adrenalin or lidocaine prevents the distal vasodilation. Vasodilation does not occur in people with brachial plexus injury. Intact nerves may be required for the vasodilatory response to nicotinic acid esters.

Although not commercially available, in investigations, an aerosol spray product (methyl nicotinate 1.6 per cent, 2-hydroxyl ethyl salicylate 5 per cent, methyl salicylate 1 per cent, and ethyl salicylate 5 per cent) produces visible redness of the skin as well as an increase in venous oxygen concentration in the arm to which the spray is applied. The opposite arm shows no such changes. The increase in local oxygen concentration is attributed to an increased local blood flow secondary to vasodilation. This spray is therapeutically active, but effects are local rather than systemic. Pain relief has not been measured.

Studies of efficacy are few. Tetrahydrofurfuryl nicotinic acid 5 per cent produces flushing, warmth and prickling when applied to the skin of healthy, normal volunteers, but fails to reduce pain resulting from intramuscular injection of hypertonic saline. The nicotinic acid ester was compared to volatile oil of mustard ointment, which produced severe irritation and was effective in reducing pain. The authors concluded that counterirritation relieved pain by producing skin pain of adequate intensity and that local vasodilation as evidenced by flushing was not important.

A liniment containing esters of salicylic acid, nicotinic acid and benzoic acid was evaluated in 146 people with degenerative or rheumatoid arthritis. The following results were reported: 83 people found the medicated liniment superior, 27 people found the placebo superior, 33 people found them equally effective, and 4 people derived no benefit from either preparation. The only adverse effect reported was mild skin irritation. This finding suggests an important placebo component to application and massage of a liniment. Many people in this study requested the liniment be added to their previous medication regimen.

Esters of nicotinic acid penetrate the skin well. Fainting, caused by a drop in blood pressure, has been reported in some people who applied the product over large areas of the body. This effect is due to generalized vasodilation.

Methyl nicotinate is used as a counterirritant in concentrations of 0.25 to 1 per cent applied 3 to 4 times daily.

Dimethyl Sulfoxide

Dimethyl sulfoxide (DMSO) is not approved for topical use to relieve pain in inflammatory conditions. However, public interest in DMSO

External Analgesics

persists and a number of trials have evaluated this agent. DMSO is approved in Canada by prescription only for use in treating scleroderma and chronic inflammatory genitourinary disorders, but not as an external analgesic.

DMSO has a number of pharmacologic properties including analgesic, anti-inflammatory and connective tissue modification effects. It passes easily through membranes and makes tissues permeable to other topical drugs. DMSO is detected in the plasma within 5 minutes of topical application. It may be useful in treating acute inflammatory musculoskeletal conditions and soft tissue injury. Use in chronic conditions such as arthritis has also been suggested. Proposed mechanisms of action include: action as a free-radical scavenger; chemical block of small nerve fibres; stabilization of lysosomal membranes; enhancement of blood flow; and decreased prostaglandin production.

Two large studies are commonly cited to support claims for the beneficial effects of DMSO. These two studies are merely summaries of clinical observations in heterogeneous populations in uncontrolled trials, making it difficult to evaluate and interpret results. In one study a 90 per cent aqueous solution of DMSO was evaluated in 4,180 cases of unspecified acute and chronic musculoskeletal injuries. Eighty-six per cent of people with acute conditions showed complete or partial remission. The response rate in chronic conditions was 84 per cent. People with rheumatoid arthritis had the poorest response. Common adverse effects of DMSO were seen, of which local skin reactions were most frequent. The degree of reaction varied; 3.5 per cent were severe and required discontinuation of therapy.

The second paper compiled the results of the use of 90 per cent DMSO in aqueous solution in 1,900 people suffering from acute and chronic musculoskeletal conditions. In the acute musculoskeletal condition group, 72 per cent exhibited an excellent or good response, compared to 52 per cent in the chronic group. As in the previously mentioned study, people with rheumatoid arthritis had the poorest response. Therapy was discontinued in 6 per cent of the people due to local skin reactions.

A 10 per cent DMSO ointment compared to placebo in people with rheumatoid arthritis resulted in no difference in response rate (50 per cent DMSO versus 58 per cent placebo). A 10 per cent concentration of DMSO is not thought potent enough to provide pharmacologic benefits. However, the high placebo response rate should be noted.

There was no difference in response to DMSO 50 per cent ointment or placebo in people with arthrosis; an equal number of people responded to either treatment. A double blind placebo control design is essential for evaluation of treatments for musculoskeletal disease.

Side effects with DMSO are common although not always serious. Local skin reactions include warmth, burning, stinging, dermatitis, redness, hives and blistering. The skin may become dry and scaling or thickened. A musky, garlicky breath and skin odor occurs in all people due to the metabolite dimethylsulfide. Other common side effects include nausea, vomiting, anorexia, headache, sedation and dizziness. Many of these adverse effects may be more common when DMSO is used systemically rather than topically. The incidence of adverse effects may increase if commercial or veterinary grades are used topically on humans, due to the presence of impurities and toxic byproducts. Damage to the lens of the eye has been reported in animals and has been of major concern regarding use of this drug in humans. However, human evidence of such damage is lacking.

DMSO may provide temporary relief of pain in acute and chronic

musculoskeletal disorders including arthritis, but it does not reverse the inflammatory process. It should not be recommended as an external analgesic agent, as it is not currently approved for such use.

Clinical Considerations and Dosage Forms

Nonprescription counterirritants are available in a number of dosage forms including liniments, gels, lotions and ointments. As mentioned previously, the massaging action of application may be an important component of efficacy. The desired effect is local rather than systemic. Ideally, absorption through the skin should be minimal, so the vehicle used in the product formulation is of some importance. Factors that influence absorption are skin condition (intactness), skin age (fetal and infant skin are more permeable than adult skin), regional skin site, skin hydration, drug concentration, solubility and molecular characteristics of the drug, and vehicle characteristics. The amount of rubbing performed and the period of time the medication is permitted to remain in contact with the skin also may have an effect.

Liniments may be defined as solutions or mixtures of various substances in oil, alcoholic solutions of soap, or emulsions. They are applied to the affected area with friction or rubbing. The oil or soap base allows for ease of application and is preferred for massage. Alcoholic liniments are commonly used for rubefacient, counterirritant or astringent properties. They penetrate the skin better than the oily liniments. Liniments should not be applied to broken skin or bruised areas.

Ointments are semisolid dosage forms for external application. They may be greasy (oleaginous) or water-soluble. Water-soluble ointments are easier to remove after application. Because ointments soften when applied to the skin, massage is easy to perform.

Lotions are liquid suspensions or dispersions for external application. They require shaking before use to disperse the active ingredients. Gels are semisolid systems that are easy to apply and remove. Gels often provide a faster release of drug than ointments.

Choosing a suitable dosage form depends on the individual. Some people prefer water-washable or greaseless preparations; others find the greasier, heavier preparations more soothing. Lanolin (wool fat) produces a number of allergic reactions, which should be considered when choosing a product.

External analgesics should not be used for children younger than 2 years of age without first consulting a physician. No information is available about how long these preparations can remain on the skin. The FDA recommends these preparations be applied not more than 3 or 4 times daily. However, many Canadian products are labelled "Use as required", "May be reapplied when needed" or "May be used every 2 hours." If excessive burning, redness, irritation or a rash occurs, the product should be washed off immediately with soap and warm water or removed with olive oil. Overzealous application may lead to severe irritation and blistering, and consumers should be warned against excessive use. The use of heat in the form of heat lamps, heating pads and hot water bottles in combination with counterirritants may lead to severe burning and blistering or to systemic effects as a result of enhanced absorption. This combination should be used cautiously if at all.

No rationale exists for combining the use of more than one counterirritant product. If the condition worsens, fails to clear up or recurs within a few days of discontinuing the product, the individual should be referred to a physician. Seven days of use is a reasonable length of time for most products except capsaicin.

Other information that should be provided to the consumer includes the following:
- The product is for external use only.
- Avoid contact with the eyes.
- Do not apply to wounds or damaged skin.
- Do not bandage tightly.

For capsaicin, the following additional information should be provided.
- Application less than 3 times a day may not provide optimal pain relief and may cause the initial burning sensation to persist.
- With regular use, the transient burning sensation diminishes.
- Continued application for 3 to 4 weeks is necessary for optimal response.
- Discontinue use if condition worsens or does not improve after 28 days and consult a physician.

All external analgesic products should be stored in a cool, dry, dark place. They must be stored out of reach of children, as ingestion leads to severe toxicity.

Summary

External analgesic products have a place in the self-treatment of local pain. Some studies suggest a high placebo component, which may be due, in part, to the subjective nature of pain. External analgesics are effective for many people for symptomatic pain relief. They have the advantage of avoiding the adverse effects of systemic analgesic products. When used appropriately, external analgesics have limited toxicity, but consumers should be warned that significant toxicity may result from overzealous application and that these agents are extremely toxic if accidentally ingested. External analgesics should be stored where children cannot get into them.

The user should fully understand that these products provide short-term symptomatic relief. No claims are made on speed of healing of sprains and strains or relief from underlying disease processes involved in rheumatoid arthritis or osteoarthritis. The pharmacist has the opportunity to assist consumers in selecting the most appropriate product and to advise them on proper use, including instructions regarding application, duration of therapy and expected degree of pain relief.

Ask the Consumer

Q. What is the nature and location of the pain?
- It is necessary to identify individuals who need referral to physicians. To self-medicate, consumers should be able to specify the location of pain in a muscle, joint or bone. Pain that radiates to other areas should not be treated with external analgesics.

Q. How long has the pain been present?
- External analgesic products are used for short-term, self-limiting conditions such as sprains or strains or as temporary adjunctive treatment of chronic conditions such as rheumatoid arthritis. If the pain has persisted for longer than one week, the consumer should be referred to a physician.

Q. Is the occurrence of pain associated with a particular event such as strenuous exercise, recent injury or particular work?
- This information is used to assess the need for referral to a physician. If the condition is associated with broken or irritated skin, external analgesics should not be recommended. External analgesics may be recommended for muscle aches and pains associated with strenuous exercise or work.

Q. If the pain is associated with a joint, is the joint red, swollen or hot to touch? Is the pain worse in the morning, but lesser as the day progresses?
- Rheumatoid and other types of arthritis should be diagnosed by a physician. Redness and swelling of a joint may be associated with many conditions, including septic arthritis, gout and rheumatoid arthritis. The characteristic pattern of improvement as the day progresses is suggestive of rheumatoid arthritis; worsening of pain and swelling might occur with an untreated infection. If infection of the joint or gout is a possibility, the person should be referred to a physician. If the individual has been diagnosed as having an arthritic condition, adjuvant therapy with external analgesics can be recommended for temporary relief of pain.

Q. Does the person have signs and symptoms of a flu-like illness?
- Viral infections may be associated with muscle aches and pains as well as fever. Systemic analgesic/antipyretic products may be more appropriate than external analgesics in this situation.

Q. What is the age of the individual?
- Children may absorb topical products to a much greater extent than adults. External analgesics are not recommended for children less than 2 years of age.

Q. Does the individual have any allergies?
- Look specifically for acetylsalicylic acid hypersensitivity. Systemic absorption of salicylates does occur, and agents containing methyl salicylate and triethanolamine salicylate should not be recommended to people with salicylate allergies.

Q. Has the individual attempted to treat the condition before? What was tried and did it work?
- The answers to these questions help the pharmacist choose products to recommend or to reinforce the appropriate use of specific products. The need to refer the person to a physician also may be ascertained.

References
Introduction

Crossland J, ed. Lewis's pharmacology. New York: Churchill Livingstone, 1970:560–4.
Food Drug Cosmetic Reporter. Vol. 1 Drugs/Cosmetics. Drug Monograph. Commerce Clearinghouse Inc, 1986;Sec:a)72,068;b)72,091.3;c)72,291.2; d)72,295.
Gammon GD, Starr I. Studies on the relief of pain by counterirritation. J Clin Invest 1941;20:13–20.
Grollman A, ed. Pharmacology and therapeutics. Philadelphia: Lea & Febiger, 1965:825–32.
Lewis JJ, ed. Introduction to pharmacology. Edinburgh: E and S Livingstone, 1965:581–8.

External Analgesics

Uses

Anonymous. Sprains, strains and bruises. Drug Ther Bull 1976;14:66–8.

Appenzeller O, Atkinson R, eds. Sports medicine. Baltimore: Urban and Schwarzenberg, 1983:284–347.

Barker LR, Burton JR, Zieve PD, eds. Principles of ambulatory medicine. Baltimore: Williams and Wilkins, 1986:835.

Hoffman GS. Tendinitis and bursitis. Am Fam Physician 1981;23(6):103–10.

Hurst JW, ed. Medicine for the practicing physician. Toronto: Butterworths, 1983;227,242,367–80.

Jacknowitz AI. External analgesic products. In: Feldmann EG, ed. Handbook of nonprescription drugs. Washington: American Pharmaceutical Association, 1990:871–87.

General Treatment

Sherman M. Hot or cold: which treatment to recommend? Am Pharm 1980;NS20(8):46–9.

Mechanism of Action

Anonymous. The pain paradox (Editorial). Lancet 1976;1:945–6.

Behbehani M. Physiology of pain. In: Prithvi Raj P, ed. Practical management of pain. Chicago: Yearbook Medical Publishers, 1986:61–77.

Collins AJ, Notarianni AJ, Ring EFJ, Seed MP. Some observations on the pharmacology of "deep-heat", a topical rubefacient. Ann Rheum Dis 1984;43:411–5.

Crockford GW, Hellon RF, Heyman A. Local vasomotor responses to rubefacients and ultraviolet radiation. J Physiol (Lond) 1962;161:21–9.

Dowd PM, Whitefield M, Greaves MW. Hexyl-Nicotinate-induced vasodilation in normal human skin. Dermatologica 1987;174:239–43.

Guy RH, Wester RC, Tur E, Maibach HI. Noninvasive assessments of the percutaneous absorption of methyl nicotinate in humans. J Pharm Sci 1983;72:1077–9.

Hannington-Kiff JG. Counterpains. Nurs Times 1977;73(9):312–3.

Hoskins-Michel T, ed. International perspectives in physical therapy I: pain. New York: Churchill Livingstone, 1971:560–4.

Lange K, Weiner D. The effect of certain hyperkinemics on the blood flow through the skin. J Invest Dermatol 1949;12:263–9.

Maciewicz R, Martin JB. Pain: pathophysiology and management. In: Braunwald E, Isselbacher KJ, Petersdorf RG, et al, eds. Harrison's principles of internal medicine. Montreal: McGraw-Hill, 1987:13–7.

Melzack R, Wall PD. Pain mechanisms: a new theory. Science 1965;150(3699):973–9.

Morison RAH, Woodmansey A, Young AJ. Placebo responses in an arthritis trial. Ann Rheum Dis 1961;20:179–84.

Peterson JB, Farber EM, Fulton GP. Responses of the skin to rubefacients. J Invest Dermatol 1959;35(2):57–64.

Post BS. Effect of percutaneous medication on muscle tissue: an electromyographic study. Arch Phys Med Rehabil 1961;42:791–8.

Post BS, Forster S, Benton JG. The effect of percutaneous medication on motor nerve conduction velocity. Arch Phys Med Rehabil 1964;45:460–5.

Roskos KV, Bircher AJ, Maiback HI, Guy RH. Pharmacodynamic measurements of methylnicotinate percutaneous absorption: the effect of aging on microcirculation. Brit J Dermatol 1990;122:165–71.

Traut EF, Carstens HP, Thrift CB, Clark HM. Topical treatment in rheumatic disease. IMJ 1962;121:257–60.

Traut EF, Passarelli EW. Placebos in the treatment of rheumatoid arthritis and other rheumatic conditions. Ann Rheum Dis 1957;16:18–21.

Traut EF, Passarelli EW. Study in the controlled therapy of degenerative arthritis. Arch Intern Med 1956;98:181–6.

Vuopala U, Vesterinen E, Kaipainen WJ. The analgesic action of dimethylsulfoxide (DMSO) ointment in arthrosis. Acta Rheum Scand 1971;17:57–60.

Vuopala U, Isomaki H, Kaipainen WJ. Dimethylsulfoxide (DMSO) ointment in the treatment of rheumatoid arthritis. Acta Rheum Scand 1969;15:139–44.

Wang JK. Stimulation-produced analgesia. Mayo Clin Proc 1976;51:28–30.

White JR, Sage JN. Topical analgesic on induced muscular pain. Phys Ther 1970;50:166–72.

White JR, Sage JN. Effects of a counterirritant on muscular distress in patients with arthritis. Phys Ther 1971;51:36–42.

White JR. Effects of a counterirritant on perceived pain and hand movement in patients with arthritis. Phys Ther 1973;53:956–60.

Allyl Isothiocyanate

Gennaro AR, ed. Remington's pharmaceutical sciences. Easton: Mack Publishing, 1985:780–1,1286,1291,1301,1506,1512-3.

Macarthur JG, Alstead S. Counter-irritants. A method of assessing their effects. Lancet 1953;2:1060–2.

Reynolds JEF, ed. Martindale: the extra pharmacopoeia. London: The Pharmaceutical Press, 1989:1064.

Strong Ammonia Solution

Reynolds JEF, ed. Martindale: the extra pharmacopoeia. London: The Pharmaceutical Press, 1989:1542.

Methyl Salicylate

Brown EW, Scott WO. The absorption of methyl salicylate by the human skin. J Pharmacol Exp Ther 1934;50:32–50.

Chow WH, Cheung KL, Ling HM, See T. Potentiation of warfarin anticoagulation by topical methyl salicylate ointment. JR Soc Med 1989;82:501–2.

Gordon RR. Poisoning by oil of wintergreen (Letter). Br Med J 1968;1:769.

Gosselin RE, Smith RP, Hodge HC, eds. Clinical toxicology of commercial products. Baltimore: Williams and Wilkins, 1984:III–368.

Heng MCY. Local necrosis and interstitial nephritis due to topical methyl salicylate and menthol. Cutis. 1987;39:442–4.

Hindson C. Contact eczema from methyl salicylate reproduced by oral aspirin. Contact Dermatitis 1977;3:348–9.

Littleton F. Warfarin and topical salicylates (Letter). JAMA 1990;263:2888.

Morgan JK. Iatrogenic epidermal sensitivity. Br J Clin Pract 1968;22(6):261–4.

Roberts MS, Favretto WA, Meyer A, Reckmann M, Wongseelashote T. Topical bioavailability of methyl salicylate. Aust NZ J Med 1982;12:303–5.

Trapnell K. Salicylate intoxication. J Am Pharm Assoc 1976;16(3):147–9.

Yip ASB, Chow WH, Tai YT, Cheung KL. Adverse effect of topical methyl salicylate ointment on warfarin anticoagulation: an unrecognized potential hazard. Postgrad Med J 1990;66:367–9.

Triethanolamine Salicylate

Algozzine GJ, Stein GH, Doering PL, Araujo OE, Akin KC. Trolamine salicylate cream in osteoarthritis of the knee. JAMA 1982;247:1311–3.

Golden EL. A double-blind comparison of orally ingested aspirin and a topically applied salicylate cream in the relief of rheumatic pain. Curr Ther Res 1978;24:524–9.

O'Brien WM. Trolamine salicylate cream in osteoarthritis (Letter). JAMA 1982;248:1577–8.

Rabinowitz JL, Feldman ES, Weinberger A, Schumacher HR. Comparative tissue absorption of oral ^{14}C aspirin and topical triethanolamine ^{14}C salicylate in human and canine knee joints. J Clin Pharmacol 1982;22:42–8.

Turpentine Oil

Morgan JK. Iatrogenic epidermal sensitivity. Br J Clin Pract 1968;22(6):261–4.

Reynolds JEF, ed. Martindale: the extra pharmacopoeia. London: The Pharmaceutical Press, 1989:1067.

Willis GA, Freeman DA. Poison management manual 1989. Ottawa: Canadian Pharmaceutical Association, 1989:439–40.

Capsicum Preparations

Crismon JM, Fox RH, Goldsmith R, MacPherson RK. Forearm blood flow after inunction of rubefacient substances. J Physiol 1959;145:47P–48P.

Lynn B. Capsaicin: Actions on nociceptive C-fibres and therapeutic potential. Pain 1990;41:61–9.

Nolte MJ. Topical capsaicin for postherpetic neuralgia. Drug Intell Clin Pharm 1988;22:488–9.

Rumsfield JA, West DP. Topical capsaicin in dermatologic and peripheral pain disorders. DICP 1991;25:381–7.

Camphor

Aronow R. Camphor poisoning. JAMA 1976;235:1260.

Gosselin RE, Smith RP, Hodge HC, eds. Clinical toxicology of commercial products. Baltimore: Williams and Wilkins, 1984:III–84.

Phelan WJ. Camphor poisoning: over-the-counter dangers. Pediatrics 1976;57:428–31.

Trestrail JH, Spartz ME. Camphorated and castor oil confusion and its toxic results. Clin Toxicol 1977;11:151–8.

Menthol

Papa CM, Shelley WB. Menthol hypersensitivity. JAMA 1964;189:546–8.

Esters of Nicotinic Acid

Nassim JR, Banner H. Skin response to local application of a nicotinic acid ester in rheumatoid arthritis. Lancet 1952;1:699.

Dimethyl Sulfoxide

American Academy of Pediatrics. Dimethyl sulfoxide (DMSO). Committee on Drugs & Committee on Sports Medicine. Pediatrics 1983;71:76.

Anonymous. Dimethyl sulfoxide. Med Lett Drugs Ther 1980;22:94–5.

Demos CH, Beckloff GL, Donin MN, Oliver PM. Dimethyl sulfoxide in musculoskeletal disorders. Ann NY Acad Sci 1967;141:517–23.

Jimenez RAH, Willkens RF. Dimethyl sulfoxide: a perspective of its use in rheumatic diseases. J Clin Lab Sci 1982;100:489–500.

John H, Laudahn G. Clinical experiences with the topical application of DMSO in orthopedic diseases: evaluation of 4180 cases. Ann NY Acad Sci 1967;141:506–16.

Parker WA, Bailie GR. Current therapeutic status of DMSO. Can Pharm J 1982;115:247–51.

Clinical Considerations and Dosage Forms

Idson B. Percutaneous absorption. J Pharm Sci 1975;64:901–24.

4

Sunscreens

Sanna G. Pellatt

The ultraviolet components of solar radiation can cause the acute effects of sunburn, tanning and photosensitivity and such chronic effects as skin aging, hyperplasia and cancer. Physical and chemical sunscreens protect the skin against these effects. The choice of a sunscreen depends, in part, on the agent's sun protection factor (SPF). Particular care must be taken in recommending sunscreens for children. Tanning effects are often sought through the use of pigmenting agents; other consumers may request depigmenting agents to lighten hyperpigmented areas caused by freckling, medical disorders or drugs.

As outdoor sports and leisure activities become more popular, many Canadians spend more time in the sun, both at home and abroad. For a large part of the population, outdoor leisure activities are essential to leading a normal, healthy life. Others are exposed to sunlight as part of their occupation.

Until a few generations ago, affluent men and women of the western world carefully protected themselves from exposure to sunlight. White skin was considered the beautiful ideal. Modern fashion has reversed this trend. A year-round tan now connotes leisure, wealth, health and beauty.

Exposure to ultraviolet (UV) light rays from the sun can cause both acute and chronic effects. The acute effects include sunburn and photosensitivity reactions; chronic UV light exposure can result in premature aging, changes to the skin's immune system, damage to the eyes, and skin malignancies. To reduce health risks posed by sunlight, the public must be aware of sunburn prevention and treatment and the appropriate use of sunscreens for various skin types.

Solar Radiation

Sunlight consists of electromagnetic radiation of various wavelengths ranging from gamma rays to radio waves (see Figure 1). The UV component of sunlight induces normal and abnormal changes in the skin. Ultraviolet radiation is subdivided into UVA, UVB and UVC.

The shortest wavelength in the UV spectrum is UVC (200 to 290 nm), also referred to as germicidal radiation. UVC radiation from sunlight does not reach the earth's surface; it is effectively screened by the ozone layer in the atmosphere. The radiation is also emitted by artificial sources such as germicidal lamps, welding arcs, and high and low pressure mercury arc lamps. Individuals exposed to UVC radiation from artificial sources can experience a mild reddening of the skin.

The next longest radiation, UVB (290 to 320 nm), is responsible for sunburn and for delayed tanning (melanogenesis). The energy from UVB radiation has also been implicated in causing skin cancer and wrinkling.

The UVA region extends from 320 to 400 nm. It penetrates well into the dermis causing both an immediate tanning reaction, known as immediate pigment darkening reaction, and delayed tanning. It can also evoke a weak sunburn reaction. UVA radiation is responsible for photosensitivity reactions to certain chemicals and drugs and can enhance the acute and chronic effects of UVB radiation.

Several factors modify the intensity of UV radiation reaching the skin. UVA radiation is present all day and throughout the year whereas the intensity of UVB radiation varies according to the time of day and the season. About 30 to 50 per cent of the total daily sunburning energy is received between 11 a.m. and 1 p.m. At this time, the angle of incoming radiation is perpendicular to the earth's surface. In the early morning and late afternoon more UVB radiation is filtered out because it passes through the ozone layer at a lower angle, thus travelling through a greater distance of atmosphere. At latitudes other than the equator, the thickness of the ozone layer varies with the season of the year. It is thickest in late winter and thinnest in late summer and early fall. Currently, much concern surrounds the integrity of the ozone layer, which is endangered by the fluorocarbons released from such sources as aerosols and air conditioners.

Higher altitudes result in greater UV intensities. In general, sunburning effectiveness of sunlight increases by 4 per cent for every 300 metres increase in altitude. This intensity also increases as one travels toward the equator. Clouds and air pollution can filter out infrared and visible radiation while letting through as much as 90 per cent of UV radiation as scattered light. Sunburn can therefore occur on a relatively cool, sunless day. High humidity and air movement across the skin surface can increase the severity of sunburn. The components of this "windburn" effect are not yet known. Window glass filters out UVB radiation while allowing UVA rays to pass through.

Sunlight can be reflected from a variety of sources. A covered porch or beach umbrella does not protect against reflected radiation and sunburn may occur. Reflected light can be damaging because it often strikes parts of the body that are normally shaded, such as the eyes. A green lawn scatters about 3 per cent of incident radiation, dry sand reflects about 25 per cent, and fresh snow may reflect 80 per cent or more of incident sunlight. White paint and sheets of aluminum reflect 70 to 90 per cent of UV radiation. Reflection from water is

Figure 1 *Solar Spectrum*

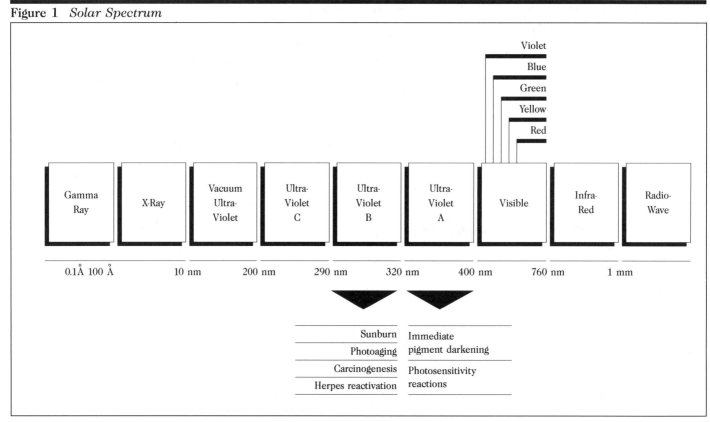

Adapted from: Warshauer DM, Steinbaugh IR. Sunlight and protection of the skin. Am Fam Physician 1983;27(6):109-15.

usually minimal (4 per cent) unless the sun is directly overhead. Ultraviolet light passes through water, with at least 40 per cent of incidental UV radiation transmitted through 50 cm of clear water. Hence, swimming in either the sea or an outdoor pool offers little protection against sunburn. Figure 2 illustrates important environmental factors that affect UV radiation.

Acute Effects of UV Radiation
Sunburn

Sunlight acts on normal skin to produce a variety of short term effects. The most common effect is sunburn, which in the mildest form appears as a reddening of the skin (erythema). Sunburn is usually evident 2 to 12 hours after initial exposure to UV light. It reaches a maximum in 20 to 48 hours and gradually subsides over the following 3 to 5 days.

Skin responds to solar injury in two phases: an early inflammatory phase followed by a delayed repair phase. The inflammatory phase is characterized by redness and tenderness. The sunburn response is complex and not fully understood. It has been suggested that several vasoactive substances such as histamine, prostaglandins, kinins and arachidonic acid metabolites may be responsible for the inflammatory response. Epidermal changes evoked by UV injury involve the formation of "sunburn" cells. These damaged cells form within 24 hours of exposure and are eliminated by phagocytosis within 72 hours after UV exposure. With longer exposure, the

initial erythema may be accompanied by edema, itching, fever and pain. Blistering occurs in more severe reactions. Systemic symptoms such as nausea, chills, abdominal cramping and headache may also accompany the local reactions if large areas of the body are involved.

Treatment of sunburn depends on its severity. Mild cases can be treated like any other minor burn with the application of cool water soaks or compresses for 20 minutes, followed by an oil-in-water moisturizing lotion to relieve dryness. Acetylsalicylic acid is recommended as an effective analgesic and as a mild anti-inflammatory agent. Studies have shown that topical indomethacin (not commercially available), applied in the early stages of sunburn, may decrease erythema by preventing the formation of "sunburn" cells and inhibiting prostaglandin synthesis. However, pretreatment with topical indomethacin has not been shown to suppress the erythema response. Topical anesthetic sprays should be avoided because they pose the risk of contact sensitization. Mild sunburn is self-limiting and usually heals without scarring.

More severe sunburn calls for immediate medical attention. Systemic steroids can abort extreme inflammation before it occurs. Oral prednisone, starting with 40 to 60 mg daily and gradually reduced over 4 to 8 days, may be used to control the severe sunburn reaction. It is controversial whether topical corticosteroids speed recovery from sunburn. Systemic antibiotics may be initiated if bacterial superinfection occurs. General therapeutic measures are the same as for mild sunburn except that more potent analgesics may be required.

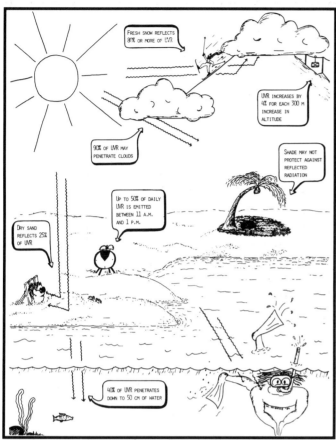

Figure 2 *Environmental Factors Affecting Ultraviolet Radiation.*

Tanning

The tanning reaction that follows sun exposure involves two distinct processes. Immediate pigment darkening (IPD) is due to photo-oxidation of the skin pigment melanin. This "tan" due to UVA radiation usually disappears in 1 to 4 hours. Delayed hyperpigmentation, the classic suntan, is caused by increased melanin formation (melanogenesis) in the lower epidermal layer and takes several days to become noticeable.

Individuals demonstrate different degrees of burning and tanning. Whether a person burns or tans after a single sun exposure depends on the amount of melanin in the skin and on the individual's capacity for melanogenesis. Since the degree of sunburn is inversely proportional to the amount of melanin in the dermal layers of the skin, darker skinned individuals, who have more melanin, are rarely affected by sunburn, whereas those with fairer complexions are highly susceptible.

Human skin is categorized into six types. This classification is not based on the genotype (hair and eye color), but on the individual's tendency to burn and the subsequent ability to suntan (see Table I).

After repeated exposure to sunlight, the skin becomes less sensitive to sunburn. This effect occurs as a result of increased melanin production (tanning) and increased thickening of the stratum corneum that accompanies epidermal hyperplasia. The skin feels rough and dry—an effect that may persist for months.

The photoprotective role of thickened stratum corneum is evident in albinos and individuals with vitiligo who do not produce melanin and yet become resistant to sunburn on repeated exposure to sunlight. An individual can increase the resistance of unprotected skin to solar radiation by gradually increasing exposure to sunlight. This approach also stimulates melanin pigmentation of the skin.

Commercial tanning units are promoted and used to induce a suntan for cosmetic purposes. Tanning booths are small rooms in

Table I *Skin Types* and Recommended Sun Protection Factor (SPF)*

Skin Type	Sunburn/Suntan History	Examples	SPF
I	Poor ability to tan; burns easily and severely, then peels	Very fair skin, freckles Unexposed skin is white Blue, green or grey eyes Blonde, red or brown hair	15 or more
II	Tans minimally or lightly following exposure; usually burns easily resulting in a painful burn	Fair skin Unexposed skin is white Blue, green, grey or brown eyes Blonde, red or brown hair	15 or more
III	Tans gradually following exposure; burns moderately	"Average" Unexposed skin is white Eye and hair color usually brown	10 to 15
IV	Tans well with initial exposure; burns minimally	Unexposed skin is white or light brown Dark eye and hair color (Mediterraneans, Orientals, Hispanics)	6 to 10
V	Tans easily and profusely; rarely burns	Unexposed skin is brown (American Indian, East Indian, Latin American)	4 to 6
VI	Deeply pigmented; never burns	Unexposed skin is black (African and American blacks, Australian and South Indian Aborigines)	none indicated

*Determined by the reaction to the first 30 minutes of sun exposure after winter season or no sun exposure.
Adapted from: Pathak MA. Sunscreens and their use in the preventative treatment of sunlight-induced skin damage. J Dermatol Surg Oncol 1987;13(7):739–50.

Sunscreens

which a patron is exposed to several lamps emitting UV radiation. Most of these lamps produce more than 95 per cent UVA and less than 5 per cent UVB. The radiation emitted has no known benefit to human health, but does pose potential short-term and long-term hazards to the eyes and skin. Cataracts and retinal damage as well as degenerative skin changes are associated with this type of UV radiation.

The age of the bulb emitting radiation can be an important factor in the severity of an individual's reaction. As UV bulbs age they emit less radiation, so a safe exposure time with an old bulb may no longer be safe with a new one. Patrons should be aware of the maximum exposure time recommended for a particular unit, and timers should be used to prevent overexposure. Protective eyewear should be worn while the lamps are in operation.

Another concern with the use of high intensity UVA sunlamps is the risk of photosensitivity reactions occurring in susceptible individuals. Because of these serious concerns, the use of tanning booths for cosmetic tanning should be discouraged. Anyone using these booths should be advised of the potential hazards to the eyes and skin as well as possible photosensitivity reactions.

Photosensitivity

Photosensitivity is an adverse reaction to the sun and encompasses both phototoxicity and photoallergy. Drug photosensitivity reactions are adverse skin responses resulting from the combination of UVA radiation and topical or systemic exposure to a chemical. Often, these chemicals are prescription and nonprescription medications. These longer wavelengths are readily transmitted through window glass and are produced by fluorescent lamps commonly found in offices and factories. A person susceptible to these reactions is not necessarily protected by being indoors.

Phototoxic reactions can occur in almost anyone if the photosensitizing agent absorbs enough of the appropriate radiation to result in cellular damage. A phototoxic reaction can occur on first exposure to the drug, is dose related and is confined to exposed areas of the skin. The reaction can occur within a few minutes to several hours after UV exposure and can reach a maximum from several hours to several days later. It resembles an exaggerated sunburn reaction characterized by erythema, edema and blister formation. Most phototoxic reactions can be treated the same way as an ordinary sunburn.

Photoallergic reactions are less common. They occur in a small proportion of people exposed to the drug and require administration of small amounts of the drug to elicit a response. They are allergic reactions involving the immune system and require prior sensitization to the drug and to UV radiation. Photoallergens can combine with proteins in the skin to form complete antigens, which then initiate the immune response. Photoallergic reactions may look like urticarial lesions developing within a few minutes after exposure or may resemble papular or eczematous lesions appearing within

Table II   Agents That May Cause Photosensitivity Reactions

Anticancer drugs	Sulfacytine+	Trimeprazine	Sulindac
Dacarbazine*	Sulfadoxine-pyrimethamine	**Diuretics**	
Fluorouracil	Sulfamethazine+	Acetazolamide	**Sunscreens**
Methotrexate	Sulfamethizole+	Amiloride	6–acetoxy–2,4,–dimethyl–m–dioxane
Procarbazine	Sulfamethoxazole	Bendroflumethiazide	(preservative in sunscreens)
Vinblastine	Sulfamethoxazole-trimethoprim	Benzthiazide	Benzophenones
	Sulfasalazine	Chlorothiazide	Cinnamates
Antidepressants	Sulfathiazole	Cyclothiazide+	Oxybenzone
Amitriptyline	Sulfisoxazole	Furosemide	Para-aminobenzoic acid (p-ABA)
Amoxapine	Tetracycline	Hydrochlorothiazide	p–ABA esters
Clomipramine		Hydroflumethiazide+	
Desipramine	**Antiparasitics**	Methylclothiazide	**Others**
Doxepin	Bithionol+	Metolazone	Amiodarone*
Imipramine	Pyrvinium pamoate	Polythiazide+	Benzocaine
Isocarboxazid	Quinine	Quinethazone	Bergamot oil, oils of citron, lavender,
Maprotiline		Trichlormethiazide+	lime, sandalwood, cedar (used in
Nortriptyline	**Antipsychotics**		many perfumes and cosmetics; also
Protriptyline	Chlorpromazine	**Hypoglycemics**	topical exposure to citrus rind oils)*
Trimipramine	Chlorprothixene	Acetohexamide	Captopril
	Flupenthixol	Chlorpropamide	Carbamazepine
Antihistamines	Fluphenazine	Glipizide+	Coal tar and derivatives (acridine,
Cyproheptadine	Haloperidol	Glyburide	anthracene, phenanthrene)*
Diphenhydramine	Loxapine	Tolazamide+	Contraceptives, oral
	Perphenazine	Tolbutamide	Disopyramide
Antimicrobials	Piperacetazine		Gold salts
Demeclocycline*	Prochlorperazine	**Nonsteroidal**	Hexachlorophene
Doxycycline	Promethazine	**anti-inflammatory drugs**	Isotretinoin
Griseofulvin	Thioridazine	Ketoprofen	6–methylcoumarin (used in perfumes,
Methacycline+	Thiothixene	Naproxen	shaving lotions and sunscreens)
Minocycline	Trifluoperazine	Phenylbutazone	Musk ambrette (used in perfumes)
Nalidixic acid	Triflupromazine+	Piroxicam	Quinidine sulfate and gluconate
Oxytetracycline+			

*Reactions often occur.
+Not available in Canada.

Photo-allergy

24 hours or later. Itching usually occurs before the appearance of lesions and often subsides in an hour. These reactions usually show cross-sensitivity with chemically related compounds. Avoiding further contact with the agent usually results in complete clearance of the eruption. Persons taking medications or using topical agents known to cause photosensitivity reactions should avoid exposure to sunlight and to artificial sources of UVA radiation.

Various drug products and chemicals cause photosensitivity reactions (see Table II). The same agent can cause both a phototoxic and photoallergic reaction. Several chemicals added to soaps, cosmetics and perfumes for their antibacterial properties have been implicated in photosensitivity reactions.

Certain disease states can be caused or exacerbated by exposure to sunlight. The abnormal reactions to light range from photosensitivity reactions to degenerative and neoplastic changes (see Table III). The wavelengths implicated in a particular reaction may be used as a guide in selecting an appropriate sunscreen.

Table III *Action Spectra of Various Normal and Abnormal Responses of Human Skin to Solar Radiation*

Condition	Range of effectiveness wavelengths (nm)	Maximum reaction (nm)
I *Normal individuals*		
Sunburn reaction (solar)	290-320	305-307
Sunburn reaction (artificial light source)	250-320	250-275
Immediate pigment darkening (IPD) or tanning reaction	320-700	340-380
Delayed tanning (melanogenesis)	290-480	290-320
II *Photosensitivity*		
A. Phototoxic reaction		
Oral or internal (drugs) (see Table II)	300-400	320-380
Topical or external (drugs) (see Table II)	300-400	320-380
Phytophotodermatitis (plants)	320-400	320-360
Phototoxicity in chemically induced porphyria or hematoporphyrins	380-600	380-420
B. Photoallergic reaction		
Drug photoallergy (delayed hypersensitivity, topical or systemic) (see Table II)	290-450	320-380
Certain solar urticarias (immediate hypersensitivity)	290-380	290-320 320-400
C. Persistent photosensitivity (persistent light reactions or actinic reticuloid)	290-400	290-320

Condition	Range	Max
III *Degenerative and neoplastic*		
Chronic actinic elastosis	290-400	290-320
Actinic keratosis	290-320	290-315
Basal cell epithelioma	290-320	290-315
Squamous cell carcinoma	290-320	290-315
Malignant melanoma (?)	290-320	290-315
IV *Genetic and metabolic*		
Xeroderma pigmentosum	290-320	290-320
Albinism	290-400	290-320
Ephelides (freckles)	290-400	290-320
Erythropoietic porphyria	390-600	390-420
Erythropoietic protoporphyria	390-600	390-420
Porphyria cutanea tarda	390-600	390-420
Variegate porphyria	390-600	390-420
Vitiligo (macules)	290-320	290-315
Hartnup syndrome	290-320	
Cockayne's syndrome	290-320	
Darier-White disease	290-320	
Bloom's syndrome	290-320	
Rothmund-Thomson syndrome	290-320	
Hailey-Hailey disease	290-320	
V *Nutritional*		
Kwashiorkor	290-400	
Pellagra	290-400	
VI *Infections (viral)*		
Lymphogranuloma venereum	290-320	
Herpes simplex	290-320	
VII *Miscellaneous (light and normal skin or diseases)*		
Hydroa aestivale	290-400 infrared	290-320
Hydroa vacciniforme	290-400 infrared	290-320
Polymorphous photodermatoses, including variants such as papular, plaques, papulovesicular and eczematous eruptions	290-400	290-320
Disseminated superficial actinic porokeratosis	290-320	290-320
Discoid lupus erythematosus	290-320	290-320
Systemic lupus erythematosus	290-320	
Dermatomyositis	290-320	
Photosensitive eczema	290-320	

Adapted from Pathak MA. Sunscreens: topical and systemic approaches for protection of human skin against harmful effects of solar radiation. J Am Acad Dermatol 1982;7(3):285–312.

Chronic Effects of UV Exposure

Long-term exposure to sunlight causes considerable cumulative damage to the skin. The major changes, which are in pigment and skin texture, are known as photoaging and are commonly called actinic damage or skin aging. These changes are manifested as atrophy, wrinkling, dryness, telangiectasia (capillary dilation) and the splotchy hypo-hyperpigmentation often seen on sun-exposed areas of middle-aged or older persons.

Sunscreens

Solar elastosis refers to the loss of normal elastic and connective tissue in the upper dermis. This loss often results in easy bruising and stellate scar formation due to degeneration of the supportive structures. The "turkey skin" pattern is characteristic of this condition. Solar lentigo is a flat, evenly pigmented macule commonly referred to as an age spot or liver spot. Fair-skinned individuals are more susceptible to skin changes caused by chronic exposure to sunlight, although pigmented skin only partly resists photoaging.

Abnormal epidermal hyperplasia, known as actinic or solar keratosis, develops after years of sun exposure. These lesions are reddened patches often covered with a coarse scale that can be pulled off but quickly returns. They cause burning or stinging of the skin after washing or sun exposure and are considered pre-malignant. People who exhibit such lesions should be referred to a physician. These lesions are most common in older persons but may occur in younger individuals who have prolonged exposure to sunlight (e.g., sailors, farmers, beach lifeguards).

Cancer is the most serious long-term effect of sunlight on the skin. The incidence of skin cancer is higher when UV radiation exposure is greater. The risk of skin cancer is inversely proportional to the amount of natural pigmentation. Most skin cancers occur on sun-exposed areas.

The most common skin cancers are basal cell carcinoma, squamous cell carcinoma and malignant melanoma. These carcinomas are most often seen on sun-exposed areas, such as the head, neck, rim of the ears, chin and back of the hands of fair-complexioned individuals. They seem to occur less in black populations living in the same geographic area.

In recent years the incidence of malignant melanoma of the skin has increased markedly. In Canada, this incidence has escalated from 735 in 1980 to an estimated 2 600 in 1990 in both males and females. In the United States, the lifetime risk of developing malignant melanoma is 1:1 500 for a person born in 1935 in contrast to 1:105 for someone born in 1991. The projected risk for a person born in the year 2000 is 1:90. Investigators have concluded that this increase is related to increased sun exposure.

Studies show that the risk of developing skin melanoma is associated with an individual's tendency to burn easily and tan poorly. A history of repeated sunburn also correlates with a higher risk of melanoma. It has been suggested that if sunburn contributes to the risk of melanoma, the use of sunblocking agents to prevent sunburn may well reduce this risk. One study showed that sunscreen used during childhood and adolescence can substantially lower the risk of skin cancer and provide other beneficial effects.

Melanomas, which usually form from pigmented moles, can spread easily once they reach a certain size. It is therefore important to differentiate them from normal moles. The characteristic features of early malignant melanoma can be remembered by the mnemonic ABCD: A for Asymmetry; B for Border irregularity; C for Color variegation; and D for Diameter greater than 6 mm. Early melanomas have an irregular shape and border, may become inflamed and have a reddish edge and may bleed, ooze or crust. A melanoma is often itchy, grows in size, is usually greater than 6 mm in diameter and is irregularly colored in shades of brown or black. These signs are not characteristic of ordinary moles. A person who displays such lesions should seek medical advice. Regular spot checks of moles can increase early detection of both melanoma and non-melanoma skin cancers.

Changes in the immune system due to habitual sun exposure may

Table IV *Sunscreen Agents Recognized as Safe and Effective by the FDA Advisory Review Panel*

Sunscreen agent	Concentration
Chemical Agents	
UVA Absorbers	
Avobenzone (Parsol 1789)	
Dioxybenzone	3%
Menthyl anthranilate	3.5–5%
Oxybenzone	2–6%
Sulisobenzone	5–10%
UVB Absorbers	
Cinoxate	1–3%
Diethanolamine p-methoxycinnamate	8–10%
Digalloyl-trioleate	2–5%
Ethyl 4-bis(hydroxypropyl)aminobenzoate	1–5%
2-ethylhexyl 2-cyano-3,3-diphenylacrylate	7–10%
Ethylhexyl p-methoxycinnamate	2–7.5%
2-ethyl hexyl salicylate	3–5%
Glyceryl p-aminobenzoate	3%
Homosalate	4–15%
Lawsone with dehydroxyacetone (DHA)*	0.25% lawsone 3% DHA
Para-aminobenzoic acid (p-ABA)	5–15%
Padimate A	1–5%
Padimate O	1.4–8%
2-phenylbenzimidazole-5-sulfonic acid	1–4%
Triethanolamine salicylate	5–12%
Physical Agents	
Red Petrolatum	30–100%
Titanium Dioxide	2–25%

*DHA, except in combination with lawsone, has no appreciable sunscreen activity.
Adapted from: Fed Reg 1978;43(Pt 2):38213 and Lowe. J Dermatol Surg Oncol 1990;16(10):936–8.

contribute to the risk of skin cancer. A lifetime exposure to UV radiation may also cause eye damage resulting in decreased transmittance of visible light by the lens and an increase in cataract formation.

Pharmaceutical Agents

Sunscreens can be grouped into two broad categories: topical and systemic. Topical sunscreens can be subdivided further into two groups: physical and chemical sunscreens. Table IV lists the sun-protection agents considered safe and effective by the United States Food and Drug Administration (FDA) advisory review panel.

Topical Protection
Physical Sunscreens

Physical sunscreens (sunblocking agents) form an occlusive barrier that reflects and scatters light in both the visible and UV spectrum. They include zinc oxide, talc (magnesium trisilicate), titanium dioxide, kaolin and red veterinary petrolatum. These formulations are cosmetically unacceptable, may stain clothing and are often messy to use. However, they help protect particularly sun sensitive areas such as the nose and lips and may be more appealing to use now that they are available in a variety of bright colors. Physical sunscreens do not wash off easily when the skin is immersed in water,

Sunscreens

but melt with the heat of the sun. They offer limited protection when sunbathing extends for more than 2 hours.

Chemical Sunscreens

Chemical sunscreens absorb, reflect or scatter a certain portion of UV light away from the skin to prevent its penetration into the dermis. They are usually colorless because they do not contain any visible-light absorbing chemicals. They are therefore cosmetically acceptable to most individuals.

The molar absorptivity of a chemical sunscreen refers to its ability to absorb UV radiation. A large molar absorptivity at a particular wavelength indicates good absorption at that wavelength. To be effective against sunburn, a sunscreen agent should have a range of maximum absorption that overlaps the range of UV radiation responsible for sunburn. An agent with a low molar absorptivity may be made more effective by increasing its concentration in a formulation.

Para-aminobenzoic acid (p-ABA) and its esters absorb light in the burning region of the UV spectrum (UVB, 290 to 320 nm) but not in the tanning region (UVA), thereby permitting immediate pigment darkening but offering no protection against sun photosensitivity reactions. p-ABA is most effective in a concentration of 5 per cent in a 70 per cent ethanol solution. Its use has declined in recent years because of a significant number of incidences of irritation and hypersensitivity reactions. Its main advantage is its ability to penetrate the stratum corneum and bind to proteins. Esters of p-ABA, amyldimethyl p-ABA (padimate A) and octyldimethyl p-ABA (padimate O)—have low water solubility and are poorly removed by water. They can be incorporated into lotion or cream bases, which are less irritating than alcohol bases and more resistant to removal by water. Sunscreens with p-ABA and p-ABA ester should be applied 1 to 2 hours before sun exposure to allow for binding to the stratum

Table V *Examples of Drugs That Cross-React with p-ABA and Its Esters*

Sulfonamide antibiotics
  sulfamethoxazole
  sulfisoxazole

Sulfonamide-based oral hypoglycemics
  chlorpropamide
  glyburide
  tolbutamide

Thiazide diuretics
  chlorothiazide
  hydrochlorothiazide

Ester-type anesthetics
  benzocaine
  procaine
  tetracaine

Artificial sweeteners
  saccharin
  sodium cyclamate

Para-amino type azo dyes
  aniline
  paraphenylenediamine

Adapted from: Mathias CGT. Commentary and update: cutaneous sensitivity to monoglyceryl para-aminobenzoate. Cleve Clin Q 1983;50(2):85–6.

corneum. To assure maximum protection, it is best to reapply sunscreens after swimming or profuse sweating.

p-ABA can stain clothes yellow, especially after exposure to sunlight; the esters are less likely to stain. Allergic contact dermatitis may develop from the use of p-ABA and certain esters, mainly glyceryl p-ABA. In addition, certain drugs have been reported to cross-react with p-ABA and its esters (see Table V). People with a history of hypersensitivity to these agents should avoid sunscreens containing p-ABA and its derivatives.

Benzophenone derivatives, such as oxybenzone, dioxybenzone and sulisobenzone, absorb light in the complete UV spectrum (290 to 400 nm). Since they absorb radiation within the UVA range, they are indicated for persons who exhibit photosensitivity reactions or for conditions exacerbated by sunlight. They are applied 30 minutes before sun exposure and, because they wash off easily, must be reapplied after swimming or profuse sweating.

Products containing benzophenones in combination with p-ABA or p-ABA esters are more water resistant and provide better protection than either agent used alone. Adverse effects are rare, but contact dermatitis may occasionally develop.

Cinnamic acid derivatives commonly used are cinoxate (2-ethoxyethyl p-methoxycinnamate) and 2-ethylhexyl p-methoxycinnamate. They absorb primarily in the UVB region (270 to 328 nm). They do not bind to the stratum corneum, so they wash off easily and must be reapplied frequently. Cinnamic acid derivatives used in combination with benzophenones appear to be effective sunscreens in protecting against UVB and UVA radiation up to 360 nm.

Salicylic acid derivatives, such as homosalate (homomenthyl salicylate) and 2-ethylhexyl salicylate, absorb primarily in the UVB region, but have about one-third the absorbency of p-ABA. Since they are weak in absorbing UV, they have to be used in relatively high concentrations (4 to 12 per cent). They have low potential for sensitization, do not bind to the skin and are easily removed by sweating or swimming.

Menthyl anthranilate is the only anthranilic acid derivative currently available in sunscreen products. It has the weakest molar absorptivity of all sunscreen agents. It absorbs UV radiation in the range of 300 to 360 nm; maximum absorption is between 332 and 345 nm. It has about one-twentieth the absorbency of p-ABA and is used in combination with other sunscreens to provide an effective product.

Dibenzoylmethane derivatives such as Parsol 1789 (butyl methoxy-dibenzoylmethane or avobenzone) and Eusolex 8020 (4-isopropyl dibenzoylmethane) are a new class of sunscreens recently introduced into Canada. They absorb radiation in the entire UVA region (310 to 400 nm). They are formulated in concentrations of 2 to 3 per cent and have been used extensively in Europe. Since these agents offer no protection from UVB radiation, they are usually formulated in combination with benzophenones or p-ABA esters. They are indicated for persons who suffer from photosensitivity reactions or conditions exacerbated by sunlight. They should be applied prior to sun exposure and reapplied after swimming or sweating. Allergic reactions and photocontact dermatitis have been reported with these agents especially with isopropyl dibenzoylmethane.

Sun Protection Factor

To compare the degree of protection offered by preparations available in Canada, the sun protection factor (SPF) is now stated by most manufacturers on the labels of their products. This value is the quotient of the dose of UV radiation necessary to produce perceptible redness (minimal erythemal dose or MED) using a sunscreen, to the

amount necessary to produce this erythema without the sunscreen.

$$SPF = \frac{\text{MED of sunscreen-protected skin}}{\text{MED of unprotected skin}}$$

The higher the SPF, the more protection the product offers. In practical terms, the SPF means that if a person can stay in the sun unprotected for 15 minutes before experiencing erythema, a sunscreen with an SPF of four extends this period to one hour. Reapplying the sunscreen after the first hour does not extend protection for another hour since the skin has already received enough UV radiation to begin a sunburn.

SPF values are determined experimentally under ideal conditions with indoor solar simulators. In natural sunlight the protective efficacy of a sunscreen product may vary considerably due to differences in individual characteristics, environmental conditions and sunscreen properties. These factors are summarized in Table VI.

Choice of a Sunscreen

Sunscreen products are available in creams (oily or vanishing), lotions (clear or milky) or gels. In counselling people in the prevention of sunburn, skin cancer, aging and various forms of sun sensitivity, the choice and recommendation of a sunscreen depend on several factors.

Skin type: People with fair complexions and blue, green or grey eyes who burn easily and tan poorly (skin types I and II) should use sunscreens with an SPF of 15 or more. Individuals with skin types III and IV who burn moderately or minimally but tan well may use a sunscreen with an SPF of 6 to 15. Darker-skinned people (skin type V) who tan profusely and rarely burn may use a sunscreen with an SPF rating of 4 to 6. Individuals with skin type VI do not generally require a sunscreen (see Table I).

Type of activity: Before recommending a sunscreen product, consideration should be given to the type of activity and duration of sun exposure. A person engaging in water sports (for example, swimming, waterskiing or windsurfing) or who sweats profusely due to exercise or prolonged sunbathing should use a product that is not washed off easily by water. An individual who requires a sunscreen for snow-skiing or mountain climbing might benefit from a higher SPF product because of the added effects of UV radiation due to higher altitude and reflection off snow.

Site of application: The lips and nose are particularly sensitive to UV radiation. Normal skin has a thick stratum corneum containing melanin, keratin and protein, which protect against moderate exposure to UV light. The stratum corneum on the lips is thin and melanin is absent, so maximum protection is required. Physical sunscreens, such as zinc oxide, may be used on these vulnerable areas. However, these agents are not cosmetically acceptable to most people. Taste and substantivity are problems for lip protection since much of the sunscreen is removed by constant licking. While in the sun, reapplication is required hourly and immediately after swimming. Gel-based products offer best protection for the lips (93 per cent protection after one hour). Women may use an opaque lipstick after applying the sunscreen. Some people with recurrent sunlight-induced herpes labialis may benefit from using a high SPF sunscreen to eliminate recurrence.

Condition of skin: People with dry skin often benefit from a cream or lotion base; those with oily skin, especially if prone to acne, do better with an alcohol solution or gel. Some alcohol-based vehicles

Table VI *Factors Affecting Sunscreen Efficacy*

Individual characteristics

Test subjects:	Variations in skin type, melanin content, skin thickness, degree of vascularity, amount of hair on test site, age of subject
Sweating:	Skin temperature, rate of production and evaporation of sweat, amount of urocanic acid (a natural sunscreen present in sweat)
Swimming:	Duration of swimming, water (whether chlorinated or salted), state of hydration of the skin

Environmental conditions

UV intensity:	Irradiation dose of UVA and UVB, season, latitude, altitude, clouds, air pollution, time of day, reflectivity of the ground
Temperature	*Snow*
Degree of humidity	*Sand*
Direct and scattered radiation	*Wind velocity*

Sunscreen properties

Concentration:	Differences in the concentration of the UV-absorbing active ingredients
Vehicle:	Composition, chemical properties (lipophilic or hydrophilic nature), pH, emollient properties
Thickness of applied film:	Uniform application of about 2 mg/cm² or 2 mcL/cm² (equivalent to a film thickness of 0.02 mm on the skin) has been recommended. It takes about nine 2.5 mL measures of sunscreen to achieve that thickness of film on the skin. On average, one measure (2.5 mL) is to be used for the face and neck, one for each arm and shoulder, one for the front of the torso, one for the back and two for each leg and top of the foot. Studies examining the effect of film irregularities on sunscreen efficacy report discrepancies of approximately 50 per cent in SPF values.
Other ingredients:	Some impurities or additives can act as photo-sensitizers (for example, ortho and meta esters of p-ABA, and 6–methylcoumarin, a fragrance).
Substantivity:	It refers to the ability of a sunscreen to maintain efficacy when subjected to moisture (such as swimming and sweating). This property is a function of both the sunscreen agent and the vehicle. Sunscreen substantivity varies with its hydrophilic and lipophilic properties, pH, heat stability, emollient nature, percutaneous absorptivity, ionized state and diffusion capacity, and with ingredient absorption and conjugation to the stratum corneum proteins. Products with cream, oil or gel bases are more resistant to removal by water than those with alcohol bases. In addition, a water-in-oil base has a greater resistance to water removal than gel or oil-in-water emulsion. Combination products are more substantive than those containing a single ingredient. Emollients in creams or lotions lower the substantivity of the sunscreen agent.

may irritate individuals engaged in energetic activity. In addition, sunscreens with an alcohol base should not be used on eczematous or inflamed skin.

Sun sensitivity: Individuals who exhibit a photosensitivity reaction or who have a condition that is exacerbated by exposure to sunlight need protection against both UVA and UVB radiation. Products containing p-ABA or p-ABA esters alone are not suitable since they do not absorb the UVA radiation responsible for photosensitivity reactions. A combination product, containing butyl methoxydibenzoylmethane and an UVB absorbing agent, with a high SPF should be used. People with skin carcinomas require maximum protection from UV radiation. Nonpharmacologic methods may also be used. Broad-brimmed hats partially protect the ears, nose and cheeks. Tighter weaves of clothing, preferably dyed, allow less radiation to penetrate the skin. The most effective preventive measure is avoiding sun exposure.

Cross-sensitivity: Certain drugs (for example, sulfonamides and thiazide diuretics) may show cross-sensitivity with p-ABA and its derivatives. Individuals who have previously experienced hypersensitivity reactions to these agents should not use sunscreens containing p-ABA or its esters. Products containing benzophenones or cinnamates are better choices. In rare instances, individuals may be sensitive to an ingredient other than the active sunscreen in the product. There have been reports of allergic contact dermatitis to the vehicle (for example, triethanolamine stearate), the preservative (for example, parabens) and the lubricant (for example, phenyl dimethicone) present in a sunscreen product. New users can test the product by applying a small amount to a small patch of skin at least 24 hours before using it on a larger area.

Other factors that may influence the choice of a sunscreen are past experience with various products, motivation for its use, ease of application, cosmetic acceptability, fragrance and cost. In prophylactic programs against photoaging, some dermatologists are recommending daily use of a low SPF (4 to 6) sunscreen in the form of facial makeup for women and after shave lotion for men.

Sunscreens on Children Do not keep over 1 yr.

To date, the Health Protection Branch of Health and Welfare Canada has not issued any guidelines regarding the use of sunscreens on young children. In the United States, the FDA recommends that products with an SPF of less than 4 not be used on children under the age of 2 since these sunscreens do not provide adequate protection. No sunscreen should be used on children under the age of 6 months, since different absorptive characteristics have been noted in this age group. Alcoholic lotions and gel sunscreens can cause stinging, irritation and burning of the eyes and are not recommended for children under 12 years of age. p-ABA and its esters should also be avoided. The recommended sunscreen for children is a high SPF (10 to 15) milky lotion for total body application and a physical block for sun-sensitive areas such as the nose and shoulders. Educating children to practise sun protection early in life is an important step in reducing sun-related skin damage since damage begins with the first exposure and accumulates over a lifetime.

Systemic Protection

The desire for systemic photoprotectants to reduce reaction of the skin to solar radiation has inspired much research. Agents such as p-ABA, antihistamines, vitamins A, C and E, acetylsalicylic acid, unsaturated fatty acids and steroids have been investigated but not proven successful. Three systemic agents that have shown limited efficacy are beta-carotene, antimalarials and some of the psoralen derivatives.

Beta-carotene (Solatene Roche) absorbs radiation in the visible spectrum of light (360 to 500 nm) with a maximum absorption at 450 and 475 nm. It is an effective systemic photoprotective agent for people with erythropoietic protoporphyria, erythropoietic porphyria and variegate porphyria, who are extremely sensitive to visible radiation. Beta-carotene should not be used to protect against UVB radiation.

Beta-carotene is a natural constituent of many plants such as carrots, tomatoes and oranges. It is a precursor of vitamin A and is virtually nontoxic. Recommended doses for photoprotection are 120 to 180 mg per day for adults; 90 to 120 mg per day for children 9 to 16 years of age; 30 to 60 mg per day for children 1 to 8 years of age. People usually take beta-carotene during the spring and summer. Maximal effects of the drug, as measured by increased tolerance to sunlight, occur after one to two months of therapy and may persist for one to two months after cessation of therapy. All people exhibit a slight yellowing of the skin (carotenemia). The safety of beta-carotene use during pregnancy and in people with renal or hepatic dysfunction has not been established. Beta-carotene is believed to act by becoming preferentially photo-oxidized by the free radicals generated in photosensitivity reactions, thereby sparing cell components.

Antimalarials such as chloroquine, hydroxychloroquine and quinacrine have been used to reduce photosensitivity reactions associated with lupus erythematosus, polymorphous light eruptions and solar urticaria. They are not first-line drugs and should be used only after trials with topical sunscreens. The recommended maintenance dose is 250 mg per day for chloroquine, 200 mg per day for hydroxychloroquine and 100 to 300 mg per day for quinacrine.

People should not use antimalarials indefinitely; the drugs should be discontinued as the skin condition improves. Prolonged treatment with these drugs can result in retinopathy. Therefore, a complete ophthalmic examination should be performed before initiating therapy and at 4- to 6-month intervals during treatment.

The mechanism of action of antimalarials in treating photosensitizing disorders is unknown. It is doubtful that they act as a sunscreen that filters radiation. They have been shown to inhibit histamine and various enzyme systems and to possess anti-inflammatory properties.

Oral psoralens such as 8-methoxypsoralen (methoxsalen or 8-MOP) and 4,5,8-trimethylpsoralen (trioxsalen, as in Trisoralen) may be useful in increasing resistance to solar damage in people with polymorphous light eruptions, people with vitiligo and albinos. The protective action of 8-MOP is probably due to epidermal hyperplasia and an increased formation and melaninization of pigment-producing cells. The recommended dose is 20 to 30 mg of 8-MOP or 20 mg of trioxsalen 2 hours before exposure to sunlight. This approach should be restricted to people sensitive to topical sunscreens and who have a significant need for this type of therapy.

Pigmenting or Tanning Agents

In Europe, 5-methoxypsoralen, a constituent of oil of bergamot (5-MOP or bergapten), has recently been incorporated into suntan formulations to stimulate the tanning response. The claim is that the product can stimulate tanning, which subsequently provides photoprotection due to increased melanin production. Topical application of sunscreen products containing 10 to 50 mcg/mL of 5-MOP results in photosensitization caused by UVA radiation; this sensitization in turn leads to enhanced pigmentation. In addition to being cytotoxic and phototoxic to melanocytes, 5-MOP has been shown to be mutagenic and carcinogenic to epidermal keratinocytes and melanocytes. Its use and promotion for a cosmetic tan should be seriously questioned and discouraged.

Quick-Tanning Products

The term "suntan lotions" is misleading, since these products, unless they contain a known photosensitizer (for example, 5-MOP), do not promote a tan. Enhanced tanning following sun exposure results from increased melanin production due to stimulation of melanocytes by UV rays. The quick-tanning products, none of which stimulate melanogenesis, can be divided into three groups.

Low SPF sunscreens or products containing no sun-protective agent in oil or emollient-rich bases are promoted as "suntan" products. Because of their low SPF values (less than 3), these formulations provide minimal protection for the skin. The oily base makes the skin more permeable to UV radiation. This minimal protection results in inflammation and post inflammatory hyperpigmentation, and not tanning.

Systemic agents that modify skin color are beta-carotene and canthaxanthine; their use has declined in recent years. Canthaxanthine is a carotenoid, but unlike beta-carotene it possesses no vitamin A activity. It is commonly used in low concentrations as a coloring agent for foods such as cheese and ketchup.

Canthaxanthine is dosed by body weight using a 20-day dosing schedule; subsequent maintenance doses are necessary to maintain the color. Its use to produce an artificial suntan has been associated with retinal deposits and in some cases has resulted in impaired vision. Another concern with this product is the development of brick-red stools that can mask lower gastrointestinal tract bleeding.

After ingestion, beta-carotene and canthaxanthine accumulate in subcutaneous fat and in the epidermis. In individuals with skin types I, II and III, the skin becomes orange-brown in color. People with erythropoietic protoporphyria or generalized vitiligo may find this color more appealing than the yellowish color produced by beta-carotene alone. Some people do not like the resulting unnatural color of the palms, soles and skin behind the ear lobes.

Since the photoprotective ability as well as the long-term systemic effects of the canthaxanthine/beta-carotene mixture have not been fully evaluated, recommendation for its use must await further investigation.

Agents that oxidize and bind to the stratum corneum contain 3 to 5 per cent dihydroxyacetone (DHA) and 0.25 per cent lawsone (1,4-dihydroxynaphthaquinone). The topical formulation containing DHA becomes oxidized and stains the skin. These agents bind to the keratin of the stratum corneum to form a dark pigment that looks like a suntan. No new melanin is produced. The resulting color washes off with soap and water or with solvents such as acetone or alcohol. These formulations offer no photoprotection against UVA or UVB radiation, but protect from the visible spectrum (400 to 500 nm). Such a stain may be useful for people with erythropoietic protoporphyria who require protection from visible radiation.

Dihydroxyacetone (DHA) in concentrations of 0.2 to 5 per cent has been used in creams and lotions. The presence of 20 per cent water is recommended. An acid medium and the presence of a surfactant speeds the color reaction; no reaction occurs above pH 8. DHA is incorporated into camouflaging creams for use by people with

vitiligo. A single application of DHA may result in a patchy appearance, especially when applied to large areas of vitiliginous skin. Repeated application after the lotion dries results in progressive darkening of the skin. Although products are available in only one color, most people find they can adequately camouflage lesions once they know how many applications are required to achieve the desired skin tone. When treatment is stopped, the color fades after about 2 days and disappears completely within 8 to 14 days as the epidermal cells of the stratum corneum are lost by normal sloughing.

Depigmenting Agents

Depigmenting agents lighten hyperpigmented areas caused by excessive or persistent freckling, medical disorders or drugs. Freckles (ephelides) occur most often in fair-skinned individuals. They darken considerably in the summertime and may fade almost completely in the winter.

Disorders of melanin pigmentation can be due to a number of factors, including genetic, metabolic, endocrine, inflammatory, neoplastic and nutritional disorders. Increased pigmentation results from an increase in the activity, number or size of the melanocytes. Drugs associated with hyperpigmentation are tetracyclines, antimalarials, hormones and chemotherapeutic agents such as busulfan, 5-fluorouracil, cyclophosphamide, nitrogen mustard and bleomycin. Melasma, or brownish macules on the face, may occur in pregnant women, women on oral contraceptives or in people taking phenytoin or mephenytoin. Its cause is unknown, but sunlight is necessary for its development.

Hydroquinone is an antioxidant that inhibits the conversion of tyrosine to dihydroxyphenylalanine (a precursor of melanin). It does not injure or decrease the number of melanocytes and is available without prescription in concentrations of 2 to 4 per cent in bleaching creams and ointments. It should be applied only to intact skin and kept away from the eyes. Since its action is only temporary, repeat applications are needed at frequent intervals, usually 2 to 3 times a day for weeks to months. Hydroquinone should not be used on children or on sunburned or irritated skin. It is best stored in airtight containers and protected from light.

Hydroquinone is relatively safe in low concentrations (2 per cent); the incidence of side effects greatly increases at higher concentrations. Adverse reactions include stinging sensations, erythema, and allergic and contact dermatitis. Toxic reactions resulting in complete depigmentation of the treated areas instead of a mere lightening have been reported. Using sunscreens and avoiding prolonged sun exposure during treatment with hydroquinone achieves best results and prevents repigmentation.

Monobenzone is the monobenzyl ether of hydroquinone. It, too, inhibits the conversion of tyrosine to dihydroxyphenylalanine, preventing formation of melanin pigment in the skin. Its pigment-decreasing action is irreversible and somewhat erratic and unpredictable. It should be used only when permanent depigmentation is desired.

Monobenzone is used topically in concentrations of up to 20 per cent in the form of a lotion. It is applied to hyperpigmented areas 2 or 3 times daily until a satisfactory result is obtained. Twice weekly applications are then sufficient to maintain the desired degree of depigmentation. It may take several months to achieve results since depigmentation becomes apparent only after pre-existing pigments are exhausted. If the condition does not improve after 4 months of treatment, the drug should be discontinued. Monobenzone is not effective against pigmented moles.

Vitiligo individuals with more than 50 per cent depigmentation have been treated with monobenzone to bleach their normal skin. Therapy starts with topical application of a 5 per cent preparation of the drug. The concentration is increased every 2 to 3 months until a 20 per cent preparation is used. Total depigmentation requires one to two years of therapy. These people must use high SPF sunscreens, since monobenzone treatment irreversibly destroys residual melanocytes.

Monobenzone can irritate and sensitize skin. This effect is usually transient and does not necessitate withdrawal of the drug. Lower concentrations may be used to decrease the incidence and severity of adverse reactions, although depigmentation then occurs more slowly.

Summary

Excessive exposure to sunlight can lead to serious short-term and long-term effects. Preventing the adverse effects of sunburn—drying, wrinkling and possibly skin malignancies—starts at an early age.

Fair-skinned people have a higher incidence of sun-damaged skin. Exposure to the sun should be gradual. Avoiding outdoor activities between 10:00 hours and 15:00 hours during the summer months reduces the risk of sunburn. Increased UV exposure can occur at higher altitudes and from reflection off snow, sand and water.

The choice of sunscreen depends primarily on the individual's skin type. Other factors influencing selection are cross-sensivitiy to an ingredient, substantivity, type of vehicle (alcohol or cream base) and staining properties of the product. A combination product that protects against both UVA and UVB radiation is preferred for people who may exhibit photosensitivity to sunlight.

For maximum effectiveness, sunscreens should be applied at least 30 minutes before exposure (1 to 2 hours for p-ABA and its esters) and reapplied after swimming or sweating. If a tan is desired, a slow and cautious approach is best. Initial overexposure should be avoided, since a severe sunburn leads to peeling, never to a tan.

Pharmacists have the opportunity to expand public awareness about acute and chronic effects of sun exposure. Educating the public especially children and adolescents about sun-protective measures decreases the incidence of severe sunburn reactions and limits the long-term effects of UV radiation.

Ask the Consumer

Q. Are you requesting a sunscreen product for yourself or someone else? Will exposure to the sun be intense or limited?
■ It is important to determine the skin type of the person using the sunscreen (see Table I). Does the person sunburn easily or tan? Depending on the sunburning/suntanning history of the individual and the degree of sun exposure, an appropriate sunscreen product with a high or low sun protection factor (SPF) may be selected.

Q. Do you require the sunscreen for outdoor work or for recreational activities? Do you plan to swim, ski, climb mountains or participate in strenuous activities while using the product?

■ The type of activity for which a sunscreen is required helps determine the product to recommend. An individual who swims or sweats requires a product that is not washed off easily by water.

Q. What sunscreens have you used in the past? Have you ever reacted to a sunscreen product?
■ A person's past experience (successful or unsuccessful) with a certain product may help in selecting an appropriate sunscreen. Individuals who have experienced any allergic reactions to a sunscreen formulation should choose a product containing different ingredients.

Q. Have you had any allergic reactions to oral or topical medications?
■ Although sunscreens do not generally produce hypersensitivity reactions, p-ABA has shown cross-sensitivity with chemically related drugs. A person who reports an allergic reaction to drugs such as sulfonamide antibiotics, sulfonamide hypoglycemics, thiazides or ester-type anesthetics should be cautioned against using products containing p-ABA and its derivatives (see Table V).

Q. What medications are you currently taking?
■ Certain drugs may cause photosensitivity reactions (see Table II). A person taking a medication that may be photosensitizing requires a sunscreen that protects against both UVB and UVA radiation.

Q. Do you have any medical conditions that predispose you to skin problems (such as a rash or severe sunburn) on exposure to sunlight or ultraviolet radiation? Has your physician advised you to use a sunscreen when exposed to sunlight?
■ Certain medical conditions may be caused or aggravated by skin exposure to sunlight (see Table III). A person with abnormal responses to sunlight should be referred to a physician. A sunscreen product should offer protection against the radiation responsible for precipitating the skin reactions.

Q. Is your skin dry or oily?
■ The condition of a person's skin should be considered when recommending a sunscreen. Individuals with dry skin often benefit from a cream-based formulation; those with oily skin may benefit from an alcohol-based product.

Q. Have you ever had cold sores caused by sun exposure?
■ Sunlight is a precipitating factor of recurrent herpes labialis. An adequate lip sunscreen may block the effect of solar radiation to eliminate cold sore recurrence in some people.

References
Solar Radiation
Anonymous. Sunscreens. Med Lett Drugs Ther 1984;26(663):56–8.
Cavallo J, DeLeo VA. Sunburn. Dermatol Clin 1986;4(2):181–7.
Council Report. Harmful effects of ultraviolet radiation. JAMA 1989;262(3): 380–4.
Diffey BL, Larkoe O. Clinical climatology. Photodermatol 1984;1(1):30–7.
FDA Formulating Guidelines. Which sunscreens offer the best protection against UVA radiation? Primary Care and Cancer 1991;July-August:30–2.
Lowe NJ. Photoprotection. Seminars in Dermatology 1990;9(1):78–83.
Menter JM. Recent developments in UVA protection. Int J Dermatol 1990; 29(6):389–94.

Pathak MA. Sunscreens: topical and systemic approaches for protection of human skin against harmful effects of solar radiation. J Am Acad Dermatol 1982;7(3):285–312.

Pathak MA. Sunscreens: topical and systemic approaches for the prevention of acute and chronic sun-induced skin reactions. Dermatol Clin 1986; 4(2):321–34.

Shear NH. Year-round safe sun. Pharmacy Practice 1990;July-August: 10–4.

Taylor CR, Stern RS, Leyden JJ, et al. Photoaging/photodamage and photoprotection. J Am Acad Dermatol 1990;22(1):1–15.

Sunburn

Anders JE, Leach EE. Sun versus skin. Am J Nurs 1983;83(7):1015–20.

Bickers DR. Sun-induced disorders. Emerg Med Clin North Am 1985;3(4):659–77.

Gschnait F, Schwarz TH, Seiser A. Topical indomethacin protects from UVB and UVA irradiation. Arch Dermatol Res 1984;276(2):131–2.

Pathak MA, Fitzpatrick TB, Parrish JA. Photosensitivity and other reactions to light. In: Petersdorf RG, Adams RD, Braunwald E, Isselbacher KJ, Martin JB, Wilson JD, eds. Harrison's principles of internal medicine. New York: McGraw-Hill, 1983:273–82.

Pathak MA, Fanselow DL. Photobiology of melanin pigmentation: dose/response of skin to sunlight and its contents. J Am Acad Dermatol 1983; 9(5):724–33.

Warshauer DM, Steinbaugh JR. Sunlight and protection of the skin. Am Fam Physician 1983;27(6):109–15.

Tanning

Boger J, Araujo OE, Flowers F. Sunscreens: efficacy, use, and misuse. South Med J 1984;77(11):1421–7.

Kligman LH. Photoaging: manifestations, prevention, and treatment. Dermatol Clin 1986;4(3):517–28.

Photobiology Task Force of the American Academy of Dermatology. Risks and benefits from high-intensity ultraviolet A sources used for cosmetic purposes. J Am Acad Dermatol 1985;12(2Pt1):380–1.

Photosensitivity

Anonymous. Drugs that cause photosensitivity. Med Lett Drugs Ther 1986; 28(713):51–2.

Diffey BL, Farr PM. An evaluation of sunscreens in patients with broad action-spectrum photosensitivity. Br J Dermatol 1985;112(1):83–6.

Elmets CA. Drug-induced photoallergy. Dermatol Clin 1986;4(2):231–41.

Epstein JH. Phototoxicity and photoallergy in man. J Am Acad Dermatol 1983;8(2):141–7.

Photobiology Task Force of the American Academy of Dermatology. Risks and benefits from high-intensity ultraviolet A sources used for cosmetic purposes. J Am Acad Dermatol 1985;12(2Pt1):380–1.

Chronic Effects of UV Exposure

Canadian Cancer Statistics 1990. Toronto: National Cancer Institute of Canada, 1990:14–5.

Cancer in Canada 1980. Ottawa: Statistics Canada, 1983:12–3.

Elwood JM, Gallagher RP, Davison J, Hill GB. Sunburn, suntan and the risk of cutaneous malignant melanoma: the Western Canada melanoma study. Br J Cancer 1985;51(4):543–9.

Epstein JH. Photocarcinogenesis, skin cancer and aging. J Am Acad Dermatol 1983;9(4):487–502.

Friedman RJ, Rigel DS, Silverman MK, et al. Malignant melanoma in the 1990's: The continued importance of early detection and the role of physician examination and self-examination of the skin. CA-A Cancer Journal for Clinicians 1991;41(4):201–26.

Green A, Siskind V, Bain C, Alexander J. Sunburn and malignant melanoma. Br J Cancer 1985;51(3):393–7.

Kopf AW, Friedman RJ, Rigel DS. The many faces of malignant melanoma. The Skin Cancer Foundation, 1987.

Kopf AW, Kripke ML, Stern RS. Sun and malignant melanoma. J Am Acad Dermatol 1984;11(4Pt1):674–84.

Pownall M. Suntanning: skin scare. Nurs Times 1985;81(32):19.

Stern RS, Weinstein MC, Baker SG. Risk reduction for nonmelanoma skin cancer with childhood sunscreen use. Arch Dermatol 1986;122(5):537–45.

Physical Sunscreens

Fed Reg 1978;43(Pt2):38213.

Chemical Sunscreens

Anonymous. Photoplex—a broad spectrum sunscreen. Med Lett Drugs Ther 1989;31(794):59–60.

Dromgoole SH, Maibach HI. Sunscreening agent intolerance: contact and photocontact sensitization and contact urticaria. J Am Acad Dermatol 1990;22(6):1068–78.

English JSC, White RI, Cronin E. Sensitivity to sunscreens. Contact Dermatitis 1987;17:159–62.

Harvey SC. Topical drugs. In: Gennaro AR, ed. Remington's pharmaceutical sciences. Easton: Mack Publishing, 1985:790–1.

Lowe NJ. Sunscreens and the prevention of skin aging. J Dermatol Surg Oncol 1990;16(10):936–8.

Mathias CGT. Commentary and update: cutaneous sensitivity to monoglyceryl para-aminobenzoate. Cleve Clin Q 1983;50(2):85–6.

Motley RJ, Reynolds AJ. Photocontact dermatitis due to isopropyl and butylmethoxy dibenzoylmethanes (Eusolex 8020 and Parsol 1789). Contact Dermatitis 1989;21:109–11.

O'Donoghue MN. Sunscreen—the ultimate cosmetic. Dermatol Clin 1991; 9(1):99–104.

Pathak MA. Sunscreens and their use in the preventative treatment of sunlight-induced skin damage. J Dermatol Surg Oncol 1987;13(7):739–50.

Thune P. Contact and photocontact allergy to sunscreens. Photodermatol 1984;1(1):5–9.

Sun Protection Factor

Azizi E, Kushelevsky AP, Schewach-Millet M. Efficacy of topical sunscreen preparations on the human skin: combined indoor-outdoor study. Isr J Med Sci 1984;20(7):569–77.

Canadian drug identification code. Ottawa: Health and Welfare Canada, 1991.

Garmyn MA, Murphy GM, Gibbs NK, Hawk JLM. Are the protection factors assigned to proprietary sunscreen products misleading? Photodermatol 1986;3(2):104–6.

Watson A. Sunscreen effectiveness: theoretical and practical considerations. Aust J Dermatol 1983;24(1):17–22.

Choice of a Sunscreen

Basler RSW. Sunscreens. Nebr Med J 1983;68(6):162–5.

Brasier S, Baker K, Mattson K. Screening summer sun. Canadian Consumer 1982;12(6):25–7.

Edwards EK Jr, Edwards EK. Allergic reaction to triethanolamine stearate in a sunscreen. Cutis 1983;31(2):195–6.

Edwards EK Jr, Edwards EK. Allergic reaction to phenyl dimethicone in a sunscreen (Letter). Arch Dermatol 1984;120(5):575–6.

Farr PM, Diffey BL. How reliable are sunscreen protection factors? Br J Dermatol 1985;112(1):113–8.

Gilmore GD. Sunscreens: A review of the skin cancer protection value and educational opportunities. J School Health 1989;59(5):211–3.

Leroy D, Deschamps P. Influence of formulation on sunscreen water resistance. Photodermatol 1986;3(1):52–3.

Lundeen RC, Langlais RP, Terezhalmy GT. Sunscreen protection for lip mucosa: a review and update. J Am Dent Assoc 1985;111(4):617–21.

O'Neill JJ. Effect of film irregularities on sunscreen efficacy. J Pharm Sci 1984;73(7):888–91.

Relling MV, Dorr RT. Choosing a sunscreen. Ariz Med 1983;40(8):550–4.

Stenberg C, Larkoe O. Sunscreen application and its importance for the sun protection factor. Arch Dermatol 1985;121(11):1400–2.

Sunscreens on Children

Fed Reg 1978;43(Pt2):38217.

Systemic Protection

Kenney JA, Grimes PE. How we treat vitiligo. Cutis 1983;32(4):347–8.

Pigmenting or Tanning Products

Anonymous. Colouring agents. In: Wade A, ed. Martindale: the extra pharmacopoeia. London: Pharmaceutical Press, 1989:857.

Sunscreens

Anonymous. Dermatological agents. In: Wade A, ed. Martindale: the extra pharmacopoeia. London: Pharmaceutical Press, 1989:919.

Natow AJ. Corrective cosmetics. Cutis 1985;36(2):123–4.

Depigmenting Agents

Anonymous. Dermatological agents. In: Wade A, ed. Martindale: the extra pharmacopoeia. London: Pharmaceutical Press, 1989:928.

Anonymous. Hyperpigmentation and hypopigmentation. In: Arndt KA, ed. Manual of dermatologic therapeutics. Boston: Little, 1983:107–13.

Boyle J, Kennedy CTC. Hydroquinone concentrations in skin lightening creams. Br J Dermatol 1986;114(4):501–4.

Fisher AA. Hydroquinone uses and abnormal reactions. Cutis 1983;31(3):240–4,250.

Fitzpatrick TB, Mosher DB. Pigmentation of the skin and disorders of melanin metabolism. In: Petersdorf RG, Adams RD, Braunwald E, Isselbacher KJ, Martin JB, Wilson JD, eds. Harrison's principles of internal medicine. New York: McGraw-Hill, 1983:265–73.

Gossel TA. Skin lighteners. US Pharmacist 1985:10–6,18–20,22.

Lerner EA, Sober AJ. Chemical and pharmacological agents that cause hyperpigmentation or hypopigmentation of the skin. Dermatol Clin 1988;6(2):327–37.

Vasquez M, Sanchez JL. The efficacy of broad spectrum sunscreen in the treatment of melasma. Cutis 1983;32(1):92,95–6.

5
Dermatitis

Debra J. Ricciatti-Sibbald

The clinical manifestations of dermatitis vary for atopic, contact and hand dermatitis, and dry skin. Some non-pharmacologic treatments help relieve dermatitis, but a number of pharmacologic products are available as bath oils, bath salts, soaps, emollients and wet dressings. The products include hydrating agents, keratin softeners, anti-inflammatory agents and antipruritic agents.

Dermatitis accounts for a very large proportion of all skin disease. It may be argued that all eczema is dermatitis, but not all dermatitis is eczema. These terms are often used interchangeably. Although the word eczema (boiling over) has been used synonymously with atopic dermatitis, most dermatologists use the term eczema to describe an acute non-specific skin reaction that exhibits erythema (redness), scaling, and a variable number of vesicles (small blisters) and crusts. It does not describe dry, lichenified (hardened) chronic lesions. The term dermatitis is less specific and describes both acute and chronic

skin reactions with corresponding clinical patterns and history. The causes of dermatitis are varied and include allergic and toxic reactions, simple irritations and infections. There are also several distinct forms of dermatitis of which the origins are still unknown.

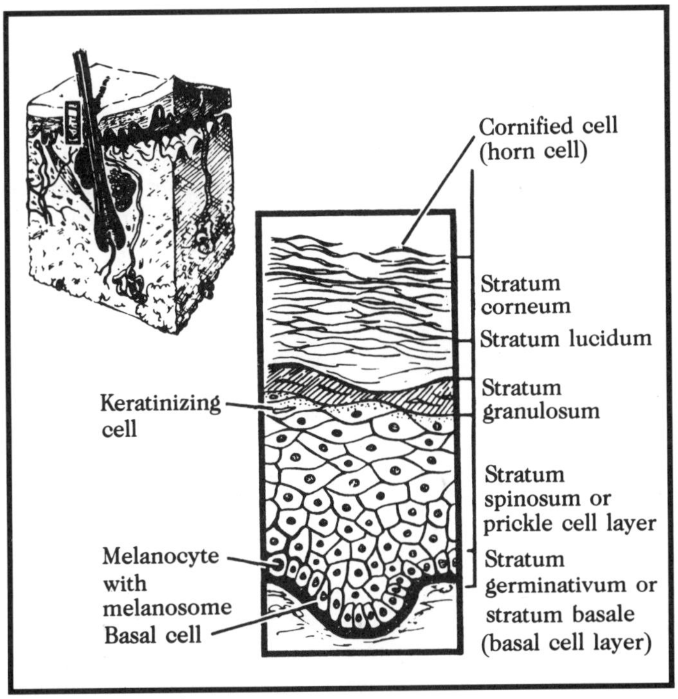

An understanding of the nature and treatment of dermatitis is based upon knowledge of the structure and function of normal and abnormal skin.

Normal skin consists of three layers: a stratified, cellular epidermis; an underlying vascular dermis of connective tissue; and a fatty layer beneath the dermis known as subcutaneous fat. There are two main kinds of human skin: a thick, hairless skin on the palms of the hand and the soles of the feet and a hairy skin on all other body surfaces.

The epidermis is composed of several different cell types. The basal, or deepest layer, consists of dividing cells. As the cells move upward, they synthesize an insoluble protein, keratin, which gradually fills them. Within these ascending cells, the keratin becomes granular. The cells lose their water content and nuclei and then die. The stratum corneum, the "horny" or uppermost layer of the epidermis, is constantly shed as scales that are not normally visible. A complete cellular turnover requires about 28 to 45 days. Pigment-forming cells are present in the basal layer of the epidermis and in the hair follicles (see Figure 1).

The dermis supports the epidermis and separates it from the subcutaneous fat. The main component of the dermis, apart from water, is collagen, a fibrous protein embedded in a ground substance primarily comprised of mucopolysaccharides. Elastic fibres are scattered throughout the dermis. Hair follicles extend from the epidermis into the dermis, and sebaceous glands empty into these follicles through a short canal. Follicles in the axilla (armpit) contain apocrine or scent glands. Eccrine sweat glands appear throughout the dermis (see Figure 2).

Two main layers divide the dermis. A superficial layer beneath the epidermis is rich in blood vessels that bring nutrients near the epidermis but not across the dermo-epidermal junction. A deeper underlying layer contains coarser tissue. A network of nerves runs through the dermis and into the epidermis. The itch sensation is generated in the superficial dermis, the sting sensation at the mid-dermis and the pain sensation at the border of the subcutaneous fat.

The most important function of the skin is to act as a two-way barrier. It prevents loss of water, electrolytes and other body constituents and retards the entry of foreign materials, chemical poisons and radiation. It is the crucial regulator in the percutaneous absorption of drugs. It also mediates sensation, moderates heat loss and resists

Figure 1 *Epidermis*

Cornified cell (horn cell)
Stratum corneum
Stratum lucidum
Stratum granulosum
Stratum spinosum or prickle cell layer
Stratum germinativum or stratum basale (basal cell layer)
Keratinizing cell
Melanocyte with melanosome
Basal cell

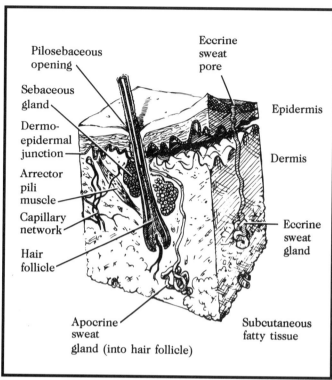

Figure 2 *Dermis*

mechanical shocks. The dermis is involved in pigment development and in synthesis of some vitamins.

These barrier functions are of the utmost importance in governing the use of topical and cosmetic therapy. Before a chemical penetrant coming into contact with the skin surface can reach the blood circulation, it must pass through surface hair, the skin surface lipid film,

Table I *Natural Moisturizing Factor (NMF)*

Component	%
Free amino acids	40.0
Pyrrolidine carboxylic acid (PCA)	12.0
Urea	7.0
NH_3, uric acid, glucosamine, creatinine	1.5
Sodium	5.0
Calcium	1.5
Potassium	4.0
Magnesium	1.5
Phosphate	0.5
Chloride	6.0
Lactate	12.0
Citrate, formate	0.5
Sugars, organic acids, peptides, unidentified materials	8.5

Adapted from: Fisher AA. Irritant reactions from topical urea preparations used for dry skin. Advantages of a urea-free "Dead Sea salt" cream. Cutis 1976;18:761–7.

the stratum corneum and the dermis. There are three potential pathways through the skin: via sweat ducts and hair follicles, intercellular spaces, or across the cells.

The stratum corneum serves as the principal barrier to the environment through an interplay of three distinct mechanisms. First, the lipid component of the semipermeable cell membrane may store lipid-soluble substances (for example, corticosteroids) rather than allowing them to pass through the aqueous epidermis. Cell membranes are highly resistant to physical and chemical insults, but removal of their lipid content destroys their semipermeable nature. The second mechanism involves water retention through the action of keratin, a protein that swells and absorbs its weight in water many times over. Third, intercellular spaces contain hygroscopic substances —collectively termed natural moisturizing factor (NMF)—which can hold water and allow passage of water-soluble drugs.

The flexibility and cohesiveness of the stratum corneum depend on the water content bound intercellularly by NMF. By lowering the surface tension of the skin, NMF overcomes normal water repellency and absorbs water on the skin from perspiration or from outside sources (see Table I).

Water can move freely in and out of corneal cells under the influences of environmental humidity, temperature and hygroscopic substances. Under average environmental conditions, the corneum contains between 10 and 20 per cent water by weight. If the water content drops below 10 per cent, the corneum becomes brittle and cracks easily, allowing irritants to penetrate. This penetration leads to mild inflammation and impairs proper cell maturation. Chapping results.

The following external and internal influences may be responsible for decreasing the water content of the corneum. A combination of these factors may cause irreversible loss of cell function by permitting hygroscopic substances to escape.

Ambient humidity: Water is the primary plasticizer of the skin. The rate of surface loss of water into the environment varies with the ambient humidity. The moisture content of the stratum corneum reaches 10 mg per 100 mg of dry weight when relative humidity is 60 per cent. As relative humidity increases, transepidermal water loss falls. A drop in ambient humidity may result in increased transpiration and water loss from the skin; thus, dry skin is usually seen in cold, dry weather.

Temperature: Even if water content is kept constant, skin pliability decreases with lower skin temperature. Surface ventilation also accelerates water evaporation. Although of less clinical importance, skin becomes drier with decreasing "dewpoint." The dewpoint temperature is the temperature at which visible condensation of water vapor appears under a constant pressure. The stratum corneum becomes brittle at a dewpoint temperature of 15 °C. Clinically, the skin begins to chap when the dewpoint temperature falls below −7 °C. Increased ambient or body temperature or stress causes water loss through sweat gland perspiration.

Surface active agents: Soaps remove oil and dirt, but their degreasing effects may lead to excessive drying. Overexposure to soaps, detergents and solvents destroys the semipermeable nature of the skin membranes by removing lipid.

Physical and chemical trauma: Repeated minor trauma, such as contact with an article of clothing, a cosmetic or a detergent, leading to inflammation can increase percutaneous absorption of contact irritants and sensitizers, which can damage the skin further. Keratolytics such as salicylic acid, also loosen the outer layers of the stratum corneum, especially if it is abnormal, as in dermatitis. Chemicals that irritate the basal layer may cause cells to mature abnormally, making them unable to retain water.

Conversely, external influences can also increase water content of the skin. Occlusion impairs barrier function by hydrating the stratum corneum and raising its temperature. This enhances aqueous intercellular channels for water-soluble molecules. The penetration of corticosteroids is greatly enhanced by hydration, a principle used in occlusive therapy. Drug absorption is increased in moist body fold areas in which the stratum corneum is more hydrated. Vehicles may increase drug penetration if they have occlusive properties, for example ointments. Bacteria may also proliferate rapidly under these circumstances.

Water diffusion through the epidermis doubles with a rise in temperature from 26° to 35°C. Skin resistance diminishes, increasing the permeability to foreign substances.

Barrier resistance may be altered by age. Absorption through the skin of very young children, particularly neonates, is thought to be increased. Although it has been thought that the skin of the aged is more permeable than that of younger adults, evidence of reduced transepidermal water diffusion implies greater barrier resistance.

Barrier efficiency varies with body site. The face, forehead and backs of the hands may be more water-permeable than the trunk, arms and legs. The scrotum and body folds are particularly permeable, but the palms of the hands are impermeable to nearly all molecules except water, perhaps contributing to the decreased incidence of contact dermatitis at this site.

Barrier function is affected by skin diseases that involve the stratum corneum. The degree of impairment reflects the severity of the disease condition. Diseases such as dermatitis unequivocally impair barrier function. Transepidermal water diffusion is always increased at the site of acute dermatitis and therapeutic agents penetrate these areas more easily than normal skin. The thickened stratum corneum of chronic dermatitis still depresses barrier function because this layer is qualitatively abnormal.

Barrier efficiency begins to regenerate within 24 hours of damage, owing to the formation of a temporary barrier of parakeratotic cells and dried exudate. The normal horny layer reforms slowly over the next 12 to 25 days. Treatment must reflect these regenerative processes.

Clinical Manifestations

Skin changes in dermatitis reflect the pattern of inflammatory response. They therefore are much the same in all forms of dermatitis, regardless of cause, and are easily recognized as functions of the time during which the reaction has occurred.

When dermatitis is acute, the earliest and mildest changes are erythema (redness) caused by engorgement and dilatation of the small blood vessels and, usually, swelling (edema) resulting from fluid

Table II *Basic Differentiating Features and Treatment Measures*

Condition	Symptoms	Location	Description	Trigger factors	Aims of therapy
Atopic dermatitis	Cycles of itching and scratching	2 months: chest, face 2 years: scalp, neck, extremities	Red, raised blisters with oozing, dry skin	Extreme heat or cold, rapid change in temperature, sweating, irritant or occlusive clothing (wool or nylon), greases, oils, soaps and detergents, environmental, allergens, anxiety, infections	Decrease trigger factors and pruritus; suppress inflammation; lubricate the skin; alleviate anxiety.
		4–10 years: scattered, neck, wrist, elbow, knee	Less acute and oozing, dry papules, thickening, periorbital edema and erythema		
		12–20 years: flexor areas, hands	Dry, thickened, hyper-pigmented plaques		
Contact dermatitis (primary irritant and allergic)	Acute: itching, pain in fissures Chronic: stiffness, dryness	Irritant—in contact area Allergic—in exposed or contact area; transferred by touch	Irritant—mild, acute: red, blisters, oozing; mild, chronic: dry, thick, fissured; strong: ulcers, blisters, erosions Allergic—unusual pattern, sharp, straight margins, acute angles, straight lines; grouped or linear tense vesicles and blisters	Irritant—contact time and concentration of irritant; friction, heat and cold, occlusion, pressure, maceration, disease states Allergic—contact time and concentration of allergen; genetic predisposition	Decrease contact exposure to irritants and allergens; if dry, wet it; if wet, dry it.
Hand dermatitis (dishpan hands)	Itching, dryness, fissures, inelasticity	Sides of the fingers; less often throughout palms	Redness, dryness, chapping; small vesicles; excess sweating	Repeated contact with primary irritants, soap and water, solvent and detergents; family history of atopic dermatitis or psoriasis	Decrease contact exposure.
Dry skin (chapping, xerosis, winter itch, asteatotic eczema)	Usually none, sometimes itching may be severe	Lower legs (shins); dorsa of hands; forearms	Dry skin with fine scale; diffuse or round patches; severe cracks and fissures in diamond pattern with redness	Increasing age; decreased humidity (increased room heat and cold, dry winter air, repeated contact with solvents, soaps, disinfectants; hypothyroidism.	Replace water in the skin and in the immediate environment.

leaving the damaged blood vessels and accumulating in the tissue. If swelling is severe, the skin cells form vesicles that fill with the edema fluid; this process is called vesiculation or blistering. When the blisters break, the skin oozes or weeps. Evaporation of this fluid causes crusting and scaling.

Dermatitis may progress to a chronic stage. The skin becomes dry, fissured and cracked. With prolonged itching and scratching, it thickens, and the normal skin markings become more prominent. This process is called lichenification. The skin may show damage through scratching and hyperpigmentation or hypopigmentation.

The pattern of dermatitis and its trigger factors influence clinical classification and therapy. Dermatitis can be caused by an infection, or seborrhea. These forms will not be discussed in this chapter. Some of the most common presentations include atopic dermatitis, contact dermatitis, hand dermatitis and dry skin. Table II outlines the differentiating features and treatment measures for each condition.

Atopic Dermatitis

Atopic dermatitis is a genetically predetermined disease. This intensely pruritic and chronic eruption is seen in characteristic patterns in infants, children and adults. It begins in infancy, but is rarely present at birth, and it decreases in intensity with age. In approximately 80 per cent of cases of atopic dermatitis, the problem develops during the first year of life, and in up to 90 per cent of cases the onset occurs before 5 years of age. Atopic dermatitis affects 10 to 20 per cent of the population. These people and their families also show an increased incidence of hay fever, asthma and chronic rhinitis.

The symptoms and signs of atopic dermatitis are numerous, but usually nonspecific. One expert describes atopic dermatitis as an "itch that rashes, not a rash that itches." The primary symptom is pruritus with its accompanying scratch response. People with this type of dermatitis have a low itch threshold and a longer duration of itch. In rare cases, babies present with what appears to be atopic dermatitis and the parents say the baby is not pruritic. Some clinicians maintain there are no specific lesions in atopic dermatitis and that it is scratching the itchy skin that produces the eczematous lesions. They equate the beginning of atopic dermatitis around the age of 3 with the fact that it is at this time that infants are first old enough to scratch. Others say the lesions occur even before the area is scratched. The familiar redness and chapping of a baby's cheeks can be the earliest sign of atopic dermatitis. This chapping usually begins at 2 to 3 months of age and persists for 2 years. An infantile eruption shows all the features of acute eczema, but scalp and neck involvement is generally limited to infants.

A 3 to 4 week old infant with an eruption probably does not have atopic dermatitis, but may have seborrheic dermatitis, which can be present from birth. If children present for the first time with eczematous lesions after 5 years of age, it is important to look for other disease states such as scabies.

A remission usually occurs between 2 and 4 years of age. Visual signs include less redness, increased dryness and early lichenification. Involvement of the back of the arms and the front of the legs is seen first and later a transition occurs to the elbows and knee folds. Frictional areas such as wrists and ankles are regular sites of involvement. Localization to the toes is often misinterpreted as a fungus infection. Dermatitis of the toes is now referred to as the nylon shoe syndrome, secondary to excessive sweating and drying of the feet by shoes that are completely occlusive. As the child reaches adulthood, recurrent outbreaks diminish or disappear.

Itch is the dominating complaint and may be most intense during evening and nights. It is usually intermittent and leads to vigorous itch-scratch cycles. Itching may be limited to the lesions or, if the skin is dry, may involve all skin surfaces.

Most patients with atopic dermatitis are colonized with coagulase positive *Staph aureus* especially in wet lesions. Some patients have demonstrated a relationship between skin lesions and colonization with the yeast, *Pityrosporum ovale*. Patients may have an increased susceptibility to cutaneous herpes infections and to warts. They are less likely to develop contact sensitivity reactions, such as poison ivy dermatitis, due to a decrease in cellular (T cell) immunity.

For many years, atopic dermatitis was considered purely an allergic disease, encouraging the use of traditional therapy. Attempts were made to desensitize people suffering from atopic dermatitis with injections, to eliminate food and inhaled materials thought to provoke symptoms and to prolong or increase breastfeeding.

Recent reports using improved experimental designs have resurrected some of the old and controversial ideas of dietary factors in atopic dermatitis. The concept of a nutritional basis for eczema began with observations in 1933 that eczematous children had decreased serum unsaturated fatty acids. Subsequent investigations found no benefit from feeding eczematous children various unsaturated oils. The issue remained in dispute until 1982, when researchers showed clinical improvement in atopic people treated with oral evening primrose oil (EPO). This substance, widely distributed in health food stores, contains linoleic acid and gamma-linolenic acid. Adult patients had clinical improvement while the results in children were far less significant or no better than placebo. A similar study also substantiated a decrease in inflammation, dryness and itch in patients receiving EPO. Other authors have not been able to duplicate beneficial clinical effects or have had unimpressive results. EPO has been used as a dietary supplement in patients with atopic dermatitis. Two potential problems associated with its use are its high cost and the possibility of purchasing adulterated brands which may not have the same composition (in some cases simply corn oil) and effect. At present, the efficacy of EPO in atopic dermatitis is unconfirmed and awaits the support of independent studies.

More controversy has arisen about the role of food allergy in atopic dermatitis. A number of current reports using convincing methodology show that hypersensitivity to such foods as milk products, eggs, wheat and nuts may be more common and relevant than realized.

Table III *Major Treatment Principles*

Acute (wet) dermatitis: measures which dry
Compresses—Burow's, tap water, saline
Warm baths—with or without baking soda or oatmeal colloids
Avoid ointments and powders

Resolving dermatitis: oozing has stopped
Discontinue wet dressings
Soothing lotion or oil-in-water cream
Prescription corticosteroid

Chronic (dry) dermatitis: measures which lubricate
Warm water soaks—containing or followed by bath oil
  application
Hydrating ointments—with or without keratin softeners

Figure 3 *Suggested Approach for Treating Atopic Dermatitis*

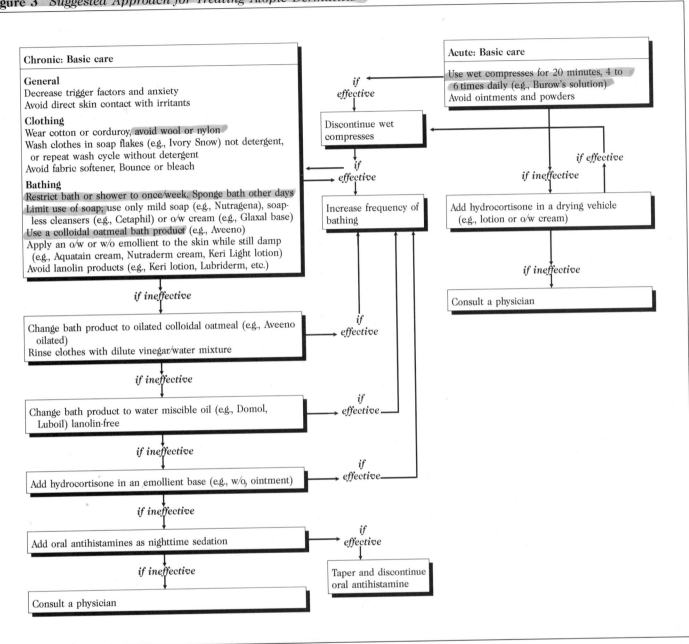

It is difficult to apply this information to practical management of atopic children. Although some children showed marked initial improvement after strict avoidance of offending food, none cleared completely. The best results were in children between 2 and 8 years of age. Over the long term, the benefits decreased drastically. Tremendous compliance problems exist in the dietary management of atopic dermatitis. In children, strict food elimination diets present the danger of malnutrition.

These new studies have not greatly influenced therapy for most people with atopic dermatitis. Dietary management of established atopic dermatitis is not routinely indicated for the majority of patients. Food allergen elimination and double blind challenges are

so difficult they should be reserved for only the most severely symptomatic and unresponsive individuals and should not be continued long term. Gradual reintroduction of the offending foods is often appropriate.

Lack of success with these types of treatment indicates more complex origins of atopic dermatitis. Major principles of treatment for acute and chronic phases are summarized in Table III.

The acute phase is relatively easy to manage. Wet, oozing lesions are compressed for 20 minutes every few hours or dried out by warm bathing, which reduces pruritus and inflammation. Although hot baths and soap are contraindicated, a processed oatmeal colloid may be added to the bath. Topical hydrocortisone, 0.5 per cent or greater, in a drying vehicle, such as a lotion, or oil-in-water cream, helps combat itch as the oozing subsides. Steroids should not be applied more than 2 to 3 times a day. Oral antihistamines may relieve itch, and, if given at bedtime, may help a child sleep. Tolerance may develop. The person should consult a physician if the condition remains unresponsive, if the dermatitis continues to involve larger body areas or if itching is so severe it disrupts normal daily functioning or sleep patterns. Stronger corticosteroid therapy, or antibiotics for a secondary infection, may be necessary. Topical mupirocin and imidazoles have been used successfully, but the problem of resistant organisms should be borne in mind, as well as their relatively high cost.

Long-term management is more difficult. People with dry, chronic lesions should keep the skin lubricated and attempt to decrease possible trigger factors including anxiety. They must avoid direct skin contact with irritants. Baths should be restricted, and bath oils added near the end of each bath. If necessary, a mild soap can be used to cleanse the anus, groin and underarms, but a nonlipid cleanser may be preferred. A child who becomes filthy at play needs a bath. However, the general advice is to wash regularly and take a bath only once a week. Emollients are used whenever possible, to alleviate dryness, but no oily or greasy lubricant should be allowed. Skin is patted dry, as rubbing increases irritation. Topical lubrication is applied while the skin is damp. Use of a cool air humidifier may help in a dry, winter environment. Cotton and corduroy clothing is preferred, as wool or nylon is often too irritating and sweating leads to itch.

Hydrophilic, oil-in-water preparations or cold cream preparations are suitable lubricants. Preparations containing urea or lactic acid produce superior results. More resistant cases may respond to mild tar compounds applied to the skin or in a bath. As this condition can become extremely stressful, a physician should be consulted if these measures produce little response. For dry, chronic cases, hydrocortisone is applied in vehicles that provide the greatest lubrication to the skin—such as ointments or water-in-oil creams—in as weak a concentration as adequately controls symptoms. Stronger steroids available only by prescription may become necessary.

Wearing cotton gloves or mittens to prevent scratching and secondary infection allows healing of affected hands. Keeping fingernails clean and short is also essential. Sunlight is usually beneficial. If environmental influences such as diet or inhalants (for example, dust) seem to be a factor in the worsening of the dermatitis, the person should seek a physician's counsel.

Atopic dermatitis is subject to spontaneous exacerbations and remissions. Claims for any particular therapy must always be assessed with this unpredictability in mind. Reports of response to therapy with topical cyclosporin A, phosphodiesterase inhibitors (papaverine) and Chinese herbs are all inconclusive to date.

The first discussion with a patient should be devoted to developing compliance with basic therapy. Complex verbal instructions are usually too overwhelming and confusing. Information sheets or algorithms are very useful for patients and for parents. Focus counselling upon 3 or 4 principles: mild corticosteroids; bath products and avoidance of harsh soaps; the use of emollients to alleviate dryness; and oral antihistamines for bedtime sedation. The key is to prevent scratching.

Atopic dermatitis affects the individual but influences the whole family. Treatment must be directed toward the parents as well as the child. Constant support is necessary to encourage the affected person and decrease family tension associated with this disease. Often a parent is more distressed than the child. The family can be reassured that the disease does not scar, is not contagious and that any pigment changes are temporary. This long-term condition can be controlled, but not cured. The major principles of treatment for atopic dermatitis are summarized in Figure 3.

Contact Dermatitis

Contact dermatitis can be produced by primary irritants or allergic sensitizers. Acute reactions are often red, blistered and oozing; in chronic reactions the skin may be dry, thick and fissured. As with other forms of acute and chronic dermatitis, itching is the primary symptom and the degree of inflammation determines severity. The area involved usually resembles the pattern of the contacting substances and may have sharp, straight margins or unusual shapes. Allergic sensitizers or strong irritants may be transferred from the primary site by touch. Palms of the hands, soles of the feet and scalp areas are more resistant.

Primary irritant contact dermatitis is a nonallergic reaction that can be produced by exposure to any substance, including chemical, physical and biological agents, if the concentration and duration of contact are sufficient. Mild irritants (for example, soaps, detergents and most solvents) require repeated or sustained contact to produce inflammation; strong irritants (for example, acids and alkalis) may injure the skin immediately. Irritant effects may be considerably enhanced by occlusion.

Allergic contact dermatitis is a delayed or cell-mediated hypersensitivity reaction resulting from exposure of sensitized individuals to contact allergens. Most of these reactions produce sensitization in only a small percentage of those exposed. The incubation period after initial sensitization is 5 to 21 days and after subsequent re-exposure is 12 to 48 hours.

The five most common contact allergens, in order of frequency, are as follows: *Rhus* (poison ivy, oak or sumac); paraphenylenediamine (hair dyes); nickel compounds (such as found in costume jewelry and metal buckles); rubber compounds (such as found in adhesives, gloves and synthetic plastics); and ethylenediamine. Other substances commonly implicated are topical antihistamines, local "caine"-containing anesthetics, iodine, mercury-containing antiseptics, antibiotics such as neomycin and sulfonamides, lanolin, and additives such as parabens and perfume. Cross-reactions can occur between benzocaine and paraphenylenediamine, sulfonamides and aminobenzoic acid sunscreens. Cross-reactions can also occur between ethylenediamine and aminophylline and certain antihistamines containing the ethylenediamine structure (for example, tripelennamine).

Allergic rashes are frequently caused by cosmetics or self-medication with topical nonprescription preparations. People whose skin is already inflamed due to an initial contactant may worsen their condition following exposure to a secondary allergen or irritant to which they might not normally react; such an irritant may be a topical preparation containing neomycin or antihistamines. Discomfort and itch may lead to increased use of anti-itch lotions, starting a vicious cycle that may obscure the initial problem.

How should any irritant or allergic contact dermatitis be treated? An excellent rule of thumb is, "if it's dry, wet it; if it's wet, dry it." The primary recommendation in contact dermatitis is to decrease contact exposure to irritants and allergens. A good history is essential in identifying the cause, especially any previous treatments that may have exacerbated symptoms or cross-reacted with the contactant. Table IV lists a few contact allergens to suspect in dermatitis involving different body areas. Other treatment objectives are simple and safe. Protect the damaged skin against secondary infection until the acute stage subsides. Do not allow debris due to oozing, scaling and crusting to accumulate. Relieving itch prevents damage due to scratching. A change of environment may be helpful.

A person with irritant contact dermatitis is advised to avoid such irritants as soaps, detergents, bleaches and moist vegetables (for example, onions or garlic). Rings should be removed while working. A bland cream or emollient lotion can be applied throughout the day as a lubricant. Waterless hand cleansers can also be used. Hands can be protected with plastic or vinyl gloves worn with cotton liners, but rubber gloves should be avoided.

A person who develops acute allergic or irritant contact dermatitis should immediately wash the area thoroughly. If the area is wet or oozing, astringent compresses (for example, Burow's) can be applied for 20 to 30 minutes, 4 to 6 times daily. Oral antihistamines and tepid baths with oatmeal can be recommended for itch. Topical hydrocortisone reduces inflammation and pruritus. A lotion or gel preparation is best for drying wet dermatitis. If the condition does not respond to these measures, a physician should be consulted. Once the area has dried, a cream or lotion (for example, Calamine) with or without an antipruritic or hydrocortisone can be used.

Chronic contact dermatitis that is dry or fissured should be soaked for 5 minutes rather than compressed. This therapy can be followed immediately by treatment with an occlusive ointment. Hydrocortisone may be used intermittently to control symptoms.

Poison Ivy Contact Dermatitis

Poison ivy *(Toxicodendron radicans)* and other members of the *Rhus* genus of plants, poison oak *(Toxicodendron diversilobum)* and poison sumac *(Toxicodendron vernix)* are responsible for many cases of allergic contact dermatitis each year. An estimated 70 per cent of the population could acquire the allergy if exposed. People at risk include workers in logging, agriculture, forest fire fighting, construction and utility maintenance, as well as outdoor enthusiasts.

The allergenic component of poison ivy is an oleoresin known as urushiol contained in the leaf, stem and root of the plant. It consists of four pentadecyl catechols. Poison oak and poison sumac have a chemically similar antigen resulting in immunologic cross-reactivity. True poison oak is not found in Canada, but grows only in the southern and Pacific states of the United States. Poison sumac is indigenous to the swampy southern United States. The leaf containing oleoresin must be broken before a reaction can occur. Poison sumac leaves are antigenic throughout the growing season but become less potent after they dry out and fall off the plant.

Plant particles in smoke may be a problem for extremely sensitive persons. Indirect contact from pet fur or clothing may also cause the dermatitis. Cross-reactivity may occur to substances that are

Table IV *Contact Allergens*

Area	Suspect
Eyelids	Perfume Nail polish Hand cream Cosmetics Eye medication Eyelash curlers
Ears	Earrings Glasses Perfume Hair products
Mouth	Lipstick Gum Food dyes Mouthwashes Toothpaste Pen or pencil
Face	Cosmetics Hair products Soap Aerosol sprays
Hands	Jewelry Foods Soaps Cosmetics Occupational contacts
Feet	Leather Glue Nickel Chromium Rubber Dyes

Adapted from Walzer RA. Dermatitis and eczema: a few rash statements. Skintelligence: how to be smart about your skin. New York: Appleton-Century-Crofts, 1981:71–87.

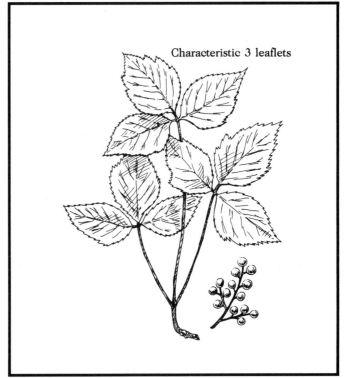

Characteristic 3 leaflets

Figure 4 *Poison Ivy*

Figure 5 *Suggested Approach for Treating Contact Dermatitis*

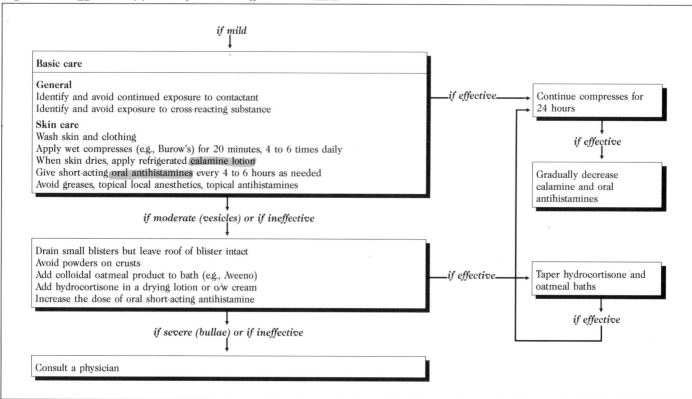

members of the same plant family, such as mango rind, cashew nut shells and lacquer from the Oriental *Rhus vernicifera* tree.

Sensitization occurs readily in persons over 3 years of age and rarely in those under 1 year. The first episode of allergic dermatitis occurs 14 to 21 days after contact, but subsequent episodes occur 8 hours to 3 days after contact. The reaction is a red, itchy eruption characterized by linear streaks of small blisters called vesicles.

Prevention of *Rhus* dermatitis involves recognizing the plant and avoiding contact with it. It is a low-growing plant or vine; each compound leaf consists of three leaflets (see Figure 4). Barrier creams advocated in the past to protect the skin before exposure are impractical and do not work. Once exposed, clothing should be changed. Highly sensitive individuals may benefit by washing the skin immediately after contact (within 5 minutes) whereas mildly sensitive persons benefit by washing up to 30 minutes after contact. Beyond this time, the oleoresin becomes fixed to the skin. The dermatitis occurs only where the oleoresin contacts the skin; it does not spread by vesicle fluid.

An organoclay preparation (the quaternary ammonium salt of sodium bentonite) has been evaluated for topical protection against experimental poison ivy and poison oak. It was more effective than comparable preparations of bentonite, kaolin or silicone. However, the observations were made in highly sensitive volunteers with weak dilutions of urushiol. It would be surprising if the same protection were achieved against exposure to poison ivy leaves.

Generalization can occur from an immune enhancement of severe local reactions. *Rhus* antigen fixed to the skin is processed in the epidermis by Langerhans' cells. These antigen-containing cells then migrate to the local lymph nodes, stimulating recruitment of lymphocytes and a systemic response.

For over 40 years, various detoxicants have been investigated to try to chemically inactivate the antigen. Among these are exchange resins, such as Amberlite, which absorb urushiol by an ion exchange; oxidants such as hydrogen peroxide, potassium permanganate and sodium perborate; and complexing agents such as iron, zirconium and silver ions, which chelate urushiol to a metal ion. This testing procedure is difficult as the antigen is rapidly absorbed. None have proven effective. Zirconium oxide may produce granulomas—nodules of chronic inflammation that remain focal and heal with fibrotic scarring.

Treatment of poison ivy dermatitis includes tap water or antiseptic compresses, and calamine lotion to dry the vesicular stage. Topical hydrocortisone benefits mild cases. No greasy preparation should be applied to oozing skin. If the blisters drain, the surface should be left intact to prevent secondary infection. Topical agents containing sensitizers should be avoided (for example, neomycin, benzocaine or antihistamines). Oral antihistamines are seldom sensitizers and may reduce the itch. In moderate to severe cases or when the face, eyelids or large areas of the body are involved, the person should be referred to a physician, as systemic corticosteroids may be necessary. The major principles of treatment for contact dermatitis are summarized in Figure 5.

Hand Dermatitis

Hand dermatitis is not a specific disease, but an inflammatory pattern of response to a variety of stimuli. It may have an acute presentation characterized by erythema, papules, blisters, oozing and scaling, or

Dermatitis

Figure 6 *Suggested Approach for Treating Hand Dermatitis*

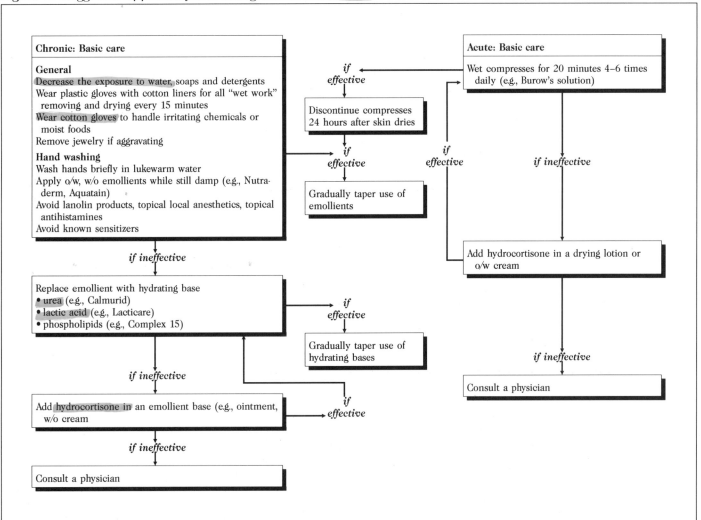

a chronic appearance with dry, thickened, lichenified skin. Only its location and frequency of occurrence justify its consideration as a separate entity.

Hand dermatitis must be distinguished from several other itchy skin conditions: psoriasis, tinea infections and scabies. In psoriasis, vesicles, the key sign of acute dermatitis, are absent. Fungal infections usually predominate on one hand and can be cultured. Evidence of scabies can usually be found elsewhere on the body, such as the penis, scrotum, axillae and breasts. Hand dermatitis is generally due to either exogenous causes, such as irritant or allergic contact sensitivity, or to endogenous causes, related to unknown constitutional factors. Misdiagnosis of an acute contact hand dermatitis as an endogenous eczema may allow the problem to become chronic if the offending contactant is not identified and avoided.

Hand dermatitis is a common chronic pruritic disorder, also known as "dishpan hands." Housewives, medical personnel, bartenders, dishwashers, hairdressers, food handlers and others involved in work that necessitates frequent immersion of the hands in water are susceptible to this type of dermatitis. It frequently begins under a ring, especially on the left fourth finger, and typically several weeks post-

partum. This site may result from several interplaying factors. Soaps, detergents, waxes and polishes that accumulate and concentrate under the ring act as primary irritants. Rings, especially alloys of copper and silver, can corrode to form a primary irritant when exposed to an adequate concentration of salt. The metal of the ring, usually nickel, can produce allergic contact dermatitis.

After being limited to the ring area for several weeks, the dermatitis begins to enlarge. Several weeks later the eruption may extend to adjacent fingers. Ultimately, both hands may be affected to a varying degree. It appears on the sides of the fingers and, less often, throughout the palms, as red, dry, chapped skin that may blister and sweat excessively.

Although hand dermatitis is most often a reaction to repeated contact with mild irritants such as soap, detergents and solvents, other causes include atopic dermatitis, fungal infections and allergic dermatitis, usually from nickel.

Hand dermatitis may be complicated by secondary bacterial infection. A unilateral, dry, red scaling of the palm is usually a fungal infection. Interdigital infections in people who do a great deal of "wet work" may be due to yeast organisms.

Dermatitis

People with hand dermatitis often find it difficult to rest their hands because, generally, they depend on using them. Hand dermatitis tends to be chronic and recurrent; the longer the chronic phase of the disease, the longer the convalescent period away from irritants.

Preventive measures for acute and chronic hand dermatitis parallel those for contact dermatitis. Affected people should decrease exposure to irritants and maintain an even temperature, avoiding heat in all forms. Hands should be washed briefly in lukewarm water, without soap, rinsed well and dried between the fingers. Strong household cleansers should not be used; if they are necessary, they must not be too concentrated, but should be measured accurately and the packages wiped clean. Alkaline soap should be replaced with a soap substitute when possible. For all "wet work," plastic gloves with cotton liners should be worn for 15 to 20 minute intervals, then turned inside out, rinsed and sprinkled with talc. Gloves must be worn to shampoo hair or apply hair products, to handle citrus fruits, tomatoes or potatoes or when using polishes, solvents or stain removers. Rings should not be worn during handwashing or housework. Gloves should be worn in cold weather.

Treating hand dermatitis depends on the stage of the disease. A good history is important in determining the cause and in eliminating or reducing any irritant or allergenic contact. The acute stage, characterized by redness, oozing and swelling, is best managed by applying continuous or intermittent wet dressings. Large cotton gloves soaked in the solution are a convenient method. The gloves are wrung out well before application, and removed and rewet every 2 to 3 minutes. The wet dressings are continued for an extra 24 hours after the lesions dry. This procedure is repeated for 20 to 30 minutes every 3 to 4 hours.

The subacute stage, characterized by erythema, scaling and some blistering but no weeping, is treated by applying intermittent wet dressings (for a half-hour, 3 to 4 times daily) followed by the application of a hydrocortisone cream. The effect of the cream can be enhanced by occlusion with disposable plastic gloves. For convenience, the plastic gloves are usually applied at night and removed in the morning. Creams containing neomycin should not be used since they are of doubtful efficacy and are known to have sensitizing capabilities.

The chronic stage, characterized by dryness, scaling and fissuring, is best treated by applying a protective and lubricating water-in-oil hand cream or an ointment regularly during the day, especially after washing hands or removing gloves. Barrier creams that protect the skin from specific chemicals or solvents are greasy and tend to interfere with manual dexterity. If inflammation is still present, a water-in-oil hydrocortisone preparation or an ointment can be used. If dryness is severe, the hands are soaked for a few minutes in cool water before applying a lubricant.

Hand activity that involves friction, pressure, squeezing, or twisting should be avoided. If infection due to bacteria, fungus or yeast is suspected, the person should be referred to a physician for diagnostic culture and treatment. Patients with hand dermatitis should avoid irritants for several months after complete healing. The major principles of treatment for acute and chronic stages are summarized in Figure 6.

Dry Skin (Asteatotic Eczema, Xerosis)

Dry skin refers to roughened, flaky or scaly skin that is less flexible than normal and dry to the touch. Follicles are often prominent on exposed areas, especially on the front of the lower legs. The syndrome is aggravated by cold, dry climates or seasons and is more common in elderly individuals. It has also been called "winter itch". This subacute, superficial dermatitis is caused by dehydration of the epidermis. It can occur in the general population, and particularly affected are areas exposed to the environment, such as legs, arms and hands.

Important factors in its production include a naturally dry skin with a lack of obvious seborrhea and a life-long tendency to chapping. Reduction in lipid production with age, illness, malnutrition and hormonal decline are all contributing factors. Environmental influences are extremely important, including low humidity, sudden skin cooling by air conditioning, dry heat, cold weather and wind.

People with dry skin must replace water in the skin and in the environment. Rooms should be kept cool; humidifiers are recommended. Excessive bathing is one of the common causes of dry skin. Alternatives are daily sponge baths, with tub baths (10 to 20 minutes) or showers once a week, or a quick, daily shower, limiting the use of soap to underarm, genital and foot areas. Warm water is preferable to hot water. Bath oil or oil application after bath is advised. For the elderly, non-oily colloidal products are less slippery in the bath.

Emollients containing antipruritic agents can be applied frequently while the skin is still damp. A slight dryness may require only emollients with glycerin or propylene glycol; more severe cases may require urea or lactic acid creams. Healing should occur within 5 to 10 days. When the dermatitis shows chronic inflammation, hydrocortisone water-in-oil creams or ointments can be used. If pruritus is excessive, antihistamines can also be used. If the itching or rash does not respond to these measures within one to two weeks, a physician should be consulted. The major treatment principles for dry skin are summarized in Figure 7.

Pharmacologic Agents

General measures to treat particular dermatitis conditions have been discussed. In each instance, the regimen is individualized with close attention to the aims of therapy (see Table II).

In most dermatitic conditions, a degree of dryness at some stage initiates or exacerbates the course and symptoms of the dermatitis. The skin is dry not because it lacks grease or skin oils, but because it lacks water. The primary means of correcting dryness is to add water to the skin and then to apply a hydrophobic substance to keep it there.

Bath Products

Bath oils applied during or after bathing help to reduce the rate of water loss through the epidermis. They help control dry skin symptoms, particularly in asteatotic dermatitis, and chronic atopic dermatitis, but should be considered a supplement to other, more effective measures such as lotions and creams applied directly to wet skin. Oil is not particularly effective because it is diluted with water. If added at the beginning of the bath, it may prevent rather than enhance hydration. Moreover, it is in contact with the skin for only a short period of time. As well, most oil deposited on the skin during bathing is wiped off when drying with a towel. Some of these problems can be circumvented by adding oil near the end of the bath to produce a water-trapping effect. Oil can also be applied as a topical treatment after the bath, using 5 mL of oil per 50 mL of water applied with a cotton swab while the skin is still damp.

Figure 7 *Suggested Approach for Treating Dry Skin*

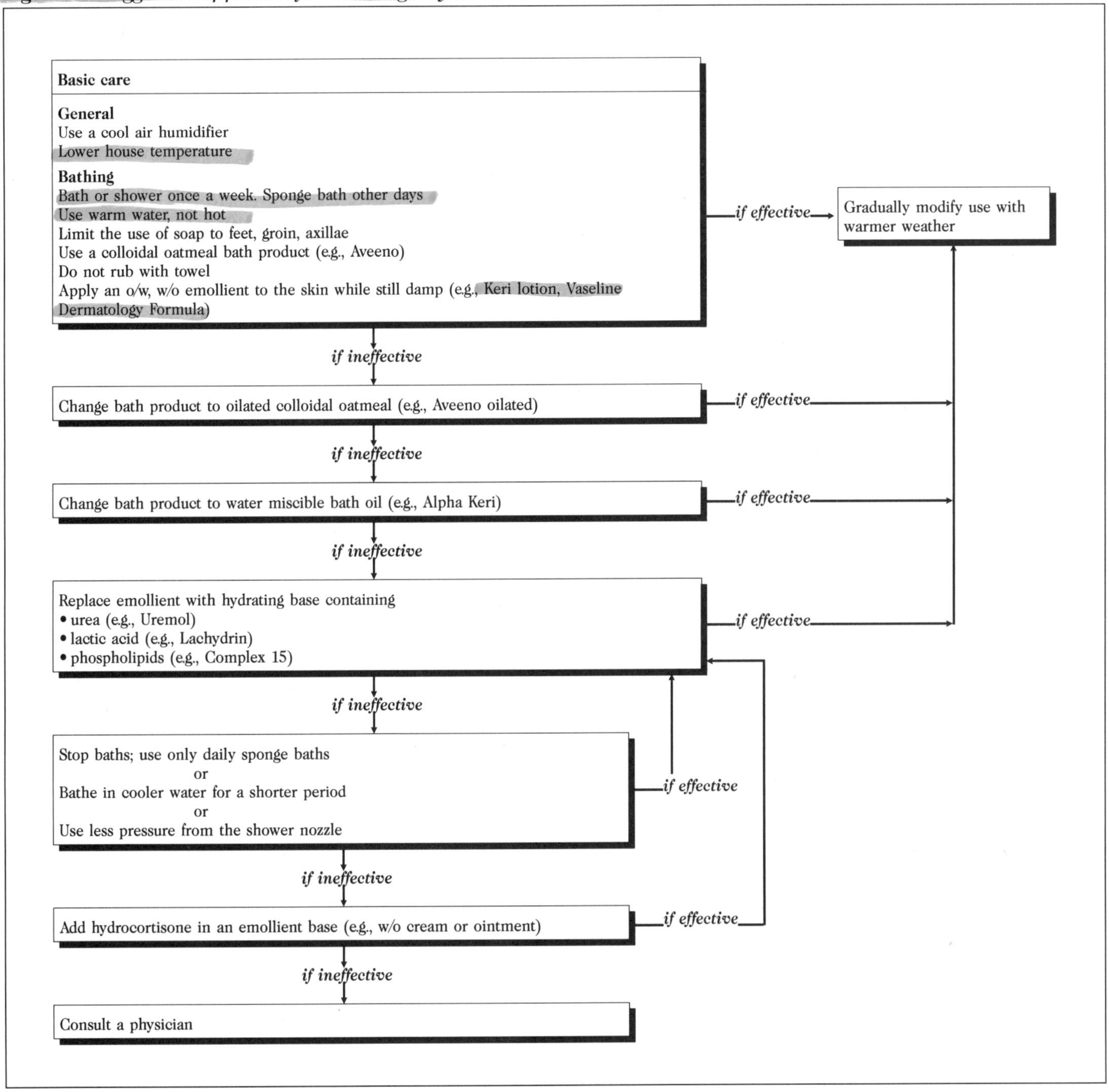

Basic care

General
Use a cool air humidifier
Lower house temperature

Bathing
Bath or shower once a week. Sponge bath other days
Use warm water, not hot
Limit the use of soap to feet, groin, axillae
Use a colloidal oatmeal bath product (e.g., Aveeno)
Do not rub with towel
Apply an o/w, w/o emollient to the skin while still damp (e.g., Keri lotion, Vaseline Dermatology Formula)

if effective → Gradually modify use with warmer weather

if ineffective

Change bath product to oilated colloidal oatmeal (e.g., Aveeno oilated) — *if effective*

if ineffective

Change bath product to water miscible bath oil (e.g., Alpha Keri) — *if effective*

if ineffective

Replace emollient with hydrating base containing
• urea (e.g., Uremol)
• lactic acid (e.g., Lachydrin)
• phospholipids (e.g., Complex 15)

if effective

if ineffective

Stop baths; use only daily sponge baths
or
Bathe in cooler water for a shorter period
or
Use less pressure from the shower nozzle

if effective

if ineffective

Add hydrocortisone in an emollient base (e.g., w/o cream or ointment) — *if effective*

if ineffective

Consult a physician

Many bath oils are available as mineral or vegetable oils that float on top of the water; others combine surfactants that disperse the oil throughout the bath. Concentrations of surfactants above 4 per cent reduce the affinity of oil for the skin. Products containing fragrance should be avoided when allergy is suspected. It has not been established clearly that any type of bath oil is superior to another. One characteristic all bath oils share is that they make the bathtub slippery, and everyone, especially older people, should be aware of this.

Bath oil capsules consist of small amounts of bath oil enclosed in soft, flexible gelatin capsules that dissolve in hot water. Essentially, they produce the same effects on the skin as liquid bath oils. The perfume content, often 10 per cent or more, is usually higher in capsules than in liquid oils.

Bath salts provide fragrance while softening the water. They present a potential hazard because they sometimes make the water too alkaline, causing itching or redness, especially to sensitive skin. Bubble baths which are based on detergents should be avoided by patients with dry or pruritic skin.

Oatmeal products are less effective in hydration than mineral and vegetable oil products. These colloidal preparations contain starch and protein. They benefit most in cases of asteatotic eczema, whereas acute eczematous states require the additional hydrating effect of bath oils. Some preparations combine the two effects in an oilated oatmeal product, which is more lubricating and more beneficial than a colloid alone in chronic dry conditions, such as atopic dermatitis. Users measure the required amount of oatmeal product into a small strainer that is held under the tap, allowing the running water to dissolve it quickly.

Soaps

Soaps are made from animal or vegetable fat and alkali. Fatty acid plus sodium or potassium hydroxide produce a water-soluble soap. Toilet soaps are usually made from palmitic, stearic or oleic acids. The hard sodium soaps are suitable for bars, flakes and powders, whereas the more soluble potassium soaps are used for liquid preparations.

Soap and water cleansing removes most substances from the skin surface. Excessive washing may remove lipids and water that normally keep the stratum corneum soft and pliable. In general, deodorant and germicidal soaps tend to irritate eczematic skin. Sensitivity may occur to the perfume, germicide or other additive in a soap. There is little difference in the drying effects of various types of toilet soap. No well-substantiated evidence demonstrates that the addition of neutral fats or cold cream to a soap counteracts the drying effect of soaps. It is highly improbable that such a simple cleansing agent can achieve two diametrically opposed tasks at one time: removal of soil from the skin and deposition of a fat or cream on the skin, especially since the soap is rinsed off.

Transparent soaps, sometimes called glycerin soaps, differ from opaque soaps in their content and method of manufacture. Opaque soap is usually prepared from a mixture of tallow and a lesser proportion of coconut or olive oil. In transparent soap, the fat content is increased by including castor oil or resin and other ingredients, such as alcohol, glycerin and sugar. Since these soaps are softer and more water-soluble, they do not last as long or lather as well as opaque soaps. However, many transparent soaps claim to be "neutral" and less drying or irritating to the skin than opaque soaps, which are generally more alkaline. Although objective evaluations are lacking, transparent soaps are advertised as more acceptable for people with skin problems.

Soapless cleansers, devoid of lipid, have been developed in lotion and gel form. Lotions can be applied liberally and have a foaming action. They are removed gently, leaving a thin film on the skin, thus aiding water retention in the horny layer.

The choice of soap depends primarily on skin condition. In acute eczematous states, soap should be avoided. For milder cases of dermatitis and dry skin, either a mild, nonalkaline soap, an aqueous cream or a soap-free cleanser can be used alternately. Soap is applied only to intact skin to avoid further irritation, and vigorous rubbing or massaging with soaps should be discouraged. Sufficient water should be used to rinse away all traces of the soap.

Emollients

Emollients or moisturizers are externally applied materials that tend to prevent or counteract the signs and symptoms of dry skin. They are designed to soften or give the impression of softening or smoothing the surface of the skin. It is not possible for externally applied oils or even the skin's natural oils to keep skin soft and flexible without the use of water. Very little water from emollients is absorbed by the skin: most water evaporates when the emollient is applied. It is important, therefore, to apply a hydrophobic preparation while the skin is still damp from bathing. This preparation leaves an oily film on the skin surface, retarding evaporation of moisture from the outer layer of skin and thus maintaining hydration and flexibility. Cosmetically, it makes the skin look and feel soft and smooth by smoothing down the rough scaly surface and by decreasing the "drag" or resistance to motion felt when touching the skin.

The wide selection of such bases available includes lotions, creams and ointments. Most of these products are either oil-in-water or water-in-oil emulsions. The greater the oil content, the greater the occlusive effect and the less drying through evaporation. However, users are often intolerant of oil or water-in-oil products because the greasy texture increases discomfort. In addition, a greasy application is unsuitable for an oozing skin dermatitis. In contrast, evaporating water from oil-in-water creams, or especially the more liquid oil-in-water lotions, produces a cooling effect, which alleviates pruritus. The quantities of oil contained are calculated to leave a certain liquid residual film to accomplish hydration.

Other ingredients, such as preservatives, emulsifiers and fragrances, may aggravate an allergic condition through their sensitization potential (for example, parabens, cresols, sodium lauryl sulfate and perfumes). Also, excessive hydration or maceration resulting from too frequent application may damage the skin further.

In treating dermatitis, emulsion bases are selected for their drying or lubricating properties. For a wet dermatitis that has been treated with compresses, a lotion or cream base should be applied after the oozing stops. This base facilitates drying as well as depositing any active medication. In a less acute, drier dermatitis, choose an oil-in-water emulsion base. In the chronic, very dry and scaly dermatitis, a water-in-oil emulsion gives maximum lubrication. Hairy areas may require gels or lotions.

The term "hydrating agents" describes the action achieved when a humectant (moisturizer) is added to an emollient base. These active compounds have hygroscopic (water-attracting) properties, which enable them to draw water into the stratum corneum and hydrate the skin. Examples of such agents include glycerin, propylene glycol, urea, lactic acid and phospholipids. Some provide additional benefits such as the ability to soften keratin (for example, urea). These compounds are discussed individually.

The distinction should be stressed between emollients, which do not draw water but merely trap water present on the skin, and hydrating bases, which attract water to the skin by incorporating humectants.

Compounds in Emollient Bases

Petrolatum, or paraffin, is a derivative of petroleum. It is available in liquid form as mineral oil (liquid paraffin), ointment form as white or yellow soft petrolatum (soft paraffin) and solid form (hard paraffin). It provides an occlusive effect but is cosmetically unacceptable as it feels greasy and does not wash off the skin easily. Paraffins are used as the basis of most greasy or oleaginous ointments. They maintain active ingredients in contact with the skin when prolonged action is required. They provide suitable bases for water unstable drugs. When used alone, they tend to be stable because of the lack of water. One problem associated with petrolatum is the tendency to irritate, particularly erythematous or sensitized skin. Its occlusive effect,

Dermatitis

especially on warm skin, may lead to sweat retention, producing a "prickly heat" type of reaction that can aggravate existing dermatitis.

Yellow petrolatum, or petroleum jelly, can be refined to white petrolatum, which may be more acceptable cosmetically.

Lanolin is derived from the sebum of sheep. A crude grease is recovered from the wool, cleaned with detergent to rid it of dirt and extraneous matter and further refined to give anhydrous lanolin or "wool fat." Lanolin and its derivatives are used widely in cosmetic and pharmaceutical bases. Lanolin is also present in such diverse products as paints, polishes and, occasionally, soaps. Lanolin fatty acids are added to lubricants for their water-repellant properties. Lanolin is a semi-solid, greasy preparation that facilitates spreading of mixtures and adheres well to the skin. It resembles the sebaceous secretion of the human skin and will absorb about 30 per cent of water. It is therefore a useful water-in-oil emulsifier. It is occlusive and has excellent emollient properties. It is added to creams and lotions to impart a smooth and soft texture to the skin. It is less acceptable for use alone because of its odor, its difficulty in removal and its propensity to sensitize. However, derivatives have been prepared to overcome these difficulties since lanolin is more soothing than petrolatum. Eucerin, a wool fat alcohol fraction, makes water-in-oil emulsions that are less sticky and have less color and smell, yet retain the emollient properties of lanolin. Eucerin can also be a sensitizer. Acetylated lanolin also shows a reduced sensitization capacity.

Sebum replacements have been developed with the chemical composition and the physical properties of human sebum. Such a product is recommended as a moisturizing emollient and protectant for dry, flaking skin. Although comparative trials are too few to adequately assess the efficacy of this treatment, these products are available on the cosmetic market.

Hydrating Agents

Caffeine, a methylxanthine, inhibits phosphodiesterase, thereby increasing the levels of cyclic adenosine monophosphate (cAMP) and blocking histamine release induced by antigenic challenge. Concentrations of 10 and 30 per cent have been effective in treating chronic atopic dermatitis. Caffeine has also been combined with hydrocortisone. It is suggested that its presence improves the bioavailability of the steroid. Studies of the hydrating effect of caffeine are still ongoing. The potential of adverse effects from percutaneous absorption should be noted.

Hormone creams, most of which contain estrogen, claim to cause a "plumping" of the skin by retaining water. Dry skin changes, especially those caused by aging, are counteracted by hydration and deposition of an oily film. There is no proof that adding hormones increases the oil activity or the effectiveness of the emollient base in relieving dry skin.

Phospholipid products contain lecithin, which upon hydrolysis yields oleic, palmitic and stearic fatty acids. Lecithin is a water-binding agent that occurs naturally in the skin. Each phospholipid molecule forms a complex with 15 molecules of water. Water is drawn to and kept in the skin to hydrate it and keep it soft and resilient. These preparations also contain emollients such as lanolin and mineral oil in addition to humectants such as glycerin.

Glycerin is an important ingredient in many products. As a result of its humectant or water-attracting properties, glycerin helps keep the product moist and facilitates spreading. However, when applied too liberally and in high concentrations (for example, over 60 per cent), glycerin can increase moisture loss by drawing water from the skin and drying it out further. In such products as glycerin and rose water, glycerin concentration is 50 per cent or less. In these concentrations, glycerin helps retard water evaporation by keeping the water in close contact with the skin. There is no evidence that glycerin is absorbed through the skin.

Propylene glycol is a viscous, colorless, odorless, hydroscopic liquid used as a solvent and vehicle for water-insoluble or unstable compounds. It is less viscous than glycerin, and like alcohol is bactericidal and inhibits mould and fungal growth. Because of its humectant properties, it is incorporated into nongreasy applications for dry skin. Some topical steroid preparations contain about 60 per cent propylene glycol. These preparations can remove scale from the skin by partly denaturing the epidermal proteins and making them more soluble. They also hydrate the stratum corneum through an osmotic effect. A strong aqueous solution (40 to 60 per cent) is effective with occlusion for softening the skin in patients with ichthyosis, a hereditary disorder characterized by the accumulation of large amounts of scale on the skin. The solution produces local irritation on application to mucous membranes and damaged skin surfaces or when occluded. The pH can vary from 4 to 8 among these products, and an acid pH may result in an irritant reaction. On occasion, individuals may develop hypersensitivity to propylene glycol; the incidence has been reported as 0.3 to 2 per cent.

Polyethylene occlusive dressings (for example, plastic wrap) exclude air and hydrate the keratin. Studies show that occlusion helps alleviate dryness of the skin only when the stratum corneum has functionally adequate hydroscopic components to retain the endogenous water. Occlusion is most often used in combination with a topically applied medication to enhance penetration into the horny layer. It has been shown to increase the absorption of topical corticosteroids tenfold.

Keratin Softeners

Urea (carbamide) is an important component of NMF and is included in many dry skin remedies. Anesthetic, antipruritic, bactericidal, antifungal and keratolytic properties have been claimed, but urea's effect on skin disorders probably depends on increased hydration. Urea increases water uptake in the stratum corneum. Although this effect was first described in 1943, urea's initial instability in aqueous creams and lotions deterred incorporation into commercial products. When adjusted to pH 4 with lactic acid, aqueous oleaginous urea preparations are stable and resist hydrolysis.

The concentration of urea affects its action. Concentrations of 10 per cent hydrate dry skin and 15 per cent accelerate fibrin digestion. Concentrations of 20 to 30 per cent are antipruritic, break down keratin, decrease the thickness of the stratum corneum and are used in severe scaling conditions, such as ichthyosis. Concentrations of 40 per cent are proteolytic and have been used to dissolve and peel dystrophic nails.

Urea preparations sometimes cause stinging or burning sensations and may irritate inflamed skin or exudative lesions. This irritation may be due to either the low pH or its hypertonicity at greater concentrations. In preparations with a polysaccharide powder matrix and pH of 6, urea is stable and produces less stinging. Urea has also been combined with other active ingredients, such as corticosteroids, anthralin and benzoyl peroxide, to accelerate skin penetration. Combinations with hydrocortisone are useful for the dry, itching skin of atopic or asteatotic dermatitis.

Dermatitis

Allantoin, a synthetic preparation, may be valuable in treating chronic, scaling dermatoses, including psoriasis, because of its keratin-dispersing activity. It is a relatively safe compound without such disadvantages as staining, burning and discoloration. There are few controlled reports about its use. The United States Food and Drug Administration Advisory Panel recommends allantoin as a safe and effective skin protectant. It may be able to bind to a sensitizing substance, rendering it nonsensitizing.

Alpha-hydroxy acids or closely related substances (for example, lactic, citric, glycolic, malic, pyruvic and glucuronic acids) in concentrations of 5 per cent were evaluated with more than 60 substances that decrease keratin and were found most effective after two weeks. These products may increase biosynthesis of mucopolysaccharides, which are part of intracellular cementing substances for normal keratinization, thus contributing to the natural control of keratinization. In the future, alpha-hydroxy acids may benefit other keratinization disorders such as acne and dandruff. As these compounds may produce irritation at a concentration of 10 per cent, concentrations of 2 to 5 per cent applied twice daily are better for use on large areas or on the whole body. Lactic acid has been combined with urea to stabilize the preparation and to produce an additional hydrating effect. Lactic acid (3 per cent) in emulsifying ointment is valuable for people with dry skin or ichthyosis.

Wet Dressings

Solutions for wet dressings may include ordinary tap water and saline, in addition to astringent and antiseptic compounds. Astringents precipitate protein, thereby decreasing oozing. They are primarily salts of aluminum, zinc, lead, iron, bismuth, tannins or other polyphenols. Wet dressings may be used as compresses or soaks.

Applied as compresses, wet dressings cool and dry the skin through evaporation. They reduce the augmented blood flow in inflammation, cleanse the skin of exudates, crusts and debris, and help maintain drainage of infected areas through vasoconstriction. For these reasons, they are indicated in acute eczematous conditions with oozing and crusting.

The affected person should understand the proper procedure involved in compressing a weeping dermatitis. A nonirritating cloth (for example, facecloth) is soaked with warm or tepid solution, then wrung gently so it remains wet but not dripping. The compress is applied to the skin, then removed, remoistened and reapplied every few minutes for 20 to 30 minute periods, 4 to 6 times daily. After removal, a lotion may be applied to the skin, but occlusion with an ointment should be avoided. Powders are not applied to any exudative lesion as they tend to crust, which may cause bleeding on removal and increase the risk of infection.

Water or saline is often equally effective since the primary benefit of compressing derives from the mechanical cooling, evaporating and cleansing techniques. Cold water compresses often help reduce pruritus in skin that is otherwise nonsymptomatic.

Wet dressing solutions can also be applied as warm soaks to soften hardened crusts in non-oozing scaling conditions. The saturated cloth is applied to the area for 15 to 20 minutes. This procedure occludes and breaks down the tissue below. Soaks are never used for acute, exudating dermatitis as they may macerate the skin and cause further damage to barrier function.

Burow's solution (aluminum acetate) contains approximately 5 per cent aluminum acetate and is diluted 1:10 to 1:40 for use. It is easy to use, comes in tablets or powders, does not stain, and is drying, soothing and mildly antiseptic. It is available alone or with an antiseptic.

Potassium permanganate is a germicidal oxidizing agent as well as an astringent. It is inactivated rapidly by body fluids such as pus and is not effective in oozing conditions. It stains the skin and clothing. Undissolved crystals may cause a chemical burn. It is little better than water as a wet dressing and is now seldom used. A 1:4,000 to 1:6,000 dilution is used for weeping or denuded areas (65 mg in 250 mL or 1,000 mL). For baths of 1:25,000, 650 mg of potassium permanganate are dissolved in 16.25 L of water or a full tub. Skin stains can be removed with a weak solution of oxalic acid.

Anti-inflammatory Agents

Hydrocortisone was the first topical steroid to be clinically effective in dermatitis by virtue of both anti-inflammatory and immunosuppressive activity.

Its nonspecific, anti-inflammatory action is exerted in widely different kinds of inflammation including infective, physical and allergic types. In inflammation, certain white blood cells (polymorphs and monocytes) stick to the walls of small blood vessels (marginate), then penetrate and migrate to the focus of disease (chemotaxis). Dilatation of these vessels and an increase in their permeability result in tissue swelling. Hydrocortisone reverses these processes. This effect is achieved through a number of mechanisms:

- Prevention of margination and chemotaxis appears to be a direct effect on leukocytes.
- Attachment to tissue receptors decreases membrane permeability and inhibits the release of toxic substances.
- Vasoconstriction decreases seepage of serum through the vessel wall and into the surrounding tissue (extravasation) and lessens swelling and associated discomfort, including pruritus.

Thus, hydrocortisone alleviates itch as well as the four cardinal signs of inflammation (redness, heat, pain and swelling).

The immunosuppressive effect of hydrocortisone is distinct from its action on inflammation. With the exception of dry skin, dermatitis is a cell-mediated immune reaction involving T-lymphocytes. This type of reaction is known as delayed hypersensitivity. Hydrocortisone produces a clinical response in such disorders by suppressing the action of the lymphocytes on the target cell.

The anti-inflammatory and immunosuppressive actions of hydrocortisone allow it to achieve good clinical response in suppressing both the reactive symptoms and the underlying mechanism in atopic dermatitis, allergic and irritant contact dermatitis, and the inflammatory phase of dry skin.

Unlike more potent corticosteroids, hydrocortisone does not affect protein synthesis of human skin. It is therefore ineffective in proliferative disorders such as psoriasis in decreasing cell multiplication and keratin formation, although it suppresses inflammation. This lack of antiproliferative action enables hydrocortisone to be the only topical corticosteroid free of undesirable antiproliferative side effects, such as striae (stretch marks), acne, bruising, thinning of the skin and telangiectasis (spider-like markings).

A number of factors influence the degree of response to hydrocortisone therapy, including concentration, quantity, frequency, occlusion, vehicle, combination with other agents and condition of the skin.

Concentration: There is no doubt a dose-response relationship exists. Higher concentrations have more drug available for absorption per unit area. Evidence is inconclusive on the efficacy of hydrocortisone preparations of less than 0.5 per cent potency.

Table V *Amount of Topical Steroid Required for a Single Daily Application*

Body area	Amount (grams)
Head (not scalp)	1–2
Trunk (anterior)	3–6
Trunk (posterior)	3–6
Arms (each)	1–2
Legs (each)	3–6
Genito-anal area	1–2
Total body	15–30

Adapted from: Schlagel CA, Sanborn EC. The weights of topical preparations required for total and partial body inunction. J Invest Dermatol 1964;42:253–6.

Quantity: Statistical analysis shows no correlation between the quantity of cream applied and the penetration of the steroid. The uppermost layer of skin can accumulate only a limited amount of steroid and a saturated state is reached rapidly. For therapeutic and economic reasons, it is generally recommended that hydrocortisone be applied sparingly. The appropriate amounts of steroid required for a single daily application to specific body areas have been determined and are shown in Table V.

Frequency: Response to topical steroid therapy decreases after continued use for some weeks. Clinical response can be induced again by choosing an alternative prescription steroid or by allowing a rest period before resuming treatment. Tolerance may occur less often to hydrocortisone than to more potent steroids. Nevertheless, it is rational to apply hydrocortisone in intermittent courses rather than as continuous treatment. The best clinical result is obtained if hydrocortisone is initially applied more often; once the condition begins to respond, the daily frequency is limited to the least number of applications necessary to maintain control. They are ideally applied immediately after a bath, while the skin is still damp.

Occlusion: Anything that covers the site of hydrocortisone application (bandages, dressings or natural body folds) excludes air and hydrates the skin, making it more permeable to drug absorption. Occlusive dressings enhance penetration and potency of topical steroids tenfold.

Vehicle: The choice of vehicle in which hydrocortisone is applied to the skin should be determined by the physical action desired for the skin. Gels and lotions tend to be the driest preparations, and ointments the most lubricating. Water-miscible creams are for moist, weeping areas. Ointments are best for dry, scaly or lichenified skin as they are more occlusive than creams. Lotions are sometimes useful for large areas when minimal application is needed. They are also useful on the scalp.

Combinations: A variety of other agents have been combined with hydrocortisone to enhance its topical potency. Combinations with urea increase the hydration of keratin, thereby improving steroid availability and penetration. Incorporating a surface-active agent (sodium lauryl sulfate) mobilizes hydrocortisone from the vehicle onto the skin, significantly increasing its therapeutic activity. Pretreatment with a keratolytic gel (salicylic acid-propylene glycol) enhances response by removing thickened stratum corneum. Salicylic acid may be added to the base to increase epidermal penetration.

Condition of the skin: It has been demonstrated that dermatitis influences the skin barrier to glucocorticoids. One study has shown that the percutaneous absorption of labelled hydrocortisone was higher in children with atopic dermatitis than with normal skin. Another investigator found topically applied hydrocortisone caused an increment in plasma cortisol levels in both the acute and convalescent phases of dermatitis. This decreased significantly as the dermatitis improved despite excessive application of hydrocortisone, reflecting the restoration of the skin barrier.

An incidence of allergy (4.8 per cent) to hydrocortisone in patients with suspected allergic contact dermatitis has been reported. Any dermatitis that does not improve or deteriorates after administration of hydrocortisone should be referred to a physician.

Antipruritic Agents

Although pruritus is a symptom rather than a disease, its intense discomfort should not be underestimated. It is the predominant complaint in atopic dermatitis, and prevention of the damage from scratching is a key point of therapy. The success of topical antipruritic agents can be attributed partially to substitution: a new sensation, such as cold, replaces the itch. Refrigerating the product increases this effect. The cause of the itch governs selection of a topical antipruritic. For a contact or atopic dermatitis, it is best to avoid products that may cause further sensitization.

Phenol is an antiseptic and caustic agent that decreases itch by anesthetizing the cutaneous nerve endings. It is used in concentrations of 0.5 to 2 per cent. The antibacterial and caustic effects are reduced if phenol is dissolved in alcohol, glycerin or fixed oils. Phenol is a local irritant and should not be used in concentrations greater than 4 per cent. Its toxicity depends on the magnitude and location of the area exposed. Moist areas, such as underarms, groin and feet, are more absorptive and more susceptible to irritation. Infants are most susceptible to percutaneous absorption. Phenol may also cross-sensitize to hydroquinone. Water, oil or alcohol can be used to remove phenol from the skin.

Thymol is obtained either from thyme and ajowan oils or prepared synthetically. It is a more powerful disinfectant than phenol, and its antipruritic effect is similar. However, thymol irritates tissues and is inactivated by bacterial proteins. It has a more agreeable odor than phenol. Thymol is used in concentrations of 0.25 to 1 per cent and is incorporated into antifungal preparations due to its fungicidal effects.

Camphor is a ketone derived from the camphor tree. It has mild antipruritic effects through its anesthetic properties when applied in concentrations of 1 to 3 per cent. It is a local irritant and a weak antiseptic. It is often combined with phenol to form a complex that impedes the percutaneous absorption and decreases the corrosiveness of phenol. Camphor is present in nail polishes as a plasticizer.

Menthol is a cyclic alcohol derived from peppermint and other mint oils or prepared synthetically. Applied to the skin, it dilates the vessels, causing a sensation of coldness followed by an analgesic effect. It is used in concentrations of 0.25 to 2 per cent, and is sometimes combined with camphor, phenol, thymol or chloral hydrate to form a semi-solid mass. It is used as a flavoring agent in such products as cosmetics, toothpastes, candy, cigarettes and mouthwashes. It has been reported to be a sensitizer, but widespread use makes its avoidance as a contact allergen difficult.

Calamine is a basic zinc carbonate colored with ferric oxide. It has a mild astringent action on the skin and is used as a dusting powder,

Dermatitis

cream, lotion, liniment or ointment in concentrations of 4 to 20 per cent to relieve pruritus. It also has been combined with phenol to retard absorption.

Witch hazel (hamamelis water) is found in nonprescription antipruritic preparations, especially those for hemorrhoids. It has a mild astringent effect but is also a contact sensitizer.

Antihistamines have been classified as those which bind to an H_1 receptor site and those which bind to an H_2 receptor site. Antihistamines of the H_1 receptor type may be used orally for their antipruritic and sedative properties. They are most effective for acute urticaria (hives), chronic urticaria and other allergic skin reactions, including drug reactions. They have not been shown more effective than acetylsalicylic acid for relief of nonhistamine-related itching. However, they provide significant relief for pruritus through the placebo effect (especially oral preparations). Individuals may react differently to the several chemical classes of antihistamines. One or several antihistamines may be tried to achieve the best therapeutic effect if sensitization occurs.

The most effective antihistamine in suppressing histamine-induced pruritus is hydroxyzine, a prescription drug. The sedative properties of antihistamines should be mentioned to any person taking other central nervous system depressants, consuming alcohol, driving a car or operating machinery. Antihistamines free of sedative effects are terfenadine, astemizole and loratadine. The ethanolamine type of antihistamine, such as diphenhydramine, is the most sedating. The long-acting, nonsedating antihistamines are not as effective for pruritus. Results have been disappointing with mast cell stabilizers such as ketotifen but better with oxatomide. (For more information on the sedative properties of antihistamines, see the chapter on sleep disorders and sleep aids.)

Topically administered antihistamines are contained in many nonprescription combination products. Their use should be avoided because of possible sensitization and questionable efficacy. Any benefit is overshadowed by the risk of inducing an allergic contact dermatitis.

Coal tar is a complex, natural substance distilled from bituminous coal. The chief constituents are hydrocarbons, such as benzene, naphthalene, phenols and pitch, combined with small quantities of pyridine and quinoline. It may be that the phenols are responsible for the antipruritic effect. Coal tar is a black, viscous liquid with a strong odor. The keratoplastic and reducing effect resides chiefly in the heavy oil and pitch fraction. Its astringent and antipruritic properties make it effective in treating atopic dermatitis, chronic eczema and psoriasis.

Tar is a relatively weak photosensitizer. Although it may be combined with ultraviolet light to augment its effects in psoriasis, it also acts independently. Tar couples with DNA in rapidly dividing cells, preventing mitosis in active dermatitis. The tar promotes a return to normal keratinization in eczematous and hyperplastic diseases. It can be a primary irritant, especially on hairy areas of the skin, and may cause an acneiform or pustular reaction.

Users rub medication containing tar in the direction that hair normally lies, avoiding circular motion. The tar product can be covered with a protective soft dressing, such as stockinette or old flannel pyjamas, to prevent excessive smearing. The color, odor, and photo sensitizing properties of coal tar limit its cosmetic acceptance.

Liquor carbonis detergens (LCD), a coal tar solution, is prepared by extracting coal tar with polysorbate and alcohol. Thus refined, it is much weaker than coal tar. LCD may be incorporated in concentrations from 2 to 20 per cent in creams, ointments or shampoos or added to the bath (50 mL) for therapeutic effects in various dermatitic conditions.

Wood Tars. Oils of cade, beech, birch and pine are widely used in 1 to 10 per cent strengths in ointments, pastes or solutions. They are not photosensitizers and lack the pyridine, quinoline and quinaldine rings of coal tar.

Bituminous Tars. These tars were first derived from the distillation of shale deposits containing fossilized fish, giving rise to the name of the compound, "ichthyol". About 10 per cent of ichthyol is sulphur. Bituminous tars are less effective than coal tar; are not photosensitizers and may have a different mechanism of action.

Summary

In recommending the most appropriate treatment to the person with dermatitis, the pharmacist should follow these guidelines:

- Whereas acute dermatitis may require a short and temporary course of therapy, chronic conditions may need continual treatment to maintain control. To ensure compliance and proper response, pharmacists should recommend the easiest, most effective, least costly and most tolerable regimen.
- One of the most effective and safest antipruritics in topical form is bland calamine lotion or cream, applied cold. Oral antihistamines are an alternative treatment and may be safer than a topical form, although not always effective.
- Avoid preparations that may cause allergic or irritant reactions because of fragrance, dyes, preservatives or sensitizers.
- Some forms of dermatitis may become severe or infected and should be referred to a physician. All treatments should be discontinued.

Ask the Consumer

Q. Is the rash painful or itchy? How often do you scratch your skin? Do you scratch only when itchy, often out of habit, or perhaps unconsciously during sleep?

■ The itch sensation is generated near the skin surface (superficial dermis) and is usually a symptom of dermatitis. The severity of the itch, reflected by the amount of scratching, varies with the type of dermatitis and influences the choice of therapy.

Severe itching, such as occurs in acute atopic or contact dermatitis, is treated with topical antipruritics, oral antihistamines or both. Dry skin is relatively less itchy and may not require treatment for this symptom. The sensation of pain is most often generated deep down in the skin, near the fat layer, and is not usually a symptom of dermatitis. It may reflect another cause for the rash, such as infection.

Q. At what age did this condition begin? How has it changed?

■ Atopic dermatitis appears in different patterns in sequential order in infantile, childhood and adult forms of the disease. Contact dermatitis can appear at any age. Hand dermatitis is not a function of age but rather is related to the individual's occupation. Dry skin is most common in the elderly. Appropriate treatment corresponds to the appearance of the symptoms.

Dermatitis

*Q. Does anyone in your family have a similar condition?
Does anyone in your family have asthma, hay fever or
other allergies?*

■ Dermatitis is not generally contagious. Poison ivy dermatitis may result from indirect contact with pet fur or clothing. Any other contagious rash may be an infection or infestation (for example, impetigo or scabies) contracted from a family member or pet who should also be treated.

Atopic dermatitis has genetic predispositions and may be associated with a family history of asthma, hay fever or rhinitis.

Q. What areas are involved? Describe how the skin looks and feels.

■ Appropriate nonprescription treatment cannot be chosen until the type of dermatitis is determined. Types are distinguished by symptoms, location, description and trigger factors. Any undiagnosed rash unresponsive to rational nonprescription therapy should be referred to a physician.

Wet, crusting lesions, such as those present in acute contact dermatitis, require the drying effect of compresses, but dry skin requires lubrication. Broken skin is more susceptible to infections and is more absorptive, increasing the likelihood of side effects from topical medication. A lesion that is warm generally indicates inflammation and requires anti-inflammatory and possibly anti-infective treatment. Contact dermatitis usually resembles the pattern of the contacting substance.

*Q. Do any of these factors make the rash worse: dryness or
dampness, time of year or day, diet, work or household
routines, chemicals or soaps, cosmetics, clothing,
jewelry or anxiety?*

■ Possible aggravating factors must be reduced as much as possible or eliminated.

*Q. What treatments have you tried? Has the rash improved
or become worse?*

■ Some nonprescription or prescription medications may exacerbate a person's symptoms, elicit an allergic response or cross-sensitize to an allergic contactant. A person whose dermatitis is unresponsive to reasonable nonprescription measures should be referred to a physician.

References

Dermatitis

Allen BR, Parkinson R. Chinese herbs for eczema. Lancet 1990;336 (8708):177.

Allen R. Diet. Br Med J 1988;297(6661):1459–60.

Aly R, Maibach HI, Shinefield HR. Microbial flora of atopic dermatitis. Arch Dermatol 1977;113:780–2.

Arndt KA, ed. Manual of dermatologic therapeutics. Philadelphia: Little, 1978:50–7,74–5.

Atherton DJ. Dietary antigen avoidance in the treatment of atopic dermatitis. Acta Derm Venereol (Stockh) 1980;(Suppl 92):99–102.

Atherton DJ. Allergy and atopic eczema II. Clin Exp Dermatol 1981;6:317–25.

Atherton DJ. Role of diet in treating atopic eczema. Br Med J 1988;297 (6661):1458–60.

Atherton DJ, Sewell M, Soothill JF, et al. A double-blind controlled crossover trial of antigen-avoidance diet in atopic eczema. Lancet 1978;1:401.

Atherton D, et al. Chinese herbs for eczema. Lancet 1990; 336(8725):1254.

Ayres SJ. Atopic dermatitis—a new therapeutic regimen. JAMA 1983;250 (2):2926–7.

Ayres SJ. The report by Dr. Alan Shalita on dermatitis and eczema. Cutis 1986;38(3):174,182.

Baer R. Papaverine therapy in atopic dermatitis. J Amer Dermatol Assoc 1985;13(5):806–8.

Baker H. The skin as a barrier. In: Rook A, Wilkinson DS, Ebling FJ, eds. Textbook of dermatology. Oxford: Blackwell Scientific, 1986:355–66.

Baker H, Kligman AM. Measurement of transepidermal water loss by electric hydrometry. Instrumentation and responses to physical and chemical insults. Arch Dermatol 1967;96:441–52.

Berth-Jones J, Graham-Brown RAC. Treatment of itching in atopic eczema. Br Med J 1989;6671:461.

Bamford J, et al. Atopic eczema unresponsiveness to evening primrose oil (linoleic and linolenic acids). J Amer Acad Dermatol 1985;13(6):959–65.

Bettley AR, Grace KA. Influence of ambient humidity on transepidermal water loss. Br J Dermatol 1967;79:575–81.

Blank IH. Factors which influence the water content of the stratum corneum. J Invest Dermatol 1952;18:440–3.

Blank IH. Further observations on factors which influence the water control of the stratum corneum. J Invest Dermatol 1953;21:259–69.

Calnan CD. Eczema for me. Trans St Johns Hosp Dermatol Soc Lond 1968;54:54–64.

Caputo RV, et al. Diet and atopic dermatitis. J Amer Dermatol Assoc 1986; 15(3):543–5.

Dahl M. Research on atopic dermatitis. Arch Dermatol 1986;122(3):265–6.

Dahl MV, Cates KL, Quie PG. Neutrophil chemotaxis in patients with atopic dermatitis without infection. Arch Dermatol 1978;114:544–6.

de Prost, et al. Double-blind randomized placebo-controlled trial of local cyclosporine in atopic dermatitis. Arch Dermatol 1989;125(4):570.

Doherty V, et al. Treatment of itching in atopic eczema with antihistamines with a low sedative profile. Br Med J 1989;298(6666):96.

Ebling FJ. The normal skin. In: Rook A, Wilkinson DS, Ebling FJ, eds. Textbook of dermatology. Oxford: Blackwell Scientific, 1986:5–38.

Fisher AA. Irritant reactions from topical urea preparations used for dry skin. Advantages of a urea-free "Dead Sea salt" cream. Cutis 1976;18:761–7.

Fromer JL, Goehas MC. Cutaneous manifestations in lymphoma. New York Med 1963;63:3222–8.

Gaul LE, Underwood GB. Relation of dewpoint and barometric pressure of chapping of normal skin. J Invest Dermatol 1952;19:9–19.

Hanifin JM. Atopic dermatitis. J Allergy Clin Immunol 1984;73(2):211–22.

Hanifin JM, Lobitz WC Jr. Newer concepts of atopic dermatitis. Arch Dermatol 1977;113:663–70.

Hanifin JM. Diet, nutrition and allergy in atopic dermatitis. J Am Acad Dermatol 1983;8:729–31.

Hansen AE. Study of iodine number of serum fatty acids in infantile eczema. Proc Soc Exp Biol Med 1933;30:1198–9.

Hathaway MJ, Warner JO. Compliance problems in the dietary management of eczema. Arch Dis Child 1983;58:463–4.

Horrobin DF, Stewart C. Evening primrose oil in atopic eczema. Lancet 1990; 336(8706):50.

Hoxtell E, Dahl MV. Xerosis from lithium carbonate (Letter). Arch Dermatol 1975;111:1073–4.

Jacobi OK. About the mechanism of moisture regulation in the horny layer of the skin. Proc Sci Sect Toilet Goods Assoc 1959;31:22.

Jensen P. Use of alternative medicine by patients with atopic dermatitis and psoriasis. Acta Derm Venereol (Stockh) 1990;70(5):421–4,425–8.

Kajosaar M, Saarinen UM. Prophylaxis of atopic disease by six months total solid food elimination. Acta Paediatr Scand 1983;72:411–4.

Krafchik BR. Atopic dermatitis. Pediatric Clin North Am 1983;30:669–85.

Lever WF, Schaumberg-Lever G. Histology of the skin. In: Lever SF, Schaumberg-Lever G, eds. Histopathology of the skin. Philadelphia: JB Lippincott, 1975:9–45.

Lithell H, Bruce A, Gustafsson IB, Hoglund NJ, Karlstrom B, Ljunghall K, Sjolin K, Vessby B. A fasting vegetarian diet treatment trial on chronic inflammatory disorders. Acta Derm Venereol (Stockh) 1983;63:397–403.

Melin L, et al. Behavioural treatment of scratching in patients with atopic dermatitis. Br J Dermatol 1986;115(4):467–74.

Dermatitis

Mercer EH, Jahn RA, Maibach HI. Surface coats containing polysaccharides on human epidermal cell. J Invest Dermatol 1968;51(3):204–14.

Middleton JD. Pathways of penetration of electrolytes through stratum corneum. Br J Dermatol 1969;81(Suppl):56–61.

Middleton JD. The mechanism of water binding in stratum corneum. Br J Dermatol 1968;80:437–50.

Moeller H. Clinical aspects of atopic dermatitis in childhood. Acta Derm Venereol (Stockh) 1981;(Suppl 95):25–8.

Nield VS, Marsden RA, Bailes JA, Bland JM. Egg and milk exclusion diets in atopic eczema. Br J Dermatol 1986;114:117–23.

Rasmussen RE. Recent developments in the management of patients with atopic dermatitis. J Allergy Clin Immunol 1984;76(6):771–6.

Rasmussen JE. Advances in nondietary management of children with atopic dermatitis. Pediatr Dermatol 1989;6(3):210–5.

Reed ML, et al. A usage safety study of 2 new dry skin formulations in patients with atopic dermatitis. Cutis 1983;32:180–4.

Rokugo M, et al. Contact sensitivity to P. ovale in patients with atopic dermatitis. Arch Dermatol 1990;126(5):627–32.

Rook A, Wilkinson DS. Atopic dermatitis. In: Rook A, Wilkinson DS, Ebling FJ, eds. Textbook of dermatology. Oxford: Blackwell Scientific, 1986:419–34.

Roth HL. Atopic dermatitis revisited. Int J Derm 1987;26(3):139–44.

Scholtz JR. Atopic dermatitis (Letter). Arch Dermatol 1979;115:110.

Sharpe GR, Farr PM. Evening primrose oil and eczema. Lancet 1990;335(8700):1283.

Uehara M. Atopic dermatitis and tuberculin reactivity. Arch Dermatol 1977;113:1226–8.

Van Asperen PP, Lewis M, Rogers M, Kemp AS, Thompson S. Experience with an elimination diet in children with atopic dermatitis. Clin Allergy 1983;13:479–85.

Van Joost T, et al. Efficacy of low dose cyclosporin in severe atopic skin disease. Arch Dermatol 1987;123(2):166–7.

Verbov J. Modern management of atopic eczema. Practitioner 1984;228:1013–7.

Verbov J. Treatment of atopic eczema. Arch Dis Child 1986;61:518–21.

Vickers CF. The management of the problem atopic in 1988. Acta Derm Venereol 1989;Suppl 144:23–5.

Villaveces JW, Heiner DC. Experience with an elemental diet (Vivonex). Ann Allergy 1985;55:783–9.

Walzer RA. Dermatitis and eczema: a few rash statements. Skintelligence: how to be smart about your skin. New York: Appleton-Century-Crofts, 1981:71–87.

Wolfram LF. Some thoughts on skin "moisturization". Cutis 1978;21:148.

Wright S, Burton JL. Oral evening-primrose-seed oil improves atopic eczema. Lancet 1982;2:1120–2.

Contact Dermatitis

Fergusson DM, Horwood LJ, Beautrais AL, Shannon FT, Taylor B. Eczema and infant diet. Clin Allergy 1981;11:325–31.

Golding J, Butler NR, Taylor R. Breastfeeding and eczema/asthma. Lancet 1982;1(8272):623.

Thomson AW, et al. Topical cyclosporin in alopecia areata and nickel contact dermatitis. Lancet 1986;8513:971–2.

Wilkinson JD, Rycroft RJG. Contact dermatitis. In: Rook A, Wilkinson DS, Ebling RJ, eds. Textbook of dermatology. Oxford: Blackwell Scientific, 1986:435–532.

Poison Ivy Contact Dermatitis

Alex JF, Seitzer CM. Poison ivy. Ontario Ministry of Agriculture and Food. Fact sheet. 1981;November 1–4.

Caserio RJ. Bites, rashes and itches. Postgrad Med 1983;73(5):267–73.

Epstein WL. Topical prevention of poison ivy/oak dermatitis. Arch Dermatol 1989;125(4):499–501.

Guin JD. Poison ivy (Rhus) dermatitis. J Indiana State Med Assoc 1978;71:774–5.

Hall NA. OTC Products for Rhus dermatitis: zirconium containing topical applications. J Am Pharm Assoc 1972;NS12:576–7.

Orchard S, Fellman JH, Storrs R. Poison ivy/oak dermatitis. Arch Dermatol 1986;122:783–9.

Parish LC, Haviland TN. The saga of poison ivy. Trans and Studies of the College of Phys of Philadelphia 1974;42:88–93.

Hand Dermatitis

Fisher AA. Contact dermatitis. Philadelphia: Lea & Febiger, 1973:49–65.

Fisher AA. Contact dermatitis due to topical medications. In: Maddin S. Current dermatologic therapy. Philadelphia: WB Saunders, 1982:100–3.

Provost T. Hand eczema. Demis Clin Dermatol 1985;3:13–19,1–7.

Rycroft, RJG. The management of hand eczema. The Practitioner 1984;228(Nov):1019–23.

Dry Skin

Baughman RD, Porter PS. Eczema hiemalis. Demis Clin Dermatol 1985;3:13–14,1–2.

Fine JD, Arndt K. Dry skin. Demis Clin Dermatol 1985;1:1–19,1–3.

Bath Products

Fisher AA. Contact dermatitis due to topical medications. In: Maddin S, ed. Current dermatologic therapy. Philadelphia: WB Saunders, 1982:103–5.

Soaps

Cronin E. Soaps. In: Cronin E, ed. Contact dermatitis. New York: Churchill Livingstone, 1980:814–5.

Cronin E, Kullavanijaya P. Hand dermatitis in hairdressers. Acta Derm Venereol (Stockh) 1979;59(Suppl 85):47–50.

Emollients

Blank IH. Factors that influence the water content of the skin. J Invest Dermatol 1958;29:433.

Boccanfuso SM, Cosmet L, Volpe AR. Skin xerosis. Clinical report on the effect of a moisturizing soap bar. Cutis 1978:703–7.

Cronin E. Lanolin. In: Cronin E, ed. Contact dermatitis. New York: Churchill Livingstone, 1980:771–84.

Griffiths WAD, Ive FA, Wilkinson DS. Topical therapy—cleansing agents. In: Rook A, Wilkinson DS, Ebling FJ, eds. Textbook of dermatology. Oxford: Blackwell Scientific, 1986:2529–73.

Maisey AR, Brook JHR. Initial experience with Natuderm, a new skin film emulsion analogue cream. Br J Clin Pract 1980;34:178–81.

Hydrating Agents

Cronin E. Propylene glycol. In: Cronin E, ed. Contact dermatitis. New York: Churchill Livingstone, 1980:809–11.

Fisher AA, Pasher R, Kanol NB. Allergic contact dermatitis due to ingredients of vehicles. A "vehicle tray" for patch testing. Arch Dermatol 1971;104:286–90.

Fisher A.A. Propylene glycol dermatitis. Cutis 1978:21:166.

Flesch P, Jackson-Esoda EC. Deficient water binding in pathologic horny layers. J Invest Dermatol 1957;28:5–13.

Goldsmith LA, Badin HP. Propylene glycol with occlusion for the treatment of ichthyosis. JAMA 1972;220:579.

Kaplan RJ, Daman L, Shereff R, et al. Treatment of atopic dermatitis with topically applied caffeine. Arch Dermatol 1976;112:880–1.

Kaplan RJ, Daman L, Rosenberg EW. Topical use of caffeine with hydrocortisone in the treatment of atopic dermatitis. Arch Dermatol 1978;114:60–2.

Kaplan RJ, Daman L, Rosenberg EW. Treatment of atopic dermatitis with topically applied caffeine: a follow-up report (Letter). Arch Dermatol 1977;113:107.

Marks R. Techniques for the evaluation of emollients and keratolytics. J Soc Cosmet Chem 1978;29:433.

Powers DH, Fox C. A study of the effect of cosmetic ingredients, creams and lotions on the rate of moisture loss from the skin. Proc Sci Sect Toilet Goods Assoc 1957;28:21.

Rothman S. Physiology and pathology of keratinization. Soc Cosmet Chem 1978;29:433.

Schoen LA. Skin and hair care. London: JB Lippincott, 1976:32,36.

Wilkinson DS. Topical therapy—bases. In: Rook A, Wilkinson DS, Ebling FJ, eds. Textbook of dermatology. Oxford: Blackwell Scientific, 1972:2063–8.

Dermatitis

Urea

Farber EM, South DA. Urea ointment in the nonsurgical avulsion of nail dystrophies. Cutis 1978;22:689–92.

Sneddon IB. Clinical use of topical corticosteroids. Drugs 1976;11:193.

Wilkinson DS. Topical agents commonly used in dermatological therapy. In: Rook A, Wilkinson DS, Ebling FJ, eds. Textbook of dermatology. Oxford: Blackwell Scientific, 1979:2293–328.

Allantoin

Anonymous. Today's drugs—allantoin. Br Med J 1967;iv:535.

Alpha-hydroxy Acids

McKenzie AW, Wilkinson DS. Topical therapy. In: Rook A, ed. Recent advances in dermatology IV. London: Churchill Livingstone, 1977:307.

Van Scott EJ, Yu RJ. Control of kertinization with alphahydroxy acids and related compounds. Arch Dermatol 1974;110:586–90.

Wet Dressings

Arndt KA. Wet dressings. Manual of dermatological therapeutics with essentials of diagnosis. Philadelphia: Little, Brown, 1978:330–3.

Hydrocortisone

Almeyda J, Burt BN. Double blind controlled study of atopic eczema with a preparation of hydrocortisone in a new drug delivery system versus betamethasone 17 valerate. Br J Dermatol 1974;92:579–83.

Baden HP. Therapy with keratolytic gel and corticosteroid ointment (Letter). Arch Dermatol 1975;111:1536.

Bush IE. Proceedings of the second international congress on hormonal steroids. 1967:60–7.

Goodwin P. The effect of corticosteroids on cell turnover in the psoriatic patient. Br J Dermatol 1976;94(Suppl):95–100.

Liston AJ. Availability of nonprescription topical preparations containing hydrocortisone. Information letter no 714. Ottawa: Health Protection Branch, Health and Welfare Canada, 1986:Sep 10.

Morley N. Minimizing the use of topical steroids in children. Practitioner 1988;232:949–51.

Norin P, et al. The effect of combined topical steroids and habit-reversal therapy in patients with atopic dermatitis. Brit J Dermatol 1989;121(3):359–66.

Polano MK. Factors influencing the penetration of corticosteroids through the epidermis. Adv Biol Skin 1972;12:325–38.

Polano MK, Ponec M. Dependence of corticosteroid penetration on the vehicle. Arch Dermatol 1976;112:675–80.

Ricciatti D, Lester RS. Topical corticosteroid therapy. Mod Med Can 1977;32:546–54.

Schlagel CA, Sanborn EC. The weights of topical preparations required for total and partial body inunction. J Invest Dermatol 1964;42:253–6.

Schopf E. Side effects from topical corticosteroid therapy. Ann Clin Res 1975;79:353–67.

Sneddon IB. Clinical use of topical corticosteroids. Drugs 1976;11:193–9.

Snell ES. The pharmacological properties of corticosteroids. Br J Dermatol 1976;94(Suppl):15–23.

Spearman RIC, Jarrett A. The mouse tail test for evaluation of topically applied corticosteroids. Arch Dermatol 1975;111:581–3.

Turpeinen R, et al. Percutaneous absorption of hydrocortisone during and after the acute phase of dermatitis in children. Pediatr Dermatol 1988;5(4):276–9.

Whitfield M, McKenzie AW. A new formulation of 1% hydrocortisone cream with vasoconstrictive activity and clinical efficacy. Br J Dermatol 1975;92:585–8.

Wilkinson SM, Cartwright PH, English JSC. Hydrocortisone: an important cutaneous allergen: Lancet 1991;337(March 30):761–2.

Wilson L. The clinical assessment of topical corticosteroid activity. Br J Dermatol 1976;94(Suppl):33–42.

Antipruritic Agents

Adveneir C, et al. Rational use of antihistamines in allergic dermatological conditions. Drugs 1989;38(4):634–44.

Arndt KA. Manual of dermatological therapeutics with essentials of diagnosis. Philadelphia: Little, Brown, 1978:306–11,319–26.

Fisher AA. Contact dermatitis. Philadelphia: Lea & Febiger, 1973:20.

Maisey AR, Brook JHR. Initial experience with Natuderm, a new skin film emulsion analogue cream. Br J Clin Pract 1980;34:178–81.

6

Psoriasis, Seborrheic Dermatitis and Dandruff

Dale E. Wright

The several types of psoriasis, most of which are suitable for self-medication, respond to different pharmacologic and nonpharmacologic treatments. Nonprescription drug treatments include keratolytics, coal tar and anthralin. Prescription treatments include glucocorticoids, antimetabolites, etretinate, psoralens and cyclosporine. Dandruff and most cases of seborrhea are highly responsive to nonprescription treatment with cytostatic, antifungal, keratolytic and antiseptic agents in easy-to-use shampoos, lotions, gels, ointments and pastes.

Psoriasis, seborrhea and dandruff are a group of chronic, scaly dermatoses. They may present simply a cosmetic problem (dandruff) or a significant emotional and economic burden (psoriasis). Nonprescription treatment is the cornerstone of therapy for dandruff and seborrhea, and is an important adjunctive therapy for psoriasis. In general, mild or chronic noninflamed psoriasis is suitable for self-

medication. Unresponsive lesions or involvement of the face or intertriginous region should be referred to a physician. Nonprescription drug therapy alone is suitable for dandruff and adequately controls most cases of seborrhea. Each of these conditions is dealt with separately (see Table I).

Psoriasis

Psoriasis is a chronic, scaly, erythematous disease of unknown etiology, for which there is no cure. In North America, the prevalence ranges from 0.5 to 1.5 per cent of the population. Psoriasis occurs equally in males and females, with onset most frequently in the 20s. Usually it follows an irregular, chronic course marked by remissions and exacerbations of unpredictable onset and duration. Forty per cent of people with the condition experience a remission at some point and 30 per cent find the disease disappears without medical intervention.

Table I *Differential Diagnosis of Dandruff, Seborrhea and Psoriasis*

	Dandruff	Seborrhea	Psoriasis
Location	Scalp	Adults and children: scalp, eyebrows, forehead, nose, ears, trunk Children only: back, intertriginous areas	Scalp, elbows, knees, trunk, lower extremities
Aggravating factors	Relatively stable. May be exacerbated by inadequate washing, dry climate	Exacerbated by stress, low relative humidity, low temperature	Exacerbated by stress, mechanical irritation, infection, endocrine factors, climate, drugs
Appearance	Thin, white or greyish flakes spread evenly on scalp	Patchy lesions with indistinct margins, mild inflammation, oily, yellowish scales	Usually symmetrical, red patchy plaques with sharp border, silvery-white scale. May be difficult to distinguish from seborrhea in early stages or in intertriginous zones
Treatment	Cytostatic/Antiyeast shampoos	Cytostatic/Antiyeast shampoos Topical steroids Systemic agents	Keratolytics Coal tar Topical steroids

Psoriasis, Seborrheic Dermatitis and Dandruff

Psoriatic lesions are characterized by increased epidermal cell turnover, the presence of inflammatory cells, and vascular alterations. The immune system is thought to play an important role in the pathogenesis of psoriasis, possibly inducing a primary defect in the skin cell which allows uncontrolled growth to occur, or by the activation of other cells which produce skin cell growth-promoting mediators. Environmental factors that affect the immune system play a role in precipitating active psoriasis. These include streptococcal and HIV infections, reactions to medications, and stress. In addition, there appears to be a genetic predisposition to psoriasis, with a familial pattern in 30 per cent of patients. Genetic markers for psoriasis have been detected, although the gene (or genes) responsible for the disease have not been identified.

Onset or exacerbation of psoriasis is often attributed to stress, although trauma, infection, endocrine factors and climate, particularly in a country like Canada, have also been implicated. Drugs may influence the onset or course of psoriasis by exacerbating pre-existing psoriasis, precipitating new psoriasis or promoting treatment resistance. The drugs most frequently reported to affect psoriasis include lithium, beta-blockers (including ophthalmic timolol), the antimalarials and nonsteroidal anti-inflammatory drugs. Abrupt withdrawal of corticosteroids in individuals with psoriasis can precipitate acute pustular psoriasis. Drugs applied topically, such as tar or anthralin, as well as systemic agents, such as etretinate, have been reported to worsen psoriasis in some patients as a result of irritation or hypersensitivity reactions. Other drugs rarely implicated in the exacerbation of psoriasis are listed in Table II.

Table II *Drugs That May Trigger or Exacerbate Psoriasis*

Well documented	Case reports
Antimalarials	Alpha interferon
Beta-blockers	Amiodarone
Corticosteroids	Cimetidine
Lithium	Clonidine
Nonsteroidal anti-inflammatory agents	Digoxin
	Potassium iodide
	Tetracycline

The typical psoriatic lesion is rounded with a sharply defined border, bright red color and loosely adherent silvery-white scale. In addition to visible lesions, other areas of the skin may have histologic and biochemical changes characteristic of psoriasis or be susceptible to visible psoriasis upon injury without detectable cellular abnormalities. Thus, any site on the skin of a person with psoriasis can form visible psoriasis after trauma.

Lesions can occur anywhere on the body, but are most common at sites of regular trauma or irritation: scalp, elbows, knees, trunk and lower extremities. The face is usually spared. Rarely, the mucous membranes are involved. Pruritus is unusual and most lesions are asymptomatic, although psychological distress may be profound.

Variations

The most common form of the disease is psoriasis vulgaris, or chronic plaque-type psoriasis, in which the typical psoriatic lesion occurs in plaques of any size.

Guttate psoriasis, characterized by tear-shaped lesions, arises in children or young adults, often after a streptococcal upper respiratory tract infection. Treatment, though minimal, may take time. Occasionally, hospitalization may be necessary.

In pustular psoriasis, the psoriatic lesions are associated with pustules, usually on the palms and soles. In the most severe acute form of pustular psoriasis, the entire skin becomes hot, red and studded with pustules. It is also accompanied by high fever, leukocytosis and prostration.

Flexural psoriasis involves the intertriginous folds of the axillary, inguinal, inframammary, intergluteal and perianal areas with or without other generalized lesions. Because of the maceration produced by wetness and rubbing in these areas, flexural psoriasis may present a stubborn therapeutic problem. In addition, it may be difficult to distinguish from seborrheic dermatitis if no other areas are involved.

Exfoliative erythroderma is a severe complication of generalized psoriasis, sometimes secondary to withdrawal of steroids or irritation by topical agents.

Psoriatic arthritis occurs in about 5 to 7 per cent of people with psoriasis. It is recognized as a distinct clinical entity, in which joint inflammation is asymmetrical and commonly affects the distal joints of the fingers and toes. Involvement of the sacroiliac joint is present in 20 per cent of affected individuals. Nail psoriasis may be present in up to 80 per cent of affected individuals. The prognosis is generally better than with rheumatoid arthritis, although 5 per cent of the people may progress to arthritis mutilans. Onset of skin lesions may not correspond to onset of arthritis, and activity of skin and joint involvement do not parallel each other in most cases. Effective topical treatment of the psoriasis has little impact on the joint disease, which is usually managed with nonsteroidal anti-inflammatory agents.

General Treatment

As a prophylactic measure, people with psoriasis are instructed to avoid known precipitating factors such as stress, local trauma and skin irritation. Rest and mild sedation may be useful adjuncts. Since psoriasis can be controlled, optimism is justified and may encourage compliance with a prolonged, sometimes awkward and messy treatment course. (See Table III for a summary of the treatment for psoriasis.)

Excessive dryness of the skin, sometimes accompanied by painful fissures or pruritus, is common in psoriasis. Local application of bland emollients alone, or combined with other pharmacologic agents, is the basis for most treatments in psoriasis. Emollients form a protective coating over the skin, reducing the formation of new plaques caused by injury to the skin. Scaling and pruritus are reduced by the slight occlusive effects of emollients and by the presence of added water-binding ingredients such as propylene glycol, sodium chloride or lactic acid. Occlusion alone can reduce cellular turnover in mild psoriatic plaques, possibly by increasing water content.

Warm water baths, with or without the addition of other agents, are moisturizing and may be soothing, antipruritic and mildly anti-inflammatory. They may also facilitate removal of scales. A bath oil free of unnecessary perfumes or additives that might sensitize the skin may be added for an emollient effect. If an antipruritic effect is desired, individuals can use Aveeno oatmeal or Oilated Aveeno. Since many soaps can irritate the skin, pharmacists should recommend a mild soap such as Dove. After soaking the skin, rubbing it

Table III *Treatment for Psoriasis*

Treatment	Route	Indications	Comments
Keratolytics	Topical	Psoriasis vulgaris Seborrheic psoriasis Localized pustular psoriasis	To help remove very thick scales Gels, creams, lotions, ointments Nonstaining
Coal Tar	Topical	Psoriasis vulgaris Seborrheic psoriasis	Creams, ointments, pastes, lotions, gels, shampoos, bath products Easier to apply & less staining than anthralin Offensive odor Patient acceptance of crude coal tar products poor Refined products more acceptable but less effective May be combined with keratolytics
Anthralin	Topical	Psoriasis vulgaris Guttate psoriasis Seborrheic psoriasis	Often used as stiff paste, which is difficult to apply Creams more acceptable, but may spread Stains skin, hair and clothing, and may irritate normal skin
Corticosteroids	Topical	Psoriasis vulgaris Seborrheic psoriasis Guttate psoriasis Localized pustular psoriasis Erythrodermic psoriasis	Prescription only Lotions, creams, ointments, gels Patient acceptance high Withdrawal can exacerbate disease
	Oral, IV, IM	Generalized pustular psoriasis Psoriatic arthritis Erythrodermic psoriasis	Prescription only Numerous side effects
Methotrexate	Oral, IV, IM	Recalcitrant psoriasis vulgaris Erythrodermic psoriasis Pustular psoriasis Psoriatic arthritis	Prescription only Usually given once weekly Liver and renal function tests must be monitored
Etretinate	Oral	Recalcitrant psoriasis	Prescription only Multiple side effects on skin/mucous membranes Teratogenic Increased blood lipids
Psoralens	Oral	Recalcitrant psoriasis Generalized pustular psoriasis Erythrodermic psoriasis	Prescription only Used with UV light Patient acceptance high Long-term risks not well defined Caution advised in children
Cyclosporine	Oral	Not approved for use. Restricted to persons with severe disease.	Prescription only Immunosuppressive Withdrawal can exacerbate disease

gently with a cloth or applying a cream may help remove scales. Vigorous scrubbing, which can exacerbate the lesions, must be avoided.

Occlusive dressings often enhance the efficacy of other topical agents by softening and hydrating the skin and increasing penetration of topical drugs. Usually, small areas are occluded initially under medical supervision. Occlusion of tar, steroids or salicylates can be irritating and increases the risk of systemic side effects. The following procedures can produce good results with bland emollients:
- Hydrate the skin by soaking it in water for 5 to 10 minutes (for example, in a bath) or washing it well.
- Rub the cream or medication into the lesions while the skin is still moist.
- Cover the area with an occlusive film such as plastic wrap, plastic gloves for hands, plastic bags for feet, bathing cap for scalp, or an exercise suit for large areas of the legs or torso.

- To minimize moisture loss, seal the dressing with tape, stockings, pantyhose or any dressing that ensures close adherence to the skin. Leave it in place for at least 6 hours. Overnight application is probably the most convenient.

Nonprescription Drug Treatment
Keratolytics

Thick plaques and scaling present a cosmetic problem and prevent pharmacologic agents from reaching their site of action. Keratolytics alone may be effective in mild psoriasis. In more serious cases, keratolytics remove scales to allow specific antimitotic therapy to reach the site of action. Because keratolytics irritate, acutely inflamed lesions are treated first with general measures and prescription topical corticosteroids until the acute stage has subsided.

Salicylic acid 3 to 6 per cent dissolves intercellular cement (which holds cells together), softening the outer skin layer (stratum

Psoriasis, Seborrheic Dermatitis and Dandruff

corneum) and shedding scales. In concentrations greater than 10 per cent, salicylic acid can destroy tissue. Combining it with sulfur may achieve a synergistic keratolytic effect. Propylene glycol in high concentrations (40 to 60 per cent) may also augment the keratolytic action of salicylic acid.

Commonly used formulations of salicylic acid include salicylic acid ointment, gel, soap or shampoo in concentrations of 2 to 6 per cent. They can be used alone or with sulfur, corticosteroids or a combination of sulfur and coal tar. Treatment with salicylic acid is best initiated in a low concentration and gradually increased as tolerance allows. It is applied after hydrating the lesions for 10 to 20 minutes in warm water (for example, in a bath). Occlusion may enhance efficacy, but because of the risk of excessive absorption, should be done only under medical supervision. For example, Keralyt gel, applied under occlusion to hydrated skin overnight, effectively removes thick, adherent scaling. Salicylic acid may reduce scaling in 7 days, but a reduction in erythema may not be noticed for 3 weeks.

Urea compounds are hydrophilic substances that enhance the ability of the stratum corneum to hold water. They are also mildly keratolytic, as they disrupt the normal hydrogen bonds of epidermal proteins. Concentrations of 10 to 22 per cent are used in creams, lotions or ointments to soften and moisturize the stratum corneum and to help remove adherent scales. They should not be used on open or abraded skin. Urea compounds are applied to damp skin for the best effect.

Lactic acid in a concentration of 5 to 10 per cent exerts a moisturizing/keratolytic effect similar to that of urea. Often, it is used with urea or salicylic acid for additive effects.

Coal Tar

Coal tar is a byproduct of the chemical extraction of coal at high temperatures. It is a heterogeneous mixture of over 10,000 different compounds, of which 400 (55 per cent of the total coal tar) have been chemically identified. The composition of coal tar is extremely variable depending on the origin of the tar and the distillation processes. This variability may account for the differing opinions on its therapeutic value. Crude coal tar is more active than the more refined tars, of which liquor carbonis detergens (LCD) is the least active. For example, 4 per cent crude coal tar has the same effect as 20 per cent LCD. Coal tar is available in ointments, lotions, gels, shampoos and bath preparations. Gels contain refined coal tar, which is less active than crude coal tar, although the gel vehicle may enhance penetration. The possible phototoxicity of coal tar is usually more pronounced in emulsions and creams than it is in petrolatum or polyethylene glycol.

The mode of action of coal tar is not clearly understood. Coal tar has been claimed to have antiseptic, antipruritic, antiparasitic, antifungal, antibacterial, keratoplastic and vasoconstrictive activities, although few of these have been substantiated. Coal tar reduces RNA and DNA synthesis, inhibiting mitotic activity and protein synthesis in psoriatic lesions. It may produce a photosensitivity that lowers the minimal erythema dose required to produce a therapeutic effect with ultraviolet (UV) light. Dermatologists often take advantage of this effect by advising the user to spend time in the sunlight after having applied the coal tar the previous evening. Before advising people to avoid the sun after applying coal tar, pharmacists should check what the consumer's dermatologist has advised.

Coal tar is suitable for chronic plaque-type psoriasis. It should not be used in red, irritated psoriasis until topical prescription corticosteroids reduce the acute phase. In addition, pre-existing folliculitis, severe acne, or concomitant administration of other photosensitizing drugs are possible contraindications. Coal tar baths may be used alone for mild psoriasis or before other therapies such as salicylic acid or anthralin. Lotions, creams and gels are suitable for application to lesions on the trunk and extremities. They may be combined with salicylic acid for a keratolytic effect. Since prolonged use of gel vehicles leads to drying and irritation at the site of application, the gel is often used alternately with vegetable oil or white petrolatum, both of which act as emollients and help remove scales. No treatment with coal tar is required on alternate days, since the penetrating vehicle of the gel produces a reservoir of coal tar in the stratum corneum that persists for up to 4 days.

In more severe psoriasis, coal tar is used in association with ultraviolet B (UVB) light in the Goeckerman regimen. In the classic regimen, the individual receives applications of 2 to 5 per cent crude coal tar cream or ointment, which is wiped off with vegetable or light mineral oil after 24 hours. The person is then treated with UVB light, followed by a bath and a further application of coal tar. Some dermatologists prefer to recommend a tar bath the night before or the day of the UV light exposure, since a tar bath leaves a thin film of tar on the skin for 24 hours. Coal tar cream or ointment is applied after UV light exposure. With the Goeckerman regimen, 3 weeks is usually required to clear psoriasis. Traditionally, this regimen has required hospitalization. However variations using tar gel, crude coal tar in hydrophilic ointment, or LCD have been adapted for outpatient treatment. In the Goeckerman regimen, the therapeutic effect of coal tar appears to be independent of the concentration between 1 per cent and 25 per cent.

Scalp psoriasis is common, cosmetically unappealing and may be difficult to treat. Mild scalp psoriasis may respond to tar shampoos alone. When coal tar shampoos do not effectively clear scalp lesions, a daily application of a coal tar gel may induce a remission. The remission can be maintained by shampooing twice weekly with a coal tar shampoo. Coal tar gel may stain light-colored and grey hair yellow. In more severe scalp psoriasis, application of a warm mineral oil compress for 20 minutes before shampooing helps remove extremely thick, crusty scales. Alternatively, use of a keratolytic overnight may loosen scales, after which a tar shampoo is used in the morning.

Irritation, folliculitis—particularly of hairy regions—and tar acne are the most frequent side effects of tar treatment. To prevent folliculitis, pharmacists instruct the user to apply the medication only in the direction of hair growth, and not in a circular motion. Contact allergic dermatitis and induction of generalized pustular psoriasis are seen occasionally. Side effects can be minimized by starting with a low concentration and gradually increasing the strength. Sunburn, photocontact dermatitis, actinic herpes and flat warts have been reported when coal tar is combined with UV light. Unless the dermatologist has specified otherwise, consumers should be warned to avoid excessive sunlight or to apply a sunscreen with a high sun protection factor. (See the chapter on sunscreens.) The association of skin cancer with tar, with or without UV light, is not well established and should not represent a contraindication to its use.

Anthralin

Anthralin reduces cell turnover in psoriatic plaques, possibly by interacting with DNA, inhibiting cellular metabolism or mitochondrial function, or altering other mediators of cell proliferation. Anthralin is reserved for moderately severe to severe plaque-type psoriasis. The best response is observed in lesions of the scalp, palms and soles. It must not be applied to inflamed areas, active lesions, pustular psoriasis, facial lesions or intertriginous zones.

Bioavailability is highest from an ointment vehicle, although spreading to uninvolved skin and staining may be significant problems. Creams and stiff pastes are available that minimize these problems. Staining of uninvolved skin may be used by dermatologists as evidence of therapeutic effect.

Anthralin was popularized in 1953 as the major component of the Ingram regimen. Anthralin 0.2 to 0.8 per cent in a stiff zinc oxide paste with 2 per cent salicylic acid is applied after a tar bath and increments of UV light exposure. It is left on for 24 hours, then removed with mineral oil or baby oil before the procedure is repeated. A stiff paste is used to prevent spread of the anthralin to normal skin, and salicylic acid prevents the oxidation of anthralin by impurities in the zinc oxide. Clearing is noted in 15 to 40 days in outpatients, and 10 to 20 days in inpatients, with few people failing to respond.

This regimen includes a number of modifications. The tar baths and UV light are sometimes removed, as some studies show these elements play only a minor role. The concentration of anthralin is often lowered to 0.1 to 0.4 per cent in a less stiff paste and applied overnight only. The anthralin concentration can also be increased to 5 per cent and the contact period shortened (10 to 20 minutes). Short-contact anthralin may be as effective as 24-hour contact, with less staining of skin and clothing. This method may be more suitable for home use than conventional anthralin regimens. However, the standard regimen produces a more rapid and complete improvement. Anthralin cream is as effective as similar concentrations of ointment with less staining of clothes and linen, but equal irritation. Remission induced with anthralin is maintained by twice-weekly anthralin applications, or topical corticosteroids.

Palms and soles respond well to low-strength paste formulations alternated with topical corticosteroids under occlusion. Psoriasis of the scalp is effectively treated with anthralin 0.4 per cent cream massaged into the scalp and left overnight. It is removed the next morning using any standard shampoo.

Irritation or inflammation of normal skin and staining of skin, clothes and other materials are two major problems with anthralin which are related to its clinical efficacy. Oxidation to anthraquinone byproducts stains skin, hair, clothing and bathroom surfaces a purple-brown color. Lemon juice and acidic soaps help remove the stain, whereas alkaline solutions tend to increase staining. Consumers should rinse contaminated clothes in water without using soap. Acetone, trichloroethylene or chlorine bleach may help remove stains from clothing. Individuals with gray or light-colored hair should use anthralin with caution. The psoriasis is clear when it cannot be felt, even though the brown stain is present. After treatment is stopped, the brown discoloration clears in 2 to 3 weeks. Anthralin stain may be removed from the skin with 3 to 6 per cent salicylic acid cream or ointment.

Anthralin can cause significant skin irritation and burning when applied to normal skin. Users may want to wear plastic disposable gloves or use a tongue depressor for application. Contaminated fingers must be kept away from eyes, and hands must be washed after application. Use of zinc oxide ointment around the lesions may help protect normal skin. If irritation or burning occurs, use of the

anthralin should be stopped until the irritation settles; petrolatum (for example, Vaseline) is then applied and application cautiously resumed at a lower strength. If no irritation occurs, the anthralin strength is increased every 3 to 7 days to individual tolerance. This should be done under consultation of a dermatologist.

Prescription Drug Treatment
Glucocorticoids
Topical glucocorticoids are one of the most frequently used treatments of psoriasis. The mode of action is unknown, although topical steroids are anti-inflammatory, vasoconstrictive and antiproliferative, and have a modulatory effect on the immune system. In psoriasis, topical steroids are the treatment of choice for acutely inflamed lesions and for use on the face, neck, flexures and intertriginous areas where irritants such as coal tar and anthralin cannot be applied.

In general, low-potency nonfluorinated steroids are preferred where skin is thin or penetration is greatest (for example face, groin and intertriginous areas). "Super potent" fluorinated compounds (for example, clobetasol, betamethasone dipropionate) are reserved for resistant lesions and areas where the epidermal barrier is thickened (for example, palms and soles). A wide range of fluorinated steroids can be used on other skin areas in the weakest effective preparation. In acute inflammation, potent steroids can be used for a short period (up to 2 weeks), then substituted with lower potency products as symptoms improve. Ointments are more occlusive than lotions or creams and exert a greater effect. They are generally chosen for thick dry plaques. Creams are therapeutically weaker than their respective ointments and can be used anywhere except heavy hair-bearing areas or in the ear canal. Lotions are convenient for use on the scalp. Gel vehicles release the steroid as effectively as ointments but are irritating and therefore restricted to use on the scalp or hairy areas of the trunk. Plastic wrap occlusion increases penetration of the steroid ten-fold but can also promote systemic absorption and side effects. Its use is restricted to thick, dry plaques or recalcitrant psoriasis of the scalp, hands or feet. Occlusion should not be maintained for more than 12 hours per day.

Not only are topical steroids expensive, but continued use renders them less effective. Withdrawal after prolonged use can precipitate pustular psoriasis. Topical corticosteroids can cause striae, redness, visible blood vessels on the face, thinning of the skin or aggravation of underlying nonsteroid responsive dermatoses. Systemic absorption is possible, particularly when occlusion is used, and may lead to adrenocortical suppression.

Systemic steroids should be used only to treat life-threatening pustular psoriasis, exfoliative erythroderma or rapidly progressing, destructive, psoriatic arthritis unresponsive to other agents. Intralesional steroids may effectively treat isolated patches of psoriasis and nail involvement.

Antimetabolites
Antimetabolites inhibit DNA and RNA synthesis, thereby reducing mitosis and decreasing epidermal proliferation to normal. In addition, some, such as methotrexate, suppress cellular immune function which may help normalize immune system defects in psoriasis. Antimetabolites pose considerable acute (nausea, vomiting, stomatitis) and long-term (leukopenia, thrombocytopenia, anemia) risks. Consequently, their use in psoriasis is reserved for severe cases which are resistant to intensive topical therapy and is physically, emotionally

Psoriasis, Seborrheic Dermatitis and Dandruff

Figure 1 *Suggested Approach for Treating Psoriasis*

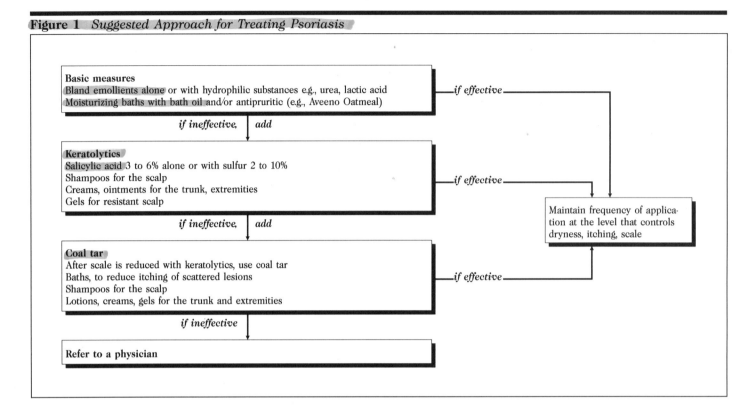

or economically disabling. Hospitalization is usually required for initiation of therapy. Methotrexate is the most effective antimetabolite in treating psoriasis and remains the antimetabolite of choice despite its potential toxicity. Other less-effective antimetabolites used in the past include hydroxyurea, 6-mercaptopurine, azathioprine, 5-fluorouracil, azarabine and thioguanine.

To minimize toxicity, methotrexate is given weekly as a single oral, intravenous or intramuscular dose, or in 3 equally divided oral doses at 12-hour intervals. When the disease is cleared adequately, the dose is gradually reduced to the lowest level required to maintain a remission, or stopped if possible. The most commonly reported adverse reactions to methotrexate include nausea, malaise, leukopenia and thrombocytopenia with possible hemorrhage and bruising. The most significant long-term problem is liver toxicity; liver biopsy is recommended before and at periodic intervals during treatment. Many drugs displace methotrexate from plasma protein binding sites, increasing the toxicity potential. In particular, users must be cautioned to avoid salicylate-containing products.

Etretinate

Etretinate is an aromatic retinoic acid derivative that inhibits excessive keratin production and cell differentiation, possibly by an effect on DNA synthesis or polyamine formation. Good to excellent results have been achieved in 60 to 70 per cent of individuals with palmoplantar, pustular and erythrodermic psoriasis and those unresponsive to other therapy. Maintenance therapy with lower doses has a high incidence of relapse. The incidence of side effects is high, outweighing possible benefits in mild psoriasis. The most common side effects are dry lips (80 per cent), dry oral/nasal mucous membranes, conjunctivitis, desquamation and increased skin fragility. The most important cause of withdrawal from treatment is hair loss. More

than 75 per cent of affected individuals may detect some hair loss, but objective alopecia occurs in only 20 per cent. Etretinate is teratogenic and is contraindicated in women of child-bearing age. In addition, because of prolonged persistence in tissues, women should not become pregnant for at least 1 year following cessation of the drug.

Psoralens/PUVA

Methoxsalen is used in combination with long-wave ultraviolet light (UVA) to treat psoriasis unresponsive to other forms of treatment. Interaction of the psoralen molecule with light energy inhibits DNA synthesis or affects the immune system. Methoxsalen is given 2 to 3 times weekly as a single oral dose, followed by UVA exposure 2 hours later at the peak reactivity to UV light. After users have taken their medication, they require protection from light exposure for the rest of the day. Acute, minor side effects include redness, itching, headache, nausea and dizziness. Documented long-term risks include increased risk of skin cancer; premature aging, wrinkling or atrophy of skin; impaired immunological function; and ocular changes resulting in an increased risk of cataracts. Careful selection of individuals, weighing benefits and risks, is essential.

Cyclosporine

Cyclosporine is an immunosuppressive which is effective in suppressing both antibody- and cell-mediated immunity, and in inhibiting chronic inflammatory reactions. It has proven to be a useful tool in attempting to define the immunologic abnormality in psoriasis, as well as an effective therapeutic agent. Cyclosporine causes a dose-related, rapid and thorough clearing of psoriasis in most patients which relapses when the treatment is stopped. Of concern are the side effects of cyclosporine which include symptoms of fatigue,

Psoriasis, Seborrheic Dermatitis and Dandruff

headache, muscle or joint pain, gastrointestinal disturbance and of more concern, renal toxicity, hypertension, and with long-term use, cancer. Presently, cyclosporine is not approved for use in psoriasis and should be restricted to persons with severe disease where the benefits outweigh the potential risks.

Summary

In general, mild or chronic noninflamed psoriasis is suitable for self-medication. A variety of products are safe and effective for these individuals. Irritating products may provoke an acute exacerbation. Extensive psoriasis, inflammation, lesions unresponsive to self-medication, or involvement of the face or intertriginous areas should be referred to a physician. When advising a person on selection and use of topical agents for psoriasis, pharmacists should first check what the consumer's physician has advised, as many of these people are under a physician's care.

Seborrhea and Dandruff

Seborrheic dermatitis is an inheritable trait occurring most commonly in infants less than 3 months of age and adults from 30 to 60 years of age. Two to five per cent of the population is affected to some degree, men more frequently than women. There appears to be a higher incidence in mental retardation, idiopathic and neuroleptic-induced Parkinsonism, and endocrine states associated with obesity, zinc deficiency and severe acne. Exacerbation of seborrheic dermatitis is associated with stress, and conditions of low humidity and temperature.

Like psoriasis, seborrheic dermatitis is characterized by increased epidermal cell turnover, with scaling and underlying inflammation. Although "seborrhea" means a hypersecretion of sebum, and seborrheic dermatitis is often found in areas with high sebaceous gland concentration, increased oil production is not usually present. The etiology of seborrheic dermatitis is subject to debate. It may be due to irritation caused by an alteration in the lipid composition of sebum, a breakdown product of sebum caused by microorganisms, or infection with a yeast, *Pityrosporon ovale*. Alternatively, the finding of increased bacterial and yeast species in seborrheic dermatitis could represent a secondary infection which perpetuates the underlying inflammatory process.

Lesions consist of scaling patches with indistinct margins, slight to moderate redness of the underlying skin and dry or oily, yellowish scales. Seborrheic lesions are usually found in areas with high sebaceous gland concentration such as the centre of the chest and mid-back area, face (nose, lips, eyebrows, eyelids), ears, axilla, and groin. Pruritus is common when the scalp or ear canal are involved. When seborrheic dermatitis and psoriasis occur together, the lesions may be difficult to distinguish, giving rise to the term "sebo-psoriasis."

Dandruff, like seborrheic dermatitis and psoriasis, is associated with increased cell turnover and visible excessive scaling, which may be accompanied by itching. Unlike these conditions, dandruff is not inflammatory, is diffuse rather than patchy and is confined to the scalp. It tends to fade in the summer, wanes with age and is not influenced by emotional state. It may be exacerbated by inadequate washing and a dry climate. Dandruff scales appear as dried-up cell fragments that are thin, white or greyish, and are spread uniformly on the scalp. Although a few dandruff scales can be found in all adults, only 25 per cent of adults have a troublesome amount.

Treatment

Seborrhea and dandruff are treated in the same manner. The objective is to remove scales and crust and alleviate associated itching or inflammation. In general, nonprescription treatment adequately controls dandruff and many cases of seborrheic dermatitis. Individuals with seborrheic dermatitis who do not improve, or whose condition worsens within 2 weeks after starting appropriate nonprescription therapy, should consult a physician. Inflamed lesions may require treatment with topical corticosteroids.

Affected individuals should shampoo the scalp frequently, massaging firmly, at least 3 times a week until the scaling is under control and twice weekly thereafter. It is important to rinse well. A nonmedicated shampoo may be enough to eliminate dirt and scaliness and should be tried first.

Cytostatic/Antiyeast Shampoos

When these measures are inadequate, the next step is to try a medicated shampoo. Both selenium sulfide 0.5 to 2 per cent and zinc pyrithione 1 to 2.5 per cent reduce scale equally well, possibly by a cytostatic effect that slows cell turnover, or by an antiyeast action. Pharmacists should instruct the user to shampoo at least twice. The first shampooing (which may be with a nonmedicated shampoo) removes oil and dirt and wets the scalp. The second allows the medicated shampoo to work on the scalp. Zinc pyrithione can be used daily to maintain control of the condition. Selenium sulfide should only be used once or twice a week, and may be added to a zinc pyrithione regimen in resistant cases. Zinc pyrithione can be applied to all involved areas except the eyelid to avoid contact with the eye.

Zinc pyrithione has few reported side effects. However, numerous precautions must be taken with selenium sulfide. Consumers must remove all jewelry before its use, and wash hands thoroughly afterward. It should not be used within 2 days of applying hair tints or perm solutions. Selenium sulfide may stain blond or grey hair if rinsed inadequately. Selenium-containing shampoos do not remove oil well, and may lead to oily hair and hair loss with excessive use. Pretreatment with a nonmedicated shampoo may help minimize this problem. Selenium sulfide should not be applied to inflamed or damaged skin and its use should be discontinued if skin irritation, conjunctivitis or hair loss occurs. It is toxic if ingested orally and must be kept out of reach of children.

Keratolytics

When cytostatic/antiyeast shampoos are ineffective, keratolytic agents (for example, sulfur, salicylic acid) may be tried to soften and detach flakes of keratin. Generally, keratolytics are less effective than selenium or zinc pyrithione. Available nonprescription agents include salicylic acid 2 to 3 per cent, sulfur 3 to 5 per cent and resorcinol 1 to 2 per cent. Higher concentrations may produce faster results, but proportionally more irritation. As with other medicated shampoos, contact time of at least 5 minutes is recommended to allow the agent to soften and loosen the scale. Thick adherent crusts, such as these that develop with "cradle cap" in infants, can be removed with an application of warm mineral oil or baby oil for 10 minutes prior to shampooing. This should be repeated once or twice daily until all crusts are removed.

Other Medicated Shampoos

Tar shampoos may be suggested for people who experience itching,

Psoriasis, Seborrheic Dermatitis and Dandruff

Figure 2 *Suggested Approach for Treating Seborrhea and Dandruff*

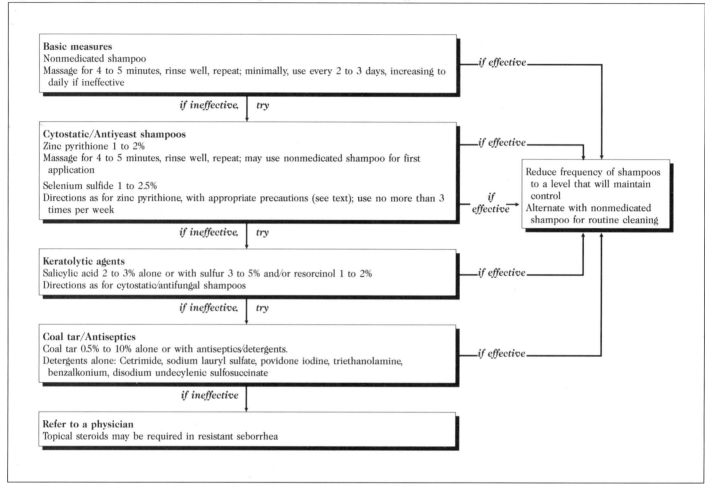

but these shampoos are unlikely to be as effective as other agents in removing scale. Many people find these products cosmetically unacceptable because of color and odor. Some people may experience phototoxicity or hypersensitivity reactions.

Antiseptic shampoos containing cetrimide, povidone-iodine, triclosan or quaternary ammonium compounds have been recommended to lower the population of bacteria or yeast on the scalp. Their efficacy in seborrhea and dandruff has never been proven and they are not recommended as first-line treatment. Combination products containing coal tar plus an antiseptic are available.

Other Treatments

Ketoconazole, an oral/topical antifungal agent active against *Pityrosporon ovale*, is effective in treating both seborrheic dermatitis and dandruff. The risk of the drug may outweigh its benefits in these relatively benign conditions.

Topical corticosteroids may be necessary for resistant seborrheic dermatitis, where significant inflammation is present or for areas inadequately treated with available nonprescription products.

Summary

Nonprescription drug therapy is suitable for dandruff and adequately controls most cases of seborrheic dermatitis. People with seborrheic dermatitis that is inflamed or does not respond to an adequate trial of self-medication should be referred to a physician.

Ask the Consumer

Q. Has your condition recently developed or worsened?
- Certain factors may trigger the development of psoriasis. These factors include skin trauma, hormonal changes, seasonal changes, emotional stress and infection.

Q. Has anyone else in your family had a skin condition similar to this?
- Information on family history can help pinpoint the diagnosis. Psoriasis and sometimes seborrhea have a genetic predisposition.

Q. What areas are affected? What do the lesions look like?
- The lesions of psoriasis, seborrhea and dandruff may have a different appearance (see Table I). They respond to different therapies. Product recommendation or referral to a physician depends on the location of the lesions, the extent of the problem, the degree of hydration of the skin and the presence or absence of inflammation or pustules.

Psoriasis, Seborrheic Dermatitis and Dandruff

Q. Are you taking medications for other conditions?

- Numerous drugs exacerbate or trigger a psoriasis-like reaction (see Table II).

Q. Has your condition been diagnosed by a doctor? Have you used any treatments previously? If so, were they effective?

- These questions can generate discussion about the severity and nature of the problem, and assist the pharmacist in either recommending a product or referring the individual to a physician. Consumers already under the care of a physician may have been given specific instructions that should not be contradicted by the pharmacist.

References

Psoriasis
Abel EA, DiCicco LM, Orenberg EK. Drugs in exacerbation of psoriasis. J Am Acad Dermatol 1986;15:1007–22.

Anderson TF, Voorhees JJ. Psoriasis. In: Provost TT, Farmer ER, eds. Current therapy in dermatology. Philadelphia: BC Decker Inc, 1985:1–6.

Baadsgaard O, Fisher G, Voorhees JJ, et al. The role of the immune system in the pathogenesis of psoriasis. J Invest Dermatol 1990;95(5):325–45.

Bergner T, Przybilla B. Psoriasis and tetracyclines. J Am Acad Dermatol 1990;23(4Pt1):770–1.

Farber EM, Nall L. Psoriasis: a review of recent advances in treatment. Drugs 1984;28:324–46.

Gardner SS, McKay M. Seborrhea, psoriasis and the papulosquamous dermatoses. Prim Care 1989;16(3):739–63.

Gottlieb A. Immunologic mechanisms in psoriasis. J Invest Dermatol 1990;95(5):185–95.

Puig L, et al. Psoriasis induced by ophthalmic timolol preparations. Am J Ophthalmol 1989;108(4):455–6.

Quesada JR, Gutterman JU. Psoriasis and alpha-interferon. Lancet 1986;1:1466–8.

Wuepper KD, Silvija NC, Haberman A. Psoriasis vulgaris: a genetic approach. J Invest Dermatol 1990;95(5):25–45.

Yates VM, Kerr REI. Cimetidine and thrombocytopenia. Br Med J 1980;280:1453.

General Treatment
Arndt KA. Manual of dermatologic therapeutics. Boston: Little, Brown, 1983:145–9,303–9.

Arndt KA. Manual of dermatologic therapeutics. Boston: Little, Brown, 1989:120–5.

Bond C. Skin diseases. In: Katcher BS, Young LY, Koda-Kimble MA, eds. Applied therapeutics, the clinical use of drugs. San Francisco: Applied Therapeutics, 1983:1163–65.

Fredriksson T, Lundberg M. A blind controlled comparison between a new cream ("12+12"), its vehicle and salicylic acid in petrolatum on psoriatic plaques. Curr Ther Res 1985;37:805–9.

Keratolytics
Baker H. Psoriasis. In: Rook A, Wilkinson DS, Ebling FJG, Champion RH, Burton JL. Textbook of dermatology. Oxford: Blackwell Scientific Publications, 1986:1469–532.

Canadian drug identification code. 17th Edition. Ottawa: Health and Welfare Canada, 1991.

Gip L, Lundberg M. A double-blind controlled trial of a new antipsoriatic cream containing urea and sodium chloride. Curr Ther Res 1985;37:797–804.

Watson W. Psoriasis: topical and systemic therapy. Rational Drug Ther 1979;13(4):1–7.

Coal Tar
Grupper C. The chemistry, pharmacology and use of tar in the treatment of psoriasis. In: Farber EM, Cox AJ, eds. Proceedings of the first international symposium on psoriasis. Stanford: Stanford University Press, 1971:347–56.

Hjorth N, Jacobsen M. Coal tar. Semin Dermatol 1983;2(4):281–6.

Langner A, Wolska H, Hebborn P. Treatment of psoriasis of the scalp with coal tar gel and shampoo preparations. Cutis 1983;32:290–6.

Anthralin
Ashton RE, Andre P, Lowe NJ, Whitefield M. Anthralin: historical and current perspectives. Semin Dermatol 1983;2(4):287–303.

Freeman K, Warin AP. Staining of baths by short-contact dithranol therapy (Letter). Br J Dermatol 1984;110:246–7.

Gip L, Zador G. Treatment of psoriasis with dithranol cream 0.1% and 0.25% in comparison with dithranol ointment 0.1% and 0.25%. Curr Ther Res 1984;36:421–5.

Harris DR, Ferrington RA. The chemistry, pharmacology, and use of anthralin in the treatment of psoriasis. In: Farber EM, Cox AJ, eds. Proceedings of the first international symposium on psoriasis. Stanford: Stanford University Press, 1971:357–65.

Ryatt KS, Statham BN, Rowell NR. Short-contact modification of the Ingram regime. Br J Dermatol 1984;111:455–9.

Statham BN, Ryatt KS, Rowell NR. Short-contact dithranol therapy—a comparison with the Ingram regime. Br J Dermatol 1984;110:703–8.

Glucocorticoids
Trozak DJ. Topical corticosteroid therapy in psoriasis vulgaris. Cutis 1990;46:341–9.

Antimetabolites
McDonald CJ. Cytotoxic agents for use in dermatology. J Am Acad Dermatol 1985;12(5):753–75.

Etretinate
Ward A, Brogden RN, Heel RC, et al. Etretinate—a review of its pharmacological properties and therapeutic efficacy in psoriasis and other skin disorders. Drugs 1983;26:9–43.

Psoralens
Helm TN, Dijkstya MD, Ferrara RJ, Glanz S. PUVA therapy. Am Fam Phys 1991;43(3):908–12.

Cyclosporine
Anonymous. A concensus report: cyclosporin A therapy for psoriasis. Br J Dermatol 1990;122(Suppl 36):1–3.

Borel J. Mechanism of action and rationale for cyclosporin A in psoriasis. Br J Dermatol 1990;122(Suppl 36):5–12.

Ellis C, et al. Cyclosporine for plaque-type psoriasis. N Engl J Med 1991;324(5):277–84.

Seborrhea and Dandruff
Binder RL, Jonelis FJ. Seborrheic dermatitis: a newly reported side effect of neuroleptics. J Clin Psych 1984;45:125–6.

Dubois M. Dandruff and seborrheic dermatitis of the scalp. Can Pharm J 1985;118:434–6.

Kligman AM, Leyden JJ. Seborrheic dermatitis. Semin Dermatol 1983;2(1):57–9.

Cytostatic/Antiyeast Shampoos and Keratolytics
Dubois M. Dandruff and seborrheic dermatitis of the scalp. Can Pharm J 1985;118:434–6.

Ford GP, Farr PM, Ive FA, Shuster S. The response of seborrhoeic dermatitis to ketoconazole. Br J Dermatol 1984;111:603–7.

McEvoy GK, McQuarrie GM, eds. American hospital formulary service drug information. Bethesda: American Society of Hospital Pharmacists, 1986:1778.

Reynolds JEF, ed. Martindale: the extra pharmacopoeia. London: Pharmaceutical Press, 1982:502.

Shore RN. Seborrheic dermatitis. In: Provost TT, Farmer ER, eds. Current therapy in dermatology. Philadelphia: BC Decker Inc, 1985:14–7.

7
Acne Therapy

Reviewed by Paul Brisson. Based on the original chapter by Cheryl M. Anderson

Acne and similar conditions include acne keloidalis, acne neonatorum, acne excoriée, occupational acne (acne cosmetica, McDonald's acne, tropical acne and chloracne), acneiform drug eruptions, acne rosacea, perioral dermatitis and acne vulgaris. Acne vulgaris is treated by removing excessive sebum, drying comedones and using retinoic acid, antibiotics, tetracycline, erythromycin, clindamycin or a combination of these or nonprescription drugs to reduce inflammatory reactions and minimize scarring. Other treatments include dermabrasion, ultraviolet light therapy and collagen implants.

Acne is a term often associated with one medical condition—acne vulgaris. However, several acne or acne-like conditions exist: acne keloidalis, acne neonatorum, acne excoriée, occupational acne, acne rosacea and acne vulgaris. Occupational acne includes acne cosmetica, McDonald's acne, tropical acne and chloracne.

Acne or acne-like lesions may present in association with endocrinopathies or drug therapy. It is important to understand the similarities and differences of the conditions to provide effective counselling and selection of nonprescription products.

Types of Acne
Acne Keloidalis

Acne keloidalis is most common in people with tight, curly hair, particularly black males. Small, firm, red, dome-shaped, follicular papules at the nape of the neck may indicate this condition. The hairs penetrate through the follicular wall into the dermis. The follicular orifice may become plugged, resulting in inflammatory and fibrotic response. There may be comedones. *Staphylococcus aureus* is found within the lesion. Nonprescription products are not recommended. The consumer should be referred to a physician, because treatment includes taking oral antibiotics for several months, applying topical antibiotics or retinoic acid, plucking hair or injecting intralesional steroids. The following instructions are given:
• Keep the area clean.
• Do not pick or scratch the lesions since they contain bacteria.
• Avoid sharing hats and helmets.

Acne Neonatorum

Acne neonatorum appears in children. It is associated with several types of lesions, dependent on the age of the child. At birth, infants with acne neonatorum may have blackheads, pustules and papules on their cheeks and face. Picking or squeezing the lesions is not recommended. Nonprescription products are not necessary. The face should be kept clean and dry. The lesions disappear in a few months.

Blackheads on the face of an infant may signify the use or abuse of oils (baby oil or lotions). The caregiver is counselled to discontinue the use of oils such as baby oil, olive oil, mineral oil, bath oil, jelly and lotions on the face of the infant. The face should be kept clean and dry.

At 3 or 4 months of age an infant may have temporary gonadal activation resulting in extensive inflammatory acne. Nonprescription products are not recommended. A physician must be consulted. This is a serious medical condition. Oral antibiotics are required. Tetracycline is not recommended during the time of teeth formation as it is deposited in the teeth, discoloring them. It may be used after the teeth are fully formed, usually after the child is at least eight years old. Topical antibiotic products are not effective.

Acne Excoriée

Young females may present with acne excoriée or mild to severe acne associated with facial itching, papules, pustules and blackheads. Small, bloody, serous crusts develop due to repeated squeezing, picking, scratching and rubbing. Medical assistance should be sought. The individuals should be reminded that picking and squeezing increases scarring. Drying lotions and antibiotics—either oral or topical—are prescribed. Other names for this condition are picker's acne and premenstrual acne, as it tends to flare at that time.

Unsuspected Endocrinopathies

A female presenting with severe treatment-resistant inflammatory acne should be referred to a physician. She may be obese, suffer facial hirsutism and have infrequent menses. Endocrinopathies have been associated with ovarian 11-hydroxylase deficiency. Prednisone may be prescribed by the physician.

If a woman has severe treatment-resistant acne, amenorrhea and virilization of external genitalia, she should be investigated for an androgen-secreting tumor.

Occupational Acne

Occupational acne encompasses several conditions: acne cosmetica, McDonald's acne, tropical acne and chloracne. When large numbers of follicular papules, comedones and pustules appear on the arms and thighs, occupational exposure should be examined during the counselling session. Exposure to heavy oil and tar coats the clothing of people employed as machinists, rubber workers, textile mill workers, coke oven workers, road pavers, printers, and coal tar and pitch handlers. Oil-soaked clothing should be removed frequently, and the worker should immediately bathe or shower. Particle or gritty cleansers such as SNAP may help remove oil and tar from arms. People with occupational acne should avoid greasy pommades, including petroleum jelly.

Acne Cosmetica

Any individual using oil-based cosmetics may develop acne cosmetica, a condition common among male and female actors, cosmetologists and teenagers. Oily make-up contains lanolin, petrolatum, vegetable oils, castor oil, butyl stearate, lauryl alcohol and oleic acid. A water-based make-up from Clinique, Estée Lauder, Max Factor or Revlon may be recommended. Hair oils and pommades may be associated with acne cosmetica on the forehead, particularly when used on bangs and long hair.

McDonald's Acne

McDonald's acne is common to young people who work in restaurants grilling hamburgers. Grease and oil contact their facial area, causing facial pustules and papules. Treatment includes good personal hygiene and frequent facial washing with a soap free of oil and grease. This condition is not limited to McDonald's or other restaurants; mechanics have similar acne.

Tropical Acne

Adolescents to senior citizens may present with nodulocystic inflammatory lesions on the neck, back and buttocks. Occupational and recreational exposure to heat and humidity should be investigated.

Heat, humidity and hydration of the skin produce swelling and sweating, thus decreasing the size of the follicular orifices. This obstruction leads to follicle wall ruptures.

People at risk are military personnel, athletes or participants in vigorous sports, coke oven workers, employees in laundries or dry cleaning establishments, and people working in hot, humid, poorly ventilated environments. Antiperspirants should be recommended along with loosely fitting cotton clothes, cool showers and, if possible, improved ventilation and avoidance of hot, humid environments.

Chloracne

Chloracne lesions may present as straw-colored cysts, comedones, inflammatory pustules or abscesses. The lesions may be mild, localized eruptions or widely distributed on covered and exposed areas of the body.

People at risk for chloracne are electric cable assemblers, manufacturers or farmers handling cutting oils, chlorinated biphenyls (paint) and pesticides, and handlers of polychlorinated biphenyls. Exposure to the chemicals (contact or inhalation) provokes a proliferation of follicular epithelium in the sebaceous duct and follicular orifice. The orifice becomes plugged, resulting in comedones and keratin cysts filled with sebaceous lipid. People at risk should avoid contact and inhalation of the chemicals. Splash guards should be installed. Therapy may include benzoyl peroxide, retinoic acid and oral antibiotics.

Acneiform Drug Eruptions

Papules and pustules may appear suddenly in a teenager or older adult. The cause may be topical exposure to industrial chemicals or ingestion of drugs or chemicals.

Medications associated with acneiform eruptions include halogens (bromides, iodides), antitubercular agents (isoniazid, ethambutol), anticonvulsants (phenytoin, trimethadione, phenobarbital), hormones (systemic and topical corticosteroids, androgens, oral contraceptives), lithium salts, vitamin B_{12}, thiouracil, quinine (a source of quinine is tonic water), disulfiram, maprotiline and psoralens.

Halogens (iodides, bromides, chlorides and halothane) are incorporated in prescription and nonprescription medications. Ethnic products sold in specialty stores and health food shops may be a hidden source of halogens. Cough and cold medications and multiple vitamins with minerals are sources of iodine. Topical antiseptics such as tincture of iodine and complexed iodine solution (Proviodine and Betadine) liberate free iodine. Prescription medications such as Darabid and Stelabid contain iodine.

Radiopaques used in diagnostic imaging or radiology departments may contain iodine. Elimination of the iodine may take 48 hours. Another source of iodine is kelp, which can be purchased in health food shops and pharmacies.

Bromides are found in sleeping products, digestants and some well water and may aggravate acne. Halothane is an inhalation anesthetic agent. Operating room personnel may experience exacerbations of acne, but properly functioning and maintained anesthetic equipment has reduced the risk of halothane-induced acneiform eruptions.

Acneiform eruptions are inflammatory and pustular. Comedones are not present. The halogens (iodine, bromide and halothane) are excreted in sebaceous glands with a resultant inflammatory reaction.

Isoniazid and ethambutol are antitubercular agents. Isoniazid may produce sebaceous gland hypertrophy (abnormal enlargement). Lesions may appear first on the cheeks, chin, nose and forehead, and then spread over the whole body. The initial keratotic plugs may evolve into inflammatory plugs.

Phenytoin, trimethadione and phenobarbital may increase surface lipids. The mechanism for induction of acneiform lesions in unknown.

Corticosteroids and adrenocorticotropic hormone induce acneiform lesions after puberty due to follicular occlusion. The lesions are found on the forehead and chin a few weeks after initiation of treatment. Unlike acne vulgaris, there are no comedones and fewer pustules.

Testosterone, progesterone, oxymetholone and oral contraceptives may produce lesions resembling acne vulgaris. Hypertrophy of the sebaceous gland is produced by testosterone and progesterone.

Acne Rosacea

A person with acne rosacea presents with a chronic, acneiform eruption of the face in the area of the nose, cheeks, brow and chin. A slight flush is noted initially, and with time the flush deepens, the superficial capillaries dilate, and follicular greasy plaques form. The blush becomes permanent, with pustules, papules and telangiectasia (dilation of a group of small blood vessels). The blush is initiated by hot beverages, alcohol, emotion, stress, spices, exposure to fluorescent and infrared light, and drugs.

The drugs associated with acne rosacea are topical corticosteroids, glyceryltrinitrate and pentaerithrityl tetranitrate. Adverse effects associated with the use of potent or fluorinated steroids on the face include atrophy (loss of fat and protein) and telangiectasia.

Treatment includes low-dose oral antibiotics and topical metronidazole applied at bedtime on a regular basis. Since acne rosacea is not acne but an acne-like condition, the microcomedone formation of sulfur is not a concern. Drying lotions with sulfur may be useful.

Perioral Dermatitis

Young females and occasionally males present with papular, erythematous, scaly eruption in the nasolabial folds and sides of the chin. The usual cause is fluorinated steroids. The treatment is discontinuation of the fluorinated steroid, oral antibiotics and hydrocortisone lotion.

Acne Vulgaris

Twenty to 25 per cent of people between puberty and the late twenties develop the lesions of acne vulgaris. Although it is a self-limiting condition, the psychological trauma, scars and disfigurement continue for life. The condition is not found in hairy mammals nor on the human scalp, since these sebaceous glands are associated with large draining hair follicular ducts. Lesions cover the face, neck, parts of the upper torso and arms.

Sebum

The sebaceous glands of the skin secrete an oily material—sebum—which lubricates the hair and skin. Comedones are epithelial plugs. They are either solid plugs within the pores (whiteheads), called a closed comedone, or extend outside the pore (blackheads) and contain oxidized lipids. The open comedone persists for long periods of time. The closed comedone obstructs the drainage of sebum.

Two main factors in developing lesions are increased sebum production and sebaceous duct blockage. When gonadal and adrenal glands produce androgenic hormones in sufficient quantities, the sebaceous glands of the acne-prone or sensitive areas produce sebum in large quantities, which in turn fuels the acne. Adrenal glucocorticoids influence the formation of comedones. Comedones are formed when the cells in the pilosebaceous follicle become sticky and do not desquamate; an active testosterone receptor or binding site is found within the follicle.

Sebum is associated with a heavy colonization of anerobic bacteria, *Corynebacterium acnes*. Excessive and abnormal keratinization of the follicle blocks the path, partly due to the irritant effects of bacteria products. Some of the bacteria products are free fatty acids, which are comedogenic and inflammatory agents. When the follicle ruptures, papules and pustules form. In the repeatedly damaged follicles, granulomatous inflammatory reactions may occur and sterile abscess cysts result.

Exacerbating factors are heat, humidity, excessive sweating,

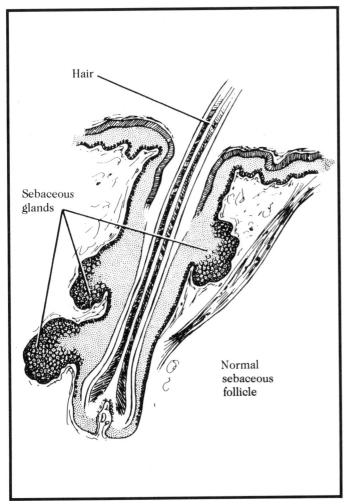

Figure 1 *Pilosebaceous Unit*

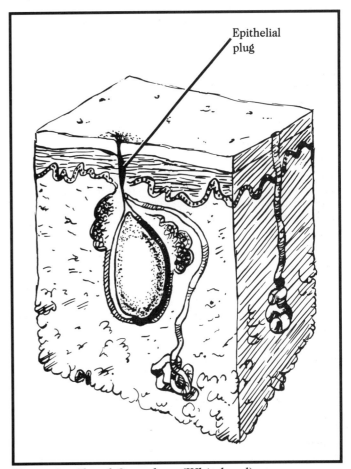

Figure 2 *Closed Comedone (Whitehead)*

Acne Therapy

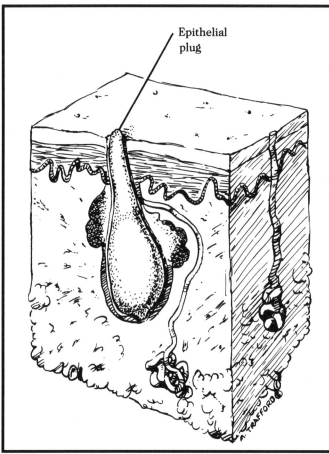

Epithelial plug

Figure 3 *Open Comedone (Blackhead)*

exposure to halogens, prolonged use of glucocorticosteroids, androgens (progesterones) in oral contraceptives and heredity. The size and reactivity of the sebaceous glands are hereditary.

Sebum production is affected by selenium and increased surface temperature. When selenium is incorporated into shampoo, sebum output is increased in one-third of the users. Increased surface temperature liquefies the sebum in the follicular reservoir and increased quantities flow out.

Diagnosis

A correct diagnosis is critical. Sweat gland tumors, follicular pustules following hyperalimentation, rhinophyma (redness, sebaceous hyperplasia, and nodular swelling and congestion of the skin of the nose), drug reactions, perioral dermatitis and contact dermatitis have been misdiagnosed as acne vulgaris.

Acne vulgaris is described as grade I, II, III or IV, or as mild, moderate or severe. Grade I has comedones; II, comedones and papules; III, comedones, papules, pustules and scars; IV, comedones, papules, pustules, scars and cystic lesions with sinus tracts.

Treatment

In the 1960s, treatment included oral tetracycline, glucocorticosteroids, estrogens, ultraviolet light, drainage, peeling agents, dermabrasion, large doses of vitamin A, superficial X-rays, restricted diets

and cleansing agents. Currently, the aim of therapy is to remove excessive sebum, prevent comedone formation, reduce inflammatory reactions, minimize scarring and improve compliance through counselling.

Excessive Sebum

Skin cleansers such as Neutrogena, Basic Soap, Night Cast Tersaseptic, Acnex or Phygiene may be used.

Excessive sebum should not be removed with harsh detergents or soaps, abrasive scrubs (plastics or aluminum pellets) or brushes. The effectiveness of scrubs has not been proven. Some physicians believe scrubs, gritty soaps and other abrasives aggravate acne. Cold creams, petrolatum and moisturizers must be avoided. Hair should be shampooed daily to remove excess oil, dirt and hair conditioners.

To remove excess sebum, a daily washing routine is imperative. The affected area should be washed at least twice daily with soap and warm water. Facial soaps that do not contain moisturizers can be recommended.

Comedonal Therapy

Comedonal therapy includes exfoliants, drying and peeling agents, and counterirritants. Exfoliants cause scaling and peeling.

The traditional drying agents incorporated into nonprescription products are mostly ineffective, although they have been used since the time of the Babylonians. These drying agents act as primary irritants and incite an inflammatory response; mitosis is stimulated, and the epidermal layer thickens and scales. Although the skin appears dry, sebum output is not diminished. Reduced sweating creates the illusion of drier skin.

Zirconium salts, sodium thiosulfate, phenol, resorcinol, and sulfur are ineffective in concentrations found in most nonprescription products. Benzoyl peroxide is now available as an effective nonprescription drug; however, special instructions should be given to the user.

Phenol is incorporated into acne products as a 0.1 per cent strength that is not a hazard. However, it may be used as a chemical face peel and is dangerous if handled by inexperienced persons. It penetrates the skin and produces systemic reactions such as tachycardia. Free phenol is conjugated with glycuronic and sulfuric acid and hence excreted by the kidneys. It may be detoxified by oxidation to hydroquinone pyrocatechia. If phenol crystals touch the skin, a severe burn results.

Sulfur is a counterirritant used to dry the lesions. However, it is reported to incite comedones that may take many months to become visible; *Corynebacterium acnes* is found within the treated comedones. Sulfur is used as a short-term treatment for rapid drying. Treatment then switches to a benzoyl peroxide. Sulfur is available as a mask in Night Cast products. The product is applied to the affected area according to directions. In 30 minutes the mask is washed off with water, skin cleanser and washcloth. The Casts contain sulfur and either resorcinol or salicylic acid. Both Casts contain at least 30 per cent alcohol. These products should be used cautiously by people receiving metronidazole or disulfiram. The manufacturer states that Night Cast products are alternatives for people who find products containing benzoyl peroxide irritating.

Salicylic acid in a concentration of 2 to 3 per cent is ineffective. It may be effective at 5 per cent or greater concentration in an alcohol or propylene glycol base. Occlusion and the release of the drug from the vehicle are important factors. Salicylate toxicity (tinnitus, dizziness and flushing) is a serious consequence of high concentrations, but disappointing results accompany low concentrations. Salicylic acid is slightly less potent than benzoyl peroxide in equal strengths.

Benzoyl peroxide is a powerful agent. When applied, it releases oxygen. Benzoyl peroxide produces good peeling, and pustules dry up more quickly than with retinoic acid. Benzoyl peroxide suppresses *Corynebacterium acnes* and is a comedolytic agent in the prevention of new lesions. It stimulates production of granulation tissue and epithelial cell proliferation. Benzoyl peroxide has been on the prescription market since the early 1980s as a nonprescription drug at 5 per cent and lower concentrations. Formulation problems such as separation of liquid and solid phases in the package and non-homogeneous preparation may cause treatment failure.

A 5 per cent concentration should be used for the first 1 or 2 months. If irritation does not occur, the 10 per cent concentration may be prescribed. Positive results usually occur in 3 months. A 10 per cent concentration can reduce free fatty acids and suppress *Corynebacterium acnes* by 50 per cent in 2 weeks.

Disadvantages include a 2.5 per cent risk of contact sensitization and a fairly high incidence of irritation. Cross-reactions are then possible with cinnamon, cocaine, benzoic acid derivatives, surfacaine, metacaine and stabilizers in flour. It may bleach hair, eyebrows, pillow slips and colored fabrics.

Benzoyl preparations are applied and allowed to dry before using a sunscreen. Benzoyl peroxide may inactivate the sunscreen if they are applied in combination. If retinoic acid is prescribed as part of the therapy, benzoyl peroxide is applied in the morning, and retinoic acid is applied in the evening and washed off in the morning. Benzoyl peroxide attacks the unsaturated bond of retinoic acid if the two products are used in combination. Benzoyl peroxide should not be applied to eyes, eyelids, mucous membranes or lips, or inside the nose or in creases.

Benzoyl peroxide was studied to determine if it can cause cancer. In one study, benzoyl peroxide and UV light did not alter epidermal cellular proliferation. Although benzoyl peroxide can promote tumor development in animals, benzoyl peroxide is considered a useful and safe product for treating acne.

Retinoic Acid

Retinoic acid is an effective but irritating compound. It is available as a cream, lotion or gel. The cream produces less irritation. Fair-skinned individuals in a dry climate respond best to the cream formulation. Dark-complexioned brunettes with oily skin prefer the solution or gel. The preparation should be applied after the skin has been cleaned and dried; a moist surface allows greater penetration. Harsh soaps and ultraviolet light should be avoided. Retinoic acid may potentiate the carcinogenic effect of ultraviolet light, as it thins the horny layer and allows more light to penetrate. Cold creams must be avoided, although a water-base make-up or moisture cream may be used. Non comedogenic sunscreens must be applied.

Consumers should be instructed how to properly apply retinoic acid and informed of the expected reactions. Treatment must be adjusted to the individual. Retinoic acid is applied once a day at bedtime to the entire face, using enough to produce a mild blush. Stinging and burning sensations are common. If erythema and peeling are not evident within 5 days, the product may be applied twice a day.

If the reaction is too intense, treatment should be withheld for a few days. The user may tolerate the therapy for only 1 to 2 hours per day.

Retinoic acid inhibits hyperkeratosis and prevents the formation of new obstructive and inflammatory lesions. It loosens the obstructive lesions for easier removal. In 30 per cent of cases, pustulation is noted within 3 to 4 weeks of starting therapy. These are microcomedones. Maximum inflammatory reactions occur in 3 to 4 weeks. Within 8 weeks, the desired initial clinical effects are obtained; maintenance therapy continues for years.

An application of retinoic acid on alternate days or twice weekly usually keeps the skin clean once all the comedones have been eradicated.

Disadvantages of retinoic acid include hyperpigmentation if used for prolonged periods by black-skinned individuals, and a diffuse pigment lightening in dark-complexioned individuals.

Antibiotics

Severe cases of acne vulgaris—grades III and IV—are treated with oral antibiotics in addition to other therapies. Once a clinical response is achieved, a lower maintenance dose is prescribed. Prophylactic prevention and grade II lesions are managed with topical antibiotics in a 1 to 2 per cent concentration in a hydroalcoholic vehicle with or without propylene glycol. The agent chosen must be safe for chronic therapy. Laboratory tests, complete blood counts and urinalysis should be performed at regular intervals if therapy continues for 2 years or longer.

Antibiotics are transported into the follicular canal via the sebaceous gland or infundibular (funnel-shaped) epithelium. The concentrations of *Corynebacterium acnes* and free fatty acids are reduced. Clinical effects are observed in at least 4 weeks. Comedone counts are reduced in 6 months. In general, side effects associated with antibiotic therapy are gastrointestinal upsets and monilial superinfections.

Antibiotics prescribed for oral and topical therapies include minocycline hydrochloride, tetracycline hydrochloride, erythromycin base and salts, and clindamycin hydrochloride. The stability of the various topical antibiotic preparations varies.

Tetracycline

Tetracycline hydrochloride is prescribed more frequently than minocycline hydrochloride since the latter product is associated with headaches and tinnitus and is more expensive. Initially, tetracycline is prescribed in the range of 0.5 to 1 g daily in divided doses. In a few cases, selected individuals may require 2 to 3 g daily. Within 4 weeks the dose is reduced to 250 mg daily, or every 2 or 3 days, to maintain control. The amount and rate of dosage reduction depend on the clinical response.

Tetracycline suppresses *Corynebacterium acnes* (reduced by 95 per cent) and inflammation by inhibiting chemotaxis. Free fatty acids are reduced in sebum as an indirect result of the inhibition of lipase producing organisms.

Tetracycline can cause photosensitivity. Larger doses are associated with nephrogenic diabetes insipidus and hepatotoxicity. The drug should not be administered with food, dairy products, antacids, zinc sulfate or products containing zinc or iron, including multiple vitamins with minerals. Oral tetracycline should be taken at least 1 hour before or 2 hours after the ingestion of other agents or food.

Tetracycline should not be prescribed to pregnant women. Tetracycline may reduce the effectiveness of oral contraceptives by reducing the enterohepatic circulation of the estrogen.

Tetracycline is available as a topical antibiotic preparation. However, erythromycin and clindamycin are prescribed more often than tetracycline.

Erythromycin

Erythromycin base and salts (estolate, stearate and lactobionate) are available for oral and topical administration. The base is used most commonly for topical therapy. Oral therapy is initiated at 0.5 to 1 g daily in divided doses. Maintenance dosage is 250 mg daily. Within 2 weeks, free fatty acid concentrations are reduced by 50 per cent. A side effect associated with erythromycin is gastrointestinal upset. All forms of erythromycin may be associated with hepatotoxicity; however, the estolate base has caused more concern than the other bases. Topical erythromycin therapy incorporates the base into the hydroalcoholic vehicle, which is stable for a maximum of 3 weeks. An application of this antibiotic preparation may be followed by tretinoin or benzoyl peroxide. Erythromycin topical preparations are applied once or twice a day.

Clindamycin

Clindamycin hydrochloride has been prescribed orally for the treatment of acne vulgaris. Because pseudomembranous colitis may develop, the drug is used topically rather than orally by most people. A severe and persistant diarrhea, with blood and mucus in the stools, may occur during or several weeks after discontinuing the oral clindamycin. The treatment includes discontinuation of the oral therapy in mild cases and medical intervention in severe cases. Pseudomembranous colitis is usually associated with an oral dosage greater than 200 mg per day. When a 1 to 2 per cent concentration of the drug is applied topically in the hydroalcoholic vehicle, less than 10 per cent of the clindamycin penetrates the skin. Over 500,000 people have applied this drug topically without one reported case of pseudomembranous colitis. After topical application, the drug has been found in small quantities in the urine of users.

Clindamycin eliminates *Corynebacterium acnes* from open comedones. After 2 months to 2 years, about 20 per cent of users develop resistant *Corynebacterium acnes* strains. If the therapy is switched to oral tetracycline for 2 months, the clindamycin preparation can be resumed, since the *Corynebacterium acnes* will be sensitive once again. Clindamycin is applied once or twice a day. It is stable in a hydroalcoholic vehicle for 1 year at room temperature.

Other Treatments

Other modes of treatment for selected cases of acne vulgaris include sulfones, intralesional triamcinolone acetonide, cyclic estrogen-progesterone therapy, isotretinoin, dermabrasion, ultraviolet light therapy and collagen implants. Each therapy has indications, side effects and contraindications.

Diaphenylsulfone, or **dapsone**, is associated with agranulocytosis. It is used with an antibiotic and exfoliant, and is rarely prescribed.

Triamcinolone acetonide is diluted with sterile normal saline to a concentration of 2.5 mg/mL and injected into the large nodulocystic lesions. Injections are made every 2 weeks. Atrophy is a side effect; the defect fills in within 6 to 12 weeks.

Isotretinoin (Accutane) is helpful in treating cystic acne or severe cases of acne resistant to oral antibiotics. The exact mechanism of action is not known, but sebum secretion is decreased in relation to the dose and duration of treatment with isotretinoin. One course of treatment is 4 months. If a second course is required, it is advisable to wait 8 weeks after the first treatment since many individuals continue to improve.

Adverse effects reported with isotretinoin therapy include dryness of the skin and mucous membranes (almost universally), musculoskeletal pains, pseudotumor cerebri (a benign intracranial hypertension), headache, papilledema and visual disturbances. Night vision may be diminished; users should be warned about driving at night. Laboratory monitoring of liver function and blood lipids is recommended. Fetal abnormalities have been reported; users should be counselled to start contraceptive measures 1 month before and continue for 1 month after isotretinoin therapy. Other products containing vitamin A should be avoided.

Dermabrasion is a procedure in which the skin is frozen and quickly planed down to remove the epidermis. Postoperative edema swells the tissue to make the scar less conspicuous. The full results are not evident for at least 6 months, when the edema has disappeared. The procedure is useful for shallow scars, but of no benefit for icepick scars.

Tretinoin may be beneficial after dermabrasion has been performed. One study shows tretinoin suppresses milia and post-inflammatory hyperpigmentation and increases proliferation. A sunscreen is recommended when tretinoin is prescribed. A 1:1 mixture of tretinoin and a sunscreen lotion with sun protection factor 15 does not compromise the effectiveness of the tretinoin.

Collagen implants have been available since the early 1980s for selected individuals. The implant is an adjuvant in the restoration of soft tissue contour defects or deformities, including acne scars. The implant becomes colonized by host connective tissue cells. This treatment is expensive, has a limited time benefit and may cause allergic reactions.

Summary

There is no cure for acne. However, improvement of lesions and prevention of iatrogenic (drug-induced) causes are realistic goals of therapy.

Ask the Consumer

Q. Do you have fewer lesions in the summer?
- Exposure to ultraviolet light may be effective treatment for acne vulgaris. The primary value may be the tanning effect, which may reduce the visibility of the lesions. The long-term effects of ultraviolet light exposure include an increased number of comedones, skin aging and solar keratosis. However, the acne may worsen if it is a very humid summer, because although the ultraviolet light helps acne, humidity aggravates it.

Q. Does stress exacerbate your acne?
- Some exacerbations of acne may relate to increased mechanical manipulation as a result of stress. The person may subconsciously pick, squeeze or handle the face, back or shoulders. Recognition of the manipulations may be helpful. Picking and squeezing may

Acne Therapy

rupture the follicle and lead to scarring lesions.(See the section on acne excoriée.)

Q. *Do you know how to apply the benzoyl peroxide when used with a sunscreen?*

■ Advise the consumer to apply the benzoyl peroxide product and allow it to dry, then apply the sunscreen. If applied at the same time, the benzoyl peroxide may inactivate the sunscreen.

Q. *Do you know how to apply the benzoyl peroxide when used with retinoic acid?*

■ The benzoyl peroxide is applied in the morning and the retinoic acid is applied in the evening and washed off in the morning. The benzoyl peroxide attacks the unsaturated bonds of the retinoic acid if they are applied in combination.

Q. *Do you know how to apply the topical steroid you have been prescribed for your acne?*

■ The medication is applied to clean skin that has been patted dry. A thin, even layer is applied to the affected area. If it is applied at night, the person should use a pillow and not lie flat. The medication must not be applied to infected areas or to lesions other than acne.

References

Types of Acne

Adams RM. Occupational skin disease. New York: Grune & Stratton, 1983:70–80,159–60.

Bruinsma W. The guide to drug eruption. Amsterdam: Excerpta Medica, 1982:17–9.

Fry L, Cornell MNP. Dermatology. Boston: MTP Press, 1985:75–80.

Jackson R. Morphological dermatology, a study of the living gross pathology of the skin. Springfield: CC Thomas, 1979.

Mailbach HI, Gellin GA. Occupational and industrial dermatology. Chicago: Year Book Medical Publishers, 1982.

Moschella SL, Hurley HS. Dermatology. Toronto: WB Saunders, 1985:1319–21.

Sheard C. Treatment of skin diseases, a manual. Chicago: Year Book Medical Publishers, 1978.

Sulzberger ME, et al. Tropical acne. Bull US Army Med Dept 1946;6:149.

Tucker SB. Occupational tropical acne. Cutis 1983;31:79–81.

Sebum

Roenigk HH Jr. Office dermatology. Baltimore: Williams and Wilkins, 1981:69–73.

Shuster S. Dermatology in internal medicine. Toronto: Oxford University Press, 1978:6,11,42–5,219.

Treatment

Andrew WC. Enterohepatic circulation of oral contraceptives. Clin Obstet Gynecol 1976;6(1):3–11.

Burks JW. Dermabrasion and chemical peeling in the treatment of certain cosmetic defects and diseases of the skin. Springfield: CC Thomas, 1979.

Culen SI, Childers RC. Tretinoin-sunscreen mixture in the treatment of acne vulgaris. Cutis 1988;411:289–91.

Duke EE. Does benzoyl peroxide cause cancer? The Canadian perspective. Contemporary Dermatol 1987;Dec/Jan:15–9.

Fisher AA. Contact dermatitis. Philadelphia: Lea & Febiger, 1973.

Leyden J. How dangerous is benzoyl peroxide as an anti-acne agent? Contemporary Dermatol 1987;Dec/Jan:22–5.

Maddin S. Current dermatologic therapy. Toronto: WB Saunders, 1982.

Mailbach HI, Gellin GA. Occupational and industrial dermatology. Chicago: Year Book Medical Publishers, 1982.

Mandy SH. Tretinoin in the preoperative and postoperative management of dermabrasion. J Am Acad Dermatol 1986;15(Suppl):878–9.

Peck GL, et al. Prolonged remissions of cystic and conglobata acne with 12-cis retinoic acid. N Engl J Med 1979;300:329–33.

Plewig G, Kligman AM. Acne: morphogenesis and treatment. New York: Springer-Verlag, 1975.

Shalita AR. Treatment of mild and moderate acne vulgaris with salicylic acid in an alcoholic-detergent vehicle. Cutis 1981;28:556-9.

Stoughton RB. Topical antibiotics for acne vulgaris. Arch Dermatol 1979;115:486–9.

USP dispensing information—advice for the patient. Easton: United States Pharmacopeial Convention, 1985.

8
Ophthalmic Products

Lynn R. Trottier

The complex physiology of the eye permits numerous common eye disorders, including glaucoma, dry eye and disorders of the eyelids, conjunctiva, cornea and uveal tract as well as complications of trauma and systemic disease. Nonprescription ophthalmic agents used to treat these disorders include decongestants, antihistamines, anti-infectives, artificial tears, astringents and local anesthetics. These agents may be combined with preservatives or other ingredients and may be formulated in solutions or ointments.

Any eye problem is potentially vision-threatening. Pharmacists need basic knowledge of the anatomy and physiology of the eye as well as knowledge of etiology, signs and symptoms, potential complications and management of common eye disorders. This knowledge is crucial to realizing the limitations and acceptability of a consumer self-medicating with nonprescription ophthalmic products.

Nonprescription medications can be used safely only when there is no pain, inflammation, bleeding, injury or major pathology (for example, glaucoma), that is, when vision is not threatened. Some symptoms can be self-medicated (see Table I). Others must be referred to a physician or ophthalmologist (see Table II).

Table I *Conditions for Which Self-medication May Be Appropriate*

•No pain
•Eyestrain
•Burning
•Itching
•Stinging
•Mild tearing

Table II *Conditions for Which Medical Referral is Essential*

•Pain
•Photophobia
•Altered vision
•Redness immediately around the cornea
•Excessive discharge
•Abnormal pupils
•Trauma
•Conditions lasting longer than 48 hours

Perhaps the most frequent ocular problems for which people seek help involve "red eye" (see Table III). These problems must be properly diagnosed, as they can range in severity from insignificant to blinding. If in doubt, pharmacists should refer the individual to an ophthalmologist or a physician.

Table III *Ocular Conditions Associated With "Red Eye"*

•Dryness
•Eyelid problems
•Conjunctival problems
•Corneal or uveal tract disorders
•Glaucoma
•Trauma

Anatomy and Physiology

The eyeballs are contained within the bony orbital cavities (see Figure 1). These cavities, which are thicker at the rim, protect the

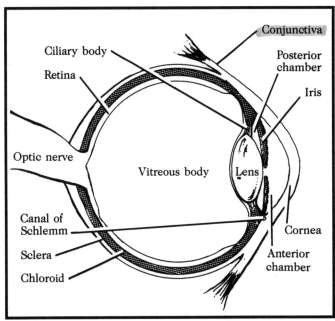

Figure 1 *The Eye Cut in a Horizontal Section.*

Ophthalmic Products

eye from injury. Muscles, ligaments and a cushion of fat suspend the eyes in the orbit.

The eyelids are thin, movable "curtains" that cover the exposed anterior surface of the eyeball. If any loud noise, sudden movement or excessive light is interpreted as potentially harmful, an involuntary blink reflex closes the lids. Regular blinking distributes the tears over the anterior portion of the eye. Eyelashes protect the eye from dust and perspiration. Dense connective tissues (tarsal plates) give the eyelids their stiffness. A number of glands are contained within the tarsal plates (see Table IV).

Table IV *Glands Contained Within the Tarsal Plates*

- Meibomian glands (secrete an oily substance which is part of the tear film)
- Glands of Zeis (modified sebaceous glands)
- Glands of Moll (modified sweat glands)

The conjunctiva, a thin, vascular, mucous membrane, lines the inner surface of the eyelids and covers the anterior surface of the eyeball (except for the cornea).

The eyeball itself is like an inflated basketball. It has three outer layers surrounding liquid-filled chambers (see Table V). If the outer layer is cut (for example, by injury), the inner contents may escape and the structure may collapse.

Table V *Outer Layers of the Eyeball*

- Sclera
- Uvea (choroid, ciliary body, iris)
- Retina

The outer, opaque, fibrous layer—the sclera, or white of the eye—is protective and gives shape to the eye when inflated by internal pressure. The sclera covers the posterior three-quarters of the eyeball and joins anteriorly with the thin, transparent cornea or "window" of the eye. At the corneoscleral junction, a vessel called the canal of Schlemm completely encircles the cornea. This canal is covered with connective tissue called the trabecular meshwork. The canal and its meshwork form a drainage system for the liquid in a small chamber behind the cornea (the anterior chamber) and thus maintain a constant intraocular pressure.

The middle layer (uvea) has three sections. The choroid is a darkly pigmented, highly vascular tissue lining the posterior portion of the sclera. Anteriorly, the choroid thickens to form the ciliary body. This smooth muscle structure attaches to the lens of the eye via thin, zonular ligaments that allow the eye to focus by controlling the shape of the lens. The ciliary body also produces liquid (the aqueous humor). The iris, a delicate, pigmented muscular tissue, projects from the front of the ciliary body. Its pigmentation gives the eye its color (for example, blue or brown eyes). The iris is a doughnut-shaped structure. The "hole" in the middle of the "doughnut" is the pupil, which appears black. By adjusting the pupil size, the iris controls the amount of light entering the eye.

The inner layer—the retina or nervous layer—covers the choroid and extends to the posterior portion of the ciliary body. It transmits nervous impulses to the optic nerve and onward to the brain. Light is detected at the retina.

The chambers of the eye aid the cornea and lens in focusing light correctly on the retina. The anterior chamber lies between the cornea and iris and the posterior chamber is between the iris and lens. Both chambers are filled with aqueous humor, which bathes the lens, then flows anteriorly through the pupil. It is filtered through the trabecular network into the canal of Schlemm, which returns it into the circulation via various blood vessels. The fluid pressure exerted by the aqueous humor gives the eye its intraocular pressure.

The vitreous chamber located behind the lens is filled with transparent, colorless, gel-like material. It fills most of the space inside the eye. If the vitreous humor is lost, it cannot be regenerated and the structure of the eye can be seriously altered.

Table VI *The Three Layers of the Tear Film*

- Oily (outer) layer
- Aqueous (middle) layer
- Mucoid (inner) layer adhering to the surface of eye

Another important part of the eye is the tear film, which covers the corneal and conjunctival surfaces. The tear film is comprised of three layers, which normally completely cover the most superficial cells of the cornea and conjunctiva (the corneal epithelial cells and conjunctival epithelial cells) (see Table VI). The thickest layer, the aqueous tear fluid, is produced by the lacrimal gland located at the upper, outer angle of the lid and by the accessory lacrimal glands located in the conjunctiva (see Figure 2). An oily (lipid) film, produced mainly by the Meibomian glands, covers the surface of the

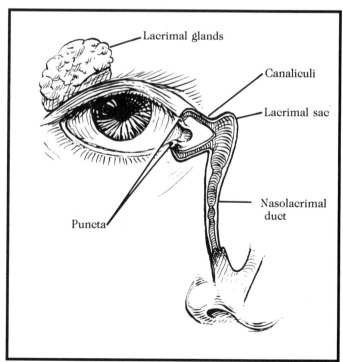

Figure 2 *Lacrimal Apparatus*

Ophthalmic Products

aqueous layer; it helps spread the tear film over the eye and may help reduce the evaporation rate of tears. Between the aqueous layer and the epithelial cells of the eye is a viscous material called the mucoid layer. Principally produced by special conjunctival cells, the function of this layer is less well known. It may help spread the aqueous tear phase over the lipid-bearing corneal epithelial cells and may help stabilize the tear film. The tear film serves several functions (see Table VII).

Table VII   Functions of the Tear Film

- Formation of an almost perfectly smooth surface on the cornea
- Lubrication for the eyes and lids
- Protective bactericidal action for the sensitive corneal epithelium (e.g., lysozymes destroy bacteria; IgA assists in controlling infection)
- Moistening and oxygenation of the cornea

Ten per cent of the tear film is lost by evaporation. The remainder is constantly drained from the eye via two lacrimal puncti (orifices at the nasal end of the upper and lower lids). The tears are carried via lacrimal canaliculi to the lacrimal sac. They exit through the nasolacrimal duct and are discharged as part of the nasal secretions (thus, the runny nose associated with crying) (see Figure 2). Eyedrops or eye ointments can be absorbed into the rest of the body from the eye via this route either by absorption through the nasal mucous membrane or by swallowing into the gastrointestinal tract. Eye preparations can also be absorbed via the vascular system in the conjunctiva.

Common Eye Disorders

The following are brief descriptions of the etiology, signs and symptoms, potential complications and management (see also Treatment) of common eye disorders (see Table VIII). Table IX summarizes the differential diagnosis of some of these conditions.

Table VIII   Common Eye Disorders

Disorders of the eyelids blepharitis hordeolum (sty) chalazion
Disorders of the conjunctiva conjunctival hyperemia subconjunctival hemorrhage conjunctivitis
Disorders of the cornea (keratitis)
Disorders of the uveal tract (uveitis)
Glaucoma
Trauma
Dry eye syndrome

Disorders of the Eyelids

Blepharitis, an acute or chronic inflammation of the eyelid margin, is one of the most common causes of eye disease. It may begin in early childhood and continue throughout life. Common etiological factors are listed in Table X. Seborrhea and *Staphylococcus aureus*

Table IX   Differential Diagnosis of Common Causes of Inflamed Eye

	Acute conjunctivitis	Acute iritis[1]	Acute glaucoma[2]	Corneal trauma or infection
Incidence	Extremely common	Common	Uncommon	Common
Discharge	Moderate to copious	None	None	Watery or purulent
Vision	No effect on vision	Slightly blurred	Markedly blurred	Usually blurred
Pain	None	Moderate	Severe	Moderate to severe
Conjunctival injection[3]	Diffuse; more toward fornices	Mainly circumcornea	Diffuse	Diffuse
Cornea	Clear	Usually clear	Steamy	Change in clarity related to cause
Pupil size	Normal	Small	Moderately dilated and fixed	Normal
Pupillary light response	Normal	Poor	None	Normal
Intraocular pressure	Normal	Normal	Elevated	Normal
Smear	Causative organisms	No organisms	No organisms	Organisms found only in corneal ulcers due to infection

[1]Acute anterior uveitis
[2]Angle-closure glaucoma
[3]Term used to mean congestion of ciliary or conjunctival blood vessels
Adapted from: Vaughan D, Ashbury T, Tabbara KF, eds. General ophthalmology. Los Altos: Lange, 1989.

Ophthalmic Products

Table X *Common Causes of Blepharitis*

- Seborrhea
- *Staphylococcus aureus*
- *Staphylococcus epidermidis*
- Parasites
- Irritation
- Allergy

either alone or in combination are the most frequent causes. *Staphylococcus epidermidis* may be underdiagnosed as a causative pathogen.

With blepharitis, a person often complains of unsightly hyperemia along the lid margins, photophobia, edema, burning and irritation. Vision usually remains normal.

Staphylococcus aureus is usually found at low levels along the healthy lid margin. Researchers theorize the toxins secreted by the organism often attack the epithelial cells when a person is in a debilitated state (for example, recovering from measles). The toxins can cause ulceration of the lid margins. A purulent discharge forms crusts along the lashes, and the individual often complains that the eyelashes are stuck together in the morning on awakening. If this ulcerative condition is improperly treated, the lashes may become distorted, grow inward to irritate the cornea, or fall out. Treatment includes use of antibiotic eyedrops or ointments and occasionally, systemic antibiotics. If there is an associated dry eye syndrome, artificial tears and lubricants may be needed. Contaminated cosmetics can be a source of reinfection.

When treating blepharitis, the aim is to eliminate etiological factors. Thorough cleansing of the lids is essential. Warm moist compresses (a clean facecloth or gauze pads) applied 5 to 15 minutes several times a day (for example, 4 times a day tapering to once daily) softens crusts. A cotton-tipped applicator or cotton pledget dipped in warm water or mild baby shampoo (diluted 1:1 with tap water) removes scales and crusts. Lid hygiene is particularly important in the morning as debris collects and builds up on the lids while the eyes are closed during sleep. If the physician recommends selenium sulfide 1 per cent to remove scales, the suspension should be diluted 1:5 or 1:10. If seborrhea coexists, an antiseborrheic shampoo should be used; ocular contact must be avoided as it may result in toxic conjunctivitis. When the scalp is treated, the blepharitis often clears.

Pubic lice (crabs) can thrive in the eyelashes. The nits attach to the lashes and cause an irritative blepharitis. Treatment of pubic lice infestations in the eyelashes and other areas of the body is discussed in the chapter on topical antiparasitics.

Irritant or allergic blepharitis may be provoked in numerous ways (see Table XI). One of the primary symptoms of this allergic reac-

Table XI *Items That May Provoke Irritant or Allergic Blepharitis*

- Smoke
- Drugs (e.g., atropine, neomycin, pilocarpine, tetracaine, timolol)
- Cosmetics
- Plants (e.g., poison ivy)
- Metal (e.g., nickel spectacle frames)
- Rubbing the eyes (i.e., in response to local irritation, congestion or attempts to clear vision)

tion is itching. Treatment requires removing the offending agents. Antihistamine drugs (given orally) and corticosteroid eyedrops or ointments, along with cold compresses saturated with Burow's 1:40 or normal saline, may be useful. An ordinary washcloth moistened with cold water and applied to the eyelids for several minutes also can be used as a cold compress.

Hordeolum, or sty, is a frequently encountered condition. An acute, pus-producing inflammation, it begins in the follicle of an eyelash or in one of the glands of Moll or Zeis. The causative organism is usually *Staphylococcus aureus*. Sties are often associated with people who have lowered resistance (for example, debility or diabetes) or local predilection (for example, concomitant blepharitis or acne vulgaris).

Initial symptoms are tenderness, edema and redness, which may be diffused over the lid. In a few days, a small collection of pus appears along the eyelid margin. Until the pustule ruptures, usually in 3 to 4 days, the person experiences considerable pain. Sometimes the sty spontaneously resolves without discharging its contents. As the infection may spread along the lid margin, directly or via fingers, sties often appear in "crops." If this condition is not appropriately treated, particularly in a severely debilitated person, the end result may be orbital cellulitis.

Sties are usually treated by applying warm compresses or dry heat several times over 10 to 15 minutes, thus encouraging drainage by opening the pores. The warmth also draws more blood to the area, increasing the inflammatory and repair mediators. These mediators close off and clean up the infection. The lesions must not be squeezed between the fingers due to the possibility of spreading the bacteria in pus, causing cellulitis. Antibiotic eye ointments applied following the heat treatments may prevent secondary or recurrent infection. If heat treatment is ineffective, if the sty persists for more than 48 hours or if there are multiple sties, the person should be referred to a physician. It may be necessary to incise the lesion or use prescription medications such as antibiotics or topical steroids.

Chalazion (Meibomian or tarsal cyst) is a chronic, granulomatous inflammation of a Meibomian gland due to retention of normal secretions. It is not infected. It may occur spontaneously or it may be associated with seborrhea and acne rosacea. The cyst develops over several weeks. It most commonly occurs in the upper lid and feels like a small pebble. It bulges externally, but points toward the conjunctival side of the eyelid. Usually, the lid margin is not involved. The lesion is often painless, but is cosmetically embarrassing. Secondary infection can occur.

Treatment may involve use of warm, moist compresses 4 times a day, excision by an ophthalmologist or application of antibiotic eye preparations to prevent secondary infection. In severe cases, ophthalmologists may inject corticosteroids directly into the cyst. For recurrent chalazions, the physician must rule out the possibility of carcinoma.

Disorders of the Conjunctiva

Conjunctival hyperemia involves dilation of the conjunctival blood vessels in both eyes. It may result from numerous causes (see Table XII). The person is usually symptomless, but may complain of a gritty foreign body sensation.

The only way to cure conjunctival hyperemia is to eliminate the cause. The person should have adequate rest. Temporary relief may be provided by cold compresses, weak "eye whitener" (vasoconstrictor) drops (if they are not the cause), astringent-containing eye-

Ophthalmic Products

Table XII *Some Causes of Conjunctival Hyperemia*

Dust	Poor ventilation
Smoke	Alcohol (after several drinks)
Chlorine	Prolonged instillation of decongestant
(in swimming pool)	eyedrops
Wind	Blepharitis
Air pollution (fumes)	Dry environment
Heat	

drops or artificial tears. Vasoconstrictor eyedrops do not cure blood-shot eyes. When self-medicating, the person must be cautioned that long-term use of vasoconstrictor eyedrops may aggravate the hyperemia or, after abrupt discontinuation of the preparation, cause the vessels to dilate further and appear even redder than before. (See the section on decongestants).

Subconjunctival hemorrhage appears when a conjunctival vessel ruptures. A bright red patch appears on the white sclera, usually in only one eye, and can alarm the person experiencing it. The rupture may be due to numerous causes (see Table XIII). The hemorrhage may occur spontaneously in healthy people, because the fragile conjunctival vessels are relatively exposed.

A person presenting with a subconjunctival hemorrhage should be referred to a physician to rule out serious disorders and treat the problem accordingly. In most instances of subconjunctival hemorrhage, no treatment is required; the hemorrhage gradually fades over a period of 2 weeks.

Table XIII *Some Causes of Subconjunctival Hemorrhage*

- Severe or minimal trauma (e.g., following a severe blow or after rubbing the eye)
- Sudden rise in venous pressure, particularly in the elderly (e.g., coughing, straining, sneezing, vomiting)
- Systemic disease (e.g., hypertension, blood dyscrasias)
- Adenovirus/bacterial conjunctivitis
- Spontaneous

Table XIV *Common Causes of Conjunctivitis*

- Bacterial
- Viral
- Chlamydial
- Allergic
- Chemical (e.g., fumes, preservatives in contact lens solutions)

Pink eye – extremely contagious

Conjunctivitis—inflammation of the conjunctiva—is one of the most common ocular conditions in North America. It is characterized by diffuse redness in both eyes, but may first appear in only one eye. Vision is almost normal. The person may complain of discharge, burning, stinging or a gritty sensation. The common forms of conjunctivitis can be classified according to etiology (see Tables XIV and XV).

Bacterial conjunctivitis has an acute onset and is usually characterized by mucopurulent or purulent discharge. The eyelids can be stuck together on awakening. A wide variety of organisms are responsible for this disease. The most common organisms involved are *Staphylococcus aureus*, *Streptococcus pneumoniae* and *Hemophilus influenzae*. Although less common, conjunctivitis may be due to *Neisseria gonorrhea*, *Pseudomonas aeruginosa* or Proteus species. These bacterial infections are usually self-limiting and often resolve spontaneously in 7 to 10 days.

As bacterial conjunctivitis may resemble serious corneal infection, accurate diagnosis is important. Although bacterial conjunctivitis is self-limiting, numerous practitioners indicate that treatment with antibiotic eye preparations reduces the duration of infection to 2 to 3 days. Some nonprescription antibacterials are used for this purpose (administered every 1 to 2 hours initially or 5 times a day for 1 week). Eye patches must be avoided as they produce an incubatory environment. With the more serious infections (for example, *Neisseria gonorrhea*), oral antibiotics are required to prevent dangerous complications.

Viral conjunctivitis may be a symptom of systemic infection (for example, respiratory tract infections, particularly in children) or may be limited to infection of the corneal and conjunctival epithelium. Symptoms and contagion vary according to the virus. Some

Table XV *Differential Diagnosis of the Common Types of Conjunctivitis*

Clinical findings and cytology	Bacterial	Viral	Chlamydial	Atopic (Allergic)
Itching	Minimal	Minimal	Minimal	Severe
Hyperemia	Generalized	Generalized	Generalized	Generalized
Tearing	Moderate	Profuse	Moderate	Moderate
Exudation	Profuse	Minimal	Profuse	Minimal
Preauricular adenopathy	Uncommon	Common	Common only in inclusion conjunctivitis	None
In stained scrapings and exudates	Bacteria, PMNs[1]	Monocytes	PMNs,[1] plasma cells, inclusion bodies	Eosinophils
Associated sore throat and fever	Occasionally	Occasionally	Never	Never

[1]Polymorphonuclear cells
Adapted from: Vaughan D, Ashbury T, Tabbara KF, eds. General ophthalmology. Los Algos: Lange, 1989.

Ophthalmic Products

adenoviruses produce a watery discharge, and the preauricular lymph nodes may become enlarged. Viral conjunctivitis can be treated symptomatically using artificial tears to provide comfort for the duration of the disease (2 to 3 weeks).

Chlamydia is an organism that can cause **inclusion conjunctivitis** in individuals with genital chlamydial infections. The eye is red and exudative. Treatment includes use of special eye preparations and sometimes oral antibiotics.

Table XVI	*Types of Allergic Conjunctivitis*
Atopic	immediate hypersensitivity antibody mediated
Contact	delayed hypersensitivity lymphocyte mediated

Allergic conjunctivitis may arise from numerous allergens (see Table XVI). Symptoms include itching, tearing and swelling. Photophobia or a purulent, stringy discharge may indicate the presence of one of the more serious forms of allergic conjunctivitis (for example, vernal or phlyctenular keratoconjunctivitis). Atopic conjunctivitis usually occurs in people who have hayfever; it is an acute seasonal or environmental problem. Contact conjunctivitis can result from local instillation of some medications (see Table XVII).

Table XVII	*Possible Offenders Causing Ocular Contact Conjunctivitis*	
Antihistamines	Local anesthetics	
Atropine	(proparacaine, tetracaine)	
Benzalkonium chloride	Neomycin	
Cyclopentolate	Pilocarpine	
Gentamicin	Sulfonamide	
Idoxuridine	Thimerosal	
Lanolin	Timolol	

[1]In ophthalmic eye drops, eye ointments, or eye gels

When there is an atopic allergic component to conjunctivitis, the condition usually responds to oral or topical antihistamines. Short-term use of vasoconstricting or astringent eye preparations may offer temporary relief. Cold compresses offer comfort. Contact lens wear, during the allergy season, may be poorly tolerated and the person may need to temporarily stop wearing the lenses. If there is a stringy discharge, photophobia or reduced vision, the person may require desensitization or treatment beyond the scope of nonprescription medications (for example, corticosteroid eyedrops or cromolyn sodium eyedrops).

Disorders of the Cornea and Uveal Tract

Keratitis is an inflammation of the cornea that can result in blindness if not properly treated. It can be due to numerous causes (see Table XVIII). Damage to the cornea is serious because its natural defence mechanisms are poor. The cornea is well supplied with sensitive nerve fibres, so damage generally causes pain. Corneal ulcers may be accompanied by purulent discharge and blepharospasm.

Table XVIII *Some Causes of Keratitis*

- Systemic disease
- Trauma
- Corneal infection
- Chronic exposure of cornea due to inadequate lid closure
- Exposure to high-density ultraviolet sources (e.g., welding arcs)

A common cause of blindness in industrialized countries is herpes simplex keratitis. The individual complains of blurred vision, photophobia, mild foreign body sensation, circumcorneal redness and watery discharge, usually in one eye. Severe pain is absent because the organism usually decreases corneal sensation.

Corneal ulcers caused by infection with *Pseudomonas aeruginosa* usually progress rapidly and can be highly destructive within 24 to 48 hours. The increased incidence of these ulcers may be associated with the inappropriate use of some extended-wear contact lenses. Depending on the cause, treatment involves the use of one or several of the following: antibiotic eyedrops, atropine eyedrops or ointment, mechanical debridement of the surface and the fitting of special contact lens bandages.

Uveitis is an inflammation of the middle layer of the eye. The iris, ciliary body, choroid or any combination of the three may be affected as the result of endogenous or exogenous mechanisms. The person presents with blurred vision, photophobia, redness around the cornea, tearing and small pupils. Pain may be absent or severe.

When dealing with corneal or uveal problems, early diagnosis by an ophthalmologist is essential; these conditions can lead to blindness. The ophthalmologist uses antibiotics (as eyedrops, direct subconjunctival injections or oral preparations) and corticosteroid eye preparations. Pharmacists should be aware of the special care needed when corticosteroid therapy is used. If the keratitis is due to herpes simplex virus, corticosteroid eye preparations may aggravate the keratitis by enhancing the activity of the virus. They may also cause or aggravate open-angle glaucoma, promote fungal infection, or produce cataracts, particularly with long-term use.

Glaucoma

Although nonprescription medications are not used to treat glaucoma, pharmacists must be knowledgeable about this disease. Consumers may request a nonprescription medication to treat reduced vision or ocular pain resulting from glaucoma.

Glaucoma is usually characterized by an increased intraocular pressure (IOP), which damages the optic nerve and causes visual defects. It may be classified as congenital, primary (for example, open-angle or angle-closure) or secondary (for example, due to trauma, changes in the lens of the eye or changes in the uveal tract).

Primary open-angle glaucoma is the most common type of glaucoma and is responsible for at least 90 per cent of primary glaucoma cases; angle-closure causes less than 5 per cent. This figure differs in various surveys and is probably overweighted in terms of the prevalence of open-angle compared to angle-closure glaucoma.

The pathology of open-angle glaucoma (simple, chronic, or wide-angle glaucoma) continues to be debated. The anterior chamber angle is normal, but it seems the aqueous outflow is blocked, as the openings in the sieve-like trabecular meshwork and canal of Schlemm are abnormal. This condition produces an elevated IOP. Initially, the disease is symptomless; there is rarely pain or redness.

Ophthalmic Products

Table XIX *Prescription Medications Used to Treat Open-Angle Glaucoma*

- Miotics (e.g., carbachol, echothiophate iodide, pilocarpine)
- Sympathomimetics (e.g., dipivefrin, epinephrine)
- Carbonic anhydrase inhibitors (e.g., acetazolamide, methazolamide)
- Adrenergic blocking agents (e.g., betaxolol, levobunolol, timolol)

Table XX *Factors That May Indicate Increased Susceptibility to Angle-Closure Glaucoma*

- Family history of narrow-angle glaucoma
- Over 50 years of age
- Far-sighted
- Current therapy with a medication that may precipitate an attack (usually by causing pupillary dilation)

Vision is gradually destroyed and the individual is often unaware of any problem until partial blindness occurs. Ophthalmic examination is essential to detect the disease early, especially because visual defects can occur before the IOP is significantly elevated. Examination is particularly important for people over 40 years of age and for those with a family history of glaucoma. Open-angle glaucoma requires chronic therapy with prescription drugs (see Table XIX).

To assist a person with open-angle glaucoma, the pharmacist can do the following:

- Advise the person on the proper administration of eyedrops.
- Check for compliance with the regimen by monitoring refill frequency.
- Emphasize the importance of compliance (especially important in a disease that usually has no initial major symptoms).
- Keep dosage adjustment records up-to-date.
- Question people about side effects. (If severe, suggest they contact their physician. If therapy has just been initiated, explain the side effect may become less bothersome in several weeks.)
- Explain the decrease in night vision if a person is using miotic drugs and warn about driving at night.

Primary angle-closure glaucoma (acute, narrow-angle, congestive glaucoma) is a rare disease that presents only when the anterior chamber angle is shallow and when the iris blocks the trabecular drainage meshwork and the peripheral cornea. This mechanical blockage results in a rapid rise of IOP. Individuals may be predisposed (for example, they may have a shallow anterior chamber) and be free of symptoms for years. With age, the lens size increases, pushing the iris forward, narrowing the angle and increasing the chances of an attack. An acute attack of angle-closure glaucoma may be precipitated by an increase in pupil size (mydriasis) resulting from emotional upset, prolonged exposure to the dark, or following the use of drugs that increase pupil size (mydriatics). The attacks usually occur late in the day or evening. They may become fully developed in 30 to 60 minutes. The person may complain of sudden onset of pain around the eyes, tearing, blurred vision and colored halos around lights. Marked conjunctival hyperemia is seen. Nausea, vomiting, and even abdominal pain may be present due to reflex vagal nerve stimulation.

Although an acute attack of angle-closure glaucoma requires immediate medical attention, the pharmacist can participate in a glaucoma alert program by carefully questioning the person who requests nonprescription eyedrops.

Eyedrops may be requested for ocular pain associated with headache, blurring vision, redness of the eyes and colored halos around lights. Consumers may associate these symptoms with "tired eyes." Nausea, vomiting and sweating can also occur. Upon questioning, individuals may admit to ocular discomfort in the evening, when watching television or a movie in a darkened room, or during periods of anxiety.

Attacks of ocular discomfort are self-limiting, especially when the person is exposed to light. For example, an individual may have ocular pain while watching television, but the symptoms are relieved upon entering a well-lit room. The ocular discomfort probably has subsided by the time the person seeks help, but a product for future use may be requested.

In conjunction with the above symptoms, a number of factors may indicate increased susceptibility to angle-closure glaucoma attacks (see Table XX).

Trauma

Trauma to the eye requires immediate attention. Bleeding, pain, photophobia and decreased vision indicate serious eye injury. Immediate steps should be taken to implement appropriate first-aid measures that may prevent blindness.

Contusion from a blunt instrument (for example, fist, baseball, hockey puck, squash ball or champagne cork) is characterized by the familiar black eye (edema, lid discoloration, lid closure) and sometimes double vision. Immediate ocular examination is necessary to rule out severe underlying damage. During transport to medical aid, cold compresses can reduce the swelling and provide comfort.

Laceration caused by high-velocity blunt objects (for example, car steering wheel) or sharp objects (for example, a knife or flying metal) is a medical emergency. With these injuries, it is important to avoid applying pressure as this can further damage the eye. Even wiping away tears or blood may increase the damage. Protruding objects (for example, a fishhook) should not be removed. The person should be immobilized and transferred to the nearest emergency room or ophthalmologist. The longer the delay, the greater the risks of damage and infection.

Foreign body damage varies in severity. If the particle is on the conjunctiva, blinking and tearing may be enough to remove the object. If these processes are ineffective, the particle may be wiped out using a spindle of facial tissue or washed out using a solution of normal saline. The person should avoid rubbing the eye, because rubbing may embed the particle further. If the individual continues to experience pain, if there is still a foreign body sensation or if the particle is seen on the cornea, there may be corneal abrasion. This situation is potentially dangerous for two reasons. The particle may penetrate the cornea and cause loss of the fluid in the anterior chamber as well as permanent damage to the cornea (as it deflates and creases). Alternatively, continued abrasion by a foreign body can predispose the eye to infection—especially by opportunistic pathogens that cause severe corneal ulceration (for example, Pseudomonas). The eye must be lightly covered, and the person transferred for ocular examination.

Chemical burns require first aid within seconds. They may result from splashing household or industrial products into the eye. Immediate, prolonged (20 to 30 minutes) washing of the surface of

Ophthalmic Products

the eye with cold tap water prevents permanent scarring more effectively than any other treatment. This washing is best achieved by firmly holding an individual's eye under a slow, steady stream of water for at least 20 minutes. The individual may strongly resist such washing, since it is uncomfortable and gradually produces a numbing coldness of the eye. The washed eye can be expected to be bloodshot after the washing. The first aider should not search for an antidote. After copious washing for at least 20 minutes, medical attention is essential.

Radiant energy may damage the cornea, iris or retina. Ultraviolet (UV) radiation can injure the cornea, resulting in pain, photophobia, tearing, blurred vision and foreign body sensation 6 to 12 hours after exposure. Welders refer to the condition as flashburn and snow-skiers call it snow-blindness. Other sources causing UV ocular damage include sunlamps and reflections from bright sand or sea when protective sunglasses are not worn. The condition is self-limiting, but requires medical attention for instillation of antibiotic eyedrops and mydriatic eyedrops or eye ointment , as well as administration of oral analgesics and eye patching. Anesthetic eyedrops relieve pain, but should be administered by an ophthalmologist because these medications can damage the corneal epithelial layers after just one day's frequent use. This damage can result in severe corneal scarring and ulceration.

Other types of radiant energy damage occur on exposure to infrared radiation (for example, watching a total eclipse of the sun without eye protection) or excessive x-ray radiation. People with this kind of damage should be referred to an ophthalmologist.

Under certain conditions (usually associated with poor contact lens care and poor fitting) certain types of **contact lenses** worn for periods in excess of suggested routines may cause severe pain and photophobia several hours after the contacts are removed. (See the chapter on contact lens care.) The person should see a physician, as therapy may involve use of oral analgesics, eye patching and possibly mydriatic eyedrops and antibiotic eyedrops. The problem usually resolves in 8 to 36 hours and leaves no permanent damage. The contact lenses should not be reinserted for at least a day or two afterward, and preferably only after a complete eye exam and check of the contact lens by an ophthalmologist or optometrist.

Dry Eye — common in elderly

Dry eye can be a serious problem. It may lead to corneal ulceration, secondary bacterial infection (blepharitis, conjunctivitis) and reduced visual acuity. People often complain of itching, excessive mucus secretion, inability to produce tears, burning sensation, photosensitivity, redness, pain, difficulty moving lids and a scratchy or sandy (foreign body) sensation. This condition may be caused by numerous items (see Table XXI).

When a consumer asks for "something for dry eyes," frequent instillation of artificial tears (every 1 to 6 hours) for a trial period of 72 hours can be recommended. Cold, moist compresses may also give symptomatic relief to burning, dry eyes. Environmental changes (for example, reduction of room temperature, use of humidifiers, wearing of protective spectacles with side pieces) may be beneficial. If these procedures are unsuccessful or if the condition persists for more than 72 hours, the person should seek medical advice. Consumers should not use artificial tears for prolonged periods unless medically supervised, as early diagnosis and appropriate therapy may be necessary to prevent irreversible ocular surface damage. Mucolytics (eyedrops that change the character of the mucus layer of the

Table XXI *Some Causes of Dry Eye*
Aqueous deficiency caused by hypofunction of the lacrimal gland e.g. aging medications (antihypertensives, anticholinergics, diuretics, sympatholytics) Sjoegren's syndrome (a chronic connective tissue disease that occurs predominantly in middle-aged women and is characterized by a triad of dry mouth, dry eyes and arthritis) excessive evaporation (dry climate or lipid deficiency)
Lipid deficiency caused by hypofunction of the sebaceous glands
Mucin deficiency caused by hypofunction of special conjunctival cells e.g. Stevens Johnson syndrome chemical burns chronic conjunctivitis
Impaired lid function e.g. altered blink reflex ectropion
Altered corneal surface
Contact lens wear

tear film), ocular inserts containing a lubricating polymer, soft contact bandage lenses, systemic therapy or surgical intervention may also be necessary.

Systemic Disease

"Red eye" may be a manifestation of serious systemic disease (see Table XXII). Consumers should seek medical advice if systemic disease is a possibility.

Treatment

In general, nonprescription ophthalmic medications offer symptomatic relief; they are not curative. Self-medication is limited to ocular problems where vision is not threatened (see Table I). In some cases, nonprescription medications are used for infections, allergies, hyperemia (for example, chemical irritants, tired eyes), dry eyes and first aid. **These products generally should not be used for unsupervised self-medication if the condition lasts more than 48 hours or if vision-threatening problems are present** (see Table II).

When infectious disease processes are suspected, especially if the condition is recurrent, not limited to the eyelids or if the individual has an underlying systemic disease (for example, diabetes), the person must be treated by a physician or ophthalmologist. The specialists, by using clinical expertise and laboratory facilities, can accurately identify the infectious agents and prescribe appropriate treatment. Although most bacterial and viral infections are self-limiting (7 to 10 days and 2 to 3 weeks respectively) and pose a minor threat to vision, there is a possibility of vision-threatening fungal infection, herpetic keratitis or pseudomonal infection. Self-treatment of conjunctivitis carries greater risk than self-treatment of blepharitis or hordeolum. Overuse of ophthalmic solutions may disrupt the tear film layer—the first line of defence of the eye—leading to further inflammation and irritation.

Individuals with infections of the eye should be advised to use

Table XXII *Some Systemic Diseases Associated With Red Eye*

Disease	Major external ocular findings
Rheumatic disorders	
Ankylosing spondylitis	Iridocyclitis, scleritis
Juvenile rheumatoid arthritis	Iridocyclitis without redness
Reiter syndrome	Conjunctivitis, iridocyclitis
Adult rheumatoid arthritis	Scleritis, keratoconjunctivitis sicca
Systemic lupus erythematosus	Keratoconjunctivitis sicca
Ulcerative colitis	Iridocyclitis
Skin diseases	
Acne rosacea	Blepharoconjunctivitis, keratitis
Cicatricial mucous membrane pemphigoid	Conjunctival and corneal scarring
Seborrhea	Blepharitis
Psoriasis	Blepharitis, conjunctivitis, episcleritis
Atopic dermatitis	Conjunctivitis, keratitis
Noninflammatory diseases	
Carotid—cavernous fistula	Conjunctival and episcleral vascular engorgement
Polycythemia	Conjunctival and episcleral vascular engorgement
Ataxia—telangiectasia	Conjunctival telangiectasia
Other	
Sarcoidosis	Iridocyclitis, keratoconjunctivitis sicca, conjunctival nodules
Endocrine exophthalmos	Vascular dilatation over horizontal rectus muscles, exophthalmos
Gout	Conjunctivitis (tophi in lids)

Adapted from: Waring GO, Boda BI. Problems in family practice—the red eye. J Fam Pract 1977;7(4):825–37.

separate face cloths and towels from other family members since the infection may be transmitted. If a cold or the flu accompanies eye symptoms, artificial tears can provide comfort. (Eye patches should not be used, as they can act as incubators for microbial growth.)

One condition for which the pharmacist can recommend short-term use of a nonprescription antibiotic (for example, polymyxin B/bacitracin/gramicidin) is a sty along the lid margin of an otherwise healthy individual. The antibiotic may prevent the infection from spreading. The person must be warned not to squeeze the lesion (due to the possibility of cellulitis), but to wait for the sty to point and discharge its contents. To encourage the sty to point, dry or moist heat may be used. Heat draws more blood to the area, increasing inflammatory and repair mediators, which close off and clean up the infection. If the sty persists longer than 48 hours or if there are multiple sties, the person should be referred to a physician.

In cases of obvious atopic allergic conjunctivitis (for example, a person with hayfever whose eyes are red, itching, tearing and swollen and whose nasal passages are congested and runny), eyedrops containing vasoconstrictors can be instilled into the eye on a short-term basis (less than 4 days). Eyedrops containing antihistamines may help, but can cause contact conjunctivitis. Oral antihistamines, particularly when used prior to subsequent allergen exposure, are effective. Cold compresses may offer comfort since they contract blood vessels and reduce swelling. Wearing cotton gloves may prevent rubbing and scratching. When feasible, the individual should avoid the offending agent.

As with atopic conjunctivitis, cold compresses and local vasoconstrictors can offer symptomatic relief for conjunctival hyperemia (for example, tired eyes or chemical conjunctivitis due to chlorine in a swimming pool, smoke or smog). Artificial tears may also be of value, particularly for tired eyes or eye strain.

As mentioned previously, people who seek treatment for dry eyes may be advised to try frequent instillation of artificial tears for a period of 72 hours along with applying cold compresses. If these measures are unsuccessful, medical referral is indicated.

When called upon to administer or recommend first aid, health professionals often deal with household or industrial chemical burns. Recommendations for these burns include immediate washing of the eye with tap water or one of the ophthalmic normal saline solutions for 20 to 30 minutes. Further treatment at an emergency room or ophthalmologist's office is necessary.

When dealing with children, all ocular conditions should be treated by an ophthalmologist or a physician.

Pharmacologic Agents
Decongestants (Eye Whiteners, Vasoconstrictors)
Ocular congestion indicates the presence of abnormal amounts of blood in the vessels of the eye. This condition can occur during inflammatory and allergic reactions.

During inflammation, the body attempts to counteract and remove any irritants, as well as repair resultant damage. This process can be elicited by disease (for example, microbial infection) or injury (for example, chemical, radiant energy or mechanical). Disease or injury traumatizes ocular tissue, causing release of various mediators. The principal mediators are thought to be natural substances produced by the body, such as histamine and prostaglandins. These mediators primarily result in two changes. The first change, vascular, occurs as blood vessels and capillaries dilate, resulting in greater blood flow reaching the damaged area, which then becomes red and hot. Increased vessel permeability allows various constituents to enter the irritated tissue. The second change involves formation of inflammatory exudate consisting of plasma and white blood cells. The exudate causes swelling, and the tension exerted on the surrounding tissue stimulates pain receptors.

Ophthalmic Products

The ophthalmic decongestants act both in inflammatory and allergic conditions by reversing dilation of blood vessels (that is, causing vasoconstriction) which decongests and whitens the area (thus leading to the term "eye whitener").

Decongestants are generally used for cosmetic reasons and should be used only for short-term treatment (less than 4 days). Treatment beyond this time must be under the direction of the physician. Caution must be exercised, as use of decongestants may mask potentially serious disorders and delay appropriate medical treatment.

Sympathomimetic (epinephrine/adrenaline-like) drugs are used as ophthalmic decongestants (vasoconstrictors) (see Table XXIII). In general, the concentrations used in decongestant self-medication products are considered safe. However, these drugs are potentially capable of widening the pupil (mydriasis), particularly if there are any corneal defects which allow penetration through the cornea. This can cause photophobia. More importantly, if these agents are misused, they may produce sufficient mydriasis in susceptible individuals to exacerbate or precipitate angle-closure glaucoma. There are case reports where blindness resulted when patients suffered angle-closure glaucoma and misused decongestant eyedrops in an attempt to whiten the eye. Because of these effects, some authorities recommend these agents be prescription medications. Nonprescription sympathomimetics must be avoided in individuals predisposed to angle-closure glaucoma, particularly if the cornea is damaged as the damage can increase the effect of the drug—or if the person is elderly as the lens may be enlarged.

Table XXIII *Sympathomimetic Agents Used in Ophthalmic Decongestant Products*

- Ephedrine
- Phenylephrine
- Imidazole derivatives (e.g., naphazoline, oxymetazoline, tetrahydrozoline)

Another problem associated with the use of any such ophthalmic decongestants is rebound (or reactive) hyperemia (similar to rebound nasal congestion). With too frequent or prolonged use, hyperemia may become worse. The preparation continues to whiten the eye when the drops are instilled, but the redness quickly returns and the individual instils more solution. This pattern continues and the condition worsens; the medication must then be discontinued. When discontinued, the reaction subsides. Additionally, after instilling

---

Table XXIV *Populations For Which Ophthalmic Sympathomimetic Decongestants Must Be Used Cautiously Due to Potential Systemic Effects*

- Chronic disease states (e.g., severe hypertension, hyperthyroidism, cardiac disorders, diabetes)
- Medication usage (e.g., tricyclic antidepressants, MAO inhibitors, adrenergic beta-blocking agents, general and local anesthetics, reserpine, guanethidine, methyldopa)
- Pediatric or geriatric groups
- Lactation

---

decongestants, some people may develop "red eye" due to an allergic reaction to the preservative.

Since these decongestants are sympathomimetic amines, they can elicit systemic effects associated with elevation in epinephrine if absorbed into systemic circulation (for example, via conjunctival vessels or via absorption following drainage through the nasolacrimal system). Usually the concentrations used in such nonprescription eyedrops are insufficient to cause serious problems; however, precautions must be taken for certain individuals (see Table XXIV). Safety for use in pregnancy has not been established.

Epinephrine, used primarily to decrease IOP in glaucoma therapy, blanches reddened conjunctival vessels when used in a 1:1,000 or 1:100 solution. It is not used as a vasoconstrictor because the effect generally lasts for less than an hour and may be followed by reactive hyperemia. It has been reported to cause deposits in the conjunctiva and cornea after prolonged use. Eye pain or ache, conjunctival hyperemia and allergic reactions may occur.

Phenylephrine, like epinephrine, is a direct-acting sympathomimetic drug but has a longer duration of action (0.5 to 4 hours). Onset of action is rapid. It can cause transient stinging when instilled into the eye. The concentration in nonprescription preparations is 0.125 per cent. Rebound hyperemia may occur. The higher concentrations in prescription preparations have been reported to cause severe adverse effects, such as hypertension and significant drug interactions. Allergies may develop and there may be cross-sensitivity with epinephrine. It may cause rebound miosis and decreased mydriatic response to glaucoma therapy in older persons. It may cause temporary blurred or unstable vision so patients should be warned to be cautious while driving or performing other hazardous tasks. Solutions of phenylephrine may oxidize on exposure to air and bright light, resulting in reduced efficacy. These solutions may cause a brown discoloration of certain soft contact lenses.

Naphazoline, an imidazole derivative with sympathomimetic activity, provides rapid, prolonged vasoconstriction (2 or 3 hours), which decreases swelling and congestion. It should not be instilled more frequently than every 4 hours. Although rebound hyperemia following prolonged use was not officially documented in a benchmark report on ophthalmic products, it certainly does occur in some individuals. It has been reported to cause redness, irritation, discomfort, punctate keratitis, lacrimation and increased IOP. Naphazoline may also cause systemic side effects such as headache, nausea and dizziness. Some individuals, especially children, may experience sedation. It should be used cautiously in all conditions discussed previously for decongestants.

Oxymetazoline is chemically similar to naphazoline. Its duration of action ranges from 6 to 12 hours. It tends to dilate pupils less than phenylephrine 0.12 per cent. Eye irritation and lid retraction have occasionally been observed.

Tetrahydrozoline (tetryzoline) is also chemically similar to naphazoline. Duration of action is 4 to 8 hours. It can cause mydriasis, blurred vision and irritation. Accidental ingestion may cause adverse effects. As with naphazoline, rebound ophthalmic hyperemia and sedation may be experienced.

Antihistamines

During allergic reactions, various mediators are released. As with inflammation, these substances alter blood vessels, causing redness and edema; stimulate nerve endings, causing itching; and directly stimulate lacrimal glands, causing tearing. Antihistamines compete

Ophthalmic Products

with the histaminic mediator for receptor sites. The effect of anti-histamines depends on the role of histamine in the allergic process. These drugs are of value in immediate-response allergies (for example, atopic hay fever) where histamine is released from mast cells. Competitive antagonism is of no value in contact allergies (for example, allergy to nail polish) where lymphokines are released from sensitized lymphocytes, but the mild local anesthetic effect of a topical antihistamine may provide symptomatic relief.

Systemic administration of antihistamines may be preferred over topical instillation. Although systemic side effects (for example, drowsiness) are avoided, hypersensitivity reactions may be associated with the use of antihistamine-containing eyedrops. If a sensitivity reaction to these topical agents occurs, the reaction may not be detected, as symptoms are similar to the pre-existing condition. Oral antihistamines may be more successful in treating ocular allergic symptoms. Symptomatic relief of redness, swelling, itching and tearing accompanying atopic allergy may be obtained by treating with topical antihistamines, although there is controversy regarding the efficacy of these agents for this condition. Some authorities state they are of questionable value, while other authorities indicate they may be excellent therapeutic agents for mild to moderate allergic disease.

Topical antihistamines marketed in nonprescription ophthalmic preparations include antazoline, pyrilamine maleate and pheniramine maleate. They are available commercially in combination with the sympathomimetic drugs discussed above. This combination may provide more relief than either agent alone.

Antazoline, an ethylenediamine antihistamine, appears to be much less sensitizing than other topical antihistamines. Upon instillation, there may be mild stinging. The drug has a short duration of action, and is usually instilled every 3 to 4 hours as required. Antazoline is often combined with naphazoline; the antihistamine competitively antagonizes histamine, while the vasoconstrictor physiologically blocks vasodilation. The combination may be more effective than either component alone. As with other antihistamines, antazoline may cause mydriasis; when combined with vasoconstrictors, which may also cause mydriasis, the risk of precipitating an angle-closure glaucoma attack increases.

Pyrilamine maleate, another ethylenediamine antihistamine, is used in low concentration (0.1 per cent) in a commercial product available in Canada. As with other antihistamines, it may be sensitizing.

Pheniramine maleate, an alkylamine antihistamine, is available in some Canadian antihistamine-decongestant products.

Anti-infectives

Indiscriminate use of anti-infectives is unwise. Their use may delay proper diagnosis resulting in serious ocular damage. Various antibac-

terials and antibiotics are marketed in commercial nonprescription preparations (see Table XXV).

Boric acid appears safe for use as an ophthalmic product; its efficacy as an anti-infective has not been established. It has been classified as a weak bacteriostatic and fungistatic agent, but is recognized officially only as a buffering agent. When used as a buffer, it is effective and well-tolerated.

One author recommends that solutions for topical use not exceed a concentration of 2 per cent, as greater concentrations exert a phagolytic effect that may depress a primary defence mechanism against bacterial invasion. Since absorption of boric acid through extensive areas of broken skin or through inadvertent oral ingestion may result in potentially fatal poisoning, commercial preparations (particularly large volume ones) should be kept out of reach of children.

As some commercial boric acid preparations are marketed with an eyecup, care must be taken to clean the eyecup thoroughly to prevent contamination and to avoid washing skin bacteria into the eye. For these reasons, use of an eyecup is criticized by some authorities.

Salicylic acid, found in some commercial products, has a slight antiseptic action. It irritates when applied topically. Its value in ophthalmic preparations has not been substantiated.

Mild silver protein (19 to 23 per cent) is primarily bacteriostatic. Efficacy as an ocular anti-infective has not been established. Unlike silver nitrate, used for prophylaxis of ophthalmia neonatorum, it is relatively nonirritating. Long-term use may result in slate-grey deposits of metallic silver (argyrosis) especially in the fornices of the conjunctiva. Prolonged use is not recommended. Safety in children, pregnancy and lactation has not been established. The solution is unstable when exposed to light.

Yellow mercuric oxide 1 per cent is antibacterial. It has been shown to reduce eyelid bacterial colony counts. It has been recommended for short-term treatment (for example, 1 week) of blepharitis. Generally, with short-term use, the medication is well tolerated although there may be hypersensitivity and transient local irritation upon instillation. Frequent or prolonged use may cause serious mercury poisoning or bluish-gray discoloration of the eyelids, conjunctiva and peripheral cornea.

Bacitracin, gramicidin and **polymyxin B** are available without prescription. When these bactericidal polypeptides are combined, the result is a preparation with broad-spectrum activity. As these agents are not commonly used systemic medications, they are preferred by many ophthalmologists. Avoiding commonly used systemic antibiotics, especially when there is a viable alternative, decreases the risk of sensitizing the individual to valuable antibiotics and decreases the risk of developing resistant strains of organisms. With topical use of these antibiotics, hypersensitivity and side effects are rare.

Bacitracin is available as an ophthalmic ointment either alone or in combination with another antibiotic. It is active primarily against a variety of gram-positive organisms (for example, *Staphylococcus aureus* and *Streptococcus pneumoniae*). Bacterial resistance develops slowly if at all.

The action of bacitracin is not affected by blood, pus, necrotic tissue or bacterial enzymes. It rarely causes hypersensitivity. It does not readily penetrate the intact cornea in therapeutic amounts. As bacitracin solutions are unstable, only ophthalmic ointments are available commercially. These ointments are stable for more than 1 year at room temperature.

Gramicidin is available in combination antibiotic preparations.

Table XXV	*Nonprescription Anti-infectives*	
Antibacterials:	• boric acid
	• salicylic acid
	• mild silver protein
	• yellow mercuric oxide
Antibiotics:	• bacitracin
	• gramicidin
	• polymyxin B

Ophthalmic Products

It shows activity toward common gram-positive ocular pathogens. It must not be used on recently traumatized areas as bleeding may recur due to hemolysis.

Polymyxin B is available as either an ophthalmic ointment in combination with bacitracin or as an ophthalmic solution in combination with gramicidin. Polymyxin is active against numerous gram-negative organisms, including Pseudomonas; it is not active against *Proteus vulgaris* or most strains of Neisseria and Serratia. Bacterial resistance is infrequent. Polymyxin B does not readily penetrate an intact cornea. Hypersensitivity reactions are rare.

Artificial Tears

Many agents, particulary water-soluble polymers, have been introduced over the past 40 years as potential tear substitutes or supplements (see Table XXVI). They attempt to promote tear film stability.

Table XXVI *Polymers Used in Artificial Tears*

- Polyesters (e.g., polyethylene glycol)
- Polyvinyls (e.g., polyvinyl alcohol, povidone)
- Cellulose derivatives (e.g., methylcellulose, hydroxypropyl methylcellulose)
- Dextrans

When **artificial tears** were first introduced, the main problem was the short duration of action. Initially, researchers thought retention time was prolonged by higher concentrations of the polymers. In more recent years this theory has been challenged. Effectiveness, as far as retention and contact time is concerned, is not dependent on the change in concentration. Various researchers suggest the change in flow (Newtonian versus pseudoplastic), viscosity (optimal centipoise) and adsorptive properties (polymers have multiple points for adsorption) are of greater significance.

When a drop of methylcellulose 1 per cent or other cellulose ester (for example, hydroxypropylmethylcellulose or hydroxyethylcellulose) or polyvinyl alcohol 1.4 per cent is instilled, the effect lasts 30 to 45 minutes. Combinations of cellulose derivative and povidone, as well as cellulose derivative and dextran, have effects lasting up to 90 minutes, apparently due to mucomimetic adsorptive activity. Inserts of artificial tear polymers (hydroxypropylcellulose) dissolve slowly over about 6 hours to produce a viscous hydrophilic solution.

In addition to increased retention time and mucomimetic activity, some formulations claim efficacy due to the synergistic effects of two polymeric components at a certain concentration. Other formulations claim efficacy due to alteration of tear tonicity; tears of dry-eyed individuals are hyperosmolar, so hypotonic products may help restore a balanced tonicity.

Artificial tears generally do not have significant side effects. Products that are highly viscous (for example, polyvinyl alcohol 3 per cent) may have a tendency to form crusts at the lid margins which may be uncomfortable for the user. Polyvinyl alcohol 1.4 per cent is less viscous than methylcellulose 0.5 per cent. The cellulose derivative and dextran combination noted above is less viscous than the cellulose derivative and povidone. The main disadvantages of artificial tears are short duration of action, development of sensitivity to the preservatives (for example, benzalkonium chloride or thimerosal), and possible corneal epithelial damage associated with

the use of preservatives (especially benzalkonium chloride). Polymer inserts may cause blurred vision and irritation after a few hours. Some people have difficulty applying and retaining the insert in the eye. They are generally inserted into the lower cul-de-sac daily. Correct insertion techniques for these products should be supervised by an ophthalmologist or optometrist.

Although in vitro testing may suggest one product is preferable to another, the testing does not necessarily parallel in vivo efficacy. Clinically, user acceptance varies widely and the consumer selects the most suitable and least irritating preparation by trial and error. No one preparation is consistently more efficacious and better tolerated; individual consumer preferences may change, probably reflecting the fluctuating nature and different etiologies of dry eyes. The search for an ideal tear substitute continues.

Ocular lubricant (emollient) ointments—containing white petrolatum, mineral oil and lanolin derivatives—are commercially available, although not advocated as tear substitutes. These constituents are in most ophthalmic ointment bases. The products are promoted for lubrication following surgery, for reducing inflammation of the eyelids and for application to the eye after removal of a foreign body. Some practitioners prescribe these ointments for use at bedtime as an adjunct to treatment with artificial tears. They should not be used during the day as they may further aggravate the dry eye condition—blinking spreads the ointment over the tear film and may promote formation of dry spots. Major disadvantages are blurred vision, poor mixing with the hydrophilic tears and formation of a coating on contact lenses. There is also a resent case report of aspiration-induced lipoid pneumonitis associated with bedtime use of an ocular lubricant ointment; if a cough develops, this potential complication should be considered. If ocular irritation occurs, the ointment should be discontinued.

For the person who complains of dry eyes, the frequent use (from every hour to every 6 hours) of artificial tears for a period of 72 hours can be recommended. If this treatment is ineffective or if the condition persists, the person should consult an ophthalmologist; more elaborate treatment may be required to prevent irreversible ocular damage (for example, hydrophilic bandage lenses, eyedrops containing mucolytic agents or surgical alterations).

Astringents

Zinc sulfate (0.25 per cent) is a mild astringent that precipitates protein, causing tissues to contract or secretions to stop. Zinc sulfate, in concentrations used in nonprescription products, has little ability to penetrate tissues, so it is considered safe for use in the eye. It is doubtful if a solution of zinc sulfate 0.25 per cent does more than clear mucin from the outer surface of the eye, although it may provide subjective relief from minor eye irritations. There is no evidence that astringents are indicated for treatment of sty or allergic conjunctivitis (for example, hayfever). Zinc sulfate does not produce vasoconstriction of conjunctival blood vessels; it may actually cause vasodilation.

Local Anesthetics

Local anesthetic ophthalmic solutions and ointments (for example, tetracaine and proparacaine) are available without a prescription in some provinces. These medications are helpful when used by the ophthalmologist or optometrist. Individuals should never self-medicate with these preparations because of their inherent toxicities.

Ophthalmic Products

With loss of corneal sensation following instillation of a local anesthetic, the ophthalmologist or optometrist can examine the eye without causing discomfort. The following problems may arise upon use of a local anesthetic in the eye: self-inflicted corneal damage to the open eye, caused by loss of the blink reflex combined with a numbing sensation, particularly if a foreign body is lodged on the surface; local allergic reactions particularly with proparacaine (due to differences in chemical structure, cross-sensitization may not be a problem); corneal edema; blurred vision; increased rate of tear evaporation; and mild to intense ocular pain if instillation is repeated. Additionally, with decreased reflex secretion of tears and resultant increased length of time required for tear washout, anesthetics allow topically applied agents to be in contact with the eye for a prolonged period of time.

With excessive dosage or chronic misuse, the following sequence of events can occur. Delayed corneal epithelial healing produces corneal edema and epithelial erosions. The increased pain causes the individual to apply the local anesthetic more frequently. The increased applications may lead to secondary infection, corneal scarring and reduced vision.

If the local anesthetic is used on an extensively traumatized area, it may enter the blood stream and cause central nervous system toxicity, cardiotoxicity and respiratory toxicity. This is a potential problem with ocular local anesthetics, but is mainly seen when these agents are applied to nasal or oral passages. If ingested, 20 mL of a tetracaine solution 0.5 per cent (100 mg) is potentially toxic therefore this agent should be kept out of reach of children.

Because of the chemical toxicity, loss of blink reflex and loss of corneal sensation, local anesthetics should never be used for self-treatment. If dispensed under close medical supervision (for example, following ultraviolet corneal burn), the consumer must use the product sparingly. Most ophthalmologists prefer oral analgesics for outpatients.

Tetracaine (amethocaine) (0.5 per cent) and **proparacaine** (proxymetacaine) (0.5 per cent) are commonly used ester-type local ocular anesthetics. They are approximately equipotent, although proparacaine does not penetrate the cornea or conjunctiva as well as tetracaine. Onset of action is about 20 seconds and duration is 10 to 20 minutes; the ointment formulation causes prolonged anesthesia. Proparacaine is used more commonly in clinical practice, as it may produce less irritation than tetracaine when instilled; tetracaine may cause a burning sensation for 30 seconds after it is instilled into the conjunctival sac. When tetracaine, a para-aminobenzoic acid ester, is metabolized, it may inhibit the action of sulfonamide (antibacterial) drugs; if only 1 or 2 drops of tetracaine are used for a local procedure, this effect is probably minimal. Due to delayed metabolism, circulating blood levels of these local anesthetics may increase in individuals using anticholinesterase drugs such as echothiophate.

Amylocaine and **butacaine** are less commonly used ester-type local anesthetics.

Preservatives

Preservatives are used to maintain sterility of eye preparations after the container is opened. This precaution prevents instillation of microbiologically contaminated drugs into the eye and maintains the potency of active ingredients.

The organism most frequently implicated in reports of contaminated ophthalmic solutions is *Pseudomonas aeruginosa*, an organism that can destroy the eye within 24 to 48 hours.

Preservatives currently used in Canada include benzalkonium chloride (BAC); disodium edetate (EDTA); chlorobutanol; organomercurials such as phenylmercuric acetate (PMA), phenylmercuric nitrate (PMN) and thimerosal; and parabens (methylparaben and propylparaben). Most ophthalmic products are preserved with BAC (50 per cent), chlorobutanol (25 per cent) or organomercurials (20 per cent).

BAC, a quaternary ammonium surfactant, is used as a preservative in a concentration of 0.004 to 0.01 per cent. It acts rapidly against organisms, but its effect against Pseudomonas is limited.

BAC may disrupt the corneal epithelium, increasing the penetration of drugs across the cornea. This effect may be beneficial (for example, with carbachol, which penetrates the cornea with difficulty) or undesirable (for example, with local anesthetics and their chemical toxicities). Some authorities stress the potential danger (toxic corneal damage) of prolonged use of topical medications containing BAC as a preservative particularly in the presence of extensive ocular surface disease. BAC may also disrupt the stability of the lipid layer of the tear film. Adverse reactions may occur (for example, irritation) but are usually reversible when the preparation is discontinued. BAC is not used in soft contact lens solutions as it binds to the soft lenses after prolonged exposure; this action can provide toxic levels of BAC at the cornea.

EDTA potentiates the activity of BAC by chelating divalent calcium and magnesium ions, which compete with BAC for sites on the organism. EDTA itself has some antimicrobial effect. It may be a weak sensitizing agent.

Chlorobutanol in a concentration of 0.5 per cent has bacteriostatic activity against gram-negative and gram-positive organisms; it also inhibits Pseudomonas and fungi. Its major disadvantage is its slow action. There are no reports of allergic reactions with topical use. Its efficiency is enhanced when used with BAC. Chlorobutanol may sting on application, but does not have major toxic effects. It adsorbs to soft contact lenses.

Organomercurials are normally used at concentrations of 0.002 to 0.004 per cent. They have slow, weak antibacterial and antifungal action, but are active against *Pseudomonas aeruginosa*. PMN is considered by some to be more active and less irritating than PMA and thimerosal. Contact sensitivity can be a problem, particularly with thimerosal. The action of thimerosal is potentiated by EDTA.

Parabens are more effective against molds and fungi than against bacteria; they are considered slow and ineffective bacteriostatic agents. They may also cause painful ocular irritation and allergic reactions.

Miscellaneous Ingredients

Allantoin, a xanthine alkaloid, has been used in the past to stimulate tissue repair, primarily in dermatological infections. Its value in ophthalmic preparations is unknown.

Antipyrine, a pyrazolone derivative, is no longer an official drug. When used locally, it may act as a mild anesthetic, feeble antiseptic and mild styptic (constricts superficial blood vessels). One source indicates that an anesthetic effect, no matter how slight, can mask symptoms of serious ocular disorders and may ultimately injure the eye.

Hamamelis (witch hazel) is used well-diluted in eye products. It has mild astringent properties.

Hydrastine and **berberine** are alkaloids obtained from the hydrastis plant. Their use in catarrhal conditions is based entirely on empirical observation.

Ophthalmic Products

Table XXVII *Comparison of Characteristics of Ophthalmic Solutions vs. Ophthalmic Ointments*

Characteristic	Solutions	Ointments
Instillation	Easier	More difficult
Frequency of instillation[1]	More	Less
Contact time[2]	Shorter	Longer (slower movement through the nasolacrimal drainage)
Irritation on instillation[3]	Frequent	Rare
Discharge retention[4]	No	Yes
Skin reactions	Few	More frequent (contact dermatitis)
Blurred vision	No	Yes (film spreads over eye)
Systemic reactions	More frequent	Less frequent (see text)
Inhibition of corneal epithelial regeneration	No	Unlikely (see text)
Readily contaminated (requires preservatives)	Yes	Unlikely (see text)
Stability a problem with storage[5]	Yes	Less likely

[1]Polymers in solution enhance contact time (see Artificial Tears). Ointments have traditionally been used for bedtime therapy to avoid instillation during sleeping hours; since ointments are less readily washed out with tears, they are also valuable in children who are crying
[2]Generalization
[3]"Stinging, burning"
[4]Discharge experienced with bacterial infection
[5]Hydrolysis, oxidation, heat degradation

Lanolin or **cetyl alcohol** 5 per cent is often added to emulsify ointment formulations, thus increasing the absorption of water-soluble drugs and water. Purified lanolin also helps distribute the drug throughout the ointment base.

Mineral oil, when added to white petrolatum during formulation of an ointment base, allows the vehicle to melt at or below conjunctival temperature.

Sodium bisulfite is used as an antioxidant (for example, for solutions of phenylephrine).

Other ingredients are used as tonicity agents (for example, sodium chloride) or buffers (for example, phosphates, citric acid, sodium borate or boric acid). Ophthalmic solutions can be buffered at a pH of approximately 7.4 (tear pH), although the eye can usually tolerate the slightly acidic character (pH 6.2 to 6.5) of many nonprescription eyedrops. This acidity may be partly responsible for the transient stinging on instillation.

Formulations

Advantages and disadvantages are associated with the use of an ophthalmic solution or ointment (see Table XXVII).

Although systemic effects may occur, they are lessened with ointments because conjunctival absorption is slower than with drops and nasolacrimal draining is minimal; the effect is comparable to depot administration versus bolus administration identified with drops.

Studies show no evidence that commercial ointment bases interfere with wound healing. Current ointment bases differ from those used in the past, as they are nonemulsive and do not contain the stiffer grades of petrolatum. They are less viscous and probably do not interfere with healing. Also, the base melts rapidly and floats above the tear film, so epithelial mitosis continues without interference. Ointments are generally the preferred form for treatment of blepharitis, as they are usually more effective.

Some authors point out that microbes can survive in a non-aqueous medium (for example, ointment), but are unlikely to multiply. In the past, authorities have stated that manufacturers' sterilization of ophthalmic ointments is necessary, but formulation with preservatives is not required. Contamination of ointments can occur, but is minimized by three trends: use of simple bases (for example, petrolatum jelly plus paraffin or mineral oil) rather than compound bases (oil in water or water in oil); use of small (3.5 g), disposable ointment tubes; and increased consumer counselling to avoid nozzle-to-finger-to-conjunctival contact.

The *British Pharmaceutical Codex* (BPC; an official British publication recognized in Canada) recommends discarding multidose ophthalmic solutions for home use 4 weeks after opening. Writing the date on the container when it is opened facilitates this practice. The BPC also recommends these solutions be used for not more than 1 week with hospitalized individuals and not more than 1 day with clinic use. One authority recommends discarding opened ophthalmic tubes 1 month after opening. Another authority recommends discarding ophthalmic preparations within 3 months of opening.

The use of eye lotions and eyecups for home use is generally discouraged. The BPC recommends "not more than 200 mL should be supplied in a container;" even if a preservative is used, the lotion should not be used at home for more than 7 days after opening. First aid irrigating agents without preservatives should be used for a maximum of 24 hours.

Although products may have the same type and concentration of active ingredients, variation in tonicity, pH or preservatives may produce different effects. For example, if one product produces discomfort on instillation, there may be tearing and the active ingredient may be washed away.

Consumer Information

Anyone experiencing severe eye pain, headache, rapid change in vision, the sudden appearance of floating spots, acute redness of the eyes, photophobia or double vision should consult an ophthalmologist, optometrist or physician immediately. If self-medication does

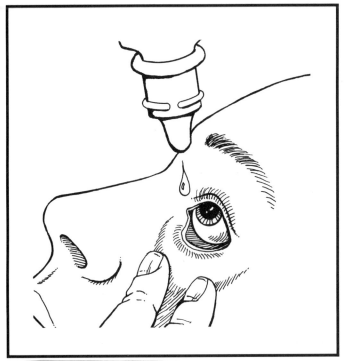

Figure 3 *Instilling Eye Drops*

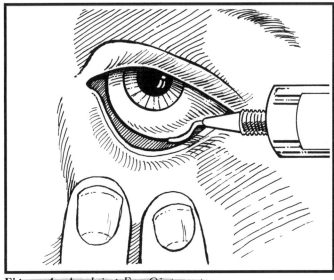

Figure 4 *Applying Eye Ointment*

not clear up the problem in 48 to 72 hours, the individual should seek an eye examination.

Eye preparations that belong to another person should never be used. The product container should be tightly closed and stored in

Figure 5 *Suggested Approach for Treating Blepharitis/Conjunctivitis/Dry Eye*

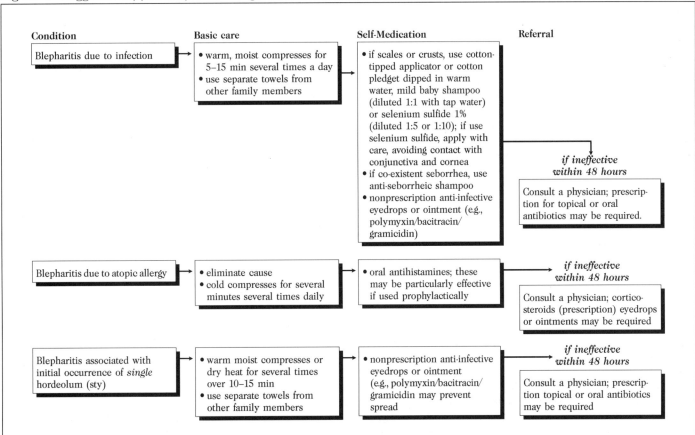

Figure 5 *(Cont'd) Suggested Approach for Treating Blepharitis/Conjunctivitis/Dry Eye*

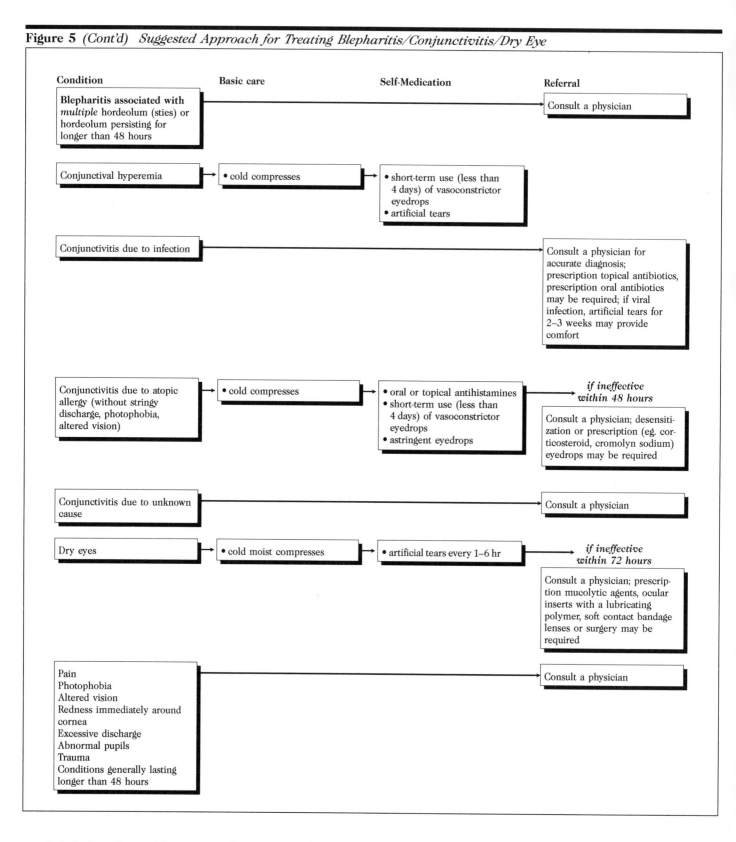

Condition	Basic care	Self-Medication	Referral
Blepharitis associated with *multiple* **hordeolum (sties) or hordeolum persisting for longer than 48 hours**			Consult a physician
Conjunctival hyperemia	• cold compresses	• short-term use (less than 4 days) of vasoconstrictor eyedrops • artificial tears	
Conjunctivitis due to infection			Consult a physician for accurate diagnosis; prescription topical antibiotics, prescription oral antibiotics may be required; if viral infection, artificial tears for 2–3 weeks may provide comfort
Conjunctivitis due to atopic allergy (without stringy discharge, photophobia, altered vision)	• cold compresses	• oral or topical antihistamines • short-term use (less than 4 days) of vasoconstrictor eyedrops • astringent eyedrops	*if ineffective within 48 hours* Consult a physician; desensitization or prescription (eg. corticosteroid, cromolyn sodium) eyedrops may be required
Conjunctivitis due to unknown cause			Consult a physician
Dry eyes	• cold moist compresses	• artificial tears every 1–6 hr	*if ineffective within 72 hours* Consult a physician; prescription mucolytic agents, ocular inserts with a lubricating polymer, soft contact bandage lenses or surgery may be required
Pain Photophobia Altered vision Redness immediately around cornea Excessive discharge Abnormal pupils Trauma Conditions generally lasting longer than 48 hours			Consult a physician

a cool, dark place. Some might recommend storage in a refrigerator after opening. Refrigerated solutions must be allowed to come to room temperature before instillation; ointments should always be applied at room temperature. Ophthalmic preparations lose potency with age and may become contaminated. They must be discarded if the expiry date has passed, the solution is discolored, the solution contains particles or the product was opened more than 1 to 3 months ago. All ophthalmic preparations are for external use only. These medications must be kept out of reach of children as they may be toxic. Prescription ophthalmics can be particularly toxic.

Pharmacists can suggest to the consumer that someone else (for example, another family member) administer the medication. Consumers should be instructed to wash their hands before and after using eyedrops or eye ointments—particularly when the eye is infected. The towels and other personal items of the person with the infection should not be used by other household members. Any discharge should be cleaned from the eye with gauze or a facecloth.

Expired, discolored or used products must be discarded so the bottles or tubes cannot be found by children or infants (either in home garbage or the local dump).

Instillation of Ophthalmic Solutions

The following is a list of instructions pharmacists can give to consumers using ophthalmic solutions:
- Wash hands thoroughly.
- Tilt the head back or lie down.
- While eyes are open, gently pull the lower lid below the eyelashes away from the eye to form a pouch. Approach the eye from the side, with the long axis of the dropper or bottle parallel to the lid margin.
- Hold the container near the lid (at least 2 cm away). Do not touch the lids or lashes.
- Look toward the ceiling. Looking up moves the cornea away from the instillation site, minimizing the blink reflex.
- Instil 1 drop into the pouch (see Figure 3). Hold this position to let the drop fall as deep as possible into the cul-de-sac.
- Look down for several seconds and then slowly release the lower lid. Looking down brings the cornea into maximum contact with the instilled drug.
- Gently close (do not squeeze) the eyes for 1 to 2 minutes while applying gentle pressure to the bridge of the nose for 30 to 60 seconds. A tissue may be used to blot around the eye, but do not rub. Closing the eye helps prevent loss of solution caused by blinking. If the eye is closed too tightly, the medication may be expelled. Gentle pressure on the bridge of the nose may help prevent systemic absorption via the nasolacrimal duct and increases retention of the solution over the eyes. If the individual has recently undergone ophthalmic surgery, the ophthalmologist should be asked whether pressure should be applied to the bridge of the nose.
- Do not rub the eye. Try not to blink.
- If multiple drops are prescribed, wait 3 to 5 minutes between the instillation of each drop. This ensures the first drop is not flushed away and the second drop is not diluted by the first.
- Never contaminate the dropper tip by allowing it to touch the eye, eyelid, eyelashes, finger or counter surface. This applies to the top of the container as well.

Instilling eyedrops into a child's eye can be a traumatic experience both for parent and child. Pharmacists can give parents the following instructions:
- Have the child sit, tilt the head backward and close the eyes.
- Approach the eye holding the long axis of the container parallel to the lid margin, resting the hand on the child's cheek. The approach prevents injury to the eye if the child moves suddenly.
- Pull the lower lid down and instil the drop through the lashes, avoiding touching the bottle to the lashes. Alternatively, place the drop on the eyelid in the inner corner of the eye, then have the child open the eye so that the drop falls in by gravity.

For infants and small children who may not cooperate in such a procedure, an alternative method can be tried.
- Have the child sit on your lap—legs astride yours—facing you. While supporting the back and head, gently lower the child backward until he or she is lying along your legs. You have the option of having your own legs at an angle toward your body. Several options are then available, according to the control desired. With the child supine, all that may be necessary is to hold the head with one hand and instil drops with the other on the same side as you are holding the head. In very resistant cases, the child's head may be gently clamped between your legs, and the feet wedged against your body under your arms. Either procedure can be done with the assistance of a third individual.
- If the instillation of drops or ointment application is important (for example, to deal with an infected eye), it is better to get some drops or ointment on the lids and lashes (keeping the lids closed momentarily) and allow the preparation to seep onto the surface of the eye, than for no drops or ointment to be used at all.

Elderly individuals and those with tremors or arthritis often find it difficult to self-administer eyedrops. A number of devices have been described which attempt to improve self-administration of eyedrops for these individuals. These include various plastic support devices, modified sunglasses, a system of mirrors and a "squeezing" device for the bottle.

Application of Ophthalmic Ointments

For ophthalmic ointments, consumers follow the same method of administration as used for drops except after the ointment is instilled into the eye and while the eye is closed for 1 to 2 minutes, roll the eyeball in all directions (see Figure 4).

In addition:
- Hold the tube in the hand for a few minutes to warm the ointment and facilitate flow.
- When opening the tube for the first time, squeeze out and discard the first 0.5 cm of ointment as it may be too dry.
- Apply a small ribbon of ointment, about 1 cm in the same area as for drops. It is not necessary to apply the ointment along the entire length of the conjunctiva or the lower lid.
- After the ointment is applied, vision may be blurred for a few minutes; do not drive or operate machinery until blurriness disappears. (If blurred vision is a problem, reducing the amount of ointment instilled can resolve it.)
- If both an ointment and solution are used, instil the solution first. Wait at least 5 minutes before instilling the ointment. If different types of ointments are to be used, wait about 10 minutes before instilling the second ointment.
- If ointments are to be applied to the outer eyelids, place the ointment on a sterile cotton-tipped applicator and apply to the lid.

Some authorities prefer to use ophthalmic ointments for children; unlike an adult, a child rarely complains of blurring after an ointment is applied. Ointments also tend to control morning "stickiness" associated with bacterial conjunctivitis and are more effective when treating blepharitis.

Ophthalmic Products

Summary

Armed with a basic knowledge of the anatomy and physiology of the eye, as well as common ocular disorders and their management, pharmacists can determine the acceptability and limitations of nonprescription self-medication. If potentially serious eye problems are suspected, the person must see an optometrist, physician or opthalmologist immediately. If use of a nonprescription medication is acceptable and safe, the person can be counselled concerning products, precautions and instructions for use.

Ask the Consumer

Q. Is this problem with your eyes, or another person's? Tech
- Age is important, particularly in the case of an infant (due to the possibility of congenital disorders or low resistance to infection) or an elderly person (due to the increased risk of angle-closure glaucoma). These individuals may also be more sensitive to vasoconstrictors used in ophthalmic decongestants.

Q. How are your eyes bothering you?
- Ask consumers to describe problems using their own words. Depending on the reply, the following questions may be applicable.

Q. Is there pain? Are your eyes burning and itchy? Does it feel as though something is in your eye (foreign body sensation)?
- Pain or photophobia (eye discomfort induced by bright lights) may indicate a severe disease process. Superficial foreign body sensation may indicate the presence of a lesion on the eyelid, something on the conjunctiva or cornea, or inflammation of the conjunctiva or cornea. Sharp pain is usually associated with corneal disease; dull, severe aching pain can be associated with scleral disease or other severe disorders. All these conditions require medical attention.
  Herpes simplex keratitis is an exception to the rule. It is a dangerous organism because it reduces corneal sensation so pain is not a prominent symptom. It can cause blindness.
  Burning, stinging and an uncomfortable feeling in the eye are seldom characteristic of serious eye disease. Usually these symptoms are only annoying and may be treated with nonprescription medications; however, microbial conjunctivitis requires medical treatment.
  Itching is a sign of ocular allergy. If the symptoms are mild, nonprescription medications can provide symptomatic relief.

Q. Is your vision normal? Blurred? Double? Spotty?
- Vision may be normal in blepharitis, conjunctivitis and systemic disease. Sudden or gradual vision loss can indicate ocular disease (for example, hemorrhage, infection, glaucoma or cataracts) or systemic disease (for example, diabetes, hypertension, transient ischemic attacks, cerebral artery occlusion or blood dyscrasias). Double vision indicates the eyes are not pointing in the same direction (for example, in ocular muscle disorders or following trauma). Spotty vision may indicate the presence of debris in the vitreous humor (floaters). This problem may be due to serious disease (for example, retinal detachment). The person should be referred for an eye examination, particularly if elderly.

Q. Are your eyes red?
- Depending on the characteristics and location of redness, the problem may be extremely serious. Medical attention is necessary.

Q. Is there discharge? Excessive tearing?
- Discharge that is purulent (eyelashes may be stuck together on awakening), foamy or stringy may signify bacterial—including chlamydial—infection, or severe allergic conjunctivitis. Clear, watery discharge may indicate viral infection.
  Excessive tearing appears in most inflammatory (for example, glaucoma or uveitis) and allergic conditions of the eye. It also accompanies photophobia. Tear overflow can result from blockage of the lacrimal drainage system or abnormality of the eyelid.

Q. Do you have dry eyes?
- Alteration of the tear film may result in permanent eye damage. Persistent dry eyes must be referred for medical treatment.

Q. Are the pupils of the eyes normal?
- Constricted pupils can be a sign of iritis. Semi-dilated or oval-shaped pupils accompany acute angle-closure glaucoma. Unequal pupils may indicate injury to the iris.

Q. Where were you and what were you doing when you first noticed the symptoms?
- The person may have been exposed to pollutants (dust or wind), may have splashed a chemical in the eye, may have had a small piece of metal penetrate the eye or may have been exposed to excessive ultraviolet radiation (skiing or welding-arc flash). The last three are all medical emergencies.

Q. Do you wear contact lenses? Which contact lens products do you use? Tech
- Some contact lenses, when worn for prolonged periods, may cause pain and photophobia several hours after they are removed. Many nonprescription ophthalmic medications should not be used when lenses, particularly soft lenses, are in the eye. Some people may be sensitive to ingredients in the contact lens products. (See the chapter on contact lens care.)

Q. Do you have any allergies? Tech
- Anyone who suffers from hayfever may have accompanying allergic conjunctivitis. The person may be sensitive to cosmetics and have an allergic blepharitis. Components in nonprescription ophthalmic products may cause allergic reactions.

Q. Have you had similar episodes before?
- If this problem is recurrent, it may have serious complications and should be treated by an ophthalmologist.

Q. How long have you had the problem? Have you used any medications for it? Which one(s)?
- In general, any condition that persists for more than 48 hours should be examined by a physician. The person may have rebound conjunctival hyperemia due to overuse of topical vasoconstrictors.

Q. Are you under the care of a physician for any medical conditions (for example, diabetes, cardiovascular

Ophthalmic Products

disease, hyperthyroidism, glaucoma or ulcer disease)? Are you taking prescribed medication?

■ The person may have lowered resistance to infection. These disease conditions may place limitations on self-medication. The person may be using a prescribed medication that is causing an ocular problem. (For example, oral antihistamines taken for seasonal allergies can cause blurred vision due to an action on the focusing mechanism of the eye and the muscles that make both eyes move together. One drug used to prevent travel sickness-the Transderm V patch—can cause blurred vision for the same reason.)

References

General

Bartlett JD, et al, ed. Ophthalmic drug facts. St. Louis: Lippincott, 1990.

Bartlett JD, Jaanus SD, eds. Clinical ocular pharmacology. Boston: Buttersworth, 1984.

Baum JL, Barza M. Common eye infections—treat or refer? Drug Ther 1981;Jul:119–31.

Ellis PP. Handbook of ocular therapeutics and pharmacology. St. Louis: CV Mosby, 1985.

Falcon MG. The infected eye. Practitioner 1982;226:839–44.

Fraunfelder FT, Roy FH, eds. Current ocular therapy. Philadelphia: WB Saunders, 1990.

Freidlaender MH. Ocular allergy—scratching the surface of the red eye. Postgrad Med 1986;79(5):261–71.

Gennaro AR, et al, eds. Remington's pharmaceutical sciences. Easton: Mac Publishing, 1990.

Gilman AG, Rall TW, Nies AS, Taylor P, eds. Goodman and Gilman's the pharmacological basis of therapeutics. New York: Macmillan, 1990.

Havener WH. Ocular pharmacology. St Louis: CV Mosby, 1983.

Havener WH, Sander W, Keith C, et al. Nursing care in eye, ear, nose, and throat disorders. S Louis: CV Mosby, 1974.

Jose JF, Polse KA, Holden EK. Optometric pharmacology. Orlando: Grune and Stratton, 1984.

Kanski JJ. Clinical ophthalmology—a systematic approval. Toronto: Buttersworths, 1989.

Krogh CME, ed. Compendium of pharmaceuticals and specialties. Ottawa: Canadian Pharmaceutical Association, 1991:683.

Martin-Doyle JL, Demp MH. A synopsis of ophthalmology. Bristol: J Wright, 1975.

Newell FW. Ophthalmology: principles and concepts. St Louis: CV Mosby, 1986.

O'Connor-Davies PH. The actions and uses of ophthalmic drugs. London: Buttersworths, 1981.

Ophthalmic drug products for over-the-counter human use. Fed Reg 1980; 45(89):30002–50.

Reynolds J, ed. Martindale: the extra pharmacopoeia. London: Pharmaceutical Press, 1989.

Robbins SL, Angell M. Basic pathology. Toronto: WB Saunders, 1976.

Robin JS, Ellis PP. Ophthalmic ointments. Surv Ophthalmol 1978;2:335–40.

Rose FC, ed. Medical ophthalmology. London: Chapman & Hall, 1976.

Smiith MB. Handbook of ocular pharmacology. Acton Mass: Publishing Sciences Group, 1974.

Stein HA, Slatt BJ. The ophthalmic assistant; fundamentals and clinical practice. St Louis: CV Mosby, 1982.

Stock EL. External eye diseases. Postgrad Med 1985;78(8):102–11.

Trevor-Roper PD. The eye and its disorders: conjunctiva. Int Ophthalmol Clin 1974;14(1–2):394–421.

Vaughan D, Ashbury T, Tabbara KF, eds. General ophthalmology. Los Altos: Lange, 1989.

Waring GO, Boda BI. Problems in family practice—the red eye. J Fam Pract 1977;7(4):825–37.

Wybar K, Muir MK. Ophthalmology: London: Bailliere Tindall, 1984.

Anatomy and Physiology

Fatt I. Physiology of the eye. Toronto: Butterworths, 1978.

Jacob SW, Francone CA, eds. Structure and function in man. Toronto: WB Saunders, 1970.

Disorders of the Eyelids

Alexander KL. Some inflammations of the external eye and adnexa. J Am Optom Assoc 1980;51:142–6.

Bohigian GM. Chalazion—a clinical evaluation. Ann Ophthalmol 1979; 11:1397–8.

Cantania LJ. Lumps and bumps of the eyelids or "what is that thing?" South J Optom 1979;21(5):16–9.

Diegel JT. Eyelid problems—blepharitis, hordeola, and chalazia. Postgrad Med 1986;80(2):271–2.

Furgiuele FP. Eye and eyelid infections: treatment and prevention. Drugs 1978;15:310–6.

Jacobs PM, Thaller VT, Wong D. Intralesional corticosteroid therapy of chalazia: a comparison with incision and curettage. Br J Ophthalmol 1984;68:836–7.

Jones DB, Liesegang TJ, Robinson NM. Laboratory diagnosis of ocular infections. Washington: American Society for Microbiology, 1981:8–10.

McCulley JP, Dougherty JM, Deneau DG. Classification of chronic blepharitis. Ophthalmology 1982;89:1173–80.

Perry HD, Serniuk RA. Conservative treatment of chalazia. Ophthalmology 1980;87:218–21.

Smolin G, Okumoto M. Staphylococcus blepharitis. Arch Ophthalmol 1977;95:812–6.

Trevor-Roper PD. The eye and its disorders. Diseases of the eyelids. Int Ophthalmol Clin 1974;14(1–2):362–93.

Watson AP, Austin DJ. Treatment of chalazions with injection of a steriod suspension. Br J Ophthalmol 1984;68:833–5.

Wilson LA, Julian AJ, Ahearn MS, Ahearn DG. The survival and growth of microorganisms in mascara during use. Am J Ophthalmol 1975; 79:596–601.

Disorders of the Conjunctiva

Fisher AA. Allergic reactions to contact lens solutions. Cutis 1985; 36(3):209–11.

Goren SB. The red eye. Postgrad Med 1975;57(7):179–82.

Sendele DD. Chemical hypersensitivity reactions. Int Ophthalmol Clin 1986;26(1):25–34.

Smith RS. Solving the mystery of the red eye. Am Fam Physician 1975; 12(4):144–50.

Glaucoma

Anonymous. Glaucoma alert program. Sight Sav Rev 1977;19–22.

Boger WP. The treatment of glaucoma—role of beta-blocking agents. Drugs 1979;18:25–32.

Durkee DP, Bryant BG. Drug therapy of glaucoma. Am J Hosp Pharm 1978; 35:682–90.

Soll DB, Saxon AM. Drugs and glaucoma. Am Fam Physician 1986;34(1):181–5.

Stamper RL. Epitomes of ophthalmology: acute angle-closure glaucoma. West J Med 1979;130(6):544–5.

Trauma

Appen RE, Hutson CF. Traumatic injuries: office treatment of eye injury. Injury due to foreign materials. Postgrad Med 1976;60(4):233–5,237.

Born CP. Ocular injuries—treat or refer? Postgrad Med 1983;73(2):311–7.

Gardiner PA. ABC of ophthalmology—accidents and first aid. Br Med J 1978;2:1347–50.

Goren SB. Common ocular injuries—assessing the severity. Postgrad Med 1975;58(7)99–102.

McIntire WC. Treatment of toxic agents to the eye. Acta Pharmacol Toxicol 1977;41(Suppl II):335–8.

Pattison GN. Ophthalmology for casualty departments. London: Churchill-Livingstone, 1967.

Romanchuk KG, Pollock V, Schneider RJ. Retinal burn from a welding arc Can J Ophthalmol 1978;13:120–2.

Ophthalmic Products

Taugher PJ. Eye emergency trauma—practical concepts in management of ocular trauma. Wis Med J 1976;75:586–7.

Dry Eye
Ehrlich DR, Keates RH. What to do when the elderly patient complains of external eye problems. Geriatrics 1978;33:34–8.

Holly FJ. Artificial tear formulations. Int Ophthalmol Clin 1980;20(3):171-1841.

Lamberts DW. Dry eye and tear deficiency. Int Ophthalmol Clin 1983; 23(1):123–30.

Williamson J. The rheumatic eye. Practitioner 1982;226:863–74.

Treatment
Brown CA. Common eye problems in infants and children. Practitioner 1977;219:53–8.

Mamelok AE. Allergic conjunctivitis. Cutis 1976;17:244–8.

McEvoy GK, ed. American hospital formulary service. Bethesda: American Society of Hospital Pharmacists, 1991.

Decongestants
Anonymous. Babies' blood pressure raised by eye drops. Br Med J 1974;1:2–3.

Anonymous. Vasocon (Training bulletin). Boisbriand: Cooper Laboratories.

Cass E, Kada D, Stein HA. Hazards of phenylephrine topical medication in persons taking propranolol. Can Med Assoc J 1979;120:1261–2.

Fraunfelder FT. Drug-induced ocular side-effects and drug interactions. Philadelphia: Lea & Febiger, 1989.

Mindlin RL. Accidental poisoning from tetrahydrozoline eyedrops (Letter). N Engl J Med 1966;275:112.

Norden LC. Adverse reactions to topical ocular autonomic agents. J Am Optom Assoc 1978;49(1):75–80.

Patton TF, Robinson JR. Pediatric dosing considerations in ophthalmology. J Pediatr Ophthalmol 1976;13(3):171–8.

Rumelt MB. Blindness from misuse of over-the-counter eye medications. Ann Ophthalmol 1988;20(1):26–30.

Vale J, Cox B. Drugs in the eye. Toronto: Butterworths, 1978.

Antihistamines
Abelson MB, Allansmith MR, Friedlaender MH. Effects of topically applied ocular decongestant and antihistamine. Am J Ophthalmol 1980;90:254–7.

Abelson MB, et al. Effects of Vasocon-A in the allergen challenge model of acute allergic conjunctivitis. Arch Ophthalmol 1990;108(4):520–4.

Miller J, Wolf EH. Antazoline phosphate and naphazoline hydrochloride, singly and in combination for the treatment of allergic conjunctivitis; a controlled, double-blind clinical trial. Ann Allergy 1975;35(1):81–6.

Anti-infectives
Hyndiuk RA, Burd EM, Hartz A. Efficacy and safety of mercuric oxide in the treatment of bacterial blepharitis. Antimicrob Agents Chemother 1990;34(4):610–3.

Kastl PR, et al. Placebo-controlled, double-blink evaluation of the efficacy and safety of yellow mercuric oxide in suppression of eyelid infections. Ann Ophthalmol 1987;19(10):376–9.

Artificial Tears
Flora MR. Dry eye syndrome—a case report. J Am Optom Assoc 1977; 48(8):1063–4.

Gilbard JP, et al. Stimulation of tear secretion and treatment of dry-eye disease with 3-isobutyl-1-methylxanthine. Arch Ophthalmol 1991;109(5):672–6.

Gilbard JP, Farris RL. New concepts in the therapy of keratoconjunctivitis sicca. In: Srinivasan D, ed. Ocular therapeutics. New York: Masson Publishers, 1980:213–7.

Gilbard JP, Kenyon KR. Tear diluents in the treatment of keratoconjunctivitis sicca. Ophthalmology 1985;92(5):646–50.

Göbbels M, Spitznas M. Influence of artificial tears on corneal epithelium in dry-eye syndrome. Graefe's Arch Clin Exp Ophthalmol 1989; 227(2):139–41.

Holly FJ, Lemp MA. Tear physiology and dry eyes. Surv Ophthalmol 1977; 22(2):69–87.

Lemp MA, Goldberg M, Robby MR. The effect of tear substitutes on tear film break-up time. Invest Ophthalmol 1975;14(3):255–8.

Lemp MA. Design and development of an artificial tear. Paper presented at 80th annual meeting AAOO Dallas, 1975;Sep:21–5.

Limberg MB. Topical application of hyaluronic acid and chondroitin sulfate in the treatment of dry eyes. Am J Ophthalmol 1987;103(2):194–7.

Liotet S, et al. A new hypothesis on tear film stability. Ophthalmologica 1987;195(3):119–24.

Motolko M, Breslin CW. The effect of pH and osmolarity on the ability to tolerate artificial tears. Am J Ophthalmol 1981;1:781–4.

Moudgil SS, et al. Effect of methylcellulose on tear film break-up-time in health and disease. Acta Ophthalmologica 1987;65(4)397–9.

Nelson JD, Farris RL. Sodium hyaluronate and polyvinyl alcohol artificial tear preparations. Arch Ophthalmol 1988;106(4):484–7.

Patton TF, Robinson JR. Ocular evaluation of polyvinyl alcohol vehicle in rabbits. J Pharm Sci 1975;64(8):1312–6.

Prakash UBS, Rosenow EC. Pulmonary complications from ophthalmic preparations. Mayo Clin Proc 1990;65(4):521–9.

Rieger G. Lipid-containing eyedrops: a step closer to natural tears. Ophthalmologica 1990;201(4):206–12.

Versura P. Dry eye before and after therapy with hydroxypropyl methylcellulose. Ophthalmologica 1989;198(3):152–62.

Wright P. The dry eye. Practitioner 1975;214:631–5.

Wright P, Cooper M, Gilvarry AM. Effect of osmolarity of artificial tear drops on relief of dry eye symptoms: BJ6 and beyond. Br J Ophthalmol 1987; 71(2):161–4.

Wright P. Other forms of treatment of dry eyes. Trans Ophthalmol Soc UK 1985;104:497–8.

Local Anesthetics
Duffin RM, Olson RJ. Tetracaine toxicity. Ann Ophthalmol 1984;16(9):836–8.

Fraunfelder FT. What's new in ocular toxicology? Sight Sav Rev 1978:53–8.

Henkes HE, Waubke TN. Keratitis from abuse of corneal anaesthetics. Br J Ophthalmol 1978;62:62–5.

Kintner JC, et al. Infectious crystalline keratopathy associated with topical anesthetic abuse. Cornea 1990;9(1):77–80.

Norden LC. Adverse reactions to topical ocular anesthetics. J Am Optom Assoc 1976;47(6):730–3.

Rosenwasser GOD. Complications of topical ocular anesthetics. Int Ophthalmol Clin 1989;29(3):153–8.

Smith RB, Everett WG. Physiology and pharmacology of local anesthetic agents. Anesthesia in ophthalmology. Int Ophthalmol Clin 1973;13:35–60.

Preservatives
Burstein NL. The effects of topical drug and preservatives on the tears and corneal epithelium of dry eye. Trans Ophthalmol Soc UK 1985;104:402–9.

Lemp MA, Zimmerman LE. Toxic endothelial degeneration in ocular surface disease treated with topical medications containing benzalkonium chloride. Am J Ophthalmol 1988;105(6):670–3.

Mullen W, Shepherd W, Labovitz J. Ophthalmic preservatives and vehicles. Suv Ophthalmol 1973;17(6):469–93.

Stern GA, Killingsworth DW. Complications of topical antimicrobial agents. Int Ophthalmol Clin 1989;29(3):137–42.

Tan B. Hypersensitivity and allergic reactions to ophthalmic drugs. Aust J Optom 1974;57:114–21.

Tosti A, Tosti G. Thimerosal: a hidden allergen in ophthalmology. Contact Dermatitis 1988;18(5):268–73.

Miscellaneous Ingredients
Osol A, Pratt R, eds. The United States dispensatory. Toronto: JB Lippincott, 1978.

Formulations
Barnstien CH, Blake MI, DeWald AE, eds. The national formulary. Washington: American Pharmaceutical Association, 1965:59.

Feldman EG, ed. Handbook of nonprescription drugs. Washington: American Pharmaceutical Association, 1991.

Ophthalmic Products

Instillation of Ophthalmic Solutions

Anonymous. Here's how to teach the "depot" method for eye drops. Pharm Pract 1977:56.

Anonymous. How to instil ophthalmic medication in a child's eyes. Pharm Pract 1975;10(12):2.

Fritz M. Eyedrops. Alaska Med 1977:43–4.

Law S. Development and utilization of the eyedropper adaptation device: an example of interdisciplinary cooperation. Home Healthcare Nurse 1987; 5(4):50–1.

Letocha CE. Methods for self-administration of eyedrops. Ann Ophthalmol 1985;17(12):768–9.

Sheldon GM. Self-administration of eyedrops. Ophthal Surg 1987;18(5):393–4.

Winfield AJ, et al. A study of the causes of noncomplicance by patients prescribed eyedrops. Br J Ophthalmol 1990;74(8):477–80.

Application of Ophthalmic Ointments

Annable WL. Therapy for ocular infections. Pediatr Clin N Amer 1983; 30(2):389–96.

Weisbecker C, Linkewich J. Dealing with ophthalmic needs—common ocular problems. On Cont Pract 1983;10(1):33–6.

9
Contact Lens Care

David S. Wing

Many different contact lenses are now available. Care regimens are chosen on the basis of lens type and individual consumer characteristics. Important considerations in choosing solutions include safety, efficacy, cost and simplicity. Wearers must be counselled to follow exactly the care regimen prescribed by lens practitioners. The strengths and weaknesses of cleaning, disinfecting and multifunction solutions and buffers, wetting agents and viscosity agents are described. The effects on wearers of oral contraceptives, ophthalmics, systemic medications and smoking are also discussed.

The history of contact lenses dates to the late 15th century when Leonardo da Vinci theorized optical devices held on the eye by water. The idea resurfaced in 1827 when a small glass shell was suggested to protect the cornea from disease, but not until 1887 were the first contact lenses made. Since they were glass, numerous unpleasant side effects occurred.

Polymethylmethacrylate (PMMA) was introduced in 1936, and the first plastic scleral lenses of this material appeared in 1939. The first corneal contact lens (resembling modern lenses) was introduced in 1947. In 1962, the first soft (hydrogel) contact lens of hydroxyethylmethacrylate (HEMA) was developed. The gas permeable lens was developed in the late 1970s when a combination of PMMA and silicone was used to increase the oxygen permeability of hard lenses (see Table I). The extended wear lens was introduced in the late 1970s for older postcataract (aphakic) wearers due to the decreased handling required. The advantage of convenience led to its cosmetic use. The most recent development is the disposable contact lens. Trade names of selected contact lenses are listed in Table II.

From a survey conducted April 1, 1987 to April 1, 1988, 81 per cent of the patients fitted for contact lenses were in the 17 to 44 age category. Half of the patients had never worn lenses within 5 years of the survey period. Soft lenses still represent the vast majority

(85 per cent) of lens type prescribed compared to rigid lenses (14 per cent).

Contact Lenses
Hard (PMMA) Lenses

Hard (PMMA) contact lenses are almost obsolete in Canada. The term "hard lens" includes gas permeable lenses, but for this discussion, they are considered different except where indicated.

Hard lenses are custom-made from PMMA. The two types are corneal (small), which make up the vast majority of hard lenses, and scleral (large), which are not discussed since they are rarely used.

Hard (PMMA) lenses are durable, inexpensive and provide excellent visual acuity, but they cannot be worn for long periods without causing corneal edema. Maximum wear time is 15 hours for 70 per cent of users. Since the lens is hydrophobic, wetting is required for compatibility with the eye. The lens sits on a fluid cushion rather than directly on the cornea. Hard lenses inhibit oxygen flow by creating an obstruction between the atmosphere and the cornea. They are smaller than the cornea so the avascular cornea can obtain its oxygen supply from tear fluids pumped around the lens. The major cause of failure is oxygen deprivation resulting in corneal edema.

Hard (PMMA) lenses can cause the overwear syndrome. Prolonged wearing can disrupt the metabolic process that transfers water, oxygen and carbon dioxide across the corneal epithelium to the cornea. This disruption results in epithelial abrasion and ulceration and corneal edema. If the corneal edema is sufficient to cause loss of corneal sensation, the wearer feels no pain. Upon lens removal, metabolic processes and corneal sensation return. Pain and photophobia indicate epithelial damage. Although the overwear syndrome resolves in 8 to 26 hours, a lens practitioner should be consulted as treatment may be required. Lenses are not worn for 1 to 2 days after resolution. The gradual return to lens wear should be under the care of a lens practitioner.

Table I *Comparison of the Different Types of Contact Lenses*

Characteristics	Hard (PMMA)	Gas permeable	Soft	Silicone
Composition	Polymethylmethacrylate (PMMA)	Silicone/acrylate, fluorinated silicone acrylate, cellulose acetate butyrate (CAB)	Hydroxyethylmethacrylate (HEMA) is the most common polymer	Silicone

Contact Lens Care

Table I *(Cont'd) Comparison of the Different Types of Contact Lenses*

Characteristics	Hard (PMMA)	Gas permeable	Soft	Silicone
Water content	Up to 1.5%	2–3% (only slightly greater than PMMA lenses)	29–85%	Up to 2%
Life expectancy*	About 5 years	About 2–4 years (if there is no warping)	1 week—2 years	About 1.5 years
Solution requirements	Hard lens solutions	Should use gas permeable specific solutions	Soft lens solutions	Can be treated as soft lenses for care purposes although solution manufacturers often make a specific recommendation
Advantages	Excellent visual acuity; can be polished if surface is scratched; may last 15 to 20 years; relatively inexpensive to replace and maintain; both hard and gas permeable lenses are able to correct some vision problems (e.g., keratoconus, astigmatism) better than soft lenses	Over hard (PMMA) lenses: increased comfort; increased wearing time; elimination of overwear syndrome; rapid adaptation to glasses after lens removal; decreased risk of lens loss. Over soft lenses: superior optics; increased durability; decreased risk of lens discoloration with various chemicals; less likely to be contaminated; easier to care for; more prescriptions are possible; rigidity is advantageous in keratoconus	Flexibility allows easy insertion and removal; large size facilitates easy fitting and decreased risk of lens loss; close fit prevents entry of wind and dust which can scratch cornea; useful for athletes and children since they do not pop out easily; maximum wear time is achieved within days of fitting; ideal for occasional use because of short adaptation period; alternating with glasses is not a problem	Over soft lenses: increased gas permeability; increased mechanical strength; decreased polymer degradation; decreased absorption of water soluble materials
Disadvantages	Gas impermeable material, may warp, crack or chip requiring replacement; short wear time; small size and relative rigidity can lead to popping out and subsequent loss; blurred vision from corneal swelling for about one hour when glasses are used after lens removal; corneal abrasion can occur if dust or other particles are caught underneath lens; up to one month may be required to gradually establish maximum wearing time; hydrophobic; overwear syndrome	Hydrophobic-wetting required for compatibility with the eye; possibly less comfortable than soft lenses; less durable and more susceptible to protein deposits than PMMA lenses; cannot be tinted as readily as hard or soft lenses	Compared to hard lenses they are more fragile, (easily torn by fingernails) and more susceptible to protein and calcium deposits from tearfilm (due to "open matrix"); are only suitable for about 80% of potential wearers; high altitude and low humidity can decrease visual acuity; low oxygen pressures can decrease the oxygen received by cornea, resulting in corneal swelling and decreased vision; low humidity can increase the rate of tear evaporation causing lenses to dry and become uncomfortable; risk of microbial contamination	Adherence to the eye even after a short wearing period; hydrophobicity of the surface; inability to modify the surface

*When soft or gas permeable lenses are used for extended wear, the lens life averages 8–10 months although the individual life is highly variable and is dependent on length of time between cleanings, amount of ocular secretions, user handling and fragility of the lens. Gas permeable lenses are not yet widely approved for extended wear in Canada.

Contact Lens Care

Table II *Selected Trade Names of Contact Lenses According to Lens Type*

Brand Name	Manufacturer	Lens Material	% Water/Saline
Soft Contact Lenses (Daily Wear)			
Cibasoft/Thin	Ciba Vision		37.5
CSI/CSIT	Syntex		38
Durasoft	Wesley-Jensen		30–55
Hydrocurve 45	Barnes-Hind		45
Hydrocurve II 55	Barnes-Hind		55
PCL-38	Plastic C. L. Lab		38
Preflex	Optech		55
Permalens	Cooper		72
Permathin	Cooper Vision		43
Sofcon	Ciba Vision		55
Soflens	Bausch & Lomb		38
U3/U4	Bausch & Lomb		38
U4	Bausch & Lomb		38
04/06	Hydron		38
Soft Contact Lenses (Extended Wear)			
Ciba 55	Ciba Vision		55
Durasoft 3	Wesley-Jensen		55
Hydrocurve II	Barnes-Hind		45–55
Permaflex	Coopervision		74
Softcon	Ciba Vision		55
Gas Permeable Hard Lenses (Daily Wear)			
Airlens	Wesley-Jesson	Alkyl Styrene	
Equalens	Polymer Technnology Corp.	Silicone-Acrylate Fluropolymer	
GP II	Barnes-Hind	CAB	
Meso	Danker	CAB	
Optacryl 60	Optacryl	PMMA/Silicone	
Silcon VFL	Dow Corning	Silicone	
Gas Permeable Brand Names (Extended Wear)			
Advent	Bausch & Lomb	Fluropolymer	
Boston IV	Polymer Technology	Silicon/Acrylate	
Flurocon	Sola Barnes Hind	Fluropolymer	
Paraperm	Paragon Optical	Silicon/Acrylate	
Disposable Contact Lenses			
Acuvue	Johnson and Johnson		58
Nuvue	Ciba Vision		58
Renew	Bausch & Lomb		38
Surevue	Johnson and Johnson		58

Gas Permeable Lenses

The rigid gas permeable lens was developed to combine the optical qualities and durability of PMMA with the oxygen permeability and comfort of HEMA. These lenses have a sufficiently high oxygen permeability to prevent clinically observable corneal edema in normal wear. These lenses lead to fewer complications and, in general, better long-term visual acuity than either hard (PMMA) or soft lenses. Two main types of gas permeable lenses are available: silicone/acrylate and fluorinated silicone-acrylate.

Fluorinated silicone-acrylate lenses are a newer addition to the gas permeable lens market. They are similar to silicone-acrylate lenses, but the fluorine substitution allows even greater oxygen permeability.

Soft (Hydrogel) Lenses

Soft contacts are composed of a flexible polymeric material (hydrox-yethylmethacrylate is most common) with a high capacity for water absorption. Increased comfort is the main advantage and is due to flexibility (which increases with greater water content), soft thin edges and hydrophilic nature, all of which allow normal tear exchange with each blink reflex. In addition to correcting refractive errors, indications include protection of cornea (for example, exposure keratitis), prevention of corneal scarring (for example, following chemical burns) and drug administration (for example, pilocarpine for glaucoma).

Soft lenses are flexible, large, and have a short adaptation time (see Table I). Unfortunately, their open matrix allows concentration of many ophthalmic preparations, environmental pollutants, chemical vapors, oil and dust from fingers, cosmetics and some contact lens solution preservatives, all of which can lead to ocular irritation. These materials also tend to develop lens deposits more rapidly than hard or gas permeable materials.

Silicone Lenses

Silicone lenses have a high permeability for oxygen and other gases. Just as the term "hard lens" includes gas permeable lenses, the term "soft lens" includes silicone lenses. Due to production and maintenance problems that led to poor demand, silicone lenses were discontinued in 1985.

The lens is still available on a limited basis for certain aphakic prescriptions.

Extended Wear

Extended wear is defined as wearing a contact lens for 24 hours or more without removing it. The lenses are usually soft and vary in thickness relative to the water content. They were designed for older, aphakic people but their convenience made them popular with myopic consumers and lens practitioners. Consequently, more than 90 per cent of extended wear is for cosmetic reasons.

Successful extended wear depends on previous success with daily contact lens wear, pre-existing medical conditions, the working or living environment and visual needs. Potential extended wear begins with daily wear. This process, lasting up to 1 month, allows the user to gain experience handling the lens, allows the cornea to adapt and gives the lens practitioner the opportunity to evaluate lens acceptance. The actual period of extended wear varies from person to person and depends on lens tolerance and deposit build-up. Some wearers have gone as long as 18 months between cleanings, although 7 days appears to be the best compromise between convenience and safety. However, extended wear soft lenses were implicated in promoting microbial keratitis, potentially the most devastating complication of contact lens wear resulting in widespread concern about the increased risk of complications.

Early uncontrolled trials suggested that the rate of serious complications were not excessive and many consumers adopted them. Unfortunately their tremendous growth was associated with reports of microbial keratitis with *Pseudomonas aeruginosa* being the most frequent isolate causing some patients to lose vision. *Pseudomonas aeruginosa* is enviromentally widespread and has been found in high concentrations in contact lens storage solutions. It has been suggested that contamination of lenses from poor hygiene is responsible for transferring Pseudomonas to the eye and from handling. A 1987 report reviewed more than 500 cases of microbial keratitis and found 63 per cent were associated with cosmetic use of soft lenses. Of those, 60 per cent were linked with extended wear and 40 per cent to daily wear. It has been estimated that microbial keratitis affects one in 15,000 daily wearers and one in 3,000 extended wearers of soft lenses. Compared to daily wear, the overnight use of soft contact lenses carries a 10 fold increased risk for developing potentially serious corneal ulcers. The risk increases incrementally with length of extended wear. More careful lens hygiene would tend to lower the risk. With extended wear, solutions became contaminated as they are used up very slowly. There was a 22 per cent contamination rate of solutions used by extended wear compared to 6 per cent with daily wearers. For extended wear, solutions should be discarded after 21 days. Lens covers should be thoroughly cleaned before each use. Also, the risks with less serious complications may be greater due to the compromised physiology of extended wear and the adherence and colonization of new lenses by bacteria. Until the results of more studies are available, consumers and lens practitioners should be aware of the question of safety and the increasing evidence of adverse effects of extended wear lenses. To decrease the frequency of infection, the U.S. Food and Drug Administration has recommended that extended wear soft lenses be worn from 1 to 7 days before removal for cleaning or disposal in the case of disposable lenses. Frequent lens removals and replacements should help minimize the incidence of complications.

Some consumers who have encountered problems with soft lenses (such as lens deposits and side effects) have tried gas permeable lenses for extended wear. Recent data indicate they can be worn safely for extended periods. These lenses may have fewer risks than soft lenses and offer superior vision.

Disposable Extended-Wear Contact Lenses

Unlike conventional extended wear lenses which are cleaned and disinfected, disposable lenses are worn once, discarded and replaced by a new lens.

Acuvue (see Table II), a competitively priced disposable contact lens was introduced in Canada in 1988. The lens is recommended for 1 to 2 weeks of wear before replacement. Preliminary data supported the manufacturer's claims that eye health would be maintained by frequent lens replacement which decreases or eliminates the problems associated with lens deposits and allergic reactions to solutions. However, side effects such as sterile corneal infiltrates, corneal ulcers and pseudomonas keratitis have been reported. Compliance would be expected to be more readily accomplished. However, case reports exist of Acanthamoeba keratitis developing in two patients who habitually removed, irrigated and reinserted disposable lenses without disinfecting them or stored disposable lenses overnight in a case rinsed with well water. The increased cost of disposable lenses have prompted some consumers to wear them longer than recommended. Acanthamoeba keratitis has also developed from an unknown cause.

Acanthamoeba keratitis is a rare but serious infection that can result in the need for penetrating keratoplasty or enucleation. Acanthamoeba is widespread in the environment making avoidance impossible. It adheres to soft lenses and has been found in the lens cases of asymptomatic wearers. The organism exists as either a rapidly growing trophozoite or when conditions become unfavorable for growth, such as a protective cyst which can survive extremes of temperature and pH.

Lens Care Solutions

When contact lenses are purchased, the lens practitioner usually gives the consumer a starter kit containing a complete lens care system. Optometrists choose products from clinical experience and from recommendations of clinical articles in eye care literature. Other sources of recommendation include advertising, advice from colleagues and user preference.

As the number of contact lens solutions grows, selecting the best system becomes difficult. Comparisons are often outdated because manufacturers reformulate their products frequently. Four important factors are safety, efficacy, cost and simplicity. It is necessary to understand the components to determine efficacy, but not all manufacturers are willing to reveal their formulations.

Most solutions contain more than 95 per cent purified water. Solution functions are determined by adding preservatives, wetting agents, buffers, surfactants, cleaners and disinfectants. Some new solutions are made up of different combinations and concentrations of the

Figure 1 *Steps for Optimum Care of Contact Lenses*

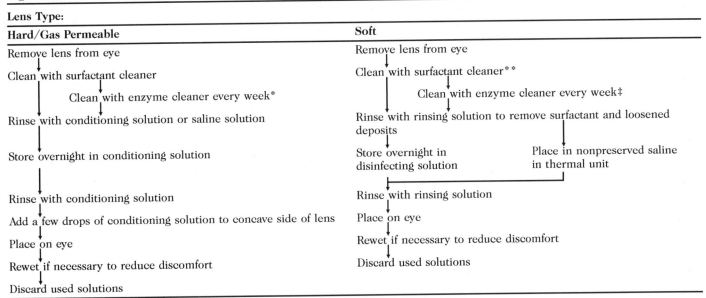

*Although not routinely recommended, weekly use of an enzyme cleaner will benefit any hard lens.
**It is important to rub the lens on the periphery first, since this is where the debris begins to accumulate, then work towards the centre; both sides should be done for at least 20 seconds each.
‡The addition of this step to chemical disinfection has decreased the incidence of red eyes, limbal injection, and discomfort in one study. This step has been incorporated into the recommendations of most manufacturers. Regular papain tablets are not recommended for extended-wear lenses but subtilisin tablets can be used.

same components. Although the efficacy and adverse effects of each component are discussed, individual consumer characteristics may be the deciding factor. Proper compliance is essential for corneal health. It is one of three areas (the other two being consumer education and responsible use of contact lenses by consumers) that needs to be improved to optimize contact lens safety. Product substitution is not recommended unless directed by the eye care practitioner. In addition, cost must be considered in long-term use of solutions.

The next section covers chemical components used for both hard and soft lenses. Ingredients used for a specific lens type are discussed in the appropriate section. Figure 1 summarizes the recommended steps for the routine care of contact lenses. The importance of each step performed in the proper sequence cannot be overemphasized.

Cleaning Solutions

Cleaning is the most important step in the proper care of contact lenses. It maintains visual acuity, comfort, wearer health and optimal lens life, and minimizes both user and lens practitioner costs. Debris from numerous sources collects on the lens surface almost from the moment of insertion (see Table III). Extended wear lenses quickly develop a thick coating because they are worn constantly. The longer the interval between cleaning, the greater is the risk of complications such as ulcerative keratitis and Acanthamoeba keratitis. Despite claims that certain contact lens materials collect certain types of debris, a mixture of debris types is usually found independent of lens composition. The proper use of surfactants reduces lens coatings which can contribute to ocular infections.

Since many contaminants of a contact lens are not water soluble,

washing the lens in water (for a hard PMMA or gas permeable lens) or rinsing solution (for a soft lens) does not remove debris. As the preservative may be inactivated by debris, the lens should be thoroughly cleaned with a surfactant before disinfecting and storing the lens. Surfactants also emulsify and suspend organisms, reducing contamination and facilitating disinfection. Proper cleaning and rinsing can remove more than 99.9 per cent of the contaminants prior to the disinfection step. Since most lens pathogens use organic

Table III *Etiology of Debris Accumulating on Contact Lenses*

Source	Composition
Ocular secretions (e.g., tears)	Protein, lipids, salts, enzymes, pigments
Handling	Protein, oils, cosmetics, salts, other particulate matter (e.g., soap, finger grease, dirt, nicotine)
Environmental	Smoke, particulate matter, volatile chemicals, airborne microbes
Cosmetics	Eyeliner, mascara, hairspray, eyeshadow, etc.
Contact lens solutions	Chemicals, salts, preservatives, solution contaminants
Contact lens cases	Bacteria, salts

Table IV *Classification of Surfactants*

Type	Charge	Examples	Comments
Nonionic	None	Poloxamer 407	Effective, compatible and generally the least toxic
Amphoteric	Positive and negative	Miranol	Depends on pH for maximum effectiveness
Cationic	Positive	BAC	Effective, but limited in usefulness, especially with soft contact lenses
Anionic	Negative	Sodium lauryl sulfate Soaps	Effective, but generally not used because of high potential for eye irritation and incompatibility with many ingredients; are generally less stable than nonionic surfactants

deposits as food, removal of the food source by effective cleaning can reduce the viability of any surviving pathogens.

Surfactants have a hydrophilic and a hydrophobic property which orients itself to the hydrophilic or hydrophobic nature of the debris, thereby softening and loosening it (see Table IV). Debris can then be removed more easily with mechanical action, such as finger rubbing or automatic agitation. Surfactants can remove oily deposits, mucus and other loosely adherent debris, such as the remnants of makeup, but they cannot remove deposits.

Daily surfactant cleaning is similar for soft and hard (PMMA and gas permeable) lenses, but the components of the solutions differ. For soft lenses, preservatives that do not concentrate in the lens are used. Immediately after lens removal, a few drops of solution are applied to both lens surfaces. The lenses are cleaned in the palm of the hand using the index finger in a circular motion. Vigorous friction rubbing between the thumb and forefinger for 30 to 60 seconds has been recommended, but ripping and tearing of the lens can occur. The surfactant is thoroughly rinsed off using a rinsing solution before disinfection. The surfactant is used before the enzyme because it acts on the lipids that may hide protein deposits and makes the enzymatic cleaner more effective.

Surfactant solutions must be rinsed thoroughly from the contact lens and hands since chemical keratoconjunctivitis, stinging, allergic reactions, conjunctival hyperemia and eyelid edema can occur. A surfactant residue may produce a permanent coating on a lens subjected to repeated thermal disinfection.

Surfactant cleaners formulated with abrasives may remove thin layers of protein film, but they are ineffective against bound protein and may damage the lens surface. It is sometimes difficult to rinse all of the abrasives off the lens which could result in corneal irritation and damage.

Enzyme cleaners are usually recommended for soft lenses but hard (PMMA and gas permeable) lenses will also benefit from their use. The use of papain as an overnight soaking solution has increased the wear time in keratoconic users with papillary conjunctivitis using either hard (PMMA or gas permeable) lenses.

Cleaning can restore hard lenses to their original appearance, but soft lenses require more than cleaning for total restoration.

Isopropyl Alcohol

Isopropyl alcohol dissolves lipid build-up. It is compatible with hard and soft lenses, but is adsorbed onto soft lenses. Severe burning and corneal epithelial damage can occur if isopropyl alcohol touches the eye. The solution must be thoroughly washed out and the lens soaked in saline solution to remove the cleaner residue.

Isopropyl alcohol 20 per cent is effective in removing nonaqueous debris from gas permeable lenses. It is very effective against Acanthamoeba cysts. However, it can alter lens parameters if used as a soaking solution. Inadvertent use of a cleaner mistaken for a lubricant, due to similarity in bottle size and shape has been reported.

Unorthodox Cleaners

Unorthodox cleaners include toothpaste, laundry detergent, hair shampoo and skin cleansers, which all have harmful effects on eyes and lenses. Some of these home remedy cleaners (baking soda and popcorn salt) have been tested against Opticlean. While as effective as Opticlean, the home remedy cleaners left long, deep, jagged scratches while Opticlean did not. The best method for cleaning lenses is a sterile regimen of known surfactants recommended by the lens practitioner.

Lens-specific cleaners, such as enzymes and oxidizing agents, are discussed under soft lenses since they are used primarily with this lens type.

Disinfection (Soaking or Storage) Solutions

Disinfecting solutions are designed to disinfect and maintain a disinfected lens, to maintain the hydrated equilibrium of the lens while it is not being worn and to prevent ocular secretions and debris from remaining after cleaning.

Disinfection destroys all vegetative bacterial cells except spores; sterilization destroys microbial activity. Contact lenses require only disinfection. Some lens practitioners question the need for disinfection since some wearers report omitting this step with no apparent problems. Others are less concerned about absolute efficacy especially compliant patients who perform regular surfactant cleaning. Thorough daily cleaning and rinsing will remove more than 99.9 per cent of the bacteria present in lenses. Yet, although the incidence of a sight-threatening eye infection is low relative to the millions of wearers, the hazard remains. As a whole, all disinfection regimens are simple, effective and convenient when weighed against the cost of not using them.

A disinfectant actively kills bacteria on lenses; a preservative maintains the sterility of a solution against outside insult. A preserved saline solution does not disinfect unless used for thermal disinfection. Most soaking solutions contain disinfectants and preservatives. Some also contain surfactants but in a lower concentration than in cleaning solutions, so soaking does not replace daily cleaning. An important issue with disinfectants is sensitivity, which is discussed under the section on soft contact lens products since solution reactions occur most often with soft lenses, which can absorb some ingredients of the solutions to which they are exposed.

Organomercurials

Organomercurials kill bacteria and fungi slowly, probably by inhibiting sulfhydryl enzymes. They are incompatible with rose bengal and benzalkonium chloride (BAC) in certain concentrations and are inhibited by EDTA and inactivated by rubber. Adverse effects include allergy, chemosis (conjunctival edema), keratitis, conjunctival hyperemia, burning, irritation and lens vacuoles.

Thimerosal, the most popular organomercurial, is generally used at 0.001 to 0.004 per cent. The maximum concentration is 0.01 per cent. Thimerosal alone successfully passes all the tests required by the United States Food and Drug Administration to qualify it as a preservative in contact lens solutions, and its combination with chlorhexidine or alkyltriethylammonium chloride yields an effective broad spectrum disinfectant. Its usefulness combined with chlorhexidine is discussed in the chlorhexidine section.

Thimerosal can be inactivated by corneal fluids and must be used in neutral or slightly alkaline conditions. The amount of thimerosal retained by HEMA lenses correlates with the water content of the lens. Storage equilibrium is reached after 1 hour, and when the lens is inserted, the thimerosal leaves the lens just as rapidly. Thimerosal can cause gray to black lens discoloration in thermal disinfection regimens.

Phenylmercuric nitrate is the other organomercurial preservative in contact lens solutions. The maximum concentrations for use in the eye is 0.004 per cent. It should not be used with soft lenses because it binds to the lenses and is precipitated by halide ions (present in debris).

Chlorhexidine

Chlorhexidine is effective against gram-negative bacteria and gram-positive bacteria, although it is less effective against the latter. It is more effective than thimerosal, but at low concentrations (for example, 0.005 per cent), clinical efficacy varies. It is more toxic to ocular tissues than thimerosal. The best results are obtained when chlorhexidine is combined with thimerosal (for its antifungal effect) and EDTA (for antimicrobial effect). This combination is effective against Acanthamoeba cysts but some chlorhexidine formulations may not be as effective. Disinfection requires at least 4 hours, preferably overnight.

Chlorhexidine is compatible with most ophthalmic products but incompatible with soaps, anions and fluorescein solutions and is inactivated by cork, starch, magnesium, zinc and calcium compounds. It binds strongly to HEMA lenses, especially in the presence of other adjuvants (such as electrolyte or hydrophilic polymers). Soft lenses store chlorhexidine and after insertion leaves slowly, exposing the eye to a decreasing concentration. The binding capacity of chlorhexidine is about one-sixth that of BAC and a large percentage is absorbed by tear proteins. The presence of protein can increase the concentration of chlorhexidine in the lens, so it is important to remove protein regularly with an enzymatic cleaner before soaking the lenses in chlorhexidine. Lenses saturated with chlorhexidine become hydrophobic and adsorb lipids to their surfaces. Chlorhexidine can eventually cause lens filming, yellowing and decreased wettability. Solutions should be discarded if they have a greenish tinge.

With extended use, a solution of 0.005 per cent appears nontoxic to eye tissue, but skin sensitivities, eye discomfort and irritation of the conjunctiva have been reported. Direct application to the eye may cause conjunctivitis.

EDTA

EDTA and its salts—edetate, disodium edetate and trisodium edetate—break down the bacterial cell wall with a detergent action. It is not a preservative, but its presence enhances the activity of preservatives. EDTA also acts as a buffer.

The usual concentrations of EDTA range from 0.01 to 0.1 per cent. These concentrations cannot prevent or remove inorganic calcium deposits from lenses, as these tasks require concentrations of 0.35 to 1.85 per cent. EDTA enhances the activity of BAC, chlorobutanol, chlorhexidine and thimerosal by chelating calcium and magnesium ions, which compete with preservatives for sites on the organism. Conjunctival edema, hyperemia and irritation are possible.

Contact Lens Cases

Contact lenses should be stored in contact lens cases. Lenses should be completely covered by the soaking solution when not worn, as they can dry out, changing the lens parameter. Soaking maintains hydration, making it wet more readily. A hard (PMMA and gas permeable) lens dries out in just 12 hours changing the lens parameter, but it requires about 72 hours to fully hydrate again. Storage cases must be kept clean by routinely boiling them in water. The lens case is allowed to cool 30 to 45 minutes before replacing the lenses. Some types of lens cases cannot withstand boiling. These types should be replaced at least monthly. To optimize disinfection and minimize potential irritation, lenses should be cleaned with a surfactant cleaner before disinfecting and soaking. The soaking solution should be replaced daily and the case flushed of old solution before adding new solution. Some manufacturers and researchers now recommend regular replacement of contact lens cases due to the risk of contamination from biofilm build-up.

Buffers

Buffers resist changes in pH from additions of small amounts of acid or base. In contact lens solutions, buffers stabilize components and improve comfort on instillation. Normal tears have a pH of about 7.3 and possess a high buffering capacity due to their protein content. Placing 1 or 2 drops of solution into the eye stimulates tear flow and rapid neutralization of excess hydrogen and hydroxyl ions within the buffering capacity of the tears. Solutions of pH 6 to 9 generally can be tolerated. Solutions that are acidic or alkaline for ingredient stability should not be buffered or should be minimally buffered so rapid neutralization by tears can occur upon instillation. It has been recommended that buffered solutions be used to ensure eye comfort unless contraindicated.

Buffers include: sodium carbonate, boric acid, sodium borate, sodium bicarbonate, sodium phosphate and disodium phosphate. The borate buffer system is advocated on the basis of user acceptance. Borate buffers react with polyvinyl alcohol to form a precipitate. Solutions with these components should not be mixed.

Wetting and Viscosity Agents

Hard (PMMA and gas permeable) lenses require wetting to reduce the foreign body sensation upon insertion. Natural saliva is an excellent wetting solution, but contains many potential pathogens and should never be used as a wetting agent.

Lubricating and rewetting drops are applied directly to relieve dry eyes when wearing a hard (PMMA and gas permeable) or soft lens. These solutions usually contain saline, preservatives and a viscosity

Table V *Wetting Agents*

Agent	Properties	Adverse effects
Polyvinyl alcohol (PVA)	Has some viscosity building effect and, unlike some viscosity agents (e.g., methylcellulose), does not retard regeneration of corneal epithelium.	All wetting agents are fairly inert, but they may slightly retard healing of the corneal epithelium.
	Some wetting solutions are adjusted to pH 5 to 6 since acetylated PVA can decompose in alkaline pH into polyvinyl alcohol and acetic acid which can irritate the eyes.	Allergic reactions to PVA have been reported.
Polyvinyl pyrrolidone (povidone)	Reduces the chemical binding characteristics of soft lenses without reducing antibacterial activity.	
	Wetting capacity is less than PVA.	
Adsorbobase povidone	Exact structure has not been released.	

agent for cushioning. In extended wear, they are also used as flushing agents before sleep and immediately upon awakening to remove debris accumulated under the lens. Most rewetting solutions designed for soft lenses are also compatible with hard (PMMA and gas permeable) lenses, but the reverse may not be true (see Table V).

Viscosity agents—large colloidal molecules—increase resistance to flow and are used to hold tears in the eyes. They produce a cushioning and lubricant effect between the lens and the eyelid and the lens and the cornea (see Table VI). They are not recommended in soaking solutions since they can retard diffusion of lens contaminants into the solution. They are not wetting agents, so they do not enhance the spread of tears over the cornea. The pH of lubricating solutions change after the expiration date and if used, may cause burning or stinging.

Multifunction Solutions

For hard lenses, the lens practitioner can recommend as many as 5 single-purpose products or as few as one all-purpose product. For convenience, numerous products combine two or more functions in a single solution. Controversy surrounds the extent of compromise of the primary functions, especially cleaning, with multifunctional solutions for hard lenses. About 80 per cent of the recommendations for hard (PMMA and gas permeable) lenses are for single-purpose solutions. The lesser use of multifunction solutions compared to single-purpose solutions is thought to be due to inadequate data and efficacy. Clinical evaluation of a nine-ingredient, all-purpose hard lens solution (clean, wet, disinfect, cushion and rewet) found consumers readily accepted the solution and it cleaned as well as single-purpose solutions. Comparative studies with single-purpose solutions in a clinical setting are required to substantiate this study.

With soft lenses, inattentive young people and elderly consumers often have difficulty with a regimen consisting of many solutions. Most noncompliance problems result from using several solutions in a certain sequence. User noncompliance (inadequate cleaning and

Table VI *Viscosity Agents*

Agent	Properties	Adverse effects
Methylcellulose (actually hydroxy-propyl methyl-cellulose in most solutions)	Viscosity range is 10 to 15,000 centipoises for 2% solutions.	Cellulose derivatives have few side effects, although granulation on the eyelids and conjunctiva is possible under dry conditions.
	Nonionic and therefore stable over a wide pH (2–12); at pH less than 2, viscosity decreases; temperatures greater than 50°C cause precipitation in water; nearly inert chemically and is entirely compatible with the drugs commonly used in the eye; will form complexes with most of the hydroxybenzoates; does not support growth of micro-organisms.	Corneal edema has been reported with methylcellulose instillation.
Ethylcellulose (actually hydroxy-ethylcellulose in most solutions)	Viscosity is not affected by pH changes between 5 and 10. Like methylcellulose, it is nonionic and water-soluble; unlike methylcellulose, it is not precipitated from water by an elevated temperature.	

Contact Lens Care

disinfection) caused about half the problems in a large study of soft lens wearers. Preliminary investigations with a multifunction solution for soft lenses have found improved compliance and good user acceptance. Multifunction soft lens care products are the fastest growing segment of the contact lens care market.

Multifunction solutions may be indicated where improved wearer compliance is the primary factor. For soft lenses, multifunction solutions can no longer be considered a compromise.

Hard Contact Lens Products
Preservatives (Antimicrobial Agents)

Benzalkonium and chlorobutanol are used in solutions for hard (PMMA and gas permeable) lenses only.

Benzalkonium chloride (BAC) probably changes the permeability of the cell membrane of the organism. It is effective against gram-negative and gram-positive bacteria. Most lens care solutions use concentrations of 0.004 to 0.01 per cent. Excessive concentrations may damage the corneal and conjunctival epithelium, but weak concentrations may be ineffective. Although a solution of 0.01 per cent is effective against resistant Pseudomonas strains of bacteria when given sufficient time, this concentration has low antibacterial activity. Other antibacterial agents, such as EDTA or chlorobutanol, are combined with BAC to produce a synergistic effect. BAC with EDTA is perhaps the best combination for hard contact lens solutions. BAC has surfactant properties and can also enhance transcorneal drug penetration.

PMMA does not carry a charge in water, so the ionic characteristics of solution components (such as BAC) are not important. It is absorbed by soft lenses which subsequently release BAC at concentrations sufficient to produce side effects. Due to BAC's ionic nature, numerous drug interactions are possible (for example, nitrate, salicylate, fluorescein solutions and some sulfonamides). The bactericidal activity decreases in the presence of cotton, methylcellulose, soaps, metallic ions and rubber. To maintain optimal activity, contact lens cases should be thoroughly rinsed of soap. Rubber ring case liners should be avoided.

Adverse reactions have been reported even with low concentrations. Although BAC can retard epithelial regeneration, most reactions (for example, epithelial damage or conjunctivitis) are superficial and reversible upon drug cessation.

Chlorobutanol above 0.35 per cent is bacteriostatic against fungi and gram-positive and gram-negative bacteria. It is bactericidal only when exposure exceeds 24 hours. It is effective only after it penetrates the bacterial cell, where it is converted to a lethal epitoxoid by the organism. It is incompatible with silicone lenses.

Chlorobutanol has no advantage over BAC. Due to its volatility, solutions exposed to air may fall below effective concentrations. It is synergistic with phenols and quaternaries, such as BAC, but requires a pH less than 6 or it breaks down to hydrochloric acid and other hydrocarbons. It does not appear to reduce the pharmacologic activity of other ophthalmic medications. It is concentrated in soft lenses and may cause a mild conjunctivitis. No allergic reactions with topical use have been reported.

Wetting Solutions

Wetting agents reduce surface interactions between tears and the contact lens or between tears and the cornea, allowing the tears to spread evenly. They generally contain large polymers that increase the tear flow over a hydrophobic lens surface and provide a brief cushion between the lens and cornea.

A hydrophobic hard (PMMA and gas permeable) lens must be wet to avoid discomfort and possible damage to the eyes. The mucin layer of the tear film contains highly hydrated polysaccharides that wet the lens but this deposition can take up to 15 minutes to develop, during which time the wearer experiences discomfort. A wetting and cushioning solution minimizes the transitional discomfort until the eyes adjust. The solution is applied to the concave side of the lens immediately before insertion.

The wetting solution serves other functions. It protects the lens surface with a viscous coating, thus avoiding direct contact with the finger during insertion. It lubricates the lid and lens surface, which cushions the lens on the cornea. It aids in lens cleaning after removal from the eye. It facilitates lens insertion by stabilizing the lens on the fingertips.

People who have surface drying of their contact lenses report blurry vision, lens dryness, scleral hyperemia and itching. Properties such as pH, osmolarity and wetting angle, are usually not included on the product label. Although irrelevant to the average wearer, these properties may be important for the atypical user with problems. When the three properties were evaluated with 10 hard lens solutions (most were for wetting), no two solutions had similar properties.

Examples of wetting agents found in hard contact lens solutions include polyvinyl alcohol, poloxamer 407 and polysorbate 80.

Accessory Solutions

The category of accessory solutions includes any combination of rewetting, lubricating and cushioning solutions. Solutions in this class have all three properties in varying degrees despite their label claims, but the clinical significance of these differences is not known.

An unusually dry environment such as one caused by air conditioning or central heating, may cause the eye or lens to dry out during wear. A few drops of rewetting solution placed in the eye every hour often relieves the discomfort.

A study of 8 solutions found that no two were alike in terms of viscosity, osmotic balance, acidity, buffering capacity and wetting angle. With such knowledge, the solution can be individualized to the wearer; certain viscosities may be more appropriate for the dry-eyed user versus the user with a thin watery tear; a more alkaline solution can be recommended for the acid-sensitive eye. The selection may be based on preservative content if the consumer is allergic to specific preservatives.

Artificial tears, also known as tear substitutes, moisturizing drops, lubricants and soothing agents, are recommended for wetting the surface of the eye once the lens is removed. They are not recommended for lubricating the lens while it is in the eye.

Cushioning agents provide an additional buffer layer between the lens, cornea and eyelid.

Tap water can no longer be recommended as a rinsing solution due to the increasing number of cases of Acanthamoeba keratitis in rigid lens wearers.

Soft Contact Lens Products

The hydrophilic nature of soft lens material requires extra attention to cleaning and disinfection. Compared to gas permeable and hard

(PMMA) lenses, soft lenses are more susceptible to protein deposits from tear film and also tend to concentrate ingredients from cosmetics and ophthalmic preparations more readily. Soft lenses are more comfortable for some people but have a higher associated risk of infection.

The care regimen for soft lenses is more complex than for hard lenses. Increased susceptibility to protein deposits require weekly use of an enzyme cleaner for most people. For disinfection, wearers can choose one of five chemical regimens or a thermal regimen. BAC and chlorobutanol should not be used in solutions for soft contact lenses because of adsorption by the HEMA polymer and subsequent rapid release, causing ocular tissue damage.

Enzymes

Most enzyme cleaners contain papain, pancreatin or subtilisin. Enzymes are used to remove protein deposits and prevent their buildup. Although little data exists on enzyme use, papain is protein specific and lipases are lipid specific. Pancreatin, a mixture of protease, lipase and amylase, is specific for protein, fats, phospholipids, starch and polysaccharides although each of these except protein can generally be removed by an effective surfactant. Enzymes catalyze the natural breakdown of debris into simple compounds, causing debris to become softer and easier to remove by mechanical action or rinsing. Since enzymes break down but do not remove protein molecules, the lens must be rubbed to effectively remove the broken down protein molecules. Enzymes cannot replace surfactants for cleaning efficiency. Furthermore, their action is slow, requiring 6 to 12 hours. However, regular use of even short soaking times can effectively prevent protein buildup. This is especially useful for high water lenses, which can take up enzyme into the lens matrix with prolonged soaking periods, sometimes resulting in irritation. Subtilisin has little capacity to bind to the lens and was thought to be safe for long soak times even with high-water content lenses. A comparison of subtilisin and pancreatin based cleaners using different soak times yielded no difference in efficacy or comfort. Longer soak times improved visual clarity but was more likely to cause discomfort. A comparison of papain, pancreatin and subtilisin found all enzyme cleaners to be effective but subtilisin soaked lenses were consistently the least deposited. Pancreatin has been found to significantly reduce the adherence of *Pseudomonas aeruginosa* to lenses.

The use of enzymes does not replace the need for daily surfactant cleaning, since nonprotein deposits are not removed. Since enzymes are specific, other debris mixed with or covering protein renders enzymes ineffective. A surfactant removes this nonprotein debris and enables the enzyme to exert its effect. Optimal lens cleaning, involves daily use of a surfactant followed by weekly treatment with an enzyme cleaner. Cleaning does not remove deposits completely. Without enzymes in the cleaning regimen, visual acuity can decrease. The build-up of protein may lead to allergic conjunctivitis as the protein acts as an antigen. It has also been demonstrated that *Pseudomonas aeruginosa* adheres more readily if a soft lens has a mucin or mucin and protein coating.

Papain is a protease (an enzyme that acts on proteins) obtained from the papaya plant. Cysteine is added as a stabilizer and reportedly aids in protein removal. Cysteine is responsible for the unpleasant odor associated with papain. Papain does not affect the lens matrix. It retards the formation of protein deposits and eases the removal of previously formed deposits. It may be more effective when used with heat disinfection since heat (40 to 60°C) denatures

protein more easily than chemical disinfection. Papain can then more readily attack the denatured protein. An enzyme cleaner added to a chemical disinfection regimen is more effective than chemical disinfection alone in preventing protein deposits. It also helps prolong lens life. Enzyme removal of protein is not the same as disinfection. Papain and pancreatin are equally effective at removing protein deposits after 24 hours although pancreatin appears to work faster.

Papain can adsorb onto HEMA lenses and cause burning, pain, photophobia, conjunctival hyperemia, punctate keratitis, corneal edema and conjunctival edema. Local ocular anaphylaxis has been reported. Thorough rinsing of the lens after enzyme cleaning is imperative. Pancreatin has been used successfully by people sensitive to papain but must also be rinsed thoroughly from the lens prior to application to prevent ocular irritation.

Pancreatin is derived from pork pancrease. It is a mixture of protease, lipase and amylase which catalyzes the breakdown of proteins, fats, phospholipids, starch and polysaccharides although each of these, except protein, can generally be removed by an effective surfactant.

Subtilisin is a protease derived from the Bacillus bacteria and is considered a GRAS (Generally Recognized As Safe) ingredient by the U.S. Food and Drug Administration. It is reported to have less specific binding characteristics and be capable of breaking more types of protein bonds than either papain or pancreatin.

Concern over potential adverse effects of enzymes prompted a comparison of chemical and thermal disinfection systems. Based on the ability to remove residual protease activity on soft lenses after enzyme cleaning, the thermal system was superior. For the few people who lack sufficient natural antiprotease activity, the thermal system can be used.

Protein begins accumulating from the first day of wear, even in users who may be asymptomatic. Eventually, these people may develop giant papillary conjunctivitis (GPC, an inflammation of the lining of the upper eyelid). The incidence of GPC can be reduced significantly by weekly enzymatic cleaning. If deposits are allowed to form, bacteria can adhere leading to ulcerative keratitis. Most lens practitioners recommend weekly prophylactic cleaning with enzymes. To ensure thorough cleaning, a second cleaning step is recommended (see Figure 1).

Chemical Disinfection Products

Chemical disinfection of soft lenses is similar to the soaking process for hard (PMMA and gas permeable) lenses, as the lenses are soaked (or stored), usually overnight, in a chemical disinfecting solution. Chemical disinfection with the appropriate solutions can be used for all soft contact lens materials. Unlike hard lens soaking solutions, disinfecting solutions for soft lenses must be rinsed off (with at least 25 mL of rinsing solution) except for some multifunction solutions before the lenses are inserted in the eyes. With hard lenses, saline solution or the disinfecting solution is used for rinsing. With all lenses, tap water is not recommended because of potential accumulation of minerals in the lens and possible contamination (for example, Acanthamoeba keratitis). Normal saline is generally used as the rinsing solution for soft lenses. Rinsing is also required after soft lens cleaning, before lens disinfection.

There are 5 chemical disinfection systems in Canada for soft contact lenses: chlorhexidine, thimerosal and an EDTA salt; alkyltriethanolammonium chloride (AKTAC), thimerosal and an EDTA salt; polyquaternium-1 (polyquad); polyaminopropylbiguanide;

Contact Lens Care

and hydrogen peroxide. Hydrogen peroxide systems must be inactivated after disinfection before the lens is worn. Sorbic acid (or potassium sorbate) combined with an EDTA salt is not a chemical disinfection system, but rather a soaking and rinsing system. Sorbic acid is gradually replacing thimerosal in these systems.

The advantages of chemical disinfectants are: ease of use (fewer products, fewer steps), greater compliance due to ease of use, lower overall cost, and no chance of forgetting to neutralize the disinfectant. Most literature on chemical disinfection concerns the first two systems. Although the hydrogen peroxide system is a chemical disinfection system, it is discussed separately and referred to by its active ingredient.

Failure rates for chemical disinfection vary from 0.63 per cent to 40.5 per cent. This wide range may be due to quality of user instruction, user selection or lens condition. Two major causes of the high rates of failure with chemical disinfection have been suggested: failure to rule out extremely fair-skinned, light-eyed users with a history of sensitivity to sun and chemicals, and improper and inadequate lens cleaning by the user. More than 95 per cent of wearers can successfully use chemical disinfection if wearers are carefully selected and instructed on the importance of thorough cleaning.

The disadvantages of chemical disinfection solutions are adverse effects from solution components, difficulty differentiating between changes produced by solutions and by lenses, and incompatibilities between chemical and thermal disinfection systems.

In addition to the preservatives for both hard (PMMA and gas permeable) and soft lenses, AKTAC and sorbic acid are used for soft lenses.

Alkyltriethanolammonium chloride (AKTAC, Quaternium 16) is a quaternary ammonium like BAC. Its antimicrobial effect outweighs its surfactant effect. Disinfection is slow but effective. It is not as effective against bacteria and fungi as chlorhexidine, and probably not effective against Acanthamoeba. A solution of 0.03 per cent alters the physical parameters of a soft lens minimally over a year, but these changes are reversible through saline soaking. Reactions similar to those of thimerosal can occur in 10 to 15 per cent of users.

In a clinical comparison of the chlorhexidine and thimerosal regimen and the AKTAC regimen, 53 soft lens wearers adapted to the former were changed to the latter. The AKTAC regimen was accepted by all but one wearer. The reasons for this finding were postulated to include differences in preservatives and increased compliance through prestudy indoctrination. In vitro bacteria testing found the chlorhexidine-based solution gave faster disinfection and more consistent results than the AKTAC-based solution.

Sorbic acid (or potassium sorbate) has limited antimicrobial activity, with weak activity against fungi and Acanthamoeba. It is most effective at a pH of 4 or less, which is enough to cause some ocular irritation. However, if the pH is raised even up to 6.5, sorbic acid loses its effectiveness as a preservative. Its use in soaking and wetting solutions may not be justified since the pH of these solutions is about 7. Preserved saline solutions containing sorbic acid are used only as a preservative. These solutions should not be used for disinfection.

Sorbic acid's fungistatic activity is increased by acids and sodium chloride; effective concentrations are 0.1 to 0.2 per cent. Concentration in HEMA lenses is minimal and it diffuses freely from the lens to the surrounding fluids. It is compatible with nonionic surfactants and is relatively nontoxic, although eye irritation and allergic dermatitis have been reported.

Sorbic acid combined with lens deposits have been implicated in lens discoloration. Lenses should not be stored in these solutions for more than 1 or 2 weeks because of discoloration (usually brownish). Minimizing the formation of deposits and following the recommendations of the lens practitioner minimizes lens discoloration. High water content lenses (55 per cent or greater), if heated with a sorbic acid system, yellow over time since they absorb significant amounts of protein, which react with heat. Gray-green discoloration has been reported when heat was used with a sorbic acid concentration greater than 0.15 per cent.

Two new disinfectants are **polyquaternium-1** and **polyaminopropylbiguanide**. The antimicrobial activities of 3 new nonperoxide soft contact lens disinfection systems: ReNu Multi-Purpose Solution (0.00005% polyaminopropyl biguanide); Opti-Soft Disinfecting Solution (0.001% polyquaternium-1); Opti-Free rinsing, disinfecting and storage solution (0.001% polyquaternium-1)) were compared to Soft Mate disinfecting solution (0.005% chlorhexidine digluconate) versus the organisms specified by the FDA for evaluating microbiological effectiveness of soft lens chemical disinfection solutions. All demonstrated excellent activity against *Pseudomonas aeruginosa* and *Staphylococcus epidermidis* with complete disinfection in 4 hours. Only Soft Mate disinfected *Serratia marcescens* and *Candida albicans* in 4 hours and reduced the spore count of *Aspergillis fumigatus*. The others reduced *Candida albicans* only slightly and had virtually no activity against *Aspergillis fumigatus*. Against *Serratia marcescens*, they were marginally effective. For newer chemical disinfection systems, diligent cleaning and rinsing are the most important steps. Polyaminopropylbiguanide and Polyquaternium-1 are less effective than thimerosal/chlorhexidine against Acanthamoeba cysts.

Oxidizing agents include peroxides (for example, hydrogen peroxide and sodium peroxide), peroxy salts (for example, sodium perborate) and chlorine-related compounds (for example, sodium hypochlorite). The only oxidizing agent used in Canada is hydrogen peroxide. Oxidizing agents are inherently unstable and, in the presence of organic debris, form free radicals that attack and disperse debris. The effervescence is a secondary means of removing debris from the lens matrix. They also act as germicides by releasing newly formed oxygen.

All oxidizing agents have a strong cleaning action independent of the nature of debris. However, all manufacturers who market hydrogen peroxide systems, recommend the use of daily cleaners and weekly enzyme cleaners. They do not affect the tint of soft lenses. Reports conflict on whether hydrogen peroxide damages lenses. Warping may result if hydrogen peroxide is used with gas permeable lenses. The safety of hydrogen peroxide systems relies entirely on adequate neutralization of the hydrogen peroxide. Neutralization methods include the use of a platinum catalyst, sodium pyruvate, catalase or rinsing and dilution. These systems are either "one step" where neutralization occurs automatically or "two step" where the consumer initiates neutralization after disinfection. Keratopathy, which developed in consumers using the one step catalytic neutralization, resolved when switched to a hydrogen peroxide system using a second catalase neutralization step. In a 4 week comparison of AOSept, Lensept, Oxysept and Consept, there were no pH changes after neutralization; Consept and Lensept were the closest to physiologic pH (7.4). A study of residual hydrogen peroxide (after neutralization) found Oxysept, Septicon, Mirasept and AOSept to have levels less than those associated with ocular discomfort. Although instillation of hydrogen peroxide (3 per cent) 3 times a day for 5 days produced no ocular damage, lenses should be thoroughly rinsed of hydrogen peroxide to prevent potential eye irritation. No permanent corneal damage due to hydrogen peroxide has been reported. However, insertion of a soft lens inadvertently stored in 3 per cent hydrogen peroxide produced an immediate, painful reaction that took 48 hours to clear. Exposure of the eyes to 3 per cent hydrogen peroxide from disinfection systems can result in stinging, tearing, hyperemia, blepharospasm, edema and possibly permanent corneal damage. No adverse effects have been observed with ocular hydrogen peroxide levels that would occur from the routine proper use of hydrogen peroxide systems. Cleaning the lens with a surfactant followed by thorough rinsing and a 2 to 3 hour soak in 3 per cent hydrogen peroxide disinfects the lens. This time is required to eradicate Acanthamoeba which is well within the recommendation of a 6 hour disinfection with AOSept. Other systems recommend disinfection times of 10 to 20 minutes. However, the addition of a cleaner to the care regimen reduces the number of cysts to which the disinfectant is exposed. Fungi require 1 to 2 hours. Oxidizing agents destroy pigments and remove color from the lens. When the pigment is oxidized and soluble, small voids remain in the lens matrix, resulting in a spongy layer at the site of pigment deposition. Oxidizing agents work most efficiently when combined with heat.

Hydrogen peroxide (3 per cent) was introduced in 1972 as the first method of chemical disinfection, but the procedure was complicated, time-consuming and prone to errors. Problems were eliminated, and newer products have simplified the regimen by decreasing the neutralization time and the disinfection time. A prolonged (6 hour) neutralization may be necessary in consumers who develop keratopathy from residual peroxide of a shorter neutralization. A neutralization time as short as 10 minutes has been effectively used. Due to problems with preserved solutions, hydrogen peroxide became the most popular chemical disinfection system. However, this segment is declining with the introduction of newer chemical disinfection systems.

Generic hydrogen peroxide is not recommended, as it is designed for topical use and meets less strict standards than ophthalmic hydrogen peroxide. Some generic hydrogen peroxide contains impurities, stabilizers or other additives that irritate ocular tissue or discolor the lenses.

Allergic Reactions

There was initial concern that retaining preservatives in the eye might eliminate normal ocular flora, leading to sterile eyes or superinfection. However, a 6 month study showed normal bacterial flora is maintained. The incidence of allergic reactions to soft lenses increased in the early 1970s when saline and cleaning solutions preserved with thimerosal were introduced. Although the concentration was similar in many brands of saline, users reported subjective differences, suggesting that buffers and pH differences were responsible.

Agreement is lacking on the proportion of chemical disinfection users who develop a sufficiently severe eye reaction to warrant cessation of the regimen. Depending on the study, the incidence ranges from 0.5 to 73 per cent although 5 to 10 per cent appears to be the most frequent estimate. Some reports do not rule out the possibility of a reaction to chlorhexidine, EDTA or sorbic acid.

Since chlorhexidine is not as widely used as thimerosal and since it attains a lower concentration in the tear film, delayed hypersensitivity reactions may be less likely. However, a diagnostic study found

a higher incidence of corneal staining (a measure of ocular damage) with a solution of chlorhexidine and thimerosal than with thimerosal alone. A subsequent clinical study found a solution intolerance rate of 33 per cent in those using chlorhexidine plus thimerosal compared to 5 to 8 per cent in those using thimerosal based solutions. A family history of allergy was not significant. Due to patient sensitivities to thimerosal and chlorhexidine, most solutions no longer are formulated to contain these compounds.

Nonallergic reactions are possible since many components can act as primary irritants. Contact lens solution components are unlikely to provoke an allergic response directly due to their small molecular size. These components can act as haptens or incomplete antigens, which bind to body proteins to form complexes that stimulate an immune reaction against the component. An allergic response is facilitated by large amounts of antigen and the antigen persisting at the reaction site. Daily use of lenses stored in an allergy-causing solution provides ideal conditions for the continuous availability of antigen to produce an allergic reaction in susceptible users, especially if a protein coating increases the amount of antigen bound to the lens.

The terms "allergy" and "sensitivity" are used loosely. An eye allergy normally involves noticeable irritation with excess physiological fluids. "Sensitivity" usually refers to the development of a physiological reaction to one or more ingredients in a formulation and usually does not include irritation. Unfortunately, the two terms are often used interchangeably in the literature.

An adverse ocular response due to allergy or toxicity encompasses a wide range of signs and symptoms. Since redness is usually present, the reaction has been called "red eye" or the red eye syndrome. Other symptoms include discomfort on lens insertion, decreased wearing time, stinging, burning, dryness, itching, irritation, tearing, discharge, swelling, blurring and nasal fullness. Signs include conjunctival hyperemia and edema, papillary follicular hypertrophy, corneal edema, pseudocysts, fluorescein or rose bengal staining, sloughed epithelial cells, limbal follicles, and ulceration and infiltrates. Tears may be excessive or may develop excess mucus secretion and present with excessive lipid-contaminated mucus threads. The lids may become swollen, and, in extreme cases, the facial derma may be affected. Corneal opacities have been reported with the use of some preserved saline.

An allergic reaction to solution components, particularly preservatives, may take days to months to develop before the onset of keratoconjunctivitis. Users who experience a reaction soon after exposure to a solution may have had a pre-existing but unrecognized sensitivity. In other wearers, sensitization or toxicity may have occurred after repeated application of exposed soft lenses to the cornea. Factors which increase the risk of developing an allergy include: allergy to intravenous pyelogram (IVP) dyes or povidone iodine, pencillin allergy, diabetic relatives, concurrent tetracycline treatment. It has been postulated that tetracycline chelates the mercury in thimerosal, precipitating the response. Discontinuing the tetracycline or the thimerosal-containing solution has cleared the reaction.

If sensitivity is suspected, the lenses and solution can be removed, allowing the eyes to return to normal. A few drops of solution containing the suspected ingredient can be instilled in the wearer's eyes. An immediate and general red eye appearance generally indicates a sensitivity reaction.

The easiest and possibly the best way to predict which consumers may react to preservatives is to take a careful history. People with a history of atopic problems tend to have more severe reactions than other users.

Lens practitioners who have witnessed adverse reactions agree that numerous reactions are due to noncompliance. However, absolute compliance may not be possible or may be too unrealistic. For non-compliant users, the best choice is a system that is difficult to use improperly.

In addition to user noncompliance, numerous other causes of adverse reactions have been postulated. These causes include the types, combinations or concentrations of preservatives, the chemical changes in residual chemicals left on lenses from thermal disinfection, cross-usage of systems in going from thermal to chemical disinfection (denatured proteins adsorb chemicals, which then become severe irritants), poor fit, defective lenses, extraneous lens deposits, environmental factors, sensitivities, allergies, incomplete care regimen, and solution-related and bacterial problems.

Allergic reactions are best treated by removing the source of antigen. A mild response may be resolved by rinsing lenses well before insertion, using more thorough surfactant cleaning techniques, rinsing the lenses well after surfactant cleaning and soaking the lenses for 5 minutes in saline before insertion.

If these procedures fail, a multipurge procedure must be performed to remove surface deposits or chemicals. An alternative system can be initiated using different chemical disinfectants and preservatives or a thermal nonpreserved system. If symptoms persist, a lens reaction should be considered.

Thermal Disinfection

Thermal disinfection uses an elevated temperature to kill heat-sensitive microorganisms. It is probably the strongest disinfecting system available. Only heat has shown to be completely effective against Acanthamoeba cysts. It applies only to soft and pure silicone lenses as other lens types cannot withstand the temperatures required. Thermal disinfection is nonspecific and works by gross protein denaturation of microorganisms. The lenses are placed in a specially designed case, which is then filled with isotonic saline and placed in a heating unit. Most units heat the lenses to $80\,^\circ C$ for 10 minutes before automatically shutting off. This time and temperature kills bacteria and fungi of potential hazard to the eye (such as *Pseudomonas aeruginosa, Staphylococcus aureus, Escherichia coli, Candida albicans,* and *Aspergillus niger*) and the cyst of Acanthamoeba. Sterilization requires $120\,^\circ C$ for 15 minutes and 103.43 kilopascals. Since the lenses are disinfected rather than sterilized, spores can germinate if the lenses are stored for a prolonged period. The lenses should be disinfected before wearing after prolonged storage. Saline intended for thermal disinfection should not contain chlorhexidine, since lenses stored in such solutions become opaque after a few boiling cycles. Thermal disinfection is not used with high water content lenses (55 per cent or greater) as this system may discolor lenses and reduce performance. The cause is unknown.

Numerous disadvantages of thermal disinfection have been cited. The initial cost of purchase is relatively high although the yearly cost is the lowest among all systems. Microorganisms can accumulate if the procedure is not performed daily and if fresh saline is not prepared daily. If heating is not performed daily to destroy vegetative forms of the bacteria, spores may survive to cause lens damage. Repeated heating may decrease lens life. It has been suggested that the lens loss rate doubles from chips, rips and cracks, but in one

study, no adverse effects occurred for 30 months from thermal disinfection. Microorganisms on the lens surface may cause lens discomfort, loss of transparency, loss of acuity, lens discoloration, conjunctival hyperemia, change in lens fitting and reduced lens porosity. If microproteins and surfactants are not adequately removed, they are baked onto the lens, decreasing lens life. With proper cleaning, the lens life with hydrogen peroxide and thermal disinfection is similar. Regular omission of cleaning before heating causes deposits to build up, decreasing visual acuity and creating discomfort. Multiple reuse of thimerosal-containing solutions with heat disinfection, may result in gray-black mercurial deposits on the lens. Usually, these deposits are first found in the lens case.

Thermal disinfection is inconvenient and likely to be neglected; electricity is required, and saline problems and mechanical failure can occur. Due to these potential problems, chemical disinfection is preferred by most wearers. Newer heat disinfection units are small, lightweight, cordless and accept various power requirements. Although popularity has dropped for these systems, thermal disinfection is still as effective as any other system.

Microwave sterilization of soft lenses has been effective but one study using a domestic microwave found a lack of effect. Efficacy against Acanthamoeba is unknown. Contact lens disinfection using ultraviolet light appears to be effective but requires further investigation.

Saline is available in two forms: preserved saline solutions and unit-dose or multi-dose unpreserved saline. Salt tablets are no longer marketed by any manufacturer in Canada.

Preserved saline minimizes the risk of contamination during repeated use. Also, the correct concentration of salt is controlled by the manufacturer. The cost is significantly higher than that of salt tablets, but safety and convenience are greater. Unfortunately, many users of preserved saline develop preservative sensitivity. The introduction of sorbic acid and polyaminopropylbiguanide preserved saline should decrease the incidence of sensitivity reactions. The introduction of thimerosal-free saline in a 120 mL unit dose size or a multi-dose aerosol form should also help overcome potential sensitivity reactions. Aerosol and other salines should be buffered to ensure that pH stays within the ocular comfort range.

Unpreserved unit dose saline overcomes potential mixing errors by the user and potential sensitivity reactions, but microbial contamination can occur if the solution stands for longer than the recommended time or if used improperly. However, multi-dose aerosol preserved saline is equally effective in preventing sensitivity reactions and remains sterile for the life of the product. The solution is maintained in a sterile environment because of the aerosol mechanism at the top of the can. Before each use, a small amount of saline should be dispensed. The saline inside the mechanism is open to the outside environment and may be contaminated. It should be dispensed before use.

A consumer developed a *Pseudomonas aeruginosa* corneal ulcer after an aerosol can, minus its cap, was stored during a trip in a washbag containing a wet face cloth.

Table VII summarizes chemical and thermal disinfection regimens. Protein films are more of a problem with thermally disinfected lenses; inorganic deposits are more frequent in chemically disinfected lenses. However, any enzyme cleaner minimizes the potential build-up of protein deposits. A switch to chemical disinfection may be valuable for consumers with problems of pigment deposits, mercurial deposits, rust deposits or microbial growth.

Table VII *Pros and Cons of Chemical and Thermal Disinfection of Soft Contact Lenses*

Factor	Chemical	Thermal
Efficacy	High	High
Convenience	High	Moderate
Restrictions on type of lens	No	No
Special apparatus and power required	No	Yes
Cost	Cheaper initially	May be cheaper eventually
Lens life	about 2.5 yr	about 1 yr
Time required	6–8 hr	about 1 hr
Debris build-up	Low to moderate	High
Compliance	Similar	Similar
Acceptability	High (85%)	High (95%)
Extended wear lenses	Tolerated better	Not tolerated well

Studies comparing the incidence of eye reactions with both methods vary from almost no irritation to a high incidence of sensitivity reactions. One study found that consumers developed more problems using chemical disinfection. In a 6 month crossover study, the chemical method produced significantly more burning, mucous protein, tiring, itching, pain, redness, watering, drying and discontinued lens wear than the thermal method. Despite the findings, the authors recommend chemical disinfection for consumers with frequent and excessive mucous protein build-up on their lenses and for those who prefer the convenience of chemical disinfection. Another study found a similar incidence of intolerance (4 per cent for chemical and 3 per cent for thermal). Due to conflicting studies and the introduction of newer disinfectants, lens practitioners should study their own practices.

There are similar and distinguishable features to allergic reactions from both forms of disinfection. Symptoms associated with chemical disinfection solutions include sting on insertion, constant low-level irritation and loss of lens tolerance (for example, since changing brands of solution). With thermal disinfection, the following symptoms may indicate an allergic response, especially if the symptoms started or worsened since the wearer stopped using an enzyme protein remover: mild itch on lens removal, increased lens awareness and blur after several hours wear, and decreased wearing time, sometimes with total loss of tolerance.

Very few consumers use heat disinfection. Almost all new patients use a chemical regimen. The advantages and disadvantages of each should be explained to the consumer. A careless person may be a better candidate for thermal disinfection since most of the work is done by the heat; however, deposits or solutions may be baked into the lens. Sloppy technique with chemical disinfection often produces problems. Statistics from a 1984 study indicate a 10 to 1 preference for chemical disinfection.

Consumer and lens practitioner preference for the chemical system may favor compliance with this regimen. However, one large study with 354 problem users found a similar noncompliance with each of the systems: 13.8 per cent for chemical and 14.7 per cent for thermal. The following problems were observed: dirty lenses and cases; soaking solution not changed; and fresh solution added to remnants of used solution. The last practice produces a more concentrated solution and precipitation of crystals on the lens surface.

Switching Disinfection Systems

If the chemical system is used first, switching to the thermal system may make lenses useless after the first boiling. Unless recommended by the manufacturer, rinsing and soaking solutions used for chemical disinfection must not be used for thermal disinfection. Lenses heated in such solutions can change shape and may turn white or opaque. This problem can be prevented by first purging the lens with thorough cleaning and repeated boiling in unpreserved saline.

Switching from the thermal to the chemical system has no harmful effects on the lenses if they are free of all protein deposits. Otherwise, preservatives can concentrate in these deposits and cause irritation and discomfort.

Wearers using thermal disinfection may wish to use a chemical method when away from home. This temporary switch is possible if the wearer has never reacted to components of the proposed chemical regimen. All solutions must be removed from the lens before the user returns to the thermal method. The lens should be cleaned with a surfactant. Chemicals can be removed by allowing the lens to remain for at least 24 hours in a preserved or nonpreserved (for example, unit dose) saline solution designed for the thermal method. After soaking, the lens is thoroughly rinsed before thermal disinfection.

Rewetting Solutions

Soft contact lenses are hydrophilic and do not require a wetting solution to adapt to the eye. However, they do tend to dry out through the day, especially in a dry or polluted environment. As many as 75 per cent of soft lens wearers experience this symptom. Rewetting solutions, artificial tears preserved with chemicals compatible with soft lenses, rehydrate the lens and the eye while the lens is worn. Other artificial tears should not be used for rewetting soft contact lenses since most contain preservatives (for example, BAC) that are incompatible with soft lenses. If they are used, the wearer should limit usage to a drop every 4 to 5 hours. If drops are used more frequently, the user may develop red, irritated eyes and a foreign body sensation.

One or more of the following can contribute to dry eye symptoms: diuretics, hormones (for example, oral contraceptives) and lack of adequate tearing due to age, certain illnesses, air conditioning or low humidity. Use of dilute saline (0.38 or 0.48 per cent) as a rinsing and soaking solution helps decrease discomfort from dry eyes. The water content of soft lenses decreases with wear, but this procedure restores the water content and prevents dryness. A 1 per cent sterile solution of saline lasts 3 hours as a rewetting and lubricating solution for people with lens surface dehydration. On average, commercially available solutions last less than 3 to 5 minutes. No one product is consistently superior to any other although nonpreserved solutions generally yield the higher comfort scores. In addition, lubricants have not been found to be significantly superior to saline.

Rewetting solutions can be used several times daily to relieve discomfort due to dehydration and partly to clean the lens. If the rewetting period is too short, the lenses may have to be removed once

Contact Lens Care

daily for surfactant cleaning and saline rinsing to increase lens wettability.

Mixing Solutions

Solutions from different manufacturers should not be used unless recommended by a lens practitioner. Manufacturers formulate each component solution of a care regimen to be compatible with each of the other components. Preclinical and ongoing research ensures their compatibility and efficacy. The effect of substituting even one solution from a different manufacturer is not predictable even if it has the same active ingredients in the same concentration. About the only solution that can be substituted by the consumer is aerosol saline.

Mixing solutions from different manufacturers is hazardous due to the proliferation of lens care products and contact lens materials. In the never ending quest to improve comfort and wear time, researchers experimented with newer and more complex lens polymers. This diversity of materials with their own individual cleaning and disinfecting requirements has stimulated solution manufacturers to become more specific in the design of solutions. If the wrong solution got into a lens that required specific solutions, the lens could be ruined.

Contact Lenses and Drugs

Oral Contraceptives

Lens intolerance has been associated with the use of oral contraceptives, but the effect appears to vary. Well-fitted users may experience fewer complications than poorly or newly fitted users. Oral contraceptives may produce two effects. One, the fluid-retaining properties of the estrogen are thought to produce corneal and lid swelling, which increase the wearer's awareness of and sensitivity to the lenses resulting in reduced wearing time, decreased visual acuity and photophobia. Two, altered tear composition may decrease the lubricating ability of tears. A sticky mucus can deposit on the lens and produce allergic conjunctivitis and uncomfortable blurry vision.

After about 3 months of oral contraceptives, a new body chemistry equilibrium is attained. Body chemistry also takes approximately 3 months to return to normal after oral contraceptives are discontinued. Reducing the wearing time for the first 3 months and cleaning the lens thoroughly may be adequate for a successful transition to or from oral contraceptives. If these measures are inadequate, the lens may have to be modified or refitted. If this is not acceptable, lens wear may have to stop until the oral contraceptive is discontinued.

Changes in brand or strength of oral contraceptive can produce further complications. Pregnancy produces the same effects as oral contraceptives.

Ophthalmics

Contact lenses attract many users with conditions other than myopia. The contact lens population includes older users with aphakia and those requiring bandage lenses for therapeutic purposes. Both groups are likely using local or systemic medications.

Dark discoloration of soft lenses has occurred with repeated use of phenylephrine, adrenaline or tetrahydrozoline, and other readily oxidizable adrenergic-containing solutions while the lens is in the eye. Diagnostic solutions containing fluorescein or rose bengal are contraindicated for wearers of soft lenses since these dyes can concentrate in the lens. Yellow-green fluorescein stains may be found on lenses if the lens is put into the eye too soon after eye examinations. These discolorations can be removed in the laboratory by heating the lens for 2 to 3 hours in 200 to 300 mL of distilled water or in a 1 per cent solution of sodium bicarbonate USP.

Drugs administered locally during contact lens wear can affect tear composition, pharmacologic responses to drugs and the lenses themselves. A lens practitioner will instruct the wearer if any local medication is to be used with lens wear. An in vitro study found that common topical ophthalmic medications did not damage a soft lens. Contact lens wearers usually report initial discomfort upon the instillation of local drugs not related to contact lens wear. The response may be due to a pre-existing corneal metabolic insult and edema directly associated with contact lens wear. The comfort and successful function of contact lenses is dependent on normal tear dynamics. Most local medication not specifically formulated for use with contact lenses affects tear dynamics. Fortunately, the effect lasts less than 10 minutes after administration.

With soft lenses, the effects of local drugs are exaggerated because the lens can increase the contact time of the medication. Absorption and concentration can occur with subsequent gradual release over a prolonged period. (This property is used to therapeutic advantage with pilocarpine in treating glaucoma.) Increased drug absorption may occur due to the compromised cornea in contact lens wearers.

The nature of the formulation can affect comfort and lens wearability. Clear solutions cause the least number of effects; suspensions can cause discomfort and lens intolerance. Inherently hypertonic solutions (for example, sodium sulfacetamide 10 per cent or pilocarpine hydrochloride 10 per cent) can cause soft lens dehydration and a change in lens shape, producing temporary discomfort. Higher water content lenses are more susceptible to this effect.

Temporary lens intolerance and decreased visual acuity can occur with solutions buffered at pH values far from the ideal of 7.4. Abnormally acidic pH can promote lens dehydration and lens steepening; abnormally basic pH has the opposite effect of promoting lens hydration and lens flattening.

Nonprescription products for the eye (for example, eye washes) should not be used without consulting the lens practitioner. Ingredients in such products may not be compatible with contact lens solutions. Such incompatibilities may be noted on the labels of eye care products. A case of film formation on lenses has been reported with an eye wash that displayed such a warning.

Acne medications that contain benzoyl peroxide can cause tinted soft lenses to fade.

Systemic Medications

A good hard-lens fit depends on the constant supply of oxygen from fresh tears moving under the lens with each blink. With soft lenses, blinking is required to maintain proper lens hydration. If a previously well-fitting hard or soft lens produces irritation and redness, the blink should be investigated. Sedatives, hypnotics and antihistamines can decrease the blink rate in susceptible people. Muscle relaxants have been reported to cause droopy eyelids. This effect may lead to incomplete blinking, which can cause wear problems.

Decreased tear volume can contribute to corneal drying in hard lens wearers and to annoying irritation and tenacious lens deposits

Contact Lens Care

Figure 2 *Suggested Approach for Questioning Contact Lens Wearers*

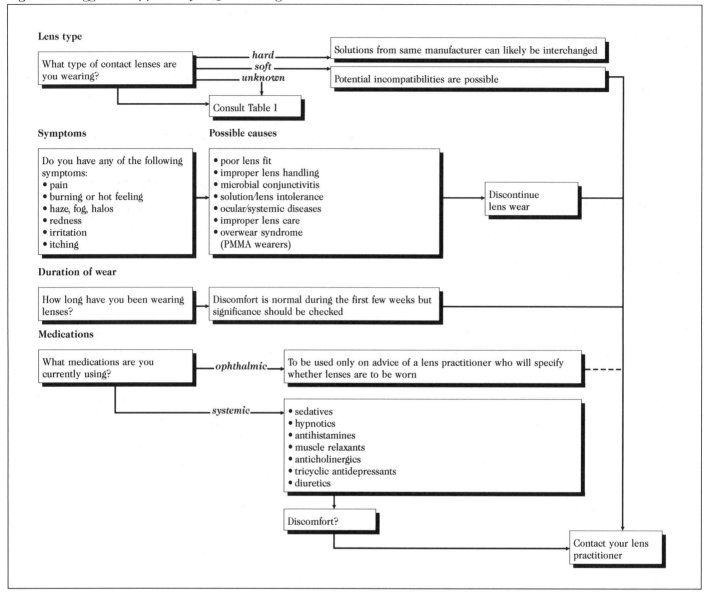

in soft lens wearers. Antihistamines, anticholinergics, tricyclic antidepressants and diuretics have been reported to decrease tear volume. Amitriptyline has produced eye irritation and blurred vision in a soft contact lens wearer. Maprotiline has caused eye irritation within 1 week after contact lenses were initiated. Darvocet-N100 (propoxyphene napsylate 100 mg and acetaminophen 650 mg) has produced soft lens adherence. Isotretinoin has produced itching and a decreased wear time within 3 days of initiating soft lenses. In the maprotiline and isotretinoin cases, initiating contact lens wear may have caused the symptoms. Salicylic acid appears in tears after oral acetylsalicylic acid administration. Salicyclic acid may be absorbed by soft lenses, resulting in an increased incidence of unexplained ocular irritation and redness in acetylsalicylic acid users.

Rifampin may cause soft contact lenses to turn orange. Although the effect varies, it might be advisable for rifampin users not to wear soft contact lenses while taking the drug. Other drugs excreted into tears and reported to discolor soft lenses include phenazopyridine, tetracycline, phenolphthalein and nitrofurantoin and sulfasalazine.

Smoking

Smokers have a higher incidence of pigmented soft lenses than non-smokers, likely from stimulation of melanin production by nicotine and other aromatic compounds present in cigarette smoke. Initially, pigmentation has little effect on visual acuity, but eventually, the deposits cause the lens to become less flexible, deforming the lens and giving it a leathery texture. For heavy smokers, chemical disinfection may have to be advocated. The user should be counselled about the potential for lens spoilage.

Finger- or smoke-transferred nicotine can reduce the physical and sometimes optical clarity of lenses. Smokers should thoroughly clean their hands before handling contact lenses. They are advised to use

Contact Lens Care

Figure 2 *(Cont'd)   Suggested Approach for Questioning Contact Lens Wearers*

Soft lens care regimen

If you wear soft lenses, what method of disinfection has your lens practitioner recommended?

chemical →
- chlorhexidine, thimerosal, EDTA salt
- alkyltriethanolamine, thimerosal, EDTA salt
- sorbic acid, EDTA salt
- polyquaternium-1
- polyaminopropylbiguanide
- hydrogen peroxide

thermal → Heating unit plus specific solutions

Product use

What products do you use for the care of your lenses?

known →
- Recommended by lens practitioner
- Not recommended by lens practitioner

unknown →

Describe how you use your lens care products →
- inadequate cleaning/inadequate disinfection
- economizing
- proper function of heating unit

Dropped lens

What would you do if you dropped your lens on the floor?

soft → Rinse with rinsing solution

Contact your lens practitioner

the third or least nicotine-stained finger and the palm of the other hand for lens cleaning and rinsing.

In a comparison of papain and an oxidizing agent on simulated nicotine and tobacco extract-stained lenses, papain was ineffective, but the oxidizing agent removed all discoloration.

Compliance

Noncompliance is the greatest threat to eye comfort and lens life. It has been suggested that more than 50 per cent of adverse reactions are due to noncompliance such as inadequate cleaning or inadequate rinsing before chemical or thermal disinfection. Economizing by using old solutions was the most common form of noncompliance in one practice. Noncompliance can lead to corneal infection which likely starts from the inoculation of a pathogenic microorganism. Lens solution contamination, inadequate lens disinfection, manipulation of the lens in the eye and poor hygiene all increase the exposure of the eye to pathogens. Storage solutions are often implicated as the source of infection as cultures from the eye and solution yield the same pathogen. The source of Acanthamoeba keratitis appears to be homemade saline or tap water used for rinsing lenses. It has been documented through epidemiologic studies that poor compliance with the care regimen increases the risk of this infection. In a recent compliance study of daily wear, a 40 per cent noncompliance rate was found which was more frequent in the 10 to 30 age group, greater than 50 age group and in those consumers

wearing lenses for more than 2 years. It was also noted that noncompliance was more common in those consumers who were not indoctrinated by the researchers. Compliance was defined as: hand washing before lens handling, correct use of an approved (FDA) care system and adherence to a recommended wear schedule. Another study found a 46 per cent noncompliance rate. Age under 30 and wearing lenses for convenience or cosmetic reasons were the two factors statistically associated with noncompliance.

It has been suggested that public awareness of the infectious complications of contact lenses has improved compliance with care regimens contributing to a decrease in Acanthamoeba keratitis since 1987. A compliance study of 100 patients found a 74 per cent noncompliance rate. Noncompliance was strongly related to signs and symptoms indicative of potential wearing problems.

Recommendations

The most important recommendations concerning the care of contact lenses are as follows:
- Follow exactly the care regimen prescribed for you.
- Follow exactly the directions for using contact lens care solutions.
- If you suspect problems or have questions, contact your lens practitioner.

The following recommendations apply to both hard and soft lenses:
- Each solution is formulated for a special purpose. Use hard lens

Contact Lens Care

solutions for hard lenses only, and soft lens solutions for soft lenses only. Never use chemical disinfection solutions for thermal disinfection.

- Thoroughly wash and dry your hands before handling your lenses. Debris on your hands can be transferred to your lenses.
- Keep your fingernails short to prevent tearing and scratching of your lenses.
- If you remove lenses over a sink, close or cover the drain to prevent possible lens loss.
- Do not wear lenses while swimming since they may wash out. In addition, soft lenses can "stick to the eye" due to the hypertonicity of swimming pool water.
- Wear protective eyegear if you participate in contact sports. Only extended wear contact lenses can be worn while sleeping.
- Do not wear lenses if your eyes are red or irritated.
- Do not use any household products—such as detergents, soaps, shampoos, skin cleansers or toothpaste—to clean your lenses.
- Do not use solutions from different manufacturers, since the solutions may not be compatible with each other.
- Do not use contact lens products beyond their expiry date.
- Keep all contact lens products out of the reach of children.
- Thoroughly rinse off cleaners or disinfectants before inserting the lens into the eye. Residues can produce adverse effects on the eye and lens.
- If you wear your lenses under a hair dryer, blink your eyes frequently and remove the lenses for cleaning if they become uncomfortable. Mucus and tears dry and harden on the lenses due to the hot air.
- Change disinfecting (soaking) solutions daily.
- Thoroughly clean and rinse the contact lens case daily.
- Daily wear lenses should not be overworn.
- Extended wear lenses should be removed overnight at least once every 7 days.
- If wearing daily wear lenses, visit your lens practitioner at least once every 6 months.
- If wearing extended wear lenses, visit your lens practitioner at least once every 2 to 3 months.

The following recommendations apply to contact lens users who wear cosmetics:

- Use a good quality mascara that does not flake off. Problems occur from mascara on or underneath lenses.
- Warn your cosmetologist that you wear contact lenses.
- Never share eye cosmetics; another person's bacteria may be dangerous to your eyes.
- If the fumes from hair dyes and bleaches cause your eyes to water, try another brand. Well-known companies wanting to maintain their reputation are more likely to have superior products due to thorough testing.
- Spray deodorants and hairsprays can irritate your eyes. Particles accumulating on your lenses may cause discomfort, and lens replacement may be necessary. Protect your lenses by closing your eyes when you spray, and walking away from the area.
- You can prevent smearing of eye makeup if lens removal is necessary by tilting your head to one side after reinsertion of your lenses. Tears then run to the side of the eye.
- Before handling lenses, scrub your hands and fingers thoroughly to remove all cosmetics, including nail polish, nail polish remover, perfumes, colognes, lotions and suntan oil.

Specific recommendations for hard lenses include:

- Never rub your eyes when lenses are in place.
- Do not rinse your lenses under hot water because warping can occur, especially in gas permeable lenses.
- Never use saliva to wet your lenses. Saliva contains bacteria that can cause an eye infection.
- Never rinse with tap water after your lenses have been cleaned or disinfected.

Specific recommendations for soft lenses include:

- Rinse your hands thoroughly after washing them. Soap residues can bind to soft lenses.
- Change boiling solutions regularly.
- Commercially preserved solutions should be discarded within 2 months.
- Do not use discoloured enzyme products.
- If you wish to change solutions, contact your lens practitioner.
- Remove your lenses before applying ophthalmic preparations. Do not reinsert your lenses for at least 1 hour unless otherwise instructed by your lens practitioner.
- When storing, carefully centre the lenses in the case and close lid tightly.
- Do not mix chemical and heat methods of disinfection.
- If your lens dries out, moisten with saline and place in its case for 1 hour.
- If your lenses become stuck, moisten with saline or daily cleaner before sliding them apart.
- If a lens tears, save the pieces as the lens practitioner will want to ensure none of the pieces have become lodged in your eye. Some companies may replace torn lenses.
- If you fall asleep with your lenses on, moisten them with lubricating drops before removing them.
- Wait 1 hour before reinserting your lenses if you have been swimming.
- Soft lenses exposed to contaminated saline or water should be thermally disinfected as current chemical disinfection solutions are ineffective against Acanthamoeba.

Ask the Consumer

Q. What type of contact lenses are you wearing?

- The lens type (hard or soft) determines the care regimen. Solutions for hard lenses from the same manufacturer can likely be interchanged. Solutions for both hard and soft lenses from a manufacturer other than the one who produced the lens may be incompatible. Consult a lens practitioner (optician, optometrist or ophthalmologist). If the person gives a lens trade name, the type of lens can be determined from Table II.

Q. Do you have any of the following symptoms: pain when inserting or wearing the lenses or after wearing them; burning that causes excessive tearing; inability to keep your eyes open; severe or persistent haze, fog or halos while wearing the lenses; redness, irritation or itching?

- These symptoms may be due to poor lens fit, damaged lenses, improper handling, microbial conjunctivitis, solution or lens intolerance, ocular or systemic disease, or improper lens care. Painful lid swelling and photophobia may be due to overwear. If

Contact Lens Care

any of these symptoms occur in a lens wearer, the person should discontinue lens wear and contact a lens practitioner.

Q. How long have you worn lenses?

■ Every contact lens wearer experiences discomfort during the first few weeks while the eyes adapt to the lenses. Since it may not be obvious at first which problems are significant, the consumer should call the lens practitioner.

Q. What medication are you using?

■ Any ophthalmic preparation should be used only on the advice of a lens practitioner who specifies if the medication is used while the lens is in place. Concurrent use of soft lenses and ophthalmic preparations can produce a reservoir effect. Other drugs, such as phenylephrine, adrenaline and tetrahydrozoline, can discolor soft lenses. Products may not be compatible with contact-lens-solution ingredients. Almost all ophthalmic preparations not specifically designed for contact lens use cause temporary discomfort. Numerous systemic medications may alter eye dynamics sufficiently to warrant therapeutic intervention. Sedatives (including alcohol), hypnotics, antihistamines and muscle relaxants can affect the eyelid, producing incomplete blinking or a decreased rate of blinking. Antihistamines, anticholinergics, tricyclic antidepressants and diuretics can decrease tear volume, leading to significant discomfort associated with contact lens wear.

Q. If you wear soft lenses, what method of disinfection did your lens practitioner recommend?

■ A chemical regimen uses one of five systems: chlorhexidine, thimerosal and an EDTA salt; polyquad; polyaminopropylbiquanide; AKTAC, thimerosal and an EDTA salt; and hydrogen peroxide. A thermal regimen uses a heating unit and saline in which the lenses are heated. Knowledge of the disinfection method makes it possible to reinforce the instructions of the lens practitioner and prevent wearers from using solutions not designed for their method of disinfection. Chemical disinfecting solutions sometimes cannot be used for thermal disinfection. If such a solution is repeatedly used for thermal disinfection, the lenses can become white or opaque. Counsel the wearer to follow specific product recommendations. Hydrogen peroxide disinfection requires two steps: disinfection with hydrogen peroxide 3 per cent; and neutralization. Most manufacturers identify the neutralizing solution with a predominantly green or blue package.

Q. What products do you use for the care of your lenses?

■ The lens practitioner recommended specific products for the lenses. The pharmacist can determine and correct inappropriate substitution of products. Refer the consumer to the lens practitioner if any products are not known or if confusion arises.

Q. Describe how you use your lens care products.

■ Noncompliance is the greatest threat to eye comfort and lens life. Inadequate cleaning and disinfection cause about 50 per cent of all problems associated with contact lenses. The attempt to economize by using solutions that should have been discarded was the most common form of noncompliance in one practice. Some consumers even forget to plug in their heating unit. To determine non-compliance, ask consumers to describe their care regimen.

Q. What measures do you take before insertion if you drop your lens on the floor?

■ Frequently, the lens is picked up and promptly inserted along with whatever the lens has collected. Rinse hard (PMMA or gas permeable) lenses with an aerosol saline solution. Rinse soft lenses thoroughly with an appropriate rinsing solution.

References

Introduction

Gordon K. A pharmacist's guide through the complexities of contact lens care. Part I. Drug Merch 1981;62:48–52.

Middleton D. Product Manager—Solutions, Barnes-Hind Inc. (Letter to D Wing, author) 1987;October 8.

Hard (PMMA) Lenses

Abel SR, Gourley DR. Eye diseases. In: Katcher BS, Young LY, Koda-Kimble MA, eds. Applied therapeutics, the clinical use of drugs. San Francisco: Applied Therapeutics, 1983:1201–37.

Appen RE, Hutson CF. Traumatic injuries: office treatment of eye injury. 1. Injury due to foreign materials. Postgrad Med 1976;60:233–5.

Cooper RL, Constable IJ. Infective keratitis in soft contact lens wearers. Br J Ophthalmol 1977;61:250–4.

Karp EJ. A guide to cosmetic contact lenses. Sight Sav Rev 1977;47:3–8.

Koetting RA. Contact lens update. J Am Pharm Assoc 1975;15:575–7,587.

Mandell RB. Contact lens practice. Springfield: CC Thomas, 1981: 296–312,383–430.

Ruben M. The pros and cons of hard and soft contact lenses. Nurs Times 1976; 72:1018–20.

Gas Permeable Lenses

Anonymous. Contact lenses now. Drug Ther Bull 1988;26:39–40.

Garnett B. Gas-permeable hard contact lenses. Can J Optom 1980;42:45–9.

Kame R, Asno G, Lee J. Hard lens solutions with the Polycon. Contact Lens Forum 1981;Aug:43–6.

Soft (Hydrogel) Lenses

Lum VJ, Lyle WM. Chemical components of contact lens solutions. Can J Optom 1981;43:136–51.

Mandell RB. Contact lens practice. Springfield: CC Thomas, 1981:495–518.

Sutherland RL, VanLeeuwen WN. Soft contact lenses. Can Med Assoc J 1972;107:49–50.

Silicone Lenses

Birdsall AA. Silicone: material of the future. Contact Lens Forum 1982; May:89–97.

Herrin S. Reliving Dow Corning's nightmare. Rev Optom 1985;122:35–44.

Mandell RB. Contact lens practice. Springfield: CC Thomas, 1981:650–1.

Extended Wear

Alfonso E, Mandelbaum S, Fox MJ, Forster RK. Ulcerative keratitis associated with contact lens wear. Am J Ophthalmol 1986;101:429–33.

Anonymous. Soft contact lenses. Med Lett Drugs Ther 1990;32:69–70.

Anonymous. Disposable extended-wear contact lenses (Editorial). Lancet 1988;1:1437.

Baldone JA, Kaufman HE. Extended wear contact lenses (Editorial). Ann Ophthalmol 1983;15:595–6.

Barr J. Extended wear with minimal corneal compromise. Int Contact Lens Clin 1984;11:10–5.

Baum J, Barza M. Pseudomonas keratitis and extended-wear soft contact lenses (Editorial). Arch Ophthalmol 1990;108:663–4.

Bennett ES, Andrasko G. Facing the hard facts. Rev Optom 1985;122:37–44.

Binder PS. Myopic extended wear with the Hydrocurve II soft contact lens. Ophthalmol 1983;90:623–6.

Bruce AS, Brennan NA. Corneal pathophysiology with contact lens wear. Surv Ophthalmol 1990;35:25–58.

Contact Lens Care

Cavanagh HD. Extended wear—what happened? CLAO J 1987;13:194.

Chalupa E, Swarbrick, HA, Holden BA, Sjostrand J. Severe corneal infarctions associated with contact lens wear. Ophthalmol 1987;94:17–22.

Cohen EJ, Laibson PR, Arentsen JJ, Clemons CS. Corneal ulcers associated with cosmetic extended wear soft contact lenses. Ophthalmol 1987;94:109–14.

Coster DJ. Medical aspects of contact lens wear. Med J Aust 1984;140:455–7.

Cuhna MC, Thomassen TS, Cohen EJ, Genvert GI, Arentsen JJ, Laibson PR. Complications associated with soft contact lens use. CLAO J 1987; 13:107–11.

Dart JK, Badenoch PR. Bacterial adherence to contact lenses. CLAO J 1986;12:220–4.

Dart JK. Bacterial keratitis in contact lens users. Br Med J 1987;295:959–60.

Dister RE, Harris MG. Legal consequences of the FDA's 7-day extended wear (Letter). J Am Optom Assoc 1990;61:212–4.

Donzis PB, Mondino BJ, Weissman BA, Bruckner DA. Microbial contamination of contact lens care systems. Am J Ophthalmol 1987;1004:325.

Duran JA, Refojo MF, Gipson IK, Kenyon KR. Pseudomonas attachment to new hydrogel contact lenses. Arch Ophthalmol 1987;105:106–9.

Farkas P, Kassalow TW, Farkas B. Parts 1 and 2. Clinical overview of the management and fitting of the extended wear patient. J Am Optom Assoc 1981;52:187–92,397–402.

Fonn, D; Holden, B. Rigid gas-permeable vs. hydrogel contact lenses for extended wear. Am J Optom Physiol Opt 1988;65:536–44.

Fontana F, Ghormley NR, Kame R, Lebow K, Silbert J, Solomon J. Targeting extended wear trouble spots. Rev Optom 1986;123:33–48.

Franks WA, Adams GGW, Dart JKG, Minassian D. Relative risks of different types of contact lenses. Br Med J 1988;297:524–5.

Galentine PG, Cohen EJ, Laibson PR, Adams CP, Michaud R, Arentsen JJ. Cornea ulcers associated with contact lens wear. Arch Ophthalmol 1984;102:891–4.

Graham CM, Dart JKG, Buckley RJ. Extended wear hydrogel and daily wear hard contact lenses for aphakia—success and complications compared in a longitudinal study. Ophthalmol 1986;93:1489–94.

Hart DE, Shih K. Surface interactions on hydrogel extended wear contact lenses: microflora and microfauna. Am J Optom Physiol Opt 1987;64:739–48.

Hirano J, Hirano M. Extended wear of our gas-permeable hard contact lenses. Contact Lens J 1989;17:213.

Holden BA, Mertz GW, McNally JJ. Corneal swelling response to contact lenses worn under extended wear conditions. Invest Ophthalmol Vis Sci 1983;24:218–26.

Holden BA, Sweeney DF, Vannas A, Nilsson KT, Efron N. Effects of long-term extended contact lens wear on the human cornea. Invest Ophthalmol Vis Sci 1985;26:1489–501.

Holden BA, Swarbrick HA, Sweeney DF, Ho A, Efron N. Strategies for minimizing the ocular effects of extended contact lens wear—a statistical analysis. Am J Optom Physiol Opt 1987;64:781–9.

Koenig SB, Solomon JM, Hyndiuk RA, Sucher RA, Gradus MS. Acanthamoeba keratitis associated with gas-permeable contact lens wear. Am J Ophthalmol 1987;103:832.

Lamer L. Extended wear contact lenses for myopes. A follow-up study of 400 cases. Ophthalmol 1983;90:156–61.

Lebow, K. The Boston IV lens. Rev Optom 1985;122:65–71.

Levy, B. Rigid gas-permeable lenses for extended wear—a 1-year clinical evaluation. Am J Optom Physiol Opt 1985;62:889–94.

Mandell RB, Liberman G. The paraperm lens. Rev Optom 1985;122:75–6.

Martin NF, Kracher GP, Stark WJ, Maumenee AE. Extended wear soft contact lenses for aphakic correction. Arch Ophthalmol 1983;101:39–41.

Mayo MS, Schlitzer RL, Ward MA, Wilson LA, Ahearn DG. Association of Pseudomonas and Serratia corneal ulcers with use of contaminated solutions. J Clin Microbiol 1987;25:1398–400.

Millodot M. Clinical evaluation of an extended wear lens. Int Contact Lens Clin 1984;11:16–20.

Nightingale SL. From the Food and Drug Administration. Maximum wearing time shortened for extended-wear lenses. JAMA 1989;262:1916.

Omerod LD, Smith RE. Contact lens-associated microbial keratitis. Arch Ophthalmol 1986;104:79–83.

Parsons MR, Holland EJ, Agapitos PJ. Nocardia asteroides keratitis associated with extended-wear soft contact lenses. Can J Ophthalmol 1989;24:120–2.

Piccolo MG. Soft lens extended wear. Rev Optom 1985;122:80–90.

Polse KA, Rivera RK, Bonanno J. Ocular effects of hard gas-permeable-lens extended wear. Am J Optom Physiol Opt 1988;65:358–64.

Rosenfeld SI, Mandelbaum S, Corrent GF, Pflugfelder SC, Culbertson WW. Granular epithelial keratopathy as an unusual manifestation of Pseudomonas keratitis associated with extended-wear soft contact lenses. Am J Ophthalmol 1990;109:17–22.

Schein O, Hibberd P, Kenyon KR. Contact lens complications: incidental or epidemic? (Editorial) Am J Ophthalmol 1986;102:116–7.

Schein OD, Glynn RJ, Poggio EC, Seddon JM, Kenyon KR. Microbial Keratitis Study Group. The relative risk of ulcerative keratitis among users of daily-wear and extended-wear soft contact lenses. A case-control study. N Engl J Med 1989;321:773–8,824–6.

Stenson S. Soft contact lenses and corneal infection (Editorial). Arch Ophthalmol 1986;104:1287–9.

Tomlinson, A. The Airlens. Rev Optom 1985;122:57–60.

Vilforth, JC. The Food and Drug Administration is requesting manufacturers of cosmetic extended-wear soft contact lenses to indicate a recommended wearing time in the product labeling (News). Arch Ophthalmol 1989;107:969.

Wilhelmus, KR. Review of clinical experience with microbial keratitis associated with contact lenses. CLAO J 1987;13:211–4.

Disposable Extended-Wear Contact Lenses

Auran JD, Starr MB, Jakobiec FA. Acanthamoeba keratitis: a review of the literature. Cornea 1987;6:2–26.

Cohen EJ, Gonzalez C, Leavitt KG, Arentsen JJ, Laibson PR. Corneal ulcers associated with contact lenses including experience with disposable lenses CLAO J 1991;17:173–6.

Doren GS, Cohen EJ, Higgins SE, Udell IJ, Eagle RC Jr, Arentsen JJ, Laibson PR. Management of contact lens associated Acanthamoeba keratitis. CLAO J 1991;17:120–5.

Dornic DI, Wolf T, Dillon WH, Christensen B, Deem CD. Acanthamoeba keratitis in soft contact lens wearers. J Am Optom Assoc 1987;58:482–6.

Dunn JP Jr, Mondino BJ, Weissman BA, Donzis PB, Kikkawa DO. Corneal ulcers associated with disposable hydrogel contact lenses. Am J Ophthalmol 1989;108:113–7.

Ficker L, Hunter P, Seal D, Wright P. Acanthamoeba keratitis occurring with disposable contact lens wear (Letter). Am J Ophthalmol 1989;108:453.

Heidemann DG, Verdier DD, Dunn SP, Stamler JF. Acanthamoeba keratitis associated with disposable contact lenses. Am J Ophthalmol 1990;110:630–4.

John T, Desai D, Sahm D. Adherence of Acanthamoeba castellani cysts and trophozoites to unworn soft contact lenses. Am J Ophthalmol 1989;108:658–64.

Kaye DB, Hayashi MN, Schenkein JB. A disposable contact lens program: a preliminary report. CLAO J 1988;14:33–7.

Kershner RM. Infectious corneal ulcer with over extended wearing of disposable contact lenses (Letter). JAMA 1989;261:3549–50.

Killingsworth DW, Stern GA. Pseudomonas keratitis associated with the use of disposable soft contact lenses. Arch Ophthalmol 1989;107:795–6.

Kotow M, Holden BA, Grant T. The value of regular replacement of low water content contact lenses for extended wear. J Am Optom Assoc 1987;58:461–4.

Larkin DFP, Kilvington S, Easty DL. Contamination of contact lens storage cases by Acanthamoeba and bacteria. Br J Ophthalmol 1990;74:233–5.

Mertz PHV, Bouchard CS, Mathers WD, Goldman J, Shields WJ, Cavanaugh HD. Corneal infiltrates associated with disposable extended wear soft contact lenses: a report of nine cases. CLAO J 1990;16:269–72.

Moore MB. Parasitic infections. In: Kaufman HE, Barron BA, McDonald MB, Waltman SR, eds. The Cornea. New York: Churchill Livingstone, 1988:271–9.

Parker WT, Wong SK. Keratitis associated with disposable soft contact lenses. Am J Ophthalmol 1989;107:195.

Rabinovitch J, Fook TC, Hunter WS, Ghosh M. Acanthamoeba keratitis in a soft-contact-lens wearer. Can J Ophthalmol 1990;25:25–8.

Contact Lens Care

Rabinowitz SM, Pflugfelder SC, Goldberg M. Disposable extended-wear contact lens-related keratitis (Case report). Arch Ophthalmol 1989;107:1121.

Serdahl CL, Mannis MJ, Shapiro DR, Zadnik K, Lightman JM, Pinilla C. Infiltrative keratitis associated with disposable soft contact lenses (Case reports). Arch Ophthalmol 1989;107:322–3.

Lens Care Solutions

Anonymous. Contact lens care: no easy solutions. Rev Optom 1980;117:24–5.

Smith RE, MacRae SM. Contact lenses—convenience and complications (Editorial). N Engl J Med 1989;321:824–6.

Cleaning Solutions

Anonymous. Contact lens questions and answers. All in good order. Rev Optom 1986;123:77.

Arons IJ. Your guide to contact lens care products. Contact Lens Forum 1978;Aug:49–55.

Bailey NJ. Contact lens coating: the effect on service life. J Am Optom Assoc 1975;46:214–8.

Bergenske P. Enzymatic cleaning of silicone co-polymer rigid lenses. Am J Optom Physiol Opt 1983;60:540–1.

Butrus SI, Klotz SA. Contact lens surface deposits increase the adhesion of Pseudomonas aeruginosa. Curr Eye Res 1990;9:717–24.

Clements L. Soft lens spoilage. Contact Lens J 1980;6:5–14.

Eriksen S. Cleaning hydrophilic contact lenses: an overview. Ann Ophthalmol 1975;7:1223–32.

Farkas P, Kassalow TW, Farkas B. The use of enzyme tablets to control grade III GPC with PMMA lenses. J Am Optom Assoc 1984;55:836–7.

Feldman GL, Bailey WR. Clinical experiences with chemical vs. thermal disinfection of hydrophilic lenses. Contact Lens J 1974;8:17–20.

Fontana FD, Meier GD, Becherer D. Opti-Clean for hydrophilic lenses. Contact Lens Forum 1982;Nov:57–65.

Fowler SA, Korb DR, Finnemore VM, Allansmith MR. Surface deposits on worn hard contact lenses. Arch Ophthalmol 1984;102:757–9.

Fowler SA, Allansmith MR. The surface of the continuously worn contact lens. Arch Ophthalmol 1980;98:1233–6.

Grosvenor TP. Contact lens theory and practice. Chicago: Professional Press, 1963:236–46.

Hathaway RA, Lowther GE. Soft lens cleaners: their effectiveness in removing deposits. J Am Optom Assoc 1978;48:259–66.

Houslby RD, Ghajar M, Chavez G. Microbiological evaluation of soft contact lens disinfecting solutions. J Am Optom Assoc 1984;55:205–11.

Jones RA. Assistant product manager, Personal Products Division, Bausch and Lomb. (Personal communication to D Wing, author) 1991;Sept 10.

Jose JG, Polse KA. Optometric pharmacology. Orlando:Grune & Stratton, 1984:69–87.

Josephson JE, Haber R, Pope CA; Caffery BE. Clinical evaluation of a new cleaner for hard and soft lenses. Can J Optom 1981;43(Suppl):179–85.

Kilvington S, Larkin DFP. Acanthamoeba adherence to contact lenses and removal by cleaning agents. Eye 1990;4(Pt 4):589–93.

Kleist F, Thorson JC. How effective are soft lens cleaners? Rev Optom 1978;115:43–9.

Koetting RA. What improved cleaning techniques can do. Contact Lens Forum 1978;Mar:33–7.

Korb DR, Greiner JV, Finnemore VM, Allansmith MR. Treatment of contact lenses with papain. Increase in wearing time in keratoconic patients with papillary conjunctivitis. Arch Ophthalmol 1983;101:48–50.

Missotten L, Maudgal PC, Houttequiet I. Surface deterioration of soft contact lenses. Contact Intraocul Lens Med J 1981;7:27–38.

Poggio EC, Glynn RJ, Schein OD, Seddon JM, Shannon MJ, Scardino VA, Kenyon KR. The incidence of ulcerative keratitis among users of daily-wear and extended-wear soft contact lenses. N Engl J Med 1989;321:779–83.

Reynolds JEF, ed. Martindale: the extra pharmacopoeia. London: Pharmaceutical Press, 1982:370.

Sibley MJ, Shih KL, Hu JC. The microbiological benefit of cleaning and rinsing contact lenses. Int Contact Lens Clin 1985;12:235–42.

Sibley MJ. Cleaning solutions for contact lenses. Int Contact Lens Clin 1982;9:291–4.

Stein H, Harrison K. The safety and effectiveness of Polyclens—an all purpose cleaner for hydrophilic soft contact lenses. CLAO J 1983;9:39–42.

Tsuda S, Ando N, Anan N. Fitting and analysis of the Menicon soft lens—part 1. Int Contact Lens Clin 1977;4:55–66.

Isopropyl Alcohol

Ghajar M, Houlsby RD, Chavez G. Microbiological evaluation of Mira-Flow. J Am Optom Assoc 1989;60:592–5.

Inns HDE. Soft contact lenses and solutions in Canada. Can J Optom 1980;42:27–37.

Lowther GE, Hilbert JA. Deposits on hydrophilic lenses: differential appearance and clinical causes. Am J Optom Physiol Opt 1975;52:687–92.

Ruben M. Ocular pathogens and contact lens hygiene. In: Ruben M, ed. Soft contact lenses: clinical and applied technology. Toronto: J Wiley & Sons, 1978:335–47.

Unorthodox Cleaners

Diefenbach CB, Seibert CK, Davis LJ. Analysis of two "home remedy" contact lens cleaners. J Am Optom Assoc 1988;59:518–21.

Hess RJ, Kneisser G, Fukushima A, Yamaguchi T. Soft contact lens cleaning: a scanning electron microscopic study. Contact Intraocul Lens Med J 1982;8:23–8.

Lutzi D. Contact lens solution compatibility. Contact Lens J 1980;6:2–4.

To K. Artificial tears or lens cleaner. Am J Ophthalmol 1989;108:610.

Disinfection (Soaking or Storage) Solutions

Ernst RR. Sterilization by heat. In: Block SS, ed. Disinfection, sterilization and preservation. Philadelphia: Lea & Febiger, 1977:481–521.

Sibley MJ. Disinfection solutions. Int Ophthalmol Clin 1981;21:237–47.

Organomercurials

Cioletti KR. Determination of thimerosal content in contact lens polymers. Int Contact Lens Clin 1980;7:3–7.

Connor CG, Hopkins SL, Salisbury RD. Effectivity of contact lens disinfection systems against Acanthamoeba culbertsoni. Optom Vis Sci 1991;68:138–41.

Harrison DP. Thimerosal and anterior crystalline lens vacuoles. Rev Optom 1985;122:55–6.

Harvey SC. Antiseptics and disinfectants; fungicides; ectoparasiticides. In: Gilman AG, Goodman LS, Gilman A, eds. Goodman and Gilman's the pharmacological basis of therapeutics. New York: Macmillan, 1980:964–87.

Johnsson J, Nygren B, Sjogren E. Disinfection of soft contact lenses in liquid. Contact Lens J 1978;6:3–10.

Kleist F. Appearance and nature of hydrophilic contact lens deposits—part 2: inorganic deposits. Int Contact Lens Clin 1979;6:177–86.

Kleist F. Appearance and nature of hydrophilic contact lens deposits—part 1: protein and other organic deposits. Int Contact Lens Clin 1979;6:120–30.

Lieblein JS. Overview of soft contact lens hygiene. Rev Optom 1978;115:29–32.

Ludwig IH, Meisler DM, Rutherford I, Bican FE, Langston RHS, Visvesvara GS. Susceptibility of Acanthamoeba to soft contact lens disinfection systems. Invest Ophthalmol Vis Sci 1986;27:626–8.

McBride RJ, Mackie MAL. Evaluation of the antibacterial activity of contact lens solutions. J Pharm Pharmacol 1974;26:899–900.

Morgan JF. Evaluation of a cleaning agent for hydrophilic contact lenses. Can J Ophthalmol 1975;10:214–7.

Norton DA, Davies DJG, Richards NE, Meakin BJ, Keall A. The antimicrobial efficiencies of contact lens solutions. J Pharm Pharmacol 1974;26:841–6.

Refojo MF. Reversible binding of chlorhexidine gluconate to hydrogel contact lenses. Contact Intraocul Lens Med J 1976;2:47–56.

Sibley MJ, Yung G. A technique for the determination of chemical binding to soft contact lenses. Am J Optom 1973;50:710–4.

Stewart-Jones JH, Hopkins GA, Phillips AJ. Drugs and solutions in contact lens practice and related microbiology. In: Stone J, Phillips AJ, eds. Contact lenses: a textbook for practitioners and students. London: Butterworths, 1980:59–90,365–75.

Wechsler S, George NC. Disinfection of hydrophilic lenses. J Am Optom Assoc 1981;52:179–86.

Contact Lens Care

Zand LM. Review: the effect of nontherapeutic ophthalmic preparations on the cornea and tear film. Aust J Optom 1981;64:44–70.

EDTA

Anonymous. Contact lens questions and answers. Read the label. Rev Optom 1986;123:61.

Anonymous. AMA drug evaluations. New York: J Wiley & Sons, 1980:402–3.

Dabezies OH. Contact lens hygiene: past, present and future. Contact Lens Med Bull 1979;3:2–15.

Kleist FD. Prevention of inorganic deposits on hydrophilic contact lenses. Int Contact Lens Clin 1981;8:44–7.

Lemp MA. Bandage lenses and the use of topical solutions containing preservatives. Ann Ophthalmol 1978;10:1319–21.

Phillips AJ. Contact lens solutions. Contact Lens J 1977;6:3–23.

Snyder AC, Hill RM, Bailey NJ. Home sterilization: fact or fiction. Contact Lens Forum 1977;Feb:41–3.

Contact Lens Cases

Benjamin WJ, Hill RM. Ultra-thins: the case for continuous care. J Am Optom Assoc 1980;51:277–9.

Buffers

Committee of revision. The United States pharmacopeia. Rockville: United States Pharmacopeial Convention, 1980:1100–1.

Demas GN. pH consistency and stability of contact lens solutions. J Am Optom Assoc 1989;60:732–4.

Lamy PP, Shangraw RF. Physico-chemical aspects of ophthalmic and contact lens solutions. Am J Optom 1971;48:37–51.

MacKeen DG, Bulle K. Buffers and preservatives in contact lens solutions. Contacto 1977;21:31–6.

Troy G. Contact lens solutions: your first aid to a successful fit. Optom Management 1975;11:49–75.

Wetting and Viscosity Agents

Carney LG, Hill RM, Habenicht BL. Ageing lubricant solutions—a clinical comment. Contact Lens J 1990;18:157–8.

Zografi G. Interfacial phenomena. In: Osol A, ed. Remington's pharmaceutical sciences. Easton: Mack Publishing, 1980:253–65.

Multifunction Solutions

Leisring J, Gill L. The clinical safety of a new generation chemical disinfecting agent. Spectrum 1990;Oct:63–7.

Marquardt R, Roth HW, Laux U. Experiences with a new large diameter soft contact lens. Contact Lens J 1975;8:9–19.

Mulford MB, Houlsby RD, Langston JB, Shively CD, Krezanoski JZ. Rigid lens care revisited. Contact Lens Forum 1980;Sept:33–43.

Roth HW. Soft hydrophilic contact lenses: results of a long-term study. J Japan Contact Lens Soc 1979;21:18–21.

Roth HW, Roth-Wittig M. Multipurpose solutions for soft lens maintenance. Int Contact Lens Clin 1980;7:92–5.

Hard Contact Lens Products

Shively CD. Accessory solutions in contact lens care and practice. In: Ruben M, ed. Soft contact lenses: clinical and applied technology. Toronto: J Wiley & Sons, 1978:383–424.

Preservatives

Burstein NL. Corneal cytotoxicity of topically applied drugs, vehicles and preservatives. Surv Ophthalmol 1980;25:15–30.

Dabezies OH. Soft contact lens hygiene. Contact Intraocul Lens Med J 1975;1:103–8.

Havener WH. Ocular pharmacology. St Louis: CV Mosby, 1978:425–37.

MacKeen DL, Green K. Chlorhexidine kinetics of hydrophilic contact lenses. J Pharm Pharmacol 1978;30:678–82.

Mandell RB. Contact lens practice. Springfield: CC Thomas, 1981:313–41.

Mondino BJ, Salamon SM, Zaidman GW. Allergic and toxic reactions of soft contact lens wearers. Surv Ophthalmol 1982;26:337–44.

Mondino BJ, Weissman BA, Farb MD, Pettit TH. Corneal ulcers associated with daily-wear and extended-wear contact lenses. Am J Ophthalmol 1986;102:58–65.

Rosenthal P, Chou MH, Salamore JC, Israel SC. Quantitative analysis of chlorhexidine gluconate and benzalkonium chloride adsorption on silicone/acrylate polymers. CLAO J 1986;12:43–50.

Wetting Solutions

Lemp MA, Holly FJ. Recent advances in ocular surface chemistry. Am J Optom 1970;47:669–72.

Mauger TF, Hill RM. A key to solution effects? Contact Lens Forum 1982;Apr:23–5.

Hill RM, Mauger TF. The solution label's phantom features. Contact Lens Forum 1981;Apr:115–7.

Mauger TF, Hill RM. Solutions that soothe. Contact Lens Forum 1982;Feb:75–7.

Accessory Solutions

Shovlin JP. Acanthamoeba keratitis in rigid lens wearers: the issue of tap water rinse. Int Contact Lens Clin 1990;19:47–9.

Weissman BA, Tari LA. A solution for the dry eye. Contact Lens Forum 1982;Feb:55–7.

Soft Contact Lens Products

Gordon K. A pharmacist's guide through the complexities of contact lens care. Part II. Drug Merch 1981;62:36–40.

Enzymes

Allansmith MR, Korb DR, Greiner JV, et al. Giant papillary conjunctivitis in contact lens wearers. Am J Ophthalmol 1977;83:697–708.

Aswad MI, John T, Barza M, Kenyon K, Baum J. Bacterial adherence to extended wear soft contact lenses. Ophthalmol 1990;97:296–302.

Baines MG, Cai F, Backman HA. Adsorption and removal of protein bound to hydrogel contact lenses. Optom Vis Sci 1990;67:807–10.

Begley CG, Paragina S, Sporn A. An analysis of contact lens enzyme cleaners. J Am Optom Assoc 1990;61:190–4.

Bellemare F. Compatibility of enzymatic cleaning with cold contact lens disinfection. Int Contact Lens Clin 1979;6:219–22.

Bernstein DI, Gallagher JS, Grad M, Berstein IL. Local ocular anaphylaxis to papain enzyme contained in a contact lens cleansing solution. J Allergy Clin Immunol 1984;74:258–60.

Bosmann HB, Gutheil RL, Anderson JA. Residual enzyme activity on soft contact lenses and its inhibition by tears. Int Contact Lens Clin 1980;7:156–61.

Breen W, Fontana F, Hansen D, Thomas E. Clinical comparison of pancreatin-based and subtilisin-based enzymatic cleaners. Contact Lens Forum 1990;15:32–8.

Davis RL. Animal versus plant enzyme. Int Contact Lens Clin 1983;10:277–84.

Fowler SA, Allansmith MR. The effect of cleaning soft contact lenses: a scanning electron microscopic study. Arch Ophthalmol 1981;99:1382–6.

Gold RM, Kaplan AI, Orenstein J. Reducing failure in cold disinfection systems. Contact Lens Forum 1979;Dec:57–65.

Gold RM, Orenstein J. Surfactant cleaners vs the enzyme cleaner. Contact Lens Forum 1980;Jan:39–40.

Hill RM, Goings J. Enhancing the enzyme action. Contact Lens Forum 1980;Sept:53–5.

Kleist FD. Soft lens cleaners compared. Contact Lens Forum 1980;Aug:47–53.

Krezanoski JZ. Contact lens products. J Am Pharm Assoc 1970;10:13–8.

Lieblein JS. How important is enzymatic cleaning? An in-office evaluation. Int Contact Lens Clin 1979;6:151–3.

Morgan JF. Maintenance and care of soft lenses. In: Ruben M, ed. Soft contact lenses: clinical and applied technology. Toronto: J Wiley & Sons, 1978:285–90.

Sibley MJ. Cleaning solutions for contact lenses. Contact Lens Clin 1982;9:291–4.

Stern GA, Zam ZS. The pathogenesis of contact lens-associated Pseudomonas aeruginosa corneal ulceration: I. The effect of contact lens coatings on

Contact Lens Care

Adherence of Pseudomonas aeruginosa to soft contact lenses. Cornea 1986;5:41–5.

Chemical Disinfection Products

Anonymous. Contact lens questions and answers. Generic peroxide. Rev Optom 1986;123:77.

Anonymous. Doctors go "cold." Rev Optom 1984;121:8.

Beattie AM, Slomovic AR, Rootman DS, Hunter WS. Acanthamoeba keratitis with two species of Acanthamoeba. Can J Opthalmol 1990;25:260–2.

Billig H, Bailey N, Fleischman W, Ghormley NR, Seger RG, Yamane SJ. A new, rapid hydrogen peroxide system for contact lens disinfection. CLAO J 1984;10:341–5.

Conn H, Langer R. Iodine disinfection of hydrophilic contact lenses. Ann Ophthalmol 1981;13:361–4.

Courtney RC, Jarantino N, Brown P. Clinical safety and acceptability of a catalase tablet for hydrogen peroxide neutralization. Int Contact Lens Clin 1990;17:67–73.

Epstein AB, Freedman JM. Keratitis associated with hydrogen peroxide disinfection in soft lens wearers. Int Contact Lens Clin 1990;17:74–81.

Fonn, D.; Anderson, R.; Sorbara, L.; Callender, M.G.E. A survey of optometric contact lens use in Canada. Can J Optom 1990;52:90.

Garnett B. A clinical comparison of two soft lens chemical disinfection regimens. Optom Monthly 1982;73:260–3.

Gasset AR, Ramer RM, Katzin D. Hydrogen peroxide sterilization of hydrophilic contact lenses. Arch. Ophthalmol 1975;93:412–5.

Gordon KD. The effect of oxidative disinfecting systems on tinted hydrogel lenses. Can J Optom 1989;51:175–6.

Gottardi W. Iodine and iodine compounds. Block SS, ed. Disinfection, sterilization and preservation. Philadelphia: Lea & Febiger, 1983:183–96.

Gregoire J. A retrospective study using Barnes-Hind Soft Mate II system. Contact Lens Forum 1989;14:51.

Harris MG, Hernandez GN, Nuno DM. The pH of hydrogen peroxide disinfection systems over time. J Am Optom Assoc 1990;61:171–4.

Harris MG, Kirby JE, Tornatore CW, Wrightnour JA. Microwave disinfection of soft contact lenses. Optom Vis Sci 1989;66:82–6.

Harris MG. Practical considerations in the use of hydrogen peroxide disinfection systems. CLAO J 1990;16(1 Suppl):S53–60.

Holden B. A report card on hydrogen peroxide for contact lens disinfection. CLAO J 1990;16(1 Suppl):S61–4.

Inns HDE. The Septicon system. Can J Optom 1979;41:144–6.

Inns HDE. The Griffin lens. Am J Optom 1973;50:977–83.

Janoff LE. The Septicon system: a review of pertinent scientific data. Int Contact Lens Clin 1984;11:274–82.

Josephson JE, Caffery BE. Exploring the sting. J Am Optom Assoc 1987;58:288–9.

Knopf HLS. Reaction to hydrogen peroxide in a contact-lens wearer. Am J Ophthalmol 1984;97:796.

Koetting RA. Cosmetics. Int Ophthalmol Clin 1981;21:185–93.

Krezanoski JZ, Houlsby RD. A comparison of new hydrogen peroxide disinfection systems. J Am Optom Assoc 1988;59:193–7.

Krezanoski JZ. Where are we in the development of pharmaceutical products for soft (hydrophilic) lenses? Contacto 1976;20:12–6.

Levy B, Gross ML. Clinical evaluation of a chlorine based disinfection system for contact lenses. Can J Optom 1988;50:16.

Lowther GE. Disinfection of extended wear lenses. Int Contact Lens Clin 1984;11:4.

Lutzi D, Callender M. Safety and efficacy of a new hydrogen peroxide disinfection system for soft lenses—In-a-Wink. Can J Optom 1985;47:30–3.

McNally J. Clinical aspects of topical application of dilute hydrogen peroxide solutions. CLAO J 1990;16(Suppl 1):S46–52.

Morgan JF. Complications associated with contact lens solutions. Ophthalmol 1979;86:1107–19.

Penley CA, Ahearn DG, Schlitzer RL, Wilson LA. Laboratory evaluation of chemical disinfection of soft contact lenses. II. Fungi as challenge organisms. Contact Intraocul Lens Med J 1981;7:196–204.

Penley CA, Schlitzer RL, Ahearn DG, Wilson LA. Laboratory evaluation of chemical disinfection of soft contact lenses. Contact Intraocul Lens Med J 1981;7:101–10.

Penley CA, Liabres C, Wilson LA, Ahearn DG. Efficacy of hydrogen peroxide disinfection for soft contact lenses contaminated with fungi. CLAO J 1985;11:65–8.

Petricciani R, Krezanoski J. Preservative interaction with contact lenses. Contacto 1977;21:6–10.

Piccolo MG, Leach NE, Boltz RL. Rigid lens base curve stability upon hydrogen peroxide disinfection. Optom Vis Sci 1990;67:19–21.

Reynolds JEF, ed. Martindale: the extra pharmacopoeia. London: Pharmaceutical Press, 1982:1232,1292–3.

Sagan W, Schwaderer KN. A new cleaning technique for hydrophilic contact lenses. J Am Optom Assoc 1974;45:266–9.

Shih KL, Raad MK, Hu JC, Gresh WJ, Jiries SI, Caldwell LJ, Bergamini MVW. Disinfecting activities of non-peroxide soft contact lens cold disinfection solutions. CLAO J 1991;17:165–8.

Sibley MJ, Shih KL, Hu J. Evaluation of a new thimerosal-free 5-minute hydrogen peroxide disinfection lens care regimen. Can J Optom 1982; 44(Suppl):5–7.

Sibley MJ, Chu V. Understanding sorbic acid-preserved contact lens solutions. Int Contact Lens Clin 1984;11:531–42.

Silvany RE, Wood TS, Bowman RW, Moore MB, McCulley JP. The effect of contact lens solutions on two species of Acanthamoeba (Abstract). Invest Ophthalmol Vis Sci 1988;29(Suppl):253.

Steel, S.A. Patient preference study compares top lens care systems. Contact Lens Spectrum 1990;5:56–9.

Tarantino N, Courtney RC, Lasswell LA. Simultaneous enzymatic cleaning and hydrogen peroxide disinfection of hydrogel lenses. CLAO J 1988;15:189–96.

Tse LSY, Callender MG, Charles AM. Antimicrobial effectiveness of some soft contact lens care systems. Am J Optom Physiol Opt 1987;64:824–8.

Wardlaw JC, Sarver MD. Discoloration of hydrogel contact lenses under standard care regimens. Am J Optom Physiol Opt 1986;63:403–8.

Wickliffe B, Entrekin DN. Relation of pH to preservative effectiveness. II. Neutral and basic media. J Pharm Sci 1964;53:769–773.

Wilson LA, McNatt J, Reitschel R. Delayed hypersensitivity to thimerosal in soft contact lens wearers. Ophthalmol 1981;88:804–9.

Wilson LA, Sawant AD, Simmons RB, Ahearn DG. Microbial contamination of contact lens storage cases and solutions. Am J Ophthalmol 1990; 110:193–8.

Allergic Reactions

Allansmith MR. Treatment of external diseases with immunological properties. Int Ophthalmol Clin 1973;13:193–210.

Anonymous. A three-eyed look at cold disinfection. Contact Lens Forum 1978;Jul:21–35.

Anonymous. Symposium: how to solve flexible lens care problems. Contact Intraocul Lens Med J 1981;7:89–100.

Binder PS. Myopic extended wear with the Hydrocurve II soft contact lens. Ophthalmol 1983;90:623–6.

Binder PS, Rasmussen DM, Gordon M. Keratoconjunctivitis and soft contact lens solutions. Arch Ophthalmol 1981;99:87–90.

Callender M, Lutzi D. The incidence of adverse ocular reactions among soft contact lens wearers using chemical disinfection procedures. Can J Optom 1979;41:138–40.

Courtney RC, Lee JM. Predicting ocular intolerance of a contact lens solution by use of a filter system enhancing fluorescein staining detection. Int Contact Lens Clin 1982;9:302–10.

Coward B, Neumann R, Callendar M. Solution intolerance among users of 4 chemical soft lens regimens. Am J Physiol Opt 1984;61:523–7.

Crook TG, Freeman JJ. Reactions induced by the concurrent use of thimerosal and tetracycline. Am J Optom Physiol Opt 1983;60:759–61.

Dabezies OH, ed. Soft contact lens care—the state of the art. Minutes of a symposium held at the 1980 Contact Lens Association of Ophthalmologists meetings; 1980 January 10; Las Vegas, NV. Princeton: Communications Media for Education, 1980.

Fagedes H. The problem with thimerosal. Contact Lens Forum 1980; Sept:45–9.

Fichman S, Baker VV, Horton HR. Iatrogenic red eyes in soft contact lens wearers. Int Contact Lens Clin 1978;5:20–4.

Contact Lens Care

Greenberger MH. A chlorhexidine-free chemical regimen for hydrophilic contact lenses. Int Contact Lens Clin 1981;8:13–5.

Harrison DP. Contact lens wear problems: implications of penicillin allergy, diabetic relatives, and use of birth control pills. Am J Optom Physiol Opt 1984;61:674–8.

Josephson JE. The "multi-purge" procedure and its application for hydrophilic lens wearers utilizing preserved solutions. J Am Optom Assoc 1978;49:280–1.

Josephson JE. Hydrogel lens statistics drawn from private practice. Int Contact Lens Clin 1978;5:99–103.

Josephson JE, Caffery BE. Hydrogel lens solutions. Int Ophthalmol Clin 1981;21:163–71.

Kline LN, DeLuca TJ. Thermal vs chemical disinfection. Contact Lens Forum 1979;Feb:28–31.

McMonnies CW. Allergic complications in contact lens wear. Int Contact Lens Clin 1978;5:182–9.

Molinari JF, Nash R, Badham D. Severe thimerosal hypersensitivity in soft contact lens wearers. Int Contact Lens Clin 1982;9:323–9.

Rahi AHS, Garner A. Immunopathology of the eye. London: Blackwell Scientific, 1976:4–5.

Rietschel RL, Wilson LA. Ocular inflammation in patients using soft contact lenses. Arch Dermatol 1982;118:147–9.

Robertson IF. Continuous-wear hydrophilic contact lenses versus intraocular lenses. Adv Ophthalmol 1978;37:150–5.

Roth HW. The etiology of ocular irritation in soft lens wearers: distribution in a large clinical sample. Contact Intraocul Lens Med J 1978;4:38–47.

Shank RA. Chemical disinfection. Contact Lens Forum 1979;Oct:57–9.

van Ketel WG, Melzer-van Riemsdijk FA. Conjunctivitis due to soft lens solutions. Contact Dermatitis 1980;6:321–4.

Yamane SJ. Complex questions surround increased allergic reactions in wearers of soft contact lenses. Int Contact Lens Clin 1980;7:152–5.

Zadnik K. Severe allergic reaction to saline preserved with thimerosal. J Am Optom Assoc 1984;55:507–9.

Thermal Disinfection

Anonymous. FDA mail alert to 50,000 eye care providers on hazards of Acanthamoeba. AOA News 1989;28:4.

Bailey NJ. Making contact (Editorial). Contact Lens Forum 1979;Nov:15.

Bailey NJ. Making contact (Editorial). Contact Lens Forum 1979;Jun:21.

Bailey NJ. Cleaning of coated soft lenses. J Am Optom Assoc 1974;45:1049–52.

Bailey NJ. Where the salt has gone. Contact Lens Forum 1980; Jan:19–23.

Bilbaut T, Gachon AM, Dastugue B. Deposits on soft contact lenses. Electrophoresis and scanning electron microscopic examinations. Exp Eye Res 1986;43(2):153–65.

Callender M, Lutzi D. Comparing the clinical findings of Soflens wearers using thermal and cold disinfection procedures. Int Contact Lens Clin 1978; 5:119–23.

Carmichael CA. Heat or chemical disinfection: does it really matter? Rev Optom 1983;121(Aug):71–4.

Chandler JW. Biocompatibility of hydrogen peroxide in soft contact lens disinfection: antimicrobial activity vs. biocompatibility—the balance. CLAO J 1990;16(1 Suppl):S43–5.

Dolman PJ, Dobrogowski MJ. Contact lens disinfection by ultraviolet light. Am J Ophthalmol 1989;108:665–9.

Donzis PB, et al. Bacillus keratitis associated with contaminated contact lens care systems. Am J Ophthalmol 1988;105:195–7.

Gold RM, Melman E. Salt tablets: what price economy? Contact Lens Forum 1981;Aug:35–9.

Gottschalk-Katsev N, Weissman BA. Disinfection: choose your weapons wisely. Here's a simple guide to today's infection fighters. Rev Optom 1990; 127:46–50.

Gritz DC, Lee TY, McDonnell PJ, Shih K, Baron N. Ultraviolet radiation for the sterilization of contact lenses. CLAO J 1990;16:294–8.

Harris MG, Higa CK, Lacey LL, Barnhart LA. The pH of aerosol saline solution. Optom Vis Sci 1990;67:84–8.

Harris MG, Rechberger J, Grant T, Holden BA. In-office microwave disinfection of soft contact lenses. Optom Vis Sci 1990;67:129–32.

Hathaway R, Lowther CE. Appearance of hydrophilic lens deposits as related to chemical etiology. Int Contact Lens Clin 1976;3:27–35.

Hill RM. Escaping the sting. Int Contact Lens Clin 1979;6:43–5.

Hill RM. How "pure" are the waters? Int Contact Lens Clin 1981;8:33–4.

Hind HW. Contact lens solutions: yesterday, today, and tomorrow. Contact Lens Forum 1979;Nov:17–27.

Houlsby RD, Ghajar M, Chavez G. Microbiological quality of water used by pharmaceutical manufacturers and soft lens wearers. Int Contact Lens Clin 1981;8:9–14.

Josephson JE, Caffery BE. The dangers of distilled water in contact lens maintenance. J Am Optom Assoc 1988;59:219–20.

Krezanoski JZ. Water and the care of soft contact lenses. Int Contact Lens Clin 1975;2:48–55.

Lowther GE, Hilbert JA. Deposits on hydrophilic lenses:differential appearance and clinical causes. Am J Optom Physiol Opt 1975;52:687–92.

Lowther GE. Hydrogel lens solutions (Editorial). Int Contact Lens Clin. 1982;9:272–3.

Lowther G. Lens material—an overview. J Am Optom Assoc 1984;55:186–7.

Lubert GP, Caplan L. Comparing thermal and chemical disinfection systems for the etafilcon A 58% water content contact lens. Am J Optom Physiol Opt 1984;61:683–8.

MacRae SM, Cohen EJ, Andre M. Guidelines fo safe contact lens wear. Am J Ophthalmol 1987;103:832–3.

Merindano MD, Marques MS, Lluch S, Gonzales M, Saona C. Domestic microwave oven in contact lens disinfection. Contact Lens J 1990;18:241–6.

Phillips AJ. Selection of contact lens solutions. Ophthalmic Optician 1969; 9:394–5.

Pitts RE, Krachmer JH. Evaluation of soft contact lens disinfection in the home environment. Arch Ophthalmol 1979;97:470–2.

Riedhammer TM, Falcetta JJ. Effects of long-term heat disinfection on Soflens (polymacon) contact lenses. J Am Optom Assoc 1980;51:287–9.

Riordan-Eva P, Eykyn SJ, Muir MGK. Pseudomonas aeruginosa corneal ulcer associated with an aerosol can of preservative-free saline. Case report. Arch Ophthalmol 1988;106:1506.

Rohrer MD, Terry MA, Bulard RA, Graves DC, Taylor EM. Microwave sterilization of hydrophilic contact lenses. Am J Ophthalmol 1986;101:49–57.

Ruben M, Tripathi RC, Winder AF. Calcium disposition as a cause of spoilation of hydrophilic soft lenses. Br J Ophthalmol 1975;59:141–8.

Spizziri LJ. Stromal corneal changes due to preserved saline solution used in soft contact lens wear: report of a case. Ann Ophthalmol 1981;13:1277–8.

Sposato P. A "bouquet" of new solutions: take your pick. Contact Lens Forum 1981;Aug:15–23.

Wilson LA, Schlitzer RL, Ahearn DG. Pseudomonas corneal ulcers associated with soft contact-lens wear. Am J Ophthalmol 1981;92:546–54.

Yamane SJ. Studies with a unit dose saline solution. Contact Lens Forum 1979;Aug:91–5.

Rewetting Solutions

Anonymous. Contact lens questions and answers. Tracks of my tears. Rev Optom 1985;122:53.

Brennan NA, Efron N. Symptomatology of HEMA contact lens wear. Optom Vis Sci 1989;86:834–8.

Caffery BE, Josephson JE. Is there a better "comfort drop"? J Am Optom Assoc 1990;61:178–82.

Efron N, Golding TR, Brennan NA. The effect of soft lens lubricants on symptoms and lens dehydration. CLAO J 1991;17:114–9.

Ghormley NR. Rewetting solutions for soft contact lenses (Editorial). Int Contact Lens Clin 1984;11:588.

Maeda AY. Discomfort from drying with hydrogel contact lenses. Int Contact Lens Clin 1982;9:143–5.

Poster MG. Optical efficacy of rewetting and lubricating solutions. Contact Lens Forum 1981;25–31.

Mixing Solutions

Sibley MJ, Shovlin JP. Are you having mixed reactions? Switching solutions can make for bad chemistry. Rev Optom 1990;127:52–6.

Contact Lens Care

Oral Contraceptives

Caron GA. Contact lenses and oral contraceptives (Letter). Br Med J 1966;1:980.

Chizek DJ, Franceschetti AT. Oral contraceptives: their side effects and ophthalmological manifestations. Surv Ophthalmol 1969;14:90–105.

De Vries Reilingh A, Reiners H, Van Bijsterveld OP. Contact lens tolerance and oral contraceptives. Ann Ophthalmol 1978;10:947–52.

Dixon JM. Twenty years and twenty thousand contact lens patients. Trans Am Ophthalmol Soc 1981;79:64–73.

Goldberg JB. A commentary on oral contraceptive therapy and contact lens wear. J Am Optom Assoc 1970;41:237–41.

Guyton AC. Basic human physiology: normal function and mechanisms of disease. Toronto: WB Saunders, 1977:242,343–51,856–66.

Kaufman A. The effects of contraceptives on contact lens performance. Contact Lens J 1980;6:15–8.

Koetting RA. The influence of oral contraceptives on contact lens wear. Am J Optom 1966;43:268–74.

Manchester PJ Jr. Hydration of the cornea. Trans Am Ophthalmol Soc 1970;68:427–61.

Petursson GJ, Fraunfelder FT, Meyer SM. Pharmacology of ocular drugs. 6. Oral contraceptives. Ophthalmol 1981;88:368–71.

Reid IS. Prenatal sex-hormone exposure and congenital limb-reduction defects (Letter). Lancet 1976;2:373.

Ruben M. Contact lenses and oral contraceptives (Letter). Br Med J 1966;1:1110.

Sabell AG. Oral contraceptives and the contact lens wearer. Br J Physiol Opt 1970;25:127–37.

Sarwar M. Contact lenses and oral contraceptives (Letter). Br Med J 1966;1:1235.

Ophthalmics

Anonymous. Contact lens questions and answers. Fading away. Rev Optom 1985;122:89.

Fraunfelder FT. Drug-induced ocular side effects and drug interactions. Philadelphia: Lea & Febiger, 1982:251.

Garber JM. "Film" solution (Letter). Contact Lens Forum 1980;Sept:15.

Krezanoski JZ. Topical medications. Int Ophthamol Clin 1981;21:173–6.

Lea SJH, Loades J, Rubinstein MP. The interaction between hydrogel lenses and sodium fluorescein. Theoretical and practical considerations. Acta Ophthalmol (Copenh) 1989;67:441–6.

Miller D, Brooks SM, Mobilia E. Adenochrome staining of soft contact lenses. Ann Ophthalmol 1976;8:65–7.

Miranda MN, Garcia-Castineiras S. Effects of pH and some common topical ophthalmic medications on the contact lens Permalens. CLAO J 1983;9:43–8.

Sugar J. Adenochrome pigmentation of hydrophilic lenses. Arch Ophthalmol 1974;91:11–2.

Systemic Medications

Aucamp A. Drug excretion in human tears and its meaning for contact lens wearers. South Afr. Optom 1980;39:128–36.

Barber JC. Management of the patient with dry eyes. Contact Intraoc Lens Med J 1977;3:10–5.

Bergmanson JPG, Rios R. Adverse reaction to painkiller in hydrogel lens wear. J Am Optom Assoc 1981;52:257–8.

Chang FW. The possible adverse effects of over-the-counter medications on the contact lens wearer. J Am Optom Assoc 1977;48:319–23.

Farber AS. Ocular side effects of antihistamine-decongestant combinations. Am J Ophthalmol 1982;94:565.

Fraunfelder FT. Drug-induced ocular side effects and drug interactions. Philadelphia: Lea & Febiger, 1982:88–97,112–31,165–70,186–7, 190–4, 206–7,297–305,306–8,311–5.

Harris J, Jenkins P. Discoloration of soft contact lenses by rifampicin (Letter). Lancet 1985;2:1133.

Koffler BH, Lemp MA. The effect of an antihistamine (chlorpheniramine maleate) on tear production in humans. Ann Ophthalmol 1980;12:217–9.

Lemp MA, Hamill JR Jr. Factors affecting tear film breakup in normal eyes. Arch Ophthalmol 1973;89:103–5.

Litovitz GL. Amitriptyline and contact lenses (Letter). J Clin Psychiat 1984;45:188.

Lyons RW. Orange contact lenses from rifampin (Letter). N Engl J Med 1979;300:372–3.

Miller D. Systemic medications. Int Ophthalmol Clin 1981;21:177–83.

Riley SA, Flegg PJ, Mandal BK. Contact lens staining due to sulphasalazine (Letter). Lancet 1986;1:972.

Simmerman JS. Contact lens fitting after Accutane treatment. Rev Optom 1985;122:102.

Troiano G. Amitriptyline and contact lenses (Letter). J Clin Psychiat 1985; 46:199.

Valentic JP, Leopold IH, Dea FJ. Excretion of salicylic acid into tears following oral administration of aspirin. Ophthalmol 1980;87:815–20.

Smoking

Stewart BV. Soft contact lens discoloration and the use of tobacco. Int Contact Lens Clin 1978;6:269–75.

Compliance

Adams C, Cohen E, Laibson, et al. Corneal ulcers in patients with cosmetic extended-wear contact lenses. Am J Ophthalmol 1983;96:705–9.

Bowden FW, Cohen E, Arentsen J, Laibson P. Patterns of lens care practices and lens product contamination in contact lens associated microbial keratitis. CLAO J 1989;15:49–54.

Chun MW, Weissman BA. Compliance in contact lens care. Am J Optom Physiol Opt 1987;64:274–6.

Collins MJ, Carney LG. Patient compliance and its influence on contact lens wearing problems. Am J Optom Physiol Opt 1986;63:952–6.

Jones DB. Acanthamoeba—the ultimate opportunist? Am J Ophthalmol 1988;102:527–30.

Kleinstein R, Stone G. Helping patients to follow their treatment plans. J Am Optom Assoc 1978;49:1144–6.

Mayo MS, Cook WL, Schlitzer RL, Ward MA, Wilson LA, Ahearn DG. Antibiograms, serotypes, and plasmid profiles of Pseudomonas aeruginosa associated with corneal ulcers and contact lens wear. J Clin Microbiol 1986;24:372–6.

Sokol JL, Mier MG, Bloom S, Asbell PA. A study of patient compliance in a contact lens-wearing population. CLAO J 1990;16:209–13.

Stehr-Green JK, Barley TM, Visvesvara GS. The epidemiology of Acanthamoeba keratitis in the United States. Am J Ophthalmol 1989;197:331–6.

Stehr-Green JK, Bailey TM, Brandt FH, Carr JH, Bond WW, Visvesvara GS. Acanthamoeba keratitis in soft contact lens wearers. A case-control study. JAMA 1987;258:57–60.

Recommendations

Bailey NJ. Making contact (Editorial). Contact Lens Forum 1978;Aug:47.

Fontana F, Weiner B. A new approach to compliance. Supply 'em, drill 'em, and grill 'em. Rev Optom 1990;127:63–5.

Weissman BA, Donzis PB, Hoft RH. Keratitis and contact lens wear: a review. J Am Optom Assoc 1987;58:799–803.

10
Otic Products

Penny F. Miller

Self-medication should be restricted to treating minor conditions of the auricle and external ear canal and to the prophylactic treatment of recurrent infections of the external ear canal. Most Canadian otic products available today are designed to treat earaches and infections involving the external ear canal. They include anti-infectives, analgesics, anesthetics, emollients, humectants and solvents, as well as cerumenolytics. Inner ear problems are not amenable to self-medication.

Disturbing symptoms arising from the ear are more common than might be expected. About 3 out of 4 children under age 3 develop infections of the middle ear that produce ear pain. Symptoms other than localized pain occurring in people of all ages are varying degrees of hearing loss, tinnitus, dizziness, vertigo, itching and discharges of many descriptions. These symptoms singly or in combination may result from ear disorders of the auricle, the external ear canal, the middle ear or occasionally from another area of the head or neck. Basic understanding of the pathophysiology of various ear ailments is essential to promoting safe and rational drug therapy and preventing complications arising from inadequately treated or misdiagnosed ear disorders.

Anatomy and Physiology

Anatomically and functionally, the ear is divided into three parts: the external ear, the middle ear and the internal ear (see Figures 1, 2, 3 and 4).

The external ear consists of the auricle, which is the outermost appendage, and the external auditory canal (meatus), which is a tube leading to the eardrum (tympanic membrane) (see Figures 1 and 2). The auricle is made of three tissue layers, which include a layer of cartilage covered by the perichondrium and a layer of skin that is thinner than most found elsewhere on the body. The lobule is the only portion of the auricle that contains no cartilage and is mainly fat.

The external auditory canal is composed of two parts: the outer one-third is an extension of the cartilage of the auricle and the inner two-thirds are formed by bone. The canal ends blindly at the tympanic membrane, which is obliquely positioned to the canal. The canal bends as if S-shaped; it must be straightened by upward traction on the auricle before the eardrum can be examined. In children, a downward traction is required. A narrowing at this bend makes it difficult to dry and clean the inner canal.

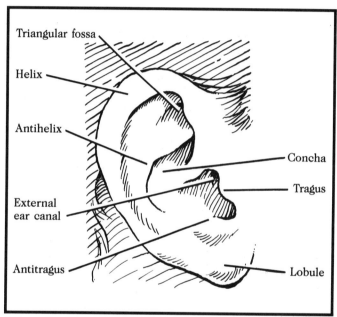

Figure 1 *Right Auricle (Pinna)*

The cartilaginous outer portion of the canal differs markedly in structure from the bony portion. The skin lining this cartilaginous portion is thick, and contains fine hairs and sebaceous and ceruminous glands. The epithelium lining the bony portion of the ear canal is thin and contains no hair or glands. The length of the external auditory canal in adults is about 24 mm, averages 7 to 9 mm in diameter, and has a capacity of 0.85 mL (17 drops).

Cerumen (earwax) is composed of the clear, colorless, watery secretions of the ceruminous glands and the oily secretions of the sebaceous glands. Chemically, it is a mixture of polypeptides, lipids, fatty acids, and amino acids. The normal pH of the external auditory canal is 5 to 7.2, whereas normal skin pH is 3.3 to 7. This acidic environment provides some antibacterial effect. Cerumen also creates a protective surface as it lubricates the skin and entraps foreign material entering the canal. Cerumen turns brown when it mixes with desquamated cells and dust. Normally, cerumen is produced in small amounts, dries in the ear canal and is forced out bit by bit during chewing and talking. The drum and bony canal skin are self-cleaning with a migrating keratin layer of epithelium from the middle of the drum outward to the cartilaginous portion.

Otic Products

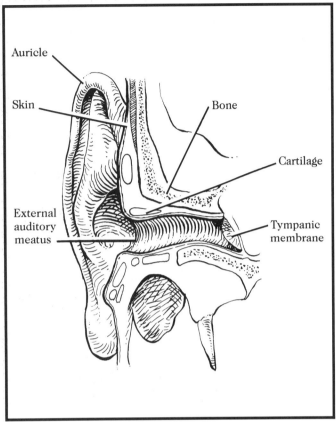

Figure 2 *External Ear*

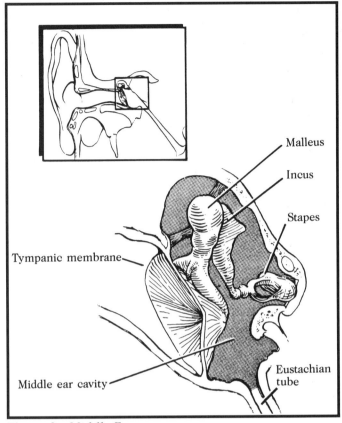

Figure 3 *Middle Ear*

The tympanic membrane is composed of three layers: skin, fibrous tissue and mucous membrane. It is set at an angle of 55° to the floor of the canal. It is a thin (0.1 mm), pearly-grey structure, elliptical in shape, and measures 8 to 9 mm in diameter. The tympanic membrane is considered anatomically with the external ear, but functionally with the middle ear (see Figure 3).

On the inner side of the eardrum lies the middle ear or tympanic cavity, a small cavity in the temporal bone. It is lined with mucosa and contains a chain of three small bones (ossicles) extending from the eardrum to an oval membrane that opens to the cochlea of the inner ear. These ossicles are called the malleus (hammer), incus (anvil) and stapes (stirrup). They represent the normal pathway of sound transmission across the middle ear space, carrying vibrations from the eardrum to the inner ear. The eustachian tube connects the tympanic cavity with the pharynx and provides an air passage from the nasopharynx to the middle ear to equalize pressure on both sides of the eardrum. The inner ear harbors the sensory apparatus of hearing and equilibrium (see Figure 4).

Common Problems of the Auricle

The common conditions of the auricle and their characteristics and management are outlined in Table I.

Trauma

Lacerations, such as minor cuts and scrapes to the skin lining the auricle, are frequent and usually heal well because of the vast blood supply. Even if the auricle is torn completely from the head, it can sometimes reattach successfully after suturing. Suggested treatment for minor lacerations is good hygiene; a more significant laceration should be repaired as soon as possible by a physician.

Hematomas, or potentially harmful or painful bruises, may be caused by any blunt trauma (blow) to the auricle. Subcutaneous blood or serous fluid accumulates between the cartilage and the perichondrium and is poorly resorbed. The perichondrium may undergo necrosis owing to the lack of normal supply of blood provided by the cartilage. The person should be seen by a physician to have this blood accumulation removed immediately.

Cauliflower ear is the result of repeated injuries to the ear. If the hematomas caused by blunt trauma are not aspirated, the blood collects, scarring occurs and the auricle becomes an ugly, shrivelled appendage. Plastic surgery may correct this deformity.

Frostbite to the auricle is particularly likely because of the auricle's exposed position and the lack of subcutaneous or adipose tissue to insulate the blood vessels from the effects of cold. Frostbite primarily damages the blood vessels. Initially, the ears appear white and hard, then red, swollen and tender. The final stage is ischemic necrosis of the involved tissue. Although treatment of frostbite is controversial, it is suggested that treatment consist of gradual warming to body temperature, beginning with streams of cool compresses (not dressings) over the affected area. Massage of any sort is avoided to prevent risk of further damage. Deep injury leads to deformity. A physician should be consulted in any case of frostbite.

Mild burns of the ear are managed with the aim of preventing

Table I *Common Problems of the Auricle*

Conditions	Characteristics	Management
Trauma		
Lacerations	Minor cuts and scrapes	Good hygiene
Hematoma	Painful bruising	Medical consultation
Cauliflower ear	Malformed earlobe due to trauma	Medical consultation for plastic surgery
Frostbite	Initially, white and hard; later, red, swollen and tender	Gradual warming and medical consultation
Burns (mild)	Red, painful	Strict hygiene, antibiotic creams, or impregnated gauze
Burns (involving deeper layers)		Medical consultation
Keloid	Excess scar tissue	Medical consultation
Infections		
Perichondritis	Red, swollen, feels hot; acutely painful auricle, fever and swollen glands	Medical consultation
Dermatitis		
Allergic	Small, raised, red, itchy and weeping lesions	Compresses of Burow's solution; bufexamac cream and medical consultation
Seborrheic	Yellow, greasy scales (usually accompanied by dandruff)	Antidandruff shampoo for scalp; medical consultation
Ear piercing		
	Minor infection	Alcohol (70%) swabs, antibiotic creams
	Minor allergic reaction	Avoid nickel earrings; bufexamac cream

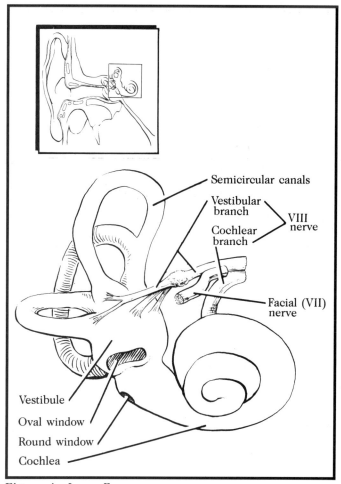

Figure 4 *Inner Ear*

infection and further trauma. Anti-infective creams or impregnated gauzes are applied. Burns involving the layers beneath the skin often result in deformity and should be treated by a physician.

Keloids are massive overgrowths of scar tissue that form after trauma to the skin. On the ear, they commonly occur on the lobule as a result of ear piercing. Suggested treatment performed by the physician is repeated injections of a long-acting corticosteroid. Keloids commonly recur.

Infections

Perichondritis is an inflammation of the perichondrium, the thin, attached lining of the auricular cartilage, and is caused by a presumed infection of *Pseudomonas aeruginosa*. This condition most often results from wound infections secondary to hematomas, burns and lacerations. It can also occur with severe external otitis involving the cartilaginous part of the external auditory canal.

At the onset of perichondritis, the auricle is red and swollen, feels hot and stiff, and is acutely painful. An elevated temperature and regional swollen glands are common. As the disease progresses, pus collects between the perichondrium and the cartilage, cutting off the blood supply to the cartilage and resulting in necrosis. The auricle becomes deformed and shrunken. Topical antibiotics are ineffective, and a physician should be consulted. Systemic antibiotics and hot moist packs are usually advised.

Dermatitis

Any inflammatory skin disorder, such as psoriasis, seborrhea, allergic conditions or contact dermatitis (poison ivy and stinging nettles), and eczema (atopic dermatitis) may also affect the skin of the auricle and external ear canal.

Allergic dermatitis appears as reddened, vesicular and weeping lesions that are extremely itchy. Contact dermatitis can be caused by topical antibiotics or vehicles, chemicals or metals used around the ear, hair sprays, earrings, detergents, perfumes or cosmetics. Scratching can proceed to a secondary infection. Because of its allergic nature, this condition tends to be recurrent or chronic. Compresses of Burow's solution may relieve the itching and dry the area involved. Topical corticosteroids may be prescribed by a physician. Alternatively, a mild condition may be helped by a nonprescription, nonsteroidal anti-inflammatory cream such as bufexamac.

Seborrheic dermatitis is a greasy, scaly eruption usually associated with seborrheic dermatitis of the scalp. Lesions have a yellowish appearance because of abnormal sebum production. Many individuals are not aware of the excess oiliness and believe the scaling results from dry skin. Treatment consists of controlling the seborrheic dermatitis affecting the scalp. Topical corticosteroid creams applied to the scalp and auricle may be necessary because of the condition's recurrent nature. (See the chapter on psoriasis, seborrheic dermatitis and dandruff.)

Ear Piercing

The pierced ear fashion is not without complications. The spring gun method of firing a pre-sterilized, gold-plated stud through the ear lobe may cause the stud to become embedded in the lobe, resulting in severe inflammation. Removing the stud allows healing to occur in 1 to 5 weeks.

Frostbite from overuse of the ethyl chloride spray used to temporarily anesthetize the ear lobe before piercing has been reported. Infants and young children have an increased risk of traumatic laceration or tear to the lobe if the earring gets caught on something and the child tries to pull away.

Table II *Common External Auditory Canal Disorders*

Conditions	Characteristics	Management
Foreign objects	May be no symptoms or a sensation of something in the canal	Medical consultation to remove object
Impacted cerumen	Hearing loss, discomfort	Glycerin, olive oil drops, syringe (and cerumenolytic) by trained personnel
Otitis externa Localized— furunculosis	Painful boil	Analgesics and local heat, medical consultation
Infectious— bacterial ("swimmer's ear")	Itching, pain when chewing or moving the auricle	If mild, use propylene glycol and acetic acid drops; otherwise medical consultation
Infectious—fungal (otomycosis)	Red, swollen canal that bleeds easily, itching, some pain	Medical consultation (antifungal medication)
Infectious—viral	Painful swelling and vesicles	Self-limiting condition (anesthetic ear drops)
Dermatitis Seborrheic	Itchy greasy scaling over inflamed areas with associated dandruff	Antidandruff shampoos for scalp, medical consultation (corticosteroid drops)
Allergic (eczema)	Itchy vesicles	Medical consultation (corticosteroid drops)
Neurodermatitis	Excoriations produced by chronic rubbing or scratching	Medical consultation (corticosteroid drops)

Another hazard is allergic contact sensitivity to nickel and, although rare, to pure gold earrings. These sensitizations can be avoided by wearing stainless steel studded earrings. Keloid formation and recurrent itching have also occurred.

Two serious consequences of ear piercing are viral hepatitis resulting from inadequately sterilized piercing instruments and life-threatening staphylococcal disease caused by insertion of foreign bodies (earrings and piercing devices), which are a source of pyogenic infections.

Good hygiene prevents most complications. This includes frequently swabbing the lobe and earrings with alcohol (70 per cent). If swelling and an exudate are present, topical antibiotics should be helpful. If no improvement occurs, a physician should be consulted.

Common External Auditory Canal Disorders

The common conditions of the external auditory canal and their characteristics and management are outlined in Table II.

Foreign Objects

Foreign objects placed in the ear by young children can obstruct the ear canal, sometimes causing no symptoms. Cotton is the most common foreign body found in the ear canal of adults. Occasionally pus may drain from the ear, indicating a secondary bacterial infection following trauma caused by a foreign object. The foreign object should be removed by a physician, since unskilled attempts may damage the sensitive lining of the external auditory canal.

Occasionally, an insect flies or crawls into the ear canal and causes great distress by beating its wings and crawling about. Before removal, insects should be drowned with lukewarm tap water or, if the canal is not inflamed, be killed with alcohol instillation.

Impacted Cerumen

A great range exists in the amount and migration speed of cerumen. Some individuals have a scanty amount, but others form masses of cerumen that periodically obstruct the canal. Repeated attempts to remove the wax with cotton-tipped applicators, pencils and hairpins merely push the cerumen deeper into the external canal. Normally, cerumen is not present in the innermost portion of the external auditory canal unless it has been pushed there. Deafness often occurs suddenly after washing or bathing when the water causes the wax to swell, producing a more profound blockage. Some discomfort is experienced.

In the elderly, an additional problem is the admixture of long hairs with the cerumen in the external ear canal. A matted obstruction forms, preventing normal expulsion.

Soft wax can be removed easily by syringing the ear with warm water or a mixture of 1:1 hydrogen peroxide and water. Syringing should be reserved for experienced persons, since too vigorous an application may perforate the tympanic membrane. Hard impacted wax requires softening by instilling warmed ear solvents—such as olive oil, glycerin, hydrogen peroxide, sweet almond oil or mineral oil—twice daily for 2 to 3 days before syringing.

Cerumen-dissolving agents containing triethanolamine polypeptide oleate condensate must be used cautiously, since their action depends on chemicals that can often irritate the canal and may cause an external otitis. These drops are best used only in a physician's office. Forceps may be required to remove the loosened cerumen.

Otic Products

Otitis Externa

Otitis externa is a broad term describing any inflammatory process involving the skin of the external auditory canal. These disorders may be classified as infectious, allergic, or seborrheic and also as acute, recurrent and chronic.

Furunculosis is caused by furuncles (boils), which form in the outer one-third of the external canal as staphylococcal infections of the hair follicles or sebaceous glands. Most of these cases are brought on by the trauma of scratching the ear canal. Even a small furuncle causes severe pain (especially if pressure is applied to the tragus or the auricle) until it breaks spontaneously or is incised. Occlusion of the external canal by swelling may cause a conductive hearing loss. Topical antibiotics are ineffective since they do not penetrate boils, but they may help prevent the spread of infection. Individuals should be referred to a physician who can incise the boil, drain it, administer local antibiotics and, if fever or cellulitis of adjacent tissues is present, order systemic antibiotics. If the boil drains spontaneously, pus may produce a diffuse otitis externa. Systemic analgesics and local heat reduce pain symptoms.

Bacterial infections, such as infectious or acute diffuse otitis externa (swimmer's ear), are the most common forms of otitis externa. The highest incidence is in warm humid climates, with the peak occurrence during the summer months.

Prolonged exposure to moisture tends to cause maceration and fissuring of the skin, raising its normal pH. These factors improve the growth media for bacteria to thrive.

Otitis externa may also occur following conditions that traumatize the skin layer, such as scratching the ears to relieve itching, vigorous cleaning with cotton swabs or forceful syringing, or introducing excessive water into the ear canal while bathing or swimming. The first symptom is itching, progressing to moderate or excruciating pain. The pain is aggravated by chewing and becomes more pronounced upon manipulation of the auricle or tragus. This feature helps distinguish between acute otitis externa and acute otitis media. Severe infection may involve some fever and decreased hearing from the edematous canal. There is usually a copious serous discharge and a noticeable absence of wax. One or both ears may be affected.

The causative organisms include *Pseudomonas aeruginosa, Proteus mirabilis, Enterobacter aerogenes, Klebsiella pneumoniae,* group A beta-hemolytic streptococci and *Staphylococcus epidermidis.* Mild cases are usually due to *Pseudomonas aeruginosa;* severe cases are apt to be caused by multiple organisms.

Acute diffuse otitis externa is managed by cleansing the ear canal, controlling pain, using appropriate medication, acidifying the canal and controlling predisposing causes.

For effective topical therapy, drops must contact the infected skin surface for an adequate time period; therefore, the canal should be cleansed. Irrigation of a mildly inflamed canal with warm water suffices. The use of cotton-tipped applicators is not advised since they may induce more trauma. For a severely inflamed and swollen ear canal, the physician may insert a cotton wick soaked with Burow's solution and have the person put additional drops of Burow's solution on the wick every 2 hours to keep it moist. The wick is left in for 24 to 48 hours or until the swelling subsides, when the canal can be cleaned.

Pain is relieved best by oral acetylsalicylic acid or acetaminophen, but codeine may be necessary. Since the pain is due to edema and inflammation, local heat and hygroscopic vehicles (for example glycerin and propylene glycol) aid in pain relief. The use of sensitizing and probably ineffective local anesthetics (for example, benzocaine) is not recommended.

Propylene glycol and acetic acid 2 per cent drops have bactericidal and fungicidal effects without the risk of developing resistant organisms and sensitizing the skin as with antibiotics. In vitro, this combination is bactericidal for Pseudomonas in less than 1 minute, but it takes 5 minutes to kill streptococcus. More than 90 per cent of all cases of otitis externa resolve with acetic acid 2 per cent solution in propylene glycol. Duration of treatment is usually 4 to 5 days. Severe nonresponsive cases of otitis externa should be referred to a physician.

In addition to providing an appropriate antibacterial agent, a product that also produces an acidic environment is ideal. The combination of propylene glycol and acetic acid 2 per cent provides a desirable acid pH of 3, which discourages bacterial growth. Many commercial products designed for use in both the ear and the eye do not offer this acidity.

Foreign objects should not enter the ear canal, since they can predispose the individual to acute otitis externa. For frequent swimmers, the preventive use of propylene glycol and acetic acid eardrops and the removal of water from the canal after swimming helps maintain a healthy ear canal.

A person with recurrent otitis externa who does not respond to these measures must be examined by a physician. Diabetics or debilitated individuals should be watched carefully for adequate control of otitis externa since a rare complication is malignant otitis externa.

Otomycosis, a fungal infection of the ear canal, is common in the tropics but can also occur in temperate climates, usually following the use of topical antibiotics that can suppress the normal bacterial flora. Fungi most commonly found are *Aspergillus niger* and *Candida albicans. Aspergillus niger* forms a black or greyish blotting-paper-like mass in the ear canal. When removed, the underlying epithelium is red, swollen and bleeds easily. *Candida albicans* produces a brownish, almost gelatinous, semisolid debris.

Not all fungal infections of the ear produce symptoms, since growth forms on wax or debris in the ear and does not invade tissue. Individuals present with itching and, at times, pain of the external canal. Some otologists maintain that severe symptoms are caused by a secondary bacterial infection.

Treatment of fungal infections should be supervised by a physician. Debris is removed from the ear canal and an antifungal regimen selected. Various treatment regimens, including nystatin drops, clotrimazole solution and clioquinol powder, have been suggested by physicians. For chronic fungal infections, a 2 per cent salicylic acid in alcohol mixture has been prescribed. In the treatment of *Candida albicans,* propylene glycol and acetic acid drops have been shown to have a fungicidal effect.

Viral infections, such as herpes zoster or herpes simplex, affect the external canal, although rarely, causing pain, and swelling and vesiculation (blistering) of the canal. The condition is self-limiting with no specific treatment other than keeping the canal dry. An anesthetic otic drop may provide some relief.

Dermatitis, including seborrheic dermatitis, contact dermatitis and neurodermatitis, commonly involves the skin of the external auditory canal. Seborrheic dermatitis of the scalp, characterized by scaling with patches of erythema visible at the hair margins, can spread to adjacent areas of the face and ear causing a diffuse otitis externa.

This condition is particularly itchy; scratching may induce a secondary infection. Suggested treatment is control of the scaling scalp with selenium sulfide or zinc pyrithione shampoo. A yeast-like fungus, *Pityrosporum ovale*, may be involved in seborrheic dermatitis and can be treated specifically with the imidazole derivative antifungal shampoo, ketoconazole. Any superimposed infection of the ear canal must be healed first and the meatus kept clean. Prescribed treatments consist of corticosteroid drops, or an ointment of salicylic acid, precipitated sulfur, and petroleum jelly applied to the meatus.

Contact dermatitis occurs in atopic individuals as a result of skin hypersensitivity to some allergen or infecting organism similar to those that affect the auricle. Topical antibiotics more commonly cause hypersensitivity reactions. Occasionally, the offending agent may include frequently used substances such as cosmetics, jewelry, hair sprays or nail polish. The appearance is one of vesiculation followed by a serous (watery) exudate. Itching and irritation promote scratching, which may lead to a secondary infection. Treatment consists of eliminating the offending substance if possible. Corticosteroid drops (with an antibiotic only if necessary) produce a rapid response.

Neurodermatitis is presumably caused by chronic rubbing or scratching of the skin, producing excoriations and scaling of the areas near the external auditory meatus. Intense itching is distressful, and the resultant scratching can lead to secondary infection. People may have a concomitant disease, such as diabetes mellitus, jaundice or a psychosomatic disturbance. Treatment consists of corticosteroid drops for itching, an antibacterial for infection and tranquilizers or psychiatric assistance when indicated.

Malignant otitis externa is an uncommon disorder that occurs almost exclusively in elderly diabetics, but it may occur in people on immunosuppressive medications. The condition manifests itself as severe pain and purulent discharge. *Pseudomonas aeruginosa* progressively invades the external canal, temporal bone, parotid space and base of the skull. Cranial nerve involvement causes death. Treatment consists of giving massive doses of antibiotics intravenously and debriding infected tissues. Otitis externa should be treated promptly in elderly diabetics to prevent this condition.

Common Middle Ear Disorders

For correct evaluation of earache symptoms, the pharmacist should understand middle ear disorders, since some symptoms may appear as an otitis externa (see Table III).

Eardrum Perforation

Traumatic perforation of the tympanic membrane may result from three causes: increased pressure in the external auditory canal accompanying an explosion, a slap or diving; a penetrating injury due to flying debris, overzealous cleaning with cotton applicators or ear syringes, or foreign objects placed in the ear canal; or burns from welding sparks. The symptoms are immediate pain and hearing loss followed by bleeding from the ear. A physician should be consulted. The use of eardrops should be discouraged in any possible eardrum perforation. Treatment consists of systemic antibiotics to prevent secondary infections.

Barotitis Media

A sudden increase in atmospheric pressure, as in airplane descent or deep sea diving, forces air to move from the nasopharynx into the middle ear to maintain equal pressure on both sides of the eardrum. If the eustachian tube is swollen due to an allergy or upper respiratory tract infection, the air pressure does not equalize, resulting in negative pressure in the middle ear. This pressure causes the eardrum to retract and fluid to fill the middle ear, causing serous otitis and pain if the pressure differential is great. Ventilation of the middle ear must be re-established using decongestants or physical methods to dilate the eustachian tubes.

Bullous Myringitis

Bullous myringitis is an inflammation of the tympanic membrane characterized by blister formation. It is thought to be of viral etiology, although bullous myringitis also occurs in 10 to 20 per cent of people with pneumonia caused by *Mycoplasma pneumoniae*. Minimal hearing loss combines with sudden onset of pain. Systemic analgesics relieve pain. The disease is self-limiting, lasting from a few days to 2 weeks.

Otitis Media
Acute (Suppurative) Otitis Media

When an infecting organism migrates along the eustachian tube from the nasopharynx to the middle ear, an inflammation of the middle ear and an accumulation of pus causes an acute suppurative otitis media. Otitis media is one of the most common infections of childhood and a frequent complication of the common cold, measles, scarlet fever or influenza.

The most common infecting bacteria in decreasing order of frequency are *Streptococcus pneumoniae* (25 per cent), *Haemophilus influenzae* (20 per cent), *Moraxella catarrhalis*, formerly called *Branhamella catarrhalis* (9 per cent), *beta-hemolytic streptococcus* (2 per cent) and *Staphylococcus aureus* (1 per cent). In children older than age 5, *Haemophilus influenzae* is rarely isolated, although one report showed an occurrence rate of 36 per cent in 5 to 9 year olds. Viral otitis media usually becomes invaded secondarily by one of these

Table III *Common Middle Ear Disorders*

Conditions	Characteristics	Management
Trauma of the eardrum	Immediate pain and hearing loss with bleeding	Medical consultation
Barotitis media	Atmospheric pressure changes cause pain	Decongestants
Bullous myringitis	Sudden pain and minimal hearing loss	Medical consultation
Acute (suppurative) otitis media	Progressing pain, mild hearing loss, malaise, occasionally fever	Medical consultation
Serous (secretory) otitis media	Fullness and crackling sensation; mild hearing loss; no pain	Decongestants, antihistamines, medical consultation
Chronic otitis media	Painless discharge from the ear	Antibiotic drops or surgery, or both; medical consultation
Mastoiditis	Fever, pain, tenderness of the mastoid	Medical consultation

organisms. Predisposing factors include poor eustachian tube function due to edema secondary to infection, large adenoids or allergy. The eustachian tube in children is shorter and on a more horizontal plane. This anatomical configuration makes it easier for bacteria and nasopharyngeal contents to enter the middle ear of children and thus explains the frequent occurrence of otitis media in children.

Rapidly progressing ear pain is the major symptom. It may be accompanied by fever, malaise and mild hearing loss as pus fills the middle ear. If the accumulating exudate exerts excessive pressure on the tympanic membrane, perforation may occur giving immediate pain relief. Fever occurs often, especially in young people. Occasionally young children pull at their ears or complain of gastrointestinal cramps that often indicate an acute suppurative otitis media.

Treatment usually consists of a 10 day course of systemic antibiotics; ampicillin or amoxicillin being the drug of choice for children less than 10 years and penicillin G or V for those 10 years old and over. Although the administration of decongestants, antihistamines or both was once widely advocated for improving eustachian tube function, there is insufficient controlled data to indicate that either drug is effective. Oral acetylsalicylic acid or acetaminophen relieves pain and fever. Benzocaine eardrops are considered ineffective as a local anesthetic or analgesic in the external ear and may cause hypersensitivities. To alleviate pain, some authors suggest applying dry local heat or instilling mineral oil or glycerin warmed to body temperature.

Recurrent Otitis Media

If 3 episodes of acute otitis media occur within 6 months or 4 episodes within 1 year, antibiotic prophylaxis with sulfisoxazole in low doses (50 mg/kg at bedtime) as well as amoxicillin (20 mg/kg at bedtime) and cotrimoxazole (half the usual dose, at bedtime) is effective. Prophylactic therapy is usually continued for about 3 months during the common cold seasons of winter and early spring.

Serous Otitis Media

With eustachian tube dysfunction, oxygen in the middle ear is absorbed leaving a relative negative pressure or vacuum, which results in a transudation of fluid into the middle ear cleft. If the serous fluid in the middle ear cavity remains sterile, the condition is referred to as serous otitis media. Other terms commonly used are secretory otitis media or otitis media with effusion.

Symptoms present as fullness, a crackling sensation in the ear and partial hearing loss. There is no pain or fever as in acute suppurative otitis media. The individual's own voice sounds different to the affected ear.

Treatment consists of inflating the eustachian tube by using the Valsalva technique (plug nose with fingertips, close mouth, and blow through the nose) or by using oral or topical nasal decongestants. If allergic rhinitis (hayfever) is the cause of the congestion, then antihistamines should be used.

If serous otitis media is allowed to persist for more than 3 months, fluid may thicken to produce what is commonly called glue ear, which can cause permanent hearing loss. The largest single factor responsible for chronic serous otitis media is inadequate treatment of acute or subacute suppurative otitis media. Since bacteria can be cultured in 21 to 48 per cent of children with this persistent middle ear effusion, a 10 day course of antibiotics effective against beta lactamase producing organisms is recommended. If this is not successful, then surgery is considered. Here the retained fluid is removed

by needle aspiration and tympanostomy tubes are inserted through the incised eardrums to equalize the pressure on both sides of the eardrum. Some tubes may extrude spontaneously within 6 or 7 months.

A recent study revealed that one-third of children who qualified for tube placement did not need surgery after 6 months of sulfisoxazole (75 mg/kg/day) therapy.

Chronic Otitis Media

This rare but potential complication of acute suppurative otitis media usually involves permanent perforation of the tympanic membrane. A chronic bacterial infection exists and is caused by the organisms *Pseudomonas aeruginosa* and *Staphylococcus aureus* in addition to those organisms involved in acute otitis media. The recurring symptom is a painless, foul-smelling or nearly odorless discharge from the ear. Medical treatment includes culturing the discharge and using suitable oral antibiotics. The use of topical antibiotic eardrops or powders remains controversial. Concerns include possible ototoxic effects from the antibiotics, neomycin, gentamicin and polymyxin B, and inflammation produced by progylene glycol. Once the draining ceases, surgery to patch the eardrum may be performed.

Mastoiditis

Persistent pain and tenderness for longer than 2 weeks accompanying an acute suppurative otitis media may indicate an acute mastoid infection. Treatment consists of large doses of antibiotics. Chronic mastoiditis results when the infection extends to the bone, as may occur after an attack of acute otitis media or more often with chronic otitis media. This condition causes no fever, pain or tenderness as in acute mastoiditis, but results in a persistent discharge of foul-smelling, purulent material. Conductive hearing loss can also occur. The discharge is treated with antibiotics, and the destroyed part is usually surgically removed. Fortunately, this complication of acute suppurative otitis media is uncommon since the advent of antibiotics.

Serious complications of middle ear infections include meningitis, brain abscess, conductive deafness and facial nerve paralysis.

Tumors

Tumors of the middle ear are rare.

Pharmaceutical Agents

Anti-infectives   *Ear drops do not have to be sterile.*

Polymyxin B sulfate exerts its antibacterial effects by altering the membrane permeability of gram-negative organisms only; it is ineffective against gram-positive organisms and fungi. Resistant organisms do not readily develop, and only slight systemic absorption occurs from topical application.

Gramicidin is a polypeptide antibiotic with action against gram-positive bacteria. Its bactericidal effect is a result of altered bioenergetic function in the bacterial cell. Hypersensitivity reactions and untoward effects are rare with the topical use of gramicidin. It is hydrolysed and therefore rendered ineffective in hydrophilic creams thus it is compounded as an ointment only.

Aluminum acetate or **Burow's solution**, is a clear, colorless liquid with a faint odor of acetic acid. It produces an acid pH of 3.6 to 4.4. Aluminum acetate solution contains 4.8 to 5.8 per cent of aluminum

Otic Products

acetate and is stabilized with 0.6 per cent boric acid. Its therapeutic use is as an astringent and antiseptic. All salts of aluminum possess astringent properties that precipitate proteins, causing contraction and wrinkling of the tissue. When applied to damaged skin, the salts form a superficial protective layer and are seldom absorbed. Local inflammation, edema and exudation are reduced since these preparations harden the skin and check secretions and minor hemorrhage. The dilute solution (1:10) is used as a wet dressing for suppurating wounds and dermatitis and any acute or subacute inflammation of the auricle. It is also applied locally in furunculosis. A 1:20 to 1:40 solution is astringent. Aluminum acetate solutions are widely used in pruritic and inflammatory disorders of the external ear. They are nonsensitizing, well tolerated and do not produce resistant organisms. They cause acidification of the canal, which helps restore normal flora. They are also useful as irrigating solutions to remove debris.

Burow's solution is available as a commercial powder. When added to 450 mL of water, the 2.36 g powder produces a 1:15 solution (Buro-Sol).

Acetic acid solution is prepared by mixing 35 mL of glacial acetic acid with sufficient water to make a total of 100 mL. When applied to the skin, a solution of 1 to 5 per cent is lethal to many microorganisms, especially *Pseudomonas aeruginosa*.

Household white vinegar contains the equivalent of 5 per cent acetic acid. The use of vinegar in medicine dates back to antiquity when it was the first anti-infective known. Comparing the bactericidal effect of acetic acid with other acids, hydrochloric and sulfuric acids are not effective, but acetic, propionic and tartaric acids inhibit the growth of organisms. This difference reveals that the bactericidal effect is not solely dependent on the acidic pH produced. In earlier days, vinegar was an effective method of clearing chronic infection of the middle ear. Acetic acid is well tolerated, nonsensitizing and does not produce resistant organisms even with routine use. For these reasons, acetic acid solutions made as a 50:50 mixture with propylene glycol, alcohol or glycerin are recommended to be instilled after swimming to prevent swimmer's ear.

1,2-Propanediol diacetate is a chemical composition of acetic acid plus propylene glycol, resulting in a loosely combined ester. When in contact with the wet skin surface, this ester readily dissociates to acetic acid and propylene glycol. It irritates less than a concentrated aqueous acetic solution. The release of acetic acid and propylene glycol is slow, so a fairly constant degree of acidity in the ear canal is maintained.

Since macerated skin is commonly found in swimmer's ear and in otitis externa occurring in hot, humid climates, avoiding aqueous solutions is advisable. In a comparative study of an aqueous acetic acid solution of 2 per cent and a nonaqueous acetic acid solution of 2 per cent, better results in uncomplicated otitis externa were achieved with the nonaqueous solution. Further maceration with an aqueous solution can cause recurrences of infection and permit the spread of bacteria deeper into the tissue.

The propylene glycol and acetic acid combination provides bactericidal and fungicidal activity. It also permits good penetration because of propylene glycol's cerumen-softening action.

Boric acid (boracic acid) has weak bacteriostatic and fungistatic properties. It is therapeutically categorized as an astringent and antiseptic in dilute solutions of 1 to 5 per cent. Both the medical profession and the public have used boric acid as a mild, nonirritating topical antiseptic to treat inflamed skin, burns and wounds. It does not readily penetrate intact skin. If used on abraded or denuded skin, it is absorbed systemically. Because this absorption has caused fatal poisonings, particularly in infants, boric acid has fallen into disrepute.

A saturated solution of boric acid in equal parts of alcohol and water has been used to treat otorrhea (purulent discharge from the ear). This solution should provide the desirable acid pH, but because boric acid has been superseded by more effective disinfectants with less toxicity, its use is not recommended.

Glycerin plus boric acid forms a complex, glyceroboric acid that is much stronger than boric acid alone. Low concentrations of boric acid are often included in commercial preparations as a preservative or solution stabilizer.

Phenol (carbolic acid) is categorized therapeutically as an antimicrobial agent with topical anesthetic properties. A solution of 0.2 to 1 per cent phenol is fungicidal and bacteriostatic against gram-positive and gram-negative organisms; stronger solutions are bactericidal. To relieve itching, a solution of 0.5 to 2 per cent provides local anesthesia. Its germicidal action diminishes slightly in the presence of proteins (for example, blood and organic matter) and by a nonacidic medium (for example, alcohol or glycerin) in which it is dissolved. A solution of 5 per cent in glycerin was once used to treat simple earache but phenol eardrops may cause necrosis and perforation of the tympanic membrane. Poisoning may occur not only by ingestion, but by absorbing phenol through unbroken skin or wounds. Also, aqueous solutions as dilute as 10 per cent may be corrosive.

Ichthammol, which contains various hydrocarbons, has only slight bacteriostatic properties and is an emollient. When applied to the skin, it irritates slightly and produces a local stimulation to improve peripheral circulation. It has been used in subacute and chronic eczematous dermatitis as a 10 per cent ointment. Ichthammol 10 per cent weight by water in glycerin has been employed in eardrops for inflammatory conditions of the external ear. It functions mainly as an emollient, not as an antibacterial.

Analgesics and Local Anesthetics

Benzocaine is a local anesthetic that acts by blocking the sensory nerve endings in the skin or mucous membranes. Local anesthetics are of two types: the older compounds are esters, usually of aminobenzoic acid, and the newer compounds are amides. Benzocaine is an ester of aminobenzoic acid. All topical anesthetics have a maximum effective concentration; any concentration above this level or combination of two drugs at optimal doses does not prolong the duration of action nor enhance the degree of anesthesia.

Benzocaine is usually employed in a concentration of 1 to 20 per cent in ointments, sprays and powders for topical use. Ear drop preparations contain 0.5 to 1.4 per cent benzocaine. Benzocaine is comparatively nonirritating and has a low systemic toxicity because of its slow absorption. It is contraindicated in infants because of the danger of methemoglobinemia after absorption.

Benzocaine may cause hypersensitivity reactions. Reports indicate that 3.3 per cent of males and 4.5 per cent of females are allergic to benzocaine. People with eczema have a higher incidence of benzocaine hypersensitivity; 5.9 per cent of these people are allergic. Sensitized skin is characterized by redness and pruritus, progressing to inflammation, swelling, vesiculation and oozing. If benzocaine causes an allergic response, lidocaine (an amide) can be substituted. However, a low incidence of allergy to lidocaine has also been encountered.

The efficacy of benzocaine in relieving discomfort of the external ear canal, tympanic membrane, and auricle has been investigated by the United States Food and Drug Administration (FDA) advisory review panel. The panel concluded that benzocaine is ineffective topically as an analgesic or anesthetic on ear canal tissue and the tympanic membrane and that it is not safe for nonprescription use. Systemic analgesics can be administered to provide adequate analgesia.

Lidocaine (lignocaine) is a potent local anesthetic of the amide type. Concentrations used topically range from 1 per cent to a maximum of 5 per cent. It is a useful anesthetic for mucous membranes. Various preparations are available to anesthetize the mouth, throat, cornea and hemorrhoidal tissue as well as the external ear canal. Onset of mucosal anesthesia is 5 minutes and the duration of action is 30 minutes or longer.

Because serious toxic effects may result if large amounts are systemically absorbed, the application of lidocaine to traumatized mucosa is contraindicated. However, toxicity is not a problem when lidocaine is used on the skin lining the ear canal, where lidocaine is generally well tolerated. The main untoward effect may be an unusual sensitization or allergic reaction. Although lidocaine has been available in ear drop preparations for many years, its effectiveness for relief of ear pain has not been clinically evaluated according to modern standards.

Camphor is classified therapeutically as a topical anti-infective and antipruritic. Applied topically as eardrops, camphor acts as a counterirritant and rubefacient with a possible numbing influence on the peripheral sensory nerves. A sensation of cold and mild analgesia follows application. It is only weakly antiseptic and is often incorporated as a preservative in pharmaceuticals. In inflammatory conditions, its counterirritant action does not affect inflammation, but the person may feel improved. Camphor 1 to 3 per cent is often used in conjunction with menthol or phenol for its local anesthetic and antipruritic effect.

Antipyrine (phenazone) is a pyrazolone derivative. Locally, it has a mild anesthetic effect on nerve endings, feeble antiseptic action and causes constriction of the superficial blood vessels (styptic action). It was formerly used for these effects to treat inflammatory conditions of mucous membranes in a solution of 5 to 15 per cent. Used topically, antipyrine acts primarily as an irritant and consequently may cause burning and itching in the ear. Blisters on the canal lining have been reported. Eardrop preparations of 5.4 per cent antipyrine plus 1.4 per cent benzocaine in dehydrated glycerin are commonly used to treat minor discomfort of the ear. The FDA Advisory Panel states that antipyrine is neither safe nor effective as a topical otic anesthetic or analgesic.

Turpentine oil is an essential oil obtained from turpentine. When applied to intact skin, it has an irritant and rubefacient action. It causes a sensation of warmth and smarting, followed by mild local anesthesia. It is a strong sensitizer; topical application has caused vesicular eruptions, urticaria and vomiting in susceptible persons. It is absorbed through the skin. Its effectiveness as a topical anesthetic on the tissue of the external ear canal and tympanic membrane has not been clinically evaluated.

Humectants and Solvents

Glycerin (glycerol) absorbs moisture from the air and mucous membranes. The main medicinal use of glycerin is as a solvent for many inorganic and organic substances. Although it is not used as an antiseptic, glycerin can prevent bacterial growth by its dehydrating

action if present in sufficient concentration. It is considered comparable to alcohol as a solvent and antiseptic. Because of its hygroscopicity, glycerin is often used as a humectant for keeping surfaces moist and as an emollient in treating various skin disorders.

In edematous stages of ear inflammation, glycerin is believed to withdraw moisture from the external meatus and tympanic membrane to relieve pressure and the resultant pain.

Glycerin is as effective as any other preparation for softening earwax. It is often effective in preventing scale development on the skin of the external canal. Glycerin is safe and nonsensitizing with topical use and is a valuable pharmaceutical used by itself or as a vehicle for other drugs.

Propylene glycol is a clear, colorless, viscous and practically odorless liquid with hygroscopic properties. It is widely used as a solvent substitute for glycerin where the resultant otic preparations are less viscous than glycerin. When drugs are insufficiently soluble in water or unstable in aqueous solutions, propylene glycol is a useful vehicle. Its effect on inhibiting mold growth and fermentation is equal to ethanol and is greater than glycerin; therefore, it provides a preservative effect. The humectant properties of propylene glycol provide nongreasy preparations that prevent drying out of the skin and ear wax.

Emollients (Wax Softeners)

The occasional instillation of olive oil, sweet almond oil, mineral oil, glycerin, hydrogen peroxide solution or urea preparations in the ear canal may soften and promote normal removal of cerumen in individuals who have chronically hard, impacted cerumen.

Olive oil (commonly called sweet oil) is a nondrying fixed oil consisting of mixed glycerides, mainly oleic acid (about 85 per cent). It becomes rancid when exposed to air. Used externally, it serves as an emollient to soothe inflamed surfaces. It is used to soften the skin and crusts in eczema and psoriasis. As well, olive oil softens ear wax, thus promoting normal removal of cerumen.

Sweet almond oil is a nondrying fixed oil consisting of glycerides, chiefly oleic acid. Used externally, sweet almond oil possesses emollient properties characteristic of fixed oils, but it has the advantage of being odorless and it does not become gummy. Sweet almond oil should not be confused with bitter almond oil, which can cause cyanide poisoning from ingestion. Sweet almond oil also softens the skin and cerumen, as does olive oil.

Urea (or carbamide) is a metabolic product of proteins. In a cream base with a 10 per cent concentration, it is used to soften the skin in dry, scaly conditions. The major effect is probably increased hydration. An aqueous solution of 50 per cent was widely used for the topical treatment of wounds and ulcers at one time. Topical applications may irritate inflamed skin or exudative lesions. The 5 per cent urea in cerumenolytic products may help soften cerumen and ear residue for easier removal.

Cerumenolytics

Hydrogen peroxide solution is a dilute 10-volume solution containing 3 per cent weight-by-volume hydrogen peroxide. The number "10-volume" indicates the volume of oxygen obtainable from one volume of solution. Its therapeutic classification is as a topical antibacterial. In the ear, it is most useful as an aid to wax removal and as an ear canal cleanser.

In contact with tissues containing the enzyme catalase, hydrogen peroxide solution releases its oxygen to destroy microorganisms by an oxidizing effect. This effervescence (release of oxygen) also affords a mechanical means for removing tissue debris and pus from inaccessible areas. Hydrogen peroxide solution has poor power of penetration and is short-acting since oxygen releases rapidly; hence, it is a relatively feeble germicide. Hydrogen peroxide solution also has a styptic effect, possibly due to the activation of a step in the blood coagulation process. Therefore, it may be useful as an application for minor wounds.

In conditions of external otitis, a solution of 3 parts water to 1 part hydrogen peroxide 10 volume solution is a valuable cleanser. If cerumen must be removed, a 1:1 ratio of water plus hydrogen peroxide 10 volume solution is effective. The occasional instillation of hydrogen peroxide 10-volume solution may soften wax in people with chronically hard, impacted cerumen. Indiscriminate use can lead to skin maceration, which is a predisposing factor for infection.

Carbamide peroxide (urea hydrogen peroxide) consists of equimolar proportions of hydrogen peroxide and urea. On contact with water, it yields about 35 per cent hydrogen peroxide. It is classified therapeutically as an antibacterial agent owing to its release of hydrogen peroxide, which is a weak germicide. Carbamide peroxide can be used as a substitute for hydrogen peroxide solution, thus providing the mechanical cleansing action and weak antibacterial effect of hydrogen peroxide solution. The proprietary and United States National Formulary (USNF) preparations of carbamide peroxide in glycerol (for example, Debrox) contain the equivalent of 2.82 to 3.98 per cent weight by water of hydrogen peroxide and produce a pH of 4.2 to 7.

The urea (carbamide) portion is effective in skin disorders because of its ability to increase hydration and soften dry scaly skin. These combined effects of hydrogen peroxide and urea help soften the cerumen and ear residue for removal by warm water irrigation.

Triethanolamine polypeptide oleate condensate (for example, Cerumenex) is a combination of an equimolar proportion of triethanolamine (an alkaline solvent with a slight odor of ammonia) plus the fatty acid, oleic acid, forming a soap. It is used as an emulsifying agent to produce a stable, fine-grained, oil-in-water emulsion yielding a pH of about 8. Several trials have been conducted to assess its effectiveness as an earwax remover. One trial with 45 people revealed that Cerumenex plus water syringing was more effective than water syringing alone in removing cerumen. Cerumenex and olive oil were equally effective after single applications in a double-blind trial of 67 ears. Cerumenex can irritate and cause severe contact dermatitis. These effects range from mild erythema and pruritus of the external canal to a severe eczematoid reaction involving the external ear and periauricular tissue. To help prevent this acute otitis externa and dermatitis, it is recommended that Cerumenex not be left in the ear canal longer than one-half hour and be used only under physician supervision.

Papain is a proteolytic enzyme from the fruit of the tropical melon tree *Carica papaya*. It is the active ingredient of modern meat tenderizers because it has protein-digesting power. In medicine, papain has been used as a cerumenolytic agent and as a topical treatment to loosen the exudate of chronic purulent otitis media. Allergic reactions are possible. The value of papain as a cerumenolytic has not been established.

Paradichlorobenzene is a pesticide used in wood preservatives, mothballs and lavatory deodorant blocks. It is an irritant volatile liquid with carcinogenic potential. The inclusion of such a substance in a cerumenolytic preparation is unwarranted.

Other Ingredients

Chlorobutanol is a preservative used in otic products at 0.5 per cent concentration with antibacterial and antifungal properties.

Consumer Instructions

For topical therapy to be effective, eardrops must contact the affected skin surface and adhere for an adequate period of time. The canal must be thoroughly cleansed before instilling the drops. In a moderately inflamed ear, gentle lavage or suction performed by a properly trained person removes the debris from the ear canal.

Ear Syringing Instructions

It is impossible for people to syringe their own ears efficiently. Any competent person may be taught to assist with this procedure. Some difficult cases demand considerable technical skill and should be seen by a physician or nurse.

Pharmacists can give consumers the following instructions:

- Use warm water (about body temperature) to fill the syringe. Expel the bubbles of air.
- With the person sitting, lay a towel over the shoulder and have the person hold a bowl immediately below the ear to catch the return of fluid.
- The person's head should be slightly inclined downward toward the bowl and the bowl should be held firmly against the neck to prevent the fluid from running down the neck.
- Pull the auricle upward and backward to straighten out the canal. (In children, the auricle should be pulled downward and backward.)
- With gentle force only, inject the fluid along the upper wall of the ear canal.
- If the wax is hard, the person should instil some glycerin or olive oil into the ears twice daily for 2 or 3 days to soften the wax before syringing.
- Any abrasion to the skin of the ear canal during this procedure may become infected if left in a moist environment; therefore, a few drops of alcohol may be instilled after syringing to help dry the canal. Antibiotic eardrops may help sterilize the canal.

Instilling Eardrops

- It is best to have a second person instil the eardrops.
- At the start of a course of treatment, the ear canal should be syringed carefully in certain cases (see above).
- Before use, the eardrops should be slightly warmed by holding the bottle in the hands for a few minutes.
- The person should bend the head to one side or lie on the side with the affected ear uppermost.
- Pull the auricle upward and backward in adults, or downward and backward for children, to straighten out the canal and instil the prescribed number of drops (up to 10) into the canal.
- Press the tragus of the auricle gently. This action milks the drops down into the canal and expels air bubbles.
- The person should remain in this position for at least 5 minutes after instillation to allow the medication sufficient time to act.

Aural Hygiene

In otitis externa, aural hygiene is often more important than the treatment itself. To assist the healing process rather than complicate the condition, consumers should be given specific instructions.

Figure 5 *Suggested Approach for Treating Ear Pain*

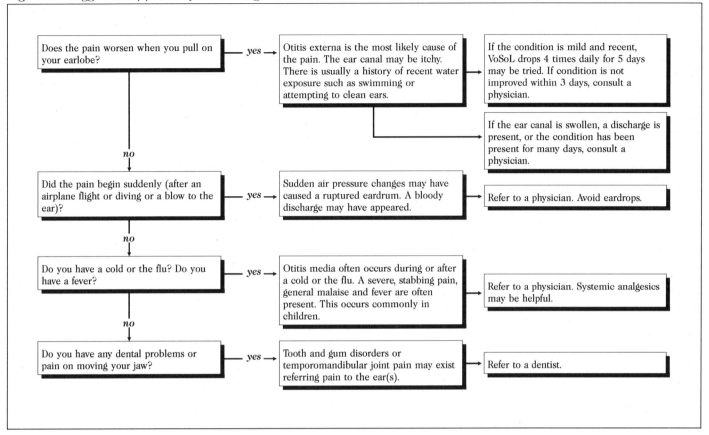

The old cliche "Never put anything in your ear that is smaller than your elbow" is good advice. Cotton-tipped applicators, hairpins, matchsticks or fingernails should not be allowed to enter the ear canal as they may cause trauma, making the ear canal more susceptible to microorganisms. During the infection, absolute avoidance of water entering the canal should be stressed, since retained moisture is a major factor in the genesis and prolongation of otitis externa. Swimming should be forbidden for at least 2 weeks after the inflammation subsides. Earplugs are not watertight seals and do not prevent water entry into the canal. They also may abrade the skin of the canal. Sealing agents (such as petrolatum-coated earplugs) and water repellents (such as silicone and artificial waxes) that coat the canal do not adequately protect it and merely add to the debris in the canal.

If self-medication is useful, symptoms begin to resolve within 1 to 2 days. A physician should be consulted if symptoms persist or increase in severity, or if an adverse reaction to the medication occurs.

Ask the Consumer

Q. Do you have an earache? Is the pain persistent? Is it aggravated by chewing?

■ The most common causes of severe earache are furunculosis (boils), acute otitis externa (inflammation of the external canal) and acute otitis media (inflammation of the middle ear). Pain upon moving the auricle or pressure on the tragus indicates inflammation of the external canal and lessens the possibility of otitis media, though they may both be present. Acute otitis media is generally a more severe illness with associated fever and malaise.

Referred pain from the temporomandibular joint, situated in juxtaposition to the ear canal, often presents as earache that occurs only while chewing or moving the jaw. In this case, refer the person to a physician or dental surgeon. Pain may also be referred from carious molar teeth. Malignant tissue involving the ear, throat or nose can cause intractable earache. Mild pain is best relieved by oral analgesics rather than local anesthetic eardrops. The underlying condition should be treated as necessary.

Q. Have you had a cold or the flu? Was there any fever?

■ Acute otitis media generally follows a cold. Particularly in children less than age 5, viral upper respiratory tract infections cause nasal stuffiness, which results in eustachian tube dysfunction. This dysfunction leads to a poorly ventilated middle ear and an opportunity for microorganisms to flourish, causing acute otitis media. Since children are more susceptible to colds, 40 per cent of those who have had acute otitis media have recurrences. Any associated fever is a sign of an infectious process and the person should be referred to a physician. Analgesics and antipyretics may be advised for fever and pain.

Otic Products

Q. Have you been swimming in the past few days?

- "Swimmer's ear" (otitis externa) usually appears 2 to 3 days after swimming so people do not relate the earache to swimming. Pain upon moving the auricle and a history of swimming are good indicators of this condition. Propylene glycol and acetic acid drops are successful both in treating the acute stage and for prophylaxis (drops instilled in the ear after swimming). Diving can cause barotrauma (an excessive imbalance of the air pressure in the middle ear compared to the external ear) resulting in a ruptured eardrum.

Q. Is the ear itchy?

- Itching in the ear canal is generally associated with otitis externa. Scratching may abrade the skin, causing a secondary infection. People with this condition must avoid scratching. Burow's solution may help relieve pruritus, but corticosteroid (and antibiotic) eardrops may be necessary for complete relief.

Q. What was the appearance and amount of discharge, if any?

- Discharge from the ear can arise from the external auditory canal or the middle ear cavity. The discharge varies in character depending upon the source. Wax is rarely the discharge. Blood-stained or foul-smelling discharge always indicates physician referral, as carcinomas and head injuries may be present.

Q. Did the pain disappear suddenly after the discharge?

- A pus-like discharge results from a ruptured boil and is accompanied by sudden pain relief. A tenacious, purulent and sometimes blood-stained discharge accompanied by reduction in pain indicates an acute otitis media has erupted through a perforated tympanic membrane. In this case, moving the tragus will not produce pain, but the person typically will be ill after recovering from a cold. Referral to a physician is necessary. Antipyretic analgesics taken orally may be useful before seeing a physician. The individual must not attempt to clean the ear or use eardrops of any kind with a ruptured tympanic membrane.

Q. Has a permanently deaf ear started to discharge again?

- If consumers report that permanently deaf ears have started to run again, the lengthy duration of the hearing loss suggests they suffer from chronic otitis media. People do not complain of being ill or experiencing any pain. The scanty discharge contains mucus and pus. A physician should be consulted.

Q. How long has this symptom of decreased hearing been present?

- A gradual loss of hearing in the elderly may be caused by arteriosclerotic deafness. A sudden loss of hearing may be due to injury of the tympanic membrane, a plug of wax or a foreign object in the ear canal, severely inflamed otitis externa, or serous otitis media (glue ear) following inadequately treated acute otitis media.

Q. Have you taken or are you now taking any medications?

- Certain ototoxic drugs, such as the aminoglycosides (neomycin, gentamicin, kanamycin and others), quinine, salicylates, ethacrynic acid and furosemide can cause deafness. The effect of salicylates on hearing is reversible on discontinuation of the drug.

Q. Do you have ringing in your ears?

- Tinnitus—ringing, buzzing or hissing noises heard only by the individual—is common, yet difficult to treat. It may be a sign of irritation of the cochlear mechanism of the inner ear. Auditory hallucinations with psychic disturbances may be reported as voices, bells or other noises. A physician should be consulted. Salicylates, aminoglycosides, ethacrynic acid, furosemide, alcohol, nicotine, quinidine and quinine all have the potential to produce tinnitus. Advise individuals to discontinue use of salicylates, alcohol and nicotine and to see a physician about other ototoxic medications they might be taking.

Q. Have you experienced dizziness?

- If the person complains of dizziness with a whirling sensation, a physician should be consulted. This symptom generally indicates some irritation of the vestibular apparatus of the inner ear. Though rare, vertigo can be produced by wax pressing against the tympanic membrane. Some cases of otitis media may cause mild dizziness; again, a referral is necessary. Antivertigo drugs, such as dimenhydrinate, are not effective for all causes of vertigo.

References

Anatomy and Physiology

Ballanger JJ, ed. Diseases of the nose, throat, ear, head and neck. Philadelphia: Lea & Febiger, 1985:877-1285.

Birrell JF, McDowall GD, McKay K, et al. Logan Turner's diseases of the nose, throat and ear. Chicago: Year Book Medical Publishers, 1977:247–387.

Bull PD. Lecture notes on diseases of the ear, nose and throat. Boston: Blackwell Scientific, 1985:1–67.

De Weese DD, Saunders WH. Textbook of otolaryngology. St Louis: CV Mosby, 1982:253–374.

English GM. Otolaryngology: a textbook. Hagerstown: Harper & Row, 1976:6–194.

Friedmann I. Pathology of the ear. London: Blackwell Scientific, 1974:3–27.

Koda-Kimble MA, Katcher BS, Young LY, eds. Applied therapeutics for clinical pharmacists. San Francisco: Applied Therapeutics, 1978:434.

Common Problems of the Auricle

Arevalo R. Ear piercing hazard of nickel-gold (Letter). N Engl J Med 1974;291:634.

Berkow R. The Merck manual of diagnosis & therapy. Rahway: Merck Sharp & Dohme, 1977:1624-7.

Cockin J, Finan P, Powell M. A problem with ear piercing. Br Med J 1977;2:1631.

Farb SN. Otolaryngology. Garden City: Medical Examiner, 1970:44–113.

Fisher AA. Ear piercing hazard of nickel-gold sensitization (Letter). JAMA 1974;228:1226.

Lazar P. Viral hepatitis prevention in ear piercing. JAMA 1975;223:1316.

Lovejoy FH Jr, Smith DH. Life-threatening staphylococcal disease following ear piercing. Pediatrics 1970;46:301–3.

Noble DA. Another hazard of pierced ears (Letter). Br Med J 1979;1:125.

Common External Auditory Canal Disorders

AMA drug evaluations. Chicago: American Medical Association, 1980;431–6.

Fed Reg 1977;42:63556–66.

Jahn AF, Hawke M. Otitis externa: a rationale for treatment. Can Fam Physician 1977;23:1388–90.

Jenkins BH. Otitis externa: prohylaxis and treatment. Eye, Ear, Nose, Throat Monthly 1964;43:47–50.

Jenkins BH. Simplified approach to otitis externa. Arch Otolaryngol 1963;77:442–3.

Jobbins D. Otitis externa. Aust Fam Physician 1986;15(6):720–6.

Otic Products

Salmon AL. Rational therapy for common ear disorders. Aust Fam Physician 1986;15(6):741–6.

Schuknecht HF. Pathology of the ear. Cambridge: Harvard University Press, 1974:215–20.

Seneca H, Avakian S. Antibacterial and antifungal spectrum of 1,2-propanediol diacetate. Antimicrob Agents Chemother 1961:807–10.

Smyth GD, Diagnostic ENT. London: Oxford University Press, 1978:22–7.

Stell PM, Pracy R, Siegler J. A short textbook, ear, nose and throat. London: English University Press, 1971:1.

Common Middle Ear Disorders

Bernard PAM, Stenstrom RJ, Feldman W, et al. Randomized controlled trial comparing long-term sulfonamide therapy for ventilation tubes for otitis media with effusion. Pediatrics 1992;88:215–22.

Bernstein JM. Recent advances in otitis media with effusion. Ann Allergy 1985;55(4):544–51.

Bluestone CD. Recent advances in the pathogenesis, diagnosis, and management of otitis media. Pediatr Clin North Am 1981;28:727–55.

Bluestone CD. Management of otitis media in infants and children: current role of old and new antimicrobial agents. Pediatr Infect Dis J 1988;7:S129–36.

Bluestone CD, Klein JO. Management. In: Bluestone CD, Klein JO, eds. Otitis media in infants and children. Philadelphia: Saunders, 1988:121–201.

Bluestone CD. Update on antimicrobial therapy for otitis media and sinusitis in children. Cutis 1985;36(5A):7–12.

Cantekin EI, Mandel EM, Bluestone CD, et al. Lack of efficacy of a decongestant-antihistamine combination for otitis media with effusion ("secretory" otitis media) in children. N Engl J Med 1983;308:297–301.

Conn HF. Conn's current therapy. Philadelphia: WB Saunders, 1982:116–9.

DeSanto LW, Stickler GB. Acute otitis media in children. Postgrad Med 1969;45(5):210–5.

Ghaffer A, Feldman W, Dolovich J. Otitis media in children. Can Fam Physician 1981;27:1399–402.

Gold R. Otitis media: current treatment controversies. Drug Ther 1988;18:26–31.

Grundfast KM. A review of the efficacy of systemically administered decongestants in the prevention and treatment of otitis media. Otolaryngol Head Neck Surg 1981;89:432–9.

Lisby-Sutch SM, Nemec-Dwyer MA, Decter RG, Gaur SM. Therapy of otitis media. Clin Pharm 1990;9:15–34.

McCracken GH. Selection of antimicrobial agents for treatment of acute otitis media with effusion. Pediatr Infect Dis J 1987;6:985–8.

McCracken GH. Management of acute otitis media with effusion. Pediatr Infect Dis J 1988;7:442–5.

Olson AL, Klein SW, Charney E, et al. Prevention and therapy of serous otitis media by oral decongestant: a double-blind study in pediatric practice. Pediatrics 1978;61:679–84.

Paradise JL. Otitis media in infants and children. Pediatrics 1980;65:917–43.

Riding KH, Bluestone CD, Micheals RH, et al. Microbiology of recurrent and chronic otitis media with effusion. J Pediatr 1978;93:739–43.

Rowe DS. Acute suppurative otitis media. Pediatrics 1975;56:285–94.

Schwartz R, Rodriguez WJ, Kahn WN, et al. Acute purulent otitis media in children older than 5 years; incidence of Haemophilus as a causative organism. JAMA 1977;238:1032–3.

Swartz MN. Infections due to mycoplasma. In: Rubenstein E, Federman D, eds. Scientific American medicine. New York: Scientific American, 1978:xii-3.

Vaughan VC, McKay RJ, Nelson WE. Nelson textbook of pediatrics. Philadelphia: WB Saunders, 1979:1182–8.

Anti-infectives

Dadagian AJ, Hicks JJ, Ordonez GE, et al. Treatment of otitis externa: a controlled bacteriological-clinical evaluation. Curr Ther Res 1974;16:431–6.

Ochs IL. Use of vinegar as an antibiotic in the treatment of chronic middle ear disease. Arch Otolaryngol 1951:935–41.

Osol A, Chase GD, Gennaro AR, et al, eds. Remington's pharmaceutical sciences. Easton: Mack Publishing, 1986.

Osol A, Pratt R, Gennaro AR. The United States dispensatory. Philadelphia: JB Lippincott, 1980.

Reynolds JEF, ed. Martindale: the extra pharmacopoeia. London: Pharmaceutical Press, 1982.

Windholz M, Budvari S, Stroumtsos L, et al. The Merck Index. Rahway: Merck Sharp & Dohme, 1976.

Analgesics and Local Anesthetics

Bandmann HJ, Calnan C.D, Cronin E, et al. Dermatitis from applied medicaments. Arch Dermatol 1972;106:335–7.

Rudzki E, Kleniewsak D. The epidemiology of contact dermatitis in Poland. Br J Dermatol 1970;83:543–5.

Humectants and Solvents

Anonymous. Wax in the ear. Br Med J 1972;4:623–4.

Emollients and Cerumenolytics

Chapu de Saintonage DM, Johnstone CL. A clinical comparison of triethanolamine polypeptide oleate condensate eardrops with olive oil for the removal of impacted wax. Br J Clin Pract 1973;27:454.

Harris PG. Solvents for ear wax (Letter). Br Med J 1968;4:775.

Instilling Eardrops

Smith DL. Medication guide for patient counselling. Philadelphia: Lea & Febiger, 1981.

Aural Hygiene

Anonymous. Swimmers' ears. Br Med J 1974;3:213.

Hutchinson JL, Wright DN. Prophylaxis of predisposed otitis externa. Ann Otol Rhinol Laryngol 1975;84:16–21.

Strauss MB, Grover-Strauss W, Cantrell RW. Swimmer's ear. Physician Sports Med 1979;7:101–5.

11
Oral Hygiene

Linda G. Suveges

The mouth and teeth are subject to numerous disorders, including dental caries, periodontal diseases, cold sores, canker sores, candidiasis, bad breath and dry mouth. Treatment must usually be provided by a dentist or physician. The pharmacist can supply information on the causes, signs and symptoms of these disorders and on preventive oral hygiene. Oral hygiene products include toothbrushes, dental floss, oral fluoride supplements, dentifrices, plaque disclosing agents, mouthwashes, fluoride mouthrinses and toothache relievers. Products are also available for cold sores and canker sores, dry mouth and denture care.

The oral health status of children in Canada and the United States appears to be generally better than that of children in other highly industrialized countries. However, dental caries or tooth decay remains the most prevalent disease among all age groups beyond infancy. Ninety-five per cent of the North American population experiences carious lesions, a frequency that has major economic and health implications. However, the combination of systemic and topical fluorides contributes to fewer dental caries: in 1979–1980, 49 per cent of 9 year old children had cavities in their permanent teeth; 71 per cent had such decay in 1971 to 1973. A 1985 study of 13 year olds in Alberta showed a further 35 per cent reduction in the number of decayed, missing or filled teeth compared to a similar group studied in 1978. In addition, the number of children whose teeth were caries-free increased from 7.5 per cent in 1978 to 24 per cent in 1985.

In adults, dental caries tend to stabilize and remain dormant until root surface caries begin to develop because of exposure of cementum from gum recession or surgery.

Periodontal diseases also afflict a significant portion of the adult population, although many causes are controllable and preventable. It has been commonly assumed that periodontal disease is the primary cause of tooth loss after age 35. However, recent studies indicate that caries, particularly in lower income individuals who have neglected their dental care, is a major reason for tooth extraction in adults. As the North American population ages and more people retain their teeth, the prevalence of periodontal diseases will remain high. Many people think that with increasing age, dentures are as inevitable as grey hair. However, natural dentition can be retained throughout a lifetime if there is proper and continuous attention to oral hygiene.

The oral cavity is also the site of conditions other than dental disease that may significantly affect an individual's overall health and welfare. These conditions include oral cancer, canker sores, cold sores and various other infections, as well as symptoms such as bad breath or dry mouth. In addition to dental practitioners, other health professionals such as pharmacists can contribute to oral health by advising consumers about appropriate self-care measures.

Anatomy and Physiology

The initial stages of food digestion are provided by mastication (chewing) and salivary secretion in the mouth. Various microorganisms make up the normal flora of the mouth; they create pathologic problems only when the host resistance is modified.

The inside of the mouth is covered by a specialized epithelial tissue called the mucosa. In its normal healthy state, the mucosa is pinkishred. It protects the underlying muscles, nerves and vascular bed from food materials and bacterial contamination. The soft gum tissue surrounding the teeth is the gingiva. It is normally coral pink, because of its keratin content. The gingiva forms sharp, well-defined points, or papillae, between the teeth. To a large extent, the teeth are not protected by any tissue.

Anatomically, the tooth has two parts—the crown and the root (see Figure 1). The crown is the part of the tooth normally completely exposed in the mouth and is responsible for mastication. The roots exist below the gingival line and are essential for support and attachment of the tooth to surrounding tissues.

The enamel covers the crown of the tooth and protects the underlying structures of dentin and pulp. Enamel is the hardest and most densely calcified tissue in the body. It is composed of crystals of a calcium phosphate compound known as hydroxyapatite. Unlike the enamel of certain animal teeth, human enamel cannot regenerate after injury or gradual loss. However, it is not an inert compound, as exchange and addition of ions can take place. This mechanism is the basis of the therapeutic application of fluoride ions, which replace hydroxy groups to form fluorapatite. This crystal is harder and more resistant to acid dissolution than hydroxyapatite. Characteristically, enamel is off-white in color, principally because of the underlying yellow dentin.

Dentin forms the bulk of the tooth. It is softer than enamel, but is a calcified tissue similar to bone. It helps to protect the pulp and also distributes nutrients from the pulp. The pulp is a delicate, highly vascular material, continuous with the surrounding tissues through

Oral Hygiene

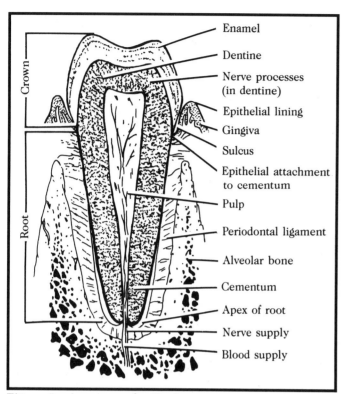

Figure 1 *Anatomy of a Tooth*

- Enamel
- Dentine
- Nerve processes (in dentine)
- Epithelial lining
- Gingiva
- Sulcus
- Epithelial attachment to cementum
- Pulp
- Periodontal ligament
- Alveolar bone
- Cementum
- Apex of root
- Nerve supply
- Blood supply

Crown

Root

an opening at the apex of the root. Any stimulus, such as pressure, heat or cold, to the free nerve endings in either the pulp or the dentin causes pain.

A cervical margin marks the joining of the root and crown of the tooth. The channel formed between the tooth and gingiva is the sulcus. Entrapment here of bacteria and debris must be minimized to prevent dental disease.

The root of the tooth is covered with a calcified tissue called cementum. The tooth is attached in its socket in the alveolar bone by periodontal ligaments. During mastication, the tooth can move slightly because of the elasticity of these fibres, but remains firmly in place in the dental arch. Collectively, the periodontium is made up of the cementum, periodontal ligament, alveolar bone and gingiva.

Normally, people are provided with two sets of teeth—primary or deciduous dentition, and permanent dentition. The deciduous teeth, commonly referred to as milk or baby teeth, begin to appear about 6 months after birth and are generally complete by the time the child is 24 to 30 months old. The first tooth to erupt is usually one of the mandibular or lower central incisors. This is followed by the fairly rapid and continuous eruption of the remaining primary teeth until the maxillary or upper second molars complete the dentition. There are 20 primary teeth, 10 in each arch. Generally, the first of the 32 permanent teeth to appear is the lower first molar, behind the primary second molar, at about 6 years of age. In some children the lower central incisors are the first permanent teeth to appear. Shedding a deciduous tooth is largely caused by root resorption stimulated by contact with the erupting permanent tooth beneath it. The permanent teeth are usually in place by age 13 except for the third molars (wisdom teeth), which usually erupt between 17 and 21 years of age.

Calcification of the crowns of the teeth begins about the fourth month of gestation and continues until a child is 7 or 8 years of age. Consequently, various environmental influences, such as inadequate nutrition or the ingestion of toxic substances, may be manifest only after tooth eruption. The relationship between light-yellow to grey-brown pigmentation of dental enamel and the ingestion of tetracycline during tooth development is firmly established. The nature of the staining depends on the form, dosage and duration of tetracycline administration. The stains darken after tooth eruption. The use of tetracycline by pregnant women or children up to the age of 8 years is not recommended.

Other oral and extraoral tissues of the head and neck may be involved in certain pathological processes. The tongue is important in mastication, speech, taste and swallowing. Its upper surface is usually irregular and rough in appearance. Taste buds are located in or around various papillae or projections on the tongue. The salivary glands in the mouth secrete saliva. Saliva is an alkaline, slightly viscous, clear secretion containing several components including enzymes, serum albumin, mucopolysaccharides, leukocytes and minerals. Normal salivary function is essential for good oral health.

Dental Caries
Etiology and Pathophysiology

Dental caries is the disease process involving the dissolution of tooth enamel, dentin and cementum, leading to the development of cavities. Formation of dental caries requires the presence and growth of cariogenic bacteria on the tooth surface. Caries susceptibility also depends on other factors such as diet, saliva composition and flow, tooth placement and the physicochemical nature of the tooth surface. Recent evidence also suggests that environmental factors such as reduction of ultraviolet light exposure may contribute to increased caries susceptibility. Systemic disorders such as bulimia may also increase the incidence of dental caries in affected individuals.

When host resistance is modified, the normal flora of the mouth may create pathologic problems. Some of these microorganisms, especially *Streptococcus mutans* and lactobacilli are cariogenic.

The pathophysiology of dental caries begins with the demineralization of tooth enamel by acid produced during fermentation of carbohydrates by the bacteria resident in dental plaque. Plaque is thought to start with formation of an acquired pellicle or protein coating that adheres to the clean tooth surface; saliva is a possible source. Bacteria and other components attach to the pellicle and tooth surface, forming a sticky mass called plaque. The high concentration of bacteria in plaque and its gel-like structure lead to acid accumulation at the tooth surface and a rapid fall in pH to a level at which demineralization can occur. Plaque also prevents the washing and buffering effects of saliva from reaching the tooth surface, thereby further enhancing caries production. Plaque also forms on dental restorations, appliances and dentures. Left unchecked, plaque thickens with food residues and proliferating bacteria. If not removed within 24 hours, plaque calcifies into calculus (tartar), which can only be removed by professional dental cleaning. Low accumulations of dental plaque are associated with significantly fewer dental caries, even in the adult population.

Not all enamel surfaces have the same potential for plaque formation and dental decay. Occlusal (top) surfaces of the molars and interproximal surfaces between the molars develop caries most often.

For caries to develop, a carbohydrate substrate must be present in the mouth. Hence, an individual's diet is thought to be an important

Oral Hygiene

determinant of susceptibility to dental decay, although one report has suggested that the link between sugar consumption and dental decay is not strong.

Carbohydrate-containing foods differ in their cariogenic potential. Those with a high concentration of sucrose are strongly cariogenic because of rapid solubilization and fermentation to acids. The amount of sucrose ingested also influences the number of cariogenic bacteria able to colonize on tooth surfaces. When dietary intake of sucrose is limited, *Streptococcus mutans* colonizes only in small numbers. Because the average North American man, woman or child consumes over one kilogram of sucrose per week, dental caries remains a significant health problem. Much of this sugar is consumed in commercially prepared foods of all types.

Other sugars such as fructose (in fruits and corn syrup) and lactose (in milk) are also cariogenic, but much less so than sucrose. As well, starchy foods that adhere to the teeth may lead to dental caries because of prolonged availability for acid formation. The cariogenic potential of snack foods that contain fermentable carbohydrates and are also sticky, such as raisins and chewy granola bars, is greater than that of chocolate candy bars or aged cheddar cheese. However, high sugar concentrations also stimulate more rapid removal of carbohydrates from the tooth environment. Thus, breakfast cereal that is not sugar coated is actually retained in the mouth longer than sugar-coated cereal. The carbohydrate content of a particular food may therefore be a more important contributor to its cariogenic potential than has been generally believed. Some foods, such as milk, cocoa and peanuts, have cariostatic effects. Their presence in a food item may therefore also modify its cariogenic potential.

Although sucrose has long been implicated as a major factor in tooth decay, the relative cariogenicity of foods depends on variations in composition, solubility, retentiveness and ability to stimulate saliva flow. The cariogenic potential of foods also depends on the frequency and timing of eating those foods. Individuals who do not eat between meals have fewer decayed teeth than those who snack frequently. In part, this effect occurs because stimulated saliva, produced at mealtimes, has a greater buffering capacity for acid. In addition, the increased flow of saliva reduces the contact time of carbohydrates with the teeth.

After primary teeth erupt, some children who are bottle-fed for extended periods, especially while lying down, may also develop extensive caries of the upper incisors. This condition, "nursing bottle syndrome," can be largely prevented by avoiding the use of milk-containing or juice-containing bottles as pacifiers.

Children who require long-term therapy with a sugar-containing liquid medication are at increased risk of developing dental caries. Ingesting such medication should be followed by correct toothbrushing or at least by rinsing the mouth thoroughly with water.

Although the human preference for sweets appears innate, it can be modified greatly by environmental factors such as restricting sugar consumption from birth. Enamel decay is most common in young persons, reaching a peak between 11 and 18 years of age. Unfortunately, children and adolescents are in the group that finds sugary foods most attractive and may resist diet modification.

Some nutritive sweetening agents, such as the sugar alcohols mannitol, sorbitol and xylitol, are less susceptible to rapid acid production by oral microorganisms, and therefore have lower cariogenic potential. These agents are used as sweeteners in a number of sugarless gums and candies. They satisfy cravings for sweet foods while

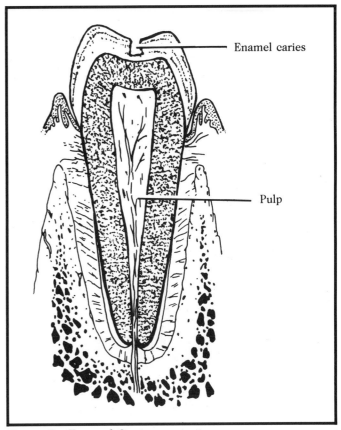

Figure 2 *Enamel Caries*

lowering the opportunity for plaque formation and caries development. In addition, chewing xylitol or sorbitol-containing gum after consuming sugary snacks may lessen the cariogenicity of such foods by stimulating saliva flow and delivering the saliva to interproximal areas of the teeth by mechanical action. The chewing of such gum for 10 minutes after consuming acidogenic foods is sufficient to return plaque pH to levels present before eating. Chewing xylitol-containing gum 3 times daily as part of a Canadian school-based dental program has also been shown to reduce the progression of dental decay over 24 months in children 8 to 9 years of age.

Other noncariogenic sweeteners include saccharin and cyclamates, but concerns exist for their safety in long-term use. Aspartame appears to be a safe and noncariogenic sugar-substitute.

Symptoms

The demineralization of a tooth's enamel surface by acids produced by bacteria in dental plaque is chronic. Initially, a carious lesion exhibits no clinical symptoms and is difficult to detect without close examination with specific diagnostic instruments (see Figure 2). Once the demineralization progresses through the enamel to the softer dentin, destruction is much more rapid and may produce a large cavity beneath only a small break in the enamel (see Figure 3). At this point the individual may become aware of the lesion and complain of toothache. Any stimulus, such as heat, cold or percussion, to the affected tooth elicits pain. The quality of the pain—sharp, stabbing, dull or pulsating—indicates the proximity of the decay process to the dental pulp. Progression of the carious damage to the pulp produces continuous, often excruciating, pain.

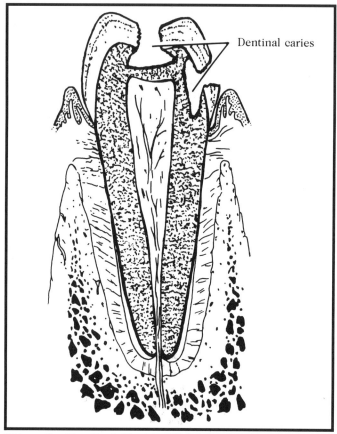

Figure 3 *Dentinal Caries—Pulpitis*

When a carious lesion is left untreated, infection of the pulp with bacteria elicits an inflammatory response, or pulpitis. Eventually, the opening at the apex of the root can become occluded and infection may spread to the periodontal ligament and bone (see Figure 4). Such abscess formation can create a variety of signs and symptoms, including severe pain, edema and erythema of tissue around the tooth, or massive cellulitis and facial swelling. Some people may develop septicemia from untreated dental caries.

Other symptoms, such as bleeding and bad breath, more often relate to poor oral hygiene and periodontal disease than to dental caries.

Treatment

Once the caries process is initiated it cannot be reversed. It can be arrested by removing the external causes. Because the sequelae of dental decay are loss of enamel and bacterial infection of underlying tissue, the treatment of choice is removing the infected hard tissue and filling the cavity with an inert material that restores the shape and function of the tooth. Such restorative treatment by a dentist is usually sufficient to relieve any associated pain. However, if the individual cannot receive such treatment immediately, nonprescription oral analgesics such as acetylsalicylic acid, acetaminophen or ibuprofen may help. Adult doses of 650 to 1,300 mg of ASA or acetaminophen or 200 to 400 mg of ibuprofen are suggested. (See the chapter on internal analgesics for more detail.) In addition, an obtundent, such as benzocaine, applied to the cavity may help reduce the pain until dental treatment is received.

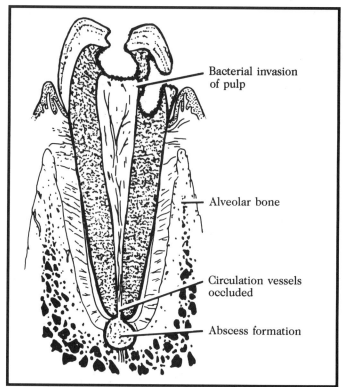

Figure 4 *Advanced Caries with Pulp Necrosis and Abscess Formation*

Because dental caries can eventually cause loss of tooth vitality and abscess formation, a pharmacist should encourage all people seeking nonprescription medication for toothache relief to see a dentist as soon as possible. They should also avoid any stimuli such as sweet, hot or cold substances, which may precipitate or aggravate pain.

Prevention

Most dental caries can be prevented. These factors must be present for dental caries to occur: a susceptible tooth; bacteria in dental plaque that can produce acids from carbohydrates; and fermentable carbohydrates in the diet. Hence, measures to prevent caries focus on attempts to increase resistance of the teeth with fluorides and fissure sealants, to lower the number or cariogenicity of bacteria in contact with teeth by mechanical means or chemical agents, and to modify dietary patterns to reduce the amount and frequency of carbohydrate ingestion.

The prospects for reducing dental caries by altering the dietary habits of the public are not promising. Although the relationship between sugar and caries activity is accepted, significant reductions in sugar intake have not occurred. Perhaps the most practical recommendations a health professional can make are to suggest that sugary and starchy foods be restricted to meals, and the teeth be brushed promptly after all meals or snacks. If brushing is not possible, chewing a sugarless gum for 10 minutes after eating may help reduce the potential for caries development.

Fluoride

The use of fluoride in various forms continues to be the most effective way to prevent dental caries. Delivery methods include systemic

Oral Hygiene

ingestion of fluoridated water or fluoride tablets and topical application via various gels, varnishes, mouthrinses or dentifrices.

The fluoride ion exerts its anticaries effects through several mechanisms. When it first touches the enamel surface, the fluoride ion combines to form calcium fluoride. In addition, it slowly replaces hydroxyl groups in hydroxyapatite to form fluorapatite. The latter is a denser, less soluble crystal that has a greater resistance toward acid. Fluoride ions are also antibacterial, particularly toward *Streptococcus mutans*, and may also remineralize early or incipient caries.

The method of fluoride therapy determines its effectiveness to a certain extent (see Table I). However, widespread availability of fluorides from various sources and the geographic mobility of society today has made it increasingly difficult to conduct additional research on the effectiveness of a single type of fluoride treatment. Perhaps the most important element in dental treatment is the frequent application of low concentrations of fluoride to the tooth and to dental plaque.

Table I *Effectiveness of Various Methods of Administering Fluorides*

Method	Concentration of dose	Percentage reduction in dental cares
Community water fluoridation	0.7–1.2 ppm	50–65
School water fluoridation	4.5 times optimum above	40
Dietary fluoride (F) supplements		
Home	Depends on age of child and F concentration in water	50–65
School only	2.2 mg NaF	30–35
Mouthrinses	0.05% NaF (daily) 0.20% NaF (weekly)	20–50
Dentifrices	0.40% SnF$_2$ 0.76% MFP 0.22% NaF	20–30
Professionally applied applications	2.0% NaF 8.0% SnF$_2$ APF (1.2% F)	30–40

NaF = sodium fluoride
SnF$_2$ = stannous fluoride
MFP = monofluorophosphate
APF = acidulated phosphate fluoride
Adapted from: Horiwitz HS. The prevention of oral disease. Established methods of prevention. Br Dent J 1980;149:311–8.

Over the past 40 years, much controversy has developed around the idea of community water fluoridation. A large body of research has found fluoride to be a safe and effective method of preventing the major health problem of dental caries. Careful analysis of epidemiologic data from fluoridated and nonfluoridated communities have consistently concluded that fluoride does not increase mortality due to heart disease, cancer or other specific diseases. No congenital malformations are associated with ingesting fluoridated water during pregnancy.

Recently, the widespread availability of fluoride ions in the environment and the increased use of fluoride-containing oral health products has led to concern regarding the risk of excessive exposure to fluoride. Over-exposure to fluoride ion can lead to both dental and skeletal fluorosis. Suggestions on controlling these risks include changes in optimal fluoride concentrations of water and the development of dentifrices with lower fluoride levels, especially for children.

Plaque Removal Products

Mechanical removal of dental plaque is probably the most well known method of caries prevention. If dental plaque is periodically dispersed and the bacteria prevented from becoming sufficiently established, the incidence of periodontal disease as well as dental caries is reduced. Aids available for plaque removal include toothbrushes, dental floss, disclosing agents, toothpicks and other devices. To clean the enamel surface completely, a mild abrasive is also usually necessary. Most dentifrices contain abrasives of varying properties. Chewing gum, rinsing the mouth with water or eating fibrous foods such as celery, carrots or apples does not remove plaque.

A wide variety of **toothbrushes** is commercially available. The selection of a toothbrush should take into account the individual's manual dexterity, oral anatomy and periodontal health. Prime functional properties of toothbrushes are flexibility, softness and diameter of the bristles, as well as the strength, rigidity and lightness of the handle.

For general adult use, multi-tufted brushes with soft, rounded nylon bristles are probably the best choice. The number of tufts per brush may vary. Brushes with 3 or 4 rows of 10 to 12 tufts or clusters of bristles are the most common. Four-row brushes tolerate increased pressure with flexing of the filaments; 2 or 3 row brushes, especially those with soft bristles, wear out the quickest. Brushes with tufts arranged in a V-shape are no better at plaque removal than straight, multi-tufted brushes.

Unless recommended by a dental practitioner, the use of hard-bristled brushes should be avoided. Although some practitioners report that more complete plaque removal is possible with hard-bristled brushes, other research suggests that soft brushes remove plaque more effectively. In addition, hard brushes can damage the gingiva, causing the gums to bleed, or to recede, exposing the cementum.

No official standard exists for use of the terms "soft" and "hard" in describing toothbrushes. Brands may vary in the bristle diameter and length that constitutes a "soft" brush. The experience of the user and dental practitioner may be the best guide for appropriate choice of a toothbrush for regular use.

Brushes with natural hog bristles are also available, but tend to be less durable. The bristles may loosen and become lodged in the gingiva and oral mucosa.

Handle shape varies among toothbrushes. Since there is no ideal handle shape, choice is a personal preference. Straight handles are the most common. Whatever shape is chosen, the handle should be long enough to fit comfortably into the hand. Dentists may recommend brushes specially adapted for certain user characteristics, such as an angled handle to reach posterior dental areas or bristles of different lengths for orthodontic appliances.

Children should use a toothbrush with a small head and a thick handle for ease of manipulation. Adults who gag easily may also find a child's brush, or one with a smaller head, more useful than an ordinary toothbrush.

Oral Hygiene

Worn toothbrushes do not remove plaque effectively. Toothbrushes should be replaced when they begin to show signs of matting or wear. This usually occurs after 3 months of daily use, but this time period may vary according to individual brushing technique and frequency of use. Most studies show that people do not replace toothbrushes as frequently as they should to achieve optimal plaque removal.

The proper frequency and method of brushing for optimal oral health have not been well established. Suggestions for toothbrushing frequency range from 5 times daily to once every other day. Once-daily brushing should be a minimum recommendation because *Streptococcus mutans* requires at least 24 hours to organize on a clean tooth; however, about 60 per cent of plaque may remain after daily brushing, lending support for more frequent and thorough brushing. The longer plaque remains undisturbed, the greater its pathogenic potential. Many dental practitioners recommend twice daily brushing to promote good oral health.

Thoroughness of brushing, without trauma, is more important than method of brushing. No one method of brushing has been proven superior to others in removing plaque. Individuals may need instructions in different brushing techniques to remove plaque completely. The scrub technique using short back-and-forth brush strokes is the most popular method of brushing and requires the least time. It may be the easiest method for children to learn and use, but may not remove plaque from the gingival sulcus. Although children should be encouraged to develop good preventive habits such as tooth-brushing at an early age, it is suggested an adult clean a child's teeth once daily to ensure complete plaque removal until the child has mastered the technique.

A brushing method developed by Bass is currently the method most often recommended by dentists and dental hygienists. In the Bass method, the bristles of the brush are placed at a 45° angle to the tooth, covering about 6 mm of the gingiva above the crown of the tooth. The brush is then vibrated gently and swept away from the gingiva as it is lifted to the next tooth area. With this placement of the brush, the bristles actually displace the marginal gingiva and reach the base of the healthy sulcus (about 3 mm depth), thoroughly removing plaque. Consumers should also be instructed to brush the areas behind the back molars, the occlusal (top) tooth surfaces and perhaps the upper surface of the tongue to remove plaque.

Professional advice on recommended brushing times range from 3 to 7 minutes. Consumers may significantly overestimate the time spent brushing their teeth. Studies of actual brushing times show that people spend an average of 1 minute brushing their teeth. The use of a gel dentifrice fails to enhance toothbrushing time or thoroughness over that found with use of a conventional toothpaste. Although frequency and pattern of brushing affects children's plaque removal, duration of brushing produces the most significant effect on plaque removal. Smokers tend to have more plaque on their teeth, before and after brushing. This condition may be partly explained by their practice of brushing for shorter periods of time than nonsmokers, although other factors may also contribute to their poorer oral cleanliness.

Powered toothbrushes may benefit individuals with dexterity problems or those who brush longer because of the novelty of the item. However, for most people these brushes do not remove plaque any better than a manual toothbrush used correctly. A rotary electric toothbrush may remove plaque more effectively in adolescents undergoing orthodontic treatment with fixed appliances, but it is not more effective than manual brushing and flossing in patients with periodontal conditions. The routine use of water irrigating devices is recommended only as an adjunctive measure for oral hygiene, as these devices do not remove subgingival plaque and may cause bacteremia in people with periodontitis.

As the toothbrush has a limited efficacy for cleaning between the teeth, **dental floss** should also be used. Frequent interdental flossing reduces the incidence of proximal caries. Continued flossing for long periods increases the beneficial effect.

Dental floss is available from various manufacturers in waxed and unwaxed forms. Both types remove plaque effectively and improve oral health. No significant differences in physiologic effects have been found in recent studies comparing waxed to unwaxed dental floss. On smooth, planed tooth surfaces, four types of dental floss (unwaxed, waxed, lightly waxed and Superfloss) removed plaque equally well. Lightly waxed floss was significantly better at removing plaque from rough "unplaned" surfaces than the other three products. In other studies, Superfloss, a three-in-one product made up of unwaxed floss, a threader and a nylon brush, was not consistently superior to dental floss alone. **Dental tape** has been shown to remove proximal plaque as efficiently as waxed dental floss; patients may prefer dental tape over floss because of ease of use.

Some people may prefer unwaxed floss because it is thinner and easier to manipulate. Most consumers in a recent study preferred waxed floss, presumably because it may pass between tight-fitting teeth more easily than unwaxed floss and without shredding. Lightly waxed floss may combine the benefits of both types. Flavored dental floss (for example, mint) has also been shown to be preferable to plain waxed floss.

Flossing technique is important to remove plaque effectively. A length of floss is wound around the index finger of each hand and placed through the contact area of the teeth by gentle pressure with the thumbs. It is then guided into the gingival sulcus, flattened against the tooth surface and moved toward the crown of the tooth. The tooth surface above and below the gingival margin is cleaned before the floss is moved across the interproximal tissue to the adjacent tooth surface for similar cleaning. When the floss is removed from between the two teeth, the individual should check it and the gums for gingival bleeding, which indicates gingivitis and the need for more effective cleaning.

Children's teeth may be difficult to floss depending on the age of the child. Adults responsible for such a procedure may wish to floss only areas of the child's mouth where there is contact between adjacent teeth. They may also find knitting yarn or interproximal toothbrushes useful in removing plaque from surfaces where there are openings between teeth.

People with dexterity problems may find a floss holder easier to use. As well, floss may be passed interdentally by a floss threader in areas where contacts at the crowns of the teeth are too tight to prevent normal flossing techniques.

Other interdental cleaning devices include interdental brushes, rubber points and toothpicks. Interdental brushes appear to clean interdental areas where the papillae are missing better than dental floss. Dental floss removes plaque much better than toothpicks for most people, although combinations of these cleaning techniques with toothbrushing does improve oral health. The rubber tips found on some toothbrushes are designed to massage the gingiva, which allegedly enhances blood flow into the area, increasing oxygen delivery and removal of waste products. However, these devices should be used only on the advice of a dentist. Above all, proper instruction and motivation of the individual are essential for effective oral hygiene.

Several chemical agents—chlorhexidine, quaternary ammonium compounds, volatile oils, enzymes and herbal extracts—have been used as antiplaque treatments. The most widely studied agent for this purpose is chlorhexidine, which reduces caries activity because of its antibacterial effect on cariogenic bacteria in plaque. Other agents, such as cetylpyridinium chloride and the combination of volatile oils in Listerine, also show antiplaque activity, but have not been evaluated for caries prevention.

Periodontal Diseases

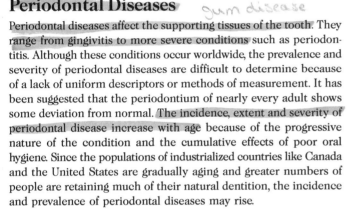

gum disease

Periodontal diseases affect the supporting tissues of the tooth. They range from gingivitis to more severe conditions such as periodontitis. Although these conditions occur worldwide, the prevalence and severity of periodontal diseases are difficult to determine because of a lack of uniform descriptors or methods of measurement. It has been suggested that the periodontium of nearly every adult shows some deviation from normal. The incidence, extent and severity of periodontal disease increase with age because of the progressive nature of the condition and the cumulative effects of poor oral hygiene. Since the populations of industrialized countries like Canada and the United States are gradually aging and greater numbers of people are retaining much of their natural dentition, the incidence and prevalence of periodontal diseases may rise.

Etiology and Pathophysiology

Bacterial plaque is the single most important external etiologic agent in inflammation of the periodontium. As plaque accumulates on the tooth at the gingival margin, it produces an inflammatory reaction in the gingivae called gingivitis. The bacteria resident in dental plaque produce various metabolic compounds, which are secreted into the gingival sulcus, activating host defence mechanisms. These metabolic products, rather than the microorganisms themselves, are thought to be responsible for the inflammatory changes in the periodontium. Further immunologic response within the gingivae enhances the destruction of the support tissue. As long as the bacterial plaque is left undisturbed, the inflammatory response continues. Eventually, alveolar bone may begin to break down and the teeth may become loose and fall out.

Although subgingival calculus does not initiate the inflammatory process, its presence can contribute to the chronicity and progression of periodontal disease. Calculus is porous enough to serve as a basis for further plaque growth. It also promotes retention of bacterial antigens and inflammatory mediators in the gingival area. Because calculus cannot be removed by normal toothbrushing, individuals must see a dentist regularly to have calculus removed from teeth.

Limited evidence suggests an association between smokeless tobacco use and gingival recession, but further research is needed on how this contributes to periodontal disease or dental caries.

The long-standing assumption that gingivitis inevitably progresses to destructive periodontitis has been challenged. Some data suggest other host-related factors may be necessary to develop severe periodontitis.

Symptoms

Healthy gingival tissue is coral pink, firm and adheres closely to the neck of the tooth. Periodontal disease begins as a marginal inflammation of the gums. The gingivae appear dark red and glossy and the interdental papillae become blunted and lose resiliency. At this stage the individual is usually unaware of the disease process, which may affect only part of the gingivae. When the disease involves most of the gum tissue, it is termed diffuse gingivitis.

As with dental caries, periodontal disease is usually a progressive or chronic disorder. Pain is not a feature until symptoms and tissue destruction are advanced. People most often complain about bleeding from the gums when they brush their teeth or chew hard foods. They may also complain about an offensive mouth odor.

The rate the disease intensifies depends on the individual's oral hygiene and oral habits. For example, mouth-breathing aggravates the symptoms around the anterior teeth due to a constant drying-wetting action. As the disease progresses to involve the rest of the periodontium, alveolar bone is resorbed and tooth attachment compromised. This stage of the disease is called periodontitis. Loss of gingival support and recession of tissue results in formation of "pockets" around the tooth, which may bleed or exude pus. The latter accounts for the outmoded term "pyorrhea" used to describe periodontal disease. The individual may feel pain at this stage when drinking hot or cold fluids or when brushing the teeth because of stimulation of the now-exposed cementum.

Eventually, the teeth become loose and bacteria may invade the support tissue, causing an acute periodontal abscess or acute periodontitis to develop. The individual can usually pinpoint the site by symptoms of deep, throbbing or radiating pain. Prognosis for teeth with advanced bone loss, extreme mobility and recurrent abscess formation is poor. The usual treatment is extraction.

Although gingivitis is more often chronic in nature, acute forms of the condition do occur. One of these, acute necrotizing ulcerative gingivitis (ANUG), also termed Vincent's stomatitis and trench-mouth, is characterized by extremely sensitive, bleeding gingival tissue. The interdental and marginal gingivae are covered with a necrotic, greyish pseudomembrane. When the necrotic tissue is removed with gauze, a painful, crater-like ulceration, which bleeds spontaneously or when touched, may be present. The individual may also complain of an offensive breath odor and a metallic taste as well as a wooden, dead or loose feeling in the teeth. Usually, fever and increased salivary secretion are associated with ANUG.

ANUG, seen most frequently in teenagers and young adults, seems to be associated with the presence of spirochete and fusiform organisms. Other predisposing factors may be anxiety and emotional stress, smoking, malnutrition and poor oral hygiene. Although it may resolve spontaneously, ANUG usually requires antibacterial therapy and a visit to the dental clinic to prevent septicemia or progressive destruction of the periodontium.

Acute gingivitis may also develop from the generally chronic course of periodontal disease as a result of physical irritation from such things as hard food particles, new or hard-bristled toothbrushes, toothpicks, hot foods or tobacco tars. The symptoms may vary from linear lacerations to eroded areas and vesicle formation.

Pregnancy gingivitis is an acute form of gingivitis usually confined to one or more sites on the gums. It is usually painless, but bleeding may occur. Inadequate oral hygiene is the primary cause of the condition, but the intensified tissue reaction is perhaps due to changes in hormone levels. Oral contraceptive use may also be associated with an increased incidence of gingivitis.

About 50 per cent of people taking phenytoin develop a condition called gingival hyperplasia within 2 to 3 months of the start of therapy. The first sign of this condition is usually enlargement of the interdental papillae, particularly in the front of the mouth. Gingival tissue may eventually cover the teeth, interfere with mastication and be esthetically unacceptable. Development of gingival hyperplasia from phenytoin does not seem to be dose-related, but is precipitated by poor oral hygiene. Surgery may be required to remove excess tissue even if the medication is discontinued.

Nifedipine and cyclosporine may also cause gingival hyperplasia in certain people. The condition can often be prevented by maintaining a high standard of oral hygiene, thus eliminating gingival irritation from such things as plaque. Pharmacists should advise all people taking these drugs about effective toothbrushing and flossing techniques.

Treatment

The most effective method of treating periodontal disease in all stages is to remove bacterial plaque. In the early stages of gingivitis, the disease process can be completely reversed by thoroughly cleaning the teeth every day to remove plaque. As periodontal disease progresses, more concentrated and sustained oral hygiene measures must be undertaken to control the disease and to limit the amount of destruction to the support tissue.

To begin and maintain an adequate program of oral hygiene may require guidance from dental practitioners and pharmacists in using preventive aids. The use of toothbrushes and dental floss are completely outlined in the section on dental caries prevention. Advanced periodontal disease may require surgical intervention and, in certain cases, systemic antibacterial therapy.

Nonprescription medications are generally of little use in treating periodontal disease. Products containing oxygenating agents, such as sodium perborate, zinc peroxide, hydrogen peroxide and carbamide (urea) peroxide in concentrations of 1 to 30 per cent have been promoted as adjunctive therapy. These products may be recommended by dentists for postoperative use or after other oral treatments. Any benefit derived from the use of oxygenating agents is thought to be due to loosening of adherent debris by the liberated oxygen. Long-term use of these agents may produce oral irritation or decalcification of teeth (due to the agents' acidity) and development of a black, hairy tongue. The use of sodium bicarbonate by individuals at home has not been shown to effectively treat periodontal disease. Because most studies on the use of sodium bicarbonate or hydrogen peroxide in periodontal therapy have also employed techniques such as root scaling and planing by the dental practitioner, the effectiveness of such adjunct therapy has been questioned.

Antibacterial mouthrinses may also be used to reduce plaque levels in individuals with periodontal disease, although they do not affect subgingival plaque found in periodontitis associated with deep pockets.

Prevention

Because periodontal diseases are closely associated with accumulations of dental plaque, reducing or removing plaque from the teeth and gingiva is the best way to prevent periodontal diseases. Gingival stimulation may play a role, but removing plaque from both hard and soft tissues is essential to prevent gingival inflammation.

Other Dental Problems
Dental Pain

Besides caries, dental pain may be caused by certain dental procedures, such as placing large restorations or fillings, or removing calculus. Both treatments may cause hypersensitive teeth.

Receding gingival tissue may expose the cementum or root of the tooth and create an area of hypersensitivity to certain stimuli. The major symptom of this condition is a short, sharp pain or shock elicited by cold food or beverages, cold air, sweet or sour substances, salt, touching the tooth surface with the fingernail or toothbrush, or, in some cases, closing the teeth together. The pain is usually transient and can be prevented by avoiding the stimuli or protecting the area with a desensitizing agent.

Individuals may also complain of a dull, mild, generalized pain in a number of maxillary teeth at the back of the dental arch. The cause of such pain is often infection in the maxillary sinuses (sinusitis). Sinusitis is most severe in the morning and is aggravated by bending over or going up and down stairs. It is less painful when lying down. The person may also describe symptoms such as tenderness, sensitivity to cold fluids, and pain when the teeth are clenched together. Mild analgesics may ease the discomfort of this type of dental pain, but complete relief requires medical assessment and proper antibiotic and decongestant therapy.

Another source of dental pain may be a tooth fracture, which may not be visually evident. The individual experiences a sudden, brief, unbearable, stabbing pain when chewing or when cold liquids contact the tooth. Avoiding such stimuli and promptly consulting a dentist are the only recommendations to give such people.

Vague tooth pain, especially in the early morning, may result from grinding the teeth together while sleeping or from an improperly contoured dental restoration. Nonprescription oral analgesics may help until the person can consult a dentist.

Dental Erosion

Although demineralization of tooth enamel is usually caused by acids produced by plaque-resident bacteria, teeth can be eroded by stomach acid when frequent vomiting occurs (for example, in bulimia) or by acidic substances taken orally. Chewing large numbers of vitamin C tablets regularly may also lower saliva pH sufficiently to cause tooth erosion. People who take chewable products containing vitamin C should use such products judiciously and, if possible, brush the teeth after chewing the product.

Broken Teeth or Misfitting Restorations

Broken teeth, besides being esthetically unappealing, can result in pulp exposure, pain, malocclusion and compromised mastication. Any break or chip in the natural dentition must be referred to a dentist for proper treatment. If a crown is chipped only slightly, restorative techniques may repair it. A large fracture may require root canal therapy or extraction. Occasionally a tooth that is knocked out, intact, from the dental arch can be reimplanted with prompt treatment. A dentist should be consulted immediately for appropriate instructions to ensure the greatest chance for possible reimplantation.

Lost or broken fillings and nonremovable prostheses such as crowns and bridges must also be evaluated and treated by a dental practitioner to prevent loss of normal function, discomfort and tooth breakdown.

Complete or partial dentures are removable prostheses used for

Figure 5 *Suggested Approach for Evaluating and Treating Dental Problems*

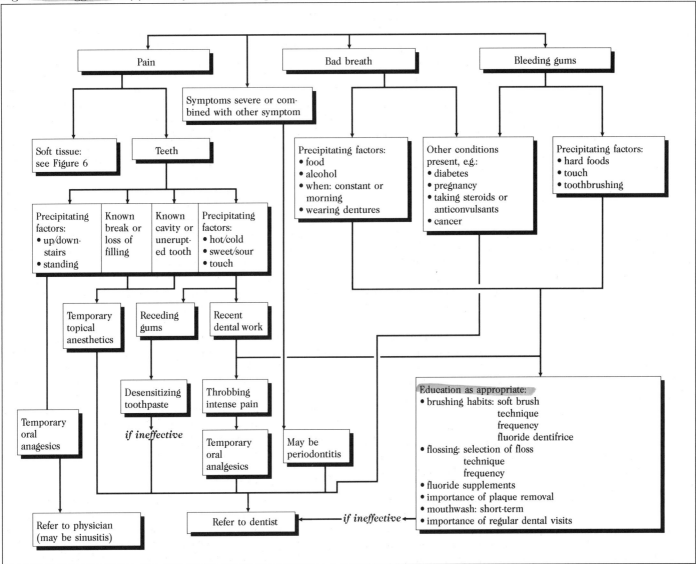

partial correction of the loss of natural dentition. Dentures modify oral tissue and, later, the anatomy and physiology of the oral cavity. As well, they may cause significant psychological effects. Wearing dentures satisfactorily requires the coordinated activity of the tongue and perioral musculature, as well as perseverance by the wearer and the clinician. To ensure maximal effectiveness, periodic professional attention is required. Although the time of useful service for a denture may be as low as 5 to 6 years, many denture wearers have had the same prostheses in place for much longer periods.

Ill-fitting or broken dentures can create several problems for the wearer, including accelerated bone loss with subsequent facial structure changes, ulceration, irritation, tumor growth and compromised oral function. Refitting, relining or repairing dentures to ensure proper functioning requires professional dental attention.

Common Oral Problems

Sore areas or ulcerations of the mouth affect about 20 to 50 per cent of the population. Although usually self-limiting, conditions such as canker sores or cold sores are painful, causing consumers to self-medicate. Other symptoms such as halitosis (bad breath) or xerostomia (dry mouth) are annoying and may also cause the consumer to try nonprescription treatments.

Cold Sores   *inherited*

The existence of disease caused by herpes simplex virus (HSV) has been known for at least 2,000 years. Despite identification of the virus in the 1940s and knowledge of its two varieties since 1960, developing effective treatment or preventive measures for herpes infections has been largely unsuccessful.

Etiology and Pathophysiology

Cold sores, or fever blisters, are usually caused by reactivation of latent herpes simplex virus Type I (HSV-I), although HSV-II has been

Oral Hygiene

Table II *Features for Differential Diagnosis of Canker Sores and Cold Sores*

	Primary herpes	Recurrent labial herpes	Recurrent aphthous ulcers
Etiology	*Herpes simplex* virus	*Herpes simplex* virus	Unknown; possibly hypersensitivity or *Streptococcus sanguis*
Predisposing factors	None	Fever; stress; trauma; sunlight; infection	Heredity; food/drug allergy; trauma; stress; physiological factors
Prodrome	Slight fever; malaise; cervical lymphadenopathy	Burning; tingling sensation	Burning; tingling sensation
Lesions	Multiple vesicles; large superficial ulcers; diffuse erythema; yellow membrane; gingival inflammation	Small papules and vesicles; red centre; yellow crust; labial swelling	Small, multiple, erosive lesions; yellow or gray membrane; erythematous halo
Location	Labial mucosa; buccal mucosa; tongue; gingivae	Mucocutaneous junction of lips and adjacent skin	Buccal mucosa; labial mucosa; tongue, soft palate
Symptoms	Fever; intense oral pain; increased salivation; halitosis	Fever (only with other illnesses); lip pain; salivation unaffected; breath unaffected	Usually no fever; intense oral pain; localized hyperesthesia

isolated from a few cases. Because the lesions commonly affect the lips or areas bordering the lips, cold sores are also known as recurrent herpes labialis (RHL). Although not as common, recurrent intraoral herpes (RIH) also occurs.

The peak incidence of primary infection with HSV-I is 6 to 36 months of age, but new cases appear in all age groups due to the contagious nature of the virus. An estimated 15 per cent of adults experience the primary infection. The disease is thought to be transmitted by direct contact, usually with an individual suffering from recurrent herpes labialis. Virus excretion persists in all body secretions for 15 to 42 days after the onset of the primary herpes infection. In most cases of primary oral herpes, symptoms are subclinical or cannot be distinguished from other viral infections. The remainder of people experience an acute gingivostomatitis during the primary infection.

After the primary infection has healed, effective immunity develops in some people, but 20 to 45 per cent have recurrent lesions. The virus apparently remains dormant in nerve cells until stimulated to reactivate. In North America, an estimated 7 per cent of the general population have 2 or more bouts of herpes labialis annually. Recurrences may be precipitated by a number of factors, including fever, emotional stress, physical trauma, sunlight, systemic infections and menses (see Table II). People whose resistance is compromised may experience more severe lesions with slower healing.

Symptoms

The onset of primary oral herpes infection is preceded by generalized systemic symptoms, including high fever, nausea, vomiting, headache and malaise for 1 to 2 days. Small vesicles that appear on the oral mucosa, tongue, lips or in the throat quickly rupture to form shallow round ulcers surrounded by inflammation. An important diagnostic feature is acute marginal gingivitis. The person may also experience severe pain when the lesions are touched, increased saliva flow, malodorous breath and swollen neck glands. Table II outlines the features of primary and recurrent herpes. Primary herpes infection is usually a self-limiting condition and lasts 10 to 14 days. The lesions heal without scarring.

Recurrent herpes labialis is often preceded for 24 to 48 hours by prodromal tingling, itching or burning of the lesion site (usually on

or near the lips). A cluster of small vesicles then appears, ruptures and crusts over to form the typical cold sore or fever blister. The base of the lesion is reddened and edematous. A yellow crust on older lesions may indicate bacterial superinfection. Cold sores generally last from 3 to 10 days and are rarely accompanied by systemic symptoms. Patients who experience frequent recurrences of RHL (such as an average of 3 recurrences within 6 months) may differ from the general population; those with frequent episodes may have multiple facial locations for their lesions.

The vesicles of RIH lesions break rapidly to form ulcers. These are typically 1 to 2 mm in diameter and cluster on the keratinized mucosa of the gingiva, palate or alveolar ridge.

Treatment

The treatment for acute herpetic gingivostomatitis is essentially symptomatic and supportive. Bed rest, adequate fluid maintenance and a soft diet supplemented by proteins are recommended. Oral analgesics such as acetylsalicylic acid, acetaminophen or ibuprofen, in recommended doses, may be required to relieve pain and fever. Severe pain not controlled by nonprescription analgesics may require use of an opiate derivative such as codeine. Because most primary herpes infections occur in children less than 6 years of age, sedation with diphenhydramine or prescribed agents may help.

Local therapy to ameliorate symptoms is also suggested. Cleansing mouthwashes with benzalkonium chloride 1:1,000, dilute hydrogen peroxide or a saline solution help clean and soothe involved mucous membranes. An appropriate saline solution can be prepared by dissolving 1/2 teaspoonful of table salt in 250 mL warm water.

Acute herpetic gingivostomatitis is one of the few conditions for which topical anesthetics are justified. Preparations containing benzocaine or lidocaine in vehicles that adhere to the oral mucosa, or that can be used as mouthrinses, are perhaps the most useful. The agents are applied as often as necessary to keep the individual comfortable, but should not be used long-term due to the possibility, although rare, of hypersensitivity. Oral lesions may also be covered with an adherent protective paste such as Orabase to relieve discomfort.

Recurrent herpes labialis is an annoying, cosmetically disfiguring
outside of lip

and uncomfortable condition for which consumers often seek a pharmacist's advice. Unfortunately, no treatment reliably shortens healing time or lowers the recurrence rate of cutaneous herpes simplex infections. Ice applied within 24 hours of the prodrome may abort a cold sore, although controlled study of this preventive method has not been undertaken. Anecdotal reports show that cold sore vesicles may be resorbed and completely healed in 1 to 2 days if ice is applied continuously for 45 to 60 minutes to the prodromal area. To be effective, this treatment must be instituted as soon as possible after the prodromal tingling or burning is noticed.

When cold sore lesions are vesicular, cool compresses with tap water or Burow's solution applied for 10 minutes 3 to 4 times daily can be used. Bland emollients such as AquaCare, Keri products or white petrolatum are recommended to prevent drying lesions from cracking or fissuring. Secondary bacterial infections can be prevented by applying a topical nonprescription antibiotic ointment. The use of caustic agents, such as phenol or silver nitrate, are contraindicated in cold sore therapy. When an attack is precipitated by sunlight, nonprescription sunscreen products may be recommended to prevent cold sore development, although some individuals may still experience reactivation of HSV. Oral acyclovir may prevent RHL during a brief, high-risk circumstance such as skiing.

Applying a topical corticosteroid to a cold sore for its anti-inflammatory action is controversial. Topical acyclovir, a prescription antiviral agent, has been shown to decrease virus titers in herpes labialis lesions if therapy is begun within 8 hours of the first signs of a lesion developing; healing time is not shortened. Oral or intravenous acyclovir may benefit immunocompromised individuals by promoting rapid healing of recurrent herpes lesions. Topical interferon applied during RHL eruptions has been shown to reduce recurrences and duration of lesions. Early application of idoxuridine in dimethylsulfoxide also appears to accelerate healing time of cold sores.

As outlined in Table III, many topical agents have not proven clearly useful for herpes labialis. Well controlled, double-blind studies have not been published for several products, such as those containing propolis 2 per cent and a combination of heparin with zinc sulfate.

Table III *Treatments Ineffective or Not Proven Clearly Useful in Herpes Labialis*

Ethyl ether	Alcohol
Chloroform	Lysine
Adenine arabinoside	Povidone-iodine
Vitamins C, E and B_{12}	Dye-light (photodynamic inactivation)
Lactobaccilus	Silver sulfadiazine
Zinc	2-deoxy-D-glucose

Canker Sores

Recurrent aphthous stomatitis (RAS) is a common disease characterized by painful oral ulcers, often called canker sores. Although it is one of the most common conditions for which people seek treatment, the course of RAS is essentially unaltered by modern medical and dental therapy. At least 20 per cent of the general population is affected, with women about twice as susceptible as men. RAS

can occur at any age but its incidence rises sharply after age 10. Susceptibility to RAS appears to be inherited, although the exact mode of genetic transfer has not yet been determined.

Etiology

Numerous etiologic factors for RAS have been suggested. These include hereditary predisposition, microbial agents, hypersensitivity, psychological factors, endocrine abnormalities, chemicals in food stuffs, trauma and foreign bodies. In particular, the pleomorphic, alpha-hemolytic *Streptococcus sanguis* may be partly responsible for canker sore development in predisposed individuals. These people seem to be hypersensitive to certain components of *Streptococcus sanguis*, although some reports do not substantiate this etiology. Most researchers have also implicated autoimmune mechanisms in the etiology of RAS. Herpes simplex virus has been ruled out as a causative factor.

Various endogenous precipitating factors have been associated with RAS (see Table II). Trauma from dental procedures, cheek-biting and hard foods commonly leads to canker sore development in susceptible people. Emotional stress and hormonal changes may also play a role for some individuals.

Deficiencies in cyanocobalamin, folic acid or iron have been reported for a small number of people. RAS may be associated with the presence of celiac disease. Consequently, dietary elimination of gluten has been suggested as a treatment. Certain other foods may precipitate or irritate canker sores, or may act as nutrients for oral streptococci. Smokers develop canker sores less frequently than do nonsmokers.

It has been suggested that RAS is caused by a complex interaction between host and environment. Apparently, a genetic component is required to establish susceptibility, but interaction with several environmental factors is essential for clinical expression.

Symptoms

RAS is characterized by painful recurrent ulcerations of the oral mucosa. Ulcers are most often found on nonkeratinized tissues of the mouth such as the buccal mucosa, lips, mucobuccal fold, tongue, floor of the mouth and soft palate. Aphthous lesions usually occur singly, although several areas of the mouth may be ulcerated simultaneously. Individuals may notice a prodromal burning or tingling sensation up to 24 hours before the ulcer appears. The lesion begins as a small macule, which enlarges and progresses to a shallow ulceration 3 to 10 mm in diameter. The ulcer is round or ovoid with sharply delineated margins surrounded by an intense erythematous halo. A gray or yellowish membrane covers the ulcer crater. Canker sores are extremely painful and may cause difficulty eating, talking, drinking or swallowing. Lesions generally persist for 7 to 14 days and heal slowly from the margins without scarring.

Treatment

Aphthous stomatitis therapy is aimed at controlling the pain, shortening the duration of lesions already present and aborting new lesions. Nondrug measures include rinsing the mouth with warm water, a saline solution (see the discussion of herpes labialis) or mouthwash as often as possible. Individuals should also avoid any known precipitating factors and irritating foods and remove any cause of trauma such as ill-fitting dentures (see Table IV).

Topical anesthetics applied as often as needed are useful in

Table IV	Foods to Avoid During an Attack of Aphthous Stomatitis	
Citrus fruits	Chocolate	Melons
Sour substances	Spices	Strawberries
Tomatoes	Vinegar	Walnuts

relieving canker sore pain. These agents should be applied to small areas only or a disturbing "cotton-mouth" feeling and total loss of taste results.

Coating the ulcers with protectants, such as emollient mixtures or denture-adhesives, often alleviates pain. Protectants may be particularly helpful if applied before eating or retiring for the night. Chlorhexidine gluconate mouthwash 0.2% used three times daily may shorten the number of days ulcers occur but it does not reduce the discomfort of lesions. Patients who experience frequent, large or numerous canker sores should be referred to a physician or dentist. Prescribed treatments for RAS include tetracycline compresses or mouthrinses, or topical corticosteroids in an emollient base (for example, Kenalog in Orabase). Beclomethasone dipropionate aerosol spray has also been shown to reduce the severity and pain of RAS lesions. Levamisole, in immunostimulant doses, is effective for some people. People with vitamin or iron deficiencies may benefit from appropriate supplements; one study has demonstrated that a vitamin supplement may prevent RAS episodes.

Oxygenating agents such as carbamide peroxide in 10 per cent glycerol, oral zinc sulfate and lactobacillus preparations are not useful in treating RAS. A toothpaste containing sodium cromoglycate 2.5 per cent was successful in healing aphthous lesions when used 3 times daily by two individuals. However, a double-blind crossover study involving 30 people with RAS showed no effect of sodium cromoglycate toothpaste on the number of ulcers, their duration, and size, the ulcer-free interval or pain severity. A sucralfate suspension has been shown to heal oral ulcers caused by antineoplastic drug therapy, but does not appear to be effective in treating RAS. Carbenoxolone sodium mouthwash reduced the average number of ulcers per day, the number of new lesions and the discomfort associated with RAS in 24 people in a double-blind crossover study. Other agents which have been used with some success in the treatment of RAS in selected patients include: thalidomide, nicotine, colchicine, alpha-interferon, and topical cyclosporine.

Candidiasis

Etiology

Candida albicans is a true fungus that is part of the normal flora of the gastrointestinal tract and oral cavity in a large percentage of the population. The tongue serves as the primary oral reservoir for the fungus, which may then colonize other parts of the mouth.

Under certain circumstances, *Candida* can change from a commensal organism to a pathogen and cause a variety of mucocutaneous conditions. Associated predisposing factors include environment (warmth, moisture, maceration or occlusion); physiology (early infancy, pregnancy, old age or diabetes mellitus); compromised immune mechanisms (malignant diseases, immunosuppressive drugs, corticosteroids, cytotoxic drugs or radiation therapy); malnutrition and malabsorption (iron-deficiency anemia, pernicious anemia or alcoholism); drugs causing xerostomia (anticholinergics, antidepressants, antipsychotics, antihypertensives or antihistamines);

and other changes in the host environment (antibiotic therapy, trauma or postoperative states).

Symptoms

Acute oral candidiasis appears as acute pseudomembranous candidiasis or acute atrophic candidiasis. The most common form of candidal infection of the oral mucosa is the acute pseudomembranous type, often called thrush. It appears as white, milk-curd plaques attached to the mucosal surface. When the plaques are removed, erythematous, bleeding erosions are seen. Thrush is associated with some pain or soreness, but systemic symptoms are generally lacking or mild.

Acute atrophic candidiasis, sometimes referred to as antibiotic sore mouth, is thought to be similar to the form taken by thrush but without the white plaques. It is characterized by reddened painful mucosal areas in the oral cavity and commonly occurs with concomitant antibiotic therapy.

Two chronic candidal infections also exist—chronic hyperplastic candidiasis and chronic atrophic candidiasis. In chronic hyperplastic candidiasis *(Candida leucoplakia)*, firm, well-attached and persistent white plaques are present on the inner cheeks, tongue, palate and lips. Individuals may complain of soreness, roughness or a white plaque that cannot be removed. This type of candidiasis may resist treatment.

Chronic atrophic candidiasis is also known as denture stomatitis or denture sore-mouth because it is commonly found in people wearing full or partial dentures. Symptoms include a diffuse inflammation of the denture-bearing area. Denture stomatitis generally can be distinguished from the trauma caused by ill-fitting dentures because the latter is localized to one spot. Individuals with chronic atrophic candidiasis may also experience soreness or a burning sensation.

An iron or vitamin B deficiency may also play a role in susceptibility to denture stomatitis, but colonization of the denture material appears necessary for it to develop. Failure to remove the denture at bedtime or to clean the denture worsens the condition. Angular cheilitis (inflammation at the corners of the mouth) is commonly associated with denture stomatitis. Cultures of these lesions frequently show *Candida albicans* or *Staphylococcus aureus* organisms.

Treatment

Treating oral candidal infection involves elimination, if possible, of such contributing factors as concurrent antibiotic or corticosteroid therapy and the use of oral nystatin suspension. Clotrimazole or miconazole vaginal suppositories may also be dissolved in the mouth to treat thrush. Gentian violet 1 to 2 per cent solution may also be used, although it is esthetically unappealing.

Because no nonprescription products are available to treat oral candidiasis, the pharmacist's role involves recognizing clinical symptoms and referring the individual to a dentist or physician. Pharmacists can also assist by providing advice on the proper use of antifungal agents. People with denture stomatitis should be reminded of the importance of regularly removing and cleaning dentures.

Other Causes of Oral Lesions

Many other diseases and conditions also have oral manifestations, including bacterial infections, blood dyscrasias, dermatoses, allergies, metallic intoxication and neoplasms. As a general rule, any person exhibiting an oral ulcer that persists for 3 weeks or longer should see a dentist or physician.

People undergoing radiation treatment or drug therapy for cancer may experience various problems affecting the mouth. Problems include inflammation of the mucosa (mucositis), ulcerations and severe dental caries precipitated by loss of normal salivary function. These people may be treated with one of several protocols that take into account the individual's disease condition and treatments, as well as oral health status. Pharmacists may assist by preparing specially compounded treatments, if they have been prescribed by a physician. Pharmacists can also help select appropriate dental care items.

Bad Breath
Etiology

Bad breath or halitosis is an unpleasant problem caused by a mixture of the breath and malodorous compounds coming from the mouth, parts of the digestive tract or the respiratory tract. It can be a benign condition, easily treated, or the symptom of a serious disease.

Up to 85 per cent of cases of bad breath are caused by disorders of the oral cavity. Halitosis is most frequently associated with poor oral hygiene, dental plaque or caries, gingivitis, stomatitis, periodontitis and oral carcinoma. Because there is no flow of saliva during sleep, putrefaction of saliva and debris in the mouth can lead to bad breath in the morning. Similarly, mouth-breathers may also experience bad breath. Other common causes of halitosis include various respiratory conditions, such as sinusitis, tonsillitis, rhinitis, tuberculosis and bronchiectasis. Gastrointestinal tract disorders above the gastroesophageal junction may also cause bad breath. In addition, the metabolism of certain foods and beverages such as alcohol, garlic, onions and pastrami produces volatile, malodorous compounds that are excreted through the lungs. The drug dimethylsulfoxide is also excreted in this manner, producing a breath odor similar to stale oysters. Other drugs can alter the senses of taste and smell and cause subjective halitosis. These drugs include lithium salts, penicillamine, griseofulvin and thiocarbamide.

Treatment

When not secondary to a specific disease, halitosis can usually be eliminated through good oral hygiene. This includes frequent brushing and flossing of the teeth and brushing of the tongue to remove bacterial plaque and food debris. Mouthwashes or other breath fresheners probably serve only to mask bad breath and to increase salivary flow. The American Council on Dental Therapeutics believes that mouthwash use does not substantially contribute to oral health and may aggravate certain conditions because of alcohol content. If a marked breath odor persists after thoroughly cleaning the teeth, the individual should see a dentist to determine the cause.

Dry Mouth
Etiology

Dry mouth or xerostomia is the subjective complaint of dryness of the mouth. Although a dry mouth is commonly thought to be due to disturbed salivary function, it may arise from multiple causes. Elderly people in particular complain of a dry mouth. The structure and function of the salivary glands do change with age, but xerostomia is unlikely to develop from the aging process alone. Four basic causes have been outlined for xerostomia: factors affecting the salivary centre (emotions, organic disease, and drugs such as levodopa or morphine); factors affecting the autonomic nervous systems (encephalitis, brain tumors, cerebrovascular accidents and drugs—see Table V); factors affecting salivary gland function (autoimmune disorders such as Sjögren's syndrome, obstruction and infection, and irradiation); and factors affecting fluid or electrolyte balance (dehydration, edema, diabetes mellitus, cardiac failure, other systemic conditions and diuretics). The most frequent causes of dry mouth are drugs, autoimmune diseases and irradiation of the salivary glands.

Symptoms

People suffering from dry mouth may also complain of generalized burning or soreness in the mouth, ulceration, difficulty in swallowing or speaking, and poor denture retention. Taste acuity may also decrease. A rapid progression of dental caries in dentate individuals may occur if effective oral hygiene is not practised. Cracks and fissures may appear at the corners of the mouth, and the tongue may be red and smooth. Bad breath and a sore throat commonly accompany xerostomia.

Treatment

Treating xerostomia effectively may be difficult and frustrating, but a multifaceted approach may be successful. Individuals should be thoroughly evaluated first to determine the causes of the condition, which may also give some insight into appropriate treatment.

In general, people with xerostomia should avoid dry and bulky foods, spicy or acidic foods, alcoholic or carbonated beverages, and tobacco. They should also sip water or thin soup throughout the day, unless medically contraindicated. They may also find that chewing dill pickles or sucking on ice chips relieves the dryness. Humidification of inspired air may provide benefit. Candy or chewing gum (preferably sugarless) may help by stimulating salivary production in people who have viable salivary glands. All these measures provide only temporary relief.

Although people often become tolerant to the xerostomic effects of drugs, a reduction in dosage or the use of an alternative therapy might be indicated.

Salivary function may also be stimulated by cholinergic medications such as pilocarpine or bethanechol or by a sialagogue (such as anetholtrithion), providing the xerostomia is not related to an underlying condition such as irradiation of the salivary glands. Citric acid and lemon oil have also been used successfully as salivary stimulants, but dentate individuals should be cautious in the chronic use of acidic solutions. Recently, saliva substitutes have proven useful in alleviating oral discomfort from a dry mouth.

Pharmaceutical Agents

Both the Canadian Dental Association and the Council on Dental Therapeutics of the American Dental Association (ADA) evaluate and recommend certain treatments for oral conditions. Products which meet established criteria may be eligible to carry a seal of recognition of either of these associations. In addition, several of the United States Food And Drug Administration (FDA) advisory review panels looking at nonprescription products have evaluated drugs used in oral health. These panels include dentifrice and dental care drug products, miscellaneous external drug products and oral cavity drug products. Publications from these panels are referred to where their recommendations are appropriate.

Table V *Drugs Causing Xerostomia*

Classification	Major effect	Minor effect
Antispasmodic	belladonna, alkaloids, glycopyrrolate, hyoscine, 1-hyoscamine, isopropamide, oxybutynin, pirenzipine, propantheline	anisotropine, dicyclomine, orphenadrine, pinaverium
Antidepressant	amitriptyline, amoxapine, doxepin, protriptyline, trimipramine	clomipramine, desipramine, imipramine, isocarboxazide, nomifensine, nortriptyline, phenelzine, trancylpromine, trazodone
Antipsychotic	chlorpromazine, chlorprothixene, promazine, thioridazine	haloperidol, fluphenazine, lithium carbonate, loxapine, mesoridazine, methotrimeprazine, perphenazine, piperacetazine, thiopropazate, thiothixene, trifluoperazine
Skeletal muscle relaxant	cyclobenzaprine	baclofen, diazepam, orphenadrine
Parkinsonism therapy	benztropine, biperiden, trihexyphenidyl	amantadine, benserazide, carbidopa, dextroamphetamine, levodopa, orphenadrine, procyclidine
Antiarrhythmic	disopyramide	
Antihistamine		antazoline, astemizole, azatadine, brompheniramine, chlorpheniramine, clemastine, cyproheptadine, dexchlorpheniramine, diphenhydramine, hydroxyzine, promethazine, trimeprazine, tripelennamine
Appetite depressant		chlorphentermine, diethylpropion, fenfluramine, mazindol, phenteramine
Anticonvulsant		carbamazepine, clonazepam, nitrazepam
Anxiolytic		alprazolam, bromazepam, chlordiazepoxide, chlormezanone, celorazepate, lorazepam, oxazepam, temazepam, triazolam
Antihypertensive	clonidine	atenolol, captopril, debrisoquine, guanethidine, labetolol, methyldopa, metoprolol, nadolol, oxprenolol, pindolol, propranolol, timolol
Diuretic (Dry mouth may be a symptom of a serious potassium loss)		amiloride, chlorothiazide, chlorthalidone, furosemide, hydrochlorothiazide, indapamide, metolazone, methychlothiazide, polythiazide, spironolactone
Miscellaneous	bleomycin, busulfan, doxorubicin, isotretinoin	cimetidine, meclizine, procarbazine, ranitidine, sucralfate

Adapted from: Grad H, Grushka M, Yanover L. Drug-induced xerostomia: the effects and treatment. J Can Dent Assoc 1985;51:296–300.

In Canada, the Bureau of Nonprescription Drugs of Health and Welfare Canada has recently revised criteria for drug and cosmetic claims of plaque and tartar removal products. Claims that point to mechanical removal of plaque or tartar are now deemed cosmetic; those suggesting a chemical or antimicrobial effect are classified as drugs.

Oral Fluoride Supplements

In Canada, 46 per cent of the population is served by optimally fluoridated water. People living in areas where water supply is not fluoridated can reduce the incidence of dental caries by giving oral fluoride supplements to children at home or in school-based programs. Maximum benefits of this anticaries program are seen when fluoride supplements are administered through pregnancy or when given from birth through to adolescence.

Although one study has shown that an almost caries-free dentition may occur in children whose mothers take 1 mg of fluoride daily during pregnancy, such supplementation is not routinely recommended for pregnant women. Instead, the Canadian and American Dental Associations recommend appropriate fluoride supplements be given to infants and children from birth through 13 years of age, who live in areas with less than optimal levels of fluoride in drinking water.

The optimal amount of fluoride necessary to reduce most dental decay, with the least amount of risk of dental fluorosis (discoloration of the enamel), is 0.7 to 1.2 mg/L (0.7 to 1.2 ppm). In areas where water is not fluoridated to this level, oral supplementation of fluoride according to the regimen in Table VI is recommended by the CDA, as well as numerous authorities in the United States.

Fluoride supplements should be given under close professional supervision to ensure their correct, consistent use. Those prescribing fluoride supplements should consider the amount of fluoride in drinking water normally consumed by the child, as well as that from dietary sources such as infant formula or foods.

Children should be instructed to dissolve or chew tablet dosage forms of sodium fluoride before swallowing, thus delivering fluoride to the teeth topically as well as systemically. Fluoride drops may be administered in fluids, except in milk, or directly onto a child's tongue. If the child is old enough, the fluoride drops should be swished around the mouth before swallowing. In addition, no food or beverages should be consumed for 30 minutes after taking the fluoride dosage.

Oral Hygiene

Table VI	*Supplemental Fluoride Dosage Schedule (in mg F/day*) According to Fluoride Concentration of Drinking Water*		
Age (years)	Concentration of fluoride in water (ppm) (mg/L)		
	< 0.3	0.3–0.7	> 0.7
Birth to 2	0.25	0.00	0.00
2 to 3	0.50	0.25	0.00
3 to 13	1.00	0.50	0.00

*2.2mg sodium fluoride contains 1mg fluoride ion.
milligram per litre (mg/L)=part per million (ppm)
Adapted from: Forsythe J. Coordinator, Committee for Consumer Products Recognition, Canadian Dental Association (Letter to L. Suveges, author).

Compounded sodium fluoride solutions should be dispensed in plastic containers, as aqueous preparations of fluoride slowly attack glass. Large quantities of fluoride should not be stored in the home. For safety reasons, no more than 264 mg of sodium fluoride (120 mg of fluoride) are dispensed at one time. Although most fatalities associated with fluoride toxicity have resulted from industrial exposure or accidental use of a fluoride compound in cooking, two fatal cases have been related to fluoride used for dental prophylaxis. Both fatalities were 3 year old children; one died after swallowing large amounts of material used in a professional prophylaxis treatment; the other child died after swallowing 200 sodium fluoride (1 mg) tablets.

Acute fluoride intoxication is associated with gastrointestinal symptoms such as nausea, vomiting, diarrhea and abdominal pain. The more serious consequences of overdose include hypocalcemia and hyperkalemia, both of which may affect the cardiovascular system. The toxic and lethal doses of fluoride reported in the literature vary considerably. Mild gastrointestinal symptoms are usually associated with doses up to 5 mg/kg of body weight, and more serious systemic toxicity with any doses greater than that.

At levels less than 5 mg/kg, treatment for fluoride toxicity is calcium given orally to relieve gastrointestinal symptoms. Milk and ice cream are suitable as calcium sources. Any fluoride ingestion greater than 5 mg/kg requires induction of vomiting and treatment in an emergency facility.

Because of the widespread use of fluoride-containing products (in addition to possible ingestion of fluoridated water), mild dental fluorosis has been reported. Young children in particular must be supervised when using fluoride products to ensure their appropriate use.

Dentifrices

Dentifrices are substances used with toothbrushes to clean teeth. Although toothbrushing alone is partly effective in controlling plaque build-up, dentifrices help remove stains, debris and dental plaque from tooth surfaces. Dentifrices have cosmetic functions (to improve the appearance of teeth and freshen breath) and they also provide therapeutic benefits, such as preventing dental caries and periodontal diseases because of plaque removal. In addition, therapeutic dentifrices may convey specific drug substances such as fluoride to the tooth.

Dentifrices are available in three forms: paste, gel and powder. Toothpastes are by far the most popular. Most dentifrice formulations contain the same types or classes of ingredients. These formulations include abrasives (cleaning and polishing agents), foaming agents and flavoring mixtures. Pastes also contain water, humectants and thickening agents or binders. Some products may also incorporate low levels of preservatives, and therapeutic dentifrices contain a drug substance.

Abrasives are the largest component of dentifrices and are responsible for physically removing plaque and debris. An ideal abrasive provides a maximum cleaning action with minimum abrasion of tooth surfaces. In addition, the abrasive agent must be physically compatible with the other dentifrice ingredients. If used correctly, dentifrice abrasives should not damage dental enamel appreciably. However, exposed cementum and dentin can be damaged by routine use of dentifrices and toothbrushes, particularly if an individual brushes the teeth aggressively.

Abrasives are pharmacologically inactive and insoluble compounds, such as silicates and calcium or phosphate salts, that vary greatly in abrasiveness. Individuals vary in the degree of abrasiveness required to keep their teeth free from stains. Some are able to keep their teeth stain-free by using only water and a toothbrush; others can achieve a similar effect using sodium bicarbonate as the dentifrice. Although low in abrasivity, a sodium bicarbonate dentifrice showed no measurable therapeutic advantage in reducing plaque or gingivitis when compared to available commercial dentifrices. A low-abrasive toothpaste containing beads of poly(methyl)methacrylate as the abrasive was as effective as conventional toothpastes in removing plaque from teeth. However, brown staining of the teeth was worse with the low abrasivity product.

Most dentifrices sold in Canada and the United States are similar in abrasivity. None of these products appreciably abrade enamel. With normal use, they do not greatly affect dentin or cementum. In general, consumers may use any of these commercially available dentifrices safely, unless advised otherwise by their dentists. Dentifrices promoted to whiten and brighten the teeth may contain harsher abrasives and probably should not be used regularly by most consumers.

Generally speaking, dentifrice powders are more abrasive than pastes. Gel dentifrices are similar to pastes, but are clear because the refractive indices of the abrasive and humectant systems have been carefully matched. Manufacturers of gel dentifrices claim that use of these products cause children to brush longer and more thoroughly. This claim was not substantiated in a study that examined toothbrushing times and patterns after initial use and after one month of use of either a gel or paste in matched groups of children aged 10 to 16 years.

Humectants are incorporated into toothpastes and gels to prevent loss of water and subsequent hardening of the product. Thickening agents or binders stabilize dentifrice formulations. Foaming agents in dentifrices are usually synthetic detergents; most consumers prefer to use a product with adequate foaming capabilities. Various flavoring systems are also used to appeal to dentifrice users. Most products use saccharin or sorbitol as their sweetening agent.

Fluoride Dentifrices

Certain dentifrices that contain stannous fluoride or sodium monofluorophosphate (MFP) have been accepted by the CDA and the ADA as providing a significant decrease in caries incidence compared to similar nonfluoride products. Formulation modifications have also produced sodium fluoride dentifrices that provide readily available fluoride ions to the tooth surface. Acceptable products bear the Seal of Recognition of the CDA (see Table VII). The FDA

Table VII *Products Bearing the CDA Seal of Recognition*

CDA statement that accompanies the Seal of Recognition:
This product contains ingredients which are, in our opinion, effective decay preventive agents/agents for the control of supragingival plaque accumulation and gingivitis, and is of significant value when used in a conscientiously applied program of oral hygiene and regular professional care.

Product	Company
MacLeans Toothpaste	SmithKline Beecham
Aquafresh Toothpaste	SmithKline Beecham
Sensodyne-F Toothpaste	Block Drugs
Colgate Junior Toothpaste	Colgate-Palmolive
Colgate Mint Toothpaste and Gels (Tartar Fighting Formula)	Colgate-Palmolive
Colgate Regular and Winterfresh Flavour Toothpaste	Colgate-Palmolive
Aim Toothpaste	Chesebrough-Ponds
Close-Up Toothpaste	Chesebrough-Ponds
Cepacol Mouthrinse	Merrell-Dow
Crest Toothpaste	Procter & Gamble
Crest for Kids Toothpaste	Procter & Gamble
Crest Tartar Control	Procter & Gamble
Listermint Mouthrinse	Warner-Lambert

As of March 1991.

approved the ingredients outlined in Table VIII as safe and effective for caries prevention. Although the safety of fluoride dental products has been questioned, the FDA stated on the basis of available evidence that toxicities do not occur with normal usage. It has been suggested that dental fluorosis is unlikely except in areas where water supplies contain excess fluoride (greater than 2 ppm) but some authors have challenged this contention. Although the quantity of dentifrice used and the proportion ingested varies, average brushing by an adult produces little systemic ingestion of fluoride. Concern has been expressed for young children who might swallow excessive amounts of toothpaste. The FDA has recommended that fluoride dentifrices be labelled for use by adults and children over 2 years of age, and that children aged 2 to 6 use these products under parental supervision. Recent reports have also called for the development of dentifrices for children which would contain less fluoride.

Table VIII *Dosages of Approved Fluoride Ingredients*

	In dentifrice	In rinse
Acidulated phosphate		0.02%
Sodium fluoride	0.22%	0.05% daily 0.2% weekly
Sodium monofluorophosphate	0.76%	
Stannous fluoride	0.40%	0.1%

Adapted from: Fed Reg 1980;45:20666.

Ad libitum toothbrushing with a recognized fluoride dentifrice reduces the incidence of dental caries up to 35 per cent. Because most people prefer to use a dentifrice while brushing their teeth, pharmacists should encourage regular use of a fluoride dentifrice by both children and adults. This recommendation holds true even in areas where drinking water is fluoridated. The use of fluoride dentifrices and mouthrinses provides added cariostatic benefits in such communities, although the cost-benefit ratio for school-based rinsing programs in fluoridated communities has been questioned. Fluoride dentifrice use has also been shown to reduce the incidence of caries, including root surface caries, in adults older than 54 years of age.

Desensitizing Agents
Dentifrices containing fluoride may reduce hypersensitivity by strengthening the tooth surface or remineralizing tiny flaws in the enamel. The FDA rates fluoride dentifrices safe but not proven effective for this purpose. These agents are currently under review by the FDA.

Dentifrices containing potassium nitrate 5 per cent, strontium chloride 10 per cent and sodium citrate have been accepted by the ADA for treatment of dentinal hypersensitivity. Products containing sodium citrate are not available in Canada. The council has also accepted Sensodyne-F, which contains a combination of potassium nitrate 5 per cent and sodium MFP 0.76 per cent, for use as "desensitizing decay preventive dentifrices."

In one study, potassium nitrate was found to provide hypersensitivity relief faster than strontium chloride. A role for other toothpaste ingredients, particularly abrasives, in reducing dental hypersensitivity has also been suggested.

Tartar Control Dentifrices
Soluble pyrophosphates are crystal-growth inhibitors that interrupt the transformation of amorphous calcium phosphate into dental calculus. Use of a dentifrice containing these compounds has been shown to reduce the build-up of calculus or tartar on teeth that were made calculus-free by professional dental cleaning. A sodium fluoride dentifrice containing a combination of soluble pyrophosphates was used ad libitum in an adult population for 6 months after dental prophylaxis. Compared to a control group using only a sodium fluoride dentifrice without the pyrophosphates, the test group showed a 32 per cent reduction in newly formed calculus. In addition, the test group had fewer sites affected by calculus. Additional studies have supported these results.

The CDA does not yet recognize any toothpaste for tartar control alone. Both Crest and Colgate Tartar Control toothpastes are recognized for their anticaries activity.

Other Dentifrices
A dentifrice containing sanguinaria and zinc chloride has been evaluated for its effectiveness in preventing plaque formation and gingivitis. Although not effective when used alone, a combination of this toothpaste and a sanguinarine mouthrinse has reduced the amount of plaque and gingival inflammation in adult and orthodontic patients.

An experimental dentifrice containing triclosan and zinc chloride has also been effective in reducing plaque and gingival bleeding when used regularly.

Tooth Whiteners
Products containing oxidizing agents such as hydrogen peroxide or

carbamide peroxide have recently been marketed as tooth whiteners. Most of these products are liquids or gels which are applied via a mouthguard tray, worn for several hours daily. Some others are toothpastes or consist of a multistep process (mouth-cleanser, gel, and polishing cream). Some products are available by prescription from a dentist, while others are over-the-counter products.

Although these products may be safe and effective, long-term safety data are not available. Concern has been expressed because of possible damage to oral soft tissues and the pulp of the teeth.

Recent decisions by the Bureau of Nonprescription Drugs of Health and Welfare Canada mean that these products are now classified as cosmetics, when labelled solely for whitening or brightening the teeth. Labelling requirements include cautionary statements regarding seeing a dentist if irritation occurs and not using the product for a child under the age of 6 years, or for longer than 14 days unless on a dentist's advice. Patients are also to be cautioned not to allow gel products to contact the gums. In addition, manufacturers must ensure that products have a pH greater than 4 if they are to be sold as cosmetics.

The Canadian Dental Association believes that the public should only use these tooth whitening products after consultation with a dentist.

Plaque Disclosing Agents

Disclosing agents make dental plaque visible. By staining plaque either at home or in the dentist's office, individuals can evaluate their oral hygiene techniques and identify areas needing improvement.

Disclosing agents are available as chewable tablets (Red Cote) or as a solution. These agents should be expectorated completely and the mouth rinsed with water, which also should be expectorated. Disclosing products commonly contain the dye FDC Red No. 3, which has the advantage of staining red to match soft tissues, and not markedly staining the teeth. However, plaque at the gingival margin may not be well differentiated. A combination of FDC Red No. 3 and FDC Green No. 3 or FDC Blue No. 1 is able to color differentiate between thick old plaque and thin plaque. All these dyes are considered safe when used at approved doses and expectorated. Disclosing agents are meant for occasional use as indicators and should not be used continuously (for example, daily).

Mouthwashes

A mouthwash is generally regarded as a medicated liquid used for cleaning the mouth or treating diseases of the oral mucosa. Such a description does not accurately define the contents of most products nor differentiate between cosmetic and therapeutic uses. General use of these products is undoubtedly for cosmetic purposes to relieve bad breath. However, a mouthwash may serve as a vehicle for a therapeutic or prophylactic ingredient such as fluoride. Other terms that are used for mouthwashes are mouthrinses, oral antiseptics and gargles.

The most popular form of mouthwash is a liquid, although troches, lozenges, concentrates and sprays also exist. The basic ingredients in commercially available liquid mouthwashes are water, alcohol, flavoring oils and coloring materials. Other ingredients, such as humectants, astringents, emulsifiers, antimicrobial agents, sweeteners and therapeutic substances, may also be included.

Although water is the principal component of mouthwashes, ethanol is present in concentrations of 15 to 30 per cent to enhance the solubility of other ingredients. A single container of mouthwash can supply an alcohol dose lethal to a small child. Pharmacists should make consumers aware that mouthwashes are not innocuous and should be stored out of the reach of children.

Claims that mouthwashes overcome mouth odors are viewed with skepticism. Consumers should be questioned first about the presence of any oral lesions or other symptoms accompanying the breath odor. In the absence of any other symptoms, proper toothbrushing and flossing techniques should be emphasized. A marked breath odor persisting after these measures should be investigated by a dentist to determine the underlying cause. Mouthwashes should not be relied on to mask odor.

The presence of antimicrobial agents in mouthrinse formulations is controversial. The most commonly used agents in this category are the quaternary ammonium compounds such as cetylpyridinium chloride (CPC), benzethonium chloride and domiphen bromide, and phenolic substances such as phenol, thymol, betanaphthol and hexylresorcinol.

The FDA and the ADA do not recognize mouthwashes as contributing substantially to the treatment of oral conditions when used unsupervised. Besides concern over lack of data on effectiveness, both groups expressed concern that use of such products might delay treatment of an underlying disease. Therapeutic use of mouthwashes should occur with appropriate evaluation and supervision of a dentist or physician.

In addition to a cosmetic breath-freshening function, some antiseptic mouthwashes have antiplaque activity. Specifically, mouth rinsing with chlorhexidine, CPC, volatile oils, benzethonium chloride or a combination of CPC with domiphen bromide may reduce dental plaque formation. Sanguinarine, an herbal extract, is also retained in the mouth and may have antiplaque activity, especially when a sanguinarine mouthrinse and dentifrice are used concurrently.

Next to fluoride, **chlorhexidine** is the most widely studied preventive agent in dentistry. Compared to most other ingredients in antiseptic mouthwashes, chlorhexidine shows much greater substantivity in the mouth. Its bactericidal effect on plaque bacteria is less important than the bacteriostatic effect provided by a slow release of chlorhexidine from its binding sites on tooth enamel. Adsorbed chlorhexidine is gradually released for up to 24 hours, although rinsing twice daily is recommended, and has been employed in most studies on its effectiveness. Chlorhexidine significantly reduces the number of plaque-resident bacteria and the amount of plaque formed on teeth.

Chlorhexidine, employed as a mouthrinse or an applied gel, has reduced the incidence of dental caries in animal models and in children. However, its major use appears to be in preventing and treating gingivitis. Mouth rinsing with 0.1, 0.12 or 0.2 per cent chlorhexidine solutions in addition to normal oral hygiene measures significantly reduced plaque and gingivitis scores when compared to placebo in both short-term and long-term studies. However, use of chlorhexidine dentifrice has generally failed to produce effects on plaque accumulation comparable to its effects as a mouthrinse. Formulation of such a dentifrice may have reduced chlorhexidine's activity. As well, toothbrushing removes the agent from areas where it needs to be retained to be active.

Brushing, rinsing or topical application of chlorhexidine has little or no effect on advanced periodontal disease because the drug cannot reach the subgingival plaque in deep pockets around the teeth. Subgingival irrigation with chlorhexidine has been effective in reducing periodontal inflammation and controlling subgingival plaque.

Oral Hygiene

Unfortunately, chlorhexidine's usefulness as an antiplaque agent may be limited by its bitter taste and such adverse effects as brownish staining of the teeth, tongue and dental restorations. Staining varies greatly among individuals and may be increased with the ingestion of tannin-containing substances such as tea and red wine. The stains may be removed by dental cleaning in the dentist's office. The bitter taste of chlorhexidine also varies among individuals, but may be masked by flavoring agents.

When chlorhexidine rinses are employed without toothbrushing, an increase in gingival bleeding may occur due to irritation from debris built up in the gingival sulcus. Desquamation of the oral mucosa has also been reported with the use of a 0.2 per cent solution of chlorhexidine. A mouthrinse concentration of 0.12 per cent has proven equally effective in reducing gingivitis and plaque accumulation to a 0.2 per cent solution, without producing adverse effects on the soft tissues of the mouth. Chlorhexidine may also temporarily affect taste sensations, and therefore should not be used before meals.

Suggested clinical indications for chlorhexidine include its short-term use as an adjunctive measure in preventing and treating gingivitis, dental infections, RAS and denture stomatitis. Long-term use as a plaque control agent might be suggested for immunocompromised or debilitated individuals, individuals unable to perform adequate mechanical cleaning, and people undergoing orthodontic therapy.

Chlorhexidine is not commercially available in North America as a nonprescription mouthwash. However, chlorhexidine gluconate 0.12 per cent solution (Peridex) is now available in the United States for treating gingivitis when prescribed by a dentist.

The mixture of **volatile oils** (eucalyptol, thymol, menthol and methyl salicylate) in Listerine has been used for over a century with little change in the basic formulation. The product has been evaluated recently for antiplaque action in several double-blind studies involving more than 700 people. Results from these studies vary, but generally indicate that the mouthwash helps reduce plaque by up to 50 per cent depending on the study design protocol.

When used as a mouthrinse against pre-existing plaque deposits, twice daily rinses with Listerine produced no reductions in plaque when compared with a placebo. In short-term studies on plaque formation over 7 to 14 days, Listerine rinses 2 or 3 times daily as the only form of oral hygiene resulted in plaque scores significantly reduced compared to those found in placebo groups. Longer studies of 21 days in which the formation of plaque was evaluated after a dental prophylaxis, and when rinsing accompanied twice daily toothbrushing, showed plaque reductions of 38 to 43 per cent. A nine-month trial of Listerine rinsing in conjunction with normal toothbrushing and flossing routines resulted in 50 to 60 per cent less plaque, by wet weight, than the placebo rinse. Therefore, this agent appears capable of reducing plaque formation on a long term basis. Its efficacy in combination with brushing is greater than that of a placebo rinse with brushing.

Listerine is also effective in helping to prevent gingivitis. Although a 21-day experimental gingivitis trial found no difference between Listerine and a placebo rinse when gingivitis development was evaluated, several studies have shown reductions of 28 to 36 per cent in gingivitis scores after daily rinsing for 6 months or longer. Listerine is the first nonprescription mouthrinse to receive the Seal of Acceptance of the ADA Council on Dental Therapeutics as safe and effective in helping to prevent and reduce supragingival plaque and gingivitis.

It is not yet known whether plaque inhibition by any chemical agent is of any long-term value in preventing periodontitis.

Quaternary ammonium compounds have shown excellent in vitro antimicrobial activity against plaque-resident bacteria. However, clinical trials of these compounds as antiplaque agents have produced variable results, perhaps because of their short retention time in the mouth. Although they rapidly adsorb to the tooth surface in a high concentration, they also release rapidly. CPC rinses have significantly reduced plaque formation by an average of 30 per cent in the absence of other oral hygiene measures. When used in addition to regular toothbrushing for 6 weeks, CPC rinsing reduced plaque wet weight by 25 per cent and was also associated with reduced gingival inflammation when compared to placebo. Both CPC and a combination of CPC with domiphen bromide (Scope) have produced significant reductions of 15 to 20 per cent in plaque accumulation, compared to rinsing with water, when used in conjunction with normal oral hygiene procedures over a 31-day period.

To prevent plaque formation to the same degree as that produced with twice-daily rinses with chlorhexidine, quaternary ammonium compounds need to be used 4 times daily.

Side effects with quaternary ammonium compounds include staining, ulcerations and discomfort. Long-term studies with Listerine generally show no soft tissue problems or extrinsic staining of the teeth or oral mucosa.

Sanguinarine is the chief constituent alkaloid found in sanguinaria extract. Studies of its activity as an antiplaque mouthrinse, used alone or in combination with a sanguinarine-zinc chloride dentifrice, indicate that it can reduce and prevent plaque formation and gingivitis. Although staining and taste alteration do not appear to be a problem with sanguinarine, the taste of the product has been subjectively rated as "poor" in one study.

A combination product (PLAX) has recently been extensively marketed as a prebrushing antiplaque rinse. However, insufficient evidence exists to substantiate claims for antiplaque activity. Although using PLAX in combination with toothbrushing has been shown to remove plaque effectively, the amount of plaque removed has not been any greater than that removed with toothbrushing alone.

Consumers who wish to use a mouthwash for plaque control should be advised to use it in addition to regular toothbrushing and flossing. It should not replace usual oral hygiene measures or visits to the dentist. A product containing cetylpyridinium chloride alone or in combination with domiphen bromide, or Listerine may help prevent plaque formation when used routinely 2 to 4 times daily along with mechanical plaque removal. Consumers should swish 30 mL of the product around the mouth for 30 to 60 seconds before expectorating. They should not rinse with water after this procedure, and should refrain from eating, drinking or smoking for at least 30 minutes after rinsing. The effectiveness of this rinsing is most significant if done immediately after brushing and/or flossing the teeth. The manufacturer of PLAX suggests it be used as a prebrushing rinse.

Products may receive the CDA Seal of Recognition if their ingredients are recognized as effective agents for the prevention of supragingival plaque accumulation and gingivitis.

Because of the widespread use of mouthwashes and a known link between frequent alcohol ingestion and oral cancer, several retrospective studies have attempted to determine if mouthwash use may also be involved in cancer development. When compared to control subjects, a small subgroup of women who had not been exposed to either smoking or alcohol use were shown to have a slightly higher risk of developing oral or pharyngeal cancer. However, these results have not been confirmed by other studies, and may be due to chance because of the small number of cases studied.

Fluoride Mouthrinses

Several mouthwashes containing fluoride and special fluoride rinses are available. The substances outlined in Table VIII have been approved as anticaries ingredients by the FDA; several may carry the Seal of Recognition of the CDA (see Table VII). Although these products appear particularly useful for people living in areas of non-fluoridated water, some cavity prevention benefits may be achieved even where water is fluoridated. Fluoridated mouthwashes for daily use currently available contain 0.05 per cent sodium fluoride. The recommended procedure is to swish a mouthful through the teeth for one minute, once daily, and then expectorate. The individual should also be cautioned not to rinse the mouth after this procedure, nor to eat and drink anything for 30 minutes. Mouthrinses containing 0.2 per cent sodium fluoride are also available for use once weekly.

In nonfluoridated areas, dentists may recommend certain fluoride rinses that must be diluted before use, or they may recommend others that are to be swallowed after rinsing. Consumers should be instructed in the appropriate use of the selected product.

Toothache Relievers

Most products marketed for relieving toothache contain eugenol or benzocaine. **Eugenol** is the essential chemical constituent of clove oil and is principally responsible for its action. Eugenol acts as an antiseptic and in concentrations of 85 to 87 per cent acts as an obtundent or analgesic. It is accepted by the Council for Dental Therapeutics for use by dentists, often as a zinc oxide paste formulation to cover exposed pulpal areas.

Because eugenol irritates, it must be applied carefully, only to the cavity in the tooth. It is so irritating that eugenol can actually destroy viable dental pulp. The FDA recommends eugenol be used only on irreparably damaged teeth (candidates for extraction or root canal therapy). People experiencing intermittent toothaches, indicating a viable and repairable tooth, should not use any nonprescription toothache product containing eugenol. Instead, they should make an emergency dental appointment, apply cold compresses or ice cubes, and take oral analgesics until the condition can be treated. If the pain is throbbing and relentless, the tooth is likely to be irreversibly damaged. When properly applied, eugenol preparations may bring some relief until dental attention is possible.

Benzocaine has been widely used for toothache relief since 1926. A recent clinical study confirmed the efficacy of 7.5 per cent benzocaine in propylene glycol for the temporary relief of toothaches. When applied as directed to the tooth, its cavity and the surrounding gingival tissue, benzocaine is safe and noncaustic. However, it should be used only temporarily until dental service can be obtained.

Other ingredients in combination products available for toothache relief include benzyl alcohol and phenolic compounds. None have been proven both safe and effective for this purpose. In addition, the alcohol present in some products may cause dehydration of the dentin. Products such as waxes, gums or cotton soaked with medication are not recommended because their occlusive properties may prevent an abscess from draining.

Cold Sore and Canker Sore Products

Nonprescription products available to treat cold sores and canker sores are primarily intended to control pain and do not alter the course of either disease. They contain various protective, drying, counterirritant, anesthetic, antibiotic and antiseptic agents (see Table IX). These products are marketed for sore mouth generally, or for canker or cold sores specifically. Many of these ingredients were evaluated by the FDA for the general treatment category of sore mouth. However, the FDA recommends that people with canker sores be treated by physicians or dentists. Because some people with an occasional canker sore or cold sore attempt to self-medicate, the following information may help pharmacists. Individuals with extensive lesions, frequent recurrences or ulcers lasting longer than 3 weeks should be referred for medical evaluation.

The most useful products to relieve canker sore discomfort are those containing a local **anesthetic** or a protective agent. Benzocaine is the most common anesthetic used. It is poorly absorbed and can be safely applied to ulcerated areas of the mucosa. Benzocaine provides local anesthesia for 5 to 10 minutes after application, although this effect may be prolonged with repeated use.

Lidocaine preparations are also available for use in the mouth. The FDA does not consider these preparations safe for nonprescription use.

Consumers should apply a local anesthetic only to the canker sore, or a "cotton-mouth" feeling occurs. If extensive areas of the oral cavity are anesthetized, individuals are unaware of such sensations as extreme heat. When eating or drinking hot food or beverages, they should be careful to prevent burning the oral mucosa and causing

Table IX *Agents Found in Nonprescription Canker and Cold Sore Remedies*

Agent	Purpose
Allantoin	Cleansing, debridement
Aluminum potassium sulfate	Astringent
Benzocaine	Anesthetic
Benzoin	Protective
Camphor	Counterirritant
Carbamide peroxide	Cleansing, debridement
Carboxymethylcellulose	Protective
Dequalinium chloride	Antiseptic
Ethanol	Antiseptic
Heparin sodium	Healing agent
Hydrogen peroxide	Cleansing, debridement
Iodochlorhydroxyquin	Anti-infective
Lidocaine	Anesthetic
Menthol	Counterirritant
Myrrh	Astringent
Para-aminobenzoic acid	Sunscreen
Polymyxin B	Anti-infective
Potassium chlorate	Astringent
Propolis	Antipruritic
Quinine bisulfate	Astringent
Sodium percarbonate	Oxidizing agent
Tannic acid	Astringent
Tyrothricin	Anti-infective
Zinc salicylate	Astringent
Zinc sulfate	Astringent

Adapted from: Popovich NG, Popovich JG. What you should know about fever blisters and canker sores. US Pharmacist 1978;3(2):35–48.

further discomfort. Prolonged use of local anesthetics may produce localized allergic reactions.

Demulcents, such as carboxymethylcellulose, benzoin or gums, are protective agents used to relieve irritation. These agents adhere to the mucosal surface and protect the lesion from friction. Consumers apply the product (such as Orabase) directly onto the lesion to create a smooth, slippery film. If the medication is rubbed in, it produces a granular, gritty sensation. These products may be applied as frequently as necessary to relieve discomfort.

An **oxidizing agent** such as hydrogen peroxide may be used as a cleansing agent for inflamed mucous membranes. When it touches the mucosa, oxygen is liberated and loosens debris. After dilution with an equal volume of water, a solution of 3 per cent hydrogen peroxide is considered safe for use as a mouthrinse, gargle or topical application in the mouth. It can be used 3 to 4 times daily, but for no longer than 2 days unless recommended by a dentist. Since hydrogen peroxide is an irritant, prolonged unsupervised use can retard the healing of ulcerated mucosa.

Carbamide peroxide is another form of peroxide that is formulated in anhydrous glycerin. The glycerin increases the peroxide's stability and also helps the product adhere to the lesion. Concentrations of 10 to 15 per cent can be used safely up to 4 times daily for 2 days. Sodium perborate and its modified forms also release oxygen, but these are considered ineffective and unsafe because of boric acid absorption and irritation to the mucosa.

Antibiotics available in canker sore products do not produce any beneficial effect. Topical tetracycline and cephalexin, which are effective against *Streptococcus mutans*, require a prescription by a physician or dentist. Antibiotics do not alter the course of recurrent herpes labialis. They may help prevent or treat a bacterial superinfection.

Antiseptics have limited use in treating RAS or herpes labialis. Agents such as benzalkonium chloride, dequalinium chloride or the phenolic compounds generally affect only a limited number of bacteria and have not been proven totally safe or effective. Ethanol (70 per cent) denatures protein to destroy bacteria. Unfortunately, this concentration also irritates mucous membranes. Ethanol or other solvents, such as ethyl ether, applied to herpes labialis may dilute virus particles and dry the lesion. However, their therapeutic efficacy has not been substantiated in well-controlled studies.

Tannic acid and other **astringents** precipitate proteins when applied to the mouth, protecting the area from irritating substances. However, their effect is temporary.

Counterirritants, such as camphor, menthol and phenol, relieve discomfort by creating another sensation such as irritation or warmth. However, they can increase irritation. They must be kept away from children, as camphor is toxic when ingested.

Silver nitrate sticks have been used in the past to cauterize canker sores. Although this procedure may relieve pain, it is not recommended because the ulcer itself may enlarge and heal slowly. The surrounding area of the gums and teeth may also be stained black.

A product containing propolis of flavenoids (Probax) has been marketed to treat cold sores, but published studies on its effectiveness are lacking. It is claimed to relieve the itching and stinging commonly associated with cold sores. Another product containing heparin sodium and zinc sulfate (Lipactin) is also claimed to provide symptomatic relief from cold sores, and may shorten the time required for the lesions to heal.

Products for Dry Mouth

Several approaches can be taken to relieve xerostomia: sialogogues may be employed to stimulate salivary flow if salivary gland function remains; a palliative mouthrinse may be used to relieve dryness; or a saliva replacement may be employed.

Mouthrinses that moisten and lubricate the mouth are effective only for short periods of time. Most examples of such mouthrinses contain water or a humectant glycerin-water mixture. Substances such as citric acid or lemon oil may be added to such mouthrinses or used alone as gustatory stimulants of salivary function. However, prolonged use of acidic substances should be avoided in dentate individuals due to their demineralizing effect on tooth enamel.

Cholinergic drugs such as bethanechol or urecholine act on the central nervous system to increase salivary flow; anetholtrithion acts directly on the salivary glands. Cholinergic drugs may be associated with significant systemic effects that may limit their usefulness in treating xerostomia. Anetheltrithion is generally well-tolerated and may be prescribed by medical or dental practitioners for some people.

Artificial saliva describes preparations whose chemical and physical properties resemble those of natural saliva. An ideal artificial saliva should be "long-lasting", inhibit colonization by cariogenic bacteria, provide lubrication and coat and protect oral tissues. Such products relieve the feeling of mouth dryness longer than mouthrinses and have proven benefit for soft tissue care.

A thickening agent such as methylcellulose or mucin is the primary ingredient in artificial saliva. It gives the product viscosity and provides sustained activity. Mucin appears to be the better lubricant, acting much like natural saliva. Ingredients such as glycerin, sorbitol and lemon oil increase palatability because of their humectant and flavoring ability.

Although sorbitol does not promote tooth decay in people with normal salivary function, oral cariogenic microorganisms can also ferment sorbitol and enhance caries formation in people who constantly use artificial saliva. The ADA therefore recommends a professionally applied topical fluoride treatment for dentate individuals using artificial saliva.

All saliva substitutes currently available have similar viscosity, pH and ion content. However, Moi-stir has the highest sodium content, which may be a consideration for people on sodium-restricted diets who wish to use the preparation frequently.

Xerolube (also known as VA-Oralube), available in the United States, is the only product that contains fluoride ion. Limited in vitro data indicate fluoride, along with the calcium and phosphate present in artificial saliva, promotes remineralization of tooth enamel. No clinical evidence exists that artificial saliva reduces caries. Fluoride rinses specifically designed to prevent caries are probably more effective for this purpose.

Artificial saliva products are used to relieve soft tissue discomfort whenever mouth dryness persists. Consumers should be encouraged to use them as often as needed to keep the mouth moist. They are particularly effective in relieving nocturnal xerostomia.

Artificial saliva may be recommended to any person experiencing a dry mouth, providing treatable causes (for example, neoplasms) have been ruled out by a physician or dentist. Dentate individuals experiencing xerostomia should be reminded also of the importance of toothbrushing and flossing, and the need for regular visits to a dentist. Denture-wearers with dry mouth should clean their dentures frequently and see a dentist regularly.

Figure 6   *Suggested Approach for Evaluating and Treating Soft Tissue Problems in the Mouth*

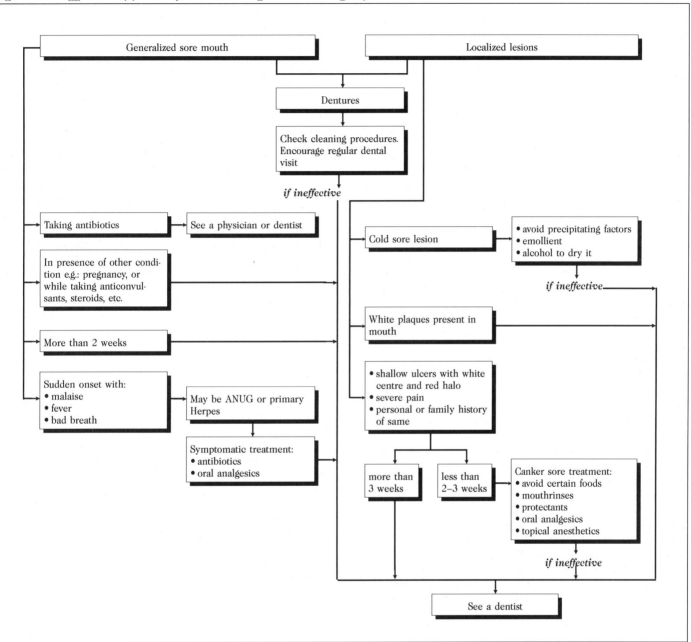

A toothpaste developed to fight xerostomia contains enzymes and other agents found in saliva (Biotene). It is said to produce antibacterial levels of hypothiocyanate and hydrogen peroxide during brushing. However, clinical trials on its effectiveness have not been published.

Denture Products
Denture Cleansers

Denture cleansing removes denture plaque, stain and debris. Regular removal of plaque and extrinsic materials from dentures helps control or prevent oral malodor and conditions such as denture stoma-titis the same way toothbrushing and flossing prevent dental caries, periodontal disease and halitosis in dentate individuals. The suggested methods of cleaning acrylic resin dentures include mechanical and abrasive action and immersion in chemical solutions.

The most common method for cleaning dentures is brushing with tap water and soap or pastes. This technique removes stain and plaque effectively when used meticulously. In general, a specialized denture brush and low-abrasive denture cleaning powder or paste should be used instead of a regular toothbrush and toothpaste. Denture-wearers should not use scouring powders to clean dentures.

The ADA has found no form of denture cleaning device or product

Oral Hygiene

superior to cleaning with a denture brush. Ultrasonic agitation devices may increase a disinfectant's effectiveness, but data conflict on their effectiveness in removing denture stains and plaque.

Chemical denture cleansers are dissolved in water and the denture immersed in the resulting solution for a period of time. Alkaline peroxide products (for example, Efferdent and Polident) are the most commonly used chemical cleansers. They provide alkaline solutions of hydrogen peroxide that release oxygen and exert the cleaning action. They seem most effective on new plaque and stains when the denture is soaked overnight or for several hours. They are not effective in the 15 to 30 minute time period recommended by manufacturers, as they remove only 30 per cent of accumulated plaque in that time. A denture brush should be used after soaking to ensure thorough denture cleaning. Alkaline peroxide solutions are safe for denture cleaning, but routine use may cause bleaching of the acrylic resin material.

When the two most popular methods of denture cleaning (Dentu-creme and Efferdent) were compared, an Efferdent soak reduced plaque bacteria levels significantly more than Dentu-creme alone. Although a combination of the cream and soak did not produce additional reductions in microflora, regular use of such a combination regimen is recommended to effectively remove plaque, bacteria and debris from dentures.

Alkaline hypochlorite and dilute acid solutions are also available to remove stains and plaque on dentures. Overnight soaking is recommended when using these solutions. They should be used only weekly or bi-weekly as either solution can corrode metal denture parts. These products remove stains better than do alkaline peroxide solutions. Consumers should not use strong hypochlorite solutions such as bleach to clean dentures, because of possible damage to the denture material. Hot water or hot soaking solutions also should be avoided to prevent distortion of the dentures.

Some denture cleansers contain enzymes such as protease or mutanase. These enzymes break down the proteins and polysaccharides in plaque on the dentures. Use of such products has been shown to significantly reduce denture plaque when compared to placebo or Steradent solutions.

All dentures should be thoroughly rinsed before reinsertion into the mouth, and all cleaning products kept out of the reach of children.

Adhesives, Reliners, Cushions and Repair Kits

Even the best-fitting dentures result in chronic bone resorption from the dental arch. If a denture becomes loose or poorly retained, the individual should see a dentist for re-evaluation to ensure proper denture fit. Although denture adhesives may improve denture retention in some people, the chronic use of such products may lead to further pathological changes in the tissues under the denture.

Denture adhesives are available in powders and pastes based on ingredients such as methylcellulose, Karaya gum, carboxymethylcellulose and gelatin.

Denture reliners and cushions damage the denture and the wearer if used for extended periods. Any person considering purchasing a denture reliner or cushion should see a dentist as soon as possible. Pharmacists should discourage the use of denture repair kits except in emergencies. Dentures can be properly fitted and repaired only by trained professionals.

Summary

Self-medication with nonprescription products is not generally recommended for most dental or oral problems. In most cases, diseases of the hard and soft tissues of the mouth require evaluation and treatment by a dentist. However, topical anesthetic preparations may provide temporary relief from toothache or teething symptoms, as well as from pain associated with canker sores or primary herpes infections. Protective agents also can be useful in relieving oral ulcer discomfort. Nonprescription mouthwashes may serve a cosmetic function, but should not be used unsupervised to treat oral conditions.

On the other hand, products available to prevent dental diseases are numerous and varied. These include nonpharmaceutical items such as toothbrushes, dentifrices and dental floss, as well as fluoridated toothpastes and mouthrinses. Because all preventive techniques require co-operation and sustained effort on the part of the individual, the pharmacist may serve a valuable function by reviewing and reinforcing instructions for good oral hygiene.

Ask the Consumer

Q. How long have you had this dental problem? Did it begin suddenly or develop gradually? Is only one tooth involved?

- A history of vague, nondescript discomfort not localized to one tooth suggests periodontal disease. Acute gingivitis may develop from trauma to the gums, but, in general, periodontal disease is a chronic disorder.

Q. How painful is it? Is the pain radiating, deep, intense or dull? Is it generalized or specific to one tooth? Is it triggered by hot or cold substances or by chewing?

- Dental pain precipitated by hot, cold or sweet substances suggests superficial dentinal caries or exposed cementum. Chronic pain that gradually becomes more intense and has deep, boring or radiating characteristics is associated with pulpitis from a deep carious lesion or the placement of extensive restorative material in one tooth. Nonprescription analgesics may provide temporary pain relief, but consumers should consult a dentist as quickly as possible for professional evaluation and treatment.

Q. How old is the individual? Have all the teeth erupted in the mouth? What other symptoms are present?

- Infants may experience discomfort from teething as well as increased salivation and restlessness. Eruption of the permanent third molars—the wisdom teeth—may be associated with pain and possible swelling if an abscess forms.

Q. Have you seen a dentist about this condition? When? What treatments have you tried?

- A dentist should be consulted for pain that may follow recent dental treatment. Nonprescription toothache remedies should only be used short-term for any dental pain, as an emergency measure before obtaining dental treatment.

Q. Is the pain altered by lying down, going up and down stairs, or by clenching your teeth?

- Symptoms such as these suggest the problem may be nondental in origin (for example, sinusitis).

Oral Hygiene

Q. Are your teeth loose? Do your gums bleed when you brush your teeth? Do you have a continuous foul breath problem? How do you clean your teeth? How often? Do you use dental floss or toothpicks?

■ Removing bacterial plaque by proper toothbrushing and flossing methods is essential for good oral hygiene. If plaque is allowed to accumulate, gingivitis and halitosis are possible. The improper use of dental floss or toothpicks may also precipitate an acute attack of gingivitis.

Q. Do you use fluoride supplements? Is your drinking water fluoridated? Is your baby breast-fed or on prepared formula?

■ The need for fluoride supplementation to prevent caries is determined by the amount of fluoride already ingested. Too much fluoride causes enamel mottling. If local water supplies contain less than 0.3 ppm fluoride, all breast-fed and bottle-fed babies should receive appropriate fluoride supplementation.

Q. Do you wear dentures? Are they loose? Do they cause sore spots? How do you clean them?

■ Improperly fitting dentures may create oral problems, such as sores, difficulty in chewing and destruction of supporting bone. Denture stomatitis may develop if dentures are inadequately cleaned.

Q. How long have you had the sore in or around your mouth? Describe the lesion. Have you ever had a similar condition before?

■ Harmless canker sores last up to 14 days. Primary herpes infections generally last from 10 to 14 days; cold sores last from 3 to 10 days. However, mouth ulcers caused by blood dyscrasias or an oral cancer persist and grow over a period of months.

Q. Do you have any other symptoms such as fever, increased salivation, bad breath or flu-like symptoms?

■ A young child with such symptoms may be experiencing a primary herpes infection. Bad breath, bleeding gums, fever and malaise, and cervical lymphadenopathy may indicate the presence of acute necrotizing gingivitis.

Q. Do you suffer from any chronic medical illness such as diabetes mellitus, rheumatoid arthritis, heart disease, or epilepsy?

■ Many diseases have periodontal manifestations, especially those of endocrine imbalances, blood dyscrasias, dermatoses and allergies. Some conditions, such as angina pectoris, have referred pain to the teeth. Sjögren's syndrome is commonly associated with rheumatoid arthritis, particularly in females, and presents as a chronic dry mouth condition.

Q. Are you allergic to any foods or medications? What are they?

■ Certain foods may precipitate recurrent aphthous stomatitis. Topical anesthetics such as lidocaine may produce localized allergic reactions in the mouth. Drugs may also produce oral lesions as manifestations of an allergic response.

Q. What medications are you taking?

■ Certain drugs may produce blood dyscrasias or allergic reactions that manifest as oral lesions. Drugs can also cause a dry mouth. Anticonvulsants such as phenytoin, and some other agents, may cause gingival hyperplasia.

References

Introduction

Anonymous. Dental caries and community water fluoridation trends—United States. JAMA 1985;253:1377,1383.

Bailit HL, Braun R. Is periodontal disease the primary cause of tooth extraction in adults? J Am Dent Assoc 1987;114:40–5.

Douglass CW, Gillings D, Sollecito W, Gammon M. National trends in the prevalence and severity of the periodontal diseases. J Am Dent Assoc 1983;107:403–12.

Evans RG. Implications of dental disease: an economist's perspective. J Can Dent Assoc 1980;46:56–9.

Legler DW, Menaker L. Etiology, epidemiology and clinical implications of caries. In: Menaker L, ed. The biologic basis of dental caries: an oral biology textbook. Hagerstown: Harper-Row, 1980:211–25.

Lizaire AL, Hargreaves JA, Finnigan PD, Thompson GW. Oral health status of 13-year-old school children in Alberta, Canada. J Can Dent Assoc 1987;53:845–8.

Locker D, Slade GD, Leake JL. Prevalence of and factors associated with root decay in older adults in Canada. J Dent Res 1989;68:768–72.

Miller MA. Odontologic diseases. In: Lynch MA, ed. Burket's oral medicine. Toronto: JB Lippincott, 1977:283–301.

Olds GE, Yanchik VA. Preventive dentistry: an educational module for pharmacists. Clin Prev Dent 1979;1:27–30.

Scott JH, Symons NBB. Introduction to dental anatomy. Edinburgh: Churchill-Livingstone, 1977.

Ship JA, Ship IJ. Trends in oral health in the aging population. Dent Clin N Amer 1989;33(1):33–42.

Stamm JW. Some indicators of the oral health status of the North American child population. J Can Dent Assoc 1980;46:21–30.

Etiology and Pathophysiology—Dental Caries

American Dental Association Council on Dental Therapeutics. Accepted dental therapeutics. Chicago: American Dental Association, 1984.

Bibby BG. Diet and nutrition and dental caries. J Can Dent Assoc 1980; 46:47–55.

Bibby BG, Mundorff SA, Zero DT, Almekinder KJ. Oral food clearance and the pH of plaque and saliva. J Am Dent Assoc 1986;112:333–7.

Catalanotto FA, Wrobel WR, Epstein DW. Sucrose taste thresholds and dental caries: implications for dietary counselling. Clin Prev Dent 1979;1:14–8.

Cooper SA. Oral analgesics used to treat dental pain. Clin Prev Dent 1981; 3:28–32.

Derkson GD, Ponti P. Nursing bottle syndrome: prevalence and etiology in a non-fluoridated city. J Can Dent Assoc 1982;48:389–93.

Feigal RJ, Jensen ME, Mensing CA. Dental caries potential of liquid medications. Pediatrics 1981;68:416–9.

Finn SB. The epidemiology of dental caries. In: Stallard RE, ed. A textbook of preventive dentistry. Philadelphia: WB Saunders, 1982:20–31.

Flemming WJ. Dental and oral hygiene. In: Krogh CME, ed. Canadian self-medication. Ottawa: Canadian Pharmaceutical Association, 1978:85–95.

Grenby TH, Bashaarat AH, Gey KF. A clinical trial to compare the effects of xylitol and sucrose chewing-gums on dental plaque growth. Br Dent J 1982;152:339–43.

Hargreaves JA, Thompson GW. Ultraviolet light and dental caries in children. Caries Res 1989;23:389–92.

Hunter PB. Risk factors in dental caries. Int Dent J 1988; 38:211–7.

Jensen ME. Responses of interproximal plaque pH to snack foods and effect of chewing sorbitol-containing gum. J Am Dent Assoc 1986;113:262–6.

Jones RR, Cleaton-Jones P. Depth and area of dental erosions and dental caries in bulimic women. J Dent Res 1989;68:1275–8.

Oral Hygiene

Kandelman D, Gagnon G. A 24-month clinical study of the incidence and progression dental caries in relation to consumption of chewing gum containing xylitol in school preventive programs. J Dent Res 1990;69:1771–5.

Kennon S, Tasch EG, Arm RN, et al. The relationship between plaque scores and the development of caries in adult dentition. Clin Prev Dent 1979; 1:26–31.

Kingman A, Little W, Gomez I, Heifetz SB, et al. Salivary levels of *Streptococcus mutans* and lactobacilli and dental caries experiences in a US adolescent population. Community Dent Oral Epidemiol 1988;16:98–103.

Klausen B, Helbo M, Dabelsteen E. A differential diagnostic approach to the symptomatology of acute dental pain. Oral Surg Oral Med Oral Pathol 1985;59:297–301.

Kleinberg I. Etiology of dental caries. J Can Dent Assoc 1979;45:661–8.

Korberly BH, Schreiber GF, Kilkuts A, et al. Evaluation of acetaminophen and aspirin in the relief of preoperative dental pain. J Am Dent Assoc 1980; 100:39–42.

Loe H, Kleinman DV, eds. Dental plaque control measures and oral hygiene practices: proceedings from a state-of-the-science workshop. Oxford: IRL Press, 1986:39–116.

Loesche WJ, Grossman NS, Earnest R, Corpron R. The effect of chewing xylitol gum on the plaque and saliva levels of *Streptococcus mutans*. J Am Dent Assoc 1984;108:587–92.

Makinen KK, Soderling E, Hurttia H, et al. Biochemical, microbiologic and clinical comparisons between two dentifrices that contain different mixtures of sugar alcohols. J Am Dent Assoc 1985;111:745–51.

Morrissey RB, Burkholder BD, Tarka SM Jr. The cariogenic potential of several snack foods. J Am Dent Assoc 1984;109:589–91.

Newbrun E. Sugar and dental caries: a review of human studies. Science 1982;217:418–23.

Newbrun E. Sugar and dental caries. Clin Prev Dent 1982;4:11–3.

Shaw L, Glenwright HD. The role of medications in dental caries formation: need for sugar-free medication for children. Pediatrician 1989;16(3–4): 153–5.

Vratsanos SM, Mandel ID. The effect of sucrose and hexitol-containing chewing gums on plaque acidogenesis in vivo. Pharmacol Ther Dent 1981;6:87–91.

Walker AR, Cleaton-Jones PE. Sugar intake and dental caries: where do we stand? ASDC J Dent Child 1989;56:30–5.

Prevention—Dental Caries

Honkala E, Tala H. Total sugar consumption and dental caries in Europe—an overview. Int Dent J 1987;37:185–91.

Horowitz HS. The prevention of oral disease. Established methods of prevention. Br Dent J 1980;149:311–8.

Fluoride

Bagramian RA, Narendran S, Ward M. Relationship of dental caries and fluorosis to fluoride supplement history in a non-fluoridated sample of schoolchildren. Adv Dent Res 1989;3:161–7.

Bayless JM, Tinanoff N. Diagnosis and treatment of acute fluoride toxicity. J Am Dent Assoc 1985;110:209–11.

Beiswanger BB, Gish CW, Mallatt ME. A three-year study of the effect of a sodium fluoride-silica abrasive dentifrice on dental caries. Pharmacol Ther Dent 1981;6:9–16.

Blahut P. Fluoride supplements. Drugs Ther Maritime Pract 1984;7(6).

Bohannan BM, Stamm JW, Graves RC, et al. Fluoride mouthrinse programs in fluoridated communities. J Am Dent Assoc 1985;111:783–9.

Carlos JP. The prevention of dental caries: ten years later. J Am Dent Assoc 1982;104:193–7.

Clark DC, Robert G, Tessier C, et al. The results after 20 months of a study testing the efficacy of a weekly fluoride mouthrinsing program. J Public Health Dent 1985;45:252–6.

Clovis J, Hargreaves JA, Thompson GW. Caries prevalence and length of residency in fluoridated and non-fluoridated communities. Caries Res 1988;22:311–5.

Driscoll WS, Swango PA, Horowitz AM, Kingman A. Caries-preventive effects of daily and weekly fluoride mouthrinsing in a fluoridated community: final results after 30 months. J Am Dent Assoc 1982;105:1010–3.

Glass RL. Caries reduction by a dentifrice containing sodium monofluorophosphate in a calcium carbonate base. Partial explanation for diminishing caries prevalance. Clin Prev Dent 1981;3:6–8.

Glenn FB, Glenn WD, Duncan RC. Fluoride tablet supplementation during pregnancy for caries immunity: a study of the offspring produced. Am J Obstet Gynecol 1982;143:560–4.

Gossel TA. The role of fluorides in preventing cavities. US Pharmacist 1986;11:28–34.

Horowitz AM. Oral hygiene measures. J Can Dent Assoc 1980;46:43–6.

Horowitz HS. Review of topical applications: fluorides and fissure sealants. J Can Dent Assoc 1980;46:38–42.

Keeping B, Canadian Dental Association. (Letter to L Suveges, author.)

Leverett DH. Fluorides and the changing prevalence of dental caries. Science 1982;217:26–30.

Leverett DH, Sveen OB, Jensen OE. Weekly rinsing with a fluoride mouthrinse in an unfluoridated community: results after seven years. J Public Health Dent 1985;45:95–100.

Levy SM. Expansion of the proper use of systemic fluoride supplements. J Am Dent Assoc 1986;112:30–4.

Lu KH, Hanna JD, Peterson JK. Effect on dental caries of a stannous fluoride-calcium pyrophosphate dentifrice in an adult population: one-year results. Pharmacol Ther Dent 1980;5:11–6.

Newbrun E. Systemic fluorides: an overview. J Can Dent Assoc 1980; 46:31–7.

Newbrun E. Effectiveness of water fluoridation. J Public Health Dent 1989; 49:279–89.

Popovich NG, Popovich JG. Fluoride dental therapy. US Pharmacist 1981; 6:37–61.

Ripa LW. Fluoride rinsing: what dentists should know. J Am Dent Assoc 1981;102:477–81.

Smith GE. Fluoride and fluoridation. Soc Sci Med 1988;26:451–62.

Swango PA. The use of topical fluorides to prevent dental caries in adults: a review of the literature. J Am Dent Assoc 1983;107:447–50.

Szpunar SM, Burt BA. Fluoride exposure in Michigan schoolchildren. J Public Health Dent 1990(Winter);50:18–23.

Szpunar SM, Burt BA. Dental caries, fluorosis, and fluoride exposure in Michigan schoolchildren. J Dent Res 1988;67:802–6.

Yanover L. Fluoride varnishes as cariostatic agents: a review. J Can Dent Assoc 1982;48:401–4.

Zacherl WA. A three-year clinical caries evaluation of the effect of a sodium fluoride-silica abrasive dentifrice. Pharmacol Ther Dent 1981;6:1–7.

Plaque Removal Products

Abelson DC, Barton JE, Maietti GM, et al. Evaluation of interproximal cleaning by two types of dental floss. Clin Prev Dent 1981;3:19–21.

Adams RA, Mann WV. Oral hygiene techniques and home care. In: Stallard RE, ed. A textbook of preventive dentistry. Philadelphia: WB Saunders, 1982:217–40.

Ashley FP, Skinner A, Jackson P, et al. The effect of a 0.1% cetylpyridinium chloride mouthrinse on plaque and gingivitis in adult subjects. Br Dent J 1984;157:191–6.

Beaumont RH. Patient preference for waxed or unwaxed dental floss. J Periodontol 1990;61:123–5.

Bergenholtz A, Olsson A. Efficacy of plaque-removal using interdental brushes and waxed dental floss. Scand J Dent Res 1984;92:198–203.

Bergenholtz A, Brithon J. Plaque removal by dental floss or toothpicks. An intra-individual comparative study. J Clin Periodontol 1980;7:516–24.

Bergenholtz A, Gustafsson LB, Segerlund N, et al. Role of brushing technique and toothbrush design in plaque removal. Scand J Dent Res 1984; 92:344–51.

Boyd RL, Murray P, Robertson PB. Effect on periodontal status of rotary electric toothbrushes vs manual toothbrushes during periodontal maintenance. I. Clinical results. J Periodontol 1989;60:390–5.

Boyd RL, Murray P, Robertson PB. Effect of rotary electric toothbrush versus manual toothbrush on periodontal status during orthodontic treatment. Am J Orthod Dentofacial Orthop 1989;96:342–7.

Brecx M, Theilade J. Effect of chlorhexidine rinses on the morphology of early dental plaque formed on plastic film. J Clin Periodontol 1984;11:553–64.

Oral Hygiene

Breitenmoser J, Mormann W, Muhlemann HR. Damaging effects of toothbrush bristle end form on gingiva. J Periodontol 1979;50:212–6.

Briner WW, Grossman E, Buckner RY, et al. Effect of chlorhexidine gluconate mouthrinse on plaque bacteria. J Periodontol Res 1986;21(Suppl 16):44–52.

Briner WW, Grossman E, Buckner RY, et al. Assessment of susceptibility of plaque bacteria to chlorhexidine after six months oral use. J Periodontol Res 1986;21(Suppl 16):53–9.

Ciancio SG. Chemotherapeutics in periodontics. Dent Clin North Am 1980; 24:813–26.

Dahlen G. Effect of antimicrobial mouthrinses on salivary microflora in healthy subjects. Scand J Dent Res 1984;92:38–42.

De la Rosa M, Guerra JZ, Johnston DA, et al. Plaque growth and removal with daily toothbrushing. J Periodontol 1979;50:661–4.

Emling RC, Flickinger KC, Cohen DW, et al. A comparison of estimated versus actual brushing time. Pharmacol Ther Dent 1981;6:93–8.

Fardal O, Turnbull RS. A review of the literature on use of chlorhexidine in dentistry. J Am Dent Assoc 1986;112:863–9.

Fine DH, Letizia J, Mandel ID. The effect of rinsing with Listerine antiseptic on the properties of developing dental plaque. J Clin Periodontol 1985; 12:660–6.

Glavind L, Zeuner E. The effectiveness of a rotary electric toothbrush on oral cleanliness in adults. J Clin Periodontol 1986;13:135–8.

Glaze PM, Wade AB. Toothbrush age and wear as it relates to plaque control. J Clin Periodontol 1986;13:52–6.

Gordon JM, Lamster IB, Seiger MC. Efficacy of Listerine antiseptic in inhibiting the development of plaque and gingivitis. J Clin Periodontol 1985; 12:697–704.

Gossel TA. Mouthwashes: how effective are they against plaque? US Pharmacist 1985;10:23–9,32.

Gossel TA. Toothbrushes. US Pharmacist 1985;10:22–8.

Graves RC, Disney JA, Stamm JW. Comparative effectiveness of flossing and brushing in reducing interproximal bleeding. J Periodontol 1989;60:243–7.

Grossman E, Reiter G, Sturzenberger OP, et al. Six-month study of the effects of a chlorhexidine mouthrinse on gingivitis in adults. J Periondontol Res 1986;21(Suppl 16):33–43.

Honkala E, Nyyssonen V, Knuuttila M, Markkanen H. Effectiveness of children's habitual toothbrushing. J Clin Periodontol 1986;13:81–5.

Hull PS. Chemical inhibition of plaque. J Clin Periodontol 1980;7:431–42.

Jackson CL. Comparison between electric toothbrushing and manual toothbrushing, with and without oral irrigation, for oral hygiene of orthodontic appliances. Am J Orthod Dentofacial Orthop 1991;99:15–20.

Kleber CJ, Putt MS, Muhler JC. Duration and pattern of toothbrushing in children using a gel or a paste dentifrice. J Am Dent Assoc 1981;103:723–6.

Kortsch WE. Challenging the soft brush (Letter). J Am Dent Assoc 1983; 106:594.

Kreifeldt JG, Hill PH, Calisti LJP. A systematic study of the plaque removal efficiency of worn toothbrushes. J Dent Res 1980;59:2047–55.

Lamberts DM, Wunderlich RC, Caffesse RG. The effect of waxed and unwaxed dental floss on gingival health. Part I. Plaque removal and gingival response. J Periodontol 1982;53:393–6.

Lang NP, Brecx MC. Chlorhexidine digluconate an agent for chemical plaque control and prevention of gingival inflammation. J Periodontol Res 1986; 21(Suppl 16):74–89.

Llewelyn J. A double-blind crossover trial on the effect of cetylpyridinium chloride 0.05% (Merocet) on plaque accumulation. Br Dent J 1980; 148:103–4.

Lobene RR, Soparker PM, Newman MB. Use of dental floss: effect on plaque and gingivitis. Clin Prev Dent 1982;4:5–8.

Macgregor IDM. Toothbrushing efficiency in smokers and non-smokers. J Clin Periodontol 1984;11:313–20.

Niemi ML, Sandholm L, Ainamo J. Frequency of gingival lesions after standardized brushing as related to stiffness of toothbrush and abrasiveness of dentifrice. J Clin Periodontol 1984;11:254–61.

Okada K. A study on the preventive effect of dental caries by chlorhexidine mouthwash. J Nihon Univ Sch Dent 1980;22:65–9.

Ong G. The effectiveness of 3 types of dental floss for interdental plaque removal. J Clin Periodontol 1990;17:463–6.

Reitman WR, Whiteley RT, Robertson PB. Proximal surface cleaning by dental floss Clin Prev Dent 1980;2:7–10.

Schifter CC, Emling RC, Seibert JS, Yankell SH. A comparison of plaque removal effectiveness of an electric versus a manual toothbrush. Clin Prev Dent 1983;5:15–9.

Schonfield SE, Farnoush A, Wilson SG. In vivo antiplaque activity of a sanguinarine-containing dentifrice: comparison with conventional toothpastes. J Periodontol Res 1986;21:298–303.

Segreto VA, Collins EM, Beiswanger BB, et al. A comparison of mouthrinses containing two concentrations of chlorhexidine. J Periodontol Res 1986; 21(Suppl 16):23–32.

Siegrist BE, Gusberti FA, Brecx MC, et al. Efficacy of supervised rinsing with chlorhexidine digluconate in comparison to phenolic and plant alkaloid compounds. J Periodontol Res 1986;21(Suppl 16):60–73.

Smith BA, Collier CM, Caffesse RG. In vitro effectiveness of dental floss in plaque removal. J Clin Periodontol 1986;13:211.

Southard GL, Boulware RT, Walborn DR, et al. Sanguinarine, a new antiplaque agent: retention and plaque specificity. J Am Dent Assoc 1984;108:338–41.

Wade AB. A clinical assessment of the relative properties of nylon and bristle brushes. Br Dent J 1953;94:260–4.

Wennstrom J, Lindhe J. The effect of mouthrinses on parameters characterizing human periodontal disease. J Clin Periodontol 1986;13:86–93.

Wieder SG, Newman HN, Strahan JD. Stannous fluoride and subgingival chlorhexidine irrigation in the control of plaque and chronic periodontitis. J Clin Periodontol 1983;10:172–81.

Wright GZ, Banting DW, Feasby WH. The Dorchester dental flossing study: a final report. Clin Prev Dent 1979;1:23–6.

Wunderlich RC, Lamberts DM, Caffesse RG. The effect of waxed and unwaxed dental floss on gingival health. Part II. Crevicular fluid flow and gingival bleeding. J Periodontol 1982;53:397–400.

Zickert I, Emilson CG, Krasse B. Effect of caries preventive measures in children highly infected with *Streptococcus mutans*. Arch Oral Biol 1982;27:861–8.

Etiology and Pathophysiology—Periodontal Diseases

Amigoni NA, Johnson GK, Kalkwarf KL. The use of sodium bicarbonate and hydrogen peroxide in periodontal therapy: a review. J Am Dent Assoc 1987;114:217–21.

Anderson DL. Etiology of periodontal disease. J Can Dent Assoc 1979; 45:669–72.

Butler RT, Kalkwarf KL, Kaldahl WB. Drug-induced gingival hyperlasia: phenytoin, cyclosporine, and nifedipine. J Am Dent Assoc 1987;114:56–60.

Capilouto ML, Douglass CW. Trends in the prevalence and severity of periodontal diseases in the US: a public health problem? J Public Health Dent 1988;48:245–51.

Dickey RP. Managing contraceptive pill patients. Durant: Creative Infomatics, 1983:68.

Fourel J, Falabregues R, Bonfil JJ. A clinical approach to gingival stimulation. J Periodontol 1981;52:130–4.

Goldhaber P. Oral manifestations of disease. In: Isselbacher KJ, Adams RD, Braunwald E et al. Harrison's principles of internal medicine. New York: McGraw-Hill, 1980:187–92.

Kornman KS. The role of supragingival plaque in the prevention and treatment of periodontal diseases. A review of current concepts. J Periodontol Res 1986;21(Suppl 16):5–22.

Mandel ID, Gaffar A. Calculus revisited. A review. J Clin Periodontol 1986; 13:249–57.

Robertson PB, Walsh M, Greene J, Ernster V, et al. Periodontal effects associated with the use of smokeless tobacco. J Periodontol 1990; 61:438–43.

Serio FG, Siegel MA. Periodontal diseases: a review. Cutis 1991;47:55–62.

Shapiro L, Stallard RE. Etiology of periodontal disease. In: Stallard RE, ed. A textbook of preventive dentistry. Philadelphia: WB Saunders, 1982:61–70.

Stallard RE. Epidemiology of periodontal disease. In: Stallard RE, ed. A textbook of preventive dentistry. Philadelphia: WB Saunders, 1982:50–60.

Weintraub JA, Burt BA. Periodontal effects and dental caries associated with smokeless tobacco use. Public Health Rep 1987;102:30–5.

Oral Hygiene

Wunderlich RC, Caffesse RG, Morrison EC, et al. The therapeutic effect of toothbrushing on naturally occurring gingivitis. J Am Dent Assoc 1985; 110:929–31.

Dental Erosion
Giunta JL. Dental erosion resulting from chewable vitamin C tablets. J Am Dent Assoc 1983; 107:253–6.

Broken Teeth or Misfitting Restorations
Burket LW. Oral medicine in the edentulous patient. In: Lynch MA, ed. Burket's oral medicine. Toronto: JB Lippincott, 1977:568–81.

Cold Sores
Anonymous. Herpes simplex: an overview of the disease and its treatment. Pharm Advis 1982;4(3).

Anonymous. Topical acyclovir for herpes simplex. Med Lett Drugs Ther 1982;24:55–6.

Anonymous. Lipactin gel, Nitrol TSAR kit, MS Contin among Rx/OTC launches. Drug Merch 1986;Feb:38.

Anonymous. Probax, Tabinil, Calsan launched. Drug Merch 1985; Dec:56.

Arndt KA. Herpes simplex. In: Arndt KA, ed. Manual of dermatologic therapeutics. Boston: Little, 1989:75–81.

Danziger S. Ice-packs for cold sores (Letter). Lancet 1978;1:103.

Davis LE, Redman JC, Skipper BJ, McLaren LC. Natural history of frequent recurrences of herpes simplex labialis. Oral Surg Oral Med Oral Pathol 1988;66:558–61.

DiGiovanna JJ, Blank H. Failure of lysine in frequently recurrent herpes simplex infection. Arch Dermatol 1984;120:48–51.

Glezerman M, Lunenfeld E, Cohen V, Sarov I, et al. Placebo-controlled trial of topical interferon in labial and genital herpes. Lancet 1988;1:150–2.

Greenberg MS. Ulcerative, vesicular and bullous lesions. In: Lynch MA, ed. Burket's Oral medicine. Toronto: JB Lippincott, 1984:163–208.

Guinan ME, MacCalman J, Kern ER, et al. Topical ether and herpes simplex labialis. JAMA 1980;243:1059–61.

Jensen JL, Kanas RJ, DeBoom GW. Multiple oral and labial ulcers in an immunocompromised patient. J Am Dent Assoc 1987;114:235–6.

Mills J, Hauer L, Gottlieb A, Dromgoole S, Spruance S. Recurrent herpes labialis in skiers. Clinical observations and effect of sunscreen. Am J Sports Med 1987;15:76–8.

Popovich NG, Popovich JG. What you should know about fever blisters and canker sores. US Pharmacist 1978;3:35–48.

Raborn GW, McGaw WT, Grace M, Percy J, Samuels S. Herpes labialis treatment with acyclovir 5% modified aqueous cream: a double-blind randomized trial. Oral Surg Oral Med Oral Pathol 1989;67:676–9.

Sketris I. Cold sore/canker sore. In: Canadian self-medication. Ottawa: Canadian Pharmaceutical Association, 1978:51–4.

Spruance SL, Stweart JC, Freeman DJ, Brightman VJ, et al. Early application of topical 15% idoxuridine in dimethylsulfoxide shortens the course of herpes simplex labialis: a multicenter placebo-controlled trial. J Infec Dis 1990;161:191–7.

Spruance, SL, Hamill ML, Hoge WS, Davis LG, Mills J. Acyclovir prevents reactivation of herpes simplex labialis in skiers. JAMA 1988;260:1597–9.

Taieb A, Body S, Astar L, du Pasquier P, Maleville J. Clinical epidemiology of symptomatic primary herpetic infection in children. A study of 50 cases. Acta Paediatr Scand 1987;76:128–32.

Wilson IJ. Self treatment of cold cores with ice (Letter). Lancet 1979;1:613.

Young TB, Rimm EB, D'Alessio DJ. Cross-sectional study of recurrent herpes labialis. Prevalence and risk factors. Am J Epidemiol 1988;127:612–25.

Zimmerman DR. Self treatment of cold sores with ice (Letter). Lancet 1978;2:1260.

Canker Sores
Antoon JW, Miller RL. Aphthous ulcers: a review of the literature on etiology, pathogenesis, diagnosis, and treatment. J Am Dent Assoc 1980;101:803–8.

Arndt KA. Aphthous stomatitis (canker sores). In: Arndt KA, ed. Manual of dermatologic therapeutics. Boston: Little, 1983:19–21.

Axell T, Henricsson V. Association between recurrent aphthous ulcers and tobacco habits. Scand J Dent Res 1985;93:239–42.

Bittoun R. Recurrent aphthous ulcers and nicotine. Med J Aust 1991; 154:471–2.

Burns RA, Davis WJ. Recurrent aphthous stomatitis. Am Fam Physician 1985;32:99–104.

Eisen D, Ellis CN. Topical cyclosporine for oral mucosal disorders. J Am Acad Dermatol 1990;23:1259–63.

Eversole LR, Shopper TP, Chambers DW. Effects of suspected foodstuff challenging agents in the etiology of recurrent aphthous stomatitis. Oral Surg Oral Med Oral Pathol 1982;54:33–7.

Ferraro JM, Mattern JQA. Sucralfate suspension for stomatitis (Letter). Drug Intell Clin Pharm 1984;18:153.

Frost M. Cromoglycate in aphthous stomatitis (Letter). Lancet 1973;2:389.

Gallina G, Cumbo V, Messina P, Caruso C. HLA-A, B, C, DR, MT, and MB antigens in recurrent aphthous stomatitis. Oral Surg Oral Med Oral Pathol 1985;59:364–70.

Greenberg MS. Ulcerative, vesicular and bullous lesions. In: Lynch MA, ed. Burket's Oral medicine. Toronto: JB Lippincott, 1984:163–208.

Hay KD, Reade PC. The use of an elimination diet in the treatment of aphthous ulceration of the oral cavity. Oral Surg Oral Med Oral Pathol 1984;57:504–7.

Hoover CI, Olson JA, Greenspan JS. Humoral response and cross-reactivity to viridans streptococci in recurrent aphthous ulceration. J Dent Res 1986;65:1101–4.

Hunter L, Addy M. Chlorhexidine gluconate mouthwash in the management of minor aphthous ulceration. A double-blind, placebo-controlled cross-over trial. Br Dent J 1987;162:106–10.

Hutchinson VA, Angenend JL, Mok WL, Cummins JM, Richards AB. Chronic recurrent aphthous stomatitis: oral treatment with low-dose interferon alpha. Mol Biother 1990;2:160–4.

Lindemann RA, Riviere GR, Sapp JP. Oral mucosal antigen reactivity during exacerbation and remission phases of recurrent aphthous ulceration. Oral Surg Oral Med Oral Pathol 1985;60:281–4.

Miller MF, Chilton NW. The effect of an oxygenating agent upon recurrent aphthous stomatitis—a double-blind clinical trial. Pharmacol Ther Dent 1980;5:55–8.

Miller MF. Use of levamisole in recurrent aphthous stomatitis. Drugs 1980; 19:131–6.

Miller MF, Garfunkel AA, Ram CA, et al. The inheritance of recurrent aphthous stomatitis. Observations on susceptibility. Oral Surg Oral Med Oral Pathol 1980;49:409–12.

Nicolau DP, West TE. Thalidomide: treatment of severe recurrent aphthous stomatitis in patients with AIDS. Drug Intell Clin Pharm 1990;24:1054–6.

Olson JA, Feinberg I, Silverman S Jr, Abrams D, Greenspan JS. Serum vitamin B_{12}, folate, and iron levels in recurrent aphthous ulceration. Oral Surg Oral Med Oral Pathol 1982;54:517–20.

Pedersen A, Hougen HP, Klausen B, Winther K. LongoVital in the prevention of recurrent aphthous ulceration. J Oral Pathol Med 1991;19:371–5.

Pimlott SJ, Walker DM. A controlled trial of the efficacy of topically applied fluocinonide in the treatment of recurrent aphthous ulceration. Br Dent J 1983;154:174–7.

Poswillo D, Partridge M. Management of recurrent aphthous ulcers: a trial of carbenoxolone sodium mouthwash. Br Dent J 1984;157:55–7.

Potoky JR. Recurrent aphthous stomatitis; a proposed therapeutic regimen. J Oral Med 1981;36:44–6.

Potts AJC, Frame JW, Bateman JRM, Asquith P. Sodium cromoglycate toothpaste in the management of aphthous ulceration. Br Dent J 1984;156:250–1.

Ricer RE. Sucralfate vs placebo for the treatment of aphthous ulcers: a double-blinded prospective clinical trial. Fam Pract Res J 1989;9:33–41.

Ruah CB, Stram JR, Chasin WD. Treatment of severe recurrent aphthous stomatitis with colchicine. Arch Otolaryngol Head Neck Surg 1988; 114:671–5.

Scully C, Porter SR. Recurrent aphthous stomatitis: current concepts of etiology, pathogenesis and management. J Oral Pathol Med 1989;18:21–7.

Thompson AC, Nolan A, Lamey PJ. Minor aphthous oral ulceration: a double-blind cross-over study of beclomethasone dipropionate aerosol spray. Scott Med J 1989;34:531–2.

Wray D, Graykowski EA, Notkins AL. Role of mucosal injury in initiating recurrent aphthous stomatitis. Br Med J 1981;283:1569–70.

Wray D, Vlagopoulos TP, Siraganian RP. Food allergens and basophil histamine release in recurrent aphthous stomatitis. Oral Surg Oral Med Oral Pathol 1982;54:388–95.

Wray D. A double-blind trial of systemic zinc sulfate in recurrent aphthous stomatitis. Oral Surg Oral Med Oral Pathol 1982;53:469–72.

Wright A, Ryan FP, Willingham SE, et al. Food allergy or intolerance in severe recurrent aphthous ulceration of the mouth. Br Med J 1986;292:1237–8.

Zissis NP, Hatzioti AJ, Antoniadis D, Ninika A, Hatziotis JC. Therapeutic evaluation of levamisole in recurrent aphthous stomatitis. J Oral Med 1983;38:161–3.

Candidiasis

Arendorf TM, Walker DM. The prevalence and intraoral distribution of *Candida albicans* in man. Arch Oral Bio 1980;25:1–10.

Arndt KA. Fungal infections—candidiasis. In: Arndt KA, ed. Manual of dermatologic therapeutics. Boston: Little, 1989:63–6.

Cohen L. Oral candidiasis—its diagnosis and treatment. J Oral Med 1972; 27:7–11.

DePaola LG, Peterson DE, Overholser CD Jr, et al. Dental care for patients receiving chemotherapy. J Am Dent Assoc 1986;112:198–203.

Hay KD. Candidosis of the oral cavity: recognition and management. Drugs 1988;36:633–42.

Holbrook WP, Rodgers GD. Candidal infections: experience in a British dental hospital. Oral Surg Oral Med Oral Pathol 1980;49:122–5.

Jones HE. Therapy of superficial fungal infection. Med Clin North Am 1982;66:873–93.

Scrafani JT. Superficial fungal infections and their treatment. US Pharmacist 1978;3:26–38.

Other Causes of Oral Lesions

Wright WE, Haller JM, Harlow SA, Pizzo PA. An oral disease prevention program for patients receiving radiation and chemotherapy. J Am Dent Assoc 1985;110:43–7.

Bad Breath

Attia EL, Marshall KG. Halitosis. Can Med Assoc J 1982;126:1281–5.

Dry Mouth

Ettinger RL. Xerostomia—a complication of aging. Aust Dent J 1981; 26:365–71.

Fox PC, van der Ven PF, Sonies BC, Weiffenbach JM, Baum BJ. Xerostomia: evaluation of a symptom with increasing significance. J Am Dent Assoc 1985;110:519–25.

Glass BJ, Van Dis ML, Langlais RP, et al. Xerostomia: diagnosis and treatment planning considerations. Oral Surg Oral Med Oral Pathol 1984;58:248–52.

Gossel TA. Dry mouth and use of saliva substitutes. US Pharmacist 1986; 11:22–8,58.

Grad H, Grushka M, Yanover L. Drug-induced xerostomia: the effects and treatment. J Can Dent Assoc 1985;51:296–300.

Navazesh M. Xerostomia in the aged. Dent Clin N Amer 1989;33:75–80.

Schubert MM, Izutsu KT. Iatrogenic causes of salivary gland dysfunction. J Dent Res 1987;66:680–8.

Spielman A, Ben-Aryeh H, Gutman D, et al. Xerostomia—diagnosis and treatment. Oral Surg Oral Med Oral Pathol 1981;51:144–7.

Sreebny LM, Valdini A. Xerostomia: a neglected symptom. Arch Int Med 1987;147:1333–7.

Pharmaceutical Agents

Anonymous. NDMAC Nonprescription Drug Digest 1991;(August):7.

Dentifrices

Addy M, Mostafa P. Dentine hypersensitivity. II. Effects produced by the uptake in vitro of toothpastes onto dentine. J Oral Rehabil 1989;16:35–48.

Anonymous. New rules for tooth whiteners, labels. NDMAC Nonprescription Drug Digest 1991;(August):7.

Council on Dental Therapeutics. Acceptance of Sensodyne toothpaste for sensitive teeth. J Am Dent Assoc 1985;110:394–5.

Council on Dental Therapeutics. Evaluation of Denquel sensitive teeth toothpaste. J Am Dent Assoc 1982;105:80.

Council on Dental Therapeutics. Acceptance of Promise with Fluoride and Sensodyne-F toothpastes for sensitive teeth. J Am Dent Assoc 1986; 113:673–5.

Dowell TB. The use of toothpaste in infancy. Br Dent J 1981;150:247–9.

Fed Reg 1980;45:20666.

Goldberg HJ, Enslein K. Effect of an experimental sodium bicarbonate dentifrice on gingivitis and plaque formation: I. in adults. Clin Prev Dent 1979;1:12–6.

Hannah JJ, Johnson JD, Kuftinec MM. Long-term clinical evaluation of toothpaste and oral rinse containing sanguinaria extract in controlling plaque, gingival inflammation, and sulcular bleeding during orthodontic treatment. Am J Orthod Dentofacial Orthop 1989;96:199–207.

Harper DS, Mueller LJ, Fine JB, Gordon J, Laster LL. Clinical efficacy of a dentifrice and oral rinse containing sanguinaria extract and zinc chloride during 6 months of use. J Periodontol 1990;61:352–8.

Harper DS, Mueller LJ, Fine JB, Gordon J, Laster LL. Effect of 6 months use of a dentifrice and oral rinse containing sanguinaria extract and zinc chloride upon the microflora of the dental plaque and oral soft tissues. J Periodontol 1990;61:359–63.

Jensen ME, Kohout R. The effect of a fluoridated dentifrice on root and coronal caries in an older adult population. J Am Dent Assoc 1988;117:829–32.

Kanapka JA. Over-the-counter dentifrices in the treatment of tooth hypersensitivity. Dent Clin N Amer 1990;34:545–60.

Kazmierczak M, Mather M, Ciancio S, Fischman S, Cancro L. Clinical evaluation of anticalculus dentifrices. Clin Prev Dent 1990;12:13–7.

Kohut BE, Rubin H, Baron HJ. The relative clinical effectiveness of three anticalculus dentifrices. Clin Prev Dent 1989;11:13–6.

Lamb DJ, Howell RA, Constable G. Removal of plaque and stain from natural teeth by a low abrasivity toothpaste. Br Dent J 1984;157:125–7.

Lobene RR. A study to compare the effects of two dentifrices on adult dental calculus formation. J Clin Dent 1989;1:67–9.

Mallatt ME, Beiswanger BB, Drook CA, Stookey GK, et al. Clinical effect of a sanguinaria dentifrice on plaque and gingivitis in adults. J Periodontal 1989;60:91–5.

Rugg-Gunn AJ. A double-blind clinical trial of an anticalculus toothpaste containing pyrophosphate and sodium monofluorophosphate. Br Dent J 1988;165:133–6.

Schiff TG. The effect of a dentifrice containing soluble pyrophosphate and sodium fluoride on calculus deposits. A 6-month clinical study. Clin Prev Dent 1987;9:13–6.

Svatun B, Saxton CA, Rolla G, van der Ouderaa F. One-year study of the efficacy of a dentifrice containing zinc citrate and triclosan to maintain gingival health. Scand J Dent Res 1989;97:242–6.

Tarbet WJ, Silverman G, Fratarcangelo PA, Kanapaka JA. Home treatment for dentinal hypersensitivity: a comparative study. J Am Dent Assoc 1982; 105:227–30.

Volpe AR. Dentifrices and mouthrinses. In: Stallard RE, ed. A textbook of preventive dentistry. Philadelphia: WB Saunders, 1982:170–216.

Winer RA, Tsamtsouris A. Effects of an experimental sodium bicarbonate dentifrice on gingivitis and plaque formation: II. in teenaged students. Clin Prev Dent 1979;1:17–8.

Zacherl WA, Pfieffer HJ, Swancar JR. The effect of soluble pyrophosphates on dental calculus in adults. J Am Dent Assoc 1985;110:737–8.

Mouthwashes

Addy M. Pre-brushing mouthrinse PLAX. (Letter) Br Dent J 1989;167:10–1.

Anonymous. Peridex oral rinse (Product Information). Cambridge: Procter and Gamble, 1987.

Asikainen S, Sandholm L, Sandman S, Ainamo J. Gingival bleeding after chlorhexidine rinses with or without mechanical oral hygiene. J Clin Periodontol 1984;11:87–94.

Axelsson P, Lindhe J. Efficacy of mouthrinses in inhibiting dental plaque and gingivitis in man. J Clin Periodontol 1987;14:205–12.

Beiswanger BB, Mallatt ME, Mau MS, Katz BP. The relative plaque removal effect of a prebrushing mouthrinse. J Am Dent Assoc 1990;120:190–2.

Oral Hygiene

Blot WJ, Winn DM, Fraumeni JF Jr. Oral cancer and mouthwash. JNCI 1983;70:251–3.

Brecz M, Netuschil L, Reichert B, Schreil G. Efficacy of Listerine, Meridol, and chlorhexidine mouthrinses on plaque, gingivitis, and plaque bacteria vitality. J Clin Periodontol 1990;17:292–7.

Etemadzadeh H, Ainamo J. Lacking anti-plaque efficacy of 2 sanguinarine mouth rinses. J Clin Periodontol 1987;14:176–80.

Fed Reg 1982;47:22760–930.

Grossman E, Meckel AH, Isaacs RL, Ferretti GA, et al. A clinical comparison of antibacterial mouthrinses: effects of chlorhexidine, phenolics, and sanguinarine on dental plaque and gingivitis. J Periodontol 1989;60:435–40.

Grossman E. Effectiveness of a prebrushing mouthrinse under single-trial and home-use conditions. Clin Prev Dent 1988;10:3–6.

Lamster IB, et al. The effect of Listerine antiseptic on reduction of existing plaque and gingivitis. Clin Prev Dent 1983;5:6.

Leung AKC. Ethanol-induced hypoglycemia from mouthwash (Letter). Drug Intell Clin Pharm 1985;19:480–1.

Mankodi S, Ross NM, Mostler K. Clinical efficacy of Listerine in inhibiting and reducing plaque and experimental gingivitis. J Clin Periodontol 1987;14:285–8.

Mashberg A, Barsa P, Grossman ML. A study of the relationship between mouthwash use and oral and pharyngeal cancer. J Am Dent Assoc 1985;110:731–4.

Minah GE, DePaola LG, Overholser CD, Meiller TF, et al. Effects of 6 months use of an antiseptic mouthrinse on supragingival dental plaque microflora. J Clin Periodontol 1989;16:347–52.

Moran J, Addy M, Newcombe R. A clinical trial to assess the efficacy of sanguinarine-zinc mouthrinse (Viadent) compared with chlorhexidine mouthrinse (Corosodyl). J Clin Periodontol 1988;15:612–6.

Overholser CD, Meiller TF, DePaola LG, Minah GE, Niehaus C. Comparative effects of 2 chemotherapeutic mouthrinses on the development of supragingival dental plaque and gingivitis. J Clin Periodontol 1990;17:575–9.

Overholser D, et al. Comparative effects of chemotherapeutic agents in the reduction of plaque and gingivitis. J Dent Res 1988;67:329.

Parsons LG, Thomas LG, Southard GL, Woodall IR, Jones BJ. Effect of sanguinaria extract on established plaque and gingivitis when supragingivally delivered as a manual rinse or under pressure in an oral irrigator. J Clin Periodontol 1987;14:381–5.

Quirynen M, Marechal M, van Steenberghe D. Comparative antiplaque activity of sanguinarine and chlorhexidine in man. J Clin Periodontol 1990;17:223–7.

Ross NM, Charles CH, Dills SS. Long-term effects of Listerine antiseptic on dental plaque and gingivitis. J Clin Dent 1989;1:92–5.

Singh SM. Efficacy of a prebrushing rinse in reducing dental plaque. Am J Dent 1990;3:15–6.

Weller-Fahy ER, Berger LR, Troutman WG. Mouthwash: a source of acute ethanol intoxication. Pediatrics 1980;66:302–5.

Wynder EL, Kabat G, Rosenberg S, Levenstein M. Oral cancer and mouthwash use. JNCI 1983;70:255–60.

Toothache Relievers

Fed Reg 1982;47:22172–59.

Hume WR. The pharmacologic and toxicologic properties of zinc oxide-eugenol. J Am Dent Assoc 1986;113:789–91.

Sveen OB, Yaekel M, Adair SM. Efficacy of using benzocaine for temporary relief of toothache. Oral Surg Oral Med Oral Pathol 1982;53:574–6.

Products for Dry Mouth

Anonymous. Fights mouth dryness: Biotene. Drug Merch 1986;Aug:47.

Fischer JM, Schwinghammer T. Are saliva substitute products available, and why would they be used? US Pharmacist 1983;8:9.

Hatton MN, Levine MJ, Margarone JE, Aguirre A. Lubrication and viscosity features of human saliva and commercially available saliva substitutes. J Oral Maxillofac Surg 1987;45:496–9.

Klestov AC, Webb J, Latt D, et al. Treatment of xerostomia: a double-blind trial in 108 patients with Sjögren's syndrome. Oral Surg Oral Med Oral Pathol 1981;51:594–9.

Levine MJ, Aguirre A, Hatton MN, Tabak LA. Artificial salivas: present and future. J Dent Res 1987;66:693–8.

Wiesenfeld D, Stewart AM, Mason DK. Critical assessment of oral lubricants in patients with xerostomia. Br Dent J 1983;155:155–7.

Denture Products

Abelson DC. Denture plaque and denture cleansers. J Prosthet Dent 1981;45:376–9.

Augsburger RHH, Elahi JM. Evaluation of seven proprietary denture cleansers. J Prosthet Dent 1982;47:356–9.

Budtz-Jorgensen E. Materials and methods for cleaning dentures. J Prosthet Dent 1979;42:619–23.

Budtz-Jorgensen E. Prevention of denture plaque formation by an enzyme denture cleanser. J Biol Buccale 1977;5:239–44.

Council on Dental Materials, Instruments, and Equipment. Denture cleansers. J Am Dent Assoc 1983;106:77–8.

Dills SS, Olshan AM, Goldner S, Brogdon C. Comparison of the antimicrobial capability of an abrasive paste and chemical-soak denture cleaner. J Prosthet Dent 1988;60:467–70.

Ghalichebaf M, Graser GN, Zander HA. The efficacy of denture-cleansing agents. J Prosthet Dent 1982;48:515–20.

Lambert JP, Kolstad R. Effect of a benzoic acid-detergent germicide on denture-borne Candida albicans. J Prosthet Dent 1986;55:699–700.

Moore TC, Smith DE, Kenny GE. Sanitization of dentures by several denture hygiene methods. J Prosthet Dent 1984;52:158–63.

Murray ID, McCabe JF, Storer R. Abrasivity of denture cleaning pastes in vitro and in situ. Br Dent J 1986;161:137–41.

Tarbet WJ, Axelrod S, Minkoff S, Fratarcangelo PA. Denture cleansing: a comparison of two methods. J Prosthet Dent 1984;51:322–5.

12

The Common Cold

Jeffrey G. Taylor

As no known cure exists for the common cold, treatment is directed at relieving symptoms. Decongestants, antitussives, expectorants and antihistamines are the main groups of agents that will, to varying degree, be useful in alleviating bothersome symptoms. Pharmacists with a knowledge of about 20 individual agents from these groups can help the cold sufferer sort through the vast assortment of cold products.

The common cold is an acute, self-limiting viral infection involving the mucous membranes of the upper respiratory tract. Various references may use the synonyms catarrh, coryza, or infectious rhinitis to describe a cold. Regardless of the term used, the common cold is one of the most common acute illnesses to affect mankind. Most can attest to the discomfort a cold creates.

While rarely serious, colds are responsible for much of the absenteeism from school and the workplace. In about half of all cases, affected individuals spend at least one day at home. Colds are also one of the major reasons for visits to the family doctor. Many other individuals choose to combat their colds with a variety of "remedies"—from hot lemonade, garlic, a spoonful of honey or chicken soup to a good shot of whiskey.

Epidemiology

As many as 90 per cent of all acute respiratory infections are caused by viruses. More than 200 distinct viruses are known to cause illness in the respiratory tract. Over 100 virus types have been identified as the causative agents of the common cold. The most common causes are rhinoviruses and coronaviruses, which respectively cause about 40 per cent and 10 to 20 per cent of colds in adults. Other viruses such as parainfluenza, respiratory syncytial, adenosackie-, echosackie- and coxsackie-viruses have also been implicated. The causative agents in 30 to 50 per cent of cases have yet to be determined; most are assumed to be viral. Generally, cold symptoms produced by the common respiratory viruses are similar and isolating the specific agent in each case would be unproductive.

The common cold is an easily spread and easily contracted illness. Surveys in the United States and England indicate colds occur at a rate of about one to three episodes per person per year. Infants typically get more colds than members of any other age group, averaging about 6 to 8 episodes per year. This group is quite susceptible as they have a relatively underdeveloped immune system. The incidence

remains high in children until around age 6, then frequency progressively decreases.

Adults experience fewer common respiratory illnesses than children. Women (especially those aged 20 to 30 years) have more colds than men, apparently because of greater exposure to children.

Colds can occur throughout the year but show peak rates of occurrence in autumn, mid-winter and early spring. The peak evident in September is possibly due to the reopening of school, but other unknown factors may be involved. Why the incidence of colds is higher in the winter remains unknown but may relate in part to people spending more time indoors.

Common beliefs that cold weather, wet feet or chilling of the body induce a cold are unlikely true. Exposure to cold temperature in itself has not lead to colds in volunteers. However, cold or wet weather may play a role. A possible explanation for this is that indoor to outdoor temperature variations often cause a vasomotor response in the nasal mucosa, which leads to a runny nose. This state may make nasal cells easier targets for viral penetration.

Whether fatigue, poor nutritional status or general state of health can lead to more cold episodes remains unclear; they may be factors in the severity of the cold. The elderly are more prone to infections, perhaps as a result of these factors. Emotional stress may be associated with higher susceptibility to colds.

Most research on the spread of the common cold has involved rhinoviruses under laboratory conditions. Cold sufferers spread the virus to other people via infected respiratory secretions. While it is a natural tendency to turn quickly away from someone sneezing or coughing, there is evidence that some cold viruses are inefficiently transmitted directly via aerosolized droplets. Droplets created by a sneeze may be more apt to cause infection if the infected droplets land on the cold sufferer's hand.

Hand-to-hand contact is therefore felt to be an important mechanism for viral transfer. Contact with an object recently handled by an infected person is also a proposed mechanism. Cold viruses can survive several hours on hands or hard surfaces and it only takes brief contact with an infected person or object for transmission to take place. The virus enters the body of uninfected persons when their hands subsequently touch their eyes or rub their nose. Virus contacting the eyes eventually are introduced into the nose by way of the nasolacrimal duct.

A study with married couples indicates saliva is poorly associated with transmission. The mucous membranes of the oral cavity have a relatively high resistance to the virus.

The Common Cold

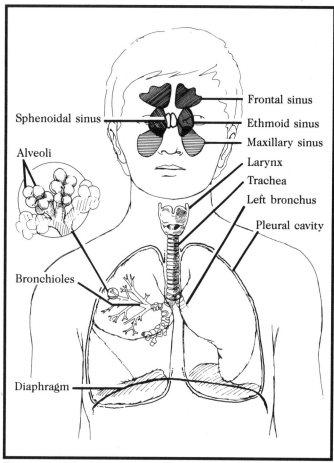

Figure 1 *The Respiratory Tract*

The Respiratory Tract

Many structures and mechanisms are present to protect the respiratory tract against infection and inhaled foreign material. Some of these structures and mechanisms are mucus, cilia, phagocytosis, cough and bronchoconstriction.

The nose marks the entrance to the respiratory tract (see Figure 1). The hairs at the entrance of the nose filter incoming air of relatively large particles and, with the sneeze reflex, provide the first line of defence for the respiratory tract. The interior cavity of the nose is lined with mucous membrane, which contains a rich network of capillaries to heat and supply moisture to inspired air. The layer of mucus that coats the internal surfaces of the nose also helps to trap inhaled particles.

Autonomic control of the local vasculature maintains the delicate balance of nasal patency; membranes shrink and expand throughout the day to vary the size of the air passages. Stimulation of sympathetic (adrenergic) nerves causes vasoconstriction and drying of secretions. Parasympathetic (cholinergic) stimulation produces vasodilation and an increase in secretions. Reflex changes may also occur in the nasal tissues to changing conditions of the inspired air, for example, a temperature change.

The nasal passages lead into the pharynx (throat). It is possible to breathe through the mouth and bypass the nose. However, as the mouth has no apparatus for conditioning air, mouth breathing often causes the throat to become dry and irritated.

Four pairs of paranasal sinuses are present in the skull. They are cavities formed by bone and are lined with mucous membrane. The names of the sinuses relate to the skull bones in which they are located: maxillary, frontal, ethmoidal and sphenoidal. Mucus produced in the sinuses is continually being swept out through small openings and into the nasal cavity by cilia. During a cold, sinus openings may become blocked subsequent to swelling of the mucous membrane. Drainage of secretions into the nasal cavity decreases, but mucus continues to form and pressure builds within the sinuses.

The eustachian tubes connect the middle ear to the nasopharynx, the part of the throat behind the nose. They are lined with mucosa and are present to equilibrate middle ear pressure. Unfortunately, they also provide pathways by which throat and nasal infections enter the middle ear.

A mucous blanket covers most of the respiratory tract. Mucus is a demulcent fluid that helps trap particulate matter and micro-organisms. It is produced by various cells and glands of the mucous membranes. Respiratory mucus is 95 per cent water. Glycoproteins give mucus its consistency and the necessary viscosity and elasticity for effective clearance by ciliary transport and by coughing. The mucous blanket is also rich in substances like lysozymes and immunoglobulins which protect the underlying cells by destroying foreign substances.

Mucus is transported up the airway and down from the nose and sinuses by the constant wavelike motion of the cilia. Healthy persons produce 100 to 150 mL of tracheobronchial fluid daily, move it to the pharynx and swallow it without being aware of doing so. Removal of the mucus covering on the ciliated cells or a change in its consistency (for example, via dry inspired air) can impair the function of the cilia. Cigarette smoke also has a detrimental effect on the activity of cilia.

Two defensive respiratory reflexes exist by which material can be expelled from the respiratory tract: the cough and the sneeze. The purpose of coughing is to help eliminate the stimulus responsible for its initiation. When coughing no longer serves this function it is of little benefit. Each cough is a complex reflex that begins with irritation of cough receptors lining the respiratory tract. Stimulus from the irritation transmits impulses along the vagus nerve to the cough centre in the medulla. Little is known about the cough centre except that it appears to summate incoming impulses, then coordinates the cough response. Impulses from the cough centre are transmitted along cholinergic pathways to the diaphragm and to the intercostal and abdominal muscles.

The mechanical events of a cough begin with the inspiration of air, for which the glottis opens widely. Glottic closure follows along with the active contraction of the expiratory muscles. This causes a rapid increase in intrathoracic pressure which creates the air speed necessary for an effective cough. Pressures as high as 300 mm Hg can be generated during this phase. Expiration occurs with the sudden opening of the glottis—the characteristic sound of a cough occurs. It is during this expulsion of high-velocity air that irritant material can be removed from the respiratory tract. Coughing is partly under voluntary control, unlike the sneeze reflex.

The sneeze reflex is a protective mechanism similar in function to the cough reflex. Irritation to the nasal tissues provides the stimulus to initiate the reflex. The outcome of events is rapid air travel through the nose, which helps clear the nasal passages of foreign material.

Pathophysiology

Colds are caused by viruses. A typical viral particle contains a core of nucleic acid (either DNA or RNA) that governs replication. Many viruses have an envelope surrounding this material, which serves a protective function and participates in the attachment to susceptible host cells. The protein content of the envelope is responsible for the antigenicity of the virus. Viruses must enter living host cells to survive because they lack metabolic activity of their own.

To produce infection, a virus must penetrate the mucous blanket covering the nasal epithelium. Only a few infectious particles need be implanted for an infection to occur. After traversing the mucous layers, viral particles will bind to cell receptor sites. Host cells appear to have specific entry sites where viruses enter the cell, replicate, and cause disease. Originally, it was theorized many sites for entry existed. Recent evidence suggests that many strains of rhinovirus use the same receptor site for cell entry. This has important implications for the research into developing receptor-blocking agents.

Once viruses penetrate the host cell, they release their nucleic acid. Following this release, the replication, transcription and translation of the viral genome occurs. These events lead to the production of new viruses.

The period from exposure to a virus to the appearance of the first symptoms of a cold is called the incubation period. The incubation period for rhinoviruses is short, generally 1 to 2 days, whereas that for coronaviruses is about 3 days.

Most respiratory viruses produce illness through the direct consequences of local multiplication that leads to host cell death and causes desquamation of the respiratory epithelium. Symptoms of colds are due in part to this respiratory epithelial injury. As the virus disseminates, the body also responds with an inflammatory reaction in the affected areas involving immunomodulators and inflammatory mediators. Kinins (potent autocoids) may contribute to the symptomatology of the inflammatory reaction. Immunoglobulins (especially IgA) become more abundant in the area. Increased perfusion brings lymphocytes to fight the infection. Histamine release is not a significant factor in upper respiratory tract infections.

Acute viral infections usually terminate when the host develops a sufficient immune response to the infecting virus. Immunity to specific cold viruses begins to fade 18 months after infection. Because so many viruses can cause a cold, exposure to a different strain of virus within this time is likely, with resultant infection. Vaccination against cold viruses is not feasible at this time due to the multiplicity of virus strains and the difficulty in preparing attenuated versions of the viruses.

Signs and Symptoms

The signs and symptoms of the common cold are primarily manifestations of inflammation of the mucous membranes of the respiratory tract. This inflammation is evident as excess blood flow to the area, abnormal fluid accumulation in the extracellular spaces, and profuse watery discharge from the nasal mucous membranes. The most common symptoms are nasal discharge and congestion (80 to 100 per cent of patients), sneezing (50 to 70 per cent), sore throat (50 per cent), and cough (40 per cent). Symptoms usually last about 7 days with peak symptoms occurring on the second and third days. Symptoms last up to 2 weeks in 25 per cent of cases.

The most bothersome symptoms of each cold and their sequence of appearance differ from person to person, but generally follow a pattern. The first symptom to appear is usually discomfort of the throat. People often describe this feeling as dryness, scratchiness, or soreness rather than as actual pain. Viral infections do not result in exudate over the pharynx or tonsils.

Varying degrees of nasal congestion and rhinorrhea follow the throat discomfort. Initially, nasal discharge is clear and watery, but becomes thicker and opaque as the infection progresses. This is due to the large number of epithelial and white blood cells being shed. The discharge may become purulent if secondarily infected with bacteria.

The inflammatory response dilates blood vessels and increases blood flow to the area. The increase in the volume of nasal secretions and the change in its consistency make breathing through the nose difficult. One nostril is often completely occluded while the other is slightly open, a situation that alternates back and forth throughout the day. Congestion may lead to sinusitis and headache or to otic symptoms (especially in children) such as pain or a plugged sensation. Congestion also causes nasal irritation that can lead to sneezing. Postnasal drip is common and can cause coughing or laryngitis. Conjunctivitis and watering eyes can be common initial manifestations.

Children may develop fever (38 to 39°C), but fever of any significant degree is seldom prominent with colds. Chill sensations, however, are common. Cervical lymph nodes may be enlarged and slightly tender.

The cough accompanying a cold usually starts as dry and unproductive. As the cold progresses, the increased bronchial secretions and cellular debris from phagocytic activity can lead to a productive cough. Either a dry or a productive cough may persist for 1 to 2 weeks.

Although these symptoms can be discomforting, they seldom cause serious complications. Complications that have occurred include sinusitis, otitis media, exacerbation of asthma, and infectious exacerbations in people with chronic obstructive pulmonary disease. Increased chest involvement with purulent sputum suggests bacterial infection. Barring complications, the common cold causes minimal residual pathological damage to the respiratory tract.

Differential Diagnosis

Other conditions are known to present with symptoms similar to those of the common cold. For example, persistent cold-like symptoms in the summertime may suggest allergic rhinitis. It is important for the pharmacist to differentiate other conditions from the common cold, assess if self-medication is appropriate and, if not, refer the individual to a physician. Suspected bacterial infections should always be referred to a physician, as should fever in small children.

Table I should assist in the assessment of symptoms involving the upper respiratory tract. Generally, the main difference between the common cold and other respiratory tract infections is the absence of fever with the common cold and their relative lack of systemic symptoms.

Pharyngitis (Sore Throat)

Acute pharyngitis (sore throat) is an inflammatory syndrome of the pharynx, generally due to viral or bacterial infections. Most cases are of viral etiology (75 to 80 per cent of episodes) and occur as part of the symptom complex evident with colds and influenza. Most

The Common Cold

Table I *Differential Diagnosis of the Common Cold*

Symptom	Common cold	Acute sinusitis	Strep throat	Influenza
Nasal discharge	Common; clear, copious rhinorrhea initially, followed by a more mucopurulent appearance; nasal congestion is common.	Purulent, often colored	Rare	Present, but overshadowed by systemic symptoms; clear discharge initially, becoming more purulent; nasal obstruction is uncommon.
Fever	Rare; low grade if any.	Over 38°C; variable with severity of the infection; present in less than one-half of sufferers; mainly children.	Over 38°C in 90% of children; spiking	39 to 40°C; sudden onset, lasting 3 to 4 days.
Sore throat	Common but mild; should be gone within 3 days.	None, unless associated with postnasal drip.	Pain onset is severe and sudden; inflamed; exudate at back of throat and on tonsils; voice could be hoarse.	Sometimes
Cough	Mild to moderate, dry, hacking cough; may change presentation during course of cold.	None, unless associated with postnasal drip.	Rare	Common; can be severe.
Headache	Rare; more frequent with sinus congestion.	Occurs via sinus congestion; pain over involved areas; typically is worse during the day and subsides in evening; varies with a change in body position.	Occurs in 70% of children.	Prominent; throbbing, frontal headache; severity is related to the level of the fever.
General aches and pain/fatigue and weakness	Mild	Rare	Malaise possible.	Common; often severe; fatigue and weakness can last up to 2 to 3 weeks.
Other		Acute maxillary sinusitis may cause a feeling of pain in the area of the teeth; chronic sinus infection may produce minimal symptoms.	Breath odor; cervical lymphadenopathy; abdominal pain in 20% of children.	Chills; GI symptoms, e.g., diarrhea, vomiting; the main symptoms are sudden and severe in onset.
Duration of illness	5 to 7 days	Days; months if not treated	Commonly 3 days; up to a week.	Approximately 10 days
Cause	Viral	Bacterial (Staphylococcus, Streptococcus, *Haemophilus influenzae*); usually follows an acute upper respiratory infection or nasal allergies, or less frequently, swimming and dental abscess.	*S. pyogenes;* note that other bacteria can cause sore throat.	Influenza virus

episodes are therefore benign and self-limiting. However, sore throat in children, alone or with other symptoms, should be referred to a physician. Throat irritation is present in about half of those suffering with a cold. Sore throat associated with nasal involvement and cough, but with mild pharyngeal discomfort suggests viral rather than bacterial infection. Acute episodes of uncomplicated viral pharyngitis usually clear within 3 days. Generally, antibiotic therapy is of little benefit in sore throats of viral origin.

Bacteria are the next most common cause of a sore throat, with the main causative agent being *Streptococcus pyogenes* (group A ß-

hemolytic streptococcus). This organism is the most frequent bacterial cause of acute pharyngitis, although it accounts for a minority of all sore throats. Infections of this type occur mainly in the young and are uncommon in adults.

Streptococcal pharyngitis (strep throat) is characterized by sore throat, fever (often greater than 38.3°C), a beefy-red pharynx and exudate over the tonsils. The onset of pain in the throat is more rapid than commonly seen with viral infections and the pain is more severe. The pain is aggravated by swallowing. The cervical lymph nodes may enlarge and become tender. Though uncommon, if cough and nasal congestion do occur, the bacterial infection may be in concert with another etiologic agent. It is often difficult to differentiate streptococcal from nonstreptococcal sore throat without a throat culture. Home diagnostic tests for *S. pyogenes* are commercially available in the United States.

Strep throat symptoms usually last about 3 days, with or without antibiotic therapy. Regardless, individuals who are suspected of having strep throat are to be referred to medical care. A decision to treat with antibiotics is partly based on the risk of the individual developing two serious sequelae to strep throat, acute rheumatic fever and acute glomerulonephritis.

Sore throat can also be a manifestation of serious illness and the pharmacist must be aware of this.

Influenza

Those suffering from cold-like symptoms may describe their condition as the "flu"; the public often incorrectly use the two terms interchangeably. The majority of patients with upper respiratory tract symptoms are not suffering from influenza, but rather the common cold. True influenza is a much more serious state.

Influenza is an acute respiratory infection caused by myxovirus A, B or C. Type A-influenza virus is the most virulent and causes outbreaks of infection almost annually. The outbreaks reach epidemic proportions every 2 or 3 years, usually in winter. The three types vary genetically and cross-immunity to them cannot be acquired. People of all ages are affected but influenza is most prevalent in school children. Symptoms are most severe in the young, the aged and those confined to bed.

Influenza is contracted by coming into contact with the respiratory secretions of a person with the virus. Symptoms occur rapidly and many people are able to pinpoint the hour of onset. Initially, systemic symptoms predominate including fever, chills, headache, myalgias (most pronounced in the back and legs) and malaise. The individual often feels extremely weak. The face is flushed and the skin is hot and moist. Diarrhea occurs in children but is rare in adults. Fever is marked and rises rapidly to a peak of 38 to 40°C within 12 hours of onset. Occasionally temperatures reach 41°C. The severity of the illness parallels the level of the fever; as the fever subsides, systemic symptoms diminish.

Symptoms such as sore throat, unproductive cough and rhinorrhea are mild at first, but become dominant later in the illness. These symptoms usually persist 3 to 4 days after the fever subsides. Cough, lassitude and malaise may linger for 2 or more weeks before full recovery. Cough is the most frequent and troublesome of these lingering symptoms. It develops in more than 75 per cent of cases and can be severe. An unproductive cough is evident more often than a productive cough.

Although the symptoms are more severe than the common cold, little can be done to reduce the effects or the duration of the infection. Symptomatic measures such as bed rest and increased fluid intake are the mainstays of therapy. Acetylsalicylic acid (ASA) should not be used to lower temperature in children and teenagers due to the association of such use with the development of Reye's syndrome. Cough suppression, once pneumonia has been ruled out, allows the patient to rest.

A major complication of influenza is pneumonia due either to an overgrowth of the influenza virus or, more commonly, bacteria. The onset of viral pneumonia is about 1 week after the individual appears to recover from the original illness. Secondary bacterial pneumonia also appears after apparent recovery from influenza, with severe respiratory symptoms and characteristic infectious symptoms. Patients with bacterial pneumonia often present with fever, chills, chest pain, and a cough that produces purulent or rust-colored sputum.

True influenza is a serious disease. An estimated 5,000 Canadians die every year due to flu-aggravated illness. Over 80 per cent of these were over 65 years of age. Annual immunization can prevent influenza and is therefore recommended for patients at high risk of complications. The National Advisory Committee of Immunization (1991) recommended that the following receive consideration for immunization: those over 65 years of age; residents of nursing homes or chronic care facilities; those with chronic lung, heart, or kidney disease; diabetics; cancer patients; and those with anemia. Health professionals and household members in contact with persons of high-risk groups should also consider vaccination. Protection as a result of the vaccine begins within 2 weeks and lasts for about 6 months. The type of vaccine used each year may change. During influenza epidemics, systemic antiviral agents may have to be considered.

Sinusitis

Sinusitis can be described as an inflammation of the mucosal lining of the nasal sinuses. It is commonly caused by Staphylococcus, Streptococcus and *Haemophilus influenzae* bacteria. The most common event leading to its appearance is the common cold. The congestion created by a cold blocks natural drainage of the sinus, thereby setting the stage for bacterial infection.

Symptoms that help differentiate sinusitis from a cold are as follows. Purulent discharge may be evident from the sinus cavities. Headache may be somewhat diagnostic if the pain can be localized to a sinus of maximum involvement. For example, acute ethmoiditis produces headache sensation between and behind the eyes. Fever occurs more often with bacterial sinusitis than with the common cold. Chronic sinus infection may produce low-grade symptoms which include post nasal discharge associated with a musty odor or a nonproductive cough.

The most common presentation of sinusitis in children is persistent cough and purulent rhinorrhea. Headache and facial tenderness, although frequently seen in adults with sinusitis, are uncommon. The child is likely to be irritable and tired.

Patients experiencing sinus headache and post-nasal drip accompanied with fever should be referred to a physician. The basic principle of therapy is to treat any infection present and facilitate drainage. Systemic antibiotics and oral decongestants are first-line therapies for sinusitis.

Bronchitis

Bronchitis is an inflammation of the tracheobronchial tree due to infection. Common etiologic agents include *S. pneumoniae*, *H. influenzae*, *M. pneumoniae*, and common cold viruses. It is usually self-limiting, lasting 1 to 2 weeks, and often follows an episode with a cold. Cough is the main symptom and it is essential to the removal of the bronchial secretions. The cough is initially dry and nonproductive but becomes productive after a few hours or days. Sputum eventually becomes abundant and mucopurulent. Wheezing after coughing is commonly noted. Fever and chest pain may be present in severe bronchitis. Persistent fever suggests complicating pneumonia.

Bronchitis in young children is best treated empirically with antibiotics. Adults should have cultures taken before beginning antibiotic therapy. A cough suppressant may be used if cough is troublesome and interferes with sleep.

Allergic Rhinitis

The symptoms of allergic rhinitis are similar to those of the common cold. Allergic rhinitis often presents as recurring cold-like symptoms such as nasal stuffiness, rhinorrhea, sneezing and watery eyes during the summer. Ocular symptoms are generally more prevalent with allergies. People whose cold symptoms persist longer than the 7 days normally seen with a cold should be suspected of having allergic rhinitis. See the chapter on allergic rhinitis for more detailed differentiation of allergic rhinitis and the common cold.

General Treatment

While known cure exists for the common cold, a surprising number of people stand by their "proven method". Cures are perhaps "discovered" in the following manner. During the winter months, people go back and forth between the cold outside and warm indoor environments. This temperature change can induce a reflex vasomotor response in the nasal tissue resulting in a runny nose. People often mistakenly think of this as the start of a cold. This is generally not the case; the runny nose soon abates, with no cold to follow. However, if a person tries some form of a remedy at this time (for example, vitamin C, garlic, any commercial cold preparation), they may incorrectly credit the agent with curative powers.

Generally, a cold runs its course in spite of the effort thrown its way. However, until the body can rid itself of the virus, a number of measures can help relieve symptoms. General approaches to treatment include bed rest, maintaining fluid intake, humidifying the air, plus other palliative steps.

Individuals should be kept comfortably warm during a cold episode. Resting in bed for a day or two is often recommended, especially if cold symptoms are harsh. No proof exists that bed rest decreases the duration of symptoms, but it may protect others from the virus. In addition, if symptoms are especially bad, efficient performance at school or work is unlikely. Some pediatricians question the value of keeping children at home when only mild symptoms are present.

Nasal obstruction in infants is a particular problem, especially when being breast- or bottle-fed. Nonmedicated saline nose drops are available to help loosen nasal congestion. Placing a few drops in each nostril is followed by nasal suction (only on a physician's advice) or, in the older child, by nose blowing. Nasal drainage during the day may be enhanced by propping up the infant's head. This can be achieved by having the child sleep in an infant car seat.

Cold sufferers should try to maintain their strength with good nutrition. Extra fluid intake is important, especially when fever is present. The tenacity of mucus may also be affected by the state of hydration. However, there is usually little need to force fluids on an individual. Hot fluids may be slightly superior to cold fluids in managing the common cold. In addition, hot fluid with spices appears to impart more benefit to respiratory mucus than is provided by plain hot water. Those bothered by colds may therefore find chicken soup to be one of the more enjoyable cold remedies available.

Vague complaints of feverishness and headache may be treated with ASA or acetaminophen. In children and teenagers, the possibility of Reye's syndrome developing after ASA use must be considered (see the chapter on internal analgesics).

Methods for treating a sore throat include the use of lozenges, gargles and various sprays. These dosage forms are generally considered mildly beneficial at best, but are often pleasant tasting and usually harmless. Oral analgesics can also be recommended for throat pain.

A warm salt water gargle is said to help clean the back of the throat and provide local relief of pain, but the benefits do not last long (up to 1 hour). Salt water gargle can be prepared at home by adding one-quarter of a teaspoon salt to 250 mL of warm water. For each use, a small amount of solution is gargled for about 15 seconds and repeated frequently during the day.

The United States Food and Drug Administration (FDA) is doubtful of the effects of medicated gargles for treating symptoms affecting the throat. The agency states it is unlikely any medication will reach the throat unless the solution is swallowed. It also states that a spray delivery system is probably more efficient than a gargle for treating throat symptoms.

Lozenges can relieve sore throat including that caused by irritation from drying of the mucosa due to mouth breathing. When dissolved in the mouth, lozenges increase salivation and exert a demulcent effect on the throat. Thus, they provide mild relief of throat pain by coating irritated or inflamed mucous membranes. This same effect can reduce the tickling sensation often apparent with a dry throat.

Lozenges available in Canada commonly contain antimicrobials, local anesthetics, aromatic compounds, demulcents, or a combination of these agents. The duration of action of a nonmedicated lozenge is generally short-lived and disappears as soon as the locally-acting agents are washed away by saliva. Lozenges of this type must be used frequently to be effective.

Lozenges containing local anesthetics can temporarily help relieve soreness in the throat and may be used when this symptom is troublesome. However, users of anesthetic-containing lozenges may feel more anesthetic effect on the tongue than in the throat. The pharmacist should keep in mind that the symptom of sore throat may be present with conditions other than a cold. Benzocaine is one of the most widely used agents for the pain of a sore throat. It can sensitize but this seldom occurs when used in lozenge form.

Volatile aromatic agents in lozenges produce a cooling sensation to partially mask minor throat discomfort. Menthol accomplishes this effect by stimulating local cold receptors. The duration of the local anesthetic effect of menthol is under 2 minutes. Eucalyptus oil (0.15 per cent) alone or in combination with menthol (0.26 per cent) is an effective antitussive when used in lozenge form. Also considered effective is menthol for nasal congestion, at a dose of 11 mg (up to 2 hours of relief).

Phenol is a disinfectant with activity against gram-positive and gram-negative bacteria and certain viruses. Aqueous solutions of up to 1 per cent are bacteriostatic, with a similar concentration used for a local anesthetic effect. Quaternary ammonium compounds (cetylpyridium, domiphen, benzalkonium chloride) have bactericidal activity against gram positive organisms, but are relatively ineffective against viruses. The topical antibacterial agents that are present in lozenges do not change the course of a viral respiratory tract infection.

Some lozenges contain therapeutic amounts of decongestants or cough suppressants. Cold sufferers (especially children) must not perceive these as candy or use them as frequently as they would a nonmedicated lozenge.

Lozenges containing zinc gluconate have been studied for their effect on the common cold with inconclusive results to date.

Humidification of room air is an adjunctive measure for treating a sore throat. It provides a demulcent action on the mucosal surfaces of the throat. Increased humidity in inspired air may also be helpful in providing symptomatic relief to those bothered by cough, chest congestion and to some extent, nasal congestion.

It is generally recognized that dry coughs may be soothed by the humidification of air. Proper humidity of the indoor environment is especially useful during the low relative humidity of winter. With the inspiration of dry air, mucus viscosity increases and irritation of the respiratory mucosa may develop. Hydration may also help relieve coughs associated with chest congestion, apparently by making expectoration of respiratory secretions easier. If nothing else, inhaled steam or cool mist provide psychological benefits to cough sufferers.

Steam kettles and commerical humidifiers (steam, cool mist, ultrasonic) are available to produce the water vapor. Steam and cool mist appear equally effective although many users say steam gives a more pampered feeling, especially for children. Cool mist vaporizers are considered the safer of the two devices as scalding is not a problem. However, the reservoirs of cool mist machines can easily become contaminated with bacteria; they must be cleaned thoroughly and regularly after use. In contrast, the reservoirs of steam vaporizers need only a rinse after each use. The boiling electrodes will need periodic cleaning to prevent mineral build-up. Electrical shocks occur more readily with steam vaporizers because of these electrodes. Hard and soft water work differently in steam vaporizers, with soft water producing less "spitting."

Either type of machine may come with a small medication cup near the outlet where the steam or mist is emitted. Aromatic vapors of any liquid placed in this cup are picked up by the water vapor and carried throughout the room. It was once thought that volatile oil products added little to hydration therapy other than to provide a medicine-like smell. However, new evidence suggests other benefits. Some of these aromatic compounds possess decongestant and antitussive activity.

Relatively new products available to cold sufferers are the Viralizer, Virotherm, and Rhinotherm. These devices are hand-held, come equipped with an electric fan and heating coil, and are designed to deliver heated (43°C) and humidified air into the nose. The idea for the devices came from studies that showed rhinoviruses grow optimally at 33°C (normal temperature of the nasal mucosa), but do so poorly at 37°C. Breathing in air at a temperature of 43°C leads to this temperature change in the local mucosa. Apparent benefits are achieved by providing a constant flow of fully saturated warm air; breathing in steam with a towel over the head has not produced the same temperature change. The Rhinotherm has been tested using three 30-minute periods of therapy at 2-hour intervals.

Proposed mechanisms by which heated air may provide relief are by the direct inhibition of viral replication and the possibility of changes in host defences, for example, the local production of antibody or increased cell resistance to the virus. Evidence of the devices' effectiveness has been hampered by a difficulty in creating suitable control groups. Regardless, Tyrrell, et al found that heated air provided immediate relief of symptoms. Symptoms were also noticeably improved for several days after the treatment. Macknin, et al found

no real advantage of steam inhalation delivered in a similar fashion. Patients that received the active treatment were, however, more likely to think the therapy helped. Side effects have been minimal, but care should be taken in their use as they do make use of heat.

While inhaling warm, moist air is a widely accepted practice for relieving cold symptoms, it is unclear whether these devices provide further benefit. More information is needed before recommendations can be made.

Antibiotics do not affect viruses and are not recommended unless a specific bacterial complication develops. The practice of using antibiotics to prevent bacterial infection is also not recommended.

As many colds are transmitted hand-to-hand with subsequent hand-to-nose or -eye contact, washing the hands after coming into contact with a cold sufferer may reduce chances of acquiring a cold.

Pharmaceutical Agents

Relief of cold symptoms can be achieved through drug therapy, but the duration of the cold is not altered. Four main classes of agents can be considered for symptom relief: nasal decongestants, cough suppressants, expectorants and antihistamines. The public frequently turn to commercial products containing these ingredients for relief. In 1988, the Canadian cough and cold market was worth $238 million. Cold remedies accounted for $78 million, cough syrups for $68 million, while nasal sprays accounted for $12 million of this value.

The Expert Advisory Committee (EAC) of Health and Welfare Canada recently reviewed the literature on the safety and efficacy of agents for use in the common cold and categorized the ingredients found in Canadian products into one of three groups (see Table II). The US FDA also performed a review with a similar mandate. Much of this material appears in the chapter.

Table II *Category of Ingredients in Cough and Cold Products*

Category I:	Generally recognized as safe and effective
Category II:	Generally not recognized as safe and effective
Category III:	Available data insufficient to permit final classification

Adapted from: Marchessault J, Boyd J, et al. First report of the Expert Advisory Committee on nonprescription cough and cold remedies to the Health Protection Branch: Antihistamines, nasal decongestants and anticholinergics. Ottawa: Health and Welfare Canada, 1988.

Nasal Decongestants

Symptomatic treatment of congestion may include the use of nasal decongestants. Included within this group are the phenylamines (sympathomimetic amines) and the imidazolines. They exert alpha-adrenergic activity on receptors within the vascular smooth muscle, thereby producing vasoconstriction. The subsequent decrease in blood flow reduces the mucosal swelling in the nasal passages, making breathing easier and possibly enhancing sinus drainage. Decongestants are useful in treating nasal mucosal congestion due to the common cold and allergic rhinitis. Their benefit in relieving sinus pressure is less well documented.

Nasal decongestants exert their sympathomimetic effects through direct- or indirect-acting mechanisms. Direct-acting sympathomimetic amines act on effector cells without involving an intermediary substance. In contrast, indirect-acting sympathomimetic amines are taken up into the adrenergic nerve terminals where they presumably replace norepinephrine in the storage vesicles. Norepinephrine then exits from the adrenergic nerve terminal and interacts with receptors to produce the sympathomimetic effect. Indirect-acting agents therefore have the same pharmacologic activity as norepinephrine—primarily alpha-receptor effects with weak beta-receptor effects.

Some nasal decongestants can be classed as mixed-acting sympathomimetics, that is, they have both direct and indirect activity. It is difficult to predict the precise characteristics of such an agent. For example, ephedrine depends on norepinephrine release for some of its effects, but also relieves bronchospasm through its beta-2 activity on bronchial smooth muscle, an effect not seen with norepinephrine.

Nasal decongestants can be applied topically (spray or drops) or be given orally. Topically-applied preparations have a faster onset of action than agents administered orally. Oral decongestants may provide more prolonged effect as respiratory tract fluids can wash topical medication away. However, xylometazoline and oxymetazoline are purported to relieve congestion for up to 10 and 12 hours, respectively. They therefore provide longer activity than all the oral decongestants (except sustained-release versions). Oral agents potentially provide a more complete decongestant action by reaching parts of the nasopharyngeal and sinus mucosa via the systemic circulation.

The main disadvantage of oral agents is their potential to cause systemic effects and/or to interact with other medication. Individuals with heart disease, high blood pressure, thyroid disease, diabetes, glaucoma, prostatic enlargement, pregnant or breast feeding should not use these products unless directed by a physician. Those taking medication for depression should also consult a physician before taking decongestants.

While topical agents tend to produce less side effects than oral agents, warnings applicable to oral decongestants might also apply to topical decongestants. For instance, if used improperly or in excess, a topically-applied agent may flow over the nasal mucosa into the pharynx to be swallowed. The active ingredient can then be absorbed

into the systemic circulation. Absorption of topical agents from the application site, though, tends to be minimal. The EAC concluded that warning statements relating to systemic effects were not necessary on packages of topical agents.

Spray formulations are recommended for adults as they are generally more convenient to use and reach a greater area of nasal mucosa. Sprays should also lead to less drug reaching the gastrointestinal tract. Drops are recommended for children under 6 years of age because children have smaller nostrils and because it may be difficult to control the amount of spray given to a child. It is also difficult for children to coordinate inhalation to the exact time a spray is administered into the nose. Either formulation for children under 12 years of age should be administered by an adult.

Overuse of topical agents can produce what is described as a rebound effect, or "after-congestion", where the nasal mucous membranes become more congested and swollen than before treatment was started. Congestion caused by any type of drug is termed rhinitis medicamentosa. The disorder is characterized by chronic swelling of the nasal mucosa.

Rhinitis medicamentosa due to a topical nasal decongestant arises when the agent is used for prolonged periods. Exactly how the rebound congestion occurs is unclear. It may be due in part to reactive vasodilation that can occur following pharmacologic vasoconstriction. In other words, after the effect of a decongestant wears off, a degree of secondary nasal congestion results. As nasal blockade re-develops, the patient returns to the decongestant which further reinforces the continued use of the product. Ultimately the blood vessels respond less to each application of vasoconstrictor. In time, the individual becomes dependent on the agent's therapeutic effect. Continued use can actually damage the nasal mucous membrane. Limiting use of these products to 3 or 7 days (depending on the agent) per cold episode is therefore recommended.

When an individual requesting a decongestant complains that the product no longer provides adequate relief, the pharmacist should be aware of the possibility of rebound congestion. Of the new patients admitted to a rhinitis clinic over a one-year period, 13 per cent presented with persistent nasal obstruction related at least in part to prolonged (greater than two months) vasoconstrictor use.

Table III *Recommended Dosages of Oral Decongestants*

Agent	Adults and Children ≥12 yrs	Children 6–11 yrs	Children 2–5 yrs	Children <2 yrs
Ephedrine	8 mg every 6–8 hr	under review	under review	under review
Pseudoephedrine	60 mg every 4–6 hr (240 mg daily max)	30 mg every 4–6 hr* (120 mg daily max)	15 mg every 4–6 hr* (60 mg daily max)	on advice of physician
Phenylpropanolamine	25 mg every 4 hr or 37.5 mg every 6 hr (150 mg daily max)	12.5 mg every 4 hr (75 mg daily max)	6.25 mg every 4 hr (37.5 mg daily max)	on advice of physician
Phenylephrine	10 mg every 4 hr (60 mg daily max)	5 mg every 4 hr (30 mg daily max)	2.5 mg every 4 hr (15 mg daily max)	on advice of physician

*Alternatively, children may receive 1 mg/kg four times daily.
Adapted from: Marchessault J, Boyd J, Crocker J, et al. First report of the Expert Advisory Committee on nonprescription cough & cold remedies to the Health Protection Branch. Antihistamines, nasal decongestants and anticholinergics. Ottawa: Health and Welfare Canada, 1989; and McEvoy GK, ed. AHFS Drug Information. Bethesda: American Society of Hospital Pharmacists, 1992:703–4.
Do not give sustained-release formulations to children less than 12 years of age.

Table IV *Recommended Dosages of Topical Decongestants*

Agent	Dose and frequency	Adults and children ≥ 12 yrs	Concentration of solution		
			6–11 yrs	2–5 yrs*	< 2 yrs
Phenylephrine	2–3 drops or sprays not more than every 4 hr	0.25–1.0%	0.25%	0.125%	on advice of physician
Naphazoline	1–2 drops or sprays not more than every 6 hr	0.05%	———————— on advice of physician ————————		
Oxymetazoline	2–3 drops or sprays not more than every 10–12 hr (max 2 applications/24hr)	0.05%	0.025–0.05%	0.025%	on advice of physician
Xylometazoline	2–3 drops or sprays not more than every 8–10 hr	0.1%	0.05%	0.05%	on advice of physician

*Drops are recommended for children under 6 years of age.
 Single-drop and -spray dosage formulations are available with some preparations.
 Adapted from: Marchessault J, Boyd J, Crocker J, et al. First report of the Expert Advisory Committee on nonprescription cough and cold remedies to the Health Protection Branch. Antihistamines, nasal decongestants and anticholinergics. Ottawa: Health and Welfare Canada, 1988.

Preventing misuse in patients with allergic rhinitis may be more difficult due to the chronic nature of the congestion.

Several measures are available to those suffering from rebound congestion. An individual who has had significant rebound congestion and who stops using the agent usually sees reversal of the congestion within a few weeks. While the simplest form of therapy, it is not the most comfortable as this action promptly results in nasal obstruction. Some people obtain relief from an oral decongestant or a topical steroid preparation during the weening off period. Oral decongestants do not cause rebound congestion as they do not possess the intense vasoconstrictor effect of topical agents. Alternatively, a patient can discontinue the medication initially in one nostril, but use as much medication as needed in the other nostril. Once the rebound phenomenum subsides in the drug-free nostril (in about 1 to 2 weeks), the individual discontinues drug use completely. Saline drops or spray can be used to keep the nasal mucosa moist. They also provide psychological assistance to individuals in the habit of using medicated versions of these formulations. Some individuals find it very difficult to discontinue use of topical decongestants on their own and are best referred to a physician.

See Table III for the dosing regimens of oral decongestants. See Tables IV and V for the dosing regimens of topical decongestants and methods for their proper administration.

Phenylamines

Chemically, phenylamine decongestants (ephedrine, pseudoephedrine, phenylpropanolamine and phenylephrine) share a structure-activity relationship with amphetamine-like compounds. Many of their side effects can be traced to this similarity. All four agents are taken orally; ephedrine and phenylephrine can also be used topically.

All the phenylamine sympathomimetics stimulate the central nervous system (CNS). Mild stimulation is apparent as excitability, nervousness, restlessness, anxiety and insomnia. Pronounced stimulation causes auditory and visual hallucinations, paranoia and delusions, symptoms that may be mistaken for psychosis.

Dosages producing nasal vasoconstriction may alter blood flow to other body regions and can increase blood pressure, although compensatory reflex changes in heart rate may forestall a measurable increase in blood pressure. Concomitant ingestion of drugs that increase heart rate might antagonize any reflex buffering effect, increasing blood pressure further. Thus, phenylamines should be used with caution and under the supervision of a physician by people with high blood pressure or cardiac problems.

Although nonprescription products containing phenylamines carry warning labels cautioning against their use by diabetics, little evidence indicates this problem is clinically significant. The adrenergic nervous system is one of many neural and hormonal factors influencing the secretion of insulin and glucagon and, ultimately, the regulation of glucose metabolism in the body. Parenterally-administered epinephrine increases blood glucose concentrations secondary to increased glycogenolysis, gluconeogenesis and other catecholamine-induced mechanisms. Nasal decongestants seldom have as potent an effect on blood glucose as epinephrine and their use usually does not pose a practical problem in diabetics. It is still advised that individuals with diabetes mellitus not use oral decongestants except under the advice and supervision of a physician.

Other patients with concurrent disease states should carefully consider the use of these products. Sympathomimetic agents can potentiate the effects of hyperthyroidism. Patients suffering from urinary retention could experience increased difficulty in urinating when using oral decongestants. Males with an enlarged prostate should only use these drugs under the supervision of a physician. Infants, children and the elderly tend to be more susceptible than adults to the systemic effects of these drugs.

Adrenergic agents should be given with caution to patients receiving monoamine oxidase (MAO) inhibitors due to the fact that MAO inhibitors increase the amount of norepinephrine in adrenergic neuron storage vesicles. If patients receiving a MAO inhibitor subsequently receive an indirect-acting oral decongestant, the increased stores of norepinephrine will be released and potentially result in an exaggerated adrenergic response. Some caution is also warranted for those receiving tricyclic antidepressant (TCA) agents. Indirect-acting phenylamines need to be taken into the adrenergic neuron

The Common Cold

Table V Administration of Topical Decongestants

Nasal sprays

1. Gently blow nose.

2. With head upright,* close one nostril by pressing a finger on the side of the nose. Spray medication into the open nostril, breathing in through the nose while squeezing the bottle sharply.

3. Repeat in similar fashion in the other nostril.

4. The nose should be blown 3 to 5 minutes after this procedure. For severe congestion, a second application of decongestant may now be applied if needed.

5. Rinse the tip of the spray bottle with hot water, but avoid getting any water in the bottle.

6. This product is for the temporary relief of nasal congestion due to the common cold, allergic rhinitis and other upper respiratory conditions. Do not use this product more than recommended. If symptoms persist, consult a doctor.

Nose drops

1. Gently blow nose.

2. Lie child on his/her back, e.g., on a bed with the child's head hanging slightly over the side.

3. Insert the dropper about 0.8cm (^{1}/3 inch) into a nostril and instil the recommended number of drops. The child should remain in this position for approximately 5 minutes. To allow greater contact with the nasal mucosa, tilt head from side-to-side.

4. The solution should then be applied to the other nostril in a similar manner.

5. The nose should be blown 3 to 5 minutes later.

6. Alternatively, drops can be administered with the head tilted backward, followed by moving the head toward the knees, holding for a few seconds, and then returning to the upright position.

7. Rinse the dropper with hot water and return it to the bottle. Although difficult to do, avoid touching the dropper into the nostril to reduce the chance of contamination.

8. This product is for the temporary relief of nasal congestion due to the common cold, allergic rhinitis and other upper respiratory conditions. Do not use this product more than recommended. If symptoms persist, consult a doctor.

*Inverting a spray bottle does not allow good control on the amount of medication administered.

to produce their effect. For this reason, their vasopressor effect is antagonized in the presence of a TCA. Direct-acting sympathomimetic amines produce increased adrenergic effects in the presence of a TCA. The cardiovascular effects of mixed acting agents depend on the ratio of direct to indirect activity.

Ephedrine is generally the agent to which all other decongestants are compared, even though its use is becoming less common. Ephedrine stimulates both alpha and beta receptors through direct and indirect mechanisms. Ephedrine possesses beta-2 effects but has a minimal role in asthma therapy. As with most oral decongestants, ephedrine has a less pronounced effect in elevating blood glucose than epinephrine.

Significant elevation in blood pressure is unlikely with ephedrine

unless amounts higher than single doses of 5 to 15 mg are given. Single doses of 60 mg have increased blood pressure while 90 mg doses have affected heart rate.. Any elevation in blood pressure is partly due to ephedrine's vasopressor effect and the result of the drug's cardiac stimulant effect.

Ephedrine's central activity is considerably less pronounced than the activity seen with amphetamines. Effects experienced include restlessness, dizziness, irritability, insomnia and anxiety. Serious CNS effects seldom occur to any great extent. Those that have occurred have usually been associated with excessive doses or prolonged usage.

Ephedrine can be used topically or orally and is considered safe and effective. Data is not available to support its use in children under the age of 12 years.

Pseudoephedrine preparations are safe and effective as oral nasal decongestants for nonprescription use. Activity begins within 30 minutes of ingestion and persists for 4 to 6 hours. Pseudoephedrine is a stereo isomer of ephedrine and to varying degrees has similar pharmacologic activity. It has fewer effects on the CNS than ephedrine and has less vasopressor activity. Pseudoephedrine's alpha-agonist effect may increase blood pressure while its beta-agonist activity can increase heart rate. This latter effect reduces the buffering effects of any reflex bradycardia in response to increased blood pressure. Fortunately, its decongestant effect is apparent at single doses of 60 mg, about half the dose required to increase blood pressure. Two studies involving a small number of subjects found that single doses of at least 120 mg of pseudoephedrine (one of the studies indicated 210 mg) was needed to increase the pulse rate and blood pressure in healthy volunteers.

The margin of safety with pseudoephedrine appears to be greater than that for ephedrine or phenylpropanolamine. Studies show that side effects are mild in people taking 60 mg three times a day. Subjects in a study by Drew received up to 240 mg without unpleasant side effects. Mild side effects reported are dryness of the mouth, sweating, nausea, insomnia and headache. Individuals using this agent should not exceed recommended dosages; at higher doses nervousness, dizziness or sleeplessness may occur. Increasing the 24-hour dosage maximum from 240 mg to 360 mg (in adults) has not proved to be a clinical advantage.

Phenylpropanolamine is a mixed-acting phenylamine and therefore is primarily an alpha-adrenergic agonist with a lesser degree of beta-agonist activity. It is said to cause less CNS stimulation than ephedrine. Despite this fact, it is used as an active ingredient (often with caffeine) in amphetamine "look-alike" preparations. Consequently, abuse of phenylpropanolamine has been reported. Most case reports of CNS reactions with decongestants involve this agent. However, it does not appear to have the reinforcing properties necessary to lead to habitual use.

A variety of psychiatric symptoms (especially in children) have been attributed to its use including paranoid psychosis, severe restlessness, irritability, sleep disturbances and aggressiveness. When they do occur, CNS effects are usually transient, subsiding within 6 hours of ingestion. Toxic effects on the CNS are rarely seen with therapeutic doses of phenylpropanolamine.

There has been much concern expressed over this agent's potential effect on the cardiovascular system. It has been reported to have a narrow therapeutic index, where recommended doses are safe but doses described as only slightly in excess of recommendations cause increases in blood pressure. The EAC addressed this concern and concluded that the dosages found in Canadian products pose no

The Common Cold

significant risk of cardiovascular side effects. Phenylpropanolamine does raise blood pressure but significant rises do not occur until single doses of 75 to 125 mg (or higher) are reached. Increases in blood pressure have been transient and tolerance to the pressor effects may develop with continued use. The agent has been classed as a category I oral nasal decongestant. A dose of 30 mg of phenylpropanolamine given to an individual receiving MAO inhibitor therapy has caused dangerously elevated blood pressure.

Phenylephrine is primarily a direct-acting alpha-agonist. This agent is considered safe and effective as a nasal decongestant and is available in topical and oral dosage formulations. It has a short duration of action when used topically (30 minutes to 4 hours). Due to this short duration, rebound congestion may occur when applied for longer periods than recommended (more than 3 days) and may be more common with the higher strength nasal formulations.

Oral absorption of phenylephrine is erratic and some reference material suggest it is best not taken by this route.

Central stimulant effects of phenylephrine are minimal. High oral doses (for example, 80 mg for 15 days) caused psychiatric symptoms in one case when other drugs were taken concomitantly. Occasionally, enough phenylephrine is absorbed after topical application to cause systemic effects.

Phenylephrine has little effect on the beta-receptors of the heart. Reflex bradycardia therefore usually counterbalances any increase in blood pressure due to its use. Recommended adult oral doses (10 mg) should not elevate blood pressure in normal individuals. However, two or three times the single dose quantity does increase blood pressure. Doses of 40 to 60 mg of phenylephrine are required for clinically significant cardiovascular effects to occur. At doses of 25 mg, blood pressure has increased by 7 mm Hg.

The effect on blood pressure is more evident when MAO levels are reduced by MAO inhibitors. Since phenylephrine is a substrate for MAO, much of an oral dose is metabolized by this enzyme in the gut wall and liver before reaching the circulation. In one volunteer who had taken a MAO inhibitor for 7 days, 45 mg of oral phenylephrine resulted in a significant rise in blood pressure. A similar dose had a minimal effect in the absence of the MAO inhibitor.

Regarding topical application, cardiac and hypertensive patients were administered 5 drops of either 0.25 or 1.0 per cent phenylephrine, with no marked changes in blood pressure readings noted over a 45-minute period.

Imidazolines

Naphazoline, oxymetazoline and **xylometazoline** are classified chemically as imidazolines. The imidazolines possess alpha-agonist activity; they do not stimulate beta-adrenergic receptors. They are used topically and are safe and effective for the temporary relief of nasal and sinus congestion due to the common cold and allergic rhinitis.

All three agents exert their effect within 10 minutes of application. Oxymetazoline possesses the longest duration of action, with the decongestant effect persisting up to 6 hours before gradually declining (total duration of activity is stated to be 12 hours).

Local reactions to topical use of the imidazolines are generally mild and infrequent and consist of stinging, burning, sneezing and dryness of the nasal mucosa. Rebound congestion may occur with prolonged or excessive use of any of these drugs but tends to occur more often with short-acting agents. Therefore, this effect occurs more often with naphazoline than with oxymetazoline or

xylometazoline. Xylometazoline use for up to 14 days has produced negligible rebound effect. Similarly, because the decongestant effect of oxymetazoline gradually declines, negligible incidence of rebound congestion should occur. To reduce the risk of rebound congestion, naphazoline should be used for no longer than 3 days per cold episode. Use of oxymetazoline and xylometazoline should not last longer than 7 days.

The imidazolines have the potential of causing systemic sympathomimetic effects such as increased blood pressure, headache, palpitations and sweating. Occasionally, enough may be absorbed of any agent to produce these effects. Generally, though, the warnings of systemic effects applicable to oral decongestants do not apply to topical nasal decongestants. Studies in healthy adults reveal that 3.6 mL of a 0.05 per cent solution was the minimum oral dose of oxymetazoline needed to produce a measurable effect on the cardiovascular system.

Unlike the phenylamines, imidazolines tend to depress rather than stimulate the CNS and overuse has caused drowsiness, deep sleep and coma, especially in young children. Naphazoline in particular has been implicated in causing adverse CNS effects and is not recommended for children less than 12 years except under the supervision of a physician. The incidence of serious adverse effects is low with correct use of these agents.

Other Nasal Decongestants

Propylhexedrine is an indirect-acting sympathomimetic amine with a decongestant effect on nasal mucosa. Despite reported deaths subsequent to misuse (intravenous or ingestion) by drug abusers, propylhexedrine is considered safe for self-medication by adults and is effective when used as instructed. It has a wide margin of safety and is relatively free of toxic effects. Side effects include rebound congestion, headache and rarely, increased blood pressure. Children should not have unsupervised access to a propylhexedrine inhaler. Adults and children older than 6 years are instructed to take 2 inhalations in each nostril not more often than every 2 hours. Use should be limited to 7 days per cold episode.

Camphor, menthol and **eucalyptus oil** have been evaluated for effectiveness as nasal decongestants. Formulations include those taken by mouth (lozenges), applied topically, and inhaled through steam.

When in lozenge form, menthol at a dose of 11 mg every 2 hours is considered a category I nasal decongestant. Menthol 2.6 per cent, camphor 4.7 per cent, and eucalyptus oil 1.2 per cent in combination as a topical rub also effectively relieves nasal congestion associated with the common cold. For patients 2 years and older, the rub is liberally applied to the throat, chest and back area. The application sites may be covered with a warm, dry cloth if desired, but clothing should be left loose to allow the vapors to rise to the nose and mouth. Application may be repeated up to 3 times daily or as directed by a physician. A physician should be consulted before use on patients less than 2 years.

When inhaled in steam, menthol 0.05 per cent, camphor 0.1 per cent, and eucalyptus oil 0.025 per cent provide relief from nasal congestion. These concentrations represent the concentrations of ingredients following dispersal in water—the stock solution contained camphor 6.2 per cent, menthol 3.2 per cent, and eucalyptus oil 1.7 per cent. For patients 2 years and older, 15 mL of the stock solution is added to each litre of water in a steam vaporizer (check manufacturer's warranty for the suitability of this practice). This may be

The Common Cold

repeated up to 3 times daily or as directed by a physician. A physician should be consulted before use for patients less than 2 years. The EAC did not recommend the use of this type of product in open containers of boiling water due to the risk of scalds occurring.

Evaluating Coughs

A cough is not an illness, but rather a symptom of an underlying stimulus or disease. Table VI lists several disease states and situations that can result in cough. The most frequent cause of transient cough is still the common cold.

Table VI *Causes of Cough*

Chronic bronchitis
Drug-related (e.g., ACE inhibitors)
Emphysema
Foreign body
Gastroesophageal reflux
Inhaled chemical irritants
Left ventricular failure
Sinusitis (postnasal drip)
Upper/lower respiratory tract infections

Coughs are common; up to 50 per cent of visits to physicians during the winter are prompted by this complaint, usually in association with the common cold. Parents are particularly apt to seek medical attention for their child's cough, perhaps for reassurance that the cough is not a manifestation of serious disease. In spite of this, many coughs are not medically treated.

Coughs associated with the common cold are described under the section on symptoms and in Table I. Coughing generally lasts no longer than 1 to 2 weeks. The pharmacist must be able to recognize when coughing indicates a more serious process that cannot be self-medicated. Questions concerning the duration of the cough, the character of any material coughed up, family history of allergy and respiratory disease, smoking history, and change in frequency or intensity of the cough will be required to determine whether referral is required. Table VII provides differential information on coughs of various etiologies.

Sinusitis can induce cough and one described that involves throat-clearing is highly suggestive of that induced by this state. The cough may be due to postnasal discharge that irritates receptors in the pharynx or to stimulation of receptors in the sinus. One authority questions the notion that postnasal drip causes the cough. Rather, he suggests that mouth breathing as a result of nasal congestion allows poorly conditioned air to dry the upper airways.

Occasionally after what appears to be a common cold, an individual may complain of a dry, unproductive cough that persists for weeks to months after the initial symptoms. Such people are likely having an exaggerated response to the virus-induced respiratory damage, which possibly leads to bronchoconstriction. These people should see their physicians who may implement bronchodilator therapy.

Many parents believe their children's cough is worse at night. If a night cough persists and is not accompanied by other cold symptoms, the child may have asthma. Cough at night may also be the result of gastroesophageal reflex, especially if heartburn or a sour taste in the mouth occur simultaneously.

Environmental irritants can cause cough by irritating receptors in the larynx, trachea and bronchi. Cigarette smoke is the most common cause of persistent cough in adults. Cigarette smokers typically cough on awakening, with minimal sputum coughed up.

More serious conditions can present with the symptom of cough. For example, a persistent unproductive cough may be the main symptom of left ventricular heart failure. Cough is also evident with lung cancer and chronic obstructive lung disease.

Cough Medicines

Two categories of agents are available to treat cough—antitussives (cough suppressants) and expectorants. Nonprescription antitussives are designed to temporarily reduce cough due to minor bronchial and/or the throat irritation often seen with the common cold. They can be classified as either centrally- or peripherally-acting, depending on whether they act on the cough centre in the medulla or at the site of irritation. Centrally-acting agents are thought to inhibit coughing by decreasing the sensitivity of the cough centre to incoming stimuli. Narcotic compounds were some of the first agents available and they continue to play a prominent role in therapy, although a number of nonnarcotic agents are available. The most important centrally-acting antitussives today are hydrocodone, codeine, dextromethorphan and diphenhydramine.

Table VII *Differential Diagnosis of Cough*

	Common cold	Influenza	Asthma	Chronic bronchitis
Cough type:	Mild to moderate severity; dry, hacking; may become productive during course of cold.	Common; often severe; unproductive.	Wheezing, shortness of breath, and/or cough; worsened by cold air.	Chronic cough; heavy sputum production
Duration:	Generally clears within 7 days	Cough may persist for 2 weeks or longer.	Chronic	Chronic
Other:			In small children with chronic cough and a negative history for infection, CF, or foreign body aspiration, asthma is the most likely cause of chronic cough.	Smoking history common; obesity

The Common Cold

The peripherally-acting group of antitussives contains agents that exert local effects in the respiratory tract, including those that anesthetize nerve endings (local anesthetics) or those that act as demulcents. Cough is normally produced by stimulation of sensory receptors of the glossopharyngeal and vagus nerves distributed in the mucous membranes of the lower pharynx, larynx, trachea, lung, and other areas of the respiratory tract. When the site of irritation is in the throat area, demulcent activity may help reduce coughing.

Expectorants help loosen phlegm and bronchial secretions, which help rid the bronchial passageways of bothersome mucus. They may also relieve irritated membranes in the respiratory passageways by preventing dryness through increased mucus flow.

Centrally-Acting Antitussives

All opiate analgesics are said to possess antitussive activity although evidence of efficacy for all agents is limited. **Codeine** has been extensively evaluated and has been proven effective in suppressing irritative cough. Codeine inhibits coughing through a direct effect on the cough centre in the medulla by raising the threshold for cough stimulus. The antitussive activity of codeine is less than that of morphine.

In general, codeine is well tolerated. Adverse reactions seldom occur with usual antitussive doses. The most common side effects are nausea, constipation after repeated doses, dizziness, sedation and pruritus. Consumers should be warned that use of codeine may impair mental alertness. The CNS depressant effects are additive to other CNS depressants. Safety has not been established in patients receiving MAO inhibitors.

Respiratory depression seldom occurs with antitussive doses of codeine, but young children are more susceptible to this effect. Eight cases of respiratory depression, apnea, coma or death in children (ranging in age from 3 months to 2 1/2 years) associated with codeine-containing drug products have been reported between 1969 and 1986. Codeine is therefore not recommended for use in children under 2 years of age. It should not be given to children 2 to 5 years without a physician's advice. Directions for use in children of this age group do not appear on product packaging. Information on dosing does appear in professional literature, that being 1 mg/kg/day in four equally divided doses.

The abuse potential of codeine is low. Prolonged use of high doses of codeine has produced dependence, however. Very high doses have produced exhilaration, excitement, delirium, somnolence, lassitude, muscle weakness, ataxia, seizures and circulatory collapse.

All opiates can cause the release of histamine and may increase the chance of bronchospasm in susceptible individuals. Codeine also appears to dry respiratory tract mucosa and can increase the viscosity of bronchial secretions. It can therefore precipitate attacks of asthma, but the risk does not seem to be high. Allergic reactions to codeine are rare and may be more common in atopic individuals.

A dose of 15 mg of codeine produces effective cough suppression (see Table VIII for dosing regimens). Complete suppression of coughing, though, is not achieved even at the high end of recommended daily dosage ranges. The degree of relief people report does not always correlate to reduced cough frequency.

Peak antitussive effect occurs within 1 to 2 hours of ingestion with antitussive activity persisting up to 4 hours. Parents should be instructed to use a calibrated measuring device (to ensure accuracy) when the product is intended for use in children 2 to 5 years of age.

Codeine-containing nonprescription liquids contain 3.3 mg of codeine phosphate per 5 mL of liquid. Most manufacturers recommend patients take a dose of 5 to 10 mL at each interval. At this dose, however, the codeine content is subtherapeutic for adults. It may be unwise to recommend a volume to achieve adequate amounts of codeine for adults because the amounts of the other ingredients would also be increased. Liquid formulations are therefore better suited for children (over the age of 2 years). Two tablets of codeine-containing nonprescription analgesics contain enough codeine for antitussive activity and are used by some diabetics to avoid the calories present in syrups and elixirs.

Dextromethorphan developed through many modifications to the narcotic analgesic nucleus. It retains the antitussive activity of the parent compounds but none of their analgesic or addictive properties. It does not substitute for opiates in dependent individuals and is therefore considered a nonnarcotic.

Dextromethorphan acts centrally on the cough centre in the medulla to elevate the threshold required for coughing. Its antitussive potency is equal (or nearly equal) to that of codeine but it produces fewer side effects. It has a low degree of sedative, gastric-irritating, constipating and addictive properties. Adverse effects are mild and infrequent and include drowsiness, nausea and dizziness. With usual therapeutic doses there are no significant effects on the respiratory or cardiovascular systems. Unlike codeine, it does not inhibit ciliary activity. Dextromethorphan should be used cautiously in asthmatics as it has the potential to release histamine. As with codeine, safe use has not been established in individuals receiving MAO inhibitors.

The safe dose range of dextromethorphan appears to be considerably higher than that for codeine. There have been a few instances of abuse of this agent, but dependence does not appear to be a factor. At high doses (greater than 225 mg), excitation, bizarre behavior, mental confusion or depression, ataxia, toxic psychosis and even opiate-like respiratory depression have occurred. There have been no fatalities even with doses in excess of 100 times the normal adult dose. Because of its low order of toxicity, dextromethorphan is probably the safest antitussive currently available. It is especially useful for children when a cough suppressant is indicated.

Dextromethorphan starts exerting its effect 15 to 30 minutes after ingestion; antitussive activity may persist for 3 to 6 hours (see Table VIII for dosages).

Diphenhydramine is an antihistamine with antitussive activity. Its mechanism of action is unclear but appears to be independent of any sedative effect.

Diphenhydramine has antitussive activity in doses of 25 to 50 mg every 4 hours and appears equivalent to 15 mg of codeine (see Table VIII for all dosing regimens). A dose of 25 mg exhibits effective cough suppression with minimal sedation; higher doses increase the incidence of drowsiness. The sedative effect may prove beneficial at times by helping patients with nighttime cough sleep more restfully.

All precautions inherent to first generation antihistamine use should be kept in mind when recommending this agent as a cough suppressant (see the chapter on allergic rhinitis). Caution should be exercised in using diphenhydramine in children 2 to 5 years without a physician's recommendation as its use may lead to paradoxical excitement.

Hydrocodone is a centrally-acting narcotic cough suppressant that requires a prescription for use. Milligram per milligram, it is slightly

The Common Cold

Table VIII *Recommended Doses of Centrally Acting Antitussives*

Agent/Age	Dosage (daily maximum)
Codeine	
<2 yrs	not recommended
2–5 yrs*	on advice of a physician; 1 mg/kg/day in 4 divided doses
6–11 yrs	5–10 mg every 4–6 hr (60 mg)
12 yrs and over	10–20 mg every 4 to 6 hr (120 mg)
Dextromethorphan	
<2 yrs	on advice of a physician
2 to 5 yrs+	2.5 to 5 mg every 4 hr or 7.5 mg every 6 to 8 hr (30 mg)
6 to 11 yrs+	5 to 10 mg every 4 hr or 15 mg every 6 to 8 hr (60 mg)
12 yrs and over	10 to 20 mg every 4 hr or 30 mg every 6 to 8 hr (120 mg)
Diphenhydramine	
2 to 5 yrs	on advice of a physician
6 to 11 yrs	12.5 mg every 4 hr (75 mg)
12 yrs and over	25 mg every 4 hr (150 mg)
Chlophedianol	
under 6 yrs	Category III
6 to 11 yrs	12.5 mg every 6 to 8 hr (50 mg)
12 yrs and over	25 mg every 6 to 8 hr (100 mg)

*Measure with calibrated measuring device.
+Alternatively, children can be given 1 mg/kg per day in 3 or 4 divided doses.
Adapted from: Marchessault J, Boyd J, Crocker J, et al. Second report of the Expert Advisory Committee on nonprescription cough and cold remedies to the Health Protection Branch. Antitussives, expectorants and bronchodilators. Ottawa: Health and Welfare Canada, 1989.

more potent than codeine, is more sedating, but has no more constipating effect. It offers little advantage over codeine. The adult dose is 5 to 10 mg every 4 to 6 hours.

Chlophedianol is a centrally-acting cough suppressant that is considered safe and effective. It is similar in structure to diphenhydramine and possesses weak local anesthetic properties. Table VIII describes dosing regimens for adults and children 6 years of age and older. The agent is considered category III for children under 6 years pending further investigation.

Several agents (noscapine, benzonatate, caramiphen and carbetapentane) have been classified as category III agents by the EAC because at the time, data was insufficient to confirm their safety or efficacy.

Noscapine is an opiate derivative that is considered a nonnarcotic for legal purposes. It has no addiction liability as it does not produce euphoria and is without analgesic or sedative properties. Side effects with use have been minimal: slight drowsiness, dizziness, headache, nausea and skin rash. There is some debate over its effectiveness in comparison to codeine and the dose required for cough suppression. The latter is generally stated as 15 to 30 mg three to four times daily for adults.

Benzonatate is a nonnarcotic oral cough suppressant that appears to have both a central and a peripheral action. It reportedly inhibits cough by anesthetizing reflexes arising from the stretch receptors within airway smooth muscles (peripheral) and by suppressing the transmission of the cough reflex at the medulla (central). Which mechanism is more important for cough suppression is unclear. It does not produce respiratory depression at recommended doses. Adverse effects of benzonatate have included sedation, headache, dizziness, nausea, gastrointestinal upset, constipation, pruritus and numbness in the chest. Hypersensitivity reactions to the drug are possible, including anaphylactic reactions. Oral formulations not swallowed quickly may lead to numbness of the mouth, tongue or throat. Single doses of 50 to 100 mg of benzonatate have been used, with the effect persisting for 3 to 8 hours.

Caramiphen is a relatively weak nonopioid antitussive that appears to have central activity rather than a peripheral site of action. However, it possesses the qualities of a local anesthetic. Adults and children 12 years and over have received 20 mg in sustained release form twice daily.

Carbetapentane, another Category III agent, is structurally related to caramiphen and is said to possess local anesthetic activity. Adults have been given 15 mg every 4 hours, to a maximum of 60 mg per day.

Peripherally-Acting Antitussives

Camphor and **menthol** used topically or as inhalants are effective antitussive agents. Both methods allow the inhalation of their aromatic vapors. The antitussive effect may work by diminishing the sensitivity of the cough receptors in the membranes lining the throat and respiratory passages, by exerting a soothing action on irritated or inflamed throat tissues, or by both mechanisms.

For topical application, camphor and menthol are formulated into a petrolatum ointment vehicle at concentrations of 5.0 and 2.6 per cent, respectively. Eucalyptus oil 1.2 per cent will contribute to the effectiveness of this formulation. For individuals over 2 years of age, the ointment is rubbed liberally on the throat, back and chest. This may be repeated up to three times daily. The area of application may be covered with a warm, dry cloth if desired, but clothing should be left loose to allow the vapors to reach the nose. It is recommended the ointment not be applied to the nose area. A physician should be consulted before use on patients less than 2 years of age.

Camphor and menthol individually are antitussives when added to the water of a hot steam vaporizer. Whether other aromatic oils have similar action is not clear. Steam containing 0.05 per cent menthol or 0.1 per cent camphor produces a significant reduction in cough counts compared to nonmedicated steam. For these studies, stock solutions of 6.2 per cent camphor and 3.2 per cent menthol were used. Fifteen mL of stock solution is added to each 1000 mL of water in a hot steam vaporizer (check manufacturer's warranty). The individual breathes in the medicated vapors and may be repeated up to three times daily or as directed by a physician. These directions are for cough sufferers 2 years of age and older. Use in children under 2 years of age should be on the advice of a physician.

Eucalyptus oil 0.15 per cent in lozenge form is considered an effective antitussive.

While local anesthetics can theoretically be considered as peripherally-acting agents, they are seldom used for the general treatment of cough. They have been used during procedures such as bronchoscopy. Local anesthetics found in lozenges are present to reduce the pain of a sore throat.

The Common Cold

Expectorants

The course of a viral infection can lead to an increase in the volume of phlegm in the upper and lower respiratory tract, often to the point where coughing becomes laborious. The volume of material present and its consistency may lead to what patients describe as a congested chest. Agents that make bronchial secretions more mobile should diminish the severity and duration of cough. However, with the decrease in sputum viscosity and subsequent ease of expectoration, they may increase the frequency of coughing for a short time.

Expectorants may be useful in irritative, nonproductive coughs associated with minimal amounts of bronchial fluid and minimal chest congestion. Respiratory tract fluid is a natural demulcent that can soothe irritated respiratory tract mucosa. Increasing the quantity of this fluid should help remove local irritants that may be part of the cough etiology. Expectorants may exert a demulcent effect on the irritated mucosa thus diminishing ineffective coughing. In this situation, an expectorant would reduce the frequency of cough.

The use of these agents has been controversial due to a lack of objective evidence of their efficacy. Part of the difficulty in accumulating evidence stems from a lack of understanding for what changes to the properties of respiratory secretions correlate best with ease of expectoration. In addition, much of the research has been on chronic coughing associated with chronic obstructive pulmonary disease rather than cough due to the common cold. On review of the agents available, both the EAC and FDA concluded that only one agent, guaifenesin, could be considered as safe and effective.

Guaifenesin (glyceryl guaiacolate) is a derivative of guiacol, an extract of tar. Both have been used in cough medicines although guaifenesin is used almost exclusively today.

It has been proposed that guaifenesin acts to cause an indirect increase in the output of respiratory tract fluid, thereby enhancing the flow of less viscid secretions, promoting ciliary action and facilitating the removal of mucus. Another suggestion is that after guaifenesin is absorbed following ingestion, it may be taken up by the bronchial glands and directly stimulate secretions by these glands.

Some studies have shown the drug to be effective while other studies have not confirmed these results. In reviewing these controversial results, the EAC concluded guaifenesin is generally safe and effective. It is recommended that adults and children 12 years and older receive 200 to 400 mg every 6 hours. Children 6 to 11 years are given 100 mg every 6 hours, while those 2 to 5 years should receive 50 mg every 6 hours. Children under 2 years of age are given guaifenesin on the advice of a physician.

Doses of guaifenesin larger than those required for expectorant action may result in emesis. Otherwise, the agent is well tolerated. Nausea or other gastrointestinal effects at ordinary doses are rare. The agent may have a transient antiplatelet effect but is of little clinical importance.

Ammonium chloride has been used in expectorant cough mixtures in the belief that it irritates the stomach and causes a reflex increase in airway mucous secretion. Little evidence supports its use as an expectorant, however. Ammonium chloride at doses purported to enhance expectoration (250 to 500 mg four to six times daily) are considered safe but of unproven efficacy. For this reason, it is considered Category III. In high doses (6 to 8 g per day) it has caused acidosis in individuals with renal failure.

Terpin hydrate may stimulate the output of respiratory tract fluid by acting directly on the mucosa of the respiratory tract secretory glands. The efficacy of this agent is not yet clearly established. Terpin hydrate is an irritant and if taken on an empty stomach may cause gastrointestinal side effects such as nausea and vomiting. Some cough preparations incorporating this expectorant contain large amounts of alcohol (up to 40 per cent) and precautions relating to this should be considered. Adults and children over 12 years of age and older have received 200 mg every 4 hours, to a maximum of 1,200 mg.

Insufficient evidence was available on the safety or efficacy of **Friar's balsam** and **tincture of benzoin** for either oral ingestion or steam inhalation and were therefore placed in Category III.

Potassium iodide is thought to act as an expectorant by increasing respiratory tract secretions, thereby decreasing the viscosity of mucus. In doing so, the drug is absorbed into the blood stream and is taken up by the mucous glands of the nose and respiratory tract. These glands are then stimulated to produce respiratory tract secretions. Another possible explanation for its activity is that potassium ions (which irritate the stomach) are responsible for a reflex stimulation of bronchial secretions. It is also proposed that iodide stimulates protease enzymes in respiratory tract secretions, thus enhancing the endogenous breakdown of viscous mucoproteins. Finally, the agent may also stimulate ciliary activity.

The drug is an emetic when given in larger doses. It has an unpleasant metallic taste. Painful swelling of the salivary and lacrimal glands can occur after a few doses of the drug; discontinuing treatment allows the pain to subside. Manifestations of iodism (the adverse effects of iodine administration) can occur with long-term therapy, but are rare with intermediate or short courses. This agent is contraindicated in pregnant or nursing women and in neonates. The EAC concluded that iodides are unsafe for nonprescription use and are of unproven efficacy (Category II).

Iodinated glycerol is a complex containing 50 per cent organically bound iodine. It appears to act on sputum in the same manner as inorganic iodides. As with the parent compound, its action is not entirely understood and it is not known whether the glycerol molecule contributes to the expectorant effect of the complex. The drug is almost tasteless and appears to irritate the gastrointestinal tract less than potassium iodide. Precautions that apply to the use of potassium iodide generally apply to iodinated glycerol. As this compound is also an iodide, it was given Category II status.

Antihistamines and the Common Cold

Antihistamines have a long history of use in the treatment of the common cold. Combinations of oral antihistamine/decongestant formulations are some of the more popular agents available for cold therapy. However, the value of the antihistamine in these products has been the subject of considerable controversy. Part of the debate stems from a lack of understanding of the role of histamine in producing cold symptoms; if histamine is not released, the presence of antihistamines in these products is questionable.

Histamine release occurs in people with allergic rhinitis and subsequently causes the classic symptoms of this condition. Histamine can also be released from cells during trauma or infection and probably occurs during a viral infection. However, information is lacking on the extent of histamine release during a cold.

A 1975 review of the literature stated that only two studies at the time were suitably designed to look at the question of antihistamines and the common cold. The data did not support the use of antihistamines to prevent or relieve the symptoms of a cold. Researchers have since found chlorpheniramine maleate superior to placebo in lessening various symptoms. One study included the total symptom picture of cold sufferers in their analysis, but focused on nasal discharge and sneezing as symptoms theoretically treatable with antihistamines (which appeared to be the case). Another study showed that chlorpheniramine, when given four times daily for at least 7 days relieved cold symptoms. At the time the researchers were not sure whether the beneficial aspects would be seen clinically.

These and other studies made available to the FDA indicated that chlorpheniramine is effective in temporarily relieving the rhinorrhea and sneezing associated with the common cold. Chlorpheniramine was not effective in relieving other symptoms. As the pharmacologic actions of all first generation antihistamines are similar, the agency concluded that other Category I (safe and effective) first generation antihistamines would also be effective for the temporary relief of runny nose and sneezing associated with the common cold. The EAC drew the same conclusion. However, as of 1992 the FDA is reevaluating their position on the effectiveness of antihistamines and the common cold.

Any beneficial effect on rhinorrhea or sneezing may be due to the drying effect of these antihistamines on the nasal mucosa. For this reason, relief may be more evident early in the cold when a runny nose is present. Later, when nasal congestion and obstruction become more prominent, a drying effect may provide little or no benefit or may even worsen the congestion. One study did however report benefits with antihistamines from the first day of therapy to as late as the seventh day. If the pharmacist recommends an antihistamine to relieve these symptoms, either alone or in combination with other agents, the precautions that apply to their use should be considered.

Anticholinergics

Cholinergic mechanisms may play a role in the pathogenesis of rhinorrhea during the common cold. Topical anticholinergic agents such as ipratropium bromide and atropine methonitrate have therefore been studied to determine their effect on this symptom. In one study, ipratropium was sprayed intranasally three times daily for 5 days. Results slightly favored the treatment group over the placebo group, with minimal adverse effects. The overall clinical value of topical anticholinergics remains to be determined. Theoretically, it is possible that excessive drying of secretions could worsen symptoms.

Nonsteroidal Anti-inflammatory Agents

Colds caused by rhinoviruses are associated with significant increases in concentrations of polymorphonuclear (PMN) leukocytes and kinins in nasal tissue. NSAIDs have inhibitory effects on PMN leukocytes and on the biologic effects of kinins. If kinin effects and/or local PMN leukocyte influx are found to be important in causing respiratory symptoms, NSAIDs could interfere with these mechanisms. In studies to date, results remain inconclusive as to whether they can reduce cold symptoms (other than headache, sore throat, and fever).

Vitamin C

The nutritional requirement for vitamin C has been set at 40 mg per day for males 16 years and over (nonsmokers) and 30 mg for females of the same age, an amount easily obtained from a medium-sized orange. Yet, many consumers take 100 to 1000 mg a day for their colds. How did this practice come about?

In the early 1970s, Linus Pauling wrote a book on vitamin C and the common cold. This small book created much of the interest that exists today for vitamin C and this illness. Pauling reported that the vitamin had only limited value against the common cold in small

amounts, but that large daily supplements could prevent most colds. He also stated that protection increased with the amount ingested, to the point where 4 to 10 g per day provided maximum protection if taken at the immediate onset of a cold.

Since that time, scientists have been trying to determine whether this vitamin could indeed meet the promises spelled out by Pauling. In the meantime, the public in general warmed to the idea of a cure for colds. Pharmacists today are still asked questions regarding the amount of vitamin C to take.

Experiments have failed to produce any clearcut evidence that vitamin C in large doses (greater than 1 g/day) protects against or ameliorates the symptoms of the common cold. Some studies have shown small benefits—up to a half day less in the duration of cold symptoms in individuals given vitamin C than groups receiving placebo. However, it is generally agreed that a recommendation for the prophylactic or therapeutic use of large doses of vitamin C for colds is unwarranted.

Several adverse effects of high dose vitamin C intake (gram quantities) have been reported. These include a risk of renal calculi due to increased oxalic acid production and increased uric acid excretion. There is little evidence these effects would occur under most circumstances, however. Intakes of 100 mg or more per day have had no appreciable influence on oxalate formation. While uric acid and vitamin C are both reabsorbed in the proximal tubule by a common transport system, vitamin C has minimal effect on uric acid excretion. Even in patients with gout or hyperuricosuria it appears doubtful that large doses of ascorbic acid would lead to increased excretion. Doses of 1 g/day or more do cause abdominal distress and diarrhea in some subjects, but have no apparent long-term effects. Still, most clinicians believe any possible benefit of using large amounts is not worth the potential risks of megadose therapy. Withdrawal reactions in the offspring of mothers who have ingested large amounts during pregnancy, interference with diabetic urine tests, and drug interactions (the effects of acidification of urine on the elimination of drugs) have also been reported.

Interferon

As the common cold is a mild illness with few complications, the need for a cure might be questioned. However, its widespread occurrence and economic effect on society appear to be stimulis enough for research to continue. One such focus of research is with interferon.

Interferons are glycoproteins produced by the body that have a variety of biological effects, including antiviral activity. Viruses themselves are potent stimulators of interferon production. Three main types of human interferon (alpha, beta and gamma) have been described.

Technological advances have allowed the clinical testing of nasally-applied interferon for the common cold. Initial trials produced unacceptable local effects, particularly nasal ulceration and bleeding. Two subsequent studies showed intranasal sprays of alpha-interferon to be effective in preventing colds, with an acceptable side effect profile. The agent had little benefit on colds after the onset of symptoms or for infections other than rhinovirus infections. A third study showed no reduction in symptom severity or duration; however, an antiviral effect was evident. The patients of the study did experience a degree of intolerance to the agent. Results are inconclusive as to the role of interferon in cold therapy.

The Common Cold

Selecting a Treatment

Hundreds of nonprescription products are marketed in Canada for the common cold. Pharmacists cannot be familiar with each product, but must know which ingredients are safe to use in various patients and at what dose they are effective.

When assessing individuals with a cold, a systematic approach should be followed. First, the patient's symptoms should be assessed. Then a brief medical history is taken. Based on this information, a suitable product (if any) is selected. This is followed by counselling on the proper use of the product and finally, advice provided on non-drug measures.

The selection of a single ingredient is possible (and good medical practice) if the individual, with the pharmacist's assistance, can isolate one most bothersome symptom. This is usually nasal congestion or a cough. Terms such as "head cold" and "chest cold" are often used by patients to describe where the major complaint lies.

For nasal congestion, topical and oral agents are available. While there are important differences in the two, the decision as to which to recommend to otherwise healthy individuals is not always easy. Often either type of formulation can be used. Patient preference for either dosage form or previous product use should be considered. Topical agents are relatively free of systemic effects. Oral agents may be more suitable for patients bothered by congestion for extended periods of time as they do not cause rebound congestion. If symptoms are accompanied by fever or do not improve after 7 days of therapy, the individual should consult a physician.

Regarding coughs, the pharmacist must determine what type of cough the patient is experiencing. The public does not always differentiate between types and may select an inappropriate cough remedy. Coughs can be divided into the following categories: congested and productive (individual complains of chest congestion and is able to expectorate phlegm); congested and nonproductive (individual has chest congestion but is unable to expectorate), and dry and nonproductive (individual has a dry, hacking cough with no apparent chest congestion).

Since a cough is a defense mechanism, blind suppression of all episodes is unwise. A productive cough is considered useful and necessary to move secretions up and out of the airway. Antitussives, if used at all in this case, should be reserved for when the cough keeps a person awake at night, is exasperating, or causes disturbance at work or school. Otherwise, the cough should be allowed to run its course. Suggesting an expectorant for a cough that is already breaking up is probably unnecessary. However, recommending increased fluid intake is appropriate.

When a cough is nonproductive and dry, suppression is indicated as it serves no beneficial purpose. The cause must still be identified, though. The use of an expectorant for this type of cough is more ambiguous. It is not entirely clear whether expectorants can soothe a cough of this type.

When a cough is nonproductive because secretions are not being raised (chest congestion), cough suppressants can prolong the illness and may have to be avoided. However, these agents do not completely eradicate cough and there may be occasions where a degree of suppression is warranted (as described above under productive cough). Expectorants given for this type of cough, on the other hand, should increase respiratory tract secretions and help aid in the development of a productive cough.

The addition of an antitussive to an expectorant formulation has long been described as a measure that counteracts the benefits of the expectorant. The EAC, however, stated the combination of antitussive and expectorant is rational under certain circumstances.

Cough preparations should not be used to treat persistent or chronic cough such as those occurring with smoking, asthma, emphysema, or if the cough is accompanied by excessive phlegm, unless directed by a physician. If a cough is due to the irritation caused by postnasal drip, the removal of the secretions may relieve the cough. A cough that persists beyond 7 days should be referred as should those with evidence of infection (yellowish-green colored sputum, fever). A physician should be involved in the treatment of coughs in small children.

When an individual complains of several symptoms, recommending treatment is more difficult. The pharmacist should determine the most annoying symptoms and choose a multi-ingredient product accordingly. Products containing decongestant-antitussive and decongestant-expectorant combinations are probably the most useful. It is best to avoid products offering a blanket approach to relieving cold symptoms, providing ingredients to cover every symptom being experienced (and often some not present). All ingredients must play a role in reducing the patient's symptoms and be present in therapeutic amounts.

While more convenient for patients, there is some degree of flexibility lost when multiple-ingredient products are selected. For example, agents are available for sinus headache that contain a decongestant and an analgesic. Both headache and sinus pain may be present for about a day until the decongestant works to relieve pressure (with subsequent reduction in pain). While decongestant therapy might be required for several days thereafter, the analgesic may not be needed. The use of the two agents as separate entities might prove more useful at times.

Some products are available that contain two antihistamines. There is little evidence to indicate increased efficacy when two are combined within one product.

The treatment algorithm provides guidelines for selecting therapy. Nondrug measures should always be provided along with any product recommendations.

The Diabetic Individual

Diabetics are often quite knowledgeable of their condition. Still, as consumers of medicinals, they must not fall into a habit of selecting cough and cold products labelled "dietetic," assuming these formulations are safe and best suited for each new cold. Cold symptoms can vary with each episode as will the active ingredients needed in a product. Also, the term dietetic does not always mean calorie free.

When consulting a cold sufferer who states he or she is a diabetic, the pharmacist needs to determine the type of diabetes the patient has. Therapy for patients with IDDM must be carefully contemplated because potential for swings in blood glucose is considerable. These diabetics also carefully monitor caloric intake. If a diabetic is not experienced with how their condition is affected by certain cold products, a physician may have to be involved in the selection process.

Patients with NIDDM experience less dramatic swings in blood glucose. They are also often on diets and monitor their intake of calories.

Once the status of the diabetes has been determined, the individual's symptoms should be evaluated and the appropriate agent(s) selected to relieve these symptoms. Of the categories of agents available, antihistamines, antitussives, and expectorants have

Figure 2 *Suggested Approach for Treating the Common Cold*

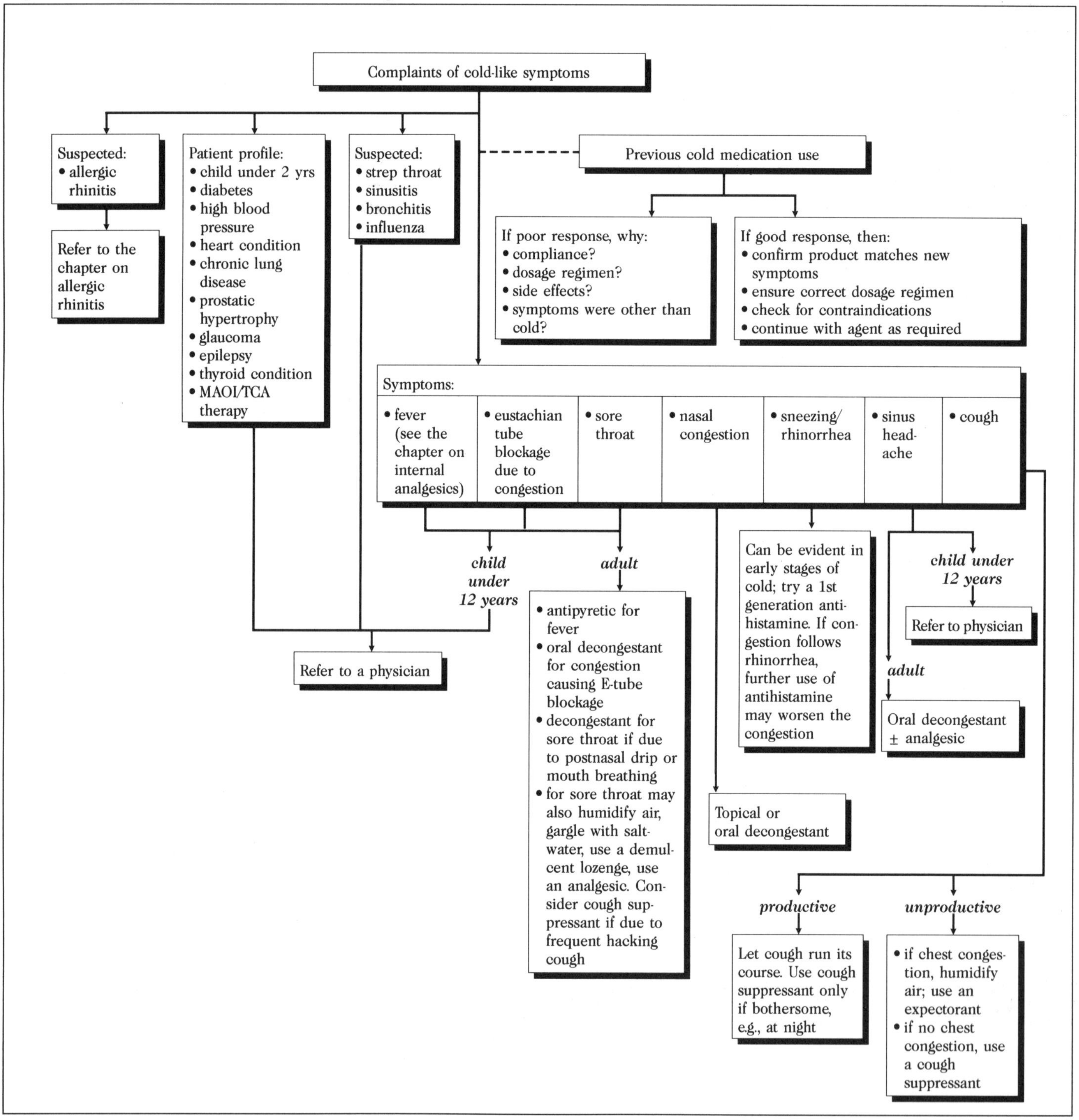

no effect on blood glucose levels. Nasal decongestants can alter blood glucose control.

The predominant effect of the sympathomimetic agents, epinephrine and norepinephrine is to inhibit insulin secretion, a response mediated by alpha-adrenergic receptors. More importantly in IDDM patients, epinephrine can also cause rapid glycogenolysis. As all nasal decongestants are sympathomimetics, they all can potentially alter control in the diabetic. However, oral decongestants generally do not affect blood glucose to the same extent as epinephrine. The decision to use an oral agent should rest with the person's physician. If an oral agent is used in a diabetic, the individual should monitor the condition more intensely with blood glucose tests. The patient should already have stepped up monitoring as the metabolic stress associated with the cold itself increases blood glucose levels.

In addition to the effects decongestants may have on blood glucose, the vascular problems that often accompany diabetes may be a further contraindication to decongestant use. In this situation, topical decongestants used correctly are safer than orally-administered decongestants for diabetics.

The caloric content of any cold preparation is of concern to the diabetic. Short-term ingestion (the duration of a cold) of liquid medications containing sugar should not be a problem for most diabetics. Still, the pharmacist should make the caloric content of the product available to the patient. The Canadian Society of Hospital Pharmacists/Connaught Novo calorie content reference provides caloric values of many cough and cold products in Canada.

Sugar-free products are often sweetened with sorbitol. Sorbitol-containing liquids are still calorigenic but the calories are released more slowly than with sucrose. The short-term use of sorbitol-containing formulations is acceptable, but long-term use poses some problems in regards to caloric intake.

The alcohol content of most liquid pharmaceuticals likely will not affect a well controlled diabetic. Still, it does add to the total caloric content of the preparation. A 10 mL dose of a product containing 4 per cent alcohol given five times a day results in the person ingesting 2 mL of alcohol. The CPS has a listing of agents that are alcohol-free.

Tablet and capsule formulations usually have minimal caloric content. Lozenges are commonly sugar-based, but low calorie versions are available.

Summary

While the common cold is a mild condition, it has a tremendous impact on society, not the least of which is economic. Millions of dollars are involved in lost days from work and in products purchased. Colds are also important to the professional role of pharmacists. Questions on cold products make up a large portion of those asked by consumers. This is due in part to the frequency of the common cold and to the fact that consumers may be taken aback by the variety of different products available to them. But, in spite of the number of products in pharmacies, only a few active ingredients find their way into formulations. Pharmacists can use their knowledge of these agents to help overcome some of the confusion cold sufferers may have. Nothing is available that can eradicate a cold but relief from symptoms is certainly possible.

Ask the Consumer

Q. *What are your symptoms?*

■ Everyone has had a cold at some time in their life. Symptoms include mild sore throat, rhinorrhea followed by nasal congestion, watery eyes, and a cough. Consumers may use terms such as head cold and chest cold to describe their symptoms.

Colds are generally easily recognized. However, other conditions exist that have similar symptoms. Greenish-colored sputum, exudate at the back of the throat, symptoms that are severe, or ones that persist for more than a week suggest more serious conditions which require medical attention.

Q. *Is a productive or nonproductive cough present?*

■ A cough may develop during a cold if the bronchial passages become irritated. A cough that brings material up from the air passages rids the body of debris and should not be suppressed by medication. Under certain circumstances, a cough suppressant may be warranted. On the other hand, a dry nonproductive cough serves little purpose, can be painful, and may perpetuate itself by further irritating the air passages. This type of cough can generally be suppressed.

Q. *What medications, if any, have you tried for your cold? What has worked well for you in the past for similar symptoms?*

■ Symptoms can change with each new cold. Knowing what has been tried and how this was taken provides insight into whether therapy was appropriate. If minimal benefits were realized for previous colds, alternative agents should be considered for the newest episode. One or two bothersome symptoms are more easily managed than three or more symptoms.

Q. *Do you have a history of allergies?*

■ Allergic rhinitis is often mistaken for the common cold. Nasal symptoms last longer with an allergy and occur with more itching of the eyes and nose. Other factors may also be present to help differentiate these two conditions.

Q. *Do you have a medical condition that is being treated by a doctor, for example, diabetes, heart condition, or asthma?*

■ Various disease states can be affected by the cold itself or by the treatment used to reduce cold symptoms. The pharmacist must be familiar with all conditions that can be affected by it. This precaution also pertains to other medications the individual may be taking.

Exacerbations of asthmatic attacks can occur during a cold. In asthmatics who do acquire a cold, secondary bacterial infections are potential complications.

Blood sugar often rises in diabetics with a cold. This effect can be enhanced with the use of oral decongestants. These agents can also affect the cardiovascular system.

References

Epidemiology

Cohen S, Tyrrell D, Smith A. Psychological stress and susceptibility to the common cold. N Engl J Med 1991;325:606-12.

D'Alessio D, Peterson J, Dick C, Dick E. Transmission of experimental rhinovirus colds in volunteer married couples. J Infect Dis 1976;133:28–36.

Douglas R Jr, Lindgren K, Couch R. Exposure to cold environment and rhinovirus common cold. Failure to demonstrate effect. N Engl J Med 1968;279:742–7.

Fox J, Cooney M, Hall C. The Seattle virus watch, V: epidemiologic observations of rhinovirus infections, 1965–1969, in families with young children. Am J Epidemiol 1975;101:122–43.

Gwaltney J Jr, Moskalski P, Hendley J. Hand-to-hand transmission of rhinovirus colds. Ann Intern Med 1978;88:463–7.

Hendley J, Gwaltney J. Mechanisms of transmission of rhinovirus infections. Epidem Reviews 1988;10:242–58.

Stickler G, Smith T, Broughton D. The common cold. Eur J Pediatr 1985; 144:4–8.

The Common Cold

The Respiratory Tract

Irwin R, Rosen M, Braman S. Cough: a comprehensive review. Arch Intern Med 1977;137:1186–91.

Kucera L, Myrvik Q. Fundamentals of medical virology. Philadelphia: Lea & Febiger, 1985:208–34.

Proud D, Naclerio R, Gwaltney J, Hendley J. Kinins are generated in nasal secretions during rhinovirus colds. J Infect Dis 1990;161:120–3.

Richardson P, Phipps R. The anatomy, physiology, pharmacology and pathology of tracheobronchial mucus secretion and the use of expectorant drugs in human disease. Pharmacol Ther 1978;3:441–79.

Pathophysiology

Dolin R. Common viral respiratory infections. In: Wilson J, Braunwald E, Isselbacher K, et al, eds. Harrison's principles of internal medicine. New York: McGraw-Hill, 1991:700–20.

Grave J, Davis G, Meyer A, et al. The major human rhinovirus receptor is ICAM-1. Cell 1989;56:839–47.

Kapikian A. The common cold. In: Wyngaarden J, Smith L Jr, eds. Cecil textbook of medicine. Philadelphia: WB Saunders, 1988;1753–7.

Levandowski R. Rhinoviruses. In: Belshe R, ed. Textbook of human virology. Littleton: Publishing Services Group, 1984:391–405.

Rabinowitz H. Upper respiratory tract infections. Primary Care 1990; 17: 793–809. Antimicrob Agents Chemother 1988;32:224–30.

Proud D, Reynolds C, Lacapra S, et al. Nasal provocation with bradykinin induces symptoms of rhinitis and a sore throat. Am Rev Respir Dis 1988;137:613–6.

Signs and Symptoms

Anonymous. Fed Reg 1983;48(203):48576–95.

Gwaltney J Jr. Rhinoviruses. In: Evans A, ed. Viral infections of humans: epidemiology and control. New York: Plenum Medical Book, 1982:491–517.

Phillpotts R, Tyrrell D. Rhinovirus colds. Br Med Bull 1985;41:386–90.

Pharyngitis

Embree J. Pharyngitis. Med North Am 1990;9:1050–3.

Huovinen P, Lahtonen R, Ziegler T, et al. Pharyngitis in adults: the presence and coexistence of viruses and bacterial organisms. Ann Intern Med 1989;110:612–6.

Lang S, Singh K. The sore throat: when to investigate and when to prescribe. Drugs 1990;40:854–62.

Lundberg C, Nord C-E. Streptococcal throat infections: still a complex clinical problem. Scand J Infect Dis 1988;57(Supp):7–11.

Influenza

Anonymous. National Advisory Committee on Immunization: Statement on influenza vaccination for the 1991–1992 season. Canada Disease Weekly Report 1991;17–24(15 June):121–6.

Dolin R. Influenza. In: Wilson J, Braunwald E, Isselbacher K, et al, eds. Harrison's principles of internal medicine. New York: McGraw-Hill, 1991:695–700.

Douglas R Jr. Influenza. In: Wyngaarden J, Smith L Jr, eds. Cecil textbook of medicine. Philadelphia: WB Saunders, 1988:1762–7.

Perlman P, Ginn D. Respiratory infections in ambulatory adults. Postgrad Med 1990;87(1):175–84.

Van Exan R. In case you're asked—Influenza in perspective. Pharm Pract 1990;6(7):9–14.

Sinusitis

Panje W. Sinusitis. In: Rakel R, ed. Conn's current therapy. Philadelphia: WB Saunders, 1991:178–80.

Shapiro G. Sinusitis in children. J Allergy Clin Immunol 1988;81:1025–7.

General Treatment

Anonymous. Disinfectants. In: Reynolds J, ed. Martindale: the extra pharmacopoeia. London: Pharmaceutical Press, 1989;949–72.

Anonymous. Fed Reg 1982;47(101):22776–81.

Eby G, Davis D, Halcomb W. Reduction in duration of common colds by zinc gluconate lozenges in a double-blind study. Antimicrob Agents Chemother 1984;25:20–4.

Farr B, Conner E, Betts R, et al. Two randomized controlled trials of zinc gluconate lozenge therapy of experimentally induced rhinovirus colds. Antimicrob Agents Chemother 1987;31:1183–7.

Kyriakos T. What's hot in self-medication. Drug Merch 1989;70(1):34–7.

Macknin M, Mathew S, Medendorp S. Effect of inhaling heated vapor on symptoms of the common cold. JAMA 1990;264:989–91.

McBean Cochran B. "What should I take for my cold?" Pharm Pract 1990; 6(9):33–8.

Saketkhoo K, Januszkiewicz A, Sackner M. Effects of drinking hot water, cold water, and chicken soup on nasal mucous velocity and nasal airflow resistance. Chest 1978;74:408–10.

Turner H, Garner W, Lanese R. A comparative study of a phenol-based mouthwash as a gargle or a spray with a saline gargle. Am Coll Health Assoc J 1980;29:129–32.

Tyrrell D. Some recent work at the Common Cold Unit, Salisbury. Infection 1988;16:261–2.

Tyrrell D. Hot news on the common cold. Ann Rev Microbiol 1988;42:35–47.

Tyrrell D, Barrow I, Arthur J. Local hyperthermia benefits natural and experimental common colds. Br Med J 1989;298:1280–3.

Nasal Decongestants

Anonymous. Fed Reg 1976;41(176):38312–423.

Anonymous. Fed Reg 1985;50(10):2200–18.

Anonymous. Decongestants and Analgesics. In: USP Convention, ed. USP DI—drug information for the health care provider. Rockville: United States Pharmacopeial Convention, 1991:1084–97.

Anonymous. Sympathomimetic Agents. In: McEvoy G, ed. American hospital formulary service drug information. Bethesda: American Society of Hospital Pharmacists, 1991:671–719.

Bale J Jr, Fountain M, Shaddy R. Phenylpropanolamine-associated CNS complications in children and adolescents. Am J Dis Child 1984;138:683–5.

Black M, Remsen K. Rhinitis medicamentosa. Can Med Assoc J 1980; 122:881–4.

Capel L, Swanston A. Beware congesting nasal decongestants. Br Med J 1986;293:1258–9.

Chaplin S. Adverse reactions to sympathomimetics in cold remedies. Adverse Drug Reaction Bull 1984;107:396–9.

Dougherty R. Pseudo-speed: look-alikes or pea-shooters. NY State J Med 1982;82:74–5.

Drew C, Knight G, Hughes D, Bush M. Comparison of the effects of D-ephedrine and L-pseudoephedrine on the cardiovascular and respiratory systems in man. Br J Clin Pharm 1978;6:221–5.

Elis J, Laurence D, Mattie H, Prichard B. Modification by monoamine oxidase inhibitors of the effect of some sympathomimetics on blood pressure. Br Med J 1967;2:75–8.

Empey D, Medder K. Nasal decongestants. Drugs 1981; 21:438–43.

Empey D, Young G, Letley E, et al. Dose-response study of the nasal decongestant and cardiovascular effects of pseudoephedrine. Br J Clin Pharmacol 1980;9:351–8.

Griffiths R, Brady J, Snell J. Relationship between anorectic and reinforcing properties of appetite suppressant drugs: implications for assessment of abuse liability. Biol Psychiatry 1978;13:283–90.

Herridge C, A'Brook M. Ephedrine psychosis (Letter). Br Med J 1968;2:160.

Higgins J, Oppenheimer E, Gershman M. Phenylpropanolamine-associated headaches (Letter). Am J Dis Child 1985;139:331.

Hoffman B, Lefkowitz R. Catecholamines and sympathomimetic drugs. In: Goodman L, Gilman A, Rall T, Nies A, Taylor P, eds. Goodman and Gilman's the pharmacological basis of therapeutics. New York: Macmillan, 1990: 187–220.

Jordan P. CNS stimulants sold as amphetamines (Letter). Am J Hosp Pharm 1981;38:29.

Marchessault J, Boyd J, Crocker J, et al. First report of the Expert Advisory Committee on nonprescription cough and cold remedies to the Health Protection Branch: Antihistamines, nasal decongestants, and anticholinergics. Ottawa: Health and Welfare Canada, 1988.

Marchessault J, Boyd J, Crocker J, et al. Third report of the Expert Advisory

The Common Cold

Committee on nonprescription cough and cold remedies to the Health Protection Branch: Phenylpropanolamine, lozenges, and combinations. Ottawa: Health and Welfare Canada, 1989.

Mueller S. Phenylpropanolamine (Letter). N Engl J Med 1984;310:395.

Pentel P. Phenylpropanolamine and blood pressure (Letter). JAMA 1985; 253:2491–2.

Pentel P. Toxicity of over-the-counter stimulants. JAMA 1984;252:1898–903.

Sankey R, Nunn A, Sills J. Visual hallucinations in children receiving decongestants. Br Med J 1984;288:1369.

Soederman P, Sahlberg D, Wiholm B-E. CNS reactions to nose drops in small children (Letter). Lancet 1984;1:573.

Waggoner W. Phenylpropanolamine issue (Letter). Neurology 1984;34:1526.

Waters B, Lapierre Y. Secondary mania associated with sympathomimetic drug use. Am J Psychiatr 1981;138:837–8.

White W, Riotte K. Drugs for cough and cold symptoms in hypertensive patients. Am Fam Physician 1985;31(3):183–7.

Evaluating Coughs

Bamer S. Cough: physiology, evaluation, and treatment. Lung 1986;164:79–92.

Braman S, Corrao W. Chronic cough: diagnosis and treatment. Primary Care 1985;12:217–25.

Chou D, Wang S. Studies on the localization of central cough mechanism: site of action of antitussive drugs. J Pharmacol Exp Ther 1973;194:499–505.

Fuller R, Jackson D. Physiology and treatment of cough. Thorax 1990; 45:425–30.

Toop L, Howie J, Paxton F. Night cough and general practice research. J Roy Coll Gen Pract 1986;36:74–7.

Cough Medicines

Anonymous. Fed Reg 1982;47(132):30002–10.

Anonymous. Fed Reg 1987;52(155):30042–57.

Anonymous. Antitussives, expectorants and mucolytic agents. In: McEvoy G, ed. American hospital formulary service drug information. Bethesda: American Society of Hospital Pharmacists, 1991:1593–607.

Anonymous. Supplementary drugs and other substances. In: Reynolds J, ed. Martindale: the extra pharmacopoeia. London: Pharmaceutical Press, 1989:1552,1586.

Boyd E. A review of studies on the pharmacology of the expectorants and inhalants. Int J Clin Pharmacol Ther Toxicol 1970;3:55–60.

Committee on drugs. Use of codeine- and dextromethorphan-containing cough syrups in pediatrics. Pediatrics 1978;62:118–22.

Domino E, Krutak-Krol H, Lal J. Evidence for a central site of action for the antitussive effects of caramiphen. J Pharmacol Exp Ther 1985;233:249–53.

Fleming P. Dependence on dextromethorphan hydrobromide. Br Med J 1986;293:597.

Krogh C, ed. Compendium of pharmaceuticals and specialties. Ottawa: Canadian Pharmaceutical Association, 1991:265,539,1097.

Lilienfield L, Rose J, Princiotto J. Antitussive activity of diphenhydramine in chronic cough. Clin Pharmacol Ther 1976;19:421–5.

Loder R. Safe reduction of the cough reflex with noscapine: a preliminary communication on a new use for an old drug. Anaesthesia 1969;24:355–8.

Marchessault J, Boyd J, Crocker J, et al. Second report of the Expert Advisory Committee on nonprescription cough and cold remedies to the Health Protection Branch: Antitussives, expectorants, and bronchodilators. Ottawa: Health and Welfare Canada, 1989.

Orrell M, Campbell P. Dependence on dextromethorphan hydrobromide (Letter). Br Med J 1986;293:1242–3.

Von Muehlendahl K, Krienke E, Scherf-Rahne B, Baukloh G. Codeine intoxication in childhood. Lancet 1976;2:303–5.

Expectorants

Anonymous. Guaiphenesin and iodide. Drug Ther Bull 1985;23(16):62–4.

Buchanan G, Martin V, Levine P, et al. The effects of "anti-platelet" drugs on bleeding time and platelet aggregation in normal human subjects. Am J Clin Pathol 1977;68:355–9.

Chodosh S, Medici T. Expectorant effect of glyceryl guaiacolate (Letter). Chest 1973;64:543–5.

Cohen B. Antitussive effect of guaifenesin (Letter). Chest 1983;84:118–9.

Hirsch S, Viernes P, Kory R. The expectorant effect of glyceryl guaiacolate in patients with chronic bronchitis. Chest 1973;63:9–14.

Kuhn J, Hendly J, Adams K, et al. Antitussive effect of guaifenesin in young adults with natural colds: objective and subjective assessment. Chest 1982;82:713–8.

Robinson R, Cumming W, Deffenbaugh E. Effectiveness of guaifenesin as an expectorant: a cooperative double-blind study. Curr Ther Res 1977; 22:284–96.

Thomson M, Pavia D, McNicol M. A preliminary study of the effect of guaiphenesin on mucociliary clearance from the human lung. Thorax 1973;28:742–7.

Antihistamines and the Common Cold

Anonymous. Fed Reg 1985;50(10):2220–41.

Bye C, Cooper J, Empey D, et al. Effects of pseudoephedrine and triprolidine, alone and in combination, on symptoms of the common cold. Br Med J 1980;281:189–90.

Crutcher J, Kantner T. The effectiveness of antihistamines in the common cold. J Clin Pharmacol 1981;21:9–15.

Gaffey M, Gwaltney J Jr, Sastre A, et al. Intranasally and orally administered antihistamine treatment of experimental rhinovirus colds. Am Rev Respir Dis 1987;136:556–60.

Howard J Jr, Kantner T, Lilienfield L, et al. Effectiveness of antihistamines in the symptomatic management of the common cold. JAMA 1979; 242:2414–7.

Pruitt A. Rational use of cold and cough preparations. Pediatric Ann 1985;14(4):289–91.

West S, Brandon B, Stolley P, Rumril R. A review of antihistamines and the common cold. Pediatrics 1975;56(1):100–7.

Anticholinergics

Gaffey M, Gwaltney J Jr, Dressler W, et al. Intranasally administered atropine methonitrate treatment of experimental rhinovirus colds. Am Rev Respir Dis 1987;135:241–4.

Gaffey M, Hayden F, Boyd J, Gwaltney J Jr. Ipratropium bromide treatment of experimental rhinovirus infection. Antimicrob Agents Chemother 1988;32:1644–7.

Nonsteroidal Anti-inflammatory Drugs

Graham N, Burrell C, Douglas R, et al. Adverse effects of aspirin, acetaminophen, and ibuprofen on immune function, viral shedding, and clinical status in rhinovirus-infected volunteers. J Infect Dis 1990;162:1277–82.

Sperber S, Sorrentino J, Riker D, Hayden F. Evaluation of an alpha agonist alone and in combination with a nonsteroidal antiinflammatory agent in the treatment of experimental rhinovirus colds. Bull NY Acad Med 1989;65:145–60.

Sperber S, Hayden F. Chemotherapy of rhinovirus colds. Antimicrob Agents Chemother 1988;32:409–19.

Vitamin C

Anderson T, Suranyi G, Beaton G. The effect on winter illness of large doses of vitamin C. Can Med Assoc J 1974;111:31–6.

Anderson T, Reid D, Beaton G. Vitamin C and the common cold: a double-blind trial. Can Med Assoc J 1972;107:503–8.

Anderson T, Beaton G, Corey P, Spero L. Winter illness and vitamin C: the effect of relatively low doses. Can Med Assoc J 1975;112:823–6.

Coulehan J. Ascorbic acid and the common cold: reviewing the evidence. Postgrad Med 1979;66(3):153–60.

Dykes M, Meier P. Ascorbic acid and the common cold: evaluations of its efficacy and toxicity. JAMA 1975;231:1073–9.

Elwood P, Hughes S, St Leger, A. A randomized controlled trial of the therapeutic effect of vitamin C in the common cold. Practitioner 1977;218:133–7.

Karlowski T, Chalmers T, Frenkel L, et al. Ascorbic acid for the common cold: a prophylactic and therapeutic trial. JAMA 1975;231:1038–42.

Murray T, Carroll K, Davignon J, et al. Nutrition recommendations: The report of the scientific review committee. Ottawa: Health and Welfare Canada, 1990:99–102.

Pauling L. Vitamin C and the common cold. San Francisco: WH Freeman, 1970:39–52.

Pitt H, Costrini A. Vitamin C prophylaxis in marine recruits. JAMA 1979; 241:908–11.

Rivers J. Safety of high-level vitamin C ingestion. Ann NY Acad Sci 1987; 498:445–54.

Interferon

Douglas R, Moore B, Miles H, et al. Prophylactic efficacy of intranasal alpha$_2$-interferon against rhinovirus infections in the family setting. N Engl J Med 1986;314:65–70.

Hayden F, Albrecht J, Kaiser D, Gwaltney J Jr. Prevention of natural colds by contact prophylaxis with intranasal alpha$_2$-interferon. N Engl J Med 1986;314:71–5.

Hayden F, Kaiser D, Albrecht J. Intranasal recombinant alfa-2b interferon treatment of naturally occurring common colds. Antimicrob Agents Chemother 1988;32:224–30.

Scott G. Interfering with the real cold. Br Med J 1986;292:1413–4.

The Diabetic Individual

Koda-Kimble MA, Rotblatt M. Diabetes mellitus. In: Young L, Koda-Kimble MA, eds. Applied therapeutics, the clinical use of drugs. Vancouver: Applied Therapeutics, 1988:1663–742.

Naylor M. Caloric and carbohydrate contents of oral pharmaceutical products in Canada. Toronto: Canadian Society of Hospital Pharmacists and Connaught-Novo, 1986.

13

Allergic Rhinitis

Jeffrey G. Taylor

Airborne allergens cause the symptoms of allergic rhinitis, with the nose, eyes and sinuses the areas most affected. Seasonal and perennial allergic rhinitis are two common forms of this disorder. Some refer to seasonal allergic rhinitis as hay fever. The mainstays of therapy are the antihistamines. Decongestants, cromolyn, corticosteroids, and immunotherapy also play a role. Active avoidance of the cause must also be part of the treatment regimen.

Allergic rhinitis is a common affliction that causes many people to view the warmer months of the year with apprehension. The symptoms characteristic of the condition occur when various cells in the body release vasoactive compounds. Symptoms can be acute, lasting only a few weeks, or individuals may suffer to varying degrees all year round.

Epidemiology

About 15 per cent of Canadians suffer from allergic rhinitis. Most individuals develop their symptoms prior to the age of 20, with peak incidence occuring in their early teens. The prognosis for spontaneous resolution of allergic rhinitis is relatively poor, but the severity of symptoms may diminish as one grows older.

Sex and race appear to have little effect on who acquires this condition. However, it does have a marked genetic predisposition.

Anatomy and Physiology

The respiratory tract is equipped with mechanisms to purify inhaled air. As we breathe air in, much of the dust and particles are removed by the special protective features of the nose. For example, just within the nostril openings are stiff hairs which serve as gross filters to remove airborne particles.

The interior cavity of the nose is lined with mucous membrane which contains an extensive network of capillaries. As air passes through the nose, the nasal cavity "conditions" the air. First, the vascular surface of the nasal cavity warms and supplies moisture to the air. This process can increase the relative humidity of inspired air from 9 to 100 per cent humidity by the time it reaches the nasopharynx. Second, any small particles passing through the nasal passageways encounter various surfaces of the nose: the turbinates (bones shaped like an inverted cone that project into the nasal cavity), the septum and the pharyngeal wall. Many inspired particles become trapped in the mucus coating these surfaces. The cilia, which are present on the epithelium of the nasal passageways, move the mucus containing the trapped particles toward the pharynx, where it is swallowed.

Neuronal control regulates airflow, blood flow and glandular secretion in the region. Stimulation of parasympathetic (cholinergic) nerves induces glandular secretions and vasodilatation. Stimulation of the sympathetic nervous system causes vasoconstriction. Neuropeptides such as substance P may also play a role.

The patency of the airways on each side of the nose are in state of flux, in what is described as the nasal cycle. As the flow in one nasal passage slightly increases, the flow in the other decreases. This occurs in approximately 80 per cent of individuals.

The sneeze reflex is another protective mechanism of the respiratory tract. Irritation to the nasal passageway provides the stimulus to initiate the reflex. When an individual sneezes, air travels rapidly through the nose, clearing passages of foreign material.

The paranasal sinuses (frontal, maxillary, ethmoid and sphenoid) open into the nasal cavity. They are lined with mucous membrane which is continuous with that of the nasal cavity. Mucus produced in the sinuses is continually being swept into the nose by the ciliated surface of the membrane. During an allergic episode, the sinus openings may become blocked, subsequent to swelling of the mucous membrane.

Pathophysiology

Allergic rhinitis is an antibody-mediated inflammatory disease of the nasal mucous membranes. When a genetically predisposed individual comes into contact with a particular substance (an allergen), the body's defence mechanisms respond by producing antibodies specific to that allergen. The antibodies involved in allergic rhinitis belong to the immunoglobulin E (IgE) class of immunoglobulins. These IgE antibodies attach to mast cells, thereby sensitizing the individual to the particular allergen.

Mast cells, with their stores of vasoactive mediators, are central to the pathogenesis of allergic rhinitis. They are generally located near small blood vessels and nerves and can be found in connective tissue, skin, lymphoid tissue and respiratory epithelium. Basophils, which circulate in the bloodstream, are also involved in this process. Like mast cells, they possess immunoglobulin receptors on their cell surface and contain histamine.

Upon subsequent challenge with the same antigenic protein, the

Allergic Rhinitis

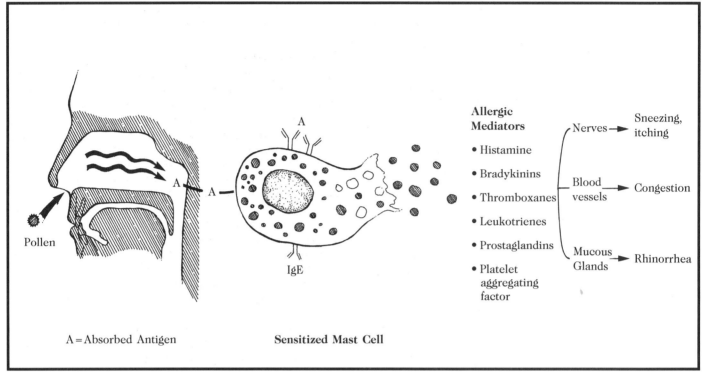

Figure 1 *Allergic Response*

antigen interacts with the IgE bound to mast cells and basophils in the nasal mucosa. The binding of 2 or more cell-bound IgE molecules by allergen subsequently occurs on the cell surface. This interaction initiates a complex chain of events leading to the degranulation of the cell and the subsequent release of mediators of immediate hypersensitivity (see Figure 1). The presence of calcium in the extracellular medium appears essential to the release of mediators. Cyclic AMP may also be involved. The chemical mediators released include histamine, prostaglandins, kinins, leukotrienes and other substances. Some, like histamine are preformed, whereas others are newly generated. *Antihistamines H₁*

The symptoms of allergic rhinitis result from the action of the chemical mediators on blood vessels, goblet cells and mucosal glands. For example, histamine produces capillary dilation which causes the surrounding tissue to swell. This effect is thought to be mediated through H_1- and H_2-receptors. Histamine also increases capillary permeability. This occurs by endothelial cells of small blood vessels contracting, thereby increasing the distance between any two cells; plasma protein and fluid can then leak out. In addition, histamine can stimulate various nerve endings which leads to an itch sensation.

Although compounds like prostaglandin D2, leukotrienes and thromboxanes do not possess the complete vasoactive profile of histamine, they are critical to the allergic reaction. Of these compounds, histamine is the least active in stimulating mucous secretion. Edema due to vascular leakage is the result of the activity of numerous mediators.

Some patients exhibit a biphasic response to allergens. The initial reaction is called the early phase of the allergic process. A second phase then occurs, about 3 to 10 hours after the initial phase, and is called the last phase. Different patterns of mediator release are seen in the two phases, which may have implications in the future approach of therapy. As part of the inflammatory process, released chemotactic mediators attract inflammatory cells to the area, including eosinophils, basophils and neutrophils.

Allergens

The allergens causing allergic rhinitis are usually airborne compounds composed mainly of protein. Common allergens include pollens, moulds, animal dander (skin scales) and house dust (see Table I).

Pollens that land on the nasal mucosa are digested and their contents released by lysozymes present in the respiratory mucus. Tree, grass and weed pollens are the most frequent causes of symptoms. The main seasonal allergen in North America is ragweed pollen. Ragweed is especially troublesome in eastern Canada, less so in the prairie provinces, and still less in British Columbia.

Grasses are second to weeds in allergenic importance, but only a few species of grasses have been singled out as significant allergens. Symptoms due to these allergens may be brought on by the individual mowing the lawn. Pollens from trees (for example, walnut, oak, elm and hickory) account for about 10 per cent of cases of allergic rhinitis. People can suffer from allergies induced by all three types of plants. Insect-pollinated plants produce sticky pollen and rarely cause allergic symptoms.

The pollen that cause problems for the individual can be identified, at least in part, by seasonal differences in their production. Trees are responsible for many cases of spring allergic rhinitis. Symptoms in late spring (April, May) and summer are commonly produced by grass pollens. Weed pollens occur in late summer and early fall.

Hot, dry, windy days are more suited to spreading pollen than cool, cloudy days. Alternatively, rainfall tends to wash it out of the air. Early

Allergic Rhinitis

Allergic Rhinitis

Table I *Allergens That Induce Allergic Rhinitis*

Allergens	Sources of exposure
Pollen	trees, grasses, weeds
Mould	outdoors—ubiquitous indoors—damp basement, barns, contaminated air conditioners, humidifiers, indoor plants, garbage receptacles, roof leaks into attics
House dust	bedding, carpeting, drapes, upholstered furniture, forced-air heating systems
Feathers	bedding, comforters, pets
Animal-derived allergens	cat, dog, horse, rodent and avian species are most common
Other plant-derived proteins Enzymes (e.g., papain)	household detergents, food and enzyme manufacturing sites
Kapok	pillows, mattresses, sleeping bags
Pyrethrum	insecticides, pediculicides
Miscellaneous—coffee bean dust, wood dusts, various grains (e.g., cotton, flaxseed)	occupational—food, lumber industries, grain handlers
Small molecular weight chemicals	chemical industries

Adapted from: Bernstein D, Bernstein I. Allergic rhinitis caused by inhalant factors. In: Rackel E, ed. Conn's current therapy. Philadelphia: WB Saunders, 1986:598–603.

morning dew may delay problems with pollen until mid-morning, when the ground warms up.

Moulds produce potential allergens in the form of airborne spores. Mould growth can occur in soil, decaying organic matter and many indoor environments. It is greatest during damp, rainy weather. Favorite areas for growth include damp, dark places (cellars, garages, attics); roof leaks behind walls; old foam rubber pillows, mattresses and furniture; rotting leaves and other vegetation; and areas continually handling water (drainage sinks, laundry tubs, washing machines, garbage cans).

Attacks that originate indoors are commonly caused by house dust, a collection of diverse particles including animal dander, vegetable material, dirt, mould, hair, wall plaster, paint chips and the dust mite. Dust mites' proteinaceous content make them an important factor in the sensitizing capacity of household dust. Dust mites eat human skin scales which they find on such things as bed sheets. Their appearance increases significantly with high humidity in the home. When searching for causes of perennial allergic rhinitis, one should diligently assess bedrooms for dust.

Another potential allergen is the dander of animals and birds. Common sources include hamsters, rabbits, gerbils, parakeets and guinea pigs. Sensitivity to dander can occur at any age and may even occur several years after a pet is introduced into the home. The length of hair or fur on the animal apparently has little effect on its poten-

tial antigenicity. Cats have been singled out as the worst offenders among domestic animals; their saliva appears to be the culprit.

Symptoms

Common signs and symptoms of seasonal allergic rhinitis are: profuse and clear rhinorrhea; nasal congestion; lacrimation, with reddened and swollen conjunctiva; periorbital swelling; palatal, nasal and ocular pruritus; sneezing (often in bouts); eustachian tube obstruction with or without earache; and frontal headaches. Physical findings are usually limited to the upper respiratory tract and eyes.

The nose, palate, pharynx and eyes usually begin to itch soon after exposure to the allergen. Lacrimation, sneezing and rhinorrhea accompany or soon follow the pruritus. Individuals with allergic rhinitis report periods of nasal congestion, intermittent sneezing and rhinorrhea lasting for at least 0.5 to 1 hour per day. Symptoms due to pollens are frequently worse in the morning and improve toward the evening. Irritability, anorexia and insomnia can be reactions to the physical discomfort the allergy creates. Secondary sinusitis may result from persistent inflammatory obstruction of the sinus cavity openings. Coughing and asthmatic wheezing may appear as the season progresses.

Symptoms in children are similar but can be more troublesome. One-third to one-half of all children who have an allergy also develop chronic serous otitis media secondary to eustachian tube blockage. Allergic shiners—dark circles under the eyes—are the result of periorbital edema. Children may also rub the tip of their nose in an upwards fashion with the palm of their hand. If done often enough, this activity can put a crease across the nose.

The severity of symptoms of allergic rhinitis correlates to allergen exposure. A rough estimate of the amount of pollen in the environment is provided with a pollen count. One way to achieve this is for specialists to collect airborne pollen particles on a greased glass slide positioned within a specially designed box; the box allows air to flow through easily. After 24 hours, the pollen grains are counted under a microscope. Symptoms in persons allergic to pollen are severest when the pollen count is highest and subside when the pollenation season begins to wane.

Primary exposure to one allergen can affect subsequent exposures, a so-called priming effect. As the nasal mucosa reacts to an allergen and the tissues become swollen, further reactivity to this or other allergens is enhanced. The priming effect increases the penetration of the new allergenic substance into the nasal mucosa. The clinical importance of this can be seen in, for example, a ragweed-sensitive person who usually responds to allergen exposure (for example, house dust) with modest swelling and rhinorrhea. During ragweed season, when priming of the tissues has occurred, the individual can develop more severe symptoms in response to the dust.

Symptoms are considered chronic when they last for more than 4 weeks. Perennial allergic rhinitis presents with a continuum of symptoms similar to acute allergic rhinitis, but at a low grade of severity. Extranasal symptoms such as conjunctivitis are less common. Chronic nasal congestion may cause hearing problems in children when it affects the function of the eustachian tube. Chronic congestion can also make people mouth breathers, with subsequent dry mouth and throat. Nasal polyps can occur as a complication of untreated cases, but are rare. Other complications of chronic rhinitis include sinusitis, otitis media, and cough due to chronic mouth breathing and/or postnasal drip. Common allergens in perennial allergic rhinitis are moulds and house dust.

Diagnosis

The diagnosis of allergic rhinitis depends upon taking a careful history to correlate symptoms to an inciting agent. The history should stress the circumstances (season, time of day and place) surrounding the onset and subsequent relief of symptoms, as well as the duration, severity and type of symptoms. A family history may reveal other members with symptoms of allergy or atopy (asthma or atopic dermatitis). Table II depicts a classification system for rhinitis.

Table II *Classification of Rhinitis*
Allergic rhinitis
Acute (seasonal; hay fever)
Perennial (chronic)
Perennial nonallergic rhinitis
Eosinophilic nonallergic rhinitis
Nasal polyps
Irritant rhinitis
Rhinitis medicamentosa
Vasomotor rhinitis
Rhinitis associated with systemic conditions

Adapted from: Meltzer E. The use of antihistamines for the treatment of airway disease. Cutis 1988;42:22–5.

If the offending allergen cannot be clearly indicated by the history, a suspected diagnosis should be confirmed by skin testing. Skin testing using suspected allergens can provide evidence of the presence of IgE antibodies. Individuals whose mast cells have been sensitized to the test allergen manifest sensitivity at the test site by wheal and flare development within 15 to 30 minutes. Indiscriminate skin testing is not warranted; the individual's history of exposure determines the substances to be tested.

Skin is tested either by injecting dilute allergen extract subcutaneously or by applying a more concentrated allergen solution to the surface of abraded or scratched skin. Usually the latter method, which is less sensitive but safer, is used first. If negative, it may be followed by intradermal testing. A positive result with the scratch test precludes further testing with the intradermal method.

Previous antihistamine use can affect skin-test results and they must be allowed to clear the body before the person is tested. A drug-free period of 48 hours has been recommneded, but this time frame has generally applied to first generation antihistamines. Antihistamines with long biologic half lives need more time to be cleared from the body before skin testing occurs. Decongestants may also decrease the skin response to an allergen.

The radioallergosorbent test (RAST) is a radioimmunoassay for measuring serum IgE antibody levels. However, total IgE serum levels are elevated in only 30 to 40 per cent of individuals with allergic rhinitis and can even be elevated in nonallergic conditions, which makes the relevance of a positive RAST unclear. It is less sensitive but more specific than a skin test. The test is usually reserved for people in whom skin testing cannot be done or should be avoided.

Differential Diagnosis of Allergic Rhinitis

Nasal congestion, rhinorrhea, and pruritus can be symptomatic of other illnesses. One such example is the common cold, but distinguishing features do exist to help differentiate between the two (see Table III). A cold should be suspect when symptoms subside within 7 days as allergy symptoms tend to continue for weeks to months. The timing of the symptoms will also be important—colds occur less often during the summer months, while symptoms of acute allergic rhinitis correspond to the appearance of various seasonal pollens.

A sore throat may occur with a cold and may also be seen with allergic rhinitis, especially if any amount of mouth breathing or postnasal drip is present. The rhinorrhea seen with allergies remains clear and watery, while secretions that occur as a result of a cold become mucopurulent. Sneezing and itchiness of the eyes, nose and throat are more evident in allergic rhinitis. The intensity of symptoms can also vary between the two illnesses: cold symptoms are bothersome throughout the day, while symptoms of allergic rhinitis will vary in intensity.

If an individual presents with a history of continuous nasal obstruction and rhinorrhea but lacks significant ocular symptoms or seasonal exacerbations, an extensive evaluation is needed to distinguish allergic from nonallergic etiologies. The physician may use nasal cytology if the cause of the rhinitis is in doubt. Eosinophils dominate nasal smears in patients with allergic rhinitis; however, their presence is relatively nonspecific.

When medications are suspected of causing rhinorrhea, cause and effect can often be confirmed when the individual's condition improves upon discontinuation of the agent. One of the most common causes of rhinitis medicamentosa is the overuse of topical decongestants. Thirteen per cent of new patients seen at a rhinitis clinic presented with chronic nasal congestion related (at least in part) to prolonged vasoconstrictor use. Antihypertensives (for example, methyldopa), antipsychotics (for example, perphenazine), ASA, oral contraceptives, and other systemic agents have been implicated in causing nasal congestion.

Congenital or acquired mechanical obstructions such as enlarged adenoids or septal anomalies may produce symptoms similar to those of allergic disease. Pregnancy and hypothyroidism are two systemic conditions that have presented with rhinitis.

Vasomotor rhinitis resembles perennial allergic rhinitis in symptom presentation: remissions and exacerbations of chronic rhinitis characterized by nasal congestion, sneezing, and rhinorrhea. It is nonallergic in nature and appears due to an increase in parasympathetic activity within the region. Symptoms are often provoked by changes in temperature or posture. It tends to respond poorly to treatment.

General Treatment

Once the offending allergens have been identified by history (and possibly skin tests), the individual must try to eliminate them from the environment, or at least avoid exposure to them. This is the simplest and most effective form of preventive therapy for the symptoms of allergic rhinitis, but is not always easily accomplished. Nevertheless, allergen avoidance must not be neglected as a method of treatment.

When attempting to reduce allergen exposure, attention must be focused on the areas where the individual spends much of their time.

Allergic Rhinitis

Table III *Differential Diagnosis of Rhinitis*

Sign/Symptom	Common cold	Acute allergic rhinitis	Perennial allergic rhinitis *allergic to dust + mold*	Vasomotor rhinitis
General symptom grade	Acute; symptoms present throughout the entire day; symptoms change somewhat over episode	Acute; symptoms wax and wane daily; usually worse in the morning	Chronic, low-grade; vary in severity, often unpredictably, throughout the year	Persistent symptoms; resembles perennial allergic rhinitis
Symptom time frame	Most episodes subside within a week	Weeks to months; symptoms correlate to seasons and to pollen count.	No distinct seasonal pattern; intermittent or continuous throughout year	Remissions and exacerbations
Nasal discharge	Initially clear and watery, then changes consistency to mucopurulent; occurs mainly during days 1 through 3 of a cold	Copious, watery; clear	Rhinorrhea mild but chronic	Rhinorrhea mild but chronic
Congestion	Nasal and sinus congestion is common	Common	Chronic nasal obstruction is often prominent and may extend to eustachian tube obstruction, especially in children	Nasal congestion alternating with watery rhinorrhea
Conjunctivitis	Not common, except initially	Common; prominent ocular lacrimation and itch	Uncommon, but lacrimation can occur; lesser grade than acute allergic rhinitis.	Uncommon, but lacrimation can occur
Sneezing	Uncommon, except at initial stages; occurs if congestion irritates nasal mucosal linings	Common, hallmark feature; sneezing often precedes appearance of rhinorrhea	Less common than with acute allergic rhinitis	Less common than with acute allergic rhinitis
Fever	Rare; more frequent in children	Absent	Absent	Absent
Pruritus	Nose and eyes can be somewhat affected	Common; nose, roof of mouth and eyes	Less common than with acute allergic rhinitis	Less common than with acute allergic rhinitis
Cough	Common, especially in later stages of cold	Coughing and asthmatic wheezing may develop as the season progresses; may be associated with postnasal drip	Rare; as for acute allergic rhinitis	Rare unless irritant-related, where inhalation of irritant induces cough reflex
Sore throat	Generally appears in early stages of cold; mild; may persist with accompanying postnasal drip or irritation via cough	Uncommon; may appear with postnasal drip	Uncommon; may appear with postnasal drip	Uncommon
Other	Mild constitutional symptoms; sinus headaches	Allergic shiners (dark circles under eyes); crease in nose from habitual rubbing; sinus headaches; recurring otitis media	As for acute allergic rhinitis	
Causative factor	Viral	Allergic; usually airborne pollens	Allergic; allergens present throughout the year, e.g., house dust	Etiology is uncertain; lacks evidence of any allergic basis; can be aggravated by dry air or inhaled irritants

Allergic Rhinitis

This is often a playroom or bedroom in the case of small children and the work environment of adults. Recommendations for changes in the home must be realistic, however. Effective and practical programs focus on the control of house dust, mould and animal dander.

Exposure to house dust can be reduced with careful housecleaning. Hot water in the wash cycle will kill mites on bedding. Studies that have looked at dust mite levels stress that efforts to reduce the problem should include rigorous cleaning of bedrooms, removal of carpets and the use of mattress covers. Careful vacuuming of existing carpets is helpful to some extent, but is not equivalent to replacing them with vinyl or wooden floors. However, before an expensive measure such as this is considered, the house should be carefully assessed to determine if dust mites could be a significant problem. Houses that have quite low humidity during the winter months may not support mite populations to a great extent and this can have a carry-over effect for the whole year. Commercial products are available in England (Actomite) and the United States (Acarosan) to kill dust mites and larvae in carpets. The American product contains benzyl benzoate powder. It is brushed on, left to dry, and vacuumed away. Another product available in the U.S. is Acarex, a dust mite test kit used to determine the level and location of dust mite infestation. Minimal information is available on the effectiveness of these products. To date these products are not available in Canada.

A baseboard heating system is the best for an allergy sufferer. Forced-air heating systems tend to disperse dust and mould spores throughout the house and may be the least desirable system. If the house has a forced-air system, filters on the furnace must be cleaned regularly to maintain maximum efficiency and the furnace and ductwork should be professionally cleaned once a year. High efficiency and electrostatic filters are available. Installing makeshift filters in each room's furnace vent is recommended.

One can reduce the activity of moulds by drying damp basements, cleaning humidifiers regularly and keeping closets dry with a constantly lit light bulb. High humidity in the home may exacerbate allergic symptoms by favoring the growth of moulds. High humidity also favors the propagation of the house dust mite. Optimum humidity for most allergy sufferers appears to be 35 to 50 per cent. Humidifiers can add to the mould count if not kept clean or if the machine's output is set too high. The ideal home temperature for allergy sufferers is estimated to be 21°C during the day and 18.5°C at night.

Animal dander in the home also may be reduced by careful cleaning and vacuuming. Unfortunately, if a child is severely sensitive to a pet, the animal should be removed from the household. Initially the pet can be given to friends or relatives to assess the effect of its removal from the home. This trial period should be of several months' duration, as the pet's dander can linger in the home several months after removal.

Indoor exposure to pollen can be reduced by filtering room air though an air conditioner. Much of the effectiveness of air conditioning, however, is simply the result of closing doors and windows. Pollen counts in closed, air-conditioned rooms approach zero; the count in an unfiltered room with the window open is usually about one-third that found outdoors.

Avoiding rural areas during pollination season and keeping windows closed when driving in the country is recommended. Mould-sensitive individuals should avoid barns, working with hay and raking leaves. Children with allergies should be discouraged from playing in open fields and should change clothes after playing outside. Weeds in the family yard should be controlled.

A change of environment is impractical for most allergy sufferers. Allergic individuals that move to avoid aggravating allergens tend to acquire new sensitivities in their new environment. If symptoms can be isolated to a well-defined seasonal appearance, such as ragweed season, an individual may choose to leave an area of exposure during peak symptomatic periods by planning a vacation for that time.

The effect of inhaled warm air on allergic rhinitis symptoms has been examined. For one study, air was administered at 43°C and was saturated with water vapor. Treatment consisted of two sessions of 30 minutes each, separated by 90 minutes, and repeated 7 days later. Some relief was evident in patients, but results are preliminary.

Figure 2 *Therapy of Allergic Rhinitis*

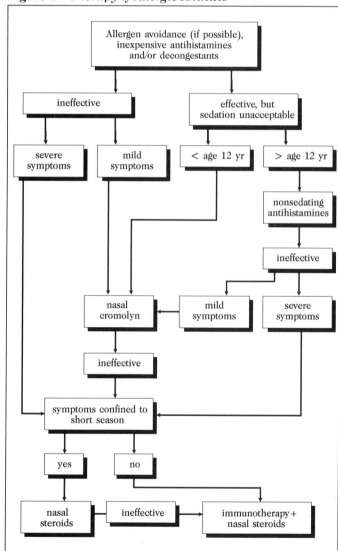

Used with permission from Schumacher M. Allergic rhinitis due to aeroallergens. In: Rakel RE, ed. Conn's current therapy. Philadelphia: WB Saunders, 1991:708–12.

Figure 3 *Suggested Approach to Treating Allergic Rhinitis*

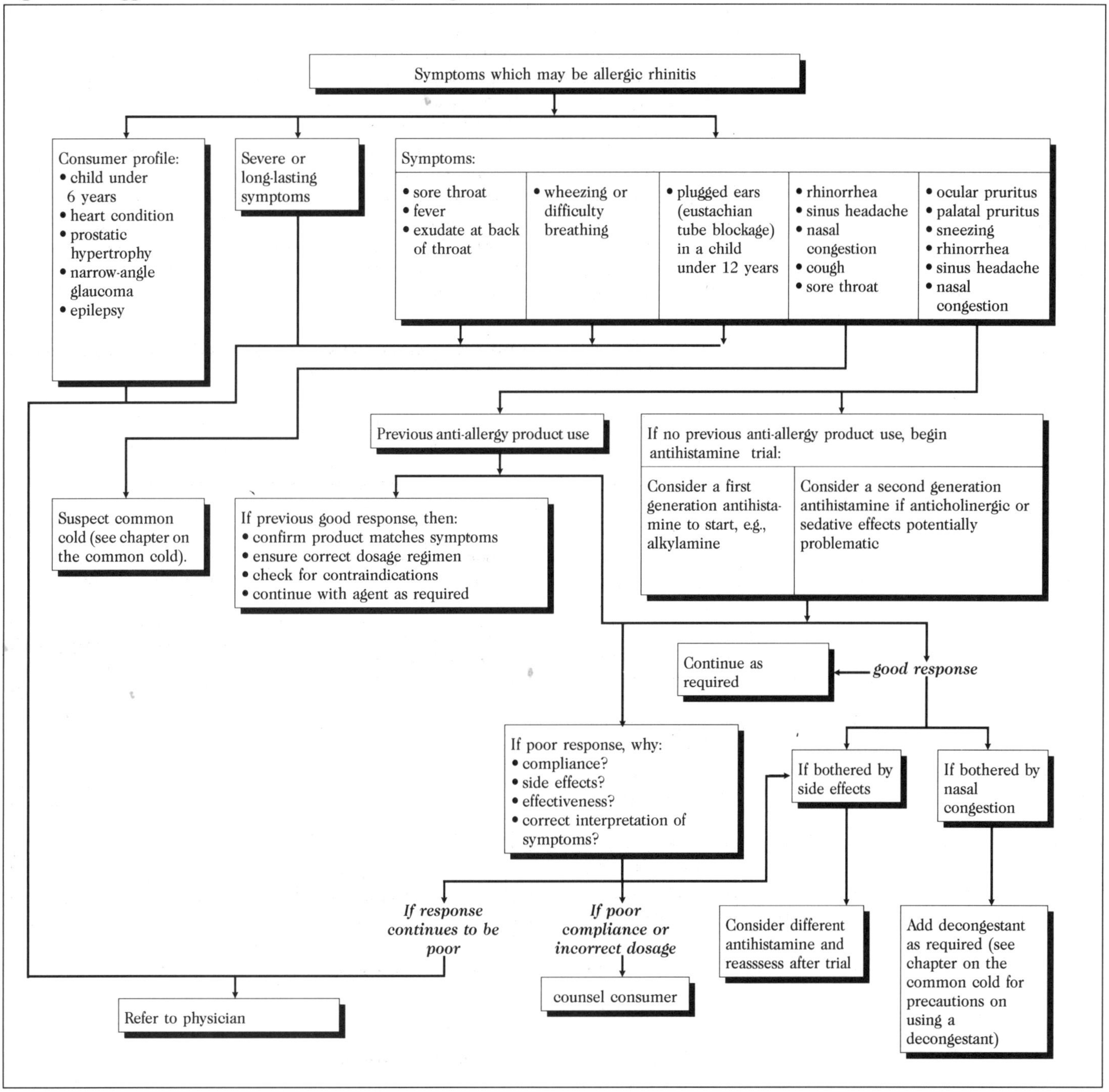

Pharmacologic Agents

Besides allergen avoidance, the other two treatment categories available for allergic rhinitis are drug therapy and immunotherapy. Drug therapy involves the use of antihistamines, decongestants, cromolyn and related compounds, anticholinergics and intranasal corticosteroids (see Figures 2 and 3).

Antihistamines

Antihistamines (H_1-receptor antagonists/blockers) are chemical enti-

ties that exert their effect primarily by preventing the action of histamine at H_1-receptor sites. They do so by occupying the receptor in a competitive and reversible manner. Antihistamines used in the treatment of allergic rhinitis do not block the effects of histamine at H_2-receptors. A third type of histamine receptor (H_3), located mainly in the brain, is thought to modulate the synthesis and release of histamine from neurons. The activity of antihistamines on these receptors, if any, is unclear. Antihistamines neither affect histamine synthesis nor do they chemically inactivate it. However, evidence suggests that some (azatadine, azelastine, terfenadine, loratadine, cetirizine, for example) may inhibit mediator release from mast cells and basophils.

There is a core structure within all antihistamines that represents the basic unit for competing with histamine at the receptor. Substitutions to this core modify the characteristics of each agent.

It has been convenient to categorize antihistamines according to their chemical structure. The classic antihistamines, now described as first generation agents, include chemical entities from several different structure groups: alkylamines, ethanolamines, ethylenediamines, phenothiazines, piperazines, and piperidines. Most are not pure H_1-receptor antagonists and tend to exhibit cross-reactivity with other receptors. This cross-reactivity may include anticholinergic, antiserotonin, and alpha-adrenergic blocking properties. The anticholinergic activity may contribute to the effectiveness of these agents by reducing the effect of cholinergic stimulation on goblet cell secretions or on fluid transfer out of capillaries. First generation antihistamines also possess antipruritic effects, which may be the result of a peripheral antihistaminic activity or local anesthetic effect.

Antihistamines considered as second generation agents include terfenadine, astemizole, loratadine, acrivastine, cetirizine, temelastine, and mequitazine. Although they contain the antihistamine nucleus, they differ enough from any first generation antihistamine structurally and pharmacologically to be classed separately. Unlike first generation antihistamines, they are generally not categorized by structure. Their lack of sedative properties is their main distinguishing feature.

Antihistamines are effective in reducing the sneezing, rhinorrhea, and itch (nasal, palatal, and ocular) associated with allergic rhinitis. They are 70 to 85 per cent effective in relieving these symptoms. Relief from congestion is less dramatic because much of the capillary vasodilatation effect is mediated through H_2-receptors, ones that are not affected by antihistamines. Both H_1- and H_2-antagonism is required to totally prevent the actions of histamine on target organs.

People with chronic symptoms are generally less responsive to antihistamine therapy. Patients using first generation agents report about a 50 per cent reduction in symptoms. Antihistamines may also be less effective when allergens are abundant—doses must be high enough to effectively compete for the receptor. Inability to achieve this concentration may mean partial therapeutic failure. Antihistamines are of limited value in vasomotor rhinitis.

Antihistamines have traditionally not been used in the treatment of asthma, but this is being re-assessed. One limiting factor has been the sedative and anticholinergic effects of the first generation antihistamines, which tend to limit the amount of drug that can be administered.

The effectiveness of antihistamines in the common cold has been a controversial issue in spite of their widespread use. Evidence now indicates that antihistamines possessing anticholinergic effects effectively reduce the symptoms of runny nose and sneezing associated with the common cold (see the chapter on the common cold).

Antihistamines are more effective in preventing the actions of histamine as they cannot reverse the effects of the mediator once receptors have been occupied and activated. They should therefore be taken before exposure to an allergen if possible.

First Generation Antihistamines

The adverse reactions of first generation antihistamines stem mainly from the multiple actions they exert on the central nervous system. These agents are liposoluble and pass easily through the blood-brain barrier. However, the side effects often disappear with continued therapy and are rarely serious. Drowsiness is the most common effect. Other possible effects on the central nervous system include altered co-ordination, dizziness, lassitude and inability to concentrate.

Drowsiness has been attributed to various central mechanisms involving histamine. Serotonin antagonism, anticholinergic activity and blockade of central alpha-adrenoreceptors may also be involved. The sedative effects can range from no effect to mild drowsiness to deep sleep. Ethanolamine- and phenothiazine-type agents are particularly prone to depressing the central nervous system. Sedation is less marked with the ethylenediamines and is least significant with the alkylamines. The incidence of sedation with brompheniramine and chlorpheniramine is about 10 to 20 per cent.

Although sedation may be desirable for nighttime use, it is a hazard for daytime activities requiring alertness and co-ordination. Most of those who do become drowsy develop tolerance to this effect within the first few days of therapy. In some people, scheduling a single dose of an antihistamine at bedtime may produce adequate symptom relief, while the individual sleeps through any sedative effect. Some people find the allergy itself leaves them drowsy even before taking medication.

Antihistamine users should be warned that alcohol and concurrent use of other central nervous system depressants can potentiate sedative effects. Counteracting any drowsiness with a decongestant (with its stimulant side effect) for daytime use has been described as a partially satisfactory solution at best.

Although these agents generally cause sedation, certain individuals may become restless, nervous, have difficulty sleeping, or experience palpitations and tremors while taking antihistamines. Children are particularly susceptible to these paradoxical reactions, which are rare but can be quite dangerous. The mechanism of this reaction is possibly due to central cholinergic blockade.

After sedation, the next most common side effects are gastrointestinal symptoms, namely gastric upset, loss of appetite, nausea, vomiting, constipation or diarrhea. The incidence of gastric upset may be reduced by administering the drug with meals or milk. Gastrointestinal effects occur infrequently with the ethanolamine group, but are common with ethylenediamine antihistamines.

First generation antihistamines exhibit anticholinergic properties, with the incidence and severity varying between the different chemical groups and from person to person. Diphenhydramine and promethazine exhibit a high potential for causing this effect. The effect is dose-dependent and large doses may cause blurred vision, urinary retention, constipation and tachycardia. These effects pose a hazard to people with difficulty in urination due to an enlarged prostate, narrow-angle glaucoma or cardiac diseases. Antihistamines should not be taken by individuals with these conditions unless so directed by a physician. Antihistamines with anticholinergic properties also potentiate similar effects of other agents.

First generation antihistamines can theoretically dry the mucous membranes of the mouth, nose, and other areas or the respiratory tract. As a result, warnings have existed to the extent where asthmatics were directed to avoid their use. However, while these agents may be contraindicated in a small group of asthmatics, warnings for the cautious use in all cases is unwarranted. First generation antihistamines have been used in many asthmatics, including those described as severe cases, with little adverse effect. It appears that

Allergic Rhinitis

the drying effect does not occur to an extent where it would exacerbate this condition. In fact, antihistamines are being re-assessed for a potential role in asthma therapy. It may still be wise for the patient to consult with their physician about the use of these agents. Dryness of mouth and nose at usual doses are still considered side effect possibilities by many references.

First generation anithistamines should be used with caution by epileptics as seizure activity may be enhanced.

These antihistamines are absorbed rapidly after ingestion. Symptom relief usually begins in 15 to 30 minutes and reaches a maximum in about 1 to 2 hours. Duration of action is generally considered in the range of 3 to 6 hours. Some researchers suggest it may be possible to administer certain agents (chlorpheniramine and brompheniramine, for example) less frequently than currently recommended, with little loss in effectiveness. Table IV outlines the current dosing schedules of various agents. Sustained-release formulations provide different drug release patterns than regular tablets or capsules and do not appear in this table. A physician should be consulted for the use of antihistamine drug products in children under 6 years of age.

First generation antihistamines are extensively metabolized in the liver. In a study done in 1963, it was theorized antihistamines could induce their own metabolism, which might in part explain how a specific antihistamine could lose effectiveness over time. Subsequent to this finding, patients complaining of a loss of effect from an antihistamine were told to switch to an agent from another chemical class. More information is needed on this issue, as some studies since have found no decrease in antihistamine levels with relatively long term use. Elimination may occur more rapidly in children than in adults.

Second Generation Antihistamines

Second generation (nonsedating) antihistamines are relatively new to the Canadian market. Although a diverse collection of chemical moieties, they all pass with difficulty through the blood-brain barrier. Substances that do enter the brain are typically small, water-, or lipid-soluble molecules unbound to protein. These newer antihistamines are large, lipophobic molecules that are extensively bound to albumin. Consequently, they are relatively (but not absolutely) excluded from passing into the brain. This characteristic leads to a class of agents that exhibits minimal central nervous system effects.

Terfenadine and **astemizole** were the first agents to reach the

Table IV *Antihistamines: Classification, Characteristics, Doses*

Class	General comments	Representative agents	Dosage (24 hour maximum)
First Generation Antihistamines			
Alkylamines	•drowsiness most common reaction, but overall incidence is low. Cause less CNS depression than members of other groups. Some CNS stimulation is possible, especially in young children	brompheniramine	Adults and children 12 yrs and over: 4 mg every 4–6 hr (24 mg) 6 to 11 yrs: 2 mg every 4–6 hr (12 mg) 2 to 5 yrs: 1 mg every 4–6 hr (6 mg) Alternatively, children less than 6 yrs: 0.5 mg/kg/day in 3 or 4 divided doses
	•low incidence of side effects	chlorpheniramine	Adults and children 12 yrs and over: 4 mg every 4–6 hr (24 mg) 6 to 11 yrs: 2 mg every 4–6 hr (12 mg) 2 to 5 yrs: 1 mg every 4–6 hr (6 mg) Alternate children's dose: 0.35 mg/kg/day in 4 divided doses
		dexbrompheniramine	Adults and children 12 yrs and over: 2 mg every 4–6 hr (12 mg) 6 to 11 yrs: 1 mg every 4–6 hr (6 mg) 2 to 5 yrs: 0.5 mg every 4–6 hr (3 mg)
		triprolidine	Adults and children 12 yrs and over: 2.5 mg every 4–6 hr (10 mg) 6 to 11 yrs: 1.25 mg every 4–6 hr (5 mg) 4 to 5 yrs: 1 mg every 4–6 hr (3.75 mg) 2 to 3 yrs: 0.625 mg every 4–6 hr (2.5 mg) Infants 4 mo to under 2 yrs: 0.313 mg every 4–6 hr (1.25 mg)

Table IV *(Cont'd) Antihistamines: Classification, Characteristics, Doses*

Class	General comments	Representative agents	Dosage (24 hour maximum)

Ethanolamines	• diphenhydramine and doxylamine can cause marked drowsiness
	
	• drowsiness is the most frequent side effect reported with clemastine but sedative effect is considered low
	
	• carbinoxamine has lowest incidence of drowsiness of this group
	
	• significant anticholinergic activity
	
	• relatively low incidence of gastrointestinal side effect
		carbinoxamine	Adults and children 12 yrs and over:
			  4–8 mg 3 to 4 times daily
			6 to 11 yrs:
			  4 mg 3 to 4 times daily
			3 to 5 yrs:
			  2–4 mg 3 to 4 times daily
			1 to 2 yrs:
			  2 mg 3 to 4 times daily
			Alternatively for children:
			  0.2–0.4 mg/kg/day in 3 or 4 doses

		clemastine	Adults and children over 12 yrs:
			  1 mg twice a day (6 mg)
			Children up to 12 yrs:
			  0.5–1 mg twice daily

		diphenhydramine	Adults and children 12 yrs and over:
			  25–50 mg every 4–6 hr (300 mg)
			6 to 11 yrs:
			  12.5–25 mg 4–6 hr (150 mg)
			2 to 5 yrs:
			  6.25 mg every 4–6 hr (37.5 mg)
			Alternatively, for children under 12 yrs:
			  5 mg/kg/day in 4 divided doses

		diphenylpyraline	Adults:
			  2 mg every 4 hr (10 mg)
			Children over 6 yrs:
			  2 mg every 6 hr (6 mg)
			2–6 yrs:
			  1–2 mg every 8 hr (4 mg)

		doxylamine	Adults and children 12 yrs and over:
			  7.5–12.5 mg every 4–6 hr (75 mg)
			6 to 11 yrs:
			  3.75–6.25 mg every 4–6 hr (37.5 mg)
			2 to 5 yrs:
			  2–3.125 mg every 4–6 hr (18.75 mg)

Ethylene-diamines	• incidence of side effects 20–35%
	
	• relatively weak CNS effects, but drowsiness may occur in some people
	
	• gastrointestinal side effects common
	
	• incidence of sedation with tripelennamine lower than with diphenhydramine, but dizziness is common
		pyrilamine	Adults and children 12 yrs and over:
			  25–50 mg every 6–8 hr (200 mg)
			6 to 11 yrs:
			  12.5–25 mg every 6–8 hr (100 mg)
			2 to under 5 yrs:
			  6.25–12.5 mg every 6–8 hr (50 mg)

		tripelennamine	Adults:
			  25–50 mg every 4–6 hr (600 mg)
			Children:
			  5 mg/kg/daily in 4 to 6 divided doses (300 mg)

Phenothiazines	• all precautions applicable to phenothiazines may apply • sedative effects prominent • significant anticholinergic activity • promethazine also used as an antiemetic	promethazine	Adults: 25 mg at bedtime; if necessary, 12.5 mg 4 times daily. Alternatively, 20–100 mg/day, in divided doses at meals, with the highest dose given at bedtime Children: 0.5 mg/kg at bedtime or 0.125 mg/kg as needed **(Note: promethazine should not be administered to children less than two years of age due to a possible association with sleep apneas.[a])**
Piperazines	• rarely used for allergic rhinitis	cyclizine hydrozyzine	

Allergic Rhinitis

Table IV *(Cont'd) Antihistamines: Classification, Characteristics, Doses*

Class	General comments	Representative agents	Dosage (24 hour maximum)
	•cyclizine and meclizine are more commonly used for treating motion sickness, although not to the same extent as promethazine and dimenhydrinate •hydroxyzine is used as a sedative and antipruritic in many dermatologic allergies. Drowsiness is the most common reaction	meclizine	

Piperadines	•drowsiness is the most common side effect; sedative potential is comparable to that of the ethylenediamine class
	•moderate anticholinergic effect
	•although cyproheptadine stimulates appetite in children, weight gain is inconsistent, transient and quickly reversible after withdrawal of the drug
		azatadine	Adults:
			  1–2 mg twice daily
			Children 6 to 12 yrs:
			  0.5–1 mg twice daily

		cyproheptadine	Adults:
			  4 mg three times a day. Most adults require 12–16 mg daily
			6–14 yrs:
			  4 mg 2 to 3 times a day
			2 to 5 yrs:
			  2 mg 2 to 3 times a day (8 mg)
			Not recommended in children less than 2 yrs

		phenindamine	Adults and children over 12 yrs:
			  25 mg every 4–6 hrs
			Children 6 to 12 yrs:
			  12.5 mg every 4–6 hr (75 mg)
			Children less than 6 yrs:
			  as directed by a physician

Second Generation Antihistamines

Class	General comments	Representative agents	Dosage (24 hour maximum)

	•although sedation is the most commonly reported side effect, it occurs at a rate similar to placebo groups
	•the CNS effects of alcohol are not enhanced by these agents
	•negligible anticholinergic effects
	•astemizole; may have a slower onset of action in relation to other agents
		astemizole	Adults and children over 12 yrs:
			  10 mg daily
			(Note: use of astemizole in children less than 12 years of age should be under the guidance of a physician.)
			Children 6 to 12 yrs:
			  5 mg daily
			Children less than 6 yrs:
			  2 mg/10 kg/day

		cetirizine	Adults and children over 12 yrs: 5–10 mg daily (20 mg)
		loratadine	Adults and children 12 yrs and over: 10 mg daily Use should be limited to no longer than 6 months unless recommended by a physician. Safety and efficacy in children less than 12 yrs have not been established.

		terfenadine	Adults and children over 12 yrs:
			  60 mg twice daily or 120 mg daily
			Children 7 to 12 yrs:
			  30 mg twice daily
			Children 3 to 6 yrs:
			  15 mg twice daily
			Children less than 3 yrs:
			  as directed by physician
			Use in children should be limited to periods of 1 week unless otherwise directed by a physician

[a]Kahn A, Hasaerts D, Blum D. Phenothiazine-induced sleep apneas in normal infants. Pediatrics 1985;75:844–7.

market. Both have relatively specific activity towards H$_1$-receptors. Terfenadine is free of serotonin and cholinergic antagonism at doses that block H$_1$-receptors and lacks anti-adrenergic effects. Astemizole also has little affinity for cholinergic receptors, but may weakly antagonize serotonin at high doses. It has shown some affinity for alpha-adrenergic receptors. In practical terms, though, astemizole's activity is limited to the antagonism of H$_1$-receptors.

Both drugs significantly reduce the frequency and severity of allergic symptoms, whether acute or chronic. Relief is seen for ocular symptoms, but less so for nasal obstruction. They are at least as effective as first generation agents. Some evidence indicates that astemizole and terfenadine dissociate more slowly from histamine receptors when compared to older antihistamines. The benefit of this characteristic may be that in periods of high histamine concentrations, the newer agents are less likely to be displaced by histamine. In some studies involving long-term use, astemizole has shown better symptom control than terfenadine.

Astemizole is more potent than the first generation antihistamines in antagonizing histamine-induced bronchoconstriction and may have a role in asthma. The role of various newer agents in asthma is currently being studied. Terfenadine has shown a degree of mast cell stabilization, an effect that is also evident in other antihistamines.

The most frequently reported side effect during terfenadine use has been sedation (12.6 per cent), but the occurrence is similar to that of placebo. Doses up to 600 mg have caused minimal sedation. Headache and gastrointestinal symptoms are also reported at similar rates to placebo groups. Both terfenadine and astemizole have prompted an increase in appetite with mild weight gain, an effect again seen in placebo-treated groups. No interaction occurs with either agent and alcohol. Cardiovascular effects have been noted with high doses of astemizole and terfenadine.

Following oral administration the antihistaminic effect of terfenadine is evident within 1 to 2 hours and is maximal in 3 to 6 hours. A dose of 120 mg daily is as effective in adults as a dose of 60 mg twice daily. The drug has a half-life of 16 to 23 hours and is metabolized in the liver. Wheal and flare reduction lasts about 24 hours, but a wash-out period of 5 to 7 days may be required if skin tests are planned.

Astemizole is rapidly absorbed from the intestinal tract. However, peak relief may not be achieved for up to 3 days. A few clinical trials (Sibbald, et al, Gendreau-Reid, et al) have used loading doses of 30 mg for 7 days in an attempt to circumvent this situation. This measure, however, has not garnered general acceptance and is not supported by the 1991 CPS monograph. Generally, therapy should begin well in advance of the pollen season.

Astemizole has a long duration of action, with an estimated half-life of up to 20 days when active metabolites are included. This fact has important implications for patients preparing for allergy skin tests after using this agent. Skin wheal and flare responses have been suppressed for 21 days after a single dose of the drug. One reference states the effect on skin tests may last for 4 to 6 weeks.

Both astemizole and terfenadine are extensively bound to plasma protein. No drug interactions of any consequence have been reported via plasma protein displacement.

Loratadine is a long-acting antihistamine that lacks sedative and anticholinergic effects. It has been found effective in the treatment of seasonal and perennial allergic rhinitis, with comparable efficacy to terfenadine. As with other antihistamines, relief from nasal congestion is not as impressive. Loratadine is a derivative of azatidine.

After ingestion, peak levels occur in 1 to 1.5 hours. The drug is metabolized in the liver with a half-life of 10 to 19 hours. Skin wheal and flare response is inhibited for about 24 hours. Loratadine is very well tolerated, with side effects no greater than the number or type seen with placebo. Loratadine has caused sedation in 8 per cent of patients. In the same reference, 6 per cent of those receiving placebo reported sedation, as did 21 per cent of those receiving clemastine. The recommended adult dose is 10 mg daily.

Acrivastine is an antihistamine that lacks the sedative effects of its parent compound, triprolidine. It has a short half-life (approximately 1.7 hours) and is dosed at a frequency of 8 mg 3 to 4 times a day.

Cetirizine is a metabolite of hydroxyzine. It is another second generation antihistamine that possesses minimal central nervous system effects. The agent shows beneficial reduction in the symptoms of seasonal and perennial allergic rhinitis at doses of 5 to 20 mg daily. Cetirizine is unique in that it inhibits the migration of eosinophils subsequent to allergen challenge; eosinophil infiltration is part of the inflammatory process of allergic rhinitis.

This antihistamine is rapidly absorbed with peak levels occurring in 1 hour. Antihistaminic effects are realized on the first day of therapy and peak by the third day. Food does not affect the extent of absorption. It is not metabolized by the hepatic cytochrome system; rather, it is excreted unchanged (70 per cent of dose) in the urine. The half-life of cetirizine is approximately 7 to 10 hours.

The incidence of side effects to date with this agent is very similar to that of placebo-treated groups: headache, gastrointestinal upset, dizziness, and cardiovascular effects have been reported.

Mequitazine and **temelastine** are agents in the development stage.

Antihistamine Selection

Pharmacists will come across patients asking for advice on product selection who have never tried a product. Many however will have self-medicated, perhaps over several seasons, and have been through the trial-and-error process of drug selection. These patients often want confirmation that what they are using is appropriate or just wonder whether there is anything "better".

Proper antihistamine selection is important as individuals may remain on an agent for extended periods of time. Pharmacists and patients should be aware, though, that several different agents may have to be tried before the most suitable agent is found. The selection of an antihistamine for allergic rhinitis rests on achieving a balance between the desired symptom relief and undesired side effects. Knowing which antihistamines an individual has tried, at what dosages they were taken, and the incidence of side effects that occurred, help determine whether the trials were appropriate and whether certain classes of antihistamines should be avoided. The antihistamines on the market are generally considered equally effective, but differ in duration of action and side effect profile.

In a typical first-time user, one may initiate therapy with an alkylamine such as chlorpheniramine or brompheniramine. These agents have a mild side effect profile. But, because they do have potential for causing drowsiness, dosage should be started off small, with the first dose taken at bedtime. Daily dose can be increased at 2- or 3-day intervals until the patient is without symptoms or attains the maximum daily dose. If not bothered by sedation, they may increase their dose at a faster rate. Higher doses than those recommended tend to show minimal increases in efficacy, with higher rates of side effects.

Those individuals who benefit from antihistamine therapy, but continue to be bothered by sedation or other effect characteristic of first generation agents, may find a nonsedating antihistamine a suitable alternative. All allergy sufferers should receive allergen-avoidance advice too.

If a preparation at recommended doses fails to provide adequate relief, an agent from a different chemical class should be tried. It should be borne in mind, however, that it is rare for any antihistamine to result in the complete eradication of symptoms. Also, pollen counts vary from day to day and an effective antihistamine may be perceived to be ineffective on days when the count is particularly high. Patients are encouraged to try an antihistamine for an adequate trial period before moving on to the next agent. It should also be noted that moderate to severe symptoms are difficult to manage effectively with a single therapeutic strategy.

Second generation antihistamines may be agents of first choice for certain patients. For example, use of a first generation antihistamine in individuals with narrow-angle glaucoma, prostatic hypertrophy, and heart problems should be carefully considered in consultation with a physician. When patients are involved in activities where drowsiness would be risky, nonsedating agents again should be considered. Indeed, many physicians and pharmacists now consider the second generation agents as drugs of first choice for the majority of allergy sufferers.

A common mistake individuals make is to take antihistamines only when symptoms are intolerable. Also, therapy is often stopped as soon as symptoms improve. In this instance, unless the discontinuation of therapy corresponds to the end of the allergy season, symptoms soon return. Patients must be wary of stopping therapy too quickly. Antihistamines should be taken regularly and for the length of the season in which the allergen is bothersome.

When an allergic response is predictable (for example, exposure to a pet), the agent should be taken before exposure to the allergen. How long before depends on the pharmacokinetic profile of the specific antihistamine.

As antihistamines are less effective in combating congestion, they are often combined with a decongestant. Combination products offer convenience to the patient and are very effective. Yet, they are still often given as separate products so the two can be adjusted for optimum relief. For example, antihistamines may be required for weeks and perhaps months. Whether a decongestant would in fact be needed at all these times should be carefully determined. Short term use of a combination product would be less of a concern.

Decongestants

Although antihistamines help control most of the symptoms of allergic rhinits, decongestants may be required when nasal congestion is part of the overall symptom complex. Nasal decongestants are alpha-adrenergic agents that act on the nasal blood vessels to cause vasoconstriction. The blood flow into tissues decreases, the tissues shrink and fluid leakage from the vessels diminishes. Breathing through the nose is thus made easier.

Oral and topical nasal decongestants are available. Topical agents provide prompt and dramatic relief from congestion. Use should be limited to 3 or 7 consecutive days (depending on the agent) as dependency can develop with continued use. Systemic reactions following topically-applied decongestants are rare when used as directed. Topical medication can be washed away by a runny nose and may lead to a shorter duration of action than normally expected.

Oral decongestants are stated to provide a more complete decongestant action because they reach deeper areas of the nose and sinuses. Their effect is slower in onset and generally less prolonged. Oral agents do not cause rebound congestion. Systemic side effects can occur and mainly affect the central nervous system and cardiovascular system.

When nasal decongestants are deemed necessary and there are no contraindications for their use, oral agents are generally chosen. Dosing antihistamines and decongestants separately will be best for many patients so that each agent can be adjusted to achieve optimal effect. Combination products containing antihistamines and decongestants are, however, less cumbersome to use than separate entities and may be less expensive. (See the chapter on the common cold for more information on nasal decongestants.)

Cromolyn

The mechanisms by which cromolyn reduces the symptoms of allergic rhinitis are not completely understood. It appears to prevent the release of chemical mediators from sensitized mast cells. Thus, not only is the release of histamine prevented, but many other vasoactive compounds as well. Current thinking on how this may be achieved is through calcium channel blockade; calcium influx is hindered, preventing the cascade of events that lead to degranulation. Cromolyn does not interfere with the binding of IgE to mast cells, nor does it possess antihistaminic activity.

Intranasal cromolyn relieves rhinorrhea, congestion, sneezing and ocular irritation. It is useful in acute or perennial allergic rhinitis. However, it is not used for acute attacks; rather, it is used prophylactically throughout allergen exposure. Therapy should be started 1 to 2 weeks before the allergy season. For patients already experiencing symptoms, cromolyn is aggressively dosed initially, then tapered to a maintenance dose. While some relief may be seen after a day of therapy, it often takes up to 2 weeks for maximum benefits to be realized.

Cromolyn is very well tolerated and has an excellent safety record. Adverse reactions are infrequent and minor. It may produce mild local irritation or sneezing immediately after use. Its lack of sedative effect makes it useful in treating children, even continuously for several years.

Nedrocromil is a new agent that is similar in activity to cromolyn. It is currently used as an adjunct in the prophylactic control of asthma. As a 1 per cent nasal spray, it has shown to be effective in seasonal allergic rhinitis with minimal side effects. Use may leave an unpleasant taste in the mouth. Headache has been reported in about a quarter of patients of one study, but this was also seen in the placebo group.

Corticosteroids

Topically-applied corticosteroids are the preferred agents for cases of allergic rhinitis that respond poorly to antihistamines or cromolyn. **Beclomethasone, flunisolide, budesonide, fluocortin,** and **triamcinolone** have been studied.

Topical steroids act mainly to prevent the late phase of the allergic response and to some extent, the early phase. Many mechanisms have been proposed to explain their beneficial action. For example, they decrease capillary permeability and mucous production. They prevent the influx of basophils into the area and reduce the intranasal concentrations of mediators of inflammation such as histamine.

Allergic Rhinitis

Direct vasoconstriction and inhibition of prostaglandin generation have also been identified.

The available agents appear to be equal in efficacy and are useful in controlling various symptoms of seasonal, perennial, and vasomotor rhinitis. Intranasal steroids do not immediately relieve symptoms, though. They are intended for prophylactic use and must be used regularly for therapeutic benefit. For best results, patients should begin therapy about 1 week before the allergy season begins. If symptoms are already present, clinical improvement is usually evident within several days. Nasally-applied steroids provide negligible relief of ocular symptoms.

These agents may not work well in cases accompanied with tenacious nasal congestion, as the nasal mucosa is not accessible. A brief course of a topical decongestant should allow the steroid greater access to the tissues.

Side effects are rarely severe enough to warrant withdrawal of treatment. Many are local effects often due to the vehicle rather than the drug. Freon-delivered aerosols (inhalers) can cause drying and crusting of the local mucosa and occasional slight bleeding (in up to 5 per cent of individuals). Some users find the inhaler triggers sneezing. Any burning that occurs usually abates after a week of continued use. Aqueous preparations administered by a pump exhibit fewer of these problems, although immediate stinging may occur. Nasal candidiasis has been reported rarely.

Suppression of the hypothalamic-pituitary adrenal axis is rare with topically-administered steroids. Evidence of mild adrenal suppression has appeared mainly when doses are raised to several times the recommended amount. These agents are rapidly degraded by enzymes in the nasal mucosa. Drug that is swallowed undergoes metabolism in the liver to relatively inactive metabolites.

Anticholinergics

Ipratropium is a derivative of atropine, but unlike atropine, has low lipid solubility and does not pass through the blood-brain barrier. In topical form it provides some relief for patients with chronic rhinitis whose predominant symptom is rhinorrhea (for example, vasomotor rhinitis). Minimal benefit is seen on symptoms such as itching, sneezing, or nasal blockage.

Although this agent has the potential of producing anticholinergic side effects, systemic effects following inhalation are very infrequent. Local effects are more common and it has produced some dryness of the nasal mucosa. It is administered at a dose of 40 μg in each nostril 2 to 4 times a day.

Immunotherapy

Immunotherapy (hyposensitization) consists of repeated subcutaneous injections of allergen extracts assumed to be causing the allergy symptoms. The extract is injected in minute doses either daily, weekly or biweekly with the dose gradually increased as tolerated by the individual. After each injection, the individual is closely observed as severe systemic reactions do occur, though rarely.

A dose of extract is sought that provides slightly more allergen than individuals are normally exposed to in the environment. After this endpoint is reached (usually 15 to 30 injections), a maintenance dose is established with the interval between injections varying from 2 to 6 weeks. The individual can then tolerate exposure to the allergen without experiencing an allergic reaction. Only clinically significant allergens should be included in the allergen-extract mixture; immunotherapy does little or nothing for symptoms due to immunologically unrelated allergens.

At least three mechanisms have been proposed for the favorable response to immunotherapy: a rise in serum IgG (IgE-blocking antibodies), which might reduce or neutralize the quantity of allergen available for interaction with mast cells; a suppression of the seasonal rise in IgE antibodies responding to the allergic stimulus; and reduced basophil reactivity and sensitivity to allergens may occur.

Immunotherapy is effective for treating allergic reactions to airborne pollens, moulds and house dust. Unfortunately, it has many drawbacks, particularly in children. The expense, pain on injection, time needed for doctor appointments, and potential adverse effects combine to make this approach a consideration only in people with severe symptoms that do not improve with drug therapy. Those who cannot avoid allergens may also be considered.

Treatment with immunotherapy is long-term. Most people experience relief within 6 months to 1 year after initiating treatment. With a good response, discontinuation is considered after 3 to 5 years. About 40 per cent of individuals relapse once maintenance therapy is stopped. *— not for under 7*

Investigational Therapy

Azelastine exhibits antihistaminic properties and is a potent inhibitor of histamine release from mast cells. It has been found effective in acute and perennial allergic rhinitis, vasomotor rhinitis and asthma. Intranasal and oral formulations have been studied. With oral administration, side effects commonly observed were altered taste and drowsiness.

A very potent topical antihistamine, **levocabastine**, has been shown to inhibit allergen-induced symptoms. **Azatadine** applied topically also inhibits the symptoms of an intranasal histamine challenge.

Ketotifen is presently used as adjunct therapy in mild atopic asthma in children. The drug has a varied pharmacologic profile: it blocks H_1-receptors, stabilizes mast cells and inhibits bronchoconstriction. Part of this drug's effect may lie in its ability to interfere with calcium influx into cells. Sedation is a common side effect experienced during the first 2 weeks of therapy.

Summary

The symptoms of allergic rhinitis can be bothersome, regardless of whether they occur acutely or chronically. These symptoms force the individual to seek relief. However, allergy sufferers often self-medicate with a number of products before seeking professional advice. Professional intervention can speed the process of finding a suitable therapeutic regimen for the individual. Treatment must also be directed toward avoiding the allergen(s). The pharmacist can provide advice on appropriate products and when to seek medical care.

Ask the Consumer

Q. Have you been experiencing many bouts of cold-like symptoms, even during the summer? Have you seen your physician?

■ The first clue to identifying allergic rhinitis is often the presentation of "summertime colds." Many people self-medicate with antihistamines or cold remedies, obtaining various degrees of relief. If relief is not achieved, a diagnosis by a physician is recommended to confirm whether the individual actually suffers from allergic rhinitis.

Q. What are your symptoms? When do they occur? How long do they persist?

■ Rhinorrhea, congestion and ocular or palatal itchiness are common complaints with allergic rhinitis. Sneezing is also common, especially several sneezes in rapid succession. Typically, symptoms last longer than the average common cold. When and where these symptoms are most bothersome helps determine the identity of the suspect allergen(s).

Q. What medications, if any, have you tried for your allergy? What was the response?

■ Antihistamines provide reasonable relief for acute allergic rhinitis if taken properly. The pharmacist should determine what agents have been tried, at what doses, for how long and the relief provided. If possible, taking antihistamines before the onset of symptoms provides better relief. A frequent practice of allergy sufferers is to use their antihistamine intermittently within the allergy season. Regular dosing is the most efficient way to control symptoms.

Q. Are you bothered by the side effects of any antihistamines?

■ First generation antihistamines are known for their effects on the central nervous system and the gastrointestinal tract. The individual has some flexibility in finding a suitable antihistamine with the pharmacist's help. The many antihistamines available possess unique side effect profiles. An individual bothered by excessive drowsiness or anticholinergic effects can switch to an agent noted for the less frequent appearance of the effect.

Q. Is your regular antihistamine still providing good results, or does it seem to be getting less potent?

■ It has long been stated that antihistamines can become less effective over time, possibly due to auto-induction of metabolism. This effect is being re-assessed. Switching to an antihistamine from a different chemical class has been suggested if effectiveness wanes. It should be determined whether the individual is still taking the original antihistamine correctly. Also, change in the allergic picture may be part of the problem. For example, pollen counts may be higher than they were the previous week, month or season.

Q. Do you suffer from narrow-angle glaucoma, heart disease, epilepsy or prostate enlargment?

■ First generation antihistamines possess effects that may potentiate the complications of these conditions. Any individual with one of these conditions should take these agents only on the advice of a physician.

References

Epidemilogy

Austen KF. Diseases of immediate type hypersensitivity. In: Wilson J, Braunwald E, Isselbacker K, et al, eds. Harrison's principles of internal medicine. New York: McGraw-Hill, 1991:1426–8.

Davies RJ, Corrado OJ, Blainey AD. Respiratory allergy. In: Lessof MH, ed. Allergy: immunology and clinical aspects. Chichester: John Wiley and Sons, 1984:253–337.

Lieberman PL, Crawford LV. Management of the allergic patient. A text for the primary care physician. New York: Appleton-Century-Crofts, 1982: 29–120,155–68.

Norman PS. Allergic rhinitis. J Aller Clin Immunol 1985;75:531–45.

Price JF. Allergy in infancy and childhood. In: Lessof MH, ed. Allergy: immunology and clinical aspects. Chichester: John Wiley and Sons, 1984:127–73.

Viner AS, Jackman N. Retrospective survey of 1271 patients diagnosed as perennial rhinitis. Clin Allergy 1976;6:251–9.

Welch M, Kemp J. Allergy in children. Primary Care 1987;14:575–89.

Anatomy and Physiology

Naclerio R, Proctor D. The anatomy and physiology of the upper airway. In: Middleton E Jr, Reed C, Ellis E, Adkinson N Jr, Yunginger J, eds. Allergy: principles and practice. St. Louis: CV Mosby, 1988:579–91.

Pathophysiology

Berman B. Allergic rhinitis: mechanisms and management. J Allergy Clin Immunol 1988;81:980–4.

Bousquet J, Chanez P, Michel F. Pathophysiology and treatment of seasonal allergic rhinitis. Resp Med 1990;84(Suppl A):11–7.

Garrison J, Rall T. Autacoids; Drug therapy of inflammation. In: Goodman L, Gilman A, Rall T, Nies A, Taylor P, eds. Goodman and Gilman's the pharmacological basis of therapeutics. New York: Macmillan, 1990:574–99.

Langer H. Allergic rhinitis: a medical insight. J Otolaryngol 1989;18:158–64.

Marone G, Casolaro V, Cirillo R, et al. Pathophysiology of human basophils and mast cells in allergic disorders. Clin Immunol Immunopath 1989; 50:S24-S40.

Marquardt DL, Wasserman SI. Mast cells in allergic diseases and mastocytosis. West J Med 1982;137:195–212.

Naclerio R. The pathophysiology of allergic rhinitis: impact of therapeutic intervention. J Allergy Clin Immunol 1988;82:927–34.

Naclerio R. The role of histamine in allergic rhinitis. J Allergy Clin Immunol 1990;86:628–32.

Smith T. Allergy and pseudoallergy: an overview of basic mechanisms. Primary Care 1987;14:421–34.

Widdicombe J. Nasal pathophysiology. Resp Med 1990;84(Suppl A):3–10.

Zweiman B. Pathogenesis of IgE-mediated allergic respiratory diseases. J Resp Diseases 1989;Nov(Suppl):S4-S9.

Allergens

Bernstein D, Bernstein I. Allergic rhinitis caused by inhalant factors. In: Rakel E, ed. Conn's current therapy. Philadelphia: WB Saunders, 1986: 598–603.

Green AR. An updated assessment of the critical environmental factors involved in the prevention of allergic disease. Ann Allergy 1979;42:372–83.

Kuo PH, Roth A. Canada. In: Roth A, ed. Allergy in the world. A guide for physicians and travelers. Honolulu: University Press of Hawaii, 1978:25–8.

Pollart S, Chapman M, Platts-Mills T. House dust sensitivity and environmental control. Primary Care 1987;14:591–603.

Schumacher M. Allergic rhinitis due to aeroallergens. In: Rakel R, ed. Conn's current therapy. Philadelphia: WB Saunders, 1991:708–12.

Weber R. Allergens. Primary Care 1987;14: 435–45.

Symptoms

Conner BL, Georgitis JW. Practical diagnosis and treatment of allergic and nonallergic rhinitis. Primary Care 1987;14:457–73.

Frazer J. Allergic rhinitis and nasal polyps. Ear Nose Throat J 1984;63:172–6.

Middleton E. Chronic rhinitis in adults. J Allergy Clin Immunol 1988;81:971–5.

Price JF. Allergy in infancy and childhood. In: Lessof M, ed. Allergy: immunology and clinical aspects. Chichester: John Wiley and Sons, 1984:127–73.

Vogt H. Rhinitis. Primary Care 1990; 17:309–22.

Wodell RA, Burg FD. Pediatric problem-solving: allergic rhinitis. Drug Ther 1984;14:136–55.

Allergic Rhinitis

Differential Diagnosis of Allergic Rhinitis

Kaslow J, Novey H. When hay fever doesn't quit. Postgrad Med 1989;85(6): 164–72.

Meltzer E. Schatz M, Zeiger R. Allergic and nonallergic rhinitis. In: Middleton E Jr, Reed C, Ellis E, Adkinson N Jr, Yunginger J, eds. Allergy: principles and practice. St. Louis: CV Mosby, 1988:1253–89.

Simons F. Allergic rhinitis: recent advances. Pediatric Clin North Am 1988; 35:1053–74.

General Treatment

Busse W. New directions and dimensions in the treatment of allergic rhinitis. J Allergy Clin Immunol 1988;82:890–900.

Jones H. Allergic rhinitis: a study on the prescribing preferences in general practice. Br J Clin Pract 1989;43:30–2.

Ophir D, Elad Y, Dolev Z, Geller-Bernstein C. Effects of inhaled humidified warm air on nasal patency and nasal symptoms in allergic rhinitis. Ann Allergy 1988;60:239–42.

Pollart S, Chapman M, Platts-Mills T. House dust sensitivity and environmental control. Primary Care 1987;14:591–603.

Reisman R, Mauriello P, Davis G, et al. A double-blind study of the effectiveness of a high-efficiency particulate air (HEPA) filter in the treatment of patients with perennial allergic rhinitis and asthma. J Allergy Clin Immunol 1990;85:1050–7.

Antihistamines

Anonymous. Antihistamines. In: Reynolds JE, ed. Martindale: the extra pharmacopoeia. London: Pharmaceutical Press, 1989:443–65.

Anonymous. Antihistamines. In: USP DI: Drug information for the health care provider. Rockville: United States Pharmacopeial Convention, 1991: 382–449.

Anonymous. Teenagers take OTC drug to induce euphoria. Can Pharm J 1987;120(1):14.

Anonymous. Antihistamine drugs. In: McEvoy GK, ed. American hospital formulary service drug information. Bethesda: American Society of Hospital Pharmacists, 1991:2–30.

Berman B. Perennial allergic rhinitis: Clinical efficacy of a new antihistamine. J Allergy Clin Immunol 1990;86:1004–8.

Bruttmann G, Charpin D, Germouty J, et al. Evaluation of the efficacy and safety of loratadine in perennial allergic rhinitis. J Allergy Clin Immunol 1989;83:411–6.

Brandon ML. Newer non-sedating antihistamines: will they replace older agents? Drugs 1985;30:377–81.

Burns JF, Conney AH, Koster R. Stimulatory effect of chronic drug administration on drug-metabolizing enzymes in liver microsomes. Ann NY Acad Sci 1963;104:881–93.

Bye CE, Cooper J, Empey DW, et al. Effects of pseudoephedrine and triprolidine, alone and in combination, on symptoms of the common cold. Br Med J 1980;281:189–90.

Callier J, Engelen RF, Ianniello I, et al. Astemizole (R 43 512) in the treatment of hay fever: an international double-blind study comparing a weekly treatment (10 mg and 25 mg) with a placebo. Curr Ther Res 1981;29: 24–35.

Campoli-Richards D, Buckley M, Fitton A. Cetirizine: A review of its pharmacological properties and clinical potential in allergic rhinitis, pollen-induced asthma, and chronic urticaria. Drugs 1990;40:762–81.

Carruthers SG, Shoeman DW, Hignite CE, Azarnoff DL. Correlation between plasma diphenhydramine level and sedative and antihistamine effects. Clin Pharmacol Ther 1978;23:375–82.

Chan K, Chan G. A study of prescribed H_1-antihistamine preparations over a period of 12 months in community pharmacy. J Clin Pharmacol Ther 1987;12:1–9.

Chiou WL, Athanikar NK, Huang S-M. Long half-life of chlorpheniramine (Letter). N Engl J Med 1979;300:501.

Chu T, Yamate M, Biedermann A, et al. Once versus twice daily dosing of terfenadine in the treatment of seasonal allergic rhinitis: US and European studies. Ann Allergy 1989;63:612–5.

Church M, Gradidge C. Inhibition of histamine release from human lung in vitro by antihistamines and related drugs. Br J Pharmac 1980;69:663–7.

Clissold S, Sorkin E, Goa K. Loratadine: a preliminary review of its pharmacodynamic properties and therapeutic efficacy. Drugs 1989;37:42–57.

Collins-Williams C. Antihistamines in asthma. J Asthma 1987;24:55–8.

Craft T. Torsade de pointes after astemizole overdose. Br Med J 1986;292:660.

Creticos P. Antihistamines in the treatment of allergic rhinitis. J Resp Diseases 1989;Nov(Suppl):S10-S12.

Crutcher JE, Kantner TR. The effectiveness of antihistamines in the common cold. J Clin Pharmacol 1981;21:9–15.

Davies AJ, Harindra V, McEwan A, et al. Cardiotoxic effect with convulsions in terfenadine overdose. B Med J 1989;298:325.

Del Carpio J, Kabbash L, Turenne Y, et al. Efficacy and safety of loratadine (10 mg once daily), terfenadine (60 mg twice daily), and placebo in the treatment of seasonal allergic rhinitis. J Allergy Clin Immunol 1989; 84:741–6.

Delafuente J, Davis T, Davis J. Pharmacotherapy of allergic rhinitis. Clin Pharm 1989;8:474–85.

Drouin MA. H_1 antihistamines: perspective on the use of the conventional and new agents. Ann Allergy 1985;55:747–52.

Evans L. Psychological effects caused by drugs in overdose. Drugs 1980; 19:220–42.

Falliers C, Brandon M, Buchman E, et al. Double-blind comparison of cetirizine and placebo in the treatment of seasonal rhinitis. Ann Allergy 1991; 66:257–62.

Fed Reg 1985;50(10):2200–18.

Fed Reg 1976;41(176):38312–423.

Fed Reg 1987;52(163):31892–914.

Feldman MD, Behar M. A case of massive diphenhydramine abuse and withdrawal from use of the drug (Letter). JAMA 1986; 255:3119–20.

Filderman R. Inhibition of skin reactivity by antihistamines. Cutis 1988; 42:19–21.

Flowers FP, Araujo O, Nieves C. Antihistamines. Int J Dermatol 1986; 25:224–31.

Hansten P, Horn J, eds. Drug interactions and updates. Malvern: Lea & Febiger, 1990.

Hays DP, Johnson BF, Perry R. Prolonged hallucinations following a modest overdose of tripelennamine. Clin Toxicol 1980;16:331–3.

Gendreau-Reid L, Simons K, Simons E. Comparison of the suppressive effect of astemizole, terfenadine and hydroxyzine on histamine-induced wheals and flares in humans. J Aller Clin Immunol 1986;77:335–40.

Girard JP, Sommacal-Schopf D, Bigliardi P, Henaver SA. Double-blind comparison of astemizole, terfenadine and placebo in hay fever with special regard to onset of action. J Int Med Res 1985;13:102–8.

Holgate S, Emanuel M, Howarth P, et al. Astemizole and other H_1-antihistaminic drug treatment of asthma. J Allergy Clin Immunol 1985; 76:375–80.

Holgate ST, Howarth PH. Treating hay fever. Br Med J 1985;291:92.

Howard JC Jr, Kantner TR, Lilienfield LS, et al. Effectiveness of antihistamines in the symptomatic management of the common cold. JAMA 1979; 242:2414–17.

Howarth PH, Emanuel MB, Holgate ST. Astemizole, a potent histamine H_1-receptor antagonist: effect in allergic rhinoconjunctivitis, on antigen and histamine induced skin wheal responses and relationship to serum levels. Br J Clin Pharmacol 1984;18:1–8.

Howarth PH, Holgate ST. Comparative trial of two non-sedative H_1 antihistamines, terfenadine and astemizole, for hay fever. Thorax 1984; 39:668–72.

Kahn A, Hasaerts D, Blum. D Phenothiazine-induced sleep apneas in normal infants. Pediatrics 1985;75:844–7.

Kaiser H. H_1-receptor antagonist treatment of seasonal allergic rhinitis. J Allergy Clin Immunol 1990; 86:1000–3.

Kemp J, Falliers C, Fox R, et al. A multicenter, open study of the non-sedating antihistamine, terfenadine (Seldane), in the maintenance therapy of seasonal allergic rhinitis. Ann Allergy 1988;60:349–54.

Krogh CM, ed. Compendium of pharmaceuticals and specialties. Ottawa: Canadian Pharmaceutical Association, 1991.

Maibach H. The relative safety and effectiveness of antihistamines. Cutis 1988;42:2–4.

Mann K, Crowe J, Tietze K. Nonsedating histamine H_1-receptor antagonists. Clin Pharm 1989;8:331–44.

McTavish D, Goa K, Ferrill M. Terfenadine: an updated review of its pharmacological properties and therapeutic efficacy. Drugs 1990;39:552–74.

Meltzer E. Antihistamine- and decongestant-induced performance decrements. J Occup Med 1990;32:327–34.

Meltzer E. The use of antihistamines for the treatment of airway disease. Cutis 1988;42:22–5.

Milavetz G, Smith J. Pharmacotherapy of asthma and allergic rhinitis. Primary Care 1990;17:685–701.

Morris E. Pharmacotherapy of allergic disease. Primary Care 1987;14:605–21.

Naclerio R, Kagey-Sobotka A, Lichtenstein L, et al. Terfenadine, an H_1-antihistamine, inhibits histamine release in vivo in the human. Am Rev Respir Dis 1990;142:167–71.

Netter KJ, Bodenschatz K. Inhibition of histamine-n-methylation by some antihistamines. Biochem Pharmacol 1967;16:1627–31.

Nicholson AN. Central effects of H_1- and H_2-antihistamines. Aviat Space Environ Med 1985;56:293–8.

Norman PS. Newer antihistaminic agents. J Aller Clin Immunol 1985; 76:366–8.

Paton DM, Webster DR. Clinical pharmacokinetics of H_1-receptor antagonists (the antihistamines). Clin Pharmacokinet 1985;10:477–97.

Richards DM, Brogden RN, Heel RC, et al. Astemizole: a review of its pharmacodynamic properties and therapeutic efficacy. Drugs 1984;28:38–61.

Schuller DE, Turkewitz D. Adverse effects of antihistamines. Postgrad Med 1986;79:75–86.

Schwartz J-C, Pollard H, Quach TT. Histamine as neurotransmitter in mammalian brain: neurochemical evidence. J Neurochem 1980;35:26–33.

Sheffer A, Samuels L. Cetirizine: antiallergic therapy beyond traditional H_1 antihistamines. J Allergy Clin Immunol 1990;86:1040–6.

Sibbald B, Hilton S, D'Souza M. An open cross-over trial comparing two doses of astemizole and beclomethasone diproprionate in the treatment of perennial rhinitis. Clin Allergy 1986;16:203-11.

Simons FE, Luciuk GH, Simons KJ. Pharmacokinetics and efficacy of chlorpheniramine in children. J Aller Clin Immunol 1982;69:376–81.

Simons F, Lukowski J, Becker A, Simons K. Comparison of the effects of single doses of the new H_1-receptor antagonists loratadine and terfenadine versus placebo in children. J Pediatrics 1991;118:298–300.

Simons FE, Simons KJ. H_1 receptor antagonists: clinical pharmacology and use in allergic disease. Pediatric Clin North Am 1983;30:899–914.

Simons F, Simons K. Optimum pharmacological management of chronic rhinitis. Drugs 1989;38:313–31.

Skassa-Brociek W, Bousquet J, Montes F, et al. Double-blind placebo-controlled study of loratadine, mequitazine, and placebo in the symptomatic treatment of seasonal allergic rhinitis. J Allergy Clin Immunol 1988;81:725–30.

Tarnasky P, Van Arsdel P. Antihistamine therapy in allergic rhinitis. J Fam Pract 1990;30:71–80.

Trzeciakowski JP, Mendelsohn N, Levi R. Antihistamines. In: Middleton E. Jr, Reed C, Ellis E, Atkinson N Jr, Yunginger J, eds. Allergy: principles and practice. St Louis: CV Mosby, 1988:715–38.

Uden DL, Huska DR, Kellenberger TA, Krenzelok EP. Antihistamines: a study of pediatric usage and incidence of toxicity. Vet Hum Toxicol 1984; 26:469–72.

Uzan A, Le Fur G, Malgouris C. Are antihistamines sedative via a blockade of brain H_1 receptors? J Pharm Pharmacol 1979;31:701–2.

Vanden Bussche G, Emanuel MB, Rombaut N. Clinical profile of astemizole. A survey of 50 double-blind trials. Ann Allergy 1987;58:184–8.

von Maur K. Antihistamine selection in patients with allergic rhinitis. Ann Allergy 1985;55:458–62.

West S, Brandon B, Stolley P, Rumrill R. A review of antihistamines and the common cold. Pediatrics 1975;56:100–7.

Woodward J. Pharmacology and toxicology of nonclassical antihistamines. Cutis 1988;42:5–9.

Decongestants

Paull B. The role of decongestants in allergic rhinitis management. J Resp Diseases 1989;Nov(Supp):S13-S17.

Storms W, Bodman S, Nathan R, et al. SCH 434: A new antihistamine/decongestant for seasonal allergic rhinitis. J Allergy Clin Immunol 1989; 83:1083–90.

Cromolyn

Anonymous. Cromolyn sodium. In: McEvoy GK, ed. American hospital formulary service drug information. Bethesda: American Society of Hospital Pharmacists, 1991:2257–61.

Druce H, Goldstein S, Melamed J, et al. Multicenter placebo-controlled study of nedrocromil sodium 1% nasal solution in ragweed seasonal allergic rhinitis. Ann Allergy 1990;65:212–6.

Schwartz H. The effect of cromolyn on nasal disease. Ear Nose Throat 1986; 65:449–56.

Sipila P, Sorri M, Pukander J. Double-blind comparison of nedrocromil sodium (1% nasal spray) and placebo in rhinitis caused by birch pollen. Clin Otolaryngol 1987;12:365–70.

Corticosteroids

Clissold S, Heel R. Budesonide: a preliminary review of its pharmacodynamic properties and therapeutic efficacy in asthma and rhinitis. Drugs 1984; 28:485–518.

McAllen MK, Langman MJ. A controlled trial of dexamethasone snuff in chronic perennial rhinitis. Lancet 1969;1:968–71.

Norman P. The role of corticosteroids in allergic rhinitis. J Resp Diseases 1989;Nov(Suppl):S22-S25.

Immunotherapy

Galant S. Allergy shots for hay fever. Postgrad Med 1989;85(6):203–9.

Thompson R, Bousquet J, Cohen S, et al. The current status of allergen immunotherapy (hyposensitization): report of a WHO/IUIs working group. Allergy 1989;44:369–79.

Tipton W. Immunotherapy for allergic diseases. Primary Care 1987;14:623–9.

Investigational Therapy

Dechant K, Goa K. Levocabastine: a review of its pharmacological properties and therapeutic potential as a topical antihistamine in allergic rhinitis and conjunctivitis. Drugs 1991;41:202–24.

Grant S, Goa K, Fitton A, Sorkin E. Ketotifen: a review of its pharmacodynamic and pharmacokinetic properties, and therapeutic use in asthma and allergic disorders. Drugs 1990;40:412–48.

Holmberg K, Pipkorn U, Bake B, Blychert L-O. Effects of topical treatment with H_1 and H_2 antagonists on clinical symptoms and nasal vascular reactions in patients with allergic rhinitis. Allergy 1989;44:281–7.

McTavish D, Sorkin E. Azelastine: A review of its pharmacodynamic and pharmacokinetic properties, and therapeutic potential. Drugs 1989; 38:778–800.

Weiler J, Donnelly A, Campbell B, et al. Multicenter, double-blind, multiple-dose, parallel groups efficacy and safety trial of azelastine, chlorpheniramine, and placebo in the treatment of spring allergic rhinitis. J Allergy Clin Immunol 1988;82:801–11.

14
Internal Analgesics and Antipyretics

Michael G. Tierney and Lesia M. Babiak

Pain and fever are commonly managed with self-medication products. Acetylsalicylic acid and acetaminophen are the two agents most often used, differentially chosen by their pharmacokinetics, efficacy and adverse effects. Ibuprofen and analgesic combinations are also used. Nonprescription muscle relaxants include methocarbamol, chlorzoxazone and orphenadrine. The assessment and management of pain depends upon whether the pain is a headache, musculoskeletal, dental, bursitic, arthritic or visceral.

All individuals experience pain and fever during their lifetime. Given the common occurrence of these symptoms, it is not surprising consumer-initiated treatment constitutes the first step in managing the vast majority of cases. Western society relies heavily on nonprescription analgesics and antipyretics for this initial step. Therefore, it is important pharmacists be familiar with the therapeutic use of these agents. This chapter reviews the approach to managing pain and fever, placing particular emphasis on the indications, efficacy, toxicity and therapeutic use of nonprescription analgesics and antipyretics. (See the chapter on feminine care products for a discussion on the management of dysmenorrhea and the premenstrual syndrome.)

Pain

Pain is the sensation of discomfort, distress or agony resulting from the stimulation of specialized nerve endings. It can be seen as a protective mechanism, which causes an individual to withdraw from a painful stimulus. Alternatively, it can be viewed as nature's earliest sign of morbidity, which should prompt investigation into the possible presence of disease. Approaches in assessing pain should include criteria for referral to a physician for further investigation.

The sensory apparatus that facilitates perception of pain is relatively complex. It originates with receptors known as nociceptors, which form a widespread network in the skin, and certain other tissues such as joints and arterial walls; deeper tissues are not as extensively supplied. These receptors are the termination points of

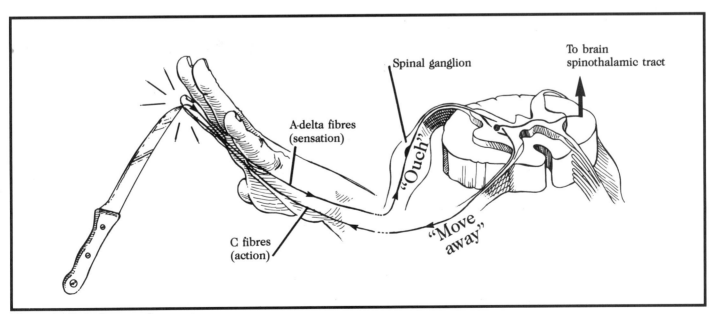

Figure 1 *Pain Sensory Apparatus*

Internal Analgesics and Antipyretics

the axons of sensory neurons. The axons originate in the cell bodies of the sensory neurons in the posterior root ganglion of the spinal cord. Specialized neural tracts, primarily the spinothalamic tract, then transmit impulses to various parts of the brain.

Pain fibres can be excited by a number of different stimuli. The free nerve endings can be directly stimulated by mechanical stress or alternatively they can be stimulated by extremes of heat or cold. The release of chemical substances such as histamine, bradykinin, prostaglandins, serotonin, acetylcholine and potassium ions can also stimulate free nerve endings as well as decrease the threshold for painful stimuli by other means such as pressure or temperature. Antagonism of these substances is an important element of therapeutic methods for treating pain.

The brain has the ability to modulate the perception of pain. The analgesic effects of morphine and other opiates are initiated by binding with specific opiate receptors in various parts of the central nervous system. The search for naturally occurring substances that bind with the opiate receptors led to the discovery of endogenous morphine-like compounds called enkephalins or endorphins, meaning "the morphine within".

Endorphins are thought to play a major role in modulating the perception of pain. The significant placebo effect described in many types of pain may be due to the stimulation of a neuronal system. This stimulation causes the release of endorphins with subsequent attenuation of the perception of pain.

Several physiological aspects of pain must be considered when attempting to locate the origin of pain.

Referred Pain

Referred pain is pain projected to a part of the body distant from the tissue where the sensory input originates. Generally, deep visceral and somatic pains tend to be referred superficially to an area more extensively supplied by sensory neurons. For example, cardiac pain can be projected superficially to the region over the heart as well as the arm and hand. In this case, a serious source of pain may be misinterpreted as benign muscular arm pain or heartburn.

Superficial Versus Visceral Pain

Superficial or skin pain consists of two main sensations. Pricking pain is usually the first sensation of pain, as it is carried by the fast myelinated type A delta nerve fibres. Burning pain, more diffuse and long-lasting, follows pricking pain by 1 to 2 seconds and is carried by the slower unmyelinated type C nerve fibres (see Figure 1). Superficial pain can be precisely localized due to the extensive overlap of nerve endings of several sensory neurons.

Deep or visceral pain arising from visceral and skeletal structures can have several qualities, such as aching and burning sensations, but it can also be sharp and penetrating. Unlike superficial pain, deep pain is usually due to diffuse stimulation rather than localized damage. Localized damage, such as surgical incision, does not cause severe pain in visceral organs whereas a diffuse inflammation does. In addition, visceral damage is generally difficult to localize; diagnostic measures other than the use of pain sensation must be used to determine the origin of the painful stimuli.

Psychology of Pain

The role of psychological factors should be considered in the overall assessment of pain. The experience and expression of pain are greatly influenced by personal factors and social context. For example, personality traits can be important in influencing the expression of pain. Some individuals, due to training or habit, remain stoic in the face of severe pain that might cause others to react in a more expressive manner. Social factors, such as race, culture and religion, are also important. Distraction, fatigue, suggestion or strong emotion such as anxiety, depression, fear or rage can alter the perception of and reaction to pain.

Fever

Fever is generally defined as an elevation of orally recorded body temperature to greater than 37.5 °C in response to a neurologic signal. Some natural variation in body temperature follows a circadian pattern, with the highest value usually reached in late afternoon or early evening. Fever is distinguished from other forms of hyperthermia (for example, heat stroke) in that the latter is often externally imposed and the hypothalamic set-point is not altered.

Body temperature is maintained at or near 37 °C by homeostatic mechanisms; the hypothalamus regulates the balance between heat production and heat loss. Fever can be caused by an abnormality or defect in any one of these three processes. Pyrogens induce an alteration in the temperature "set-point" of the hypothalamus, and body temperature is therefore regulated to a higher value. An alteration in the set-point of the hypothalamus is associated with febrile responses to infection and inflammatory conditions such as myocardial infarction, systemic lupus erythematosus and gout. Heat production is determined by the metabolic activity of the body; excessive activity (for example, vigorous physical activity and hyperthyroidism) can cause hyperthermia. Inadequate heat dissipation occurs in heat stroke and can also be caused by excessive anticholinergic effects of drugs.

Other mechanisms can be involved in drug-induced fever. For example, a drug such as bleomycin may stimulate endogenous pyrogen production or fever may be a manifestation of a hypersensitivity drug reaction. Fever can also be induced by idiosyncratic reactions such as anesthetic-induced malignant hyperthermia and the neuroleptic malignant syndrome, which is most commonly caused by antipsychotics.

The most common pathway to fever begins with an infection. In the initial step, a pathogen interacts with circulating or tissue macrophages or both. The pyrogenic polypeptide then released has

---

Table I *Considerations in Evaluating and Interpreting Fever*

1. Is the temperature a reliable reading? Was the thermometer reset before use? Was the thermometer kept in place long enough?
2. If there are no other signs of infection, is there another explanation for the fever, e.g., recent initiation of new drug therapy, vaccinations.
3. Recent administration of antipyretic drugs can mask a fever.
4. Rectal temperatures are approximately 0.5 °C higher than oral temperatures.
5. Elderly people may not show a febrile response to an infection.
6. Ovulation can induce a slight febrile response.

Internal Analgesics and Antipyretics

been identified as Interleukin-I. Interleukin-I induces production of prostaglandin E_2, believed to be one of the final steps for producing fever. This belief is consistent with the mechanism of action of many antipyretic analgesics, which inhibit the synthesis of prostaglandins.

Considerable debate surrounds the therapeutic value of fever and this topic has recently been reviewed. Fever has survival value in cold-blooded animals, but this remains to be proven in mammals, including humans. Despite the widespread use of antipyretics, no information indicates these agents have an effect on the course of an infection. On the other hand, except that it prevents febrile seizures in infants and children and relieves the malaise and discomfort associated with fever, there is little reason to believe that fever reduction is beneficial.

Pharmacists should consider several factors when interpreting fever before making a recommendation (see Table I).

Acetylsalicylic Acid   *ASA—Asprin*

As early as the middle of the eighteenth century, natural salicylates derived from willow bark were used to treat fever. By the mid-nineteenth century, sodium salicylate was synthesized and used primarily as an antipyretic to treat rheumatic fever. Since then, numerous other salicylates have been synthesized. Those for internal use include acetylsalicylic acid (ASA), choline salicylate, magnesium salicylate and sodium salicylate. Few studies have compared the relative efficacy of the various salts. However, it appears that sodium salicylate has about 60 per cent of the antipyretic potency of ASA and a less potent analgesic effect.

Pharmacology

Most of the effects of salicylates are due to inhibiting prostaglandin synthesis. ASA irreversibly acetylates the enzyme cyclo-oxygenase, thus inhibiting the conversion of arachidonic acid to prostaglandins. Salicylic acid has no acetylating capacity, although it does reduce the synthesis of prostaglandins in vivo through mechanisms not clearly understood.

Antipyretic activity is believed to be due to inhibiting prostaglandin synthesis in the hypothalamus. Although analgesic and anti-inflammatory activity is primarily explained by the inhibition of prostaglandin synthesis in the periphery, a central effect accounting for analgesic activity has been disputed.

Pharmacokinetics

Absorption of ASA is rapid; the absorption rate depends on the dissolution rate of the formulation. The rate of absorption is increased by dissolving the drug in water or combining it with an antacid. The addition of antacids to tablets of ASA causes an increase in the pH near the drug particles, thus enhancing the rate of dissolution and absorption. Enteric-coated formulations produce more delayed and prolonged absorption, which makes them unsuitable when immediate analgesic or antipyretic effect is required. Concomitant administration of food can delay absorption from both plain and enteric-coated ASA tablets, but the extent of absorption is unaffected. Rectal absorption from ASA suppositories is slow and erratic, and the bioavailability is generally less than with oral ASA.

Following oral administration, ASA is hydrolyzed by esterases to salicylate in the intestinal wall. Hydrolysis also occurs during the first

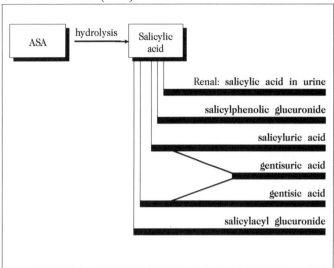

Figure 2 *Metabolic Pathways of Acetylsalicylic Acid (ASA)*

pass through the liver and by esterases present in plasma and erythrocytes. Salicylate is then metabolized by a number of pathways, some of which are saturable (see Figure 2). The plasma half-life for ASA is about 15 minutes; for salicylic acid it is 2 to 3 hours in low doses and about 12 hours in anti-inflammatory doses.

Efficacy

The salicylates, particularly ASA, have been used for many different types of pain, including muscular, vascular, arthritic and postpartum pain, the pain associated with dental extraction, headache and numerous other types. ASA and acetaminophen are equally effective except for the anti-inflammatory requirements of arthritis and bursitis. Analgesic effects increase with increasing doses to a maximum dose of 650 to 1,000 mg.

The antipyretic activity of ASA is comparable to that of acetaminophen. The peak antipyretic effect occurs about 2 hours after administration and persists 4 to 6 hours.

max 8 to 10/daily

Adverse Effects

ASA induced inhibition of prostaglandin synthesis has widespread physiological effects, which can be both therapeutic and potentially harmful. Side effects attributed to ASA, and many other nonsteroidal anti-inflammatory analgesics, affect many organ systems.

Gastrointestinal Effects

Perhaps the most widely recognized side effect of salicylate therapy is gastrointestinal irritation. Endogenous prostaglandin production has beneficial effects on gastrointestinal integrity, including inhibition of gastric acid secretion and stimulation of both gastric mucus and bicarbonate production. ASA inhibits production of these prostaglandins. This mechanism may underly the adverse gastrointestinal effects of ASA. Supporting this theory is evidence that administering a prostaglandin derivative can reduce minor, ASA induced gastrointestinal bleeding.

Other mechanisms that are likely involved in the pathogenesis of ASA induced gastrointestinal irritation include a direct topical irritation, decreased turnover of gastric epithelial cells and a breakdown

Internal Analgesics and Antipyretics

in gastric mucosal defences that allows the back-diffusion of gastric acid into mucosal cells with resultant damage. Regardless of the mechanism(s) involved, clinical evidence indicates the adverse gastrointestinal effects of ASA are primarily due to a local, rather than systemic, effect.

ASA induced gastrointestinal irritation can present as dyspepsia, occult gastrointestinal bleeding or massive gastrointestinal bleeding. Dyspepsia is common and presents as nausea, gastric pain, heartburn or vomiting. Occult gastrointestinal blood loss during ASA therapy occurs in up to 76 per cent of individuals taking 3 g daily. The blood loss can range from 2 to 12 mL daily. Although not usually clinically significant, prolonged blood loss can lead to iron-deficiency anemia.

Of more concern is the potential for ASA to induce gastric erosions and major gastrointestinal bleeding. In people who chronically take at least 2.4 g of ASA daily, gastric erosions and gastric ulcers have been reported in 40 and 17 per cent of individuals respectively. Not all individuals with ASA induced endoscopic evidence of damage complain of symptoms—29 per cent are reported to be asymptomatic despite having gastric ulcers. If allowed to progress, gastric erosions and ulcers may present as major gastrointestinal bleeding, which is a medical emergency. Data from the Boston Collaborative Drug Surveillance Program indicates 16 per cent of hospital admissions for major upper gastrointestinal bleeding are due to ASA. The presenting feature is epigastric pain with hematemesis.

Risk factors for ASA induced gastrointestinal irritation have not been well studied, but some recommendations can be made. If possible, individuals with a recent history of peptic ulcer disease should avoid ASA. Concomitant alcohol ingestion is a risk factor for upper gastrointestinal hemorrhage. Smoking, a risk factor for peptic ulcer disease, may be inclined to predispose to ASA induced gastrointestinal injury.

In an effort to reduce ASA induced gastrointestinal side effects, buffered and enteric-coated preparations have been formulated. When used in anti-inflammatory doses, enteric-coated ASA produces endoscopic evidence of gastroduodenal damage similar to placebo and significantly less than plain and buffered preparations. Buffered ASA preparations induce gastrointestinal damage as often as plain ASA, and there is little rationale for their use. Enteric-coated or sustained-release preparations are preferred when chronic ASA therapy is required, but they are not suitable when rapid analgesia is required. Patients at risk for gastric erosions who require maintenance therapy with ASA or other nonsteroidal anti-inflammatory drugs may benefit from concomitant misoprostol therapy.

Sustained-release formulations of ASA have recently been marketed. Although published literature on these formulations is limited, the incidence of gastrointestinal lesions associated with these products is presumably similar to that observed with enteric-coated preparations. Sustained-release preparations may be administered twice daily.

Platelet Effects

Prostaglandins are also important in regulating platelet function. Platelets adhere and aggregate in response to blood vessel damage and are involved in the initial step of the coagulation cascade. Platelet dysfunction impairs blood clotting, and bleeding time increases.

ASA irreversibly inhibits production of prostaglandin by platelets, thereby inducing platelet dysfunction for the life of the platelet. A single dose of ASA can significantly prolong bleeding time; this effect may persist for several days. A dose as small as 80 mg can produce this effect. Antecedent ASA use can increase blood loss associated with dental extraction, operative procedures and childbirth. Individuals should avoid ASA for one week before these events. The antiplatelet effect of ASA, combined with ASA induced gastric erosions, can also predispose to gastrointestinal bleeding.

Hypersensitivity Reactions

ASA can induce manifestations of an allergic response in certain predisposed individuals. These reactions consist of one or more of rhinitis, bronchospasm and urticarial reactions. Responses are more prevalent in individuals with chronic urticaria, nasal polyps and asthma. The mechanism underlying these reactions does not appear to be immunologically based. ASA induced bronchospasm is believed to involve the diversion of arachidonic acid metabolism from the prostaglandin pathway to the production of leukotrienes, which can cause bronchospasm.

Individuals with a history of allergic-type reactions to salicylates should avoid ASA. An individual stating an allergy to ASA should be questioned to determine the nature of the reaction; adverse gastrointestinal effects are commonly mistaken for an allergic reaction. Also, people with an allergic-type reaction to ASA may show crosssensitivity to other nonsteroidal anti-inflammatory agents and to drugs and foods containing tartrazine, a widely used yellow dye. The incidence of cross-reactivity with other anti-inflammatory drugs has been reported as high as 100 per cent; for tartrazine it is in the range of 5 to 15 per cent. Although cross-reactivity to acetaminophen has been reported, it is rare. Acetaminophen is generally considered an alternative for individuals allergic to ASA.

Renal Effects

Certain prostaglandins act as renal vasodilators if renal blood flow is reduced. Individuals at risk are those with pre-existing renal dysfunction, heart failure, and liver cirrhosis and ascites. The first two conditions occur more commonly in the elderly and may also depend on renal prostaglandins to act as vasodilators. Renal prostaglandins induce localized vasodilation to modulate the vasoconstriction caused by angiotensin II and catecholamines, which may have increased production in renal dysfunction and heart failure. Inhibiting production of renal prostaglandins by ASA and other nonsteroidal anti-inflammatory agents can interrupt this regulatory mechanism, causing an acute reduction in renal blood flow with subsequent deterioration in renal function (see section on ibuprofen).

Analgesic nephropathy refers to progressive and irreversible structural or functional (or both) renal abnormalities associated with chronic use or abuse of analgesics. Although most often linked to phenacetin (no longer available in Canada), analgesic nephropathy continues to be described in association with other nonsteroidal anti-inflammatory agents, including ASA. This syndrome is rarely seen in individuals receiving long-term therapy under medical supervision.

Salicylates can have a variable effect on the renal excretion of uric acid. In low doses of up to 2 g daily, ASA can inhibit uric acid excretion. Its use in these doses should be avoided by individuals with a history of gout. In higher doses, ASA may have no effect or may increase uric acid excretion.

Reye's Syndrome

Much attention has been focused on the association of salicylate ingestion with Reye's syndrome. Reye's syndrome, a rare but serious

Internal Analgesics and Antipyretics

illness, primarily affects children aged 5 to 15 although there have been rare cases reported in young adults. It typically occurs in a child recovering from a viral illness such as influenza or chickenpox who unexpectedly develops vomiting and abnormal behavior, such as lethargy, confusion, irritability or aggressiveness. The syndrome can progress to coma and death. Reye's syndrome is characterized by fatty infiltration of the liver associated with cerebral edema and encephalopathy. The mortality associated with Reye's syndrome ranges from 22 to 42 per cent.

Although the evidence is not conclusive, large epidemiological studies support an association between salicylate ingestion and the subsequent development of Reye's syndrome. It is now generally recommended that salicylates not be used in influenza-like illnesses or chickenpox in infants, children, teenagers and young adults. It seems reasonable to extend this recommendation to any febrile illness in this age group, except when the child is under the supervision of a physician.

ASA and Pregnancy

Because salicylates cross the placenta, the effects of ASA in pregnancy have been studied and reviewed extensively. Studies are contradictory on whether ASA is teratogenic in humans. Large studies both support and dispute this issue. However, it is apparent ASA may have deleterious effects when used in the later stages of pregnancy. When used in the last 6 months, ASA can prolong gestation and labor and cause significantly greater blood loss at birth. Additionally, two studies report a higher incidence of anemia during pregnancy, increased perinatal mortality and decreased neonatal birth weight when combination analgesics including ASA are taken daily during pregnancy. Another study failed to identify an association between ASA and either perinatal mortality or low birth weight in women who used ASA for at least 8 days per month during a minimum of 6 months during pregnancy. Conflicting results from these studies may be explained by the greater amounts of ASA ingested in the first two studies. In addition, women taking ASA in these two studies had a higher incidence of smoking than the controls.

When ingested late in pregnancy, ASA may also induce platelet dysfunction and predispose bleeding in the neonate. Use of ASA in the week before childbirth has been associated with an increased frequency of neonatal intracranial hemorrhage. If possible, expectant mothers should avoid using ASA during the latter stages of pregnancy. Ideally, ASA should be avoided throughout pregnancy. An exception to this is the use of low dose ASA (60 to 150 mg daily) to prevent pregnancy-induced hypertension after the twentieth week of gestation; ASA has been demonstrated to reduce the risk of maternal hypertension and low birth weight with little maternal or neonatal adverse effects.

Drug Interactions

Several important drug interactions with ASA have been documented. These are summarized in Table II.

Salicylate Overdose

Salicylate intoxication continues to be a common and serious problem. A survey of the Ontario Chief Coroner's records for 1984 revealed that 27 adults died from salicylate intoxication. There were no deaths in children. A detailed review of the assessment and management of salicylate overdose can be found in specialized references.

Table II *Major Drug Interactions with ASA*

Drug	Interaction
Acetazolamide	Individuals may develop lethargy and confusion. Salicylate can displace acetazolamide from protein binding sites and the acidosis induced by acetazolamide can enhance tissue penetration of salicylate.
Anticoagulants	Large doses of ASA can cause hypoprothrombinemia. Also antiplatelet and gastric effects of ASA may predispose to bleeding.
Antidiabetics	Moderate to large doses of ASA may enhance the hypoglycemia induced by insulin and sulfonylureas.
Corticosteroids	Corticosteroids may enhance salicylate elimination. Discontinuation of steroid therapy may result in salicylate accumulation and toxicity.
Ethanol	Concomitant use of ASA and ethanol may predispose to gastric bleeding.
Methotrexate	Salicylates may reduce renal elimination of methotrexate and predispose to toxicity.
Sulfinpyrazone	Salicylates can inhibit the uricosuric effect of sulfinpyrazone.

Adapted from: Hansten PD. Drug interactions. Philadelphia: Lea & Febiger, 1985.

The primary manifestations of salicylate intoxication vary. They can include any or all the following: nausea or vomiting with or without upper gastrointestinal hemorrhage; tinnitus; acid-base disturbances, which can present as metabolic acidosis, respiratory alkalosis or both; central nervous system dysfunction such as agitation, restlessness, coma and seizures; pulmonary edema; renal dysfunction; hyperthermia; and hypoprothrombinemia and platelet dysfunction, which can predispose to bleeding. A history of acute salicylate intoxication demands the individual be referred to the nearest hospital for assessment and management.

Management of a salicylate overdose is dictated by the individual's clinical condition and laboratory results, which include determination of the serum salicylate concentration. The Done nomogram (see Figure 3) is commonly used to assess the severity of an acute intoxication although it should only be used as an adjunct to clinical signs and symptoms and laboratory test results.

Therapeutic intervention in a salicylate overdose includes preventing further absorption by inducing emesis or performing gastric lavage and/or administering oral activated charcoal; correcting fluid and electrolyte abnormalities; administering bicarbonate to correct acidemia and facilitate salicylate renal excretion; and, in severe cases, use of hemodialysis to enhance salicylate elimination.

Dosage

Recommended analgesic doses for ASA and other salicylates have been developed recently. For adults, the recommended dose of ASA is 325 to 650 mg taken up to every 4 hours with a daily maximum of 4 g. Therapy using these doses should be limited to no more than

Internal Analgesics and Antipyretics

Figure 3 *Done Nomogram for Salicylate Poisoning*

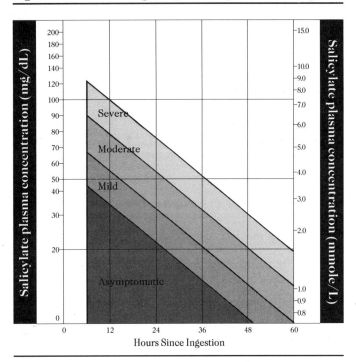

Conditions for the use of this chart:
1) The patient has taken a single acute ingestion and is not suffering from chronic toxicity.
2) The blood level to be plotted on the nomogram was drawn 6 hours after ingestion.
3) Levels in the toxic range drawn before 6 hours should be treated.
4) Levels in the nontoxic range drawn before 6 hours should be repeated to see if the level is increasing.

Adapted with permission from: Done AK. Significance of measurements of salicylate in blood in cases of acute ingestion. Pediatrics 1960;26:805.

5 days; if more prolonged therapy is required, it should be under the supervision of a physician. Children's doses for ASA are shown in Table III. Alternatively, children's doses of ASA can be determined by body weight and doses of 10 to 15 mg/kg every 4 to 6 hours to a maximum of 65 mg/kg per day have been recommended.

Doses outside those mentioned above are used for other disorders. Doses ranging from 80 mg every 2 days to 325 mg 3 times daily are used for antiplatelet effects. Anti-inflammatory doses in rheumatoid arthritis often exceed 4 g daily; dose adjustments are guided by serum salicylate concentrations.

Recently, the Food and Drug Regulations in Canada were revised for the packaging and labelling of pediatric preparations of ASA, other salicylates and acetaminophen. All package sizes of oral ASA and other salicylates, and methyl and other alkyl salicylates for external use, recommended solely for children, must be sold in child-resistant packages. If a drug is not recommended solely for children, at least one package size of each product available for sale must be child-resistant. Additionally, inner and outer labels for these products must include cautionary statements that the recommended doses not be exceeded and that the drug be kept out of the reach of children. These regulations do not apply to drugs sold by prescription or repackaged by a pharmacist at the time of sale.

Other Salicylates

Sodium, magnesium and choline salicylate are available in a variety of single-entity and combination products. Significant advantages of these products compared to single-entity ASA do not appear to exist. ASA, sodium salicylate and magnesium salicylate are all equipotent, milligram for milligram, although ASA may be more effective than sodium salicylate. Choline salicylate 435 mg is equivalent to ASA 325 mg.

Acetaminophen   Tylenol

Acetaminophen was first synthesized in 1877 but was initially discarded in favor of two structural derivatives, phenacetin and acetanilide. It was not until the 1950s that acetaminophen was introduced as a nonprescription analgesic and antipyretic. Since then its popularity has steadily increased, owing largely to its favourable side effect profile when compared with phenacetin, acetanilide and ASA. Also, as opposed to ASA, acetaminophen is available in liquid formulations. This makes it convenient to use for children.

Despite its popularity, the pharmacologic mechanisms underlying the clinical efficacy of acetaminophen have not been fully elucidated. Although acetaminophen is as effective an analgesic and antipyretic as ASA, it has no clinically useful anti-inflammatory action. This may be because acetaminophen is a selective inhibitor of prostaglandin synthesis. Presumably, acetaminophen inhibits prostaglandin synthesis in the central nervous system, which is involved in fever production and pain perception, but not in the periphery, where inflammatory processes occur. (See Table III for children's doses of acetaminophen.)

Table III *Children's Dosage Schedule for Analgesic Doses of ASA and Acetaminophen*

Age (yrs)	Recommended single dose (mg)*	Maximum daily dose (mg)	Maximum duration of use (days)
<2	Refer to text		
2–3	160	800	5
4–5	240	1,200	5
6–8	320	1,600	5
9–10	400	2,000	5
11	480	2,400	5

*Single doses may be repeated every 4 hours to a maximum of 5 times daily. Adapted from: Morrison AB. Regulatory proposals regarding nonprescription analgesics. Information Letter No. 659. Ottawa: Health and Welfare Canada, 1984;Feb 29.

Pharmacokinetics

The pharmacokinetics of acetaminophen have been well characterized. Bioavailability after oral administration appears to be dose dependent and ranges from 63 per cent after a single dose of 500 mg to 89 per cent after 1,000 mg. The time to peak serum concentrations after an oral dose is influenced by esophageal transit time, gastric emptying and perhaps the dosage form of the drug. These factors may influence the onset of action of acetaminophen. For example, administering acetaminophen to a person in the supine position

Internal Analgesics and Antipyretics

delays peak serum concentrations by more than one hour when compared to administration to a standing person. Acetaminophen suppositories are well absorbed, but the rate of absorption may be slower than with oral administration.

Acetaminophen is widely distributed in the body. It crosses the placenta and appears in breast milk, but there is little information to suggest it is teratogenic. The amounts that appear in breast milk are clinically insignificant.

Acetaminophen is eliminated from the body via hepatic metabolism (see Figure 4). With therapeutic doses, acetaminophen's elimination half-life is about 2 hours. When excessive doses are ingested, the sulfate conjugation pathway is saturated and hepatic glutathione stores are depleted. This process leads to accumulation of the toxic intermediate metabolite, which can cause hepatotoxicity.

Efficacy

The analgesic efficacy of acetaminophen has been well documented in mild to moderate pain associated with oral surgery, episiotomy, headache and cancer. Acetaminophen is as analgesic and potent as ASA in these conditions. Although ASA is clearly superior to acetaminophen in treating inflammatory bone and joint conditions, acetaminophen may possess some anti-inflammatory properties in other conditions. For example, in oral surgery, acetaminophen is not only an effective analgesic but also decreases swelling. Acetaminophen has also been shown to be as effective as ibuprofen for treatment of chronic knee pain due to osteoarthritis.

As with their analgesic effects, acetaminophen and ASA are equally effective antipyretics. Peak antipyretic effects occur about 2 to 3 hours after a dose.

Adverse Effects

In therapeutic doses, acetaminophen is extremely well tolerated. In contrast to ASA, acetaminophen does not cause gastric mucosal erosions or bleeding tendencies and has only rarely been associated with hypersensitivity reactions. Furthermore, its use has not been associated with Reye's syndrome. Isolated cases of acute renal failure in the absence of hepatotoxicity associated with acetaminophen overdose have been reported and studies implicating it in the analgesic nephropathy syndrome require confirmation. Asthmatics may experience deterioration of lung function during acetaminophen therapy, but these effects are generally less than those seen with ASA. Cross-sensitivity between ASA and acetaminophen has been reported, but the incidence is probably no greater than 10 per cent.

In addition to the hepatotoxicity associated with acute acetaminophen intoxication, evidence now exists that chronic use of high doses can induce liver damage. This effect generally requires the use of doses of at least 5 g daily for several weeks, but evidence exists that alcoholics are susceptible to hepatotoxic effects at lower doses. The threshold for toxicity may also be reduced in people with malnutrition or pre-existing liver disease, and those taking drugs that may induce microsomal enzymes.

Acetaminophen Overdose   20 tab

The potential for hepatic necrosis induced by an acute acetaminophen overdose is well documented. Specialized references exist for detailed information on this topic. The following is a brief review of some of the more important aspects of acetaminophen intoxication.

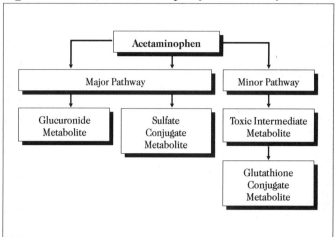

Figure 4 *Metabolic Pathways of Acetaminophen*

In an acetaminophen overdose the production of the toxic intermediate metabolite is increased (see Figure 4). Concomitantly, glutathione stores are depleted. As a result, the toxic intermediate accumulates, and binds to and destroys hepatocytes. The dose required to produce significant hepatotoxicity is generally thought to be 10 g in adults, but doses as low as 5 g have been implicated. Children appear to be more resistant to the hepatotoxic effects of acetaminophen; a proportionately higher dose is required to induce significant toxicity.

The clinical course of a significant acetaminophen overdose can be divided into four phases. In the first 12 to 24 hours postingestion, the symptoms consist primarily of nausea, vomiting, anorexia and diaphoresis. These relative benign symptoms can create a false sense of security and can belie subsequent hepatotoxicity. Biochemical evidence of liver damage is generally seen during the second phase (24 to 48 hours postingestion), and peak hepatotoxicity occurs during the third phase which is typically 72 to 96 hours postingestion. If the individual is successfully supported through this phase, the fourth phase (7 to 8 days postingestion) is characterized by recovery of liver function.

Effective antidotal therapy with N-acetylcysteine is available. Optimal results are obtained when therapy is instituted within 16 hours after the intoxication, but antidotal therapy has been reported to be successful up to 36 hours postingestion of acetaminophen. Unfortunately, symptoms of overdose in the initial 24 hours are relatively minor effects and do not adequately forewarn of subsequent severe hepatotoxicity.

Any person who has ingested a potentially toxic amount of acetaminophen should be referred to the emergency department of the nearest hospital. The severity of the overdose can be estimated by measuring the serum acetaminophen concentration on the nomogram shown in Figure 5. If the overdose is in the potentially hepatotoxic range, effective antidotal therapy with N-acetylcysteine can be instituted according to a standard protocol.

Dosage   max 8 tab/day   2-3 tabs.

The recommended adult dose of acetaminophen is 650 to 1,000 mg every 4 to 6 hours, with daily doses not to exceed 4 g. Single doses of 1 g produce greater analgesia than 650 mg. Recommended pediatric doses are shown in Table III. For children under 2 years of age,

Internal Analgesics and Antipyretics

Figure 5 *Rumack—Matthew Nomogram for Acetaminophen Poisoning*

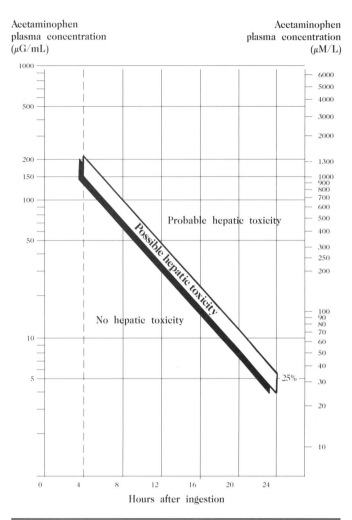

Acetaminophen plasma concentration (μG/mL)

Acetaminophen plasma concentration (μM/L)

Hours after ingestion

Conditions for the use of this chart:

1) The time coordinates refer to the time of ingestion.
2) Serum levels drawn before 4 hours may not represent peak levels.
3) The graph should be used only in relation to a single acute ingestion.
4) The lower solid line 25% below the standard nomogram is included to allow for possible errors in acetaminophen plasma assays and estimated time from ingestion of an overdose.

Adapted with permission from: Rumack BH, Matthew H. Acetaminophen poisoning and toxicity. Pediatrics 1975;55:871–6.

the dose of acetaminophen is 10 to 15 mg/kg every 4 to 6 hours with a maximum daily dose of 65 mg/kg. Alternatively, dosing may be by age: for children up to 3 months old, the maximum single dose is 40 mg; children 4 to 11 months, 80 mg; children 12 to 23 months, 120 mg.

Ibuprofen

Ibuprofen is a nonsteroidal anti-inflammatory agent that has recently been approved for sale as a nonprescription drug in the 200 mg solid dosage form. The Expert Advisory Committee to the Health Protection Branch has concluded that 200 mg of ibuprofen is a more effective analgesic than 325 mg of ASA in dysmenorrhea and dental pain. The dose of ibuprofen in adults and children over 12 years of age is 200 to 400 mg every 4 hours to a maximum daily dose of 1,200 mg.

Ibuprofen, like ASA, is a peripherally acting analgesic that inhibits cyclo-oxygenase and thus inhibits prostaglandin synthesis. Unlike ASA, inhibition of cyclo-oxygenase is reversible within 24 hours after discontinuing the drug.

The analgesic efficacy of ibuprofen has been demonstrated in a number of conditions, including dysmenorrhea, dental pain, soft tissue injury, osteoarthritis and postoperative pain. The superior efficacy of ibuprofen over ASA has been demonstrated in dysmenorrhea and dental pain. Ibuprofen has also been shown to be an effective antipyretic.

Milligram for milligram, ibuprofen is about 3.5 times as potent as ASA. Analgesic and antipyretic effects persist for up to 6 hours after a dose.

The most frequent side effects associated with ibuprofen are gastrointestinal irritation and mucosal damage. However, ibuprofen causes less gastric irritation than plain ASA. Other side effects include thrombocytopenia, skin rash, headache, dizziness, blurred vision, fluid retention and edema. Although ibuprofen is at least as effective an analgesic as ASA and appears to have a wider margin of safety, there are concerns about the widespread use of nonprescription analgesics. This is particularly pertinent for the elderly and other individuals who may be predisposed to adverse effects from these drugs. These concerns have been emphasized by evidence that ibuprofen in doses of 1,200 to 2,400 mg daily can cause acute renal dysfunction in patients with mild chronic renal failure.

Analgesic Combinations

ASA and acetaminophen are often used in combination with other analgesics as either fixed-dose combinations or as components of a multi-product treatment. Little evidence exists that combinations of two analgesic/antipyretic agents are superior to optimal dosing with either agent alone.

The most commonly used nonprescription analgesic combinations employ acetaminophen or ASA with caffeine and codeine. The amount of codeine in these nonprescription products is limited to a maximum of 8 mg per dosage form. The rationale behind combining a narcotic—which has an analgesic mechanism of action different from prostaglandin synthesis inhibition—with an analgesic/antipyretic is logical. However, little clinical evidence supports the efficacy of such a combination in the nonprescription dosage forms currently available. Studies documenting the efficacy of these combinations have used codeine doses of 60 to 65 mg combined with 600 to 1,000 mg of acetaminophen or ASA. Combinations containing codeine 30 mg were no different from either acetaminophen or ASA alone. Although codeine dependence has a relatively lower incidence and is less intense than with more potent narcotics, it is nonetheless well documented. This must always be considered in people taking codeine-containing analgesics for prolonged periods.

Caffeine can enhance the analgesic effects of ASA and acetaminophen. The dose of caffeine used in the studies (64 and 65 mg) is equivalent to that found in the usual nonprescription dosage recommendations for analgesic/caffeine combination products. This is equivalent to 2 tablets that contain 32 mg of caffeine per tablet.

Internal Analgesics and Antipyretics

Muscle Relaxants

Systemic skeletal muscle relaxants available without prescription include methocarbamol, chlorzoxazone and orphenadrine. These agents are marketed as either single-entity products or in combination with one or more of ASA, acetaminophen or codeine. The skeletal muscle relaxants are believed to work via a central effect. It is not clear if their muscle relaxant properties are a specific effect or simply an extension of their central sedative effects. The efficacy of these agents either alone or in combination products has not been rigorously established, but they appear to benefit certain situations. They are probably best reserved for short-term management of muscular pain unresponsive to ASA or acetaminophen. They may be combined with these agents for added effect.

Assessment and Management

The successful approach to the assessment and management of pain can begin with determination of the PQRST characteristics of pain (see Table IV). This information is obtained by thoroughly questioning the individual about the pain being experienced.

Table IV *The PQRST Characteristics of Pain*

		"Tell me about your pain" "Where is it?"
P	Palliative factors	"What makes it less intense?"
	Provocative factors	"What makes it worse?"
Q	Quality	"What is it like?"
R	Radiation	"Does it spread anywhere else?"
S	Severity	"How severe is it?"
T	Temporal factors	"Is it there all the time, or does it come and go?"

Adapted from: Twycross RG. Pain and analgesics. Curr Med Res Opin 1978;5:497–505.

Headache

Headache is one of the most common pain symptoms for which people seek medical attention. Headache pain may be due to serious organic disease, a vascular disorder or a psychological problem. Severe recurrent headaches are seldom caused by organic disease. About 90 per cent of these headaches are secondary to muscle contraction or vascular dilatation. Headaches with an organic basis have an underlying etiology such as sinusitis, dental problems, an acute febrile illness or an intracranial space-occupying lesion.

As with any pain, assessing a headache includes the quality, severity, location, duration and time course as well as the conditions that exacerbate or relieve the pain. The quality of headaches is usually dull and aching and not strongly localized. A throbbing, pulsatile quality indicates a vascular origin, as in migraines. Perception of intensity varies with individual attitudes to and tolerance of pain. Intensity of pain can be assessed by the degree of alteration of daily activities caused by the discomfort. A headache that interrupts or prevents sleep may have an organic basis. Localizing the pain may be difficult due to the referred nature of headaches. Mode of onset, intensity and duration may help determine the type of headache. A

severe persistent headache with stiff neck and fever indicates meningitis; without fever, subarachnoid hemorrhage. Rarely, chronic recurrent headaches of increasing intensity may be associated with organic disease such as a brain tumor.

Tension headache caused by contraction of scalp and neck muscles is the most common type of headache. Emotional factors play an important role, as tension headaches most often occur in individuals who are tense and anxious. In addition, they are strongly associated with depression. Pain is moderate, has a pressure-like quality and can be generalized or localized to the occipital-nuchal region, the bifrontal region or diffusely extended over the top of the cranium. Although analgesics may help relieve pain, the primary therapeutic modalities involve nonpharmacologic means such as stress reduction and biofeedback.

Migraine headaches affect up to 10 per cent of the population. Two main types are classic and common migraine. Both types are characterized by pulsatile headaches with nausea, vomiting, photophobia and prostration. Classic migraine is preceded by a prodromal period or aura that includes visual disturbances, speech difficulties and paresthesias. Migraine is believed to have a vascular origin, with initial vasoconstriction occurring in the prodromal period due to serotonin release. As serotonin is taken up by platelets and the spleen and excreted by the kidneys, the involved blood vessels dilate and passively distend, resulting in a pulsatile headache. Nonprescription analgesics such as ASA and acetaminophen may be useful in treating an acute migraine attack, especially if taken early. Migraines not relieved by these agents may require therapy with a vasoactive drug requiring a physician's prescription. In addition, individuals experiencing more than 2 migraine attacks per month may benefit from a prophylactic regimen, which may include propranolol or pizotyline.

Musculoskeletal Pain

Muscle pains such as those secondary to muscle spasm or after vigorous activity are commonly encountered in clinical practice. Spasms cause pain both directly and indirectly. Spasms may directly stimulate the mechanosensitive pain receptors. Muscle spasms may also compress blood vessels and decrease oxygenation to tissues, increase anaerobic metabolism, and thereby indirectly stimulate pain receptors through the evolution of chemical pain-inducing substances such as lactic acid and prostaglandins. Muscle pain occurring after vigorous physical activity often presents with pain, swelling and tenderness. Therapeutic modalities for myalgias include internal as well as external analgesics and muscle relaxants.

If muscle pain is generalized and other systemic symptoms are present, such as fatigue, insomnia and fever, an infectious process should be suspected and consideration should be given to referring the individual to a physician.

Dental Pain

Most types of dental pain have a localized inflammatory component. Tissue injury or trauma trigger the conversion of arachidonic acid to prostaglandins, resulting in pain and inflammation. Analgesics with anti-inflammatory activity may be more effective than those with only a central action. Many studies document the efficacy of both ASA and acetaminophen in preoperative and postoperative dental pain. Comparative studies support the superiority of ibuprofen over ASA and acetaminophen in dental pain. However, nonprescription use of analgesics for dental pain should be considered a temporary modality until a dentist can properly evaluate the pain.

Figure 6 *Suggested Approach for Assessing and Managing Pain*

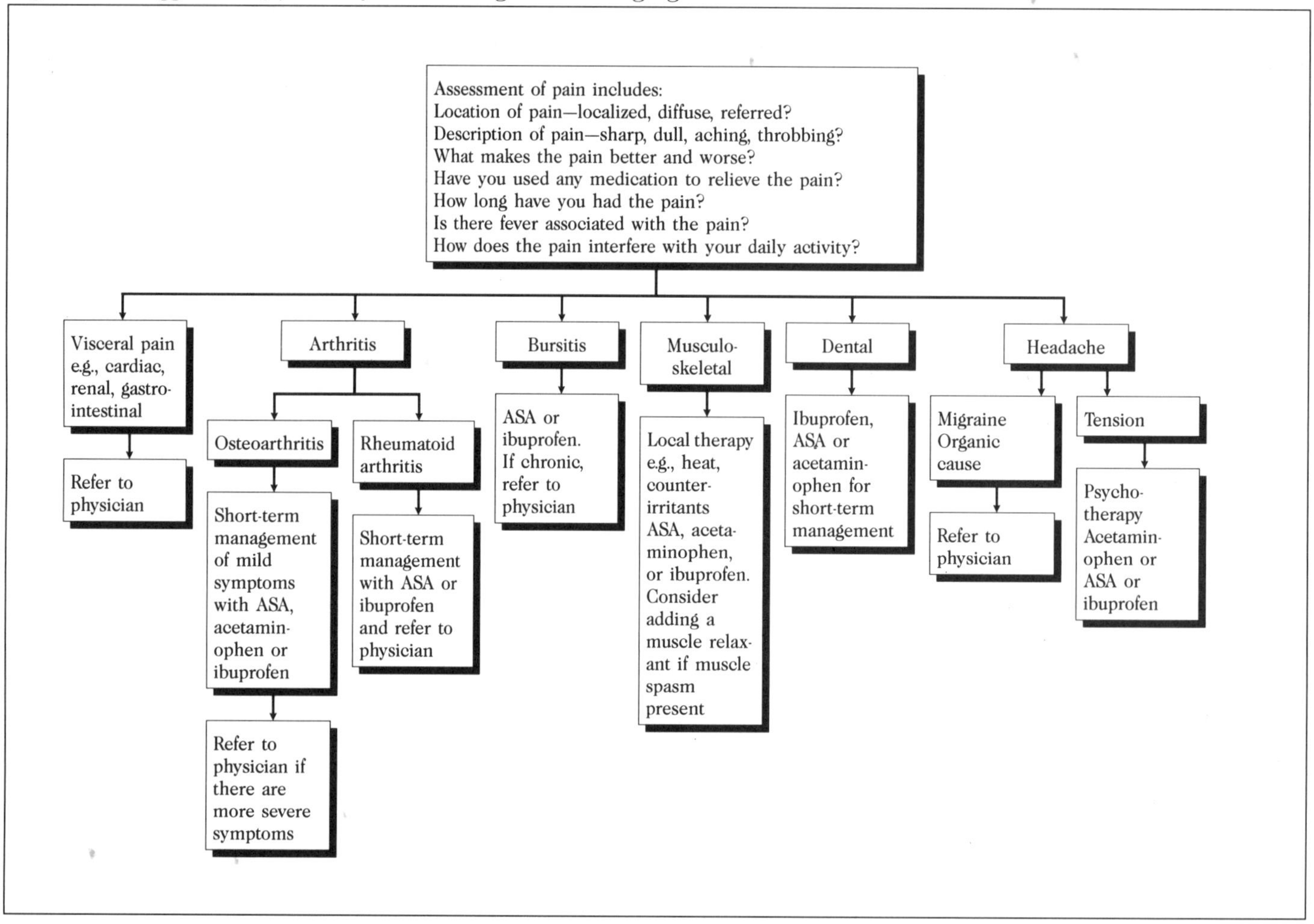

Assessment of pain includes:
Location of pain—localized, diffuse, referred?
Description of pain—sharp, dull, aching, throbbing?
What makes the pain better and worse?
Have you used any medication to relieve the pain?
How long have you had the pain?
Is there fever associated with the pain?
How does the pain interfere with your daily activity?

Visceral pain e.g., cardiac, renal, gastro-intestinal → Refer to physician

Arthritis
- Osteoarthritis → Short-term management of mild symptoms with ASA, acetaminophen or ibuprofen → Refer to physician if there are more severe symptoms
- Rheumatoid arthritis → Short-term management with ASA or ibuprofen and refer to physician

Bursitis → ASA or ibuprofen. If chronic, refer to physician

Musculo-skeletal → Local therapy e.g., heat, counter-irritants ASA, acetaminophen, or ibuprofen. Consider adding a muscle relaxant if muscle spasm present

Dental → Ibuprofen, ASA or acetaminophen for short-term management

Headache
- Migraine Organic cause → Refer to physician
- Tension → Psychotherapy Acetaminophen or ASA or ibuprofen

Bursitis

Bursitis is an inflammation of unknown cause involving any of the bursae between tendons, muscles and bony prominences. It most commonly occurs in the shoulder. Individuals experience pain upon moving the affected joint. Treatment includes rest, physical therapy and an anti-inflammatory agent such as ASA or ibuprofen. If the involved joints are warm, red, swollen, painful or, associated with shaking chills, septic arthritis should be suspected and the individual referred immediately to a physician.

Arthritis

The two major types of arthritis are rheumatoid arthritis and osteo-arthritis. Rheumatoid arthritis is a chronic disease involving inflammation of synovial membranes resulting in progressive joint damage. Osteoarthritis is characterized by loss of joint cartilage and hypertrophy of bone. It is a wear-and-tear disease as opposed to inflammatory, although progression can be complicated by periods of joint inflammation.

Treatment of rheumatoid arthritis usually starts with nonsteroidal anti-inflammatory agents such as ASA. Doses of ASA required to treat rheumatoid arthritis exceed those recommended for nonprescription use and are generally in the range of 3.5 to 5.5 g daily. When used for rheumatoid arthritis the recommended prescription dosage range for ibuprofen is 1,200 to 2,400 mg daily. Acetaminophen and analgesic doses of ASA are ineffective in treating rheumatoid arthritis. If anti-inflammatory agents fail to control the inflammation, disease-remitting drugs or elements such as gold, penicillamine and hydroxychloroquine may be prescribed by a physician.

Due to the chronic nature of arthritis and the pattern of exacerbations, people often supplement prescription therapy with nonprescription analgesics. Counselling of these individuals should strive to prevent overuse of ineffective analgesics and thereby decrease the risk of cumulative side effects. Simple analgesics, taken on demand, do have a role in osteoarthritis, particularly if the disease is localized to one or two joints and is transient. When symptoms are recurrent and affect several joints, anti-inflammatory doses of ASA or other nonsteroidal anti-inflammatory agents are indicated.

In both forms of arthritis, the individual should be referred to a physician for initial assessment. After that, simple analgesics may be used judiciously as needed, in addition to prescription therapy, after careful review of potential benefits and cumulative toxicity.

Visceral Pain

Nonprescription analgesics are not as effective for visceral pain as for specific somatic pains. Pain arising from visceral organs may

Internal Analgesics and Antipyretics

indicate the presence of organic disease. Such pain should not be masked with an analgesic but should be investigated by a physician.

As visceral pain tends to be referred, it may be difficult to distinguish from somatic pain. For example, ischemic cardiac pain is often referred to the base of the neck, over the shoulder area and pectoral muscles, and down the arms. Cardiac pain is usually referred to the left rather than the right side.

Two important epigastric pains are those secondary to gastritis and peptic ulcer disease. These are often characterized by burning pain referred to the anterior surface of the abdomen or chest, usually between the xiphoid process and umbilicus.

Pain arising from the kidney and ureters is generally referred to the area directly posterior to these structures, as in the case of pyelonephritis. Pain from the bladder, as in a urinary tract infection, is usually felt directly over the bladder.

Fever

The initial step in managing fever is to assess the cause (see Table I). Fevers that require treatment are those that are high (for example, greater than 39.5 °C) and those associated with discomfort. High fevers, especially in infants and young children, may be associated with febrile convulsions. Reducing fever in these situations is generally accepted as useful. For other situations, there is no compelling reason to treat a fever except to reduce discomfort.

Acetaminophen and ASA are the two most commonly used antipyretics; they are equally effective. Owing to a more favorable side effect profile, acetaminophen is generally preferred over ASA. Although effective as an antipyretic, there is no advantage of ibuprofen over acetaminophen. This preference is especially appropriate for children, in whom the use of ASA during episodes of influenza-like illnesses or chickenpox has been associated with Reye's syndrome. Nonpharmacologic methods of reducing fever—such as cool water baths or sponging—are effective but can be inconvenient and may not provide additional benefit to the use of antipyretics.

Summary

Successfully managing pain and fever requires that the disorder be accurately assessed. The pharmacist should take time to question the individual and obtain a description of the complaint or complaints. The pharmacist can then decide either to recommend a nonprescription treatment or to refer the individual to a physician. If the former approach is used, a treatment plan should be developed. This plan includes nonpharmacologic therapy and the choice of an appropriate analgesic or antipyretic, the dose and the endpoints of therapy. The endpoints should include both symptom relief and duration of treatment; at that time, assessment and management is reviewed.

Ask the Consumer

Q. Where is the pain? Does it travel anywhere?
■ It is important to know if the pain is localized, diffuse or referred and if it radiates. Abdominal pain can be associated with important underlying pathology (for example, peptic ulcer, gall stones, appendicitis). Flank pain may indicate kidney stones or infection.

Cardiac ischemia can present as chest, shoulder and left arm pain. In all these situations, medical referral is necessary.

Q. How would you describe the pain? Sharp? Dull? Aching? Throbbing?
■ This description helps to further characterize the pain. For example, a throbbing headache may be vascular in origin (a migraine), whereas a dull ache is more characteristic of a tension headache.

Q. What makes the pain better and worse?
■ Answers to this question may aid in the management of the pain as well as in further characterization of the cause. For example, exercise exacerbates and rest relieves angina pectoris; a recumbent position can exacerbate the pain associated with esophageal reflux.

Q. Have you used any medication to relieve the pain?
■ It is important to know the previous agent(s) used, dose and duration of treatment before implementing a new therapeutic approach.

Q. How long have you had the pain? Have you had this type of pain before?
■ Prolonged or recurrent pain may indicate chronic underlying pathology.

Q. How does the pain interfere with your daily activity?
■ Knowledge of this will indicate the importance, from the individual's point of view, of relieving the pain.

Q. How long have you had a fever?
■ Persistent fever, unresponsive to conventional management, should be referred to a physician.

Q. Are you being treated for any other illnesses?
■ Before initiating salicylate therapy, it is particularly important to identify people with peptic ulcer disease.

Q. What medications (prescription and nonprescription) are you currently taking?
■ Avoid potential drug interactions and drug duplication.

References

Pain

Adams RA, Victor M. Principles of neurology. Toronto: McGraw-Hill, 1981: 89–102.

Adams RD, Martin JB. Acute and chronic pain: pathophysiology and management. Petersdorf RG, Adams RD, Braunwald E, Isselbacher KJ, Martin JB, Wilson JD, eds. Harrison's Principles of internal medicine. Toronto: McGraw-Hill, 1983:7–15.

Baumann TJ, Lehman ME. Pain management. In: De Piro JT, Talbert RL, Hayes PE, Yee GC, Posey LM, eds. Pharmaco therapy: a pathophysiologic approach. New York: Elsevier Science Publishing Co Inc, 1989:642–59.

Craig KD. Psychology of pain. Postgrad Med J 1984;60:835–840.

Dorland's illustrated medical dictionary. Toronto: WB Saunders, 1974.

Flower RJ, Moncada S, Vane JR. Analgesic-antipyretics and anti-inflammatory agents: drugs employed in the treatment of gout. In: Gilman AG, Goodman LS, Rall TW, Murad F, eds. Goodman and Gilman's The pharmacological basis of therapeutics. Toronto: Macmillan, 1985:674–89.

Guyton AC. Textbook of medical physiology. Toronto: WB Saunders, 1986:593.

Internal Analgesics and Antipyretics

Max MB. Improving outcomes of analgesic treatment: is education enough? Ann Int Med 1990;113:885–9.

Twycross RG. Pain and analgesics. Curr Med Res Opin 1978;5:497–505.

Fever

Bartle WR. Fever—a diagnostic tool? Can Pharm J 1985;118:54–6.

Done AK. Treatment of fever in 1982: a review. Am J Med 1983; 74 (Suppl 6A):27–35.

Newman J. Evaluation of sponging to reduce body temperature in febrile children. Can Med Assoc J 1985;132:641–2.

Stitt JT. Prostaglandin E as the neural mediator of the febrile response. Yale J Biol Med 1986;59:137–49.

Styrt B, Sugarman B. Antipyresis and fever. Arch Int Med 1990;150:1589–97.

Tabor PA. Drug-induced fever. Drug Intell Clin Pharm 1986;20:413–20.

Acetylsalicylic Acid

Achong MR. Clinical pharmacology of analgesic drugs. Can Fam Physician 1979;25:179–82.

Agrawal NM, Roth S, Graham DY, et al. Misoprostol compared with sucralfate in the prevention of nonsteroidal anti-inflammatory drug-induced gastric ulcer. Ann Int Med 1991;115:195–200.

Amreim PC, Ellmun L, Harris WH. Aspirin-induced prolongation of bleeding time and perioperative blood loss. JAMA 1981;245:1825–8.

Anonymous. Reye's syndrome—United States, 1984. JAMA 1985;253:751–2.

Anonymous. Diagnosis and treatment of Reye's syndrome. JAMA 1981; 246:2441–4.

Aspirin monograph. In: Krogh CME, ed. Compendium of pharmaceuticals and specialties. Ottawa: Canadian Pharmaceutical Association, 1991.

Blackshear JL, Napier JS, Davidman M, Stillman MT. Renal complications of nonsteroidal anti-inflammatory drugs: identification and monitoring of those at risk. Semin Arth Rheum 1985;14:163–75.

Boysen G, Boss AH, Odum N, Olsen JS. Prolongation of bleeding time and inhibition of platelet aggregation by low dose acetylsalicylic acid in patients, with cerebrovascular disease. Stroke 1984;15:241–3.

Briggs GG, Freeman RK, Yaffe SJ. Drugs in pregnancy and lactation. Baltimore: Williams and Wilkins, 1986;26–31.

Capetola RJ, Rosenthale ME, Dubinsky B, McGuire JL. Peripheral antialgesics: a review. J Clin Pharmacol 1983;23:545–6.

Cohen MM, Clark L, Armstrong L, D'Souza J. Reduction of aspirin-induced fecal blood loss with low-dose misoprostol tablets in man. Dig Dis Sci 1985;30:605–11.

Collins E, Turner G. Maternal effects of regular salicylate ingestion in pregnancy. Lancet 1975;2:335–7.

Done AK. Significance of measurements of salicylate in blood in cases of acute ingestion. Pediatrics 1960;26:800–7.

Dugandzic RM, Tierney MG, Dickinson GE, Dolan MC, McKnight DR. Evaluation of the validity of the Done nomogram in the management of acute salicylate intoxication. Ann Emerg Med 1989;18:1186–90.

Dunn M. The role of arachidonic acid metabolites in renal homeostasis. Drugs 1987;33(Suppl 1):56–66.

Emkey RD, Mills JA. Aspirin and analgesic nephropathy. JAMA 1982;247:55–7.

Gibaldi M, Grundhofer B. Bioavailability of aspirin from commercial suppositories. J Pharm Sci 1975;64:1064–6.

Glen-Bott AM. Aspirin and Reye's syndrome. Med Toxico 1985;2:161–5.

Grossman MI, Matsumoto KK, Lichter RJ. Fecal blood loss produced by oral and intravenous administration of various salicylates. Gastroenterology 1961;40:383–8.

Hansten P, Horn J. Drug interactions and updates. Malvern: Lea & Febiger, 1990.

Hepsoe HU, Loekken P, Bjoernson J, et al. Double-blind cross-over study of the effect of acetylsalicylic acid on bleeding and postoperative course after bilateral oral surgery. Eur J Clin Pharmacol 1976;10:217–25.

Hurwitz ES, Barrett MJ, Bregman D, et al. Public Health Service study of Reye's syndrome and medications. JAMA 1987;257:1905–11.

Imperiale TF, Petrullis AS. A meta-analysis of low-dose aspirin for the prevention of pregnancy-induced hypertensive disease. JAMA 1991;266:261–5.

Isselbacher KJ. The role of arachidonic acid metabolites in gastrointestinal homeostasis. Drugs 1987;33(Suppl 1):38–46.

Ivey KJ, Paone DB, Krause WJ. Acute effect of systemic aspirin on gastric mucosa in man. Digest Dis Sci 1980;25:97–9.

Ivey KJ. Gastrointestinal intolerance and bleeding with non-narcotic analgesics. Drugs 1986;32(Suppl 4):71–89.

Jick H. Effects of aspirin and acetaminophen in gastrointestinal hemorrhage. Arch Intern Med 1981;141:316–21.

Kimberly RP, Plotz PH. Aspirin-induced depression of renal function. N Engl J Med 1977;296:418–24.

Lanza FL, Royer GL, Nelson RS. Endoscopic evaluation of the effects of aspirin, buffered aspirin and enteric-coated aspirin on gastric and duodenal mucosa. N Engl J Med 1980;303:136–8.

Levy G. Clinical pharmacokinetics of salicylates: a re-assessment. Br J Clin Pharmacol 1980;10:285S–290S.

Levy G. Clinical pharmacokinetics of aspirin. Pediatrics 1962;62:867–72.

Lewis RB, Schulman JD. Influence of acetylsalicylic acid, an inhibitor of prostaglandin synthesis, on the duration of human gestation and labour. Lancet 1973;2:1159–61.

Liston AJ. Child-resistant packaging (Information letter no. 705). Ottawa: Health and Welfare Canada, 1986;Mar 14.

McGuigan MA. Death due to salicylate poisoning in Ontario. Can Med Assoc J 1986;135:891–4.

Mehlisch DR. Review of analgesic efficacy of salicylates, acetaminophen and pyrazolones. Am J Med 1983;74(Suppl 6A):47–52.

Mojaverian P, Rocci ML, Conner DP, et al. Effect of food on the absorption of enteric-coated aspirin: correlation with gastric residence time. Clin Pharmacol Ther 1987;41:11–7.

Morrison AB. Regulatory proposals regarding nonprescription analgesics (Information letter no. 659). Ottawa: Health and Welfare Canada, 1984; Feb 29.

Needham CD, Kyle J, Jones PF, et al. Aspirin and alcohol in gastrointestinal hemorrhage. Gut 1971;12:819–21.

Paccioretti MJ, Block LH. Effects of aspirin on platelet aggregation as a function of dosage and time. Clin Pharmacol Ther 1980;27:803–9.

Proudfoot AT. Salicylates and salicylamides. In: Haddad LM, Winchester JF, eds. Clinical management of poisoning and drug overdose. Toronto: WB Saunders, 1983:575–86.

Rumack CM, Guggenheim MA, Rumack BH, et al. Neonatal intracranial hemorrhage and maternal use of aspirin. Obstet Gynecol 1981;58:525–65.

Sandler DP, Smith JC, Weinberg CR, et al. Analgesic use and chronic renal disease. N Engl J Med 1989;320:1238–43.

Schreiner GE, McAnally JF, Winchester JF. Clinical analgesic nephropathy. Arch Intern Med 1981;141:349–57.

Settipane GA. Aspirin and allergic diseases: a review. Am J Med 1983; 74(Suppl 6A):102–9.

Settipane GA. Adverse reactions to aspirin and related drugs. Arch Intern Med 1981;141:328–32.

Shapiro S, Monson RR, Kaufman DW, et al. Perinatal mortality and birth-weight in relation to aspirin taken during pregnancy. Lancet 1976;1:1375–6.

Silvoso GR, Ivey KJ, Butt JH, et al. Incidence of gastric lesions in patients with rheumatic disease on chronic aspirin therapy. Ann Intern Med 1979;91:517–20.

Stuart MJ, Gross SJ, Elrad H, Graeber JE. Effects of acetylsalicylic acid ingestion on maternal and neonatal hemostasis. N Engl J Med 1982; 307:909–12.

Szczeklik A, Gryglewski RJ. Asthma and anti-inflammatory drugs. Drugs 1983;25:533–43.

Temple AR. Review of comparative antipyretic activity in children. Am J Med 1983;74(Suppl 6A):38–46.

Turner G, Collins E. Fetal effects of regular salicylate ingestion in pregnancy. Lancet 1975;2:338–9.

Acetaminophen

Barker JD, de Carle DJ, Anuras S. Chronic excessive acetaminophen use and liver damage. Ann Intern Med 1977;87:299–301.

Berlin CM, Yaffe SJ, Ragni M. Disposition of acetaminophen in milk, saliva and plasma of lactating women. Pediatr Pharmacol 1980;1:135–41.

Internal Analgesics and Antipyretics

Black M. Acetaminophen hepatotoxicity. Ann Rev Med 1984;35:577–93.

Channer KS, Roberts CJ. Effect of delayed esophageal transit on acetaminophen absorption. Clin Pharmacol Ther 1985;37:72–6.

Clissold SP. Paracetamol and phenacetin. Drugs 1986;32(Suppl 4):46–59.

Cooper SA. Comparative analgesic efficacies of aspirin and acetaminophen. Arch Intern Med 1981;141:282–5.

Curry RW, Robinson JD, Sughrue MJ. Acute renal failure after acetaminophen ingestion. JAMA 1982;247:1012–4.

Expert advisory committee on the management of severe chronic pain in cancer patients. Pain: a monograph on the management of cancer pain. Ottawa: Health and Welfare Canada, 1984.

Fischer TJ, Guilfoile TD, Kersarwala HH, et al. Adverse pulmonary responses to aspirin and acetaminophen in chronic childhood asthma. Pediatrics 1983;71:313–8.

Forest JAH, Clements JA, Prescott LF. Clinical pharmacokinetics of paracetamol. Clin Pharmacokinet 1982;7:93–107.

Harrison PM, Keays R, Bray GP, Alexander GJM, Williams R. Improved outcome of paracetamol-induced fulminant hepatic failure by late administration of acetylcysteine. Lancet 1990;335:1572–3.

Hopkinson JH, Smith MT, Bare WW, et al. Acetaminophen (500 mg) versus acetaminophen (325 mg) for the relief of pain in episiotomy patients. Curr Ther Res 1974;16:194–200.

Lokken P, Skjelbred P. Analgesic and anti-inflammatory effects of paracetamol evaluated by bilateral oral surgery. Br J Clin Pharmacol 1980;10:253S–260S.

Peters BH, Fraim CJ, Masel BE. Comparison of 650 mg aspirin and 1,000 mg acetaminophen with each other and with placebo in moderately severe headache. Am J Med 1983;74(Suppl 6A):36–42.

Peterson RG, Rumack BH. Age as a variable in acetaminophen overdose. Arch Intern Med 1981;141:390–3.

Rawlins MD, Henderson DB, Hijab AR. Pharmacokinetics of paracetamol (acetaminophen) after intravenous and oral administration. Eur J Clin Pharmacol 1977;11:283–6.

Rudolph AM. Effects of aspirin and acetaminophen in pregnancy and in the newborn. Arch Intern Med 1981;141:358–63.

Rumack BH, Matthew H. Acetaminophen poisoning and toxicity. Pediatrics 1975;55:871–6.

Rumack BH, Peterson RG, Koch GG, Amara IA. Acetaminophen overdose: 662 cases with evaluation of oral acetylcysteine treatment. Arch Intern Med 1981;141:380–5.

Rumack BH. Acetaminophen. In: Haddad LM, Winchester JF, eds. Clinical management of poisoning and drug overdose. Toronto: WB Saunders, 1983:562–75.

Seeff LB, Cuccherini BA, Zimmerman HJ, et al. Acetaminophen hepatotoxicity in adults: a therapeutic misadventure. Ann Intern Med 1986;104:399–404.

Tempra monograph. Krogh CME, ed. Compendium of pharmaceuticals and specialties. Ottawa: Canadian Pharmaceutical Association, 1991.

Yaffe SJ. Comparative efficacy of aspirin and acetaminophen in the reduction of fever in children. Arch Intern Med 1981;141:286–92.

Ibuprofen

Bradley JD, Brandt KD, Katz BP, Kalasinski LA, Ryan SI. Comparison of an anti-inflammatory dose of ibuprofen, an analgesic dose of ibuprofen, and acetaminophen in the treatment of patients with osteoarthritis of the knee. N Engl J Med 1991;325:87–91.

Dawood MY. Ibuprofen and dysmenorrhea. Am J Med 1984;77(Suppl 1A):87–94.

Forbes JA, Barkaszi BA, Ragland RN, Hankle JJ. Analgesic effect of fendosal, ibuprofen and aspirin in postoperative oral surgery pain. Pharmacotherapy 1984;4:385–91.

Jain AK, Ryan JR, McMahon FG, et al. Analgesic efficacy of low-dose ibuprofen in dental extraction pain. Pharmacotherapy 1986;6:318–22.

Liston AJ. Report of the expert advisory committee on ibuprofen (Information letter no. 720). Ottawa: Health and Welfare Canada, 1987;Mar 27.

Miller RR. Evaluation of the analgesic efficacy of ibuprofen. Pharmacotherapy 1981;1:21–7.

Watson PD, Galletta G, Braden NJ, Alexander L. Ibuprofen, acetaminophen, and placebo treatment of febrile children. Clin Pharmacol Ther 1989;46:9–17.

Whelton A, Stout RL, Spilman PS, Klassen DK. Renal effects of ibuprofen, piroxicam, and sulindac in patients with asymptomatic renal failure. Ann Intern Med 1990;112:568–76.

Analgesic Combinations

Beaver WT, Feise G. Comparison of the analgesic effect of acetaminophen and codeine and their combination in patients with postoperative pain. Clin Pharmacol Ther 1978;23:108.

Beaver WT. Aspirin and acetaminophen as constituents of analgesic combinations. Arch Intern Med 1981;141:293–300.

Cooper SA, Beaver WT. A model to evaluate mild analgesics in oral surgery outpatients. Clin Pharmacol Ther 1976;20:241–50.

Eddy NB, Friebel H, Hahn KJ, Halbach H. Codeine and its alternates for pain and cough relief. Bull World Health Org 1968;38:673–741.

Gertzbein SD, Tile M, McMurty RY, et al. Analysis of the analgesic efficacy of acetaminophen 1,000 mg, codeine phosphate 60 mg, and the combination of acetaminophen 1,000 mg and codeine phosphate 60 mg in the relief of postoperative pain. Pharmacotherapy 1986;6:104–7.

Jain AK, McMahon FG, Ryan JR, et al. Aspirin and aspirin-caffeine in postpartum pain relief. Clin Pharmacol Ther 1978;24:69–75.

Laska EM, Sunshine A, Zighelboim I, et al. Effect of caffeine on acetaminophen analgesia. Clin Pharmacol Ther 1983;33:498–509.

Moertel CG, Ahmann DL, Taylor WF. Relief of pain by oral medications: a controlled evaluation of analgesic combinations. JAMA 1974;229:55–9.

Skjelbred P, Lokken P. Codeine added to paracetamol induced adverse effects but did not increase analgesia. Br J Clin Pharmacol 1982;14:539–43.

Muscle Relaxants

Elenbaas JK. Centrally acting oral skeletal muscle relaxants. Am J Hosp Pharm 1980;37:1313–23.

Headache

Atkinson R, Appenzeller O. Headache. Postgrad Med J 1984;60:841–6.

Follender AB. Chronic headache: a realistic approach to management. Postgrad Med 1983;74(5):249–55.

Peatfield R. Migraine: current concepts of pathogenesis and treatment. Drugs 1983;26:364–71.

Repschlaeger BJ, McPherson MA. Classification, mechanism and management of headache. Clin Pharm 1984;3:139–52.

Dental Pain

Korberly BH, Schreiber GF, Kilkuts A, Orkand RK, Segal H. Evaluation of acetaminophen and aspirin in the relief of preoperative dental pain. J Am Dent Assoc 1980;100:39–42.

Seymour RA. Use of analgesics in postoperative dental pain: a review. J Roy Soc Med 1984;77:949–54.

Arthritis

Hart FD. Rational use of analgesics in the treatment of the rheumatic disorders. Drugs 1987;33:85–93.

15

Antacids, Antiflatulents and Antireflux Agents

Glen R. Brown

The two disorders of the gastrointestinal tract—peptic ulcer disease and gastroesophageal reflux—are differentiated by their etiology, pathophysiology and symptoms. Self-treatment of gastric and duodenal ulcers and esophageal reflux includes nonpharmacologic measures and the use of antacids. Esophageal reflux can also be treated with alginic acid. The common problem of gastrointestinal gas can be self-treated with defoaming agents such as simethicone, but counselling in appropriate eating habits can help prevent excessive flatus.

Nonprescription products intended to treat gastrointestinal symptoms or pathology are used by a large portion of society. Although viewed as innocuous by most lay people, nonprescription medications can cause harm if they are used incorrectly, in inappropriate quantities, for irrational indications or concurrently with other specific medications. It is important for the pharmacist to know the indications, contraindications and correct therapeutic use of all nonprescription products available to treat gastrointestinal symptoms. This chapter addresses the indications and use of antacids, antiflatulents, and agents used to treat gastroesophageal reflux. It is estimated that more than one in four North American adults use one or more of these products monthly.

Peptic Ulcer Disease
Etiology

Peptic ulcer disease (PUD) includes a group of processes characterized by irritation of the mucosal surface of the gastrointestinal tract in association with exposure to gastric acid and pepsin. This situation most commonly occurs in the stomach, duodenum and esophagus, resulting in gastric ulcers, duodenal ulcers and reflux esophagitis, respectively.

About 10 per cent of the population develop PUD sometime during their lifetime. During any one year, approximately 1.7 per cent of the population suffer from PUD. Slightly more males than females experience it (1.77 per cent versus 1.72 per cent). This male/female prevalence ratio is higher for duodenal than for gastric ulcers. The prevalence of gastric and duodenal ulcers increases almost linearly with age for both men and women. The incidence of gastric ulcers rises slightly after age 40.

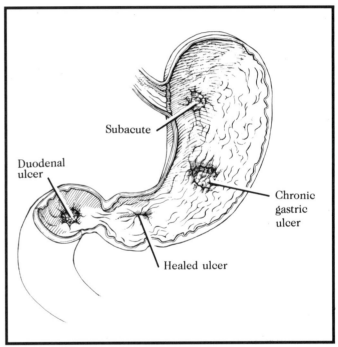

Figure 1 *Gastric and Duodenal Ulcers*

Many factors have been hypothesized as contributing to PUD. Genetic factors may predispose a person to the disease. First-degree relatives of ulcer sufferers develop PUD twice as often as relatives of disease-free people. First-degree relatives appear at increased risk of ulceration at the same site (gastric or duodenal) as the person with PUD and not at other sites. Genetic predisposition is further supported by studies showing a correlation between blood groups and duodenal ulcers. People with blood group O are about 37 per cent more likely to develop duodenal ulcers than people of other blood groups. However, genetic factors or familial tendencies do not totally explain the etiology of PUD.

Recently, considerable interest and study has centered on the possible role of an infection by *Helicobacter pylori*, a gram-negative bacillus, in the development of PUD. Patients with *H. pylori* infection of their gastric mucosa produce more acid and release more gastrin than non-infected individuals. A definite *H. pylori*-related

Antacids, Antiflatulents and Antireflux Agents

gastritis has been demonstrated. The relationship of this gastritis with the development of ulcerations with PUD is unknown, although the majority of individuals with duodenal ulcers will also be infected with *H. pylori*. The role for *H. pylori* infection in PUD development is suggested by the reduction in symptoms of gastritis and the reduced rate of PUD relapse in patients treated with antibiotics that eradicate the organism from the stomach.

A strong association appears to exist between smoking and PUD. The pathophysiologic mechanism for this association is unclear, but may involve altered pancreatic bicarbonate secretion, accelerated gastric emptying or altered acid secretion. Cigarette smokers are at about twice the risk as nonsmokers. The prevalence increases with the number of cigarettes smoked per day. PUD responds more slowly to treatment in smokers than in nonsmokers, and smoking may antagonize the beneficial effects of H_2-blockers such as cimetidine. Smokers also have a higher PUD relapse rate than nonsmokers. Alcohol may cause gastritis, but does not appear to be a risk factor for PUD. Hepatic cirrhosis, a possible consequence of alcohol abuse, may increase the incidence of PUD. Coffee consumption has not been shown clearly to influence the development of PUD.

The role of psychological stress in PUD is unclear. Studies comparing individuals with PUD and disease-free control subjects show no relationship between stressful life events and illness. This non-effect of stress appears valid for both gastric and duodenal ulcers. Despite this evidence, stress is known to cause changes to gastric mucosa, and the possible role of psychological stress in PUD cannot be ruled out totally.

Ingesting certain drugs has been implicated as a risk factor. The medications most thoroughly studied are acetylsalicylic acid (ASA), nonsteroidal anti-inflammatory drugs (NSAID) and corticosteroids. ASA in a single dose irritates the stomach, although some adaptation to this exposure occurs with chronic ingestion. Despite this ability of the mucosa to adapt partially to ASA exposure, chronic ingestion of ASA increases the risk of PUD. ASA appears to be a significant factor only when intake exceeds 22 tablets per week as reported by Cameron and by Graham in their studies. Although the milligrams of ASA in the study by Cameron were not recorded, most people used plain ASA products. The estimated threshold for developing PUD is about 7,000 mg per week. ASA may cause abdominal discomfort and heartburn at much lower doses, but these symptoms are not related to damage of the gastrointestinal mucosa. Enteric-coated ASA tablets reduce the incidence of gastrointestinal damage compared to regular ASA tablets.

Nonsteroidal anti-inflammatory drugs also increase the risk of PUD. The mechanism for developing PUD with NSAIDs is unknown, although inhibition of prostaglandin synthesis is probably involved. The risk of developing PUD from NSAID usage is greater in elderly people. The symptoms of PUD occur within three months of starting NSAID therapy. Based on available clinical trials, no particular NSAID can be singled out as particularly safe or dangerous with regard to promoting PUD.

The role of corticosteroids in PUD is uncertain. Early reviews of pooled data suggested corticosteroids increase the risk of PUD, particularly if administered for more than 30 days or if the total dose exceeds the equivalent of 1,000 mg of prednisone. A recent epidemiologic study suggests that corticosteroid use is only a risk factor for PUD when combined with concurrent NSAID therapy. Patients concurrently receiving corticosteroids and NSAIDs had a 15 times

greater risk of developing PUD than persons not receiving either medications. This suggests that prophylactic therapy for patients receiving only corticosteroids is not necessary.

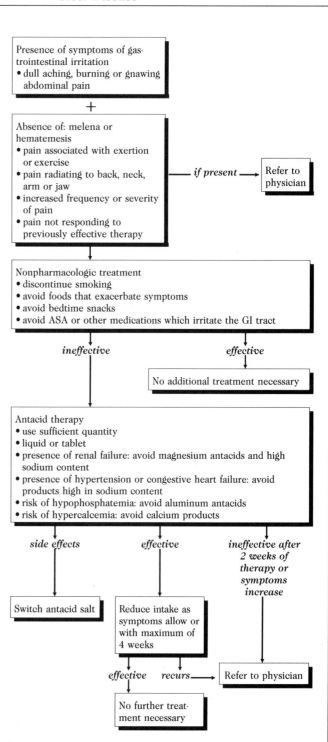

Figure 2 *Suggested Approach for Treating Peptic Ulcer Disease*

Antacids, Antiflatulents and Antireflux Agents

Pathophysiology

The changes in normal physiological processes that result in PUD are not completely understood. Recent thinking suggests PUD results from an imbalance in the gastrointestinal mucosa between aggressive factors (acid and pepsin) and defensive mechanisms. The main aggressor in PUD is hydrochloric acid, secreted from the parietal cells after stimulation by histamine, gastrin or acetylcholine. The etiology of the increased acid secretion seen in many individuals with PUD, particularly those with duodenal ulcers, is complex and variable.

Recent investigations looked at the role of alterations in the mucosal defense mechanisms in the pathogenesis of PUD. The mucosa of the stomach and duodenum are protected from autodigestion by the secretion of a mucus layer, which adheres to the mucosal surface, and by the secretion of bicarbonate under the mucus. Alterations in the mucus or bicarbonate secretion may contribute to PUD.

Cytoprotection is the protective effect on the mucosa of various agents. It is not dependent on acid reduction or neutralization. The mechanisms responsible for this protective effect are complex and variable.

Prostaglandins protect the mucosa from damage by irritants such as alcohol, NSAIDs and acids. The mechanism of protection is not clearly understood, but may involve an increase in gastric and duodenal mucus and bicarbonate secretion or alteration in mucosal blood flow. The underlying alteration in normal digestion and protection that results in PUD has not been identified yet in individuals and, no doubt, varies from person to person.

Symptoms

The discomfort of gastric and duodenal ulcers is usually described as a dull ache, burning, gnawing or exaggerated hunger sensation. A sensation of fullness, gaseous discomfort, cramping pain or nausea may be the predominant symptom. Symptoms requiring immediate assessment by a physician include constant, intense pain, radiation of the pain to the back or inadequate pain relief with previously successful therapy. Hematemesis (vomiting blood) or melena (black, tarry stools) may be the first sign of PUD and indicates a need for immediate medical attention.

Most people describe the discomfort as arising in a specific location between the umbilicus and xiphoid cartilage. Symptoms of gastric and duodenal ulcers can overlap and the ulcer location cannot be predicted with certainty by the type or location of symptoms. Originally gastric ulcer pain was thought to develop shortly after eating a meal and subsequently to recede within a few hours. In contrast, duodenal ulcer pain was thought to be relieved by food, with discomfort returning within a few hours after eating and remaining until the next meal. However, a large overlap exists between duodenal and gastric ulcers in the relationship between meals and discomfort. The rhythm of pain in relation to meals does not diagnose the location of the ulcer. Medical evaluation should be sought for persistent symptoms, any change in location or character of the discomfort, or if symptoms are related to any activity.

Gastroesophageal Reflux
Etiology

Factors contributing to gastroesophageal reflux (GER) are not clearly known. All adults have periodic reflux of stomach contents into the esophagus, but this reflux does not cause damage or discomfort since

the contents clear rapidly. People with pathologic reflux have an ineffective lower esophageal sphincter (LES), ineffective esophageal clearance mechanisms and abnormal gastric emptying.

Factors aggravating these abnormalities include posture, pregnancy, smoking, drugs and certain foods. People with GER often reflux while in the recumbent position, particularly during sleep. Esophageal clearance is less effective in the recumbent than in the upright position. Elevating the head of the bed during sleep has been shown to increase clearance of esophageal contents. Pregnancy aggravates gastroesophageal reflux by lowering LES tone and possibly by increasing intra-abdominal pressure. Cigarette smoking aggravates GER by reducing LES tone. Alcohol has been shown to reduce LES tone and inhibit esophageal clearance thereby promoting GER. Quantity and consistency of food may influence GER. Large meals result in gastric distention, which reduces LES tone allowing easier reflux.

Foods resulting in a high osmolarity of gastric contents, such as fruit juices and sherbets, may promote GER. Foods with a high fat content may also reduce LES tone. The fat content of chocolate aggravates GER in some people. Coffee has been shown to decrease LES pressure and to irritate the mucosa. Acidic foods such as citric juices and tomato products may not increase the frequency of reflux, but the pH of these foods irritates inflamed esophageal mucosa.

A number of drugs aggravate GER by either decreasing LES pressure or decreasing esophageal clearance. Pharmacologic classification of these agents varies. Drugs associated with GER include methylxanthines (theophylline), anticholinergic agents, alpha-adrenergic antagonists (phentolamine), narcotic analgesics (morphine and meperidine), beta-adrenergic agonists (isoproterenol), progesterone, diazepam and prostaglandins. Calcium channel blockers affect LES pressure and esophageal motility, which may aggravate GER in susceptible individuals.

Factors historically thought to aggravate GER but lacking supporting evidence include obesity and hiatus hernia.

Pathophysiology

The symptoms of GER develop only after prolonged or frequent reflux of gastric contents into the esophagus. The retrograde flow of gastric contents is prevented in healthy people by the LES. In people with GER, the sphincter has an abnormally low resting tone or relaxes inappropriately to allow retrograde flow. Normally, any material refluxed into the esophagus is cleared by gravity, salivation and esophageal motor activity.

People with GER tend to reflux more frequently and at night during sleep. Reflux at night results in prolonged exposure of the esophagus to the acidic gastric contents, since salivation and swallowing almost cease during sleep. The lying position also prevents gravity from clearing the esophagus. Hydrochloric acid, pepsin and possibly bile salts of the gastric fluid are the agents responsible for damaging the esophageal mucosa. The interplay of aggravating factors, such as foods or position, and altered physiologic processes, such as LES tone or gastric emptying, results in a variety of possible mechanisms for GER to develop.

Symptoms

The most common symptom of GER is heartburn, that is, a substernal or retrosternal burning sensation. Heartburn is most prominent shortly after eating, when bending over or while lying down. The burning sensation may move up the chest like a wave. GER may result in regurgitating gastric contents into the mouth. Individuals often complain of a sour or bitter taste in the throat or mouth. They may awake with a mouthful of salty fluid (waterbrash) or with a coughing, choking sensation. GER may cause fullness in the throat, difficulty in swallowing and increased swallowing to relieve throat irritation. Less commonly, pain with swallowing occurs. In many people, symptoms of GER mimic those of ischemic heart disease (angina). If symptoms occur with exertion, or if the pain radiates to the neck, jaw or down the arms, the person must be evaluated for cardiac disease.

Treatment
Gastric and Duodenal Ulcers

Nonpharmacologic treatment of gastric and duodenal ulcers consists mainly of avoiding the precipitating or aggravating factor. Smoking should be decreased and discontinued if possible. Diet therapy plays a limited role in PUD treatment. Different foods do not greatly affect the stomach's production of acid. A bland diet does not reduce acid production or improve the healing rate. Spicy or acidic foods need not be avoided unless the individual associates a particular food with the symptoms. This principle includes alcohol and caffeinated and decaffeinated coffee.

Milk may cause a temporary decrease in symptoms. Frequent and chronic use of milk for symptomatic control should be discouraged to avoid the milk-alkali syndrome. Some concern exists that milk may actually stimulate acid secretion, although it has never been shown to be a factor in developing PUD. Milk has not been shown to benefit ulcer healing.

Dietary fibre does not influence symptomatology or rate of healing of PUD, but may play a role in the prevention of duodenal ulcer relapse. People with PUD may notice an improvement in symptoms with frequent, small meals although this action may not alter acid secretion significantly. A diet of frequent small meals should not be recommended but does not need to be discouraged if the individual improves symptomatically. Food consumption at bedtime should be avoided to reduce nocturnal acid secretion.

The mainstay of self-treatment for PUD has been the use of antacids. Antacids currently available contain one or more salts of magnesium, aluminum or calcium. Antacids are believed to work by neutralizing the hydrogen ions in the gastrointestinal tract, thus reducing irritation to the mucosa. Recent work suggests antacids may also have a cytoprotective effect unrelated to acid neutralizing effects. Stimulation of prostaglandin production of the gastric mucosa by the use of aluminum-containing antacids suggests a non-acid neutralizing mechanism for the beneficial effects of antacids. However, therapeutic efficacy does not appear to vary greatly between the available antacids if taken in sufficient quantities. Side effects vary with the antacid salt.

Antacids are helpful in treating PUD, particularly duodenal ulcers. Healing rates with antacids approach 78 to 85 per cent compared to 20 to 45 per cent with placebo. The efficacy of antacids in gastric ulcer therapy is less impressive. Healing rates of gastric ulcers after six weeks of treatment with an aluminum hydroxide/magnesium carbonate product were 67 per cent compared to 25 per cent with placebo. Other investigators have been unable to demonstrate a benefit of antacids over placebo for gastric ulcers.

The choice of an antacid to treat PUD is based on neutralizing capacity, dosage form, potential side effects, palatability, sodium content and cost. Early studies suggested that for antacids to be effective, daily ingestion of quantities sufficient to neutralize 1,008 mmol of hydrogen ions were required. The acid neutralizing capacity of an antacid is determined by measuring the quantity of acid required to titrate the antacid to a pH of 3.5.

The early studies suggested antacids must be given in large doses with a large acid neutralizing capacity to be effective. More recent studies show that antacids given daily in quantities equivalent to 120 to 300 mmol of acid neutralizing capacity are as effective in healing duodenal ulcers as larger quantities. Maximum healing rates can be achieved with antacid doses of about 180 mmol of acid neutralizing capacity per day. Increasing the daily quantity of antacid above this value does not improve healing of PUD. These findings support the theory of non-acid neutralizing properties of antacids as a key factor in efficacy in treatment of PUD.

The acid neutralizing capacity of antacids varies greatly from product to product. For this reason, the quantity of each antacid product required to provide this degree of acid neutralizing capacity must be calculated. The clinical superiority of liquid antacids to tablets has been suggested but not clearly demonstrated. Early in-vivo data suggested liquids had superior acid neutralizing capacity, although recent data does not support any inferiority of tablet products. Many studies that demonstrated the benefit of antacids in PUD therapy used tablet dosage forms. These results, combined with the convenience of tablets, indicate the use of antacid tablets should not be considered inferior therapy to liquid antacids.

The minimum frequency of antacid administration required for therapeutic benefit is uncertain. Early studies suggested antacids be administered one and three hours after each meal and at bedtime for maximum effect. This administration schedule requires seven doses per day, which is inconvenient and difficult to maintain. Recent studies that achieved equivalent beneficial effects used four doses per day—one hour after each meal and at bedtime.

Potential side effects from antacids involve the gastrointestinal tract (diarrhea and constipation) and metabolic disturbances (electrolyte, mineral and acid/base imbalances). A particular side effect can be avoided by choosing an antacid with a different cation or with a combination of cations. The side effects of each cation salt are discussed individually below. Palatability of the antacid product is important to maintaining compliance. Preference in taste can guide product selection. If taste fatigue develops, an alternative product can be used. When changing antacid products, the individual must know the quantity required to provide the necessary acid neutralizing capability.

Many antacid products with low sodium content are now available. People on restricted sodium diets should avoid antacid products with a high sodium content.

Antacid preparations may contain other ingredients in addition to acid neutralizing salt. Defoaming agents, such as simethicone or dimethylpolysiloxone, ease the elimination of gastrointestinal gas through belching or flatus. Simethicone does not neutralize acid, but neither does it inhibit the acid neutralizing ability of the antacid. Defoaming agents have not been shown to benefit PUD healing rates. Antacid products containing local anesthetics, such as oxethazaine, have not been demonstrated superior to standard antacids in treating PUD.

Products containing bismuth salts such as bismuth subsalicylate (for example, Pepto-Bismol) have been promoted as treatment for

Antacids, Antiflatulents and Antireflux Agents

indigestion and upset stomach. In animal studies, bismuth subsalicylate reduced the incidence of gastric mucosal lesions after single exposures to noxious agents. Recently, bismuth salts have been shown to clear *H. pylori* infections of the gastric mucosa and to reduce the associated symptoms of gastritis. Eradication of *H. pylori* by bismuth salts has been associated with a decreased rate of relapse following discontinuation of PUD treatment. Eradication of *H. pylori* is more prolonged when bismuth salts are combined with antibiotics with antimicrobial activity for the organism. Bismuth salts have no acid neutralizing effect. Another bismuth salt, colloidal bismuth subcitrate, has been demonstrated through a number of studies to be as effective or superior to H$_2$-antagonists in the treatment of PUD. In addition to activity in eradicating *H. pylori* infections, colloidal bismuth subcitrate increases gastric mucosal prostaglandin synthesis. This medication is not yet available in Canada.

Individuals with PUD may not experience pain relief with antacid therapy. The cause of pain associated with PUD is unknown and is not directly related to exposure of irritated mucosa to acid. Placebo may produce equivalent pain relief in initial treatment of PUD. With continued antacid use, symptoms should decrease as healing occurs. People with abdominal pain after two weeks of antacid therapy should be referred for medical evaluation. The use of antacids at any time in children under the age of six should be supervised by a physician.

Antacids may not be an effective treatment for some individuals due to side effects, noncompliance or insufficient acid neutralizing capacity of administered quantities. People with PUD who do not respond to antacid therapy may benefit from other pharmacologic agents such as histamine H$_2$-receptor blockers, sucralfate, omeprazole or prostaglandins. The H$_2$-receptor blockers, cimetidine, famotidine and ranitidine, have healing rates equivalent if not superior to antacid therapy. The additional benefit obtained by continuing antacid therapy with concurrent H$_2$-blocker therapy has not been well documented. Since the H$_2$-blockers alone are effective in treating PUD, concurrent antacid therapy can be reduced to intermittent use for symptomatic relief. The additional benefit from adding antacid therapy to sucralfate or prostaglandin treatment is unknown.

Pharmaceutical Agents

Sodium bicarbonate is one of the original home remedy antacids. It has a rapid onset but short duration of action due to rapid gastric emptying. Sodium bicarbonate reacts with gastric acid to form sodium chloride, water and carbon dioxide. Any excess bicarbonate not reacting with acid is readily absorbed in the intestine. If the kidneys are unable to excrete this additional sodium and bicarbonate, fluid retention and systemic alkalosis may result. For this reason, sodium bicarbonate is contraindicated in people with renal failure or congestive heart failure and individuals on sodium-restricted diets. The use of sodium bicarbonate by elderly people who may have impaired renal function should be discouraged. Chronic use of sodium bicarbonate with calcium-containing products such as milk or antacids may result in the milk-alkali syndrome. The milk-alkali syndrome is characterized by renal failure, hypercalcemia and metabolic alkalosis. Symptoms include nausea, vomiting, mental confusion, headache and anorexia. Large single doses of sodium bicarbonate may result in increased gastric gas, belching and, rarely, stomach rupture. Since safer antacids are available, sodium bicarbonate should not be recommended.

Calcium carbonate has a high acid neutralizing capacity per gram of salt. Calcium carbonate reacts with hydrochloric acid to form calcium chloride and water, although insoluble calcium phosphate and hydroxide salts subsequently form in the intestine. Calcium is absorbed into the systemic circulation after administration of calcium carbonate. Hypercalcemia and hypercalciuria may develop with chronic use. Hypercalcemia is more likely to occur in people with renal failure or with concurrent administration of drugs that inhibit calcium excretion, such as thiazide diuretics.

Calcium carbonate has been implicated as a factor in developing the milk-alkali syndrome. Calcium carbonate produces a rebound stimulation of gastric acid, although the relative magnitude of the rebound effect following calcium versus magnesium or aluminum salts is disputed. Calcium's stimulation of gastric acid secretion does not adversely affect the therapeutic action of calcium carbonate. Although calcium carbonate is widely thought to cause constipation, evidence is lacking to support this claim.

Magnesium, in the form of magnesium hydroxide, oxide or carbonate salts, is a common ingredient of antacid products. Magnesium hydroxide reacts with hydrochloric acid to form magnesium chloride, which is subsequently converted to magnesium carbonate or phosphate in the intestine. About 5 per cent of the magnesium is absorbed into the systemic circulation after ingestion of magnesium hydroxide. This magnesium is excreted from the body via the kidney. Magnesium hydroxide may alkalinize the urine. In individuals with renal failure, hypermagnesemia may develop, resulting in neurological, neuromuscular and cardiovascular impairment. For this reason, magnesium-containing antacids should be used sparingly, if at all, in individuals with renal failure.

The most common side effect of magnesium hydroxide is diarrhea. The cathartic effect of magnesium is believed secondary to the osmotic action of the salt and secretory effects on the gut mucosa. The tendency for diarrhea with magnesium hydroxide can be partially negated either by using combination products containing both magnesium and aluminum or by alternating a combination product with antacids containing magnesium and aluminum.

Aluminum hydroxide is the most common form of aluminum in antacids, although products are formulated that contain the oxide, carbonate and aminoacetate salts. Of these salts, aluminum hydroxide has the greatest neutralizing capacity, but is considered weak compared to calcium carbonate or magnesium hydroxide. Aluminum hydroxide reacts with hydrochloric acid in the stomach to form aluminum chloride, which subsequently reacts to form insoluble phosphate salts.

The binding of phosphate is used therapeutically to treat hyperphosphatemia or renal failure. If used chronically by people with reduced phosphate intake, such as alcoholics or persons with gastrointestinal malabsorption syndromes, aluminum antacids may result in phosphate depletion and hypophosphatemia.

The insoluble aluminum phosphate salts are absorbed in negligible amounts. Any aluminum absorbed has minimal effects in normal persons although urinary aluminum excretion may increase severalfold. In people with renal failure, chronic aluminum hydroxide use results in elevated body aluminum stores. This aluminum may be a factor in dementia and changes in bone structure seen in individuals with chronic renal failure.

The most common side effect of aluminum-containing antacids is constipation. The constipating effect of aluminum salts is secondary to the binding of bile salts and the direct effects of aluminum on the intestinal smooth muscle. Products containing both magnesium and aluminum salts are intended to balance the opposing cathartic and constipating effects of individual agents. Although the side effects of magnesium and aluminum salts are believed to counteract each other, the therapeutic effect is additive. These combinations are not always successful in obtaining the correct balance and corresponding normal bowel function. As the daily dose of combination products increases, so does the tendency to develop diarrhea. This effect can be counteracted by adding or altering an aluminum hydroxide antacid. Aluminum antacids have also been reported to harden the intestinal contents. This hardening can result in total bowel obstruction.

Magaldrate is a complex hydroxymagnesium aluminate that supposedly reacts in stages to provide consistent, sustained buffering

activity. The hydroxymagnesium moiety reacts rapidly with acid and the aluminum moiety reacts more slowly to give the sustained effect. The acid neutralizing pattern is not the same as a simple mixture of aluminum hydroxide and magnesium hydroxide. This salt more closely resembles magnesium hydroxide in adverse effects and systemic action.

Although **bismuth subsalicylate** should not be considered an antacid, it may be used to treat indigestion. The use of bismuth subsalicylate may result in black stools, which can mask the appearance of blood. Bismuth absorption from these products is negligible. Salicylate absorption after bismuth subsalicylate ingestion is extensive. The recommended adult dosage of 30 mL provides salicylate equivalent to an ASA tablet of 325 mg. People with conditions or ingesting medications that may be adversely affected by salicylates should avoid bismuth subsalicylate products. The salicylate component does not increase gastrointestinal blood loss in animals. In addition to potential drug interactions with the salicylate component, bismuth subsalicylate has been shown to reduce the bioavailability of doxycycline and tetracycline.

Esophageal Reflux

The nonpharmacologic treatment of GER is to avoid factors decreasing LES tone. Foods high in fat content, including chocolate, should be reduced. Meals should be small and regularly spaced to avoid gastric distention. Food and fluid ingestion should be avoided for three to six hours before bedtime. Smoking should be reduced or discontinued, and alcohol and coffee consumption decreased. If acidic foods, such as fruit juices, aggravate symptoms, they should be avoided. Improvement in posture can reduce symptoms. Elevating the head of the bed by 15 to 20 centimetres may reduce nocturnal reflux. Using pillows to raise the head is not sufficient to reduce reflux. The individual should avoid bending over or slumping in a chair, particularly after meals.

The main components of self-medication of GER are antacids and alginic acid. Although widely used by the public and prescribed by physicians, evidence to support any beneficial effect of antacids for GER has only recently become available. Antacids increase LES pressure, which should reduce reflux episodes. Clinically, antacids provide greater symptomatic relief than placebo. The beneficial effect was demonstrated when antacid was used 7 times daily for a total acid neutralizing capacity of 595 mmol per day. A similar study using antacid 7 times daily (560 mmol per day) could not demonstrate any difference in frequency or severity of symptoms versus placebo. More recently, antacids in dosages equivalent to 120 mmol acid neutralizing capacity (1 tablet 4 times daily, 1 hour after meals and at bedtime) has been shown to produce a statistically significant reduction in symptoms of heartburn and regurgitation versus placebo over a two week treatment period. Endoscopically, antacids have not been shown superior to placebo in rate of healing of esophageal mucosa. The value of antacids in treating GER is still questionable. However, antacids appear effective in relieving symptoms of heartburn.

Alginic acid and alginate-antacid products are available for self-medication of GER. The alginate reacts with saliva to form a viscous solution that floats on the surface of the gastric contents and acts as a mechanical barrier between the esophageal mucosa and gastric fluid. Although Gaviscon tablets contain aluminum hydroxide and magnesium trisilicate, they have minimal acid neutralizing capacity and should not be considered antacids. Other alginate

Figure 3 *Suggested Approach for Treating Gastroesophageal Reflux*

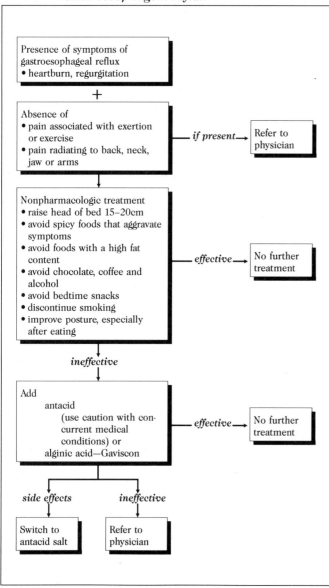

Antacids, Antiflatulents and Antireflux Agents

products may contain sufficient antacid to have significant acid neutralizing capacity. Alginic acid, such as Gaviscon, reduces heartburn after meals to a greater extent than placebo. Chronic use of Gaviscon has provided greater symptomatic relief and fewer episodes of reflux than placebo as measured by esophageal monitoring. Other studies fail to demonstrate a reduction in exposure of the esophagus to acid after Gaviscon use. The beneficial effects of Gaviscon appear equal but not superior to antacids in symptomatic relief and endoscopic evaluation of healing.

If antacids or alginic acid fail to reduce the incidence or severity of symptoms, the individual should be referred for medical evaluation. Agents that increase LES pressure, such as bethanechol or metoclopramide, or that reduce gastric acid output, such as cimetidine, famotidine or ranitidine, have been shown to reduce symptoms and aid healing of esophageal mucosa. Recent evidence to support the beneficial effects of omeprazole therapy in patients refractory to other pharmacologic treatments suggests that patients not responding to one treatment should be referred to a physician for consideration for more extensive acid inhibition.

Drug Interactions

Antacids can alter the pharmacokinetics of other drugs by altering gastric or urinary pH, or through a physiochemical reaction between the ingredients of the antacid and the drug. Depending on the interacting drug, this change can increase or decrease the amount of drug absorbed; increase or decrease the rate of drug absorption; or increase or decrease renal clearance. The effect of antacid therapy on pharmacokinetics has been evaluated for many drugs. The clinical significance of many antacid-drug interactions is questionable. Table I lists interactions that are clinically significant.

Bioavailability of captopril is reduced about 45 per cent by co-administering an antacid. This reduction may result from the change in gastric pH or by the formation of insoluble captopril-antacid salts.

Ciprofloxacin bioavailability is significantly reduced with simultaneous administration of antacids. Ciprofloxacin should be administered at least 2 hours before or 4 hours following antacid administration. Similar effects and recommendations apply to norfloxacin, enoxacin, and ofloxacin. The formation of insoluble fluoroquinolone-antacid complexes appears to be the mechanism of the interaction since gastric pH adjustments obtained with H_2-antagonists do not produce a similar reduction in bioavailability.

Diflunisal bioavailability decreases by concurrently administering aluminum hydroxide or an aluminum hydroxide/magnesium hydroxide combination, but not by magnesium hydroxide alone. This interaction is less significant if the diflunisal and antacid are taken after a meal. Antacids do not appear to interact significantly with other non-steroidal anti-inflammatory agents, specifically ibuprofen, piroxicam, ketoprofen, and tenoxicam.

Antacids were shown to reduce the absorption of single doses of digoxin. However, the digoxin was administered with quantities of antacid (60 mL) larger than those usually recommended for a single dose. The effect of smaller doses is not known. Concurrent administration of antacid with enteric-coated formulations may alter the rate of dissolution of the tablet. The rate and extent of this interaction may vary from product to product. Unless the characteristics of the interaction are known, it is best to avoid potentially altering the intended dissolution characteristics of the enteric-coated formulation by avoiding concurrent administration of antacids.

Table I *Antacid–Drug Interactions*

Drug	Antacid	Effect	Mechanism
Captopril	Mg–Al	decreased bioavailability	thought to be insoluble salt
Diflunisal	Al/Mg	decreased bioavailability	thought to be insoluble salt
Digoxin	Al/Mg	decreased bioavailability	
Enteric–coated Tabs		increased rate of dissolution	altered pH
Iron	Al/Mg	decreased bioavailability	thought to be insoluble salt
Isoniazid	Al/Mg	decreased bioavailability	
Ketoconazole		decreased bioavailability	increased gastric pH
Naproxen	Al/Mg	decreased bioavailability	
Quinolones	Al–Mg, Ca	decreased bioavailability	insoluble salt
Phenytoin	Al–Mg, Ca	decreased bioavailability	
Polystyrene Sulfonate Resin	Al/Mg	systemic alkalosis	binding of cation
Tetracycline	Al/Mg	decreased bioavailability	insoluble salt

The bioavailability of iron from various iron salts is reduced by concurrent antacid administration. Insoluble iron salts result from this interaction. Isoniazid absorption is delayed and reduced by administering 45 mL of aluminum hydroxide or magaldrate antacid. The dissolution of ketoconazole requires an acidic gastric secretion. The neutralization of the gastric contents (using sodium bicarbonate and cimetidine) reduces ketoconazole bioavailability. It is assumed other antacids have similar effects. Fluconazole does not appear to be affected by simultaneous administration of antacid.

Naproxen absorption rate and bioavailability have been reduced when administered with antacids containing magnesium or aluminum. Large doses (40 to 60 mL) of antacids can decrease the bioavailability of phenytoin. The effect of smaller doses of antacid is not consistent.

Concurrent administration of antacids and cationic exchange resins, such as sodium polystyrene sulfonate (for example, Kayexalate), may result in systemic alkalosis in people with renal failure. The antacid cation is believed to bind to the resin, increasing the intestinal bicarbonate available for absorption. In people with normal renal function, this interaction does not significantly alter the acid/base balance.

Absorption of tetracycline is greatly reduced by concurrent administration of antacids. This reduction is not related to changes in gastric pH, but is due to the formation of insoluble tetracycline salts.

The effect of concurrent antacid administration on cimetidine

Antacids, Antiflatulents and Antireflux Agents

bioavailability is not clear. Several single-dose studies show a significant decrease in cimetidine bioavailability when administered with antacids. A multiple-dose study did not demonstrate any effect of antacid on cimetidine pharmacokinetics. Avoiding coadministration of cimetidine and antacid may be unnecessary. Similarly, the bioavailability of ranitidine is not affected by antacids when administered in recommended quantities. The bioavailability of famotidine is significantly reduced by simultaneous administration of a large dose of antacid. This interaction can be avoided by spacing the administration of famotidine at least 2 hours from antacid administration.

Antacids used concurrently with rapid-release or sustained-release theophylline products does not alter the bioavailability or efficacy of the theophylline. The use of an antacid with a sustained-release theophylline product may slightly increase the rate of absorption of theophylline, but this increase is probably not clinically significant.

The effect of antacids on quinidine pharmacokinetics is complex and unpredictable. Animal data suggest antacids containing magnesium and aluminum reduce the bioavailability of quinidine sulphate and quinidine bisulphate. However, the administration of aluminum hydroxide to four people receiving quinidine sulphate did not alter the pharmacokinetics of the drug. Antacids containing magnesium and aluminum can be absorbed in quantities to alkalinize the urine. Since the excretion of quinidine is impaired in alkaline urine, antacids may result in decreased quinidine renal clearance in persons with alkalinized urine.

Urinary excretion of other weak bases, such as tocainide, may decrease if sufficient antacid is absorbed to alkalinize the urine. Urinary excretion of weak acids may increase if the urine pH rises after antacid administration. This effect can increase the rate of excretion of salicylates. The magnitude of increase in urinary excretion of salicylates is thought to be significant only when serum salicylate concentrations are greater than 1.05 mmol/L (15 mg/mL). Thus, for intermittent doses or low daily intakes of salicylates, the effect of antacid administration on salicylate kinetics is minimal.

The bioavailability of propranolol was reduced in five people administered 1,200 mg of aluminum hydroxide gel. Investigators were unable to determine the cause of this reduction. The bioavailability of valproic acid increased with a suspension of aluminum hydroxide and magnesium hydroxide, but not with a suspension of calcium carbonate or magnesium trisilicate. The mechanism and significance of this interaction are unknown. Absorption of warfarin is not altered by aluminum hydroxide or magnesium hydroxide antacids, although other coumarin derivatives may be affected.

Gastrointestinal Gas

Almost everyone has experienced the sensation of having too much gas. This condition is usually associated with frequent belching, abdominal bloating and distention, and excessive flatus. People experiencing these symptoms often seek pharmacologic treatment without consulting a physician. Symptoms of excessive gastric gas are often associated with food ingestion. Food sources of gas include carbonated beverages, whipped foods and breads. Faulty eating habits that involve swallowing air while gulping food may produce excessive gastric gas. Chewing gum may also result in swallowing air, which is subsequently expelled as a belch. One or two belches usually produce relief. People complaining of chronic, frequent belching may swallow air before the belch. Air is aspirated into the esophagus and immediately regurgitated. Some aspirated air may enter the stomach

and create a gastric air bubble. In such people, belching produces the gastric air bubble; frequent belching establishes a cycle that exacerbates the symptoms.

Many people complain of a distended or bloated abdomen that they associate with excessive intestinal gas. Studies show that the normal small and large intestine contain a total of 200 mL of gas, and that symptoms of bloating do not result from the presence of larger volumes of gas in the intestine. Bloating and distention may be symptoms of bowel irritation caused by normal quantities of intestinal gas. For people with a frequent bloated sensation, a medical workup is necessary to rule out an organic cause of abdominal symptoms.

Excessive flatus can be embarrassing. Normal flatus volume ranges from 400 to 2,400 mL per day, and 14 passages of gas per day is normal for an adult. Gases passed as flatus originate from three sources: swallowed air, production within the gut and diffusion from the blood into the gut lumen. Swallowed air travels rapidly through the gastrointestinal tract to be released as flatus. Gas can be produced in the gut through neutralization of acid by bicarbonate, resulting in carbon dioxide production. Fat ingestion results in releasing fatty acid in the intestine. Neutralization of this acid by bicarbonate can form significant quantities of carbon dioxide gas. Bacteria in the gut may produce acids when digesting non-absorbable carbohydrates. This process is thought to be the mechanism for flatus production with foods such as beans. Bacteria in the colon may also produce significant quantities of hydrogen gas if sufficient amounts of carbohydrates are present in the colon. This production may occur in people with lactase deficiency or in people who ingest foods (such as legumes) with large quantities of unabsorbable carbohydrates. Bacteria in the gut may also produce methane and other gases, but these gases rarely reach significant volumes. Nitrogen, oxygen and carbon dioxide gases can diffuse from the blood into the lumen of the intestine, although this process is unlikely to cause the symptoms.

Treatment

People who belch frequently should be alerted to the role of swallowing air in producing symptoms. They can reduce intake of carbonated beverages and avoid swallowing air with food when eating. They should closely evaluate the sequence of events before belching to detect the initial aspiration of air into the stomach resulting in the desire to belch. People complaining of only infrequent belching may not require treatment. Defoaming agents, such as simethicone, may provide symptomatic relief from excessive gas.

People complaining of excessive flatus also should avoid swallowing air. If flatus production correlates with particular foods, such as fats or legumes, individuals can avoid these foods or reduce intake. Flatus associated with ingesting milk products may indicate a lactase deficiency and should be evaluated by a physician. The benefit of simethicone in treating excessive flatus is unproven. Activated charcoal administered orally can reduce colonic hydrogen gas, which may be involved in excessive flatus in some people. Convincing proof that any pharmacologic agent is effective in reducing symptoms of excessive intestinal gas is not yet available.

Simethicone

Simethicone is a physiologically inert compound that is not absorbed from the gastrointestinal tract. It alters the elasticity of the interfaces of bubbles, causing them to break or coalesce. This process results in air bubbles that are more easily removed from the stomach

Antacids, Antiflatulents and Antireflux Agents

Figure 4 *Suggested Approach for Treating Gastrointestinal Gas*

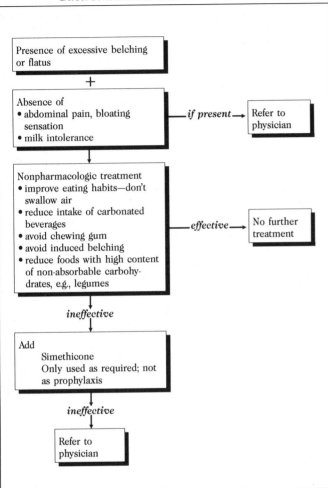

people with medical conditions other than gastrointestinal symptoms. People with hypertension or congestive heart failure should avoid antacid products with a high sodium content. Individuals with renal failure should avoid antacids containing magnesium and high in sodium content. People at risk for hypophosphatemia, such as alcoholics or those with gastrointestinal malabsorption syndromes, should avoid aluminum antacids. Persons at risk of hypercalcemia or hypercalciuria, such as those with malignancies, kidney stones or using thiazide diuretics or vitamin D, should avoid antacids containing calcium.

Q. Are you taking any medications?

■ It is important to establish if the symptoms could be caused by medication ingestion. People taking medications such as ASA or anti-inflammatory drugs should be referred to a physician for assessment of the need for continued therapy and alternative treatment. In addition, the potential for any drug interactions with possible nonprescription therapy should be determined.

Q. Do you prefer liquid or tablet medications?

■ The consumer's preference can be used to guide selection of the best formulation for the individual. Recent clinical trials using tablet formulations have demonstrated symptomatic relief and therapeutic efficacy similar to liquid antacids. The ease of handling and administering tablet products may improve compliance. The tablet antacid formulations should not be considered inferior in efficacy to liquid formulations.

Q. Have you tried any methods to relieve or prevent your heartburn?

■ Symptoms of heartburn may abate by improving posture and altering diet. Coffee, alcohol, chocolate and foods high in fat are all possible causes of heartburn. Smoking should be discontinued. Elevation of the head of the bed and improved sitting posture may reduce the incidence of heartburn.

Q. Is your excessive gas related to eating food?

■ People complaining of excessive intestinal gas should be educated about the roles of eating, swallowing air and carbonated beverages in the development of gastric gas. For people with frequent flatus, a description of normal frequency and volume may be enlightening. If the flatus can be linked to food ingestion (for example, legumes and milk products), these foods should be reduced.

through belching. Gastroscopy evaluation has demonstrated the effectiveness of simethicone in obliterating bubbles in the stomach. Clinically, simethicone was found effective in treating bloating and gas. No clinically relevant drug interactions are yet known to involve simethicone.

Ask The Consumer

Q. How long have you had discomfort? Is it associated with any other symptoms or activities?

■ A person should not attempt or continue self-treatment of gastrointestinal irritation, but should seek medical attention for any of the following: abdominal pain or discomfort associated with exertion or exercise; blood in vomitus or stools; pain radiating to the back, neck, jaw or arms; symptoms increasing in frequency and severity; and symptoms not responding to previously effective treatment.

Q. Do you have any other medical problems or dietary restrictions?

■ The ingredient(s) of the antacid product may be hazardous to

References

Introduction
Graham DY, Smith JL, Patterson DJ. Why do apparently healthy people use antacid tablets? Am J Gastroenterol 1983;78:257–60.

Etiology—Peptic Ulcer Disease
Bartle WR, Gupta AK, Lazor J. Nonsteroidal anti-inflammatory drugs and gastrointestinal bleeding: a case-control study. Arch Intern Med 1986;146: 2365–7.
Bonnevie O. The incidence of duodenal ulcer in Copenhagen county. Scand J Gastroenterol 1975;10:231–9,385–93.
Cameron AJ. Aspirin and gastric ulcer. Mayo Clin Proc 1975;50:565–70.
Conn HO, Blitzer BL. Nonassociation of adrenocorticosteroid therapy and peptic ulcer. N Engl J Med 1976;294:473–9.

Antacids, Antiflatulents and Antireflux Agents

Friedman GD, Siegelaub AB, Seltzer CC. Cigarettes, alcohol, coffee and peptic ulcer. N Engl J Med 1974;290:469–73.

Glupczynski Y, Burette A. Drug therapy for *Helicobacter pylori* infection: problems and pitfalls. Am J Gastroenterol 1990;85:1545–51.

Graham DY, Smith JL. Aspirin and the stomach. Ann Intern Med 1986; 104:390–8.

Hoftiezer JW, Silvoso GR, Burks M, Ivey KJ. Comparison of the effects of regular and enteric-coated aspirin on gastroduodenal mucosa of man. Lancet 1980;2:609–12.

Isenberg JI. Peptic ulcer. DM 1981;28(3):1–58.

Korman MG, Hansky J, Eaves ER, Schmidt GT. Influence of cigarette smoking on healing and relapse in duodenal ulcer disease. Gastroenterology 1983; 85:871–4.

Korman MG, Shaw RG, Hansky J, et al. Influence of smoking on healing rate of duodenal ulcer in response to cimetidine or high-dose antacid. Gastroenterology 1981;80:1451–3.

Kurata JH, Haile BM. Epidemiology of peptic ulcer disease. Clin Gastroenterol 1984;13:289–307.

Langman MJS, Cooke AR. Gastric and duodenal ulcers and their associated diseases. Lancet 1976;1:680–3.

Levy M. Aspirin use in patients with major upper gastrointestinal bleeding and peptic ulcer disease. N Engl J Med 1974;290:1158–62.

Messer J, Reitman D, Sacks H, et al. Association of adrenocorticosteroid therapy and peptic ulcer disease. N Engl J Med 1983;309:21–4.

Petitti DB, Friedman GD, Kahn W. Peptic ulcer disease and the tar and nicotine yield of currently smoked cigarettes. J Chronic Dis 1982;35:503–7.

Petterson WL. *Helicobacter pylori* and peptic ulcer disease. N Engl J Med 1991;324:1043–8.

Pipen JM, Ray WA, Daugherty JR, Griffin MR. Corticosteroid use and peptic ulcer disease: role of nonsteroidal anti-inflammatory drugs. Ann Intern Med 1991;114:735–40.

Piper DW, McIntosh JH, Ariotti DE, et al. Life events and chronic duodenal ulcer a case control study. Gut 1981;22:1011–7.

Siepler JK, Mahakian K, Trudeau WT. Current concepts in clinical therapeutics: peptic ulcer disease. Clin Pharm 1986;5:128–42.

Silvoso GR, Ivey KJ, Butt JH, et al. Incidence of gastric lesions in patients with rheumatic disease on chronic aspirin therapy. Ann Intern Med 1979; 91:517–20.

Somerville KW, Hawkey CJ. Non-steroidal anti-inflammatory agents and the gastrointestinal tract. Postgrad Med J 1986;62:23–8.

Sontag S, Graham DY, Belsito A, et al. Cimetidine, cigarette smoking and recurrence of duodenal ulcers. N Engl J Med 1984;311:689–93.

Spiro HM. Is the steroid ulcer a myth? N Engl J Med 1983;309:45–7.

Pathophysiology—Peptic Ulcer Disease

Ahlquist DA, Dozois RR, Zinsmeister AR, Malagelada JR. Duodenal prostaglandin synthesis and acid load in health and in duodenal ulcer disease. Gastroenterology 1983;85:522–8.

Flemstrom G, Turnberg LA. Gastroduodenal defence mechanisms. Clin Gastroenterol 1984;13:327–54.

Hawkey CJ, Rampton DS. Prostaglandins and the gastrointestinal mucosa: are they important in its function, disease or treatment? Gastroenterology 1985; 89:1162–88.

Lam SK. Pathogenesis and pathophysiology of duodenal ulcer. Clin Gastroenterol 1984;13:447–72.

Malinowska DH, Sacks G. Cellular mechanisms of acid secretion. Clin Gastroenterol 1984;13:309–26.

Robert A. Cytoprotection by prostaglandins. Gastroenterology 1979;77:761–7.

Sontag SJ. Prostaglandins in peptic ulcer disease. Drugs 1986;32:445–57.

Symptoms—Peptic Ulcer Disease

Roth JLA. Clinical aspects of peptic ulcer. In: Berk JE, ed. Gastroenterology. Philadelphia: WB Saunders, 1985:1060–88.

Etiology—Gastroesophageal Reflux

Castell DO. The lower esophageal sphincter: physiologic and clinical aspects. Ann Intern Med 1975;83:390–401.

Christensen J. Effects of drugs on esophageal motility. Arch Intern Med 1976;136:532–7.

Dennish GW, Castell DO. Inhibitory effects of smoking on the lower esophageal sphincter. N Engl J Med 1971;284:1136–7.

Dodds WJ, Dent J, Hogan WJ. Pregnancy and the lower esophageal sphincter. Gastroenterology 1978;74:1334–6.

Hogan WJ, deAndrande SRV, Winship DH. Ethanol-induced acute esophageal motor dysfunction. J Appl Physiol 1972;32:755–60.

Holloway RH, Hongo M, Berger K, McCallum RW. Gastric distention: a mechanism for postprandial gastroesophageal reflux. Gastroenterology 1985; 89:779–84.

Johnson LF, DeMeester TR. Evaluation of elevation of the head of the bed, bethanechol, and antacid foam tablets on gastroesophageal reflux. Dig Dis Sci 1981;26:673–80.

Kaufman SE, Kaye MD. Induction of gastroesophageal reflux by alcohol. Gut 1978;19:336–8.

Lloyd DA, Borda IT. Food-induced heartburn: effect of osmolality. Gastroenterology 1981;80:740–1.

Moosa AR, Skinner DB. Gastroesophageal reflux and hiatal hernia. Ann Roy Coll Surg Engl 1976;58:126–32.

Nebel OT, Castell DO. Lower esophageal sphincter pressure changes after food ingestion. Gastroenterology 1972;63:778–83.

O'Brien TF, Stroop EM. Lower esophageal sphincter pressure and esophageal function in obese humans. J Clin Gastroenterol 1980;2:145–8.

Price SF, Smithson KW, Castell DO. Food sensitivity in reflux esophagitis. Gastroenterology 1978;75:240–3.

Richter JE. A critical review of current medical therapy for gastroesophageal reflux disease. J Clin Gastroenterol 1986;8(Suppl):72–80.

Thomas FB, Steinbaugh JT, Fromkes JJ, et al. Inhibitory effect of coffee on lower esophageal sphincter pressure. Gastroenterology 1980;79:1262–6.

Traube M, McCallum RW. Calcium channel blockers and the gastrointestinal tract. Am J Gastroenterol 1984;79:892–6.

Waterfall WE, Craven MA, Allen CJ. Gastroesophageal reflux: clinical presentations, diagnosis and management. Can Med Assoc J 1986;135:1101–9.

Pathophysiology—Gastroesophageal Reflux

Dodds WJ, Dent J, Hogan WJ, et al. Mechanisms of gastroesophageal reflux in patients with reflux esophagitis. N Engl J Med 1982;307:1547–52.

Dodds WJ, Hogan WJ, Helm JF, Dent J. Pathogenesis of reflux esophagitis. Gastroenterology 1981;81:376–94.

Frazier JL, Fendler KJ. Current concepts in the pathogenesis and treatment of reflux esophagitis. Clin Pharm 1983;2:546–57.

Symptoms—Gastroesophageal Reflux

Skinner DB, Roth JLA, Sullivan BH, et al. Reflux esophagitis. In: Berk JE, ed. Gastroenterology. Philadelphia: WB Saunders, 1985:717–68.

Treatment—Gastric and Duodenal Ulcers

ACG Committee on FDA-related Matters. The use of bismuth in gastroenterology. Am J Gastroenterol 1991;86:16–25.

Barbara L, Corinaldesi R, Rea E, et al. The role of colloidal bismuth subcitrate in the short-term treatment of duodenal ulcer. Scand J Gastroenterol 1986;21(Suppl 122):30–4.

Barnett CC, Richardson CT. In vivo and in vitro evaluation of magnesium-aluminum hydroxide antacid tablets and liquid. Dig Dis Sci 1985;30: 1049–52.

Berstad A, Rydning A, Aaland E, et al. Controlled clinical trial of duodenal ulcer healing with antacid tablets. Scand J Gastroenterol 1982;17:953–9.

Berstad A, Weberg R. Antacids in the treatment of gastroduodenal ulcer. Scand J Gastroenterol 1986;21:385–91.

Brouwers JR, Tytgat GN. Biopharmaceutical properties of liquid and tablet antacids: in vivo studies using the intragastric pH-measurement technique. J Pharm Pharmacol 1978;30:148–51.

Goldenberg MM, HonKomp LJ, Castellion AW. Prevention by bismuth subsalicylate of gastric mucosal lesions in response to noxious stimuli in rats. Pharm Res Commun 1978;10:13–20.

Gorbach SL. Bismuth therapy in gastrointestinal diseases. Gastroenterology 1990; 99:863–75.

Antacids, Antiflatulents and Antireflux Agents

Hailey FJ, Newsom JH. Evaluation of bismuth subsalicylate in relieving symptoms of indigestion. Arch Intern Med 1984;144:269–72.

Hollander D, Tarnawski A. Are antacids cytoprotective? Gut 1989;30:145–7.

Isenberg JI, Peterson WL, Elashoff JD, et al. Healing of benign gastric ulcer with low-dose antacid or cimetidine. N Engl J Med 1983;308:1319–24.

Konturek SJ, Radecki T, Piastucki I, Drozdowicz D. Advances in the understanding of the mechanism of cytoprotective action by colloidal bismuth subcitrate. Scand J Gastroenterol 1986;21(Suppl 122):6–10.

Lam SK, Lam KC, Lai CL, et al. Treatment of duodenal ulcer with antacid and sulpride. Gastroenterology 1979;76:315–22.

Lanza FL, Sibley CM. Role of antacids in the management of disorders of the upper gastrointestinal tract. Review of clinical experience 1975–1985. Am J Gastroenterol 1987;82:1223–41.

MacCara ME, Nugent FJ, Garner JB. Acid neutralization capacity of Canadian antacid formulations. Can Med Assoc J 1985;132:523–7.

Orwoll ES. The milk-alkali syndrome: current concepts. Ann Intern Med 1982;97:242–8.

Peterson WL, Sturdevant RAL, Frankl HD, et al. Healing of duodenal ulcer with an antacid regime. N Engl J Med 1977;297:341–5.

Preclik G, Strange EF, Gerber K, et al. Stimulation of mucosal prostaglandin synthesis in human stomach and duodenum by antacid treatment. Gut 1989;30:148–51.

Rydning A, Weberg R, Lange O, Berstad A. Healing of benign gastric ulcer with low-dose antacids and fiber diet. Gastroenterology 1986;91:56–61.

Stemmer KL. Pharmacology and toxicology of heavy metals: bismuth. Pharm Ther 1976;1:153–5.

Sturdevant RAL, Isenberg JI, Secrist D, Ansfield J. Antacid and placebo produced similar pain relief in duodenal ulcer patients. Gastroenterology 1977;72(1):1–5.

Szelenyi I. Functional cytoprotection by certain antacids. Acta Physiol Hung 1984;64:259–68.

The United States pharmacopeia. Rockville: United States Pharmacopeial Convention, 1979:912.

Thomas JM, Misiewicz G. Histamine H_2-receptor antagonists in the short- and long-term treatment of duodenal ulcer. Clin Gastroenterol 1984;13:501–41.

Thomson ABR, Mahachai V. Medical management of uncomplicated peptic ulcer disease. In: Berk JE, ed. Gastroenterology. Philadelphia: WB Saunders, 1985:1116–54.

Weberg R, Aubert E, Dahlberg O, et al. Low-dose antacids or cimetidine for duodenal ulcer? Gastroenterology 1988;95:1465–9.

Weberg R, Berstad A, Lange O, et al. Duodenal ulcer healing with four antacid tablets daily. Scand J Gastroenterol 1985;20:1041–5.

Sodium Bicarbonate

Brismar B, Strandberg A, Wiklund B. Stomach rupture following ingestion of sodium bicarbonate. Acta Chir Scand 1986;(Suppl 530):97–9.

Walan A. Antacids and anticholinergics in the treatment of duodenal ulcers. Clin Gastroenterol 1984;13:473–99.

Calcium Carbonate

Clemens JD, Feinstein AR. Calcium carbonate and constipation: a historical review of medical mythopoeia. Gastroenterology 1977;72:957–61.

Drinka PJ, Nolten WE. Hazards of treating osteoporosis and hypertension concurrently with calcium, vitamin D, and distal diuretics. J Am Geriatr Soc 1984;32:405–7.

Holtermueller KH, Dehdaschti M. Antacids and hormones. Scand J Gastroenterol 1982;17(Suppl 75):24–31.

Texter EC. A critical look at the clinical use of antacids in acid-peptic disease and gastric acid rebound. Am J Gastroenterol 1989;84:97–108.

Magnesium

Gibaldi M, Grundhofer B, Levy G. Effect of antacid on pH of urine. Clin Pharmacol Ther 1974;16:520–5.

Graber TW, Yee AS, Baker FJ. Magnesium: physiology, clinical disorders and therapy. Ann Emerg Med 1981;10:49–57.

Stroem M. Antacid side-effect on bowel habits. Scand J Gastroenterol 1982;17(Suppl 75):54–5.

Aluminum Hydroxide

Girotti MJ, Ruddan J, Cohanim M. Amphojeloma: antacid impaction in a critically ill patient. Can J Surg 1984;27:379–82.

Harvey SC. Gastric antacids and digestants. In: Gilman AG, Goodman LS, Gilman A, eds. Goodman and Gilman's the pharmacological basis of therapeutics. Toronto: Macmillan, 1980:988–1001.

Vick KE, Johnson CA. Aluminum-related osteomalacia in renal-failure patients. Clin Pharm 1985;4:434–9.

Bismuth Subsalicylate

Ericsson CD, Feldman S, Pickering LK, Cleary TG. Influence of subsalicylate bismuth on the absorption of doxycycline. JAMA 1982;247:2266–7.

Feldman S, Chen SL, Pickering LK, et al. Salicylate absorption from a bismuth subsalicylate preparation. Clin Pharmacol Ther 1981;29:788–92.

Goldenberg MM, Brooks RR, Boise KL. Comparative evaluation of gastrointestinal blood loss in the feces of rats following Pepto-Bismol liquid and aspirin administration. Life Sci 1980;26:1335–42.

Henderson IWD. Warning against products containing bismuth subsalicylate letters. Can Med Assoc J 1980;123:848.

Pickering LK, Feldman S, Ericsson CD, Cleary TG. Absorption of salicylate and bismuth from a bismuth subsalicylate-containing compound (Pepto-Bismol). J Pediatr 1981;99:654–6.

Esophageal Reflux

Graham DY, Lanza F, Dorsh ER. Symptomatic reflux esophagitis. A double-blind controlled comparison of antacids and alginate. Curr Ther Res 1977;22:653–8.

Graham DY, Patterson DJ. Double-blind comparison of liquid antacid and placebo in the treatment of symptomatic reflux esophagitis. Dig Dis Sci 1983;28:559–63.

Grove O, Bekker C, Jeppe-Hansen MG, et al. Ranitidine and high-dose antacid in reflux oesophagitis. Scand J Gastroenterol 1985;20:457–61.

Higgs RH, Smyth RD, Castell DO. Gastric alkalinization effect on lower esophageal-sphincter pressure and serum gastrin. N Engl J Med 1974;291:486–90.

Kitchin LI, Castell DO. Rationale and efficacy of conservative therapy for gastroesophageal reflux disease. Arch Intern Med 1991;151:448–54.

Lanza FL, Smith V, Page-Castell JA, Castell DO. Effectiveness of foaming antacid in relieving induced heartburn. South Med J 1986;79:327–30.

Malmud LS, Charkes ND, Littlefield J, et al. The mode of action of alginic acid compound in the reduction of gastroesophageal reflux. J Nucl Med 1979;20:1023–8.

McHardy G. A multicentric, randomized clinical trial of Gaviscon in reflux esophagitis. South Med J 1978;71(Suppl 1):16–21.

Scobie BA. Endoscopically controlled trial of alginate and antacid in reflux oesophagitis. Med J Aust 1976;1:627–8.

Sontag SJ. The medical management of reflux esophagitis. Role of antacids and acid inhibition. Gastroenterol Clin N Amer 1990;19:683–712.

Stanciu C, Bennett JR. Alginate/antacid in the reduction of gastro-oesophageal reflux. Lancet 1974;1:109–11.

Weberg R, Berstad A. Symptomatic effect of a low-dose antacid regimen in reflux oesophagitis. Scand J Gastroenterol 1989;24:401–6.

Drug Interactions

Ambre JJ, Fischer LJ. Effects of coadministration of aluminum and magnesium hydroxides on absorption of anticoagulants in man. Clin Pharmacol Ther 1972;14:231–7.

Barzaghi N, Gatti G, Crema F, Perucca E. Impaired bioavailability of famotidine given concurrently with a potent antacid. J Clin Pharmacol 1989;29:670–2.

Brown DD, Juhl RP. Decreased bioavailability of digoxin due to antacids and kaolin-pectin. N Engl J Med 1976;295:1034–7.

Cacek AT. Review of alterations in oral phenytoin bioavailability associated with formulations, antacids, and food. Ther Drug Monit 1986;8:166–71.

Dobbs JH, Skoutakis VA, Acchiardo SR, Dobbs BR. Effects of aluminum hydroxide on the absorption of propranolol. Curr Ther Res 1977;21:887–92.

Donn KH, Eshelman FN, Plachetka JR, et al. The effects of antacid and propantheline on the absorption of oral ranitidine. Pharmacotherapy 1984;4:89–92.

Antacids, Antiflatulents and Antireflux Agents

Ekenved G, Halvorsen L, Solvell L. Influence of a liquid antacid on the absorption of different iron salts. Scand J Haematol 1976;28(Suppl):65–77.

Feldman S, Carlstedt BC. Effect of antacid on absorption of enteric-coated aspirin. JAMA 1974;227(6):660–1.

Flor S, Guay DRP, Opsahl JA, Tack K, Matzke GR. Effects of magnesium-aluminum hydroxide and calcium carbonate antacids on bioavailability of ofloxacin. Antimicrob Agents Chemother 1990;34:2436–8.

Garty M, Hurwitz A. Effect of cimetidine and antacids on gastrointestinal absorption of tetracycline. Clin Pharmacol Ther 1980;28:203–7.

Gerhardt RE, Knouss RF, Thyrum PT, et al. Quinidine excretion in aciduria and alkalinuria. Ann Intern Med 1969;71:927–33.

Grasela TH, Schentag JJ, Sedman AJ, et al. Inhibition of enoxacin absorption by antacids or ranitidine. Antimicrob Agents Chemother 1989;33:615–7.

Gugler R, Allgayer H. Effects of antacids on the clinical pharmacokinetics of drugs. Clin Pharmacokinet 1990;18:210–9.

Hurwitz A. Antacid therapy and drug kinetics. Clin Pharmacokinet 1977;2:269–80.

Hurwitz A, Scholman DL. Effects of antacids on gastrointestinal absorption of isoniazid in rat and man. Am Rev Respir Dis 1974;109:41–7.

Jonkman JHG, Upton RA. Pharmacokinetic drug interactions with theophylline. Clin Pharmacokinet 1984;9:309–34.

Kraynak Roush M, Dupuis R. Significance of the ciprofloxacin-antacid interaction. DICP 1991;25:473–5.

Lalka D, Meyer MB, Duce BR, Elvin AT. Kinetics of the oral antiarrhythmic lidocaine congener, tocainide. Clin Pharmacol Ther 1976;19:757–66.

Madias NE, Levey AS. Metabolic alkalosis due to absorption of "nonabsorbable" antacids. Am J Med 1983;74:155–8.

Mantyla R, Mannisto PT, Vuorela A, et al. Impairment of captopril bioavailability by concomitant food and antacid intake. Int J Clin Pharmacol Ther Tox 1984;22:626–9.

May CA, Garnett WR, Small RE, Pellock JM. Effects of three antacids on the bioavailability of valproic acid. Clin Pharm 1982;1:244–7.

Nix DE, Watson WA, Lener ME, et al. Effects of aluminum and magnesium antacids and ranitidine on the absorption of ciprofloxacin. Clin Pharm Ther 1989;46:700–5.

Nix DE, Wilton JH, Ronald B, et al. Inhibition of norfloxacin absorption by antacids. Antimicrob Agents Chemother 1990;34:432–5.

Remon JP, Belpaire F, Van Severen R, Braeckman P. Interaction of antacids with antiarrhythmics. Arzneimittelforsch 1983;33:117–20.

Romankiewicz JA, Rerdenberg M, Drayer D, Franklin JE. The noninterference of aluminum hydroxide gel with quinidine sulfate absorption: an approach to control quinidine-induced diarrhea. Am Heart J 1978;96:518–20.

Segre EJ, Sevelins H, Varady J. Effects of antacids on naproxen absorption. N Engl J Med 1974;291:582–3.

Shastri RA. Effect of antacid on salicylate kinetics. Int J Clin Pharmacol Ther Tox 1985;23:480–4.

Shelly DW, Doering PL, Russell WL, et al. Effect of concomitant antacid administration on plasma cimetidine concentrations during repetitive dosing. Drug Intell Clin Pharm 1986;20:792–5.

Thorpe JE, Baker N, Bromet-petit M. Effect of oral antacid administration on the pharmacokinetics of oral fluconazole. Antimicrob Agents Chemother 1990;34:2032–3.

Tobert JA, DeSchepper P, Tjandramaja TB, et al. Effect of antacids on the bioavailability of diflunisal in the fasting and postprandial states. Clin Pharmacol Ther 1981;30:385–9.

Van der Meer JWM, Keuning JJ, Scheijgrond HW, et al. The influence of gastric acidity on the bioavailability of ketoconazole. J Antimicrob Chemother 1980;6:552–4.

Walan A. Metabolic side-effects and interactions. Scand J Gastroenterol 1982;17(Suppl 75):63–8.

Gastrointestinal Gas

Levitt MD, Bond JH. Flatulence. Ann Rev Med 1980;31:127–37.

Levitt MD. Excessive gas: patient perception vs reality. Hosp Pract 1985;20(11):143–63.

Pelligrino PC, Silberner HB. Management of gastroenteric gas syndromes. Am J Gastroenterol 1961;36:450–8.

Tomlin J, Lowis C, Read NW. Investigation of normal flatus production in healthy volunteers. Gut 1991;32:665–9.

Treatment—Gastrointestinal Gas

Bernstein JE, Kasich AM. A double-blind trial of simethicone in functional disease of the upper gastrointestinal tract. J Clin Pharmacol 1974;14:617–23.

Fardy J, Sullivan S. Gastrointestinal gas. Can Med Assoc J 1988;139:1137–41.

Jain NK, Patel VP, Pitchumoni CS. Activated charcoal, simethicone, and intestinal gas: a double-blind study. Ann Intern Med 1986;105:61–2.

Rider JA, Moeller HC. Use of silicone in the treatment of intestinal gas and bloating. JAMA 1960;174:2052–4.

Rider AJ. Experience with the use of a defoaming agent in the treatment of gastrointestinal gas. Ann NY Acad Sci 1968;150:170–7.

Van Ness MM, Cattau EL. Flatulence: pathophysiology and treatment. Am Fam Physician 1985;31(4):198–206.

16
Emetics and Antiemetics

Keith Simons

Nausea and vomiting have numerous causes. Emesis, or induced vomiting, is most often done using ipecac syrup. Other emetics are less effective or unsafe. Motion sickness and adverse effects of overindulgence are the only conditions suitable for self-medication with antiemetics. Antiemetics include antihistamines (dimenhydrinate, promethazine, trimethobenzamide and cinnarizine), the anticholinergic drug scopolamine, phosphorated carbohydrate solution and bismuth subsalicylate.

Emetics are used to induce vomiting, primarily when potentially harmful or unknown substances have been ingested, or following drug overdoses. Antiemetics are used to prevent or control nausea and vomiting, which can be the symptoms of various diseases, the result of ingesting foreign substances or the outcome of well documented stimuli. Although vomiting is an important defence mechanism for ridding the body of a variety of poisons and toxins, it may also indicate a serious adverse drug reaction, be a nuisance when travelling or be extremely debilitating when induced by pregnancy.

Nausea is the imminent desire to vomit, usually experienced in the throat or epigastrium; vomiting (emesis) is the forceful oral expulsion of stomach contents; retching is the intense, rhythmic hyperventilation and abdominal spasm that usually precedes emesis; regurgitation is the eruption of stomach contents into the esophagus and mouth without oral expulsion.

Vomiting usually occurs after severe nausea and a series of retching motions. A forceful contraction of the diaphragm and abdominal musculature occurs, producing an increase in intrathoracic and intra-abdominal pressure that compresses the stomach and raises esophageal pressure. The body of the stomach and the esophageal musculature relax so the increased pressure can move the gastric contents into the esophagus and mouth.

Several cycles of reflux into the esophagus occur before vomiting takes place. Vomitus is expelled from the esophagus by a combination of increased intrathoracic pressure and reversal of the normal peristaltic waves of the esophagus. The reflex closure of the glottis over the trachea usually prevents the vomitus from entering the airways, and the reflex elevation of the soft palate keeps the vomitus out of the nasopharynx. The force of ejection of vomitus from the mouth is mainly provided by the abdominal musculature.

The act of vomiting is controlled by the vomiting centre in the medulla oblongata (see Figure 1). When the vomiting centre is stimulated, vomiting is induced by transmission through the following

efferent nerve pathways: the phrenic nerves to the diaphragm; the spinal nerves to the abdominal musculature; and the visceral nerves to the stomach and esophagus.

The vomiting centre receives its stimuli from the chemoreceptor

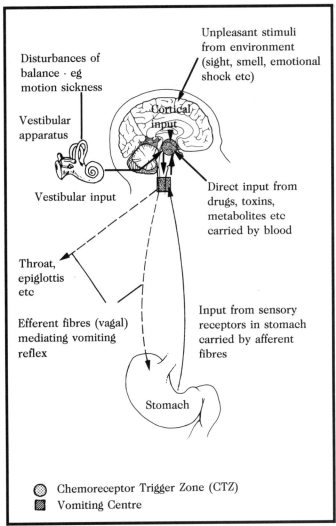

Figure 1 *The Afferent Connections of the Vomiting Centre*

Emetics and Antiemetics

trigger zone (CTZ) on the surface of the medulla close to the vagal nuclei, or from higher cortical centres such as the labyrinthine apparatus, or from the intestinal tract, or from other parts of the body such as the eyes or nose. The CTZ can be stimulated by centrally acting emetics such as apomorphine, morphine and the cardiac glycosides as well as certain chemotherapeutic agents, resulting in emesis. The antiemetic effects of centrally acting drugs such as the phenothiazines work by inhibiting the CTZ as well as the vomiting centre.

Although the cause of morning sickness in pregnancy has not been clearly established, increased levels of chorionic gonadotropin, estrogens or both, which are maximal during the first trimester of pregnancy, have been implicated. About 50 per cent of all pregnant women experience nausea, and about 30 per cent of these women suffer vomiting as well.

The central nervous system mechanisms involved with motion sickness are not completely understood. Physiologically, motion sickness appears to result from overstimulation of the labyrinth of the vestibular apparatus—the three semicircular canals on each side of the head in the inner ear—responsible for maintaining equilibrium. Under normal conditions, movement of the fluid in the semicircular canals generates nerve impulses to the brain so postural adjustments can be made. Unusual motion patterns in which the head is rotated in two axes simultaneously may induce nausea and vomiting.

Pharmacologically, competitive neural systems may be involved with motion sickness, one activated by acetylcholine and one probably mediated by norepinephrine. Motion sickness occurs when activation of the acetylcholine system disturbs the balance of these two neural systems. The anticholinergic motion sickness drugs antagonize the acetylcholine system, thus inhibiting motion sickness.

Some extremely susceptible individuals experience motion sickness by merely watching a film taken from a roller coaster or an airplane doing acrobatics. This situation is intensified by the I-Max Theatre Films. The stimulation of the vomiting centre in these circumstances appears to come from the visual senses.

The general population can be divided into about one-third highly susceptible individuals, one-third who react only to fairly rough conditions and a final third who become sick only under extreme conditions. Only deaf subjects with vestibular deficiencies are totally immune to motion sickness.

Nausea and vomiting may be induced by stimulating the sensory nerve endings in the stomach and duodenum. Overindulgence of food and alcohol may cause heartburn, eructation, stomach pain and flatulence and may even progress to nausea and vomiting. An unpleasant sight, taste or smell may be the only stimulus necessary. After ingesting one or more drugs or foreign chemicals, the medullary vomiting centre may be stimulated by gastric irritation (see Figure 1).

Nausea and vomiting may also accompany diarrhea associated with viral gastroenteritis. This may also occur in conjunction with acute respiratory tract infections with accompanying fever. In young children and geriatric individuals, excessive bronchial congestion and severe coughing spells may conclude with vomiting.

Finally, nausea and vomiting may be symptoms of severe diverse disorders, such as acute appendicitis, cholecystitis, migraine headache, cardiac diseases or drugs used to treat cardiac diseases, food allergy, radiation therapy, cancer chemotherapy, or more serious metabolic and endocrine disorders. The individual should be referred to a physician if the cause of nausea or vomiting cannot be identified (for example, motion sickness or overindulgence of food or alcohol); if the suspected cause is infection, pregnancy, or drug therapy; or if the condition has persisted for more than two or three days.

Emetics

Emetics are used to induce vomiting after ingesting potentially harmful or unknown substances. The information and training necessary to treat poisoning are beyond the scope of this chapter. (See the chapter on poisoning and overdose.) Unless a pharmacist is the local poison control consultant with special training in this area, all such emergency calls should be referred to the local poison control centre. If inducing emesis is the treatment of choice, the pharmacist should be able to recommend an emetic and describe appropriate use of such treatment. Continuing communication and follow-up with the poison control specialist is of utmost importance until the individual is considered out of danger (see Figure 2).

Ipecac Syrup

Ipecac syrup is made from a natural product, powdered ipecac, which is the powdered, dried rhizome and roots of *Cephaelis ipecacuanha* or *Cephaelis acuminata*. It contains from 123 to 157 mg/100 mL of the total ether-soluble alkaloids of ipecac, of which greater than

Figure 2 *Suggested Approach for Using Emetics*

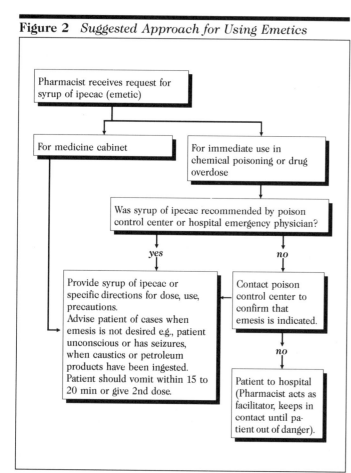

Emetics and Antiemetics

90 per cent are either emetine or cephaeline. Ipecac induces vomiting by local irritation of the gastrointestinal mucosa and by stimulating the CTZ.

The dosage of ipecac syrup is as follows: for adults and children over one year, 15 or 30 mL (the lower dose is usually adequate) with 240 to 480 mL of water depending on age; infants 9 to 11 months, 10 mL, preceded or followed by 120 to 240 mL of water; infants 6 to 8 months, 5 mL. Recent evidence shows that infants over 8 months may safely be given 15 mL. If vomiting does not occur after 30 minutes, the dose may be repeated in individuals over the age of one year. Since ipecac does not work well if the stomach is empty, the dose should be followed by the appropriate volume of water. Ambulatory individuals seem to be affected more quickly, and stimulating the posterior pharynx may help. Ipecac should not be administered to children less than one year of age without medical supervision since they do not have a well developed gag reflex. Ipecac syrup is available in 15 or 30 mL dose containers.

Ipecac syrup is 90 to 100 per cent effective, although time for emesis may be as long as 30 minutes. Even ipecac syrup past the expiry date by one month to greater than four years was 100-percent effective in a study involving 200 people, with 90 per cent of the participants vomiting after the first dose. The mean time to emesis was 24.7 minutes, the same as a control group of 200 people given unexpired drug.

Although its use is debatable, ipecac syrup has been shown to be effective even when antiemetics, for example, phenothiazines, are ingested. Milk has been shown to delay vomiting, but the effect of other protein-containing substances that might be in the stomach when ipecac is given is not known. The only well documented drug interaction involves the concurrent administration of activated charcoal and syrup of ipecac. The ipecac is adsorbed by the charcoal, and emesis is prevented while the adsorptive capacity of the charcoal is reduced. If both compounds must be used, the charcoal should be administered after emesis is induced by the ipecac.

Emesis is contraindicated if the individual has ingested caustic substances, because the esophagus is then exposed again to the caustic agent. Emesis is also contraindicated if petroleum distillates are ingested, as these agents can cause pulmonary edema or lipid pneumonia. When greater than 1 mL/kg of petroleum distillates has been ingested, ipecac syrup has been used successfully, but only under close medical supervision. Emesis is contraindicated if the individual is unconscious, expected to become lethargic within 30 minutes (for example, with a tricyclic antidepressant overdose) or having a seizure, as aspiration would inevitably occur.

The value of ipecac syrup in cases of poisoning has been questioned. The results of several studies using magnesium hydroxide, acetaminophen, aminophylline, tetracycline and salicylate as challenge agents, demonstrate that ipecac syrup given immediately before or within 30 minutes of ingesting these compounds does not cause significant recovery of the agent in the vomitus nor reduce drug absorption. In contrast, the efficacy and extent of absorption of Ipecac Syrup, USP was evaluated in dogs using acetaminophen and kanamycin as marker drugs. Recovery of acetaminophen and kanamycin in the vomitus was 42 to 50 per cent and 52 to 60 per cent respectively, while the maximum serum concentrations and area under the serum concentration versus time curves were reduced by 50 to 60 per cent when compared to values obtained following placebo emetic. Cephaeline recovery in the vomitus, as a marker of the amount of ipecac absorbed, was 41 per cent, indicating that the emetic effect was probably a result of both gastric irritation and stimulation of the CTZ. The efficacy of ipecac syrup as an emetic is not questioned, but it is recommended that in severe cases of poisoning, the individual be given activated charcoal after emesis.

Ipecac syrup is an efficient and rapidly acting emetic that only rarely produces serious sequelae. Administering 30 mL of ipecac syrup to individuals more than one year of age is safe. The only side effects observed are diarrhea and slight central nervous system depression, although prolonged vomiting may occur in some cases.

Severe toxicity and death have occurred after ingesting ipecac liquid extract that was mistaken for ipecac syrup. The liquid extract contains 14 times the alkaloid content of ipecac syrup. Symptoms were cardiovascular toxicity, including bradycardia and atrial fibrillation and hypotension.

Ipecac syrup has been used chronically by persons suffering from anorexia nervosa, and myopathies have been reported in some cases. This dangerous practice has prompted many debates on the extent of warnings required on product labels, and on regulations ensuring that pharmacists participate in all sales of ipecac syrup, allowing close monitoring of ipecac distribution and use and the control or prevention of abuse. (See the chapter on eating disorders.)

Other Emetics

Ipecac syrup is the only safe and effective nonprescription emetic. However, vomiting may be induced by a number of other compounds.

Apomorphine hydrochloride produces rapid emesis after a 0.1 mg/kg dose (maxiumum 10 mg) administered subcutaneously or intramuscularly. Since this emetic is more effective when the stomach is full, 200 to 300 mL of water should be administered just before the injection. Apomorphine acts by stimulating the CTZ. Naloxone 0.01 mg/kg is often given soon afterward to reverse any possible central nervous system and respiratory depression or to terminate protracted vomiting. For these reasons, naloxone must always be available when apomorphine is used. Indications for apomorphine are identical to ipecac syrup. It is as effective as ipecac syrup and may have a more rapid onset of action, but ipecac is considered safer and the emetic of first choice.

Copper sulfate produces emesis by irritating the gastric mucosa, which in turn stimulates the vomiting centre (see Figure 1). The emetic dose of 0.3 to 0.6 g was last reported in the 1953 *British Pharmacopoeia*. Poor recovery of doses of copper sulfate in the vomitus (54 to 67 per cent) and increased serum copper levels are indications that this agent should not be used.

Zinc sulfate as an emetic was last reported in the 1953 *British Pharmacopoeia*. The emetic dose was reported as 0.6 to 2 g every 15 minutes until emesis occurs. The lethal adult dose is about 15 g and if emesis does not occur, the zinc sulfate and the toxic agent must be removed by gastric lavage. The use of zinc sulfate as an emetic is not recommended.

Antimony and potassium tartrate (or sodium tartrate) was last listed as tartar emetic in the 1953 *British Pharmacopoeia* and the *United States Pharmacopoeia XVI*. The emetic dose listed was 30 to 60 mg orally. Tartar emetic induces vomiting by gastric irritation. This agent is considered too toxic for routine use and is not readily available in the home.

Sodium chloride as salt water (20 g or 15 mL in 250 mL of warm water), although listed as an emetic, may be toxic due to sodium absorption. Severe hypernatremia and death have occurred when vomiting was not produced. Salt water should not be used as an emetic under any circumstances.

Black mustard was listed as one of the compounds that induces vomiting. An emetic dose of 10 g should induce vomiting by gastric irritation. It is considered unpalatable and unreliable. Mustard water, prepared by dispersing powdered mustard in water, is also unsatisfactory.

Mechanical stimulation may also induce emesis. The individual is given fluids (about 180 to 240 mL of water) and gagged by gently stroking the pharynx with a blunt object (for example, a finger or the nonbristle end of a toothbrush) to stimulate the vagal sensory nerve endings. Care must be taken not to injure the person (especially a child) with this procedure. The person's body is inverted to be face down, with the head lower than the body but supported, and the feet elevated. Although this method is universally available, only a few people vomit with this procedure, and the volume of vomitus is small compared to that obtained with ipecac syrup.

Liquid dishwashing detergents (not laundry or dishwasher detergents, which may contain caustics) have been evaluated as emetics by some investigators due to lack of availability of ipecac syrup in pharmacies. In 11 out of 15 people aged 1 to 23 years who drank all or part of the prescribed solution (40 mL of detergent in 225 mL of water), 10 vomited with a mean time of emesis of 6.5 minutes (range 1 to 20 minutes). If emesis is indicated for treating drug overdose or poisoning and ipecac syrup is not available, liquid detergents seem to be a method of choice if mechanical stimulation is unsuccessful.

Antiemetics

Nausea and vomiting may be symptoms of serious organic disturbances or they may be produced by ingesting food or drugs; radiation; painful stimuli; emotional disturbances; or motion. The pharmacist must be cautious about initiating self-medication therapy for nausea and vomiting. There are many instances where supportive therapy (for example, replacing fluids and not eating solid foods) is all that is necessary until the nausea or vomiting disappears. Nonprescription antiemetic drugs should be recommended by pharmacists only to alleviate motion sickness. Careful questioning can elicit whether the situation is self-limiting and not dangerous and/or whether a physician should be consulted.

Vomiting in newborn infants should be immediately referred to a physician, as it may be the result of serious abnormalities that can be aggravated by rapidly occurring dehydration, and electrolyte and acid-base imbalance. However, the pharmacist should be able to differentiate between the infant who spits and vomits chronically and the infant who is experiencing severe, uncontrolled emesis.

There are no acceptable data on the effects of nonprescription antiemetics on vomiting with gastroenteritis. Some authors suggest that vomiting in gastroenteritis is a bodily defence that, often along with diarrhea, helps eliminate the pathogen or chemical toxic agent. In most instances, the vomiting is acute but self-limiting. Restricting solid food and increasing fluid intake may be the only treatment measures required. However, individuals in whom even a slight electrolyte imbalance may be critical, such as infants, should be referred to a physician.

Nausea may be described to the pharmacist as "upset stomach" or "tummy ache." This condition, as well as being a symptom of gastroenteritis, may be the result of overindulgence with food or alcohol.

Careful questioning can determine if hyperacidity or constipation is the possible cause. The condition could then be treated by recommending bismuth subsalicylate or other appropriate products. (See the chapters on antacids and on laxatives.)

Nausea and vomiting may be the earliest indications of pregnancy. However, this fact is so well known that women usually self-diagnose, especially if a missed menstrual cycle and weight gain are also present. Dietary management should be attempted before medication is considered. The woman can try drinking or eating only small amounts at a time and limiting herself to bland foods, such as bouillon or consommé, at difficult times. Soda crackers and a caffeine-free soft drink often relieve nausea. Only exceptionally severe cases require medication. Physicians usually approach treatment of morning sickness cautiously because of concern about the possible teratogenic effects of many drugs. Pharmacists should discourage the use of nonprescription antiemetics in pregnancy.

Since nausea and vomiting are common adverse effects of drugs, the individual's medication history should be reviewed if these symptoms are present or persistent. Under these circumstances, antiemetic therapy should not be initiated without the approval of a physician. The symptoms may be so severe that withdrawing the medication may be indicated if alternative therapy is available. However, the decision to discontinue therapy must be made on the basis of each agent, and in all cases the physician must be notified.

Motion Sickness

Motion sickness is a reaction of the central nervous system to stimulation of the vestibular apparatus. In the vestibular nuclei and reticular areas, neurons responsive to noradrenaline are intermingled with those responsive to acetylcholine. Some of the effective drugs block acetylcholine and others activate noradrenaline. The severity of motion sickness symptoms seem to result from the competing neural populations. Those mediated by acetylcholine appear to be responsible for the increase in activity resulting from vestibular stimulation, which builds up to activate the vomiting centre. Neurons responding to noradrenaline possibly produce a stabilizing influence that resists the development of motion sickness. The proper use of antimotion-sickness drugs can ensure the balance between these neuron groups is maintained to reduce symptoms of motion sickness.

Nondrug Treatment

Nondrug treatment of motion sickness includes the following recommendations. Individuals should position themselves where there is least motion, for example, amidship or over the wings in airplanes. A supine or semirecumbent position with the head braced is best. Reading should be avoided. Keeping the axis of vision at an angle of 45° above the horizontal line reduces the susceptibility of the labyrinth to motion. Excessive consumption of food or alcohol before or during travel should be avoided. If nourishment is required during extended periods of travel, small amounts of fluid and simple food should be ingested at frequent intervals; if the trip is of short duration, total abstention from food and beverage intake should be considered.

Pharmaceutical Agents

Agents proven effective in treating motion sickness include scopolamine (usually in combination with amphetamine), cyclizine, meclizine, promethazine and dimenhydrinate. Dimenhydrinate, promethazine and scopolamine are nonprescription drugs (see Figure 3).

Figure 3 *Suggested Approach for Using Antiemetics*

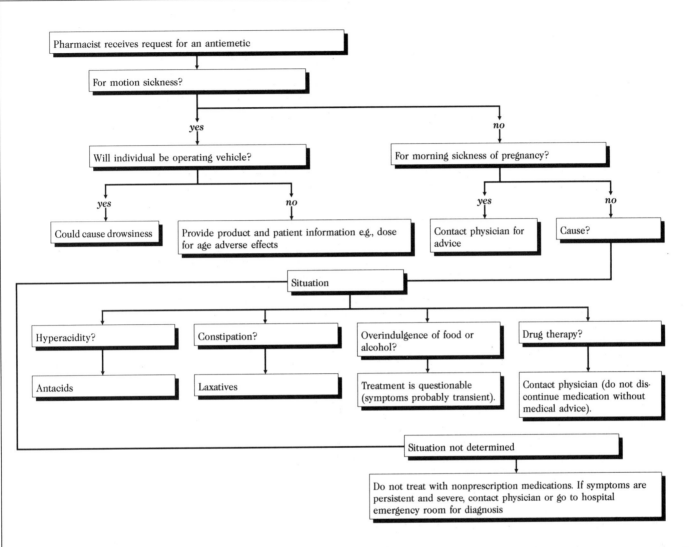

H₁-Receptor Antagonists

The mechanism of action of the H₁-receptor antagonists may be due to their anticholinergic effects.

Dimenhydrinate is the 8-chlorotheophyllinate salt of diphenhydramine. Both dimenhydrinate and diphenhydramine are effective antiemetics for motion sickness (diphenhydramine to a lesser extent). Usual adult doses of both drugs are 50 to 100 mg, 30 to 60 minutes before departure; then 2 to 4 times daily while travelling. Even though dimenhydrinate is only about 50 per cent diphenhydramine by molecular weight, similar doses of dimenhydrinate are more effective than diphenhydramine. Also, diphenhydramine is more sedating than most antihistamines. The recommended dose of dimenhydrinate for children six to eight years is 12.5 to 25 mg, up to three times daily. For children eight to twelve years, the dose is 25 to 50 mg, up to three times daily. Children over 12 years of age may receive 50 mg of dimenhydrinate three times daily. When severe vomiting prevents oral administration, suppositories should be administered. Dimenhydrinate should not be stocked for open patient access since there is evidence that it has become a drug of abuse.

Promethazine is the most effective antihistamine for treating motion sickness, but it causes marked drowsiness. It has the strongest central anticholinergic action of the drugs in this group. The normal adult dose is 20 to 100 mg per 24 hours in divided doses, with the highest dose at bedtime. The dose for infants up to one year of age is 5 to 20 mg per 24 hours according to age. For children 1 to 12 years of age, the dose is 20 to 40 mg per 24 hours, according to age. For long journeys, the dose may be halved and given every 12 hours. Recent studies have shown that promethazine depresses the arousal and respiratory mechanisms in children, inducing apneas during sleep. This information supports the hypothesis that there might be a relationship between the administration of central nervous system depressant drugs to infants and sudden infant death syndrome. The manufacturer has therefore recommended that promethazine-containing products not be administered to children less than two years of age.

Emetics and Antiemetics

Trimethobenzamide for preventing motion sickness has been questioned by some investigators, although it has been shown effective in treating nausea and vomiting due to antineoplastic chemotherapy. This drug is no longer commercially available in Canada.

Cinnarizine, a piperazine derivative, appears to antagonize the stimulated influx of calcium ions from the endolymph into the vestibular sensory cells, preventing motion sickness. An average adult dose of 15 mg three times daily prevented seasickness in several experimental studies. Extrapyramidal reactions, which disappeared when the drugs were discontinued, have been reported in five people who received cinnarizine in combination with flunarizine. Cinnarizine is an American product and is not commercially available in Canada.

Astemizole and **terfenadine** are second-generation, non-sedating H_1-receptor antagonists which have minimal central nervous system effects and no detectable anticholinergic activity. Astemizole 10 or 20 mg daily was useful in treating patients with chronic vertigo. Using the Staircase Profile Test and a 100 ft/lb rotator/chair at the Johnson Space Centre to induce motion sickness symptoms, astemizole, 30 mg daily had no effect, but terfenadine 300 mg was found to be effective in reducing motion sickness symptoms. Since these doses are higher than recommended by the manufacturer and these compounds are not yet approved for treatment of motion sickness, they should not be recommended without the direction of a physician. These H_1-receptor antagonists are known to act peripherally and possess no anticholinergic activity. Therefore the results of these studies raise additional questions regarding the etiology of motion sickness, the associated autonomic system dysfunction and the validity of assumptions that effective pharmacological agents must act centrally.

Since these drugs are H_1-receptor antagonists, the adverse effects and drug interactions common to that class of drugs are experienced. Even at recommended doses, drowsiness, vertigo and dry mouth occur; people driving or operating machinery should receive appropriate warnings. Individuals with narrow-angle glaucoma or prostatic hypertrophy may experience worsening of their symptoms.

The cholinergic-blocking effect of many H_1-receptor antagonists has an additive effect on anticholinergic drugs (for example, tricyclic antidepressants). This effect may also antagonize the miotic effect of anticholinesterase drugs (for example, neostigmine). Some H_1-receptor antagonists enhance the cardiovascular effects of epinephrine and norepinephrine (noradrenaline). The most clinically significant interaction is the additive sedative effect of H_1-receptor antagonists used with alcohol, hypnotics, narcotics or tranquillizers. Diphenhydramine may reduce the absorption of P-aminosalicylic acid.

Anticholinergic Drugs

Scopolamine's (l-hyoscine) prophylactic use for preventing motion sickness is well established, although there is no evidence of its efficacy when given to people who already feel sick. Scopolamine is thought to act on both the vomiting centre and the vestibular system.

A nonprescription dosage form takes advantage of the efficient absorption of transdermally administered scopolamine. The product is composed of a flexible disc of 2.5 cm² with an adhesive surface. It consists of a film 0.2 mm thick, made up of four layers: a backing

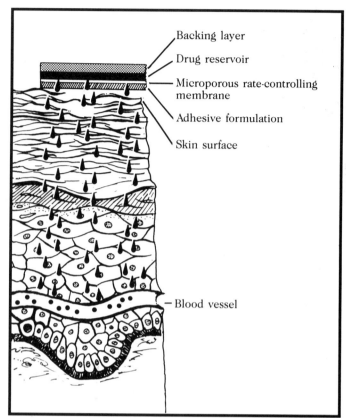

Figure 4 *Schematic Drawing Showing Cross-Section of the Skin Surface with Transdermal Delivery of the Drug Scopolamine*

layer of polyester film; a drug reservoir of scopolamine, mineral oil and polyisobutylene; a polypropylene membrane that controls the rate of delivery of scopolamine; and an adhesive formulation containing mineral oil, polyisobutylene and scopolamine (see Figure 4).

The disc delivers 1 mg of scopolamine over a three-day period. It is applied with clean, dry hands to a nonhairy area behind the ear 12 hours before exposure to motion. The disc should not be placed over cuts or abrasions. It is essential to wash the hands meticulously to remove any medication after applying the disc. If greater than 72-hour use is desired, the first disc is removed and the second placed on a different region behind the same ear or behind the opposite ear.

The effectiveness of transdermal scopolamine has been evaluated in people exposed to experimentally induced motion sickness by a variety of apparatus, and in ships at sea in weather ranging from calm to five-metre seas with two-metre swells (very rough seas). Transdermal scopolamine, in doses of 5 mcg/hr (one patch) and 10 mcg/hr (two patches) applied 4 to 16 hours before motion, has been administered alone, and in combination with oral ephedrine in doses of 12.5, 25 and 50 mg. It has been compared to dimenhydrinate 100 mg, lidocaine 100 mg intravenously followed by infusion of 2 mg/min, tocainide 250 mg intravenously followed by infusion of 17 mg/min for 30 minutes, meclizine 25 mg orally, and placebo patches and tablets. Transdermal scopolamine was significantly more effective than placebo and meclizine. The addition of oral ephedrine, at any dose, did not significantly improve the effectiveness of scopolamine. Lidocaine and tocainide provided no protection against motion sickness. Transdermal scopolamine was not significantly better than

The image labels read:
- Backing layer
- Drug reservoir
- Microporous rate-controlling membrane
- Adhesive formulation
- Skin surface
- Blood vessel

The Drug Caution Program

The Drug Caution Program as a counselling tool encourages communication between the health care professional and the consumer. Nonprescription medication can be potentially dangerous if taken incorrectly. In some disease states and in combination with other prescription and nonprescription drugs, nonprescription medication can also be harmful. The Drug Caution Program recognizes the need for greater consumer education in the area of self-medication. It provides consumers at the time of purchase of nonprescription medication, important information in a readily available and easily understood manner.

The program's mechanics involve alphabetically listing, on a large poster within the pharmacy, the most important precautions involving nonprescription medication. Products carry an alphabetical code on a special green sticker which identifies the specific Drug Caution Code that applies to the medication. A brochure that duplicates the information on the poster is available to consumers for home reference. As well, consumers are encouraged to seek further information from the pharmacist should they have any questions. Following are the code letters and the precaution they represent.

A	**Antihistamines** **Codeine**	may cause drowsiness. Consult you pharmacist if you intend to drive a motorized vehicle or operate hazardous machinery. Avoid alcohol and drugs with sedative and/or relaxing effects.
B	**Decongestants**	consult your pharmacist if you have glaucoma, diabetes, hypertension (high blood pressure), hyperthyroidism (goiter), prostate trouble, or if you take antidepressant drugs.
C	**Iron** **Antacids** **Saline laxatives** **Calcium supplements**	consult your pharmacist if you take tetracycline or related antibiotics.
D	**Acetylsalicylic acid**	contains acetylsalicylic acid (ASA). Consult your pharmacist if you have gout or use anticoagulant drugs (blood-thinners). Consult your pharmacist before giving this drug to children or adolescents (Reye's syndrome). Consult your pharmacist if you have stomach ulcers or a sensitive stomach.
E	**Sugar-containing preparations** **Wart removers** **Vitamin C**	consult your pharmacist if you are diabetic.
H	**Nasal and ophthalmic topical decongestants** **Laxatives** **Codeine**	prolonged use may be habit forming.
I	**Sugar substitutes** **Effervescent products**	consult your pharmacist if you are on a sodium restricted diet (low salt).

The Drug Caution Program *(Cont'd)*

J	**Mineral oil** **Bulk-forming laxatives** **Antidiarrheals** **Fiber products**	prolonged use of this product may alter the effect of other drugs and interfere with their effectiveness.
L	**Iron** **Acetaminophen** **Ibuprofen** **Acetylsalicylic acid**	keep out of the reach of children. A large dose may be dangerous to them.
M	**Antacids** **Antidiarrheals**	consult your pharmacist if your take digoxin (Lanoxin).
P	**Anticholinergics and ophthalmic topical decongestants** **Antihistamines (classical)**	consult your pharmacist if you have glaucoma.
S	**Vitamin A and D** **Calcium supplements with vitamin D**	do not exceed recommended dosage; taken over a long period of time in large doses, it produces harmful results.
X	**Miscellaneous** • **Acetaminophen** • **Antiparasitics** • **Benzoyl peroxide** • **Inhalers** • **Topical antibiotics, antifungals, hydrocortisone** • **Potassium-containing products** • **Ibuprofen**	may present special problems; consult the pharmacist.

General Index

The bolded phrase "**poisoning**" after a drug name indicates that emergency measures can be found on the indicated page in case of poisoning with that drug. The bold letter "**f**" indicates an illustration of the index entry. The bold letter "**t**" indicates a table concerning the index entry.

abdominal binders, compression therapy, 439
absorbents, to treat diarrhea, 323
ACE, *see* angiotensin converting enzyme (ACE) inhibitors
acesulfame potassium
  safety of, 473
  sweetness, 473
acetaminophen
  adverse effects, 237
  children's dosages, 236t
  and contact lenses, 138
  dosages, 237–38
  drug interactions, 238–39
  efficacy, 233, 237
  metabolic pathways, 237f
  with other analgesics, 238–39
  overdose, 237, 513
  poisoning, 515
  poisoning nomogram, 238f
  to treat dysmenorrhea, 303
  to treat fever and pain, 236–37
  to treat infant fever, 456
  to treat PMS, 304
acetazolamide
  affects proteinuria tests, 405
  nutrient interactions, 471
  to treat sleep apnea, 490
acetic acid
  glacial
    to treat calluses, 339
    to treat corns, 339
  solution, to treat ear disorders, 156
acetoacetic acid, in ketone tests, 404
acetohexamide, to manage diabetes, 358
acetone, in ketone tests, 404
acetylsalicylic acid (ASA)
  allergic reactions, 234
  and antacids, 233
  and blood clotting, 234
  children's dosages, 236t
  dosages, 235–36
  drug interactions, 233, 235t, 235, 238
  efficacy, 233
  enteric-coated, 233, 234
  gastrointestinal effects, 233–35
  history, 233
  metabolic pathways, 233f
  nutrient interactions, 471, 472
  with other analgesics, 238
  overdose, 235, 513
  and peptic ulcers, 246
  and pregnancy, 235
  to reduce fever, 195
  renal effects, 234
  and Reye's syndrome, 195, 196, 234–35
  sustained-release, 234

to treat colds, 196
to treat dysmenorrhea, 303
to treat fever and pain, 233
to treat PMS, 304
acne
  consumer counselling, 98–99
  diagnosis, 96
  treatment, 96–98
  types, 93–95
acne cosmetica, 94
acne excoriée, 93
acne keloidalis, 93
acne neonatorum, 93
acne rosacea, 94–95, 104
acne vulgaris, 95
acquired immunodeficiency syndrome (AIDS)
  and condoms, 292
  and contraceptives, 294
  and diarrhea, 321
acrivastine, to treat allergic rhinitis, 224
actinic damage, *see* skin aging
activated attapulgite, to treat diarrhea, 323
activated charcoal
  to treat diarrhea, 323
  to treat poisoning, 514
activity, and choice of sunscreen, 56
actors, and acne, 94
acute necrotizing ulcerative gingivitis (ANUG), 169
Addison's disease, detected through blood test, 407
adenoma of pancreas, detected through blood test, 407
adenosackie-virus, causes colds, 191
adolescents, and acne, 94, 95
adrenergic blockers, and insomnia, 485
adrenocorticotropic hormone, causes acne, 94
adsorbents, to treat diarrhea, 323
adverse reactions, and product choice, 7
agar gum, to treat constipation, 310
agranulocytes, *see* leukocytes
AIDS, *see* acquired immunodeficiency syndrome (AIDS)
airflow measurement, *see* peak expiratory flow rate measurement
air purifiers, home health care, 433–34
AKTAC, *see* alkyltriethanolammonium chloride (AKTAC)
albumin, in urine, to detect kidney disease, 354
alcohol
  as antiseptic, 30–31
  and bulimia, 479
  caffeine interaction, 487
  as cause of incontinence, 391

and diabetes, 356
drug interactions, 220
and gastroesophageal reflux, 247
herb interactions, 499
and insomnia, 485, 487
nutrient interactions, 471
and peptic ulcers, 246
alginic acid, to treat gastroesophageal reflux, 250–51
alkyltriethanolammonium chloride (AKTAC), in chemical disinfection systems, 132, 133
allantoin
  in ophthalmic products, 113
  to treat dermatitis, 76
  to treat hemorrhoids, 332
allergens
  causing allergic rhinitis, 214–15, 215t
  most common, 68
allergic reactions
  blepharitis, 104t, 104
  classification, 26
  conjunctivitis, 106t, 106
  contact dermatitis, 68–70
  to contact lens solutions, 134–35
  to food, and atopic dermatitis, 66–67
  to herbal products, 494
  to insect venom, 26
  to insulin, 363
  to ophthalmic preservatives, 113
  to ostomy products, 388
  to p-ABA, 55
  photosensitivity, 52–53
  to poison ivy, 69–70
  and product choice, 7
  skin contact, 69t
allergic response (sneeze or cough), 213–14, 214f
allergic rhinitis
  causes, 213–14
  consumer counselling, 226–27
  diagnosis, 216
  differential diagnosis, 196, 216, 217t
  immunotherapy, 226
  prevalence, 213
  symptoms, 215–16
  treatment, 216, 218f, 218–26, 219f
alloin, to treat constipation, 312
allopathic medicines
  carbenoxolone, 495
  foxglove, 495
  quinine, 495
  snakeroot, 495
  tubocurarine, 495
allyl isothiocyanate, as external analgesic, 42
almond oil, *see* sweet almond oil

aloe
as herbal medicine, 500
to treat constipation, 312
alpha-adrenergic antagonists, and gastroesophageal reflux, 247
alpha-hydroxy acids, to treat dermatitis, 76
althea, to treat diarrhea, 324
alum, exsiccated, 30
aluminum acetate
as antiseptic, 30
to treat dermatitis, 76
to treat ear disorders, 155–56
aluminum chlorhydroxyallantoinate, to treat hemorrhoids, 332
aluminum chloride, as antiseptic, 30
aluminum chlorohydrate, as antiseptic, 30
aluminum hydroxide
drug interactions, 251
to treat ulcers, 249–50
aluminum hydroxide gel
to treat diarrhea, 323
to treat hemorrhoids, 332
aluminum salts
as astringents, 30
to treat athlete's foot, 343–44
aluminum sulfate, as antiseptic, 30
ambulatory aids
canes, 419–21
crutches, 421–25
prevalence, 419
walkers, 425
wheelchairs, 426–29
amenorrhea
symptoms, 302
treatment, 302
amethocaine, see tetracaine
amides, as topical anesthetics, 34
aminophylline, drug interactions, 68
amitriptyline, affects contact lenses, 138
ammonia, to treat diarrhea, 324
ammonia solution, strong, as external analgesic, 42
ammonium chloride, to treat cough, 205
amoxicillin
and ostomy, 390
to treat otitis media, 155
amphetamines
abuse of, 479
and insomnia, 485
to treat eating disorders, 477
amphotericin B, nutrient interactions, 471
ampicillin, causes diarrhea, 321
amyldimethyl p-ABA, as sunscreen, 55
amylocaine, as ophthalmic anesthetic, 113
anal canal
anatomy, 329
arteries, 330f
cross-section, 329f
anal dilatation, to treat hemorrhoids, 333
analgesic nephropathy, 234
analgesics
and eating disorders, 479
external, see also counterirritants
and children, 41, 45

consumer counselling, 46
definition, 39
dosage forms, 45–46
mechanism of action, 40–41
purposes, 39–40
types, 41–45
user instructions, 46
internal, 233–39
opiate, 203
to treat ear disorders, 156–57
anal skin breakdown, from ostomy, 388
anaphylaxis
from insect bite, 26
treatment, 26–27
Ancylostoma duodenale, see hookworms
androgens, cause acne, 94
anemia, iron deficiency, 470
anesthetics
in antacids, 248
ophthalmic, 112–13
topical, 34–35
and dermatitis, 68
poisoning, 515
to treat canker sores, 181–82
to treat ear disorders, 156–57
to treat genital irritation, 301
to treat hemorrhoids, 331–32
to treat teething pain, 455
anetheltrithion, to treat dry mouth, 182
anethole, as medicine, 496
angelica, as herbal medicine, 500
angiotensin converting enzyme (ACE)
inhibitors, to treat diabetic nephropathy, 354
angle-closure glaucoma, see glaucoma, angle-closure
animal bites, see bites (animal)
animal dander, causing allergic rhinitis, 215
anise, see aniseed
aniseed
as herbal medicine, 496, 500
to treat diarrhea, 324
anise oil, to treat colic, 454
ankle braces, 439
anorectal region, venous drainage, 330f
anorexia nervosa
and appetite suppressant abuse, 478–79
and body image, 477
causes, 476
diagnosis, 475
and drug abuse, 476
drug treatment, 477
medical risks, 476
prevalence, 476
prognosis, 476
psychoeducational treatment, 477
symptoms, 476
antacids
and ASA, 233
drug interactions, 233, 251t, 251–52
nutrient interactions, 470
and ostomy, 390
poisoning, 515
side effects, 248

to treat gastroesophageal reflux, 250–51
to treat ulcers, 248–49
antazoline, as ophthalmic antihistamine, 111
anthelmintics, consumer counselling, 282t
anthralin
causing psoriasis, 84
to treat dermatitis, 75
to treat psoriasis, 86–87
anthranilic acid, derivatives, as sunscreen, 55
anthraquinone cathartics, to treat constipation, 311–12
antiarrhythmics, and dry mouth, 176t
antibiotics
and dermatitis, 68
and ostomy, 390
topical, 33t, 33–34
to treat acne, 97
to treat mouth sores, 182
antibiotic sore mouth, see candidiasis
anticancer drugs, drug-sunlight interactions, 52t
anticholinergics
affect contact lenses, 138
as cause of incontinence, 391
and children, 324
and gastroesophageal reflux, 247
to treat allergic rhinitis, 226
to treat colds, 206
to treat colic, 454
to treat diarrhea, 324
to treat hemorrhoids, 332
to treat motion sickness, 262–63
anticoagulants
nutrient interaction, 472
vitamin interaction, 466
anticonvulsants
cause acne, 94
and dry mouth, 176t
nutrient interactions, 471
antidepressants
affect contact lenses, 138
and dry mouth, 176t
and insomnia, 485
sunlight interactions, 52t
antidiarrheals
drug interactions, 324
user instructions, 324–25
anti-embolism stockings, 438
antiemetics
consumer counselling, 264
definition, 257
guidelines for use, 260
pharmacist's guidelines, 261f
antiflatulents, to treat colic, 454–55
antigenicity (immune response), to insulin, 362–63
antihistamines
affect contact lenses, 137, 138
characteristics, 221–23t
classification, 219–20
contraindications, 220–21
dosages, 221–23t
drug interactions, 68, 220

brain damage
    as cause of incontinence, 392
    detected through blood test, 407
bran, to treat constipation, 310
breast-feeding
    advantages, 443t
    vs bottle-feeding, 447t
    and colic, 453
    should be encouraged, 447
    supplement guidelines, 450t
bridgework, *see* dentures
bromides
    cause acne, 94
    poisoning, 516
bromphenol blue, in pH tests, 405
bronchiectasis, and bad breath, 175
bronchitis
    differential diagnosis, 195–96
    symptomatic treatment, 434
bronchodilators
    and insomnia, 485
    measuring efficacy, 409
broom, as herbal medicine, 500
bruises
    on ear, 150
    to eye (black eye), 107
    on skin, 21
buchu
    drug interactions, 499
    as herbal medicine, 501
budesonide, to treat allergic rhinitis, 225
bufexamac, as anti-inflammatory agent, 36
buffers, in contact lens solutions, 129
bulimia
    and alcohol abuse, 479
    and appetite suppressant abuse, 478–79
    and body image, 477
    causes, 476
    diagnosis, 475
    and diuretic abuse, 478
    and drug abuse, 476
    drug treatment, 477
    and laxative abuse, 478
    medical risks, 476
    prevalence, 476
    prognosis, 476
    psychoeducational treatment, 477
    symptoms, 476
bulk-forming agents
    abuse of, 478–79
    to treat constipation, 310
bullous myringitis, 154
bunionettes, 341
bunions
    causes, 341–42
    and flat feet, 342
    and hallux valgus, 341f, 342
    and metatarsus varus, 342
    symptoms, 342
    treatment, 342
burdock
    as herbal medicine, 501
    hypoglycemic action, 499

burns
    chemical, 22, 24, 107
    description, 21
    to ear, 150–51
    minor, treatment, 23–24, 24f
    serious, treatment, 24f, 24
    severity classification, 22f, 22–23, 23t
    thermal, 22, 24
Burow's solution, *see* aluminum acetate
bursitis
    definition, 39, 240
    treatment, 240
busulfan, and hyperpigmentation, 58
butacaine, as ophthalmic anesthetic, 113
butamben picrate, as topical anesthetic, 34
butterbur, dangerous medicine, 494, 499
butyl methoxy-dibenzoylmethane, as
    sunscreen, 55

caffeine
    with acetaminophen, 238
    alcohol interaction, 487
    with ASA, 238
    drug charts, 486t
    drug interactions, 487
    food and beverage chart, 486t
    and insomnia, 485, 486–87
    overdose, 487
    poisoning, 516
    and pregnancy, 487
    and smoking, 487
    to treat dermatitis, 75
    to treat PMS, 304
caffeine substitutes, safety concerns, 494
calamine
    as antipruritic, 34
    to treat dermatitis, 77–78
    to treat hemorrhoids, 332
calamus, as herbal medicine, 501
calcium
    drug interactions, 469–71
    major nutrient, 469
    to prevent osteoporosis, 469
    recommended intake, 469
calcium carbonate, to treat ulcers, 249
calcium salts, available forms, 469t
calculus (tartar)
    and gingivitis, 169
    and tooth decay, 164
calluses
    causes, 337
    definition, 337
    on diabetic foot, 345
    prevention, 339
    product formulations, 339
    product use instructions, 339
    treatment, 338–39
"calorie-reduced", definition, 357
camphor
    as external analgesic, 44
    overdose, 513
    poisoning, 516
    as topical anesthetic, 35
    to treat cough, 204

to treat dermatitis, 77
to treat ear disorders, 157
to treat mouth sores, 182
to treat nasal congestion, 201
Canada's Food Guide, 466t
Canadian Pharmaceutical Association
    (CPhA), guidelines for pharmacists, 1, 2
cancer
    caused by sunlight, 54
    colorectal
        risk factors, 408t
        screening, 409
    indication for colostomy, 383
    indication for ileostomy, 384
    indication for urostomy, 384
    and vitamin-rich food, 472
candidiasis
    causes, 174
    symptoms, 174
    treatment, 174
canes
    fitting, 420f, 420–21
    folding, 420
    forearm, 420
    gaits, 422–23f
    handle types, 420
    instructions for use, 421
    materials, 420
    monopod (standard), 419–20
    multipod (four feet), 420
    ortho, 420
    platform, 420
    purposes, 419
    tips, 420
    types, 420
canker sores
    causes, 173
    differential diagnosis, 172t
    drug treatments, 181t, 181–82
    foods to avoid, 174t
    prevalence, 173
    and smokers, 173
    symptoms, 173
    treatment, 173–74
cannulae, nasal, to deliver oxygen, 434
cantharidin, to treat warts, 341
canthaxanthine, as tanning agent, 58
capsaicin, as external analgesic, 43
capsicum
    as external analgesic, 43–44
    as herbal medicine, 501
capsicum oleoresin, as external analgesic, 43
captopril
    drug interactions, 251
    to treat diabetic nephropathy, 354
caramiphen, to treat cough, 204
carbamide, *see* urea
carbamide peroxide
    as tooth whitener, 179
    to treat canker sores, 182
    to treat ear infections, 158
carbenicillin, nutrient interactions, 471
carbenoxolone, to treat peptic ulcers, 495
carbetapentane, to treat cough, 204

drug-sunlight interactions, 52t, 52–53
  to treat psoriasis, 86, 88
drug-urine interactions, 389t
drug-vitamin interactions, 466, 470
dry eye
  and artificial tears, 112
  risk factors, 108t, 108, 136
  symptoms, 108
  treatment, 108, 109, 115–16f
dry mouth
  causes, 175, 176t
  drug treatments, 182–83
  symptoms, 175
  treatment, 175
dry skin, see dermatitis, dry skin
duodenal ulcers
  causes, 245
  cross-section, 245f
  treatment, 248–50
durable medical equipment (DME)
  ambulatory aids, 419–29
  bathroom safety products, 429, 433
  definition, 419
  pharmacy considerations, 419
  respiratory therapy equipment, 433–35
dust mites, causing allergic rhinitis, 215
dysentery, causes blood in feces, 408
dysmenorrhea
  symptoms, 302
  treatment, 302–3
dysuria, see pain, during urination

ear
  anatomy and physiology, 149–50
  auricle, 149f
  common disorders, 150–54
  consumer counselling, 158–60
  cross-section, 150f
  frostbite, 150, 152
  hygiene, 158–59
  infections, 151, 153–54
  inner, 151f
  pain, 159f
  piercing, 152
  serious complications, 155
  syringing, 158
  treatment, 155–58, 159f
eardrops, instilling, 158
eardrum
  description, 150
  perforation, 154
ear products, consumer counselling, 158–59
earwax
  definition, 119
  impacted, 152
eating disorders
  causes
    biological, 476–77
    psychosocial, 477
  consumer counselling, 480
  diagnosis, 475
  drug abuse, 477–80
  insomnia, 485
  medical risks, 476

prevalence, 476
prognosis, 476
treatment, 477
echosackie-virus, causes colds, 191
eczema, asteatotic, 72, 74
edema, see swelling
edetate, see disodium edetate (EDTA)
EDTA, see disodium edetate (EDTA)
elastic bandages, health supports, 438
elastosis, solar, 54
elbow braces, 439
elderly persons
  airflow measurement, 409–10
  colostomy, 383
  constipation, 314
  contact lens care, 130–31
  counselling, 13–14
  diabetes, 154, 353
  dry mouth, 175
  high blood pressure, 410
  hypoglycemia, 358
  hypoglycemic agents, 360
  incontinence, 391, 392
  insomnia, 487t
  lindane, 273
  mineral oil, 312
  nocturnal myoclonus, 484
  osteoporosis, 469
  phenylamines, 199
  sleep apnea, 484
  sleep-wake cycle, 484
  tooth decay, 163
electrolyte lavage solutions, for enemas, 316
electrolytes
  infant formulas, 448–49
  infant requirements, 458t
  rehydration with, 458–59
embarrassing subjects, counselling on,
  12–13
emesis, see also vomiting
  by mechanical stimulation, 260
emetics
  abuse of, 478
  antimony, 259
  apomorphine hydrochloride, 259
  black mustard, 260
  consumer counselling, 263–64
  copper sulfate, 259
  dangerous, 259
  definition, 257
  detergents, 260
  ipecac syrup, 258–59
  pharmacist's guidelines, 258f
  potassium tartrate, 259
  sodium chloride, 259–60
  sodium tartrate, 259
  zinc sulfate, 259
emollients
  as ophthalmic ointments, 112
  to soften ear wax, 157
  to treat dermatitis, 74
empathy, as assessment technique, 4
enalapril, to treat diabetic nephropathy, 354
encephalitis, 26, 175

endocrine disorders, and insomnia, 485
endotracheal tube, to deliver oxygen, 434
enemas, to treat constipation, 313
enterobiasis
  cellulose tape diagnosis, 280f
  definition, 279–80
  diagnosis, 280–81
  drug dosages, 281t
  prevalence, 279
  prevention, 282
  symptoms, 279
  treatment, 281–82
Enterobius vermicularis, see pinworms
enterocolitis, indication for ileostomy, 384
enterostomal therapist
  to consult on ileoanal reservoir surgery,
    384
  to consult on ostomy pouches, 387
  to consult on stomal fistulae, 388
  as ostomate resource, 383
enuresis alarms, see dampness detectors
environment, and ultraviolet (UV) light, 51f
enzymes, to clean contact lenses, 128, 132
ephedra, drug interactions, 499
ephedrine, to treat nasal congestion, 200
ephedrine sulfate, to treat hemorrhoids, 332
ephelides, see freckles
epidermal hyperplasia, 54
epidermis
  description, 63
  illustration, 63f
epileptics, and antihistamines, 220
epinephrine, and diabetics, 208
epinephrine hydrochloride, to treat
  hemorrhoids, 332
epithelial hyperplasia, at stoma site, 388–89
erythema, see redness
erythromycin
  causes diarrhea, 321
  to treat acne, 97, 98
esophageal reflux, see gastroesophageal
  reflux (GER)
esters, as topical anesthetics, 34
esters of nicotinic acid, as external
  analgesics, 44
esters of para-aminobenzoic acid (p-ABA), as
  sunscreen, 55
estrogens, to treat osteoporosis, 469
ethacrynic acid, nutrient interactions, 471
ethambutol, causes acne, 94
ethanol, as antiseptic, 30
2-ethoxyethyl p-methoxycinnamate, see
  cinoxate
ethylenediamine, common allergen, 68
2-ethylhexyl p-methoxycinnamate, as
  sunscreen, 55
2-ethylhexyl salicylate, as sunscreen, 55
ethyl nicotinate, as external analgesic, 44
etretinate
  causing psoriasis, 84
  to treat psoriasis, 88
eucalyptus oil
  as external analgesic, 44

foreign body sensation, contact lenses, 129
foxglove, to treat heart disease, 495
fracture
    bone, 20
    tooth, 170
frangula, to treat constipation, 312
freckles, lightening, 58
Friar's balsam, to treat cough, 205
frostbite
    description, 24–25
    to ear, 150, 152
    from burn treatment, 24
    severity classification, 25t
    treatment, 25f, 25
fructose, in diabetic diet, 356
FUO, see fever, of undetermined origin
    (FUO)
furosemide
    and diuretic abuse, 478
    nutrient interactions, 471
furunculosis, in ear canal, 153

gamma benzene hexachloride, see lindane
gargles, to treat sore throat, 196
garlic, as herbal medicine, 502
gastric lavage, to treat poisoning, 514
gastric surgery, and diarrhea, 321
gastric ulcers
    causes, 245
    cross-section, 245f
    from ASA, 234
    treatment, 248–50
gastroenteritis, causes diarrhea, 320–21
gastroesophageal reflux (GER)
    pathophysiology, 247
    risk factors, 247
    symptoms, 247
    treatment, 250f, 250–51
gastrointestinal gas
    causes, 252
    consumer counselling, 253
    in infants, 454–55
    and ostomy, 386f, 388
    symptoms, 252
    treatment, 252–53, 253f
gastrointestinal irritation
    from ASA, 233–34
    from hypoglycemic agents, 358
    and insomnia, 485
gastrointestinal tract
    detecting diseases, 408
    fluid absorption, 319f, 319
    fluid secretion, 319
    infection, 320–21
gastroparesis, caused by diabetes, 355
gate control theory of pain, 40f, 40
gaultheria oil, see methyl salicylate
gauze, for dressing, 30
GDM, see gestational diabetes mellitus
    (GDM)
gel, see also emollients
    external analgesic, 45
gelatin, as denture adhesive, 184

genital hygiene
    consumer counselling, 305
    female, 298, 300–301
    and hemorrhoids, 331
gentamicin
    nutrient interactions, 471
    and ostomy, 390
gentian, as herbal medicine, 502
gentian violet, to treat enterobiasis, 282
GER, see gastroesophageal reflux (GER)
gestational diabetes mellitus (GDM)
    definition, 350
    diagnostic criteria, 353t
giant papillary conjunctivitis (GPC), from
    contact lens wear, 132
ginger
    as herbal medicine, 502
    to treat diarrhea, 324
    to treat motion sickness, 263
gingival hyperplasia
    and cyclosporine, 170
    and nifedipine, 170
    and phenytoin, 169–70
gingivitis
    ANUG, 169
    causes, 169
    and oral contraceptives, 169
    and pregnancy, 169
    symptoms, 169
    treatment, 170
ginseng, as herbal medicine, 502
glands, within tarsal plates, 102t
glands of Moll, 102t
glands of Zeis, 102t
glaucoma
    angle-closure
        description, 107
        risk factors, 107t
        and vasoconstrictors, 110
    narrow-angle, and antihistamines, 220
    open-angle
        description, 106–7
        medications used, 107t
gliclazide, to manage diabetes, 358–59
glucagon, to restore blood glucose, 352
glucocorticoids
    and excessive sebum, 96
    nutrient interactions, 471
    to treat psoriasis, 87
glucose
    blood tests, 373–77, 375t, 407t, 407–8
    hypoglycemic levels, 352
    infant requirements, 458t
    normal levels, 351–52
    restoring, 352
    urine tests, 370–73, 371t, 403–4, 404t,
    405t
glucose intolerance, degrees of, 350–51
glucose monitors, blood, 376t
glucose oxidase tests, to measure urine
    glucose, 403–4
glucose tests
    blood, 373–77, 375t, 407t, 407–8

drug interactions, 372t
    urine, 370–73, 371t, 403–4, 404t, 405t
glucosuria
    caused by insulin deficiency, 352
    urine tests, 403
glucuronic acid, to treat dermatitis, 76
glyburide
    to manage diabetes, 358–59
    risk of hypoglycemia, 357–58
glycemic control
    monitoring with blood tests, 373–77
    monitoring with glycosylated
        hemoglobin, 369
    monitoring with urine tests, 370–73
glycerin
    in dry mouth products, 182
    to treat dermatitis, 75
    to treat ear disorders, 157
glycerin soaps, see soaps, transparent
glycerol, see glycerin
glyceryl guaiacolate, see guaifenesin
glyceryl p-ABA, as sunscreen, 55
glyceryltrinitrate, causes acne, 94
glycogen storage disease, detected through
    blood test, 407
glycolic acid, to treat dermatitis, 76
glycosides, herb interactions, 499
glycosuria, urine tests, 403
glycosylated hemoglobin, to monitor
    glycemic control, 369
gold, affects proteinuria tests, 405
goldenseal, as herbal medicine, 502
Gordolobos tea, dangerous medicine,
    497–98
GPC, see giant papillary conjunctivitis
    (GPC)
grab bars, for bathroom safety, 429
gramicidin
    as antibiotic, 33
    as ophthalmic anti-infective, 111–12
    to treat ear disorders, 155
granulocytes, see leukocytes
grasses, causing allergic rhinitis, 214
"Greenland diet", 471
gripe water, to treat colic, 454
griseofulvin, and bad breath, 175
groundsels, dangerous medicine, 499
guaiac, to detect blood in urine, 405
guaifenesin, to treat cough, 205
guanethidine, causes diarrhea, 321
gum acacia, as spermicide, 289
guttate psoriasis, 84

H₁-receptor antagonists, to treat motion
    sickness, 261–62
hair dyes, common allergen, 68
halitosis, see bad breath
hallux valgus, and bunions, 341f, 342
halogens, cause acne, 94
haloprogin, to treat athlete's foot, 343–44
halothane, causes acne, 94
hamamelis, see witch hazel

treatment, 109
rebound, 110
hyperglycemia
  caused by insulin deficiency, 352
  diabetic, 350
  signs, 352t
  treating with hypoglycemic agents, 357
hypericum, to treat diarrhea, 324
hypertension, see blood pressure, high
hyperthyroidism, detected through blood
  test, 407
hypervitaminosis
  with vitamin D, 464
  with vitamin C, 465–66
  with vitamin A, 464
  with vitamin B$_3$, 464–65
  with vitamin E, 466
hypnotics
  affect contact lenses, 137
  as cause of incontinence, 391
  herb interactions, 499
  and insomnia, 485–86
hypocalcemia, symptoms, 469
hypochlorite, to clean dentures, 184
hypoglycemia
  and alcohol, 356
  dangers of, 342
  definition, 342
  and exercise, 357
  risk factors, 358
  risk with oral hypoglycemics, 357–58
  symptoms, 352t, 352
hypoglycemic agents
  adverse effects, 357–58
  contraindications, 359
  dosages, 358t, 360
  drug choice, 358–59
  drug interactions, 358, 359t
  efficacy, 360
  sunlight interactions, 52t
  use in diabetes, 357
hypomagnesemia, 471
hypoparathyroidism, and diarrhea, 321
hypotension, caused by diabetes, 355
hypothermia, 25
hypothyroidism, detected through blood
  test, 407
hypovolemic shock, see shock

ibuprofen
  drug interactions, 303
  to treat dysmenorrhea, 302–3
  to treat fever and pain, 238
  to treat PMS, 304
ichthammol, to treat ear disorders, 156
ichthyol, to treat dermatitis, 78
IDDM, see insulin-dependent diabetes
  mellitus (IDDM)
ileoanal reservoir, as alternative to
  ileostomy, 384
ileostomy
  alternatives, 384
  discharge from, 384

reasons for, 383–84
surgical method, 383
illness, dimensions, 6t
imidazolines, to treat nasal congestion, 201
immune response, to insulin, 362–63
immunotherapy
  to treat allergic rhinitis, 226
  to treat warts, 340
imperforate anus, indication for colostomy,
  383
impotence
  caused by diabetes, 355
  caused by ostomy, 389
incontinence
  consumer counselling, 394–95, 436
  fecal, 392t, 392
  indication for urostomy, 384
  product manufacturers, 394
  products, 392–93, 435–36
  suggested reading, 394
  urinary
    causes, 391
    overflow, 391
    prevalence, 391, 435
    prevention, 392
    reflex, 391
    stress, 391
    treatment, 391–92
    types, 391
    urge, 391
incontinence garments
  disposable, 392–93, 436
  reuseable, 393, 436
incontinence products
  bedding, 436
  catheters, 435
  dampness detectors, 436
  leg bags, 435
  pharmacy consideration, 436
  undergarments, 392–93, 436
indomethacin, causes blood in feces, 408
infant formula
  carbohydrates, 448t, 448
  and colic, 453
  composition, 444–47t
  electrolytes, 448–49
  fats, 448
  instructions, 451t
  vs milk, 447t
  preparation, 450–51
  proteins, 443, 447–49
  renal solute load, 448–49
  selection, 450
  supplement guidelines, 450t
  and tooth decay, 165
  vitamin content, 450t
infants
  bathing, 451–52
  colds, 196, 455–57
  cold sores, 172
  colic, 453–55
  consumer counselling, 459–61
  cradle cap, 455
  diaper rash, 452–53

diarrhea, 320, 457–59
feeding, 443–51
fever, 455–57
finger and toenails, 452
home safety, 459
ileostomies, 384
mineral requirements, 449–50
teething, 455
tooth decay, 165
vitamin requirements, 449–50
vomiting, 260
infection
  of ear, 151, 153–54
  from burns, 23
  from skin wound, 19
  in gastrointestinal tract, 320–21
  symptoms of (SHARP), 19
inflammation, as wound heals, 20
influenza
  differential diagnosis, 195
  in infant, 456t
information-gathering skills, see assessment
ingrown toenails
  causes, 342
  development, 342f
  treatment, 342
injection
  of insulin
    by jet injector, 368
    by pen-like device, 367–68
    sites, 368f
    by syringe, 367
Injectomatic Syringe Injector, to inject
  insulin, 368–69
injuries
  musculoskeletal
    differentiating, 21t
    treatment, 20–21, 21f
    types, 20–21
  orthopedic, and health supports, 437t
inner ear, 151f
insect bites, see bites (insects)
insect-borne disease, 26
insecticides, 28
insect repellants, 28
insects
  in ear, 152
  and parasitic infections, 267
insomnia
  causes
    alcohol, 487
    caffeine, 486–87
    drugs, 485t, 485–86
    medical conditions, 485t, 485
    transient, 485
  consumer counselling, 489, 491
  definition, 484
  drug treatment, 488–89
  nondrug treatment, 487
  and pregnancy, 489
  prevalence, 484–85
  sleep-wake cycle, 484
  treatment, 487t

insulin
    absorption, 362
    abuse in eating disorders, 478
    administration, 365–69
    allergic reactions, 363
    animal vs human, 363–64
    Canadian products, 360–61t
    causes lipoatrophy, 363
    causes lipohypertrophy, 363
    choosing, 363–64
    course of action, 361–62, 362t
    course of effect, 365f
    distribution, 362
    dosing regimens, 364–65
    elimination, 362
    and exercise, 357
    formulation categories, 360–63
    how it works, 351–52
    immune response, 362–63
    indications, 364
    injection dangers, 363
    injection sites, 368f
    mixtures, 366–67
    purity of products, 363
    sources, 362
    stability, 369
    sterility, 369
    storage, 369
    subcutaneous injection, 367f, 367–69
insulin-dependent diabetes mellitus (IDDM)
    blood glucose monitoring, 374
    definition, 351
    diet, 355
    exercise, 357
    hypoglycemic agents, 359
    ketoacidosis, 352
    ketonuria, 373
    managed with insulin, 364
    nephropathy, 353
    vs NIDDM, 351t
    retinopathy, 353
insulin pumps, 369
insulin syringes
    types, 365
    user instructions, 366, 367
interactions, see drug-drug interactions
interferon, to treat colds, 206
intestinal carcinoma, and diarrhea, 321
intrauterine device (IUD), with spermicide,
    289–90
iodides, cause acne, 94
iodinated glycerol, to treat cough, 205
iodine
    as antiseptic, 32
    and dermatitis, 68
    poisoning, 517
iodochlorhydroxyquin, as antibiotic, 33–34
iodophors, as antiseptics, 32
ipecac syrup
    abuse of, 478
    dangers, 259
    guidelines for emetic use, 258–59
    to treat poisoning, 514
ipratropium, to treat allergic rhinitis, 226

iron
    causes blood in feces, 408
    drug interactions, 470–71
    major nutrient, 470
    overdose, 470, 513
    poisoning, 517
    recommended intake, 470
    supplements, 470
iron deficiency anemia, symptoms, 470
islet cell carcinoma, detected through blood
    test, 407
isoniazid
    causes acne, 94
    drug interactions, 251
    nutrient interactions, 470
isophane insulin, see neutral protamine
    Hagedorn (NPH) insulin
isopropanol, **poisoning**, 517
isopropyl alcohol
    as antiseptic, 30–31
    to clean contact lenses, 128
4-isopropyl dibenzoylmethane, as sunscreen,
    55
isoproterenol, and gastroesophageal reflux,
    247
isotretinoin
    affects contact lenses, 138
    to treat acne, 98

jaundice, detecting with urine test, 406
jequerity bean, poisonous, 494
jet injectors, to inject insulin, 368
jet-lag, and insomnia, 485
jewelry, and dermatitis, 69, 71
joints, pain in, 39–40
juniper
    drug interactions, 499
    as herbal medicine, 503
juvenile warts, see flat warts

kaolin
    drug interactions, 324
    as sunblock, 54
    to treat diarrhea, 323
    to treat hemorrhoids, 332
karaya gum
    as denture adhesive, 184
    to treat constipation, 310
karela, hypoglycemic action, 499
Kenny sticks, see crutches, forearm
keratin softeners, to treat dermatitis, 75–76
keratitis
    causes, 106t
    and contact lenses, 126, 127, 131
    description, 106
    herpes simplex, 106
    treatment, 106
keratoconjunctivitis, allergic reaction, 106
keratolytics
    traumatize skin, 64–65
    to treat dandruff, 89
    to treat hemorrhoids, 332
    to treat psoriasis, 85–86
ketoacidosis, description, 352

ketoconazole
    drug interactions, 251
    to treat seborrhea, 89–90
ketones
    affect urine glucose tests, 404
    blood tests, 408
    urine tests, 371t, 373, 404t, 404, 405t
ketonuria
    blood test for, 408
    caused by insulin deficiency, 352
    urine test for, 404
ketotifen, to treat allergic rhinitis, 226
kidney beans, poisonous, 495
kidney disease, and diabetes, 353–54
knee braces, 439
Kock, Nils G., created ileostomy, 384
kyphosis (hunchback), causes back pain,
    438

labels, dietetic products, 357
laceration, see wounds
lacrimal gland, 102f, 102–3
lactation
    and contraception, 288
    and laxatives, 314
    and vitamin supplements, 464
lactic acid
    as spermicide, 289
    to treat dermatitis, 76
    to treat psoriasis, 86
Lactobacillus acidophilus preparations, to
    treat diarrhea, 324
Lactobacillus bulgaricus preparations, to
    treat diarrhea, 324
lactoserum
    in cow's milk, 447
    in infant formulas, 443, 447–48
    in mother's milk, 447
lactulose, to treat constipation, 310, 311
lanolin
    and dermatitis, 68
    in ophthalmic ointments, 112, 114
    to treat dermatitis, 75
    to treat hemorrhoids, 332
laundromats, and acne, 94
lawsone, as tanning agent, 58
laxatives
    abuse of, 314–16, 476, 478
    cause diarrhea, 321
    and children, 314
    consumer counselling, 313, 316
    definition, 310
    and diagnostic procedures, 316
    dosages, 315t
    drug interactions, 313, 314t
    emollient, to treat constipation, 312
    and ileostomy, 390
    lubricant, to treat constipation, 312
    nutrient interactions, 471
    osmotic, to treat constipation, 310–11
    stimulant (contact), to treat constipation,
    311–12
    user instructions, 313t
LCD, see liquor carbonis detergens (LCD)

lecithin, to treat dermatitis, 75
leg bags, for incontinence, 393
lemon oil, in dry mouth products, 182
Lente insulin
 mixtures, 366–67
 products, 360t
lentigo, solar, 54
leukocytes, urine tests, 406
levocabastine, to treat allergic rhinitis, 226
levodopa
 and dry mouth, 175
 nutrient interactions, 470
levulose, in antiemetics, 263
lice
 body
  diagnosis, 269
  illustration, 267f
  transmission, 268
  treating, 271
 consumer counselling, 276
 description, 267–68
 eggs, 268f, 268
 in eyelashes, 104
 head
  definition, 267
  diagnosis, 268–69
  transmission, 268
  treating, 271
 infestations, see pediculosis
 life cycle, 268
 and parasitic infections, 267
 pubic
  diagnosis, 269
  illustration, 267f
  transmission, 268
  treating, 271
 types, 267
licorice
 drug interactions, 499
 as herbal medicine, 503
 to treat gastric pain, 495
lidocaine
 as topical anesthetic, 34
 to treat ear disorders, 157
life root, as herbal medicine, 503
lignocaine, see lidocaine
lily-of-the-valley
 drug interactions, 499
 poisonous, 495
lincomycin
 causes diarrhea, 321
 drug interactions, 324
lindane
 to treat pediculosis, 273–74
 to treat scabies, 273–74
 user instructions, 274t
linden flowers, as herbal medicine, 503
liniment, external analgesic, 45
linoleic acid
 and cholesterol, 471
 to treat PMS, 304
lipids, see fats
lipoatrophy, from insulin injection, 363
lipohypertrophy, from insulin injection, 363

lipoproteins
 high density, 471
 low density, 471
liquor carbonis detergens (LCD)
 to treat dermatitis, 78
 to treat psoriasis, 86
lithium, causing psoriasis, 84
lithium carbonate, to treat severe PMS, 304
lithium salts
 and bad breath, 175
 cause acne, 94
liver disease, detected through blood test,
  407
live yeast cell derivative (LYCD), to treat
  hemorrhoids, 332–33
lobelia, as herbal medicine, 503
loperamide, to treat diarrhea, 324
loratadine
 to treat allergic rhinitis, 224
 to treat dermatitis, 78
lordosis (swayback), causes back pain, 438
lotion, see also emollients
 external analgesic, 45
louse, see lice
lozenges, to treat sore throat, 196–97
L-tryptophan
 drug interactions, 489
 as sleep aid, 488–89
luteinizing hormone (LH), detected in
  ovulation test, 402
LYCD, see live yeast cell derivative (LYCD)
Lyme disease, 26

McDonald's acne, 94
macrovascular disease, and diabetes, 353
magnesium
 drug interactions, 470–71
 to treat ulcers, 249–50
magnesium aluminum silicate, to treat
  diarrhea, 323
magnesium citrate, to treat constipation,
  311
magnesium hydroxide
 drug interactions, 251
 to treat constipation, 311
magnesium phosphate, to treat constipation,
  310–11
magnesium salicylate, to treat fever and
  pain, 236
magnesium sulfate
 poisoning, 517
 to treat constipation, 311
magnesium trisilicate, see talc
malabsorption syndromes, and diarrhea, 321
malaria, 26
malgaldrate
 drug interactions, 251
 to treat ulcers, 250
malic acid, to treat dermatitis, 76
malnourishment, from eating disorder, 476
mandrake, dangerous medicine, 499
mannitol
 in diabetic diet, 356
 and tooth decay, 165

MAO, see monoamine oxidase (MAO)
  inhibitors
maprotiline
 affects contact lenses, 138
 causes acne, 94
massage, to ease pain, 40
mastoiditis, 155
MDI, see multiple daily injection (MDI)
mebendazole, to treat enterobiasis, 282
mechanics, and acne, 94
medroxyprogesterone acetate, to treat sleep
  apnea, 490
megacolon, indication for colostomy, 383
meibomian cyst, see chalazion
meibomian glands, 102t
melanoma, see cancer
melasma, 58
meningitis, and middle ear infection, 155
menstrual care
 consumer counselling, 306
 pads, 301
 tampons, 301
menstrual cycle, 298, 299f
menstrual problems
 amenorrhea, 302
 consumer counselling, 306
 dysmenorrhea, 302
 premenstrual syndrome, 303–4
 treatment, 302
menthol
 as external analgesic, 44
 as topical anesthetic, 35
 to treat cough, 204
 to treat dermatitis, 77
 to treat hemorrhoids, 332
 to treat mouth sores, 182
 to treat nasal congestion, 201
 to treat sore throat, 196
menthyl anthranilate, as sunscreen, 55
meperidine, and gastroesophageal reflux,
  247
mephenesin, as sleep aid, 488
mephenytoin, and pigment disorders, 58
mequitazine, to treat allergic rhinitis, 224
merbromin
 as antiseptic, 32
 poisoning, 517
6-mercaptopurine, to treat psoriasis, 88
mercuric oxide, yellow, as ophthalmic
  anti-infective, 111
mercury
 as antiseptic, 32
 and dermatitis, 68
metatarsal cushions, to prevent corns and
  calluses, 339
metatarsus varus, and bunions, 342
metformin
 adverse effects, 358
 contraindications, 359
 efficacy, 360
 to manage diabetes, 359
methotrexate
 nutrient interactions, 470
 to treat psoriasis, 87–88

and diabetics, 199
drug interaction, 199–200
and elderly persons, 199
to treat nasal congestion, 199–201
phenylephrine
as ophthalmic decongestant, 110
to treat nasal congestion, 201
phenylephrine hydrochloride, to treat
hemorrhoids, 332
phenylketonuria, from aspartame, 357
phenylmercuric acetate (PMA)
as ophthalmic preservative, 113
as spermicide, 289
phenylmercuric nitrate (PMN)
to disinfect contact lenses, 129
as ophthalmic preservative, 113
phenylmercuric salts, as antiseptics, 32
phenylpropanolamine
abuse of, 478–79
poisoning, 518
to treat nasal congestion, 200–201
phenytoin
causes acne, 94
causing gingival hyperplasia, 169–70
nutrient interactions, 470
and pigment disorders, 58
pheochromocytoma, detected through blood
test, 407
pH levels, urine tests, 404–5
phosphates, in ophthalmic products, 114
phosphate salts, to treat constipation, 311
phospholipids, to treat dermatitis, 75
phosphorated carbohydrate solution, to treat
motion sickness, 263
photoaging, 53
photoallergy, see photosensitivity
photosensitivity
and coal tar, 78
drug-sunlight interactions, 52t, 52–53
to sunlight, 52
symptoms, 52–53
phototoxicity, see photosensitivity
picker's acne, see acne excoriée
pierced ear, 152
pigment
of eye, 102
skin disorders, 58
pigmenting agents, see tanning, drug agents
piles, see hemorrhoids
pilocarpine hydrochloride, affects contact
lenses, 137
pilosebaceous unit, 95f
pinworms, cause enterobiasis, 279
piperazine, drug interactions, 281
piperazine adipate, to treat enterobiasis,
281–82
piperonyl butoxide
poisoning, 518
to treat pediculosis, 272
pituitary adenoma, detected through blood
test, 407
placebos, reduce pain, 41
plantar warts, 340–41

plants
and child safety, 459
as food, 495
as medicines, 495–98
poisonous, 494–95
plaque
chemical removal, 169
and periodontal diseases, 170
physical removal, 167–69
and smoking, 168
and tooth decay, 164
plaque disclosing agents, 179
plaques, on tongue, 174
platelet function, and ASA, 234
PMA, see phenylmercuric acetate (PMA)
p-methanylphenylpolyoxyethylene ether, as
spermicide, 289
PMMA (polymethylmethacrylate) lenses, see
contact lenses, hard (PMMA)
PMN, see phenylmercuric nitrate (PMN)
PMS, see premenstrual syndrome (PMS)
pneumonia, after influenza, 195
podophyllin, **poisoning**, 518
podophyllum, to treat warts, 341
poison control centres
and child safety, 459
must be contacted, 513
poisoning
activated charcoal treatment, 514
cathartics treatment, 514, 520
with caustics, 513
consumer counselling, 521
gastric lavage, 514
general management, 513–14
with herbal products, 494
of infants, 459
with nonprescription drugs, 515–21,
516–19t
prevention, 520–21
suggested reading, 521
via eyes, 513
via inhalation, 513
via skin, 513
vomiting treatment, 514
poison ivy
common allergen, 68
contact dermatitis, 28–29, 69–70
illustration, 69f
poison oak, see poison ivy
poisons, plants, 494–95
poison sumac, see poison ivy
poke, see pokeroot
pokeberry, see pokeroot
pokeroot
dangerous medicine, 496
as herbal medicine, 504
pokeweed, see pokeroot
pollens, causing allergic rhinitis, 214
poloxamer 407, in contact lens solutions,
131
polyaminopropylbiguanide, in chemical
disinfection systems, 132, 133

polycarbophil
to treat constipation, 310
to treat diarrhea, 323
polycarbophil calcium, to treat constipation,
310
polychlorinated biphenyls (PCBs), and acne,
94
polydipsia, caused by insulin deficiency, 352
polyethylene occlusive dressings, to treat
dermatitis, 75
polymethylmethacrylate (PMMA) lenses, see
contact lenses, hard (PMMA)
polymyxin B
as antibiotic, 34
as ophthalmic anti-infective, 111, 112
polymyxin B sulfate, to treat ear disorders,
155
polyp, indication for colostomy, 383
polyphagia, caused by insulin deficiency,
352
polyquad, see polyquaternium-1
polyquaternium-1, in chemical disinfection
systems, 132, 133
polysorbate 80, in contact lens solutions,
131
polyuria, caused by insulin deficiency, 352
polyvinyl alcohol
as artificial tears, 112
in contact lens solutions, 131
pork, parasites, 283
potassium, drug interactions, 470–71
potassium chlorate, **poisoning**, 516
potassium iodide, to treat cough, 205
potassium nitrate, in dentifrices, 178
potassium permanganate
as antiseptic, 32
to treat dermatitis, 76
potassium sorbate, in chemical disinfection
systems, 133
potassium tartrate, as emetic, 259
potatoes, poisonous, 495
pouches, for ostomy, see ostomy pouches
povidone, in artificial tears, 112
povidone-iodine
to treat dandruff, 89–90
to treat vaginitis, 305
pramoxine, to treat hemorrhoids, 332
pramoxine hydrochloride, as topical
anesthetic, 35
prazosin, as cause of incontinence, 391
pregnancy
and ASA, 235
and caffeine, 487
and constipation, 314
and contact lens use, 137
and diabetes, see also gestational
diabetes mellitus (GDM), 377–78
and fluoride, 176
and gastroesophageal reflux, 247
and gingivitis, 169
HCG levels, 401f
and hemorrhoids, 330
and herbal products, 494, 499
and insomnia, 489

and lindane, 274
nausea, 258, 260
and oregano, 497
and ostomy, 389
and parsley, 495
and piperazine adipate, 282
and vitamin supplements, 464
pregnancy tests
accuracy, 402t, 402
Canadian products, 403t
HCG, 400–401
monoclonal antibodies, 401–2
premenstrual acne, see acne excoriée
premenstrual syndrome (PMS)
causes, 304
consumer counselling, 306
symptoms, 303t, 303–4
treatment, 304
preservatives
contact lens solutions, 131
ophthalmic, 113
pressure sores
from ostomy, 388
from wheelchairs, 428
prickly heat, 25
primidone, nutrient interactions, 470
proctectomy, reason for, 383
product choice
consumer factors to consider, 7
product factors to consider, 7
product use
amount per dose, 8
doses per day, 8
duration, 8
intended benefits, 7–8
interactions, 9
method, 8
side effects, 8–9
storage, 9
timing, 8
progesterone
causes acne, 94
and gastroesophageal reflux, 247
to treat PMS, 304
prolapse, and hemorrhoids, 330–31
promethazine
to treat allergic rhinitis, 220
to treat motion sickness, 261
1,2-propanediol diacetate, to treat ear
disorders, 156
proparacaine, as ophthalmic anesthetic, 112,
113
propolis of flavenoids, to treat cold sores,
182
propoxyphene napsylate, affects contact
lenses, 138
propranolol, drug interactions, 252
propylene glycol
to treat dermatitis, 75, 77
to treat ear disorders, 157
to treat psoriasis, 86
propylhexedrine, to treat nasal congestion,
201

propylparaben, as ophthalmic preservative,
113
prostaglandins, and gastroesophageal reflux,
247
prostatitis, detecting, 406
protamine zinc insulin (PZI)
mixtures, 366
products, 361t
protectants, to treat hemorrhoids, 332
protein
in diabetic diet, 356
in infant formulas, 443, 447–48
types, 447t
urine tests, 405
proteinuria
detecting, 405
treatment, 354
protriptyline, to treat sleep apnea, 490
proxymetacaine, see proparacaine
pseudoephedrine
poisoning, 517
to treat nasal congestion, 200
pseudomembranous colitis, 321
psoralens
cause acne, 94
as sunscreens, 57
to treat psoriasis, 88
psoriasis
causes, 84t, 84
consumer counselling, 90–91
differential diagnosis, 71, 83t
symptoms, 83–84
treatment, 84–85, 85t, 88f
types, 84
psoriasis vulgaris, 84
psoriatic arthritis, 84
psychogenic diseases, detected through
blood test, 407
psyllium
to treat constipation, 310
to treat diarrhea, 323
PUD, see peptic ulcer disease (PUD)
pumps, to infuse insulin, 369
pus, symptom of infection, 19
pustulants, definition, 39
pustular psoriasis, 84
pyelonephritis
caused by diabetes, 355
detecting, 406
pyrantel pamoate
drug interactions, 281
to treat enterobiasis, 281
pyrethrins with piperonyl butoxide
to treat pediculosis, 272
user instructions, 272t
pyridoxine, see vitamin B6
pyrilamine maleate
as ophthalmic antihistamine, 111
to treat PMS, 304
pyrimethamine, nutrient interactions, 470
pyrophosphates, to control tartar, 178
pyruvic acid, to treat dermatitis, 76

pyrvinium pamoate, to treat enterobiasis,
281
PZI, see protamine zinc insulin (PZI)

quaternary ammonium compounds
as antiseptics, 33
in mouthwashes, 180
as spermicide, 289
to treat dandruff, 89–90
to treat sore throat, 196
questions
closed-ended, 3
follow-up, 3
leading, 3
multiple, 3
open-ended, 3
"why", 3
quinacrine, as sunscreen, 57
quinidine, causes diarrhea, 321
quinine
causes acne, 94
to treat malaria, 495
quinine compounds, as spermicides, 289

radiation, solar, see sunlight
radioallergosorbent test (RAST), to test for
allergies, 216
radiography, and ostomy, 390
radiopaques, causes acne, 94
ragweed, causing allergic rhinitis, 214
ragworts, dangerous medicine, 499
rapid eye movement (REM) sleep, 484
rash, see dermatitis
RAS (recurrent aphthous stomatitis), see
canker sores
RAST, see radioallergosorbent test (RAST)
Rauwolfia, to treat psychosis, 495
rebound hyperemia, 110
rebound insomnia, 485
rectum
arteries, 330f
skin breakdown, from ostomy, 388
recurrent aphthous stomatitis (RAS), see
canker sores
recurrent herpes labialis (RHL), see cold
sores
recurrent intraoral herpes (RIH), see cold
sores
red clover, as herbal medicine, 505
red eye, see also subconjunctival
hemorrhage
associated conditions, 101t, 108, 109t
and contact lenses, 134
due to decongestant, 110
is common, 101
redness, symptom of infection, 19
red veterinary petrolatum, as sunblock, 54
referral, guidelines for, 6–7
reflection, as assessment technique, 4
rehydration
during diarrhea, 322–23
formulas, 458t
home treatment, 323t

staphyloccoccal disease, from ear piercing, 152
STDs, *see* sexually transmitted diseases (STDs)
sterculia gum, to treat constipation, 310
steroids
    cause acne, 94
    cause blood in feces, 408
    and insomnia, 485
    to treat dermatitis, 77t
    to treat psoriasis, 87
stimulants, and insomnia, 486t
stings
    description, 26
    prevention, 28
    treatment, 26–28, 27f
stoma, *see* ostomy
stool, *see* feces
stool softeners, 312
stool testing, *see* fecal occult blood testing
storage, of drugs, 9
strains, 21
St. John Ambulance, first aid kit, 36
St. John's wort
    drug interactions, 499
    as herbal medicine, 505
strep throat, 194–95
stress
    causes diarrhea, 321
    detected through blood test, 407
    and peptic ulcers, 246
strontium chloride, in dentifrices, 178
strophanthus, drug interactions, 499
sty
    symptoms, 104
    treatment, 104, 109
subconjunctival hemorrhage
    causes, 105t
    symptoms, 105
    treatment, 105
subtilisin, as contact lens cleaner, 132
subungual verrucae (warts under nails), 340, 341
"sugar-free", definition, 357
sugars
    in diabetic diet, 356
    and diarrhea, 320
    and tooth decay, 165
sugar substitutes, *see* artificial sweeteners
sulfasalazine, stains contact lenses, 138
sulfate salts, to treat constipation, 310
sulfisoxazole
    affects bile pigment tests, 407
    affects proteinuria tests, 405
    to treat otitis media, 155
sulfonamides
    affect proteinuria tests, 405
    cause diarrhea, 321
    and dermatitis, 68
sulfones, to treat acne, 98
sulfonylureas
    drug interactions, 358, 359t
    efficacy, 360
    to treat diabetes, 357

sulfur
    to treat acne, 96
    to treat dandruff, 89
    to treat psoriasis, 86
    to treat scabies, 275
sulisobenzone, as sunscreen, 55
sunblocks, *see* sunscreens, topical, physical
sunburn
    caused by UVB, 50
    and eye damage, 108
    and skin type, 51t, 51
    symptoms, 28, 50
    treatment, 50
sunlamps, *see* tanning, commercial units
sunlight, *see also* ultraviolet (UV) light
    description, 49–50
    effects
        acute, 50–53
        chronic, 53–54
    and eye damage, 108
    spectrum, 50f
sun protection factor (SPF)
    and children, 57
    definition, 55–56
    in quick-tanning products, 58
    and skin type, 51t
sunscreens
    and children, 57
    consumer counselling, 59
    drug interactions, 55t, 57
    drug-sunlight interactions, 52t
    efficacy, 56t
    safety, 54t
    systemic, 57
    topical
        chemical, 55
        for children, 57
        choosing, 56–57
        physical, 54–55
        sun protection factor, 55–56
suntan, *see* tanning
support belts, for ostomates, 387
supports, *see* health supports
suppositories, to treat constipation, 312–13
surfactants
    anionic, 32–33
    to clean contact lenses, 127–28
    types, 128t
swayback, *see* lordosis (swayback)
sweet almond oil, to soften ear wax, 157
sweet birch oil, *see* methyl salicylate
sweeteners, artificial, *see* artificial sweeteners
sweetening agents
    in diabetic diet, 356
    and tooth decay, 165
sweet oil, *see* olive oil (sweet oil)
swelling
    from insect bite, 26
    as sign of dermatitis, 65
    sign of infection, 19
    as sign of sprain or strain, 21

swimmer's ear
    symptoms, 153
    treatment, 156
swimming, and ostomy care, 390
sympathomimetics
    contraindications, 110t
    in ophthalmic decongestants, 110t, 110
symptoms
    allergic rhinitis, 215–16
    amenorrhea, 302
    anorexia nervosa, 476
    assessing, 5–6
    athlete's foot, 343
    atopic dermatitis, 66
    bites and stings, 26
    blepharitis, 103–4
    bulimia, 476
    bunions, 342
    burns, 21–23
    calluses and corns, 337–38
    candidiasis, 174
    canker sores, 173
    chalazion, 104
    colds, 193
    cold sores, 172
    conjunctival hyperemia, 104
    conjunctivitis, 105
    dandruff, 89
    dental caries, 164–66
    dermatitis, 65t, 65–66
    dry eye, 108
    dry mouth, 175
    dysmenorrhea, 302
    ear disorders, 149
    enterobiasis, 279
    frostbite, 25
    gastroesophageal reflux (GER), 247
    gastrointestinal gas, 252
    gingivitis, 169
    heat-related injuries, 25–26
    hemorrhoids, 330–31
    hives, 29
    hypercalcemia, 469
    hypocalcemia, 469
    hypoglycemia, 352
    infection (SHARP), 19
    iron deficiency anemia, 470
    minor wounds, 19
    musculoskeletal conditions, 39–40
    musculoskeletal injuries, 20–21, 39
    pediculosis, 268–69
    peptic ulcer disease (PUD), 247
    periodontal diseases, 169–70
    photosensitivity, 52–53
    poison ivy, 28
    premenstrual syndrome (PMS), 303t, 303–4
    psoriasis, 83–84
    scabies, 269–70
    seborrhea, 89
    sty, 104
    subconjunctival hemorrhage, 105
    sunburn, 28, 50
    swimmer's ear, 153

toxic shock syndrome, 301
vaginitis, 305
sympto-thermal method, of contraception, 288
syringes, for insulin injection, 365–66, 367

Taenia saginata, as parasite, 283
Taenia solium, as parasite, 283
taheebo, as herbal medicine, 505
tailor's bunions, 341
talc
   poisoning, 519
   as sunblock, 54
talcum powder, and genital hygiene, 301
tampons
   for menstrual care, 301
   and toxic shock syndrome, 302
tannic acid
   as astringent, 30
   to treat diarrhea, 324
   to treat mouth sores, 182
tanning
   and beauty, 49
   commercial units, 50–51
   drug agents, 57–58
   and skin type, 51t, 51
   sunlight, 50, 51
tansy, as herbal medicine, 505
tapeworms, *see* cestodes
tarsal cyst, *see* chalazion
tartaric acid, as spermicide, 289
taste buds, 164
TCA, *see* tricyclic antidepressants (TCA)
TEA, *see* triethanolamine salicylate (TEA)
teaberry oil, *see* methyl salicylate
tear duct, *see* lacrimal gland
tear film
   functions, 102–3, 103t
   layers, 102t, 102
tears
   artificial, 112t, 112
      and contact lens wearer, 131
      and dry eye, 109
teeth, *see also* mouth
   anatomy, 163–64, 164f
   broken, 170
   color, 163, 164, 176
   demineralization, 170
   dentinal caries, 166f
   dentures, 170
   enamel caries, 165f
   fillings, 170
   pain, 170, 181, 239
   physiology, 164
   treatment, 171f
teething
   infant age, 455
   treatment, 455
temelastine, to treat allergic rhinitis, 224
temperature
   ambient, and dermatitis, 64
   basal, chart example, 400f
   body, *see also* heat
      and contraception, 288

and disease states, 397–98
and fever, 232
following burn, 23
and frostbite, 25
in infants, 456
measuring, 398–99
skin as regulator, 19
conversion chart, 397t
skin, and pain, 41
tendinitis, definition, 39
tennis elbow, health support, 439
terfenadine
   to treat allergic rhinitis, 221, 224
   to treat dermatitis, 78
   to treat motion sickness, 262
terpin hydrate, to treat cough, 205
testing strips, to test urine glucose, 371
testosterone, causes acne, 94
tetracaine
   as ophthalmic anesthetic, 112, 113
   as topical anesthetic, 34
   to treat hemorrhoids, 331
tetracycline
   allergic reactions, 134
   causes diarrhea, 321
   drug interactions, 251
   and hyperpigmentation, 58
   nutrient interactions, 469, 470
   and ostomy, 390
   stains contact lenses, 138
   and tooth color, 164
   to treat acne, 97–98
   to treat mouth sores, 182
tetracycline hydrochloride, to treat acne, 97
tetrahydrofurfuryl nicotinate, as external analgesic, 44
tetrahydrozoline, as ophthalmic decongestant, 110
tetryzoline, *see* tetrahydrozoline
theophylline, and gastroesophageal reflux, 247
thermometers
   basal, 399f, 399–400
   digital, 399f, 399
   mercury, 398t 399f, 398–99
   rectal, 398
   strips, 399
   types, 398–400
thigh braces, 439
thimerosal
   allergic reactions, 134
   as antiseptic, 32
   to disinfect contact lenses, 129, 132
   as ophthalmic preservative, 113
thiocarbamide, and bad breath, 175
thioguanine, to treat psoriasis, 88
thiouracil, causes acne, 94
thirst, caused by insulin deficiency, 352
thorn apple, dangerous medicine, 499
threadworms, *see* pinworms
throat, sore, *see* pharyngitis (sore throat)
thrush mouth, *see* candidiasis

thymol
   as antiseptic, 32
   to treat dermatitis, 77
ticarcillin, nutrient interactions, 471
ticks, and parasitic infections, 267
timolol, causing psoriasis, 84
tincture of benzoin, to treat cough, 205
tinea infection, differentiation from dermatitis, 71
tinnitus, 149
titanium dioxide, as sunblock, 54
toenails, infants, 452
tolbutamide
   adverse effects, 358
   to manage diabetes, 358
tolnaftate, to treat athlete's foot, 343–44
tongue
   anatomy, 164
   white plaques, 174
tonsillitis, and bad breath, 175
toothache, 165–66, 170, 181, 239
toothbrushes
   children, 167
   how to use, 168
   types, 167, 168
tooth decay, *see* dental caries
toothpastes, *see* dentifrices
toothpicks, 168
tooth whiteners, in dentrifices, 178–79
torticollis, causes neck pain, 438
toxic shock syndrome
   and diaphragms, 290
   symptoms, 301
   and tampons, 302
   treatment, 301–2
Toxocara canis, as parasite, 283
toys, and child safety, 459
tracheal tube, to deliver oxygen, 434
tragacanth gum, to treat constipation, 310
trauma, *see* injuries; wounds
travel
   and diabetes, 378
   and ostomy care, 390
trees, causing allergic rhinitis, 214
trematodes, as parasites, 283
trench foot, 25
trenchmouth, *see* acute necrotizing ulcerative gingivitis (ANUG)
Treponema pallidum, and antibiotics, 33
tretinoin
   to treat acne, 98
   to treat warts, 341
triamcinolone, to treat allergic rhinitis, 225
triamcinolone acetonide, to treat acne, 98
triamterene, nutrient interactions, 470, 471
triazolam, and insomnia, 485, 486
Trichinella, in pork, 283
trichloroacetic acid, to treat warts, 341
Trichuris trichiura, see whipworms
triclosan
   as antiseptic, 32
   in dentrifices, 178
   to treat dandruff, 89–90

dimenhydrinate in most trials, but was marginally better under some extreme circumstances. The scopolamine was most effective when applied from 6 to 16 hours before motion, supporting the manufacturer's recommendation of application 12 hours before exposure.

Although transdermal application of scopolamine is reputed to have virtually eliminated the adverse effects of this drug, dryness of the mouth occurs often, and drowsiness and blurred vision are also reported. These adverse effects are not significantly reduced by adding ephedrine. Other well known adverse effects of orally and parenterally administered scopolamine have been reported, such as hallucinations, confusion, disorientation, memory disturbances, restlessness and giddiness. Some of these effects have occurred with alarming frequency in unique situations, such as on cruise ships where a significant proportion of the population are using this treatment. Although these occurrences cannot be ignored, from the seven million patches sold in the period 1981 to 1984, only 139 adverse effect reports have been recorded.

A disquieting adverse effect reported is anisocoria, or bilateral difference in pupil diameter. This seems to be reversible, but may persist for several days after removing the scopolamine patch. There are also several reports of unilateral or bilateral dilated pupils due to failure to wash the hands before touching the eye or inserting contact lenses.

Transdermal scopolamine is not recommended for use in children, or in women of child-bearing age or in women who are breastfeeding. Individuals using transdermally applied scopolamine should not drive vehicles, pilot planes nor use potentially hazardous machinery, because disorientation and drowsiness can occur. People with glaucoma, intestinal obstruction and urinary bladder neck retention should use scopolamine with caution. Transdermal scopolamine should be used with caution by people taking other drugs with parasympatholytic effects. Alcohol may interfere with the metabolism of the drug, thus increasing the chances of adverse effects. Scopolamine is contraindicated in people with glaucoma or where it causes blurring of vision or pressure pain within the eye.

Other Antiemetics

Phosphorated carbohydrate solution is a mixture of levulose (fructose) and dextrose with phosphoric acid added to adjust the pH to between 1.5 and 1.6. This solution is reputed to cause a delay in gastric emptying time due to its high osmotic pressure. Its effectiveness in preventing motion sickness is questionable. There is no evidence that delay in gastric emptying time has any effect on nausea and vomiting caused by disturbance in the semicircular canals.

For control of epidemic and other functional vomiting, the usual adult dose is 15 to 30 mL at 15-minute intervals until vomiting ceases. The user should not dilute the solution nor consume other liquids within 15 minutes of taking a dose. Doses should be limited to 5 per hour, and a physician should be contacted if vomiting does not cease after five doses. Diabetics should not use this solution because of its high dextrose content. There is minimal information about this product in the literature, but there is evidence that it delays gastric emptying, the rationale by which it exerts its antiemetic properties.

Bismuth subsalicylate has been shown to be effective in relieving the symptoms of indigestion of unspecified origin. The demulcent properties of bismuth subsalicylate seems to result from complexing of bismuth to the glycoproteins and mucopolysaccharides of the gastric mucosa thus providing a protective barrier between the mucosa

and the offending agent. Healthy adult volunteers were encouraged to overindulge in food and alcohol consumption at a simulated reception and dinner. Of the 91 participants, those who experienced symptoms of gastric distress and received bismuth subsalicylate had significant relief of individual symptoms of nausea, sense of fullness, heartburn, eructation, stomach pain and flatulence as well as superior overall relief compared to those individuals who received a placebo formulation.

Bismuth subsalicylate preparations also provide some protection against ipecac syrup-induced emesis. Low doses of ipecac syrup, 5 to 7.5 mL, were used to simulate mild gastrointestinal upset in humans. Compared to placebo, bismuth subsalicylate successfully controlled the nausea and vomiting in 67 and 80 per cent of the subjects respectively. Toxicity from bismuth-containing preparations does not seem to occur, but significant serum salicylate concentrations have been reported after ingesting bismuth subsalicylate products.

Powdered rhizome of ginger (Zingiber officinale) in gelatin capsules (940 mg) reduces motion sickness under simulated experimental conditions. It is thought to work by increasing gastric motility and adsorbing or neutralizing toxins and acids, thereby blocking gastrointestinal reactions responsible for nausea feedback. This product is not available in Canada.

Sea Bands are elasticized wrist-bands that control nausea and vomiting through acupressure. These bands are worn on both wrists, three fingers' width from the uppermost crease and are fitted with a non-corrosive button which exerts pressure on the Nei-Kuan point. Sea Bands have been shown to be effective in treating nausea caused by chemotherapy, post-operative conditions, pregnancy and motion sickness as described in medical studies from the U.S. and U.K. while Canadian research is being conducted at the University of Calgary.

Summary

When emesis is indicated to treat oral poisoning, syrup of ipecac is the emetic of choice. It is effective and safe in the hospital or home. If pharmacists do not have expertise in treating poisoning, all calls for poisoning cases should be referred to the local poison control centre or consultant.

Motion sickness is the only condition suitable for self-medication with nonprescription antiemetics. Dimenhydrinate and transdermal scopolamine are the drugs of choice, but promethazine and diphenhydramine may be suggested as alternative agents. Any instances of persistent nausea or vomiting should be referred to a physician.

Ask the Consumer

Emetics
Q. Is this emetic for immediate use to treat drug overdose or poisoning?
■ If the answer is yes, the following questions should be asked.

Q. Is emesis indicated as the method of treatment?
■ Emetics are not recommended unless a poison control authority indicates that emesis is the treatment of choice.

Q. What is the toxic agent?
■ Emesis should not be induced after ingesting acids, alkalis, other caustics or petroleum products.

Q. What is the condition of the individual?
■ Emesis should not be induced if the individual is unconscious, expected to become lethargic within 30 minutes or convulsing.

Q. What is the age of the individual?
■ Emetics should not be given to children less than one year without medical supervision, since the gag reflex is not fully developed at that age. Emetic doses should also be adjusted to match the age of the individual, for example, child or adult dose.

Q. Is the emetic for possible future use?
■ The consumer should be cautioned against administering an emetic to treat poisoning without first consulting a pharmacist, physician or poison control centre. The person should be warned about possible abuse of emetics in anorexia nervosa and the dangers of children accidentally ingesting emetics.

Q. Do you know when to use emesis for poisoning?
■ Provide the consumer with a poison control chart and the telephone number of the local poison control centre.

Antiemetics
Q. Is this antiemetic for motion sickness?
■ Motion sickness is the only situation for which self-medication with nonprescription antiemetics can be safely recommended by a pharmacist.

Q. Will you be driving a vehicle?
■ Most nonprescription drugs for treating motion sickness can cause drowsiness and should not be used while operating a vehicle.

Q. What is the age of the individual?
■ This question ensures the correct dose and dosage form is recommended (that is, tablets for adults, syrup for children, and suppositories if oral administration is impossible due to severe vomiting).

Q. Is the nausea or vomiting due to pregnancy?
■ Tactful questioning of women of child-bearing age can focus attention on the possible cause, especially if the description suggests morning sickness. Self-medication with nonprescription antiemetics is contraindicated. Nondrug suggestions about diet may help. Referral to a physician is mandatory if the individual is not yet under a physician's care or if the morning sickness is severe.

Q. Can you attribute the nausea or vomiting to some situation?
■ Overindulgence in food or alcohol may induce nausea. Temporary abstinence from solid food and maintaining fluid intake may be the only treatments required. Treatment with antacids or even laxatives may be indicated if further questioning reveals that hyperacidity or constipation is an additional symptom.

Q. Could the nausea or vomiting be due to drug therapy?
■ Nausea and vomiting are potentially ubiquitous adverse effects of drug therapy. Evaluation of patient records or careful questioning may reveal that other medications could be causing these symptoms. Prescription drug therapy should not be discontinued or modified without consulting the prescribing physician. However, in certain situations if withdrawal of the medication is not life-threatening and if the symptoms are severe, the drug may be discontinued before consultation with the physician. Each situation should be treated as unique.

Q. How long has the nausea or vomiting been a problem? Are other symptoms, such as abdominal pain, headache or diarrhea, also present?
■ Chronic, severe nausea or vomiting may be a symptom of a serious medical disorder. Self-medication with nonprescription drugs is not recommended. If the cause cannot be identified, and if the symptoms are severe and have persisted for more than one or two days, the individual should consult a physician.

References

Nausea and Vomiting
Anonymous. Six-month-old persistent vomiters (Editorial). Br Med J 1979;2:459–60.
Biggs JSC. Vomiting in pregnancy: causes and management. Drugs 1975;9:299–306.
Brand JJ, Perry WL. Drugs used in motion sickness. Pharmacol Rev 1966;18:895–924.
Braunwald E, Isselbacher KJ, Petersdorf RG, et al, eds. Harrison's principles of internal medicine. New York: McGraw-Hill, 1991:140–2,252–6.
Gilman AG, Rall TW, Nies AS, Taylor P, eds. Goodman and Gilman's the pharmacological basis of therapeutics. New York: Pergamon Press, 1990: 56–7,925–6.
McEvoy GK, ed. American Hospital Formulary Service. Bethesda: American Society of Hospital Pharmacists, Inc., 1991:1739–51.
Money KE. Motion sickness. Physiol Rev 1970;50:1–39.
Norris CH. Drugs affecting the inner ear. A review of their clinical efficacy, mechanisms of action, toxicity and place in therapy. Drugs 1988;36:754–72.
Triozzi PL, Laszlo J. Optimum management of nausea and vomiting in cancer chemotherapy. Drugs 1987;34:136–49.
Wang SC. Physiology and pharmacology of the brain stem. New York: Futura Publishing, 1980:205–41.
Wang SC. Emetic and antiemetic drugs. In: Root WS, Hofmann FG, eds. Physiological pharmacology, volume II. New York: Academic Press, 1965:255–328.
Wood CD, Graybiel A. A theory of motion sickness based on pharmacological reactions. Clin Pharmacol Ther 1970;11:621–9.

Antiemetics
Anonymous. Flunarizine and cinnarizine: extrapyramidal reactions. Clin-Alert 1987;10:122.
Anonymous. Six-month-old persistent vomiters (Editorial). Br Med J 1979;2:459–60.
Anonymous. Transdermal scopolamine for motion sickness. Med Lett Drugs Ther 1981;23:89–90.
Attias J, Gordon C, Ribak J, Binah O, Rolnick A. Efficacy of transdermal scopolamine against seasickness: a 3-day study. Aviat Space Environ Med 1987;58:60–2.
Barbezat GO. The vomiting patient: a rational approach. Drugs 1981;22:246–53.
Berkow R, ed. The Merck manual. Rahway: Merck, Sharpe and Dohme, 1983:1712,1726,1850–1,2135–6.
Berkowitz JM. The efficacy of bismuth subsalicylate in relieving gastrointestinal discomfort following excessive alcohol and food intake. J Int Med Res 1990;18:351–7.

Brand JJ, Whittingham P. Intramuscular hyoscine in control of motion sickness. Lancet 1970;2:232–4.

Carlston J. Unilateral dilated pupil from scopolamine disk. JAMA 1982;248:31.

Craig DF, Mellor CS. Dimenhydrinate dependence and withdrawal. Can Med Assoc J 1990;142:970–3.

D'Arcy PF. Problems with transdermal scopolamine. Pharm Int 1984;5:290.

Dahl E, Offer-Ohlsen D, Lillevold PE, Sandvik MS. Transdermal scopolamine, oral meclizine and placebo in motion sickness. Clin Pharmacol Ther 1984;36:116–20.

Goldenberg MM, Honkomp LJ, Davis CS. Antinauseant and antiemetic properties of bismuth subsalicylate in dogs and humans. J Pharm Sci 1976;65:1398–400.

Graybiel A, Cramer DB, Wood CD. Experimental motion sickness: efficacy of transdermal scopolamine plus ephedrine. Aviat Space Environ Med 1981;52:337–9.

Hansten PD, Horn JR. Drug interactions. Philadelphia: Lea & Febiger, 1989:206,209–10,366.

Houston JB, Levy G. Effect of carbonated beverages and of an antiemetic containing carbohydrate and phosphoric acid on riboflavin bioavailability and salicylamide biotransformation in humans. J Pharm Sci 1975;64:1504–7.

Hurley JD, Eshelman FN. Trimethobenzamide HCl in the treatment of nausea and vomiting associated with antineoplastic chemotherapy. J Clin Pharmacol 1980;20:352–6.

Isaac L, Goth A. The mechanism of the potentiation of norepinephrine by antihistaminics. J Pharmacol Exp Ther 1967;156:463–8.

Jackson RT, Turner JS. Astemizole: its use in the treatment of patients with chronic vertigo. Arch Otolaryngol Head Neck Surg 1987;113:536–42.

Johnson P, Hansen D, Matarazzo D, et al. Transderm scop patches for prevention of motion sickness (Letter). N Engl J Med 1984;311:468.

Kahn A, Hasaerts D, Krogg EA. Phenothiazine-induced sleep apneas in normal infants. Pediatrics 1985;75:844–7.

Kohl RL, Homick JL, Cintron N, Calkins DS. Lack of effects of astemizole on vestibular ocular reflex, motion sickness, and cognitive performance in man. Aviat Space Environ Med 1987;58:1171–4.

Kohl RL, Calkins DS, Robinson RE. Control of nausea and autonomic dysfunction with terfenadine, a peripherally acting antihistamine. Aviat Space Environ Med 1991;62:392–6.

Krogh CME, ed. Compendium of pharmaceuticals and specialties. Ottawa: Canadian Pharmaceutical Association, 1991.

Leeder JS, Spielberg SP, MacLeod SM. Bendectin: the wrong way to regulate drug availability (Editorial). Can Med Assoc J 1983;129:1085–7.

Martin-Bouyer G, Foulon G, Guerbois H, Barin C. Epidemiological study of encephalopathies following bismuth administration per os. Characteristics of intoxicated subjects: comparison with a control group. Clin Toxicol 1981;18:1277–83.

McCrary JA, Webb NR. Anisocoria from scopolamine patches. JAMA 1982;248:353–4.

McTavish D, Goa KL, Ferrill M. Terfenadine: An updated review of its pharmacological properties and therapeutic efficacy. Drugs 1990;39:552–74.

Mowrey DB, Clayton DE. Motion sickness, ginger and psychophysics. Lancet 1982;1:655–7.

Patterson JH, Ives TJ, Greganti MA. Transient bilateral pupillary dilation from scopolamine discs. Drug Intell Clin Pharm 1986;20:986–7.

Price NM, Schmitt LG, McGuire J, Shaw JE, Trobough G. Transdermal scopolamine in the prevention of motion sickness at sea. Clin Pharmacol Ther 1981;29:414–9.

Pyykko I, Padoan S, Schalen L, et al. The effects of TTS-scopolamine, dimenhydrinate, lidocaine and tocainide on motions sickness, vertigo and nystagmus. Aviat Space Environ Med 1985;56:777–82.

Pyykko I, Schalen L, Matsuoka I. Transdermally administered scopolamine vs. dimenhydrinate. II. Effect on different types of nystagmus. Acta Otolaryngol 1985;99:597–604.

Pyykko I, Schalen L, Jantti V. Transdermally administered scopolamine vs. dimenhydrinate. I. Effect on nausea and vertigo in experimentally induced motion sickness. Acta Otolaryngol 1985;99:588–96.

Pyykko I, Schalen L, Jantti V, Magnusson M. A reduction of vestibulo-visual integration during transdermally administered scopolamine and dimenhydrinate. Acta Otolaryngol Suppl 1984;406:167–73.

Richards DM, Brogden RM, Heel RC, Speight TM, Avery GS. Astemizole: A review of its pharmacodynamic properties and therapeutic efficacy. Drugs 1984;28:38–61.

Sea-Bands relieve nausea, motion sickness. Pharmacy NB (Jan) 1991;7:1–2.

Shaw JE, Schmitt LG, McCauley ME, Royal JW. Transdermally administered scopolamine for prevention of motion sickness in a vertical oscillator (Abstract). Clin Pharmacol Ther 1977;21:117.

Shaw JE, Urquhart J. Transdermal drug administration—a nuisance becomes an opportunity. Br Med J 1981;283:875–6.

Towse G. Cinnarizine—a labyrinthine sedative. J Laryngol Otol 1980;94:1009–15.

Vargas R, McMahon FG, Ryan JR. A study of the anticholinergic activity of terfenadine in normal volunteers. J Int Med Res 1989;17:157–61.

Wood CD. Antimotion sickness and antiemetic drugs. Drugs 1979;17:471–9.

Emetics

Anonymous. Childhood poisoning: prevention and first-aid management [Editorial]. Br Med J 1975;4:483–4.

Boehm JJ, Oppenheim RC. The emergency treatment of childhood poisoning. Aust J Pharm Sci 1977;6:33–43.

Boxer L, Anderson FP, Rowe DS. Comparison of ipecac-induced emesis with gastric lavage in the treatment of acute salicylate ingestion. J Pediatr 1969;74:800–3.

British pharmacopoeia. London: Her Majesty's Stationery Office, 1988:316–7, 673–4.

Brotman MC, Forbath N, Garfinkle PE, Humphrey JG. Myopathy due to ipecac syrup poisoning in a patient with anorexia nervosa. Can Med Assoc J 1981;125:453–4.

Brushwood DB, Tietze KJ. Regulatory controversy surrounding ipecac use and misuse. Am J Hosp Pharm 1986;43:157–61.

Corby DG, Decker WJ, Moran MJ, Payne CE. Clinical comparison of pharmacologic emetics in children. Pediatrics 1968;42:361–4.

Curtis RA, Barone J, Giacona N. Efficacy of ipecac and activated charcoal/cathartic; prevention of salicylate absorption in simulated overdose. Am J Intern Med 1984;144:48–52.

Dabbous IA, Bergman AB, Robertson WO. The ineffectiveness of mechanically induced vomiting. J Pediatr 1965;66:952–4.

Dershewitz RA, Niederman LG. Ipecac at home—a health hazard. Clin Toxicol 1981;18:969–72.

Gieseker DR, Troutman WG. Emergency induction of emesis using liquid detergent products: a report of 15 cases. Clin Toxicol 1981;18:277–82.

Grbcich PA, Lacouture PG, Kresel JJ, Russell MT, Lovejoy FH. Expired ipecac syrup efficacy. Pediatrics 1986;78:1085–9.

Herfindal ET, Gourley DR, Hart LL, eds. Clinical pharmacology and therapeutics. Baltimore: Williams and Wilkins, 1988:1044–5.

King WD. Syrup of ipecac: a drug review. Clin Toxicol 1980;17:353–8.

Kulig K, Bar-Or D, Cantrill SV, et al. Management of acutely poisoned patients without gastric emptying. Ann Emerg Med 1985;14:562–7.

Manno BR, Manno JE. Toxicology of ipecac: a review. Clin Toxicol 1977;10:221–42.

Manoguerra AS, Krenzelok EP. Rapid emesis from high-dose ipecac syrup in adults and children intoxicated with antiemetics or other drugs. Am J Hosp Pharm 1978;35:1360–2.

Modell W, Schild HO, Wilson A, eds. Applied pharmacology. Philadelphia: WB Saunders, 1976:616–7.

Neuvonen PJ, Vartiainen M, Tokola O. Comparison of activated charcoal and ipecac syrup in prevention of drug absorption. Eur J Clin Pharmacol 1983;24:557–62.

Ng RC, Darwish H, Steward DA. Emergency treatment of petroleum distillate and turpentine ingestion. Can Med Assoc J 1974;111:537–8.

Reshima D, Suzuki A, Otsubo K, Aoyama T, Shimozono Y, Salta M, Noda K. Efficacy of Emetic and U.S.P. Ipecac Syrup in prevention of drug absorption. Chem Pharm Bull 1990;38:2242–5.

Taylor AT. Nausea and Vomiting. In: DiPiro JT, Talbert RL, Hayes PE, Yee GC, Posey LM, eds. Pharmacotherapy: a pathophysiologic approach. New York: Elsevier, 1989:456–67.

The United States pharmacopeia XXII/National Formutary XVII. Rockville: United States Pharmacopeial Convention Inc., 1990:717–9.

Emetics and Antiemetics

Vale JA, Meredith TJ, Proudfoot AT. Syrup of ipecacuanha: is it really useful? Br Med J 1986;293:1321.

Varipapa RJ, Oderda GM. Effect of milk on ipecac-induced emesis. N Engl J Med 1977;296:112–3.

17
Topical Antiparasitics

Kathleen F. Gesy

Lice and scabies mites are two common parasites affecting humans. Both parasitic infestations are extremely contagious with rapid transmission in environments where there is close personal contact. The clinical presentation and diagnosis of pediculosis (lice infestation) depends on whether the insects are head, body or pubic lice. Diagnosis of scabies is more difficult since the clinical signs and symptoms mimic other skin disorders. Topical antiparasitic therapy is directed at eradication of the causative parasite. Education with respect to the transmission of the parasite and institution of measures to prevent reinfestation are also essential for effective treatment of these parasitic infestations.

The most common parasitic infestations of the skin are caused by two classes of arthropods: the arachnids (spiders, scorpions, ticks and mites) and the insects (lice, bugs, flies, mosquitos, moths, beetles and fleas). The medical importance of these parasites usually relates to their ability to transmit diseases such as malaria, sleeping sickness and yellow fever, and thus directly affect human health and well-being. Efforts to control these vector-borne diseases are through prevention by host protection and destruction of the parasitic population in endemic areas. Even though many of the arachnids and insects are not vectors of disease, they can cause reactions and morbidity in the human host as a result of their bites, stings or feeding habits.

The type of association between the arthropod and the human host varies considerably. Human contact time for the mosquito is brief compared to that for some species of ticks, which may feed for several days. Fleas spend much longer periods on their host, but are not permanently attached and often hop from one host to another. Management of the bites or stings from these temporary parasitic relationships relies mainly on symptomatic treatment for the bite reaction and prevention through the use of insecticides and insect repellents. (See the chapter on topical first aid for a discussion of insect bites and insect repellents.)

True parasitic relationships exist between humans and lice and humans and the scabies mite. Lice become more or less permanently attached to humans by their hair or clothing. The scabies mite forms an even closer relationship with humans by burrowing within the outermost layers of the skin. Pediculosis and scabies are the terms used to describe the cutaneous diseases caused by infestation with lice and the scabies mite, respectively. Treatment of these two dermatoses requires the use of topical antiparasitics.

Pediculosis and scabies are highly contagious diseases commonly associated with poor hygiene, overcrowding and unsanitary living conditions that enhance their spread. After World War II, the incidence of pediculosis and scabies declined, but these parasites have made a recent and vigorous worldwide comeback. People of all socioeconomic groups are affected. Because of low morbidity and mortality, pediculosis and scabies are not reportable diseases, but they remain a major health problem in modern society. A need exists to increase awareness of these diseases and their treatment, prevention and control.

Pediculosis

Human lice are found in every climate, from the Arctic to the tropics, but are more common in temperate areas. Three species of blood-sucking lice infest humans: the head louse *(Pediculus capitis)*, the body louse *(Pediculus corporis)* and the pubic louse *(Phthirus pubis)*. They differ in morphology and, as their names suggest, the area of the body they infest.

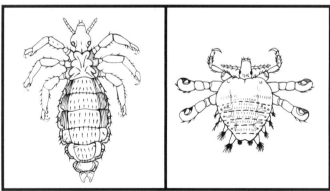

Figure 1 *Dorsal View of a Body Louse (Pediculus Humanus)*　　**Figure 2** *Dorsal View of a Pubic Louse (Phthirus Pubis)*

Lice are wingless insects with six legs (see Figure 1). Morphologically, the head and body louse are similar, except the head louse is slightly smaller. The average size of a body louse ranges from 2 to 4 mm. The pubic louse is easily differentiated because it has a broad, squat body 1 to 2 mm in length, and large claws on the middle and hind legs (see Figure 2). This appearance, together with the pubic

Topical Antiparasitics

louse's characteristically slow movement, is why the pubic louse is often called the crab louse.

Life Cycle

Lice are obligate human ectoparasites that complete their entire life cycle on the body of the host. When ready to feed, the lice puncture the skin, inject saliva into the wound and pump blood into their stomachs for digestion. Feeding can occur at any time of the day or night. The pubic louse can remain attached to the skin site for many days, sucking blood from time to time.

The adult female louse can lay 5 to 9 eggs, or nits, per day and may live up to 1 month. The eggs are firmly attached with a tenacious cement bond to the base of hair shafts or to clothing fibres. The eggs are incubated by body heat and hatch in 6 to 9 days, leaving behind the empty nits. The resulting nymphs mature to adulthood through three development stages over 7 to 10 days. The duration of the nymphal stage for body lice may be longer if the host does not wear clothing all the time, since lower temperatures slow nymph development.

Lice are acutely dependent on the host for food and warmth. The body louse is the most hardy of the species and may survive up to 10 days away from the host; survival is 2 to 4 days for the head louse and only 24 hours for the pubic louse. Lice ova can remain viable away from the host for variable periods depending on the temperature and humidity. Eggs of body lice removed from warmth through discarded clothing may take 2 to 3 weeks to hatch, but cannot survive longer than 4 weeks. Ova from other lice species survive for a shorter period of time: 6 to 7 days at 37°C and 50 per cent relative humidity, or 17 to 21 days at 24°C and 90 per cent relative humidity.

Transmission

Head lice usually transfer from one host to another by direct contact with an infested person's head. Contact with such personal items as hats, hairbrushes, combs or bedding is less commonly responsible for lice transmission. The role of fomites in transmitting head lice infestations has been challenged. Lice away from the head have a high mortality rate due to sickness, senility or injury, and thus are unlikely to infest other people or cause reinfestation. Until further work is done, public health measures such as cleaning materials that harbor lice should not be abandoned.

Contrary to popular belief, the head louse does not jump or fly from one person to another. Once present in a home, school or institutional environment, head lice usually spread rapidly. This type of louse is a major public health problem in preschool and elementary school children. Parents should be reassured that the presence of head lice is not a reflection on hygiene; indeed, head lice prefer to live on clean heads of hair.

Body lice infestation, sometimes known as vagabond's disease, is transferred from one host to another by direct contact or by contact with infested clothing or bedding. Pediculosis corporis is primarily a disease of indigent and vagrant groups, for whom crowded living conditions and poor personal hygiene are the norm. The body louse can also be an effective vector for typhus, relapsing fever and, rarely, trench fever.

Pubic lice spread rapidly through close physical contact, particularly during sexual intercourse. Only one sexual exposure is required. Pediculosis pubis is especially common in the 15 to 40 year age group and is often seen at student health services and venereal disease clinics. Besides coitus or some other close physical contact, pubic lice may be transmitted through clothing, bedding, and rarely, toilet seats. Although the crab louse is not considered a vector of disease, a diagnosis of pubic lice infestation may indicate coexisting sexually transmitted diseases. Affected individuals should see a physician for appropriate diagnostic evaluation.

Clinical Presentation and Diagnosis

Itching in the infested area is the earliest and most common symptom of lice infestation. At each feeding, lice leave behind a small purpuric puncture site. With repeated exposure over several weeks, the host develops an inflammatory hypersensitivity reaction manifested as a small red papule at each new feeding site. Pruritus, erythema and inflammation of the scalp usually indicate an infestation of several weeks duration or a recent reinfestation in an already sensitized host.

Pruritus is localized for head and pubic lice, but generalized with body lice. When pubic lice are present, itching is particularly severe at bedtime. Vigorous scratching in all cases produces increased inflammation and subsequent excoriation, which may lead to secondary bacterial infection. Itching in children often results in concomitant signs of sleeplessness, irritability and inability to concentrate in the classroom. Although pruritus is characteristic and common, some people with head and pubic lice may be asymptomatic.

Each time a louse feeds, it injects irritating saliva into the wound. The injected saliva may cause a mild fever, muscular aches (especially in the calves of the legs) and, occasionally, swelling of the cervical glands or lymph nodes. The term "feeling lousy" was aptly phrased to describe this condition.

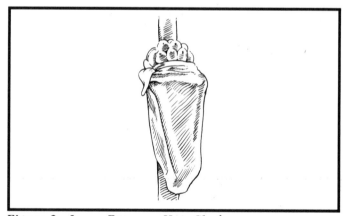

Figure 3 *Louse Egg on a Hair Shaft*

Head Lice

To diagnose head lice infestation, the hair must be inspected. On examination, live lice may be seen on the scalp, but the diagnosis is usually made by identification of nits. The nits are oval, close to the scalp and firmly attached to the hair (see Figure 3). The nits cannot be dislodged, which differentiates them from dandruff, seborrheic scales, hair spray or other artifacts that can be brushed off the hair. Nits more than 6 mm from the scalp are older than 7 days (the hair grows about 5 to 6 mm per week) and are either hatched (empty) or no longer viable. Head lice bites and eggs may be present anywhere on the scalp, but the infestation usually starts around the hairline at the back of the head and neck and around the ears. Head lice prefer these warmer, more protected spots.

Body Lice

Body lice (seam squirrels) and their nits may be identified by thoroughly searching the seams of an infested individual's clothing, particularly where there is close contact between garment and wearer, such as the waistline and armpits. Body lice visit the host's body only to feed. Tiny bites are most commonly seen on the shoulders, around the waist and on the buttocks. Due to intense pruritus, characteristic linear excoriations from scratching may be present.

Pubic Lice

Pubic lice are usually limited to the genitalia. In heavy infestations or as a result of spread through scratching, they may be found in other hairy areas, such as the short hairs of the perianal area, trunk, thighs, underarms, eyebrows, eyelids, beard and moustache. Eyelash involvement causes itching of the eyelids as well as scaling, crusting and a purulent discharge. Unique to pubic lice infestations, but not always present, are pale, bluish-gray spots called maculae cerulae on the infested parts of the body.

Scabies

Scabies is a highly contagious skin disease resulting from infestation with and sensitization to the itch mite *Sarcoptes scabiei hominis*. It is more commonly known as "the seven year itch" or simply as "the itch."

For years it was postulated that epidemics of scabies were cyclical in nature, lasting about 15 years followed by a 15-year gap between epidemics. Recent studies indicate no regular cycling in the incidence of scabies. Epidemics neither occur at constant intervals nor have constant durations. Scabies has persisted in our society now for about 20 years without signs of abating.

S. scabiei has a more or less worldwide distribution. Unlike lice, scabies mites have not been known to carry disease from one person to another. The female itch mite is a whitish, disc-shaped, eight-legged mite that is just about visible without the aid of a hand lens (see Figure 4). The female mite is twice as large as the male, being 0.4 by 0.3 mm.

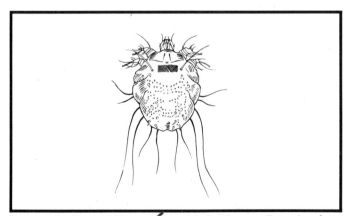

Figure 4 *Dorsal View of an Adult Mature Female of the Scabies Mite (Sarcoptes Scabiei)*

Life Cycle

The scabies mite lives in the stratum corneum and spends its entire life cycle on the host. Only the impregnated female causes infestation. The female scabies mite selects places on the body where the skin is thin and wrinkled. Within 1 hour, it digs and eats its way into the stratum corneum using specialized mouthparts and cutting edges on the front legs. Once in the superficial layers of the skin, mites excavate winding tunnels or burrows at the rate of 2 to 3 mm per day. The mite feeds on liquids oozing from the dermal cells that have been chewed.

Egg laying begins about 4 to 5 days after fertilization. The female deposits 4 to 6 large eggs per day in the burrow. Fecal pellets, called scybala, are also distributed along the path of the burrow. The eggs hatch in 3 to 5 days and the larvae crawl out of the tunnels onto the skin surface. Female mites rarely leave their burrows and may live on the human for 1 to 2 months. Hence, the potential number of mites per infestation is enormous. Fortunately, less than 10 per cent of the larvae mature to adults. The population of mites may be limited in part by hygiene, scratching and local inflammation.

A few larvae succeed in burrowing into the stratum corneum to produce not a tunnel, but a "moulting pocket." After 2 to 3 days, the larvae moult into eight-legged nymphs. A nymph destined to become a female mite moults again into a sexually immature female, which remains in the moulting pocket until fertilized by a male. She then enlarges in size to become a mature female and continues the cycle of infestation. The adult male mite probably spends most of his shorter life span wandering around on the skin surface seeking females waiting to be fertilized.

Transmission

Although scabies is commonly associated with overcrowding, poverty and poor personal hygiene, anyone can contract scabies, regardless of age, sex or socioeconomic status. Scabies is spread by close body contact with an infested individual, especially when sleeping together in the same bed. Thus, it is often seen within families, between sexual partners, among schoolaged children and in institutionalized people. Scabies can be considered a sexually transmitted disease, since prolonged intimate contact is a common means of spread. Nonsexual transmission to other household members and contacts, especially infants and children, is also common. Scabies can be transmitted through handholding games among children or between courting couples who are habitually holding hands. The transfer of mites requires about 15 to 20 minutes of close contact. Exchanging clothing or sharing a bed or towels may also spread scabies, although with much less frequency than direct contact, because the mite can survive only 2 to 4 days away from the host.

Clinical Presentation and Diagnosis

Scabies can be difficult to diagnose since the cutaneous eruptions it produces may mimic other skin disorders, such as impetigo, folliculitis, eczematous dermatitis and psoriasis. Misdiagnosis of scabies may result in prescribing of topical corticosteroids which ameliorate the signs and symptoms, but do not prevent continued infestation and transmissability. Scabies should be considered in any person presenting with a pruritic eruption of insidious onset, particularly if the eruption is common among several members of a group sharing accommodations or among close personal contacts. If scabies is suspected, the person should be referred to a physician for examination and confirmation. Self-treatment should not be recommended.

Topical Antiparasitics

The characteristic lesion of scabies is the burrow, which if found, settles the diagnosis. The burrow appears as a grayish-white, wavy, threadlike, slightly-elevated channel. The closed end is marked by a tiny, grayish speck, the resting place of the female. Burrows are often hidden by secondary lesions such as papules, nodules, vesicles, excoriations and secondary infection. It is uncommon to find a totally distinguishable, intact lesion. Diagnosis is made by lesion locale, by the polymorphic character of the lesions and by identifying the mite, ova or stool on a skin scraping.

A typical distribution pattern of scabies lesions is sometimes found and may help clinical diagnosis. The most common lesion sites in adults are the interdigital spaces of the hands, flexor surfaces of the wrists, extensor surfaces of the elbows, axillae, inframammary folds and nipples in women and the penis in men. In heavy infestations, other sites may be involved. In bedridden individuals, lesions are often concentrated over pressure points. A common misconception that scabies does not occur above the neck in adults has led to the recommendation that treatment only be applied from the neck down. Scabies lesions can be found on the scalp (commonly in the post-auricular folds) in adults, especially in those who live in warmer climates or who are bedridden.

In infants and children whose skin is soft and tender, scabies mites may be found over the entire body surface including the face and scalp. Scabies in infants and children may be more eczematous and less typical than the adult infestation. The most common lesion sites in this young group are the hands and feet, including palms and soles, intergluteal cleft, genital area, axillae, umbilicus and postauricular folds.

The primary presenting complaint is intense itching, which characteristically worsens at night or after a hot bath. A warm bed or bath may stimulate mite activity, or the mites may increase their feeding and excretion of irritating fecal pellets at night. People often scratch so vigorously, they draw blood. Besides the mite and their burrows, individuals with scabies develop a follicular, papular rash occurring mainly on areas of the body not infested with burrowing mites. If an individual has never had scabies, the onset of pruritus usually develops 2 to 6 weeks after infestation. Only after the mite population enlarges and the immune system begins to react do symptoms and rash develop. The pruritus and most eruptions in scabies result from the inflammation that accompanies the host's hypersensitivity response. The seriousness of the symptoms is not always directly related to the number of mites. Severe reactions can be found in individuals harboring a few mites.

There is no dramatic onset of pruritus and cutaneous eruption. Symptoms evolve slowly, making source identification difficult. As well, the source may be a newly infested person who is asymptomatic and capable of transmitting the disease long before he or she is aware of it. The incubation time is always shorter when an individual is reinfested; the symptoms appear within a few days.

About 5 per cent of people with scabies develop nodular scabies, presenting with pruritus and reddish lumps that can persist for months. These nodules probably result from a hypersensitivity reaction. Nodules may improve or clear with nightly application of tar gel for 2 to 3 weeks or with intralesional injections of corticosteroids.

Norwegian, or crusted scabies is a rare but highly contagious form of scabies occurring predominantly in people with physical or mental disabilities or who are immunologically compromised. Crusted scabies is manifested by thick, keratolytic crusts on the palms, soles and extensor surfaces of the extremities, and on the buttocks and ears. Minimal pruritus is associated with this form of scabies. It is highly contagious even on casual contact because of the large numbers of mites in the exfoliating scales. It has been responsible for outbreaks of scabies in both residents and staff of hospitals, nursing homes and other institutions. Normal mechanisms for destruction of mites, such as scratching and inflammation, are deficient due to the person's lack of cutaneous sensation and immune response. Crusted scabies has also been associated with extensive use of corticosteroids, which modifies the host immune response and improves the signs and symptoms of a mite infestation. This form of scabies responds slowly to treatment. It may require repeated applications of a scabicide in addition to removing the thick crusts and treating secondary infections.

Different varieties of *S. scabiei* are found in animals and may be transmitted to humans, especially canine scabies. Although they are morphologically indistinguishable from the human scabies mite, these animal mites are physiologically different and do not reproduce on the human host. Skin eruptions are usually self-limiting and resolve spontaneously within 4 to 6 weeks if the person is not exposed continually to the source of infestation. Papular and vesicular eruptions usually present where there has been contact with the infested animal. Neither burrows nor mites are found. Treatment usually requires application of a scabicide to both the person and animal.

Treatment

Primary treatment of pediculosis and scabies is always topical and directed toward killing the causative agent and its eggs. After this treatment is completed, secondary treatment may be required for residual pruritus, inflammation and secondary infection. Any treatment program for pediculosis and scabies must involve the infected individual and his or her close contacts.

Scabicides and pediculicides are curative. Their therapeutic effectiveness, as well as toxicity, depend upon adherence to correct application methods. Despite successful treatment, people often return to an environment in which they are likely to become reinfested. Thus, treatment failure may be due either to improper application or to reinfestation. Specific instructions should be given to the individual on proper application of the medication and on preventing reinfestation (see Table I).

The social stigma of scabies and pediculosis often causes people to react with shame, guilt or anxiety, and to search for someone to blame for their misfortune. They may feel self-conscious and dirty. Sensitivity is the key to dealing with these people. A matter-of-fact approach, nonjudgmental attitude and consumer education promote understanding of the disease and facilitate compliance with treatment. Unless people are aware of the nature of the disease and its transmission, adequate treatment of affected individuals and their contacts is uncertain.

Pediculosis

The two pediculicides which have been most widely used to treat head and pubic lice are lindane and pyrethrins with piperonyl butoxide. The more recent introduction of permethrin, a synthetic pyrethroid, is gaining popularity as an excellent pediculicide. Malathion lotion, an effective pediculicide used in European countries, was only briefly marketed in Canada. Malathion has an

Topical Antiparasitics

Table I *Instructions for Treating Lice and Scabies*

General information

- This recommended medication should be used as directed to prevent harmful effects.
- This medication is not for oral use. It is not effective orally and is poisonous if taken orally.
- Keep the medicine out of reach of children.
- Do not apply the medicine to the eyes, nose, mouth or urethral opening. If accidental contact with the eyes occurs, flush them thoroughly with water.
- Treatment may produce a mild skin irritation. If excessive skin irritation occurs or if a rash develops, treatment should be discontinued and the medicine washed off. Check with your doctor.
- Do not apply this medicine more often than instructed.

Specific instructions for lice infestations

- Follow the instructions carefully for the product selected.
- To prevent spreading the lice infestation, all clothing, scarves, hats, bed linen and towels should be washed in hot water and dried in the hot cycle of an automatic dryer for 20 minutes. Articles which cannot be washed may be drycleaned, pressed with a hot iron or sealed in a plastic bag and stored for about 2 weeks.
- Combs, curlers and brushes may be soaked for 1 to 2 hours in a 2 per cent Lysol solution or a solution of the medicine used to treat lice. Combs, curlers or brushes may also be heated for 10 minutes in water at 65 °C.
- A general household cleaning by carefully vacuuming mattresses, carpets and furniture helps prevent reinfestation.
- All family members and persons with whom there has been close personal contact should be examined for lice and treated if necessary.
- Children should be encouraged not to share hats or grooming aids.

Specific instructions for scabies

- After you stop using this medicine, itching may continue for a few days or weeks. This is normal and does not mean treatment has not worked.
- To prevent spreading the infestation, all clothing, bed linens and towels should be washed in hot water and dried in the hot cycle of an automatic dryer for 20 minutes. Articles which cannot be washed may be drycleaned, pressed with a hot iron or sealed in a plastic bag and stored for about 1 week.
- All family members and persons with whom there has been close personal contact must also be treated.

unpleasant odor and the application time for malathion lotion was considerably longer than other pediculicide products.

After effective treatment of head and pubic lice, the nits remain on the hair shaft. One must rely on nitpicking or thoroughly combing the hair with a fine-toothed comb to remove the nits. The space between the teeth must be less than 0.3 mm. Special nit removal combs are often supplied with the pediculicide product. Soaking the hair for 1 hour with a 1:1 solution of white vinegar and water may help loosen the nit attachment. The solution can be applied to the hair and the hair wrapped in a wet towel. A commercial solution (Step 2) containing formic acid is available for dissolving the tenacious bond between the nit and the hair shaft and thus facilitating nit removal. It must be emphasized that use of a nit removal solution does **not** replace proper pediculicide treatment. Most community public health and school regulations require that nits be removed before children can return to school.

For therapy of head lice, retreatment after 7 to 10 days should be recommended when lindane and pyrethrins with piperonyl butoxide are used. These pediculides are not completely ovicidal (ovicidal activity estimated to be about 70 per cent). Pubic lice appear to be more difficult to eradicate and two treatments are recommended regardless of the type of therapy. The interval between treatments should approximate the 1 week incubation period of the louse. If the interval is longer than 10 days, some lice may mature, lay eggs, and thus perpetuate the infestation. Permethrin, although not 100 per cent ovicidal, persists on the hair shaft for about 10 days which is sufficient to kill lice hatched from viable eggs. Because sufficient ovicidal activity may not be guaranteed for any pediculicide product (including factors of incorrect application), it is prudent to recommend nit removal in all lice treatment programs. In addition to cosmetic reasons, nit removal helps eliminates diagnostic confusion. It may be difficult for individuals to distinguish a viable nit from an empty egg case when examining for evidence of reinfestation.

Some clinicians prefer to treat all household members and close contacts of people with pediculosis capitis regardless of evidence of infestation since it may be very difficult to find a few lice or viable nits in a newly infested individual. Others examine contacts and treat them only if visibly infested. For crab lice infestations, sexual partners should receive concurrent therapy. A common cause of treatment failure in pubic lice infestation is treating only the pubic area in hairy individuals. In these individuals, the thighs, trunk and axillary regions should also be treated because of frequent involvement of these sites.

Crab lice infestations involving the eyelashes are most commonly treated with petrolatum ointment applied thickly to the eyelashes twice a day for 8 to 10 days to smother the lice and nits. This procedure is followed by mechanical removal of the nits with tweezers or fingernails.

Body lice may be treated simply by washing well with soap and water and applying a topical antipruritic, such as calamine lotion. Topical antiparasitics are not required since neither the lice nor their nits are permanently attached to the human host. Clothes must be laundered in hot water above 60 °C or drycleaned. If laundering is not feasible, clothing should not be worn for 30 days to ensure nits are no longer viable.

Scabies

The choice of a topical antiparasitic agent for scabies must take efficacy and toxicity into account. Commercially available topical scabicides from which to choose include permethrin, lindane and crotamiton. Benzyl benzoate and sulfur can be prescribed for the treatment of scabies, but must be compounded as products are not available commercially. Regardless of the scabicide used, medication must be applied to all affected body areas. Previous recommendations to apply medication only from the neck down to treat scabies in adults may not be adequate and could result in treatment failure. Appropriate evaluation of disease extent is essential. Important areas often missed during scabicide application are skin folds and creases, the umbilical area and soles of the feet. Not to be overlooked are the areas under the nails, which may harbor mites deposited by scratching. Therapy should include trimming the nails, scrubbing

Topical Antiparasitics

beneath the nails and compressing the fingertips with antiscabietic medication.

An individual is no longer contagious 24 hours after effective therapy for scabies. Most people experience dramatic relief from pruritus within 24 to 48 hours, but symptoms and rash can persist for 2 to 4 weeks after successful treatment. This postscabietic pruritus may require additional antipruritic treatment. Hypersensitivity to dead mites, eggs and feces can cause continued pruritus until these artifacts are shed from the skin surface. Treatment with oral antihistamines and topical corticosteroids is beneficial. Continuing pruritus may lead to overtreatment if people apply medication more frequently and over longer periods than prescribed. To prevent overuse of scabicides and possible toxicity, medication quantities dispensed should be sufficient for only one treatment. Individuals must be warned itching may persist despite destruction of the mite and not to exceed recommended doses of applied medication. If itching persists for longer than 4 weeks, the individual should be examined for reinfestation or treatment failure.

Effective treatment of a scabietic person must include prophylactic treatment of all asymptomatic family members, all persons contacted sexually and all persons who have had close physical contact with the infested individual, as symptoms may not develop for 4 to 6 weeks. During the incubation period, the asymptomatic infested individual is still capable of transmitting mites to others. Prophylactic treatment is especially important in institutional or long-term care settings to prevent the scabies infestation from bouncing between residents and caregivers.

Pharmaceutical Agents

Pyrethrins with Piperonyl Butoxide

The combination of pyrethrins with piperonyl butoxide is used for the topical treatment of head and pubic lice infestations. Pyrethrins are fast-acting insecticides extracted from the genus *Chrysanthemum* which act on the nervous system of the insect to cause convulsions and paralysis. Piperonyl butoxide has little or no insecticidal activity, but potentiates that of pyrethrins by inhibiting the hydrolytic enzymes responsible for the metabolism of pyrethrins in arthropods. Pyrethrins with piperonyl butoxide are available as shampoo or liquid formulations. (See Table II for correct application procedures.) Available data indicate the efficacy of pyrethrins with piperonyl butoxide is equivalent to lindane. Medical Letter consultants recommend this combination as the drug of choice for the treatment of head lice.

Table II *User Instructions—Pyrethrins with Piperonyl Butoxide*

- This medication is used to treat head and crab lice infestations.
- Apply the liquid or shampoo to dry hair in sufficient quantities to completely wet the hair of affected and adjacent areas. Massage thoroughly. Do not add water.
- Allow medication to remain on the affected areas for 10 minutes.
- **Liquid solution:** After 10 minutes, remove medication by washing the areas with warm water and soap or a shampoo.
- **Shampoo:** After 10 minutes, add small quantities of water to work the medication into a lather. Rinse thoroughly.
- Repeat treatment once in 7 days.

There is no reported evidence lice have become resistant to this combination. As with other pediculicides, pyrethrins with piperonyl butoxide are not 100 per cent ovicidal, therefore, treatment should be repeated in 1 week.

Side effects from pyrethrins are uncommon. Contact dermatitis is the most common adverse effect. This may be due to the petroleum distillates used for solvent purposes in the formulation. Very small amounts of products containing petroleum distillates can cause serious or fatal toxicity if ingested. Since these products are frequently used in small children, it is essential that appropriate cautionary and security measures be used in the home to prevent accidental ingestion. Pyrethrin containing products should not be used by individuals allergic to ragweed and *Chrysanthemum*, as cross-sensitivity can occur.

Pyrethrins with piperonyl butoxide are also available as spray formulations for use on inanimate objects. These sprays are often included in kits along with a pediculicide product. It is not clear whether use of a pediculicide spray demonstrates any advantage in terms of effectiveness in preventing reinfestation over the general household cleaning measures recommended. It is also not clear whether general cleaning measures can be abandoned in lieu of using a spray pediculicide. To avoid potential misuse, individuals using these sprays must understand they are not intended for human use.

Another shampoo formulation containing bioallethrin, a synthetic pyrethrin, in combination with piperonyl butoxide is marketed for human application in the treatment of head lice. The manufacturer of the product claims efficacy of a single application and 100 per cent ovicidal activity due to the solvent properties of isododecane in dissolving the outercovering of the louse and the nits. Current literature to support these claims is unavailable.

Permethrin

Permethrin is a synthetic pyrethroid currently marketed as a 1 per cent creme rinse for the treatment of head lice and 5 per cent dermal cream for the treatment of scabies. (See Table III for correct application procedures.) The insecticidal activity of permethrin is similar to the natural pyrethrins and causes paralysis and death by disrupting sodium transport in the nerve cell membranes of lice and mites. Permethrin has the advantage of better stability and longer shelf life

---

Table III *User Instructions—Permethrin*

Treatment of head lice—Permethrin 1% creme rinse

- With usual shampoo, wash the hair, rinse with water, towel dry.
- Apply enough permethrin creme rinse to thoroughly saturate hair and scalp.
- Leave on for 10 minutes, rinse with water, allow hair to dry.
- Nits may be removed with a comb, if desired. Discard comb.
- Shake well before using.

Treatment of scabies—Permethrin 5% cream

- Massage the cream into clean, dry skin over the entire body surface from the head to the soles of the feet, including the scalp in infants. Put on clean clothes.
- Leave cream on for 12 to 14 hours before thoroughly washing it off with soap and water. Put on clean clothes.
- If the cream is accidentally washed off during the treatment period, it should be reapplied.

---

compared to natural pyrethrins by virtue of increased resistance to heat and light degradation. Permethrin is listed as the drug of choice by Medical Letter consultants for the treatment of scabies.

A great number of studies confirming permethrin's efficacy have been done. Comparative studies with standard lindane therapy have demonstrated equivalent or superior efficacy in the treatment of both head lice and scabies. Resistance to permethrin has not yet been reported. Permethrin has been effective in treating cases of lindane-resistance. Although permethrin was as effective as lindane for pubic lice in one report, it is not yet recommended for the treatment of pediculosis pubis.

Like other pediculicide treatments, permethrin does not have complete ovicidal activity. However, unlike pyrethrins with piperonyl butoxide, permethrin demonstrates residual activity remaining on the hair shaft for 10 days following treatment regardless of the nature of shampoos, drugs or cosmetics applied to the hair. This residual activity is sufficient to kill nymphs that may hatch from eggs which were not killed with the initial application and to protect against reinfestation during the 10 day time period. Retreatment with permethrin is generally not necessary unless evidence of lice infestation is present after 7 days. If correctly applied, less than 1 per cent of patients will require retreatment. Nit removal should still be recommended for added antiparasitic control, for aesthetic and diagnostic reasons and for public health regulations.

Permethrin is poorly absorbed with less than 2 per cent of a topically applied permethrin dose absorbed through the skin. Following absorption, permethrin is rapidly inactivated by esterase hydrolysis and subsequently excreted in the urine. Fewer than 6 per cent of patients have reported adverse effects from the use of permethrin. The most commonly reported side effects are mild, transient itching, redness and swelling. Other uncommon adverse effects include burning, stinging, rash, tingling and numbness. Systemic side effects have not been reported. As with natural pyrethrin products, permethrin should be avoided in individuals allergic to ragweed and *Chrysanthemum* as cross-sensitivity reactions can occur.

Use of permethrin for the treatment of head lice in children under the age of 2 years has not been established. However, permethrin 5 per cent cream in the treatment of scabies has been used in small infants without evidence of adverse effects. Reproductive abnormalities have not been observed with permethrin in animal studies. Data on adverse reproductive effects in humans is not available, therefore, guidelines for use in pregnancy are not established. Since controlled drug studies in pregnant women are very unlikely to be performed, one must rely on medical judgement when treating pregnant patients. For lactating women, it would be prudent to advise discontinuing nursing temporarily during the application time period as it is not known whether permethrin is excreted in breast milk.

Lindane

Lindane (gamma benzene hexachloride) is a popular and effective treatment for pediculosis and scabies and has been the standard therapy for over 30 years. It is available as a 1 per cent cream, lotion or shampoo. (See Table IV for correct application procedures.) After rapid absorption through the chitinous exoskeleton of arthropods, lindane presumably stimulates the nervous system resulting in convulsions and death. As a pediculicide, lindane is as effective in killing lice as pyrethrins with piperonyl butoxide. Lindane is not completely ovicidal, therefore retreatment in 1 week is recommended for head lice therapy.

In recent years, evidence has been presented citing tolerance to lindane in the treatment of head lice and scabies. Most documented cases of resistance have occurred in areas of the developing world where lindane use has been frequent and widespread to control epidemic disease. A few scattered cases of treatment failure suspected to be caused by lindane resistance have now been reported from the United States. Although clinicians should be alert to the possibility, resistance to lindane is not generally thought to be a problem in Canada.

The Medical Letter consultants do not list lindane as the drug of choice for either pediculosis or scabies. Lindane has received much negative publicity on its safety. Reports of lindane's central nervous system toxicity following treatment for scabies have provoked concern, but these reports have usually been associated with overuse or accidental ingestion. Several studies have concluded that lindane rarely causes toxic symptoms when used appropriately. Health professionals and the public may perceive lindane to be toxic regardless of the condition treated, even though lindane has been used safely for millions of applications.

About 10 per cent of a topically applied dose of lindane is absorbed through the skin, with increased absorption when applied to inflamed or excoriated skin as is often the case in scabies and lice infestations. Infants and young children may be more susceptible to the toxic effects of topically applied lindane. Children have a larger surface area to mass ratio than adults and, therefore, absorb more lindane on a unit weight basis. Increased susceptibility to the neurotoxic effects of lindane may also occur in the elderly patient as a result of increased percutaneous absorption through thinning skin or because of a general increased sensitivity to neurotoxic chemicals.

There is no question that lindane is neurotoxic when given in large doses. Convulsions in children have been reported after lindane application. In almost all cases of suspected central nervous system toxicity, the drug has been ingested, applied repeatedly for a few to several days, applied excessively or left on the skin longer than recommended. However, one report of seizures and high serum concentrations in elderly patients occurred following appropriate topical application of lindane. Other less severe central nervous system effects are nausea, vomiting, headache, irritability and insomnia.

Lindane should be used with caution in infants, young children and the elderly because of the drug's potential for central nervous system toxicity. Lindane 1 per cent shampoo is not significantly absorbed through the scalp. No serious adverse effects have been reported in children exposed briefly to lindane for the treatment of head lice. If lindane is to be used for the treatment of scabies in infants, young children and the elderly, the following precautions might be advised. A hot bath or shower should be avoided before application since vasodilation of blood vessels in the skin facilitates absorption. The skin should be dry and cool. Lindane should be removed immediately after the recommended treatment period. Adequate supervision and protective clothing are necessary to prevent infants and children from licking the cream or lotion from their skin. A matter not to be overlooked is the potential absorption from impregnated clothes and linens not properly laundered after an application. Premature infants, and individuals with underlying skin disorders, malnourishment or existing seizure disorders should avoid the use of lindane.

In animal studies, lindane is neither a mutagen nor a teratogen. No human cases of cancer or adverse reproductive effects have been reported after exposure to lindane. The controversy exists as a result

Topical Antiparasitics

Table IV *User Instructions—Lindane (USP)*

•Lindane should be used with caution to treat lice and scabies in pregnant and nursing women, infants and children 10 years or less. Consult a health professional before use.

Treatment of head and crab lice infestations—shampoo

•Apply 15 to 30 mL of shampoo to thoroughly saturate the **dry** hair of the affected and adjacent hairy areas. Work the shampoo through the hair for 4 minutes.

•Add a small amount of water to form a rich lather. Continue shampooing vigorously for another 4 minutes. Total application time should be 8 minutes.

•Rinse thoroughly with water. Briskly towel dry hair.

•A towel should be held tightly over the eyes to prevent the eyes from coming into contact with the medication.

•This shampoo is not to be used routinely. Repeat treatment once in 7 days, unless directed otherwise by physician.

Treatment of crab lice infestations—cream or lotion

•Apply a thin layer of the cream or well shaken lotion to cover only the affected (perineal and perianal) and adjacent hairy areas. The affected area should be cool and dry. Rub the medication in thoroughly. Freshly laundered clothing should be put on.

•The lotion or cream should be left on 8 to 12 hours and removed by thorough washing. Freshly laundered clothing should be put on.

•Repeat treatment once in 7 days.

Treatment of scabies—adults

•Thinly apply the well shaken lotion or the cream to the entire skin surface from the neck down with special attention to the hands, beneath the fingernails, feet and all skin folds. If scabies is present on the face and scalp, the medication should be applied carefully to avoid contact with the eyes, nose and mouth. Rub the medication in thoroughly.

•If crusted skin areas are present, a warm bath may help soften and remove crusts. If a warm bath is taken, allow the skin to cool and dry before applying the medication.

•The lotion or cream should be left on 8 to 12 hours and removed by thorough washing. Freshly laundered clothing should be put on.

•One application is usually successful. If directed, the treatment may be repeated once in 7 days.

Treatment of scabies—infants and children

•Avoid giving a warm bath before applying the medication. A warm bath may allow some medication to be absorbed into the body, and may lead to side effects.

•Thinly apply the lotion, which should be well shaken, or the cream to the entire skin surface from the neck down. If scabies is present on face and scalp, the medication should be applied carefully to avoid contact with the eyes, nose and mouth.

•The cream or lotion should be rubbed in thoroughly, leaving no medication on the skin which may be licked off. Long-sleeved shirts, pants and mittens should also be worn to prevent any contact of the treated skin with the mouth.

•The cream or lotion should be left on for 8 to 12 hours and removed by a thorough washing. Medication left on longer may lead to harmful effects. Freshly laundered clothing should be put on.

•Any signs of nausea, vomiting, headache or restlessnes should be reported to a physician.

•One application is usually successful. If directed, the treatment may be repeated once in 7 days.

of high-dose exposure to lindane insecticide in concentrations greater than 1 per cent in some experimental animals. Lindane's product monograph advises use with caution in pregnant and lactating women. Thus, treatment of lice and scabies in pregnant and nursing women remains a perplexing clinical problem. Many clinicians would prefer to use alternative agents to lindane, especially for scabies, which requires a prolonged contact time for treatment. Other available drugs have not been as well studied nor as extensively used as lindane and cannot be recommended as proven safer alternatives for pregnant and nursing women.

Misuse of lindane by increasing the frequency or duration of application is the cause of most adverse reactions. Used as a 1 per cent concentration at recommended doses, topically applied lindane appears to be safe and effective. Slight local irritation may occur. It should not be applied to the eyes, mucous membranes or acutely inflamed skin. Lindane should not be used in individuals with extensively excoriated skin, since percutaneous absorption is enhanced and the potential for toxicity increased. Quantities prescribed and dispensed should be limited to the exact amount needed for treatment since people tend to apply this type of medication until it is finished. Adequate instructions on the proper use of lindane must be provided at the time of dispensing. Liquid preparations should be dispensed in childproof bottles.

In spite of the extensive experience with safety and efficacy of topical lindane, there is some element of risk related to abuse, overuse, failure of parents to comprehend warning instructions and similar factors not under the control of the prescribing physician or pharmacist.

Alternative Scabicides

Crotamiton, applied topically as a 10 per cent cream, is used to treat scabies. The mechanism of action of crotamiton against the scabies mite is unknown. (See Table V for correct application procedures). Current dosage recommendations warrant further study since one

Table V *User Instructions—Crotamiton*

•This medication is used externally to treat scabies.

•Apply a thin layer of cream over the skin of the entire body from the neck down. Massage the cream into the skin until dry. Put on clean clothes.

•Repeat application of the cream in 24 hours. Again, put on clean clothes.

•Take a warm bath to remove the medication 48 hours after the last application.

study suggests 5 daily applications give a higher percentage of cures than the 2 currently recommended. One author reports using twice-daily applications of crotamiton cream for 3 days in clinical practice. Available data appear to favor permethrin and lindane as more effective agents for treating scabies. Crotamiton irritates denuded skin and can induce an allergic contact dermatitis. People with acutely inflamed or excoriated skin must exercise caution in using crotamiton. Little research exists on percutaneous absorption of crotamiton, although one study of a 10 day treatment in 50 children showed no effects.

Benzyl benzoate and **sulfur preparations** have been used as alternative agents in the treatment of scabies. Prior to the introduction of permethrin, these agents were primarily recommended for the purpose of avoiding lindane use in certain individuals. It has been assumed that benzyl benzoate and sulfur were less toxic alternatives than lindane, however, little data to support efficacy and lack of toxicity exists.

Benzyl benzoate and sulfur preparations are not available commercially. If prescribed, benzyl benzoate is usually formulated in concentrations of 20 to 25 per cent and applied in a single application which is washed off after 24 hours or once nightly for 3 nights. Slight burning and stinging (especially on the male genitalia and on the scalp), itching and allergic reactions may occur. Contact with the face, eyes, mucous membranes and urethral meatus should be avoided. Concentrations of 5 to 10 per cent of sulfur in petrolatum are most commonly recommended for the treatment of scabies. Sulfur preparations are not aesthetically pleasing. They have an unpleasant odor and may stain clothing and bedding. Preparations are applied thinly to the entire skin surface below the neck once nightly after bathing for 3 nights. Irritant dermatitis has been reported. Inconvenience and cosmetic unacceptability may cause noncompliance.

Summary

Pediculosis and scabies plague our society with ever-increasing frequency. Fortunately, simple and effective therapy is readily available. If used correctly, medication usually eradicates an infestation in 24 hours.

The pharmacist plays an important role in treating and preventing pediculosis and scabies infestations because the afflicted person often seeks a nonprescription product initially. Where appropriate, the pharmacist may recommend a nonprescription medication (pediculosis) or refer the individual for medical examination (scabies).

Figure 5 *Suggested Approach for Treating Lice Infestations*

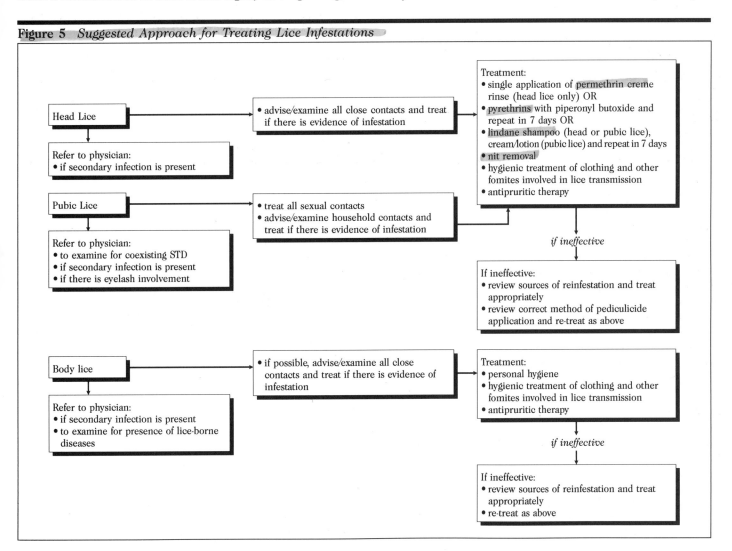

Figure 6 *Suggested Approach for Treating Scabies Infestations*

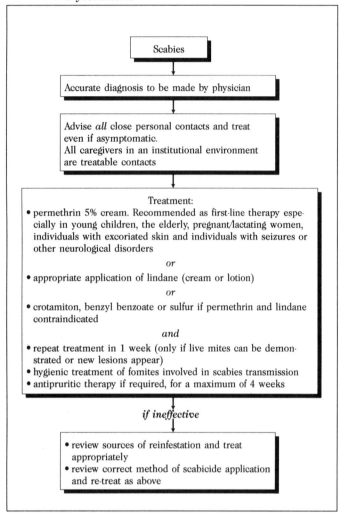

the classic burrow to papules, nodules, vesicles, wheals, pustules and excoriations. Secondary infection from scratching may be present in both cases.

Q. How long have you had symptoms of itching? Is the itching worse at a particular time?

- With scabies, itching symptoms often evolve slowly (4 to 6 weeks) while the host gradually develops a sensitivity reaction to the mite and its products. The person may describe the itch as being present for weeks or months. Itching characteristically worsens at night with scabies and pubic lice, whereas it is present during the day in head lice infestations.

Q. Are there any members of your family, close personal friends or schoolmates with a similar condition?

- If the person has close contact with others who have similar skin conditions, the probability of a scabies or pediculosis infestation rises. Both infestations are highly contagious and spread by close personal contact.

Q. What have you used to treat the skin condition?

- The person may have already been diagnosed and treated for a scabies or a pediculosis infestation. Symptoms of pruritus often remain after successful treatment, especially with scabies. Individuals may seek more medication to repeat the treatment when all they may require is reassurance and antipruritic treatment. People may also conclude treatment of head lice was unsuccessful if nits remain on the hair shaft.

  Alternatively, initial therapy may have been improperly applied, leading to treatment failure, or the person may have returned to an environment in which reinfestation occurred.

Q. Who will be involved in the treatment program?

- If treatment of scabies involves infants, young children and the elderly, modified dosage guidelines and special precautions must be recommended if using lindane (gamma benzene hexachloride). If individuals have existing skin disorders, extensively excoriated skin or seizure disorders, lindane may not be appropriate treatment.

Effective treatment of pediculosis and scabies relies on educating individuals, families and, in many cases, teachers about the nature of the disease, mode of transmission, proper methods of treatment and environmental measures to control and eradicate the infestation. Similarly, continual education of pharmacists is essential to maintain awareness of these communicable diseases.

Ask the Consumer

Q. Where are the itchy areas? Is there an associated skin rash?

- In scabies or lice infestations, pruritus is the common and predominant complaint. With lice infestations, itchy areas are localized to the infested area of the body. Local reactions to lice bites produce a papular rash as a result of hypersensitivity to the saliva injected by the lice. A characteristic pattern of skin involvement may be found in scabies, and a description helps in the diagnosis. Skin lesions described in scabies may range from

References

Pediculosis and Scabies

Altschuler DZ, Kenney LR. Pediculicide performance, profit and the public health. Arch Dermatol 1986;122(3):259–61.

Altschuler DZ, Kenney LR, Krinsky WL. More on pediculosis capitis (Letter). N Engl J Med 1984;310(25):1668–9.

Anonymous. Permethrin for head lice. Med Lett Drugs Ther 1986;28:89–90.

Burkhart CG. Scabies: an epidemiological assessment. Ann Intern Med 1983;98:498–503.

Dahl MV. The immunology of scabies. Ann Allergy 1983;51(6):560–6.

Derbes VJ. Arthropod bites and stings. In: Fitzpatrick TB, Eisen AZ, Wolff K, et al, eds. Dermatology in general medicine. New York: McGraw-Hill, 1979:1956–63.

Estes SA. Diagnosis and management of scabies. Med Clin North Am 1982;66(4):955–63.

Felman YM, Nikitas JA. Sexually transmitted diseases—scabies. Cutis 1984; 33:266,270–4.

Fine BC. Controversy about pediculosis capitis. N Engl J Med 1984;311 (12):801.

Fine BC. Pediculosis capitis. N Engl J Med 1983;309(23):1461.

Gurevitch AW. Scabies and lice. Ped Clin North Am 1985;32(4):987–1018.

Infectious Diseases and Immunization Committee, Canadian Pediatric Society. Pediculosis capitis (head lice). Can Med Assoc J 1985;133:741–2.

Lane AT. Scabies and head lice. Pediatr Ann 1987;16(1):51–4.

Leeson HS. The effect of temperature upon the hatching of the eggs of *Pediculus humanus corporis*. Parasitology 1941;33:243.

Mathias RG, Huggins DR, Leroux SJ, et al. Comparative trial of treatment with Prioderm lotion and Kwellada shampoo in children with head lice. Can Med Assoc J 1984;130:407–9.

Maunder JW. Human lice: biology and control. R Soc Health J 1977;97:29–32.

Meinking TL. Taplin D, Kalter DC, et al. Comparative efficacy of treatments for *Pediculosis Capitis* infestations. Arch Dermatol 1986;122:267–71.

Nienhius M, Rowles B. Update: treatment of pediculosis and scabies. US Pharmacist 1980;5(8):41–53.

Orkin M. Today's scabies. JAMA 1975;233:882–5.

Orkin M, Epstein E Sr, Maibach HI. Treatment of today's scabies and pediculosis. JAMA 1976;236:1136–9.

Orkin M, Maibach HI. Current views of scabies and pediculosis pubis. Cutis 1984;33:85–96.

Orkin M, Maibach HI. This scabies pandemic. N Engl J Med 1978;298:496–8.

Parish LC, Millikan LE, Witkowski JA, et al. Scabies in the extended care facility. Int J Dermatol 1983;22(6):380–2.

Plourde JJ. Scabies, chiggers and other ectoparasites. In: Isselbacher KJ, Adams RD. Braunwald E, et al, eds. Harrison's principles of internal medicine. New York: McGraw, 1980:919–20.

Sauer GC. Manual of skin diseases. Am J Dis Child 1973;126:226–8.

Sauer GC. Manual of skin diseases. Philadelphia: JB Lippincott, 1980:196.

Service MW. A guide to medical entomology. New York: MacMillan, 1980: 1–4, 136–41,167–70.

Taplin D, Meinking TL. Scabies, lice and fungal infections. Prim Care 1989;16:551–68.

Weidhass DE, et al. Lice. Geneva: World Health Organization, 1982: WHO/VBC/82.858.

Witkowski JA, Parish LC. Scabies: subungual areas harbor mites. JAMA 1984;252(10):1318–9.

Pyrethrins with Piperonyl Butoxide

Pediculicide drug products for over-the-counter human use: establishment of a monograph. Fed Reg 1982;47:28316.

Shivji A. Letter to the editor. Can Pharm J 1989;122:442.

Smith DE, Walsh J. Treatment of pubic lice infestation: a comparison of two agents. Cutis 1980;26:618–9.

Taplin D, Meinking TL. Pyrethrins and pyrethroids in dermatology. Arch Dermatol 1990;126:213–21.

Permethrin

Anon. Permethrin for head lice. Med Lett Drug Ther 1986;28:89–90.

Anon. Permethrin for scabies. Med Lett Drug Ther 1990;32:21–2.

Anonymous. Permethrin for head lice. Med Lett Drugs Ther 1986;28:89–90.

Bowerman JG, et al. Comparative study of permetrin 1% creme rinse and lindane shampoo for the treatment of head lice. Pediatr Infect Dis J 1987;6:252–5.

Brandenberg K, Deinard AS, DiNapoli J, et al. 1% permethrin cream rinse vs 1% lindane shampoo in treating pediculosis capitis. Am J Dis Child 1986; 140:894–6.

Brandenburg K, et al. 1% permethrin cream rinse vs 1% lindane shampoo in treating Pediculosis capitis. Am J Dis Child 1986;140:894–6.

Carson DS, et al. Pyrethrins combined with piperonyl butoxide (RID) vs 1% permethrin (NIX) in the treatment of head lice. Am J Dis Child 1988; 142:768–9.

Kalter DC, et al. Treatment of pediculosis pubis: Clinical comparison of efficacy and tolerance of 1% lindane shampoo vs 1% permethrin creme rinse. Arch Dermatol 1987;123:1315–9.

Mazas EA, Porto MC, Perez MCS, et al. The efficacy of permethrin lotion in pediculosis capitis. Int J Dermatol 1985;24(9):603–5.

Schultz MW, et al. Comparative study of 5% permethrin cream and 1% lindane lotion for the treatment of scabies. Arch Dermatol 1990;126:167–70.

Taplin D, et al. Permethrin 5% dermal cream: A new treatment for scabies. J Am Acad Dermatol 1986;15:995–1001.

Taplin D, et al. Community control of scabies: a model based on use of permethrin cream. Lancet 1991;337:1016–8.

Taplin D, et al. Permethrin 1% creme rinse for the treatment of Pediculosis humanus var capitis infestation. Pediatr Dermatol 1986;3:344–8.

Lindane

Anonymous. Drugs for parasitic infestations. Med Lett Drugs Ther 1986; 28:9–18.

Ginsburg CM, Lowry W, Reisch JS. Absorption of lindane (gamma benzene hexachloride) in infants and children. J Pediatr 1977;91:998–1000.

Kligman AM. Percutaneous absorption and gamma benzene hexachloride (GBH) agents. Cutis 1981;27(Suppl):17–9.

Kramer MS, Hutchinson TA, Rudnick SA, et al. Operational criteria for adverse drug reactions in evaluating suspected toxicity of a popular scabicide. Clin Pharmacol Ther 1980;27:149–55.

Pramanik AK, Hansen RC. Transcutaneous gamma benzene hexachloride absorption and toxicity in infants and children. Arch Dermatol 1979; 115:1224–5.

Rasmussen JE. Lindane: a prudent approach. Arch Dermatol 1987;123: 1008–10.

Rasmussen JE. The problem of lindane. J Am Acad Dermatol 1981;5:507–16.

Schacter B. Treatment of scabies and pediculosis with lindane preparations: an evaluation. J Am Acad Dermatol 1981;5:517–27.

Telch J, Jarvis DA. Acute intoxication with lindane (gamma benzene hexachloride). Can Med Assoc J 1982;126:662–3.

Tenenbein M. Seizures after lindane therapy. J Am Geriatr Soc 1991;39:394–5.

Benzyl Benzoate and Sulfur

Arndt KA, ed. Manual of dermatologic therapeutics. Boston: Little, 1983.

Crotamiton

Cubela V, Yawalkar SJ. Clinical experience with crotamiton cream and lotion in treatment of infants with scabies. Br J Clin Pract 1978;32:229–31.

Hurwitz S. Update: scabies in childhood. Pediatr Ann 1980;11:226–7, 230–35.

Konstantinov D, et al. J Int Med Res (GB) 1979;7(5):443–8.

18
Anthelmintics

Patrick S. Farmer

The most common human helminth, the pinworm, causes enterobiasis, which can be treated with any of several non-prescription anthelmintics: pyrantel pamoate (the drug of choice), pyrvinium pamoate, piperazine adipate, as well as mebendazole, a prescription medication. Preventing reinfection is a primary concern of treatment. Other nematodes include the large roundworm, hookworm, dog heartworm, Trichinella, and nematodes from raw fish. Cestodes include the fish, beef, pork and dwarf tapeworm. Trematodes, or flukes, are uncommon in North America.

Anthelmintics are drugs used to rid the body of helminths, or parasitic worms. Parasitic worms belong to one of three classes: nematodes (roundworms), cestodes (tapeworms) and trematodes (flukes). Over half the world's population harbors one or several species of these endoparasites, and the number of individual helminth infections is believed to exceed the world's human population. Medically and economically, helminthiasis constitutes a serious problem, particularly in tropical regions of the Third World. However, there is little cause for complacency in developed countries. Pinworm, roundworm, whipworm, hookworm, anisakid and Trichinella infections are endemic in certain areas of the United States. The number of pinworm infections in the United States is estimated to exceed 42 million. Because of our colder climate, soil-borne parasites are less prevalent in Canada, and our worm burden consists overwhelmingly of pinworm. Nevertheless, jet travel for business and pleasure, and increasing numbers of political refugees have resulted in exotic parasitic infections appearing where previously they were unknown. Unlike microbial infections, helminth infections cannot yet be vaccinated against.

Enterobiasis

Infection with *Enterobius vermicularis*, previously classified as *Oxyuris vermicularis*, is called enterobiasis or oxyuriasis. The parasite is commonly referred to as pinworm, seatworm or threadworm.

Enterobiasis is not a modern phenomenon. Archeological evidence shows it existed in North America almost 10,000 years ago, and was common in about the fifth century A.D.

Today, pinworm is the most common human helminth in North America. It is more common than measles, chickenpox, mumps, rubella and pertussis combined. Estimates of the incidence of enterobiasis in the United States range from 4.5 million to 42 million; the total incidence of the above viral infections was estimated

in 1980 to be 250,000. The incidence of pinworm is highest in school age children, lowest in adults, and intermediate in preschoolers. The pinworm does not respect class or socioeconomic status. Contrary to popular belief, infection does not signify substandard hygiene. It does occur more commonly in institutional settings such as dormitories and mental institutions.

This epidemiological pattern is explained by the nature of the life cycle of *Enterobius vermicularis* and the methods of its transmission. Adult pinworms live and copulate in the cecum and adjacent areas of the intestinal tract. The gravid female worm migrates to the anal canal and the perianal and perineal areas at night to lay 5,000 to 17,000 eggs. Noninfectious at first, the eggs embryonate and become infectious within six hours. They often initiate pruritus ani, and the ensuing scratching may result in anus-finger-mouth transmission and renewed infection of the host. Alternatively, contaminated hands may deposit the embryonated eggs on food or household objects such as doorknobs, spreading the infection to other members of the family or institution. Another, often underestimated mode of transmission of the eggs is via airborne housedust (and schoolroom dust), which can be inhaled and subsequently swallowed or which might be picked up on the hands. Under favorable conditions, such as a cool, moist environment (20°C, 47 to 67 per cent relative humidity), the eggs can remain viable for up to two days. The relatively high incidence of enterobiasis among homosexual men strongly suggests venereal transmission as another route.

Fortunately, pinworm infection generally may be regarded as a nuisance rather than as a serious medical problem. Probably guilt and mental distress are the most important traumas associated with the condition. Hosts usually are asymptomatic or complain of only mild symptoms such as perianal irritation and itching. In some cases the pruritus ani presents as severe pain. Scratching may result in bacterial infection. Other symptoms, including insomnia, nightmares, anorexia, nausea and vomiting, have been ascribed to pinworm infection, but controlled studies do not support a clear cause and effect relationship. Heavy infections may be associated with diarrhea. Perineal and vaginal pinworms may cause enuresis by reflux stimulation of the bladder. Occasionally, pinworms invade the mucosa of the vermiform appendix, causing symptoms of acute appendicitis. A statistical correlation has been confirmed of pinworm infection with chronic appendicitis, but not with acute appendicitis. The overall incidence of pinworm among appendicitis patients was low. Pinworm invasion of the anal canal, possibly via an anal gland, has been reported.

Anthelmintics

Rarely, but reported with increasing frequency in recent years, pinworms are associated with ectopic lesions. These almost exclusively result from migration of the gravid female worm into the female genital tract, where the dead parasite and/or ova can cause asymptomatic granulomas of the vagina, uterus, fallopian tubes or peritoneum. Peritoneal Enterobius lesions have also been ascribed tentatively to migration through ruptured sigmoid diverticuli and a surgically traumatized colon. Sometimes the ectopic worm provokes a symptomatic inflammatory response. The wandering worm also may carry colonic bacteria, resulting in urinary tract infections. This cause of infections is probably important, and young girls with urinary tract infections should be examined carefully for pinworm infection. Even the asymptomatic granulomas can cause medical complications, since they may be misdiagnosed as such problems as carcinoma or endometriosis, leading to unnecessary surgery.

Diagnosis

Children who exhibit perianal itching, insomnia and restlessness might be suspected of having pinworm infections. For confirmed diagnosis, the adult worms or eggs must be observed. Occasionally these eggs are found in the feces, but stool examination generally is of little value in diagnosing pinworm infection. Eggs are sometimes found under the fingernails. Parents are often able to see worms with the aid of a flashlight, as the worms crawl from the anus at night. The most efficient method of diagnosis is to swab the perianal regions with a strip of cellulose tape, 7 to 10 centimetres, looped over the end of a glass microscope slide or a tongue depressor with the sticky side out (see Figure 1). The mounted tape is pressed firmly into the folds on each side of the outer margin of the anal canal, then the tape is folded back on the slide with the gummed side down for transport to the physician's office. This procedure is done first thing in

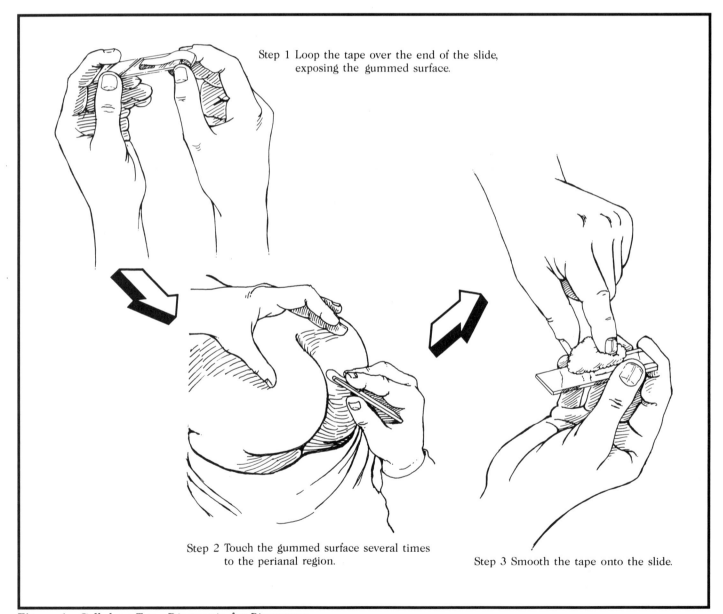

Step 1 Loop the tape over the end of the slide, exposing the gummed surface.

Step 2 Touch the gummed surface several times to the perianal region.

Step 3 Smooth the tape onto the slide.

Figure 1 *Cellulose Tape Diagnosis for Pinworms*

Anthelmintics

Table I *Dosage Information for Nonprescription Drugs for Pinworm Infection*

Drugs	Drug dose	Body weight	Product dose
Piperazine adipate	75 mg/kg* for 7 days	<13.5 kg	5 mL/day for 7 days (alternative: three 5 mL doses in 1 day only)
		13.5–27.5 kg	10–15 mL/day for 7 days (alternative: two 10 mL doses in 1 day only)
		27.5–41 kg	15–25 mL/day for 7 days (alternative: three 10mL doses or two 2 g pkts in one day only)
		>41 kg	max. 25 mL/day for 7 days (alternative: three 15 mL doses or three 2 g pkts in one day only)
Pyrantel pamoate	11 mg/kg	12–23 kg	2.5–5 mL
		23–45 kg	5–10 mL or 2–4 tablets
		45–68 kg	10–15 mL or 4–6 tablets
		>68 kg	max. 8 tablets
Pyrvinium pamoate	5 mg/kg	10–20 kg	5–10 mL
		20–40 kg	10–20 mL
		40–50 kg	20–25 mL
		50–70 kg	25–35 mL
		>70 kg	max. 35 mL

*75 mg piperazine adipate is equivalent to 65mg piperazine hexahydrate.

the morning, before the child has a bowel movement or a bath. Even with this method, only about 50 per cent of infections are confirmed by a single swabbing. Eggs are not necessarily deposited every night, particularly in a light infection where there are few gravid females. Three swabbings taken on consecutive mornings reveal about 90 per cent of infections but a suspected person cannot be considered free from infection until examinations on seven consecutive days have given negative results.

Drug Treatment

Several nonprescription anthelmintics are available in Canada to treat pinworm infection (see Table I).

Pyrantel pamoate is the drug of choice. This drug is administered as a single dose of 11 mg/kg of body weight, with a maximum dose of one gram. It may be given with or separate from meals. Dietary restrictions and use of laxatives are unnecessary. Because viable eggs in the environment may be ingested and cause reinfection, most authorities recommend routine administration of a second dose 10 to 14 days after the first. Others consider it unnecessary, as a single dose gives a cure rate of up to 97 per cent. Largely because it is poorly absorbed from the gastrointestinal tract, pyrantel pamoate causes little toxicity. The most common side effects are anorexia, nausea, vomiting and diarrhea, but these are transient. Occasionally, dizziness, headache and drowsiness are reported. One case has been reported of a possible interaction with theophylline sustained release capsules, wherein a rapid increase in the serum theophylline level was observed 2.5 hours following a single 160 mg dose of pyrantel pamoate. Although this is inconclusive, the authors speculated pyrantel may either inhibit theophylline metabolism or accelerate

its release from the dosage form. Pyrantel is not recommended for infants under one year or for pregnant women, and it should be used with caution in people with impaired liver function. It has not been detected in significant anounts in breast milk. One case has been reported of a severe possible allergic reaction to pyrantel.

Pyrantel induces a persistent nicotinic depolarization of the myoneural junction of the worms, causing spastic paralysis, and the worms are passed in the feces. The neuromuscular junction of nematodes is more sensitive than that of the host, accounting for the selective toxicity exhibited by the drug. Before a toxic dose can be reached in man, the drug causes vomiting. The action of pyrantel antagonizes that of piperazine, and the two drugs should not be taken together.

Pyrvinium pamoate is an alternative drug to treat pinworm. Like pyrantel, this drug's cure rate is over 90 per cent. It is given in a single dose of 5 mg/kg to a maximum of 350 mg. Again, retreatment after 10 to 14 days is usually recommended. Poorly absorbed, its toxicity is generally limited to gastrointestinal side effects such as occasional vomiting, cramping and diarrhea. Rarely, skin photosensitivity reactions have been reported. Pyrvinium is a cyanine dye. People using the drug or the parents of children using the drug must be counselled that the drug stains the stools bright red for several days, and staining of the underclothes may occur. If vomiting occurs, it is bright red, too. If spilled, pyrvinium suspension causes red staining.

Pyrvinium's mechanism of action is poorly understood. It inhibits oxygen metabolism and causes hyperpolarization and flaccid paralysis of the pinworm.

Piperazine adipate is a less popular alternative anthelmintic. Piperazine's major drawback is that it requires multiple doses. A two-day course of treatment gives a high cure rate, but for optimal results,

Anthelmintics

the usual regimen is 65 mg/kg (maximum 2.5 g) daily in single or divided doses for seven days. A second course of treatment begins after a respite of one week. Piperazine adipate (Entacyl) is marketed as granules in packets of 2 g, or as a suspension (120 mg/mL). The product insert advocates a single-day dosage regimen of 150 mg/kg and the packaging of the granules is difficult to adapt to a regimen of 75 mg/kg daily for seven days. Piperazine salts are water soluble and readily absorbed, with most of an oral dose appearing in the urine within 24 hours. Despite this, side effects are uncommon. Gastrointestinal disturbances such as nausea, vomiting and diarrhea may occur. Transient central nervous system effects include dizziness and difficulty in ocular focusing. Occasional allergic rashes have been reported, and cross-sensitivity to ethylenediamine has been suggested. Taken in overdose or in the presence of renal insufficiency, piperazine causes more pronounced neurotoxicity, manifested as 'worm wobble.' This is characterized by a gait instability and lack of coordination associated mainly with cerebellar ataxia, and vertigo, dysphasia, confusion and myoclonic contractions. Piperazine is contraindicated for people with renal or hepatic disease or with epilepsy. It should be used with caution in pregnancy, and avoided altogether during the first trimester. It is excreted in breast milk, and should not be taken by women who are breast feeding.

Piperazine causes a gradual flaccid paralysis of the parasite by hyperpolarization of the myoneural junction. The worms are expelled alive and active. As already mentioned, piperazine and pyrantel are mutually antagonistic, and should not be taken together.

As the other drugs are poorly absorbed from the gastrointestinal tract, piperazine seems to be the most suitable anthelmintic for eradication of pinworms from the vagina or urinary tract. Standard seven-day regimens have been used successfully. On the other hand, at least one case of pinworm-associated endometritis was treated successfully with oral pyrantel pamoate. A different approach to treating genitourinary enterobiasis is the use of intravaginal instillation of piperazine solution. No reports of use of intravaginal administration of other anthelmintics were found. Resort to this route is not likely to be warranted.

Mebendazole, a prescription drug, is also considered a drug of choice for pinworms. A single dose of 100 mg of this drug is as effective as the usual dose of pyrantel. Normally, less than 10 per cent of the dose is absorbed from the gastrointestinal tract, although fatty foods may increase this. Mebendazole is associated only occasionally with transient abdominal pain, diarrhea, fever, pruritus, skin rash and, rarely, leukopenia. This drug is teratogenic in some species and is contraindicated during pregnancy.

Mebendazole selectively and irreversibly inhibits glucose uptake by the worm, causing immobilization and death of the parasites over a period of up to three days.

Until 1986, **gentian violet** was the only nonprescription pinworm remedy available in the United States and some Canadians may request it. Use of gentian violet should be discouraged, as safer and more effective drugs are available. Gentian violet is a mitotic poison and may be mutagenic. Even though it may be detoxified by hepatic enzymes, it is potentially hazardous to exposed skin and gastrointestinal epithelial cells.

Prevention

To prevent reinfection, most authorities recommend treating all members of the household simultaneously. Others state that this measure does not affect reinfection over a four-month period. Other advice includes washing the hands carefully, taking care to scrub the nails, before meals and after visits to the toilet. Children can wear closed sleeping garments or snug underpants to prevent hand contact and contamination of bedding. Some textbooks still emphasize the importance of personal cleanliness, including such stringent measures as daily room cleaning, sterilizing bed linens, washing the perianal area on rising and covering it with ointment, twice daily showers (but avoiding tub baths), disinfecting toilet seats and even using hand restraints. These hygienic procedures do not significantly affect the spread of enterobiasis in institutions or in families, or the incidence of reinfection in individuals. One worthwhile precaution is to launder sheets and night clothes after anthelmintic treatment. Before laundering, the articles must not be shaken. Affected people and parents already feel a social stigma in harboring a parasitic infection; emphasis on "improving" personal hygiene only heightens their embarrassment and psychological trauma. Rather, counselling should include information on the prevalence of pinworm infection in all walks of life, and reassurance of its harmlessness.

Table II *Consumer Counselling Information*

General

Advisable to treat all household members
Advisable to repeat treatment within 10 to 14 days
Dosing based on body weight

Pyrantel pamoate

Administered in a single dose
Side effects include:
  anorexia, vomiting, diarrhea (transient)
  dizziness, headache, drowsiness (occasional)
Not recommended for infants under one year
Not recommended in pregnancy
Not recommended for nonprescription use in individuals with liver
  disease

Pyrvinium pamoate

Administered in a single dose
Stains the stools and vomitus bright red
Tablets should be swallowed whole to avoid staining the teeth*
Side effects include:
  vomiting, cramping, diarrhea (occasional)
  skin photosensitivity (rare)

Piperazine adipate

May be given in 3 doses over 12 hours, but is probably somewhat
  more effective if given daily for 7 days
Should not be taken together with pyrantel
Side effects include:
  nausea, vomiting, diarrhea
  dizziness, difficulty in focusing
  skin rashes (occasional)
  overdose: vertigo, ataxia, confusion

Preventive measures

Careful handwashing before meals and after defecation
After treatment—wash, do not shake, bed linens and pyjamas

*Pyrvinium pamoate is available in Canada only in suspension form.

Anthelmintics

Other Helminths

Of the three classes of parasitic worms, the most diverse and widespread are the nematodes, of which Enterobius is one. Cestodes are of less medical and economic significance than the others.

Other Nematodes

The most ubiquitous nematode is *Ascaris lumbricoides* (large roundworm), infecting approximately one billion people worldwide. *Ascaris* is most prevalent in tropical and subtropical climates and in regions with poor sanitation or where human waste is used as fertilizer.

Symptomatic Ascaris infection is most often characterized by vague abdominal pain. Serious complications include biliary and intestinal obstruction. Part of the life cycle of Ascaris includes a lung migratory larval stage associated with asthmatic attacks and other allergic manifestations, although its role in asthma is still controversial.

Although Ascaris responds well to pyrantel pamoate, piperazine and mebendazole, self-treatment must be discouraged. The symptoms of ascariasis mimic those of other, more serious conditions, and differential diagnosis is essential. Also, Ascaris infection often occurs in combination with other nematode infections; the mixed infection may require different drug therapy.

Often co-existing with Ascaris in the same person are hookworms (*Necator americanus* and *Ancylostoma duodenale*) and whipworms (*Trichuris trichiura*). Infection is via fecal-contaminated soil, food or water. These parasites are rare at latitudes north of 40 degrees north, the latitude, for instance, of Philadelphia and Columbus. Light infections are essentially benign and symptomless. Heavy hookworm infections can cause iron-deficiency anemia; whipworm may cause anemia, rectal prolapse, and peritonitis and dysentery.

In contrast to pinworms, a variety of other intestinal parasites are carried by dogs. Many helminthic infections in Canada may find their way into human hosts via man's best friend. Approximately 20 per cent of adult dogs in the United States and nearly all puppies are infected with the ascarid *Toxocara canis*. Accidental ingestion of the eggs of this parasite by children leads to the syndrome of visceral larva migrans, characterized by fever, pulmonary symptoms, hepatomegaly and eosinophilia. Toxocariasis is also associated with ocular complications and encephalitis. Additionally, dog heartworm infections, transmitted to man via the mosquito, are becoming more prevalent, especially in the New England states and, by inference, in neighboring parts of Canada.

Fortunately, better agricultural practices have resulted in satisfactory control of Trichinella-infected pork. Public education has led to general acceptance of careful cooking of pork, practically eliminating the potentially fatal trichinosis in Canada and most of the United States. However, another food source of helminth infection has received little attention, namely, uncooked or lightly cooked fish. Until recently, eating raw, marinated, salted or smoked fish was not popular in western countries. Now the western palate is accepting such delicacies and, with them, some risks. Most dangerous are the larvae of Anisakis species, which can cause human eosinophilic gastroenteritis, intestinal obstruction or peritonitis. The related cod larval nematodes, genera Phocanema and Terranova, appear to be less invasive, but several reports from such North American sites as Nova Scotia, New England, California and Alaska describe motile worms being retrieved from throats and stomachs of people suffering from this infection. It can be prevented simply by heating the fish to over 60 °C or by freezing at below −17 °C for 24 hours.

Cestodes

The fish tapeworm (*Diphyllobothrium latum*) is found in many parts of the world, including the lake regions of Canada where its most common intermediate host is the pike. The parasite is transmitted by eating inadequately cooked, infested fish or perhaps its roe. Infection can cause megaloblastic anemia. The worm competes with the host for vitamin B_{12}. The person may complain of weakness, a sore tongue and a sensation of "pins and needles" in the extremities.

Unsanitary disposal of human feces, combined with eating inadequately cooked beef or pork, can lead to contraction of the beef tapeworm (*Taenia saginata*) or pork tapeworm (*Taenia solium*) respectively. Although the more common beef tapeworm rarely produces serious disease, *Taenia solium* larvae may invade various tissue sites, causing a potentially serious condition. Both may produce abdominal pain, discomfort and anemia. Differential diagnosis is essential.

The fourth cestode found in man is the dwarf tapeworm (*Hymenolepsis nana*). It requires no intermediate host and can replicate in the gut. More common in warm climates, *Hymenolepsis nana* produces symptoms only occasionally.

Tapeworm infections can be treated only with prescription drugs.

Trematodes

Flukes are found mainly in the Far East, with some species occurring also in Russia, Spain, Africa and Central America. Most rely on snails as intermediate hosts, and most are transmitted to man via uncooked fish. These infestations can be fatal.

Summary

Although helminthiasis is a major worldwide health problem, there is little awareness of parasitic infection in Canada. Most parasitic worms are endemic in warm climates; pinworm is the only one commonly found in Canada. The North American incidence of pinworm infection is estimated to be at least 30 per cent among school age children and half that in adults. It affects people in all socioeconomic classes, although it is transmitted particularly easily in institutional environments. Rigorous hygienic measures, other than careful handwashing before meals and after defecation, do little, if anything, to prevent its spread or reinfection.

Pinworm causes little pathology, and often goes undetected. Recognized symptoms usually are limited to perianal irritation. Migration of gravid worms into the female genito-urinary tract is probably an important cause of urinary tract bacterial infections in young girls.

Several effective nonprescription drugs are available in Canada to manage pinworm infection. The drug of choice is pyrantel pamoate; alternative drugs are pyrvinium pamoate and piperazine adipate. A prescription drug indicated for pinworm infection is mebendazole. These drugs generally are well tolerated. The most common side effects are gastrointestinal disturbances. Pyrantel, pyrvinium and mebendazole are effective in single doses; piperazine therapy is most effective when administered daily for a week. In all cases, retreatment is recommended within 10 to 14 days. Most authorities also recommend treating all family members at the same time. Safety in pregnancy has not been established for any of these drugs.

No personal preparation, such as dietary measures or fasting, is necessary before anthelmintic therapy for pinworm. Use of a laxative or enema is not needed either before or after treatment.

Consumer counselling information is summarized in Table II. The

Anthelmintics

pharmacist counselling an individual or parent about pinworm infection must recognize the condition may be a source of embarrassment. Assure the person that pinworm infection is neither a sign of uncleanliness nor a serious condition. If a consulting room is not available, nonprescription remedies should be located away from the main traffic areas of the pharmacy to give the client a measure of privacy.

Ask the Consumer

Q. Has your child or another family member been bothered by itching in the anal area? When is the itching most common?

■ The most common symptom of pinworm infection is pruritus of the perianal area, particularly at night. Related symptoms might include insomnia and restlessness.

Q. If the affected child is a girl, does she have a burning sensation when urinating? Does she need to urinate more frequently than usual?

■ Migration of gravid worms into the female genito-urinary tract is probably an important cause of urinary tract infection in young girls.

Q. Have these symptoms occurred before?

■ Pinworm reinfection is common. It is best prevented by treating all family members simultaneously, by retreating at least the symptomatic person 10 to 14 days after initial treatment, and by paying careful attention to washing the hands and nails before meals and after visits to the toilet.

Q. Have you seen pinworms in the perianal area?

■ Sometimes at night, with the aid of a flashlight, pinworms may be seen in the anal area. They may also be seen in the undergarments in the morning. They are found only rarely in the feces.

Q. What other symptoms have you?

■ Heavy infections may be associated with diarrhea. There is little evidence of other symptoms due to pinworms.

Q. Have you any drug allergies?

■ People known to be allergic to any drug should avoid use of that drug again. Since they are not related chemically, cross-sensitivity among the available anthelmintics does not occur. Cross-sensitivity between piperazine and other drugs containing a piperazine ring is possible.

Q. Are you pregnant?

■ Safety for pyrantel and piperazine during pregnancy has not been established.

Q. Is there a history of liver or kidney disease?

■ Piperazine is readily absorbed from the gastrointestinal tract. In the presence of liver or kidney disease, toxic levels may accumulate.

Q. If the affected individual is a child, how heavy is she/he?

■ Dosage of nonprescription anthelmintics is based on body weight.

Ensure that the child or parent understands how to determine how much medication to administer.

References

Introduction

Anonymous. Drugs for parasitic infections. Med Lett Drug Ther 1984; 26:27–34.

Brown HW, Neva FA. Basic clinical parasitology. Norwalk: Appleton-Century-Crofts, 1983:101–29.

Cline BL. Current drug regimens for the treatment of intestinal helminth infections. Med Clin North Am 1982;66:721–42.

Harron DWG, D'Arcy PF. Helminth infestation. Pharm Int 1983;4:162–8.

Stoll NR. This wormy world. J Parasitol 1947;33:1–18.

Warren KS. Helminthic diseases endemic in the United States. Am J Trop Med Hyg 1974;23:723–9.

Webster LT. Drugs used in the chemotherapy of helminthiasis. In: Gilman AG, Rall TW, Nies AS, Taylor P, eds. Goodman and Gilman's the pharmacological basis of therapeutics. Toronto: Pergamon, 1990:959–77.

Enterobiasis

Amin OM, Nwokike FG. Prevalence of pinworm and whipworm infestations in institutionalized mental patients in Wisconsin, 1966–1976. Wisc Med J 1980;79:31–2.

Baker RW, Peppercorn MA. Gastrointestinal ailments of homosexual men. Medicine 1982;61:390–405

Beaver PC, Kriz JJ, Lau TJ. Pulmonary nodule caused by *Enterobius vermicularis*. Am J Trop Med Hyg 1973;22:711–3.

Beaver PC, Jung RC, Cupp EW. Clinical parasitology. Philadelphia: Lea & Febiger, 1984:302–25.

Beaver PC. Methods of pinworm diagnosis. Am J Trop Med Hyg 1949; 29:577–87.

Bredesen J, Falensteen Lauritzen A, Kristiansen VB, Sorensen C, Kjersgaard P. Appendicitis and enterobiasis in children. Acta Chir Scand 1988; 154:585–7.

Budd JS, Armstrong C. Role of *Enterobius vermicularis* in the aetiology of appendicitis. Br J Surg 1987;74:748–9.

Cram EB. Studies on oxyuriasis: xxviii. Summary and conclusions. Am J Dis Child 1943;65:46–59.

Dalrymple JC, Hunter JC, Ferrier A, Payne W. Disseminated intraperitoneal oxyuris granulomas. Aust NZ J Obstet Gynaecol 1986;26:90–1.

Daly JJ, Baker GF. Pinworm granuloma of the liver. Am J Trop Med Hyg 1984; 33:62–4.

El Najjar MY, Benitez J, Fry G, et al. Autopsies on two native American mummies. Am J Phys Anthropol 1980;53:197–202.

Fiumara NJ, Tang S. Folliculitis of the buttocks and pinworms: a case report. Sex Transm Dis 1986;13:45–6.

Fry GF. *Enterobius vermicularis*: 10,000-year-old human infection. Science 1969;166:1620.

Graham CF. A device for the diagnosis of Enterobius infection. Am J Trop Med Hyg 1941;21:159–61.

Jacobs AH. Enterobiasis in children. Incidence, symptomology, and diagnosis with a simplified Scotch cellulose tape technique. J Pediatr 1942; 21:497–503.

Kogan J, Alter M, Price H. Bilateral *Enterobius vermicularis* salpingo-oophoritis complicated with *Bacteroides fragilis* septicemia. Postgrad Med 1983; 73:305–10.

Kropp KA, Cichocki GA, Bansal NK. *Enterobius vermicularis* (pinworms), introital bacteriology and recurrent urinary tract infection in children. J Urol 1978;120:480–2.

Mayers CP, Purvis RJ. Manifestations of pinworms. Can Med Assoc J 1970; 103:489–93.

McMahon JN, Connolly CE, Long SV, Meehan FP. Enterobius granulomas of the uterus, ovary and pelvic peritoneum: two case reports. Br J Obstet Gynaecol 1984;91:289–90.

Mogensen K, Pahle E, Kowalski K. *Enterobius vermicularis* and acute appendicitis. Acta Chir Scand 1985;151:705–7.

Anthelmintics

Monroe LS. Gastrointestinal parasites. Berk JE, ed. Gastroenterology. Toronto: WB Saunders, 1985:4250–345.

Mortensen MJ, Thomson JP. Perianal abscess due to *Enterobius vermicularis:* report of a case. Dis Colon Rectum 1984;27:677–8.

Most H. Treatment of parasitic infection of travelers and immigrants. N Engl J Med 1984;310:298–304.

Nutting SA, Murphy F, Inglis FG. Abdominal pain due to *Enterobius vermicularis.* Can J Surg 1980;23:286–7.

Pearson RD, Irons RP Sr, Irons RP Jr. Chronic pelvic peritonitis due to the pinworm *Enterobius vermicularis.* JAMA 1981;245:1340–1.

Reyes CV, Aranha GV, Foy BK, Altergott RA. Omental oxyuriasis: case report. Milit Med 1984;149:682–3.

Sachdev YV, Howards SS. *Enterobius vermicularis* infestation and secondary enuresis. J Urol 1975;113:143–4.

Sawitz W, D'Antoni JS, Rhude K, Lob S. Studies on the epidemiology of oxyuriasis. South Med J 1940;33:913–22.

Shroff CP. Oxyuric salpingitis (Case report). Postgrad Med J 1984;30:51–2.

Simon RD. Pinworm infestation and urinary tract infection in young girls. Am J Dis Child 1974;128:21–2.

Vafai M, Mohit P. Granuloma of the anal canal due to *Enterobius vermicularis:* report of a case. Dis Colon Rectum 1983;26:349–50.

Wagner ED, Eby WC. Pinworm prevalence in California elementary school children, and diagnostic methods. Am J Trop Med Hyg 1983;32:998-1001.

Warren KS. The control of helminths: nonreplicating infectious agents of man. Ann Rev Public Health 1981;2:101–15.

Drug Treatment

Au W, Pathak S, Collie CJ, Hsu TC. Cytogenic toxicity of gentian violet and crystal violet on mammalian cells in vitro. Mutation Res 1978;58:269–76.

Au W, Butler MA, Bloom SE, Matney TS. Further study of the genetic toxicity of gentian violet. Mutation Res 1979;66:103–12.

Barrett-Connor E. Drugs for the treatment of parasitic infection. Med Clin North Am 1982;66:245–55.

Broadbent V. Children's worms. Br Med J 1975;2:89.

DelMar C. Angio-oedema after Combantrin in a six-year-old. Med J Aust 1982;2:117.

Drug Evaluations Annual. Chicago: American Medical Association, 1991: 1554–7.

Hecht L, Murray WE, Rubenstein S. Theophylline-pyrantel pamoate interaction. Drug Intell Clin Pharm 1989;23:258.

Katz M, Anthelmintics: current concepts in the treatment of helminthics infections. Drugs 1986;32:358–71.

Katz M. Adverse metabolic effects of antiparasitic drugs. Rev Infect Dis 1982;4:768–70.

Kinsella JM. Anthelmintic products. Handbook of nonprescription drugs. Washington: American Pharmaceutical Association, 1990:333–41.

Leach FN. Management of threadworm infestation during pregnancy. Arch Dis Child 1990;65:399–400.

Lefrock JL, Smith BR. Treatment of helminthic disease. Am Fam Physician 1985;32:182–8.

Matsen JM, Turner JA. Reinfection in enterobiasis (pinworm infection). Am J Dis Child 1969;118:576–81.

McKay T. Enterobius vermicularis infection causing endometritis and persistent vaginal discharge in three siblings. N Z Med J 1989;102: 56.

Parsons AC. Piperazine neurotoxicity: "worm wobble." Br Med J 1971;4:792.

Pitts NE, Migliardi JR. Antiminth (pyrantel pamoate). The clinical evaluation of a new broad spectrum anthelmintic. Clin Pediatr 1974;13:87–94.

Price ML, Hall-Smith SP. Allergy to piperazine in a patient sensitive to ethylenediamine. Contact Dermatitis 1984;10:120.

Richard A, Zhanel GG. Treatment of vaginal pinworms. Can J Hosp Pharm 1989;42:208–9.

Rosenkrantz HS, Carr HS. Possible hazard in use of gentian violet. Br Med J 1971;3:702–3.

Singh S, Samantaray JC. Topical anthelmintic treatment of recurrent genitourinary enterobiasis. Genitourin Med 1989;65:284–5.

Other Nematodes

Huntley CC. Of worms and asthma, or Tullis revisited (Letter). N Engl J Med 1976;294:1295.

Kates S, Wright KA, Wright R. A case of human infection with the cod nematode *Phocanema sp.* Am J Trop Med Hyg 1973;22:606–8.

Little MD, Most H. Anisakid larva from the throat of a woman in New York. Am J Trop Med Hyg 1973;22:609–12.

Pawlowski ZS. Ascariasis: host-pathogen biology. Rev Infect Dis 1982;4:806–14.

Scully RE, Galdabini JJ, McNeely BU. Case records of the Massachusetts General Hospital; case 13–1979. N Engl J Med 1979;300:723–9.

Seah SKK, Hucal G, Law C. Dogs and intestinal parasites: a public health problem. Can Med Assoc J 1975;112:1191–4.

Valdiserri RO. Intestinal anisakiasis. Report of a case and recovery of larvae from market fish. Am J Clin Pathol 1981;76:329–33.

Watt IA, McLean NR, Girdwood RWA, Kissen LH, Fyfe AHB. Eosinophilic gastroenteritis associated with a larval anisakine nematode. Lancet 1979; 2:893–4.

19
Contraceptives

Revised by Lynn Torsher. Based on the original chapter by Sharon E. McKinnon

ineffective as contraceptive pg 399

In addition to the basal thermometers needed for some methods of natural contraception, pharmacies carry many physical and chemical barrier contraceptives. Spermicides are available as jellies, pastes, creams, foaming tablets and aerosol foams. Diaphragms must be sized and fitted by a physician. Cervical caps are prescription items in Canada. The contraceptive sponge is a recent development. Use of the most popular contraceptive—the condom—continues to increase, partly because it protects against sexually transmitted diseases. The safety and effective use of each method requires appropriate consumer counselling.

Until 1969, the dissemination of birth control information and the sale of contraceptives were criminal offences in Canada. The law was largely ignored during the late 1950s, and contraceptives were widely prescribed by doctors and available in pharmacies. No one was ever convicted under the Criminal Code, but even with the wide publicity concerning condom use in preventing sexually transmitted diseases (STDs), the "behind the counter" atmosphere surrounding contraceptives still exists in the minds of many. Today, most pharmacies openly display a wide selection of nonprescription contraceptives. Many pharmacists willingly take an active role in contraceptive counselling. As the public becomes more aware of potential adverse effects from methods such as intrauterine devices (for example, pelvic inflammatory disease and ectopic pregnancy) and oral contraceptives (for example, increased risk of thromboembolic disease), pharmacists must become more knowledgeable about barrier methods. Given factual, unbiased information and the ready availability of the wide variety of birth control methods, all individuals and couples should be able to select the method best suited to their needs.

Birth control may be achieved in many ways, some more effective than others. One question often asked concerns the effectiveness of specific methods of birth control. The figures in Table I are an amalgamation of reported failure rates from many sources. A wide range of contraceptive effectiveness exists, but most methods provide good protection from unwanted pregnancy when used correctly and consistently. Unfortunately, many reports are biased in favor of oral contraceptives and intrauterine devices (IUDs); the safety and effectiveness possible with the diaphragm, condom or spermicide are ignored. Studies have shown that the longer these nonprescription methods are used, the lower the failure rate; therefore, statements comparing method effectiveness must give length of usage.

Table I First Year Failure Rates of Birth Control Methods

Method	Lowest Observed Failure Rate* (%)	Failure Rate in Typical Users** (%)
Tubal sterilization or vasectomy	0.4	0.4
Birth Control Pills (combined)	0.5	2
IUD	1.5	5
Condom	2	10
Diaphragm (with spermicide)	2	19
Cervical cap	2	13
Foams, jellies, creams & vaginal suppositories	3–5	18
Sponge (with spermicide)	9–11	10–20
Coitus interruptus	16	23
Fertility awareness techniques (basal body temperature, mucous method, calendar, rhythm)	2–20	24
Douche	—	40
Chance (no contraceptive used)	90	90

*Designed to complete the sentence: "In 100 users who start out the year using a given method and who use it correctly and consistently, the lowest observed failure rate has been _____."

**Designed to complete the sentence: "In 100 typical users who start out the year using a given method, the number of pregnancies by the end of the year will be _____."

Adapted from: Hatcher RA, Guest F, Stewart F, et al. Contraceptive technology 1986–87, New York: Irvington, 1986:102.

From the earliest times until the 1960s, sexual abstinence, coitus interruptus, abortion and vaginal contraception, in various combinations, effectively lowered the birth rate in many countries. In the 1960s, the advent of oral contraceptives and IUDs caused a decrease in the use of barrier contraceptive methods, a rate that was further lowered in the 1970s by the increasing popularity of surgical sterilization. In recent years, concerns about side effects and the safety of contraceptive methods have caused many men and women to reassess their contraceptive usage. According to a recent study on contraceptive use in Canada, sterilization, both male and female, accounts for well over 50 per cent of contraceptive methods currently in use. With an increase in marriage breakdown and remarriage, many individuals may regret their use of this normally irreversible method. This same study found that women with more education resorted less often to sterilization. The researchers concluded that growing levels of education among women, better general knowledge about contraceptive methods and the availability of improved methods of birth control will lower the rate of sterilization in the future. Several studies in the United States that began in the 1950s and 1960s indicate that since the mid-1970s the use of oral contraceptives and IUDs has declined while the rate of decline in the use of traditional methods, that is, barrier methods, has been less rapid. In some populations, the use of these methods even showed an increase. Since 1980, the threat of AIDS and other sexually transmitted diseases has led to a resurgence in the popularity of the condom.

Some methods widely used for birth control are ineffective. Coitus interruptus (withdrawal, "taking care" or "pulling out") is used extensively, especially by couples without access to birth control information. It is not effective since it is not always possible for the man to withdraw his penis from the vagina in time or to ejaculate well away from the vagina. Douching (with zinc or aluminum sulfate, quinine salts, vinegar, Coca Cola, laundry detergents and innumerable other solutions) has been used to remove semen from the vagina before sperm can enter the uterus. However, studies show that viable spermatozoa are in the fallopian tube within 90 seconds of ejaculation. Consequently, douching does not act as a contraceptive method and may push spermatozoa into the uterus while washing others away. (For more information on douching, see the chapter on feminine care products.)

Lactation may prevent pregnancy by delaying the return of ovulation (and menstruation) after childbirth. However, since ovulation and fertility may occur before menstruation has resumed, amenorrhea is not a reliable indicator of lack of fertility. Barrier contraceptive methods may be appropriate for lactating women since they offer protection from pregnancy without systemic effects. Consumers seeking in-depth information on any of these methods can be referred to a family planning clinic.

Natural Family Planning

Many men and women desire natural family planning for religious and other personal reasons. Some methods are effective, but this effectiveness depends on a stable sexual relationship, an extremely high degree of motivation in both partners and detailed instructions on how to use the method. These same methods may be used by couples wishing to increase their chances of conception.

Natural family planning methods depend on recognizing physiological changes that occur during the different stages of the menstrual cycle. One stage is menstruation, during which the ovaries are at a low level of activity, the circulating hormone levels are low and the lining of the endometrium, along with remnants of the unfertilized ovum, is shed with some bleeding. For most women, but not all, this stage of their menstrual cycle is infertile. The second stage is the preovulatory stage. The estrogen level rises in this stage; under its influence, follicles, each containing a primitive egg, start to develop within the ovaries. At the same time, in response to estradiol production, the cervix is stimulated to produce mucus. This clear, slippery, fertile mucus, essential in maintaining the fertilizing capacity of the sperm, protects and nourishes the sperm and provides channels for them to follow on their journey to the fallopian tubes. Without this mucus, conception does not occur. The developing follicle moving toward the surface of the ovary releases more estradiol, increasing the fertile characteristics of the mucus. The endometrial lining of the uterus begins to thicken. Ovulation occurs only one day in any particular cycle (about 14 days before menstruation) unless double ovulation occurs (within 48 hours). A woman's temperature drops slightly, then rises at the start of ovulation. The corpus luteum produces progesterone, which, with estradiol, causes the lining of the uterus to grow and thicken. During the postovulatory phase, the ovum (which has a life-span of about 12 hours after release from the ovary) moves into and along the fallopian tube toward the uterus. Fertilization may take place within the fallopian tube less than a day after ovulation. If the egg is not fertilized, it dies and disintegrates. The remnants are shed with menstruation about 14 days later.

The Billings method of natural contraception, also called the ovulation or mucous method, relies on recognizing changes in the cervix and cervical mucus to determine "safe" and "unsafe" days for sexual intercourse. During infertile days before and after ovulation, the woman may not be aware of any mucus or may find a yellow viscous mucus present. During ovulation, this mucus becomes a clear, slippery discharge, much like raw egg white. At the same time, the external opening of the cervix expands and there may be a feeling of heaviness, abdominal swelling, and rectal pain or discomfort.

The basal body temperature method relies upon determining temperature changes that occur with ovulation. (For information on the use of the basal thermometer, refer to the chapter on diagnostic aids.)

The sympto-thermal method combines the mucous and temperature methods with the chart-keeping of the traditional calendar rhythm method. Each menstrual cycle for one year is noted on the calendar to determine the average length of the cycle.

Pregnancies per 100 women in the first year of use have been reported to range from 0.6 to 25.4 for the Billings method, 3.1 to 19.5 for the basal body temperature method and 7.47 to 29.88 for the sympto-thermal method.

Barrier Methods

Other contraceptive methods available without medical intervention are the barrier methods using spermicides, diaphragms, sponges or condoms. Many factors affect the acceptability and effectiveness of these methods, including availability, comfort, ease of use, convenience, cost and cultural attitudes. Failure of barrier contraceptives is often due to inconsistent use rather than failure of the method during use. Inconsistent use may result from unease with the method or lack of understanding of proper use. Any pharmacist involved in contraceptive counselling must be knowledgeable about methods and free from personal bias to render the best education and counselling.

Spermicides

Spermicides provide a physical and biochemical block to prevent spermatozoa from reaching and fertilizing the ovum. They can be introduced into the vagina in jellies, pastes, creams, suppositories, foaming tablets or aerosol foams. The preparations generally consist of a vehicle and the spermicide. Their sole purpose is to immobilize and kill spermatozoa as rapidly as possible after ejaculation into the vagina.

The vehicle, or base, is generally inert. Its main purpose is to carry the spermicide and hold it in the vagina and against the cervix. The base may also exert contraceptive action of its own by physically blocking semen and sperm from coming into contact with the cervical mucus, thus preventing sperm from entering the uterus.

Jellies and pastes have water-soluble bases, such as polyethylene

Contraceptives

glycol, gelatin or gum tragacanth, which melt or liquefy at body temperatures. They disperse over vaginal and cervical surfaces when in contact with vaginal and cervical secretions and during sexual intercourse.

Creams are formulated from emulsions of water and fat, such as stearate, or hydrolyzed fat such as glycerin. Creams usually lubricate less and are less messy as they adhere well to the mucosa of the vagina and cervix. Since they usually do not disperse as well as jellies and pastes, the applicator must be correctly positioned in the vagina so the discharged cream covers the cervix.

Foaming tablets are usually formulated with a tartaric acid and sodium bicarbonate powder base that effervesces, releasing carbon dioxide, when in contact with acidic vaginal secretions. This release takes from 3 to 10 minutes depending on the product. Some manufacturers recommend moistening the tablet with a small amount of saliva or water before insertion to hasten the foaming action. Some warmth may be discernible in the vagina as the tablet effervesces.

Aerosol foams are generally considered one of the most acceptable of intravaginal contraceptive products available. Although the bulk of the vehicle in jellies and creams is water mixed with other fluids and solids, a large part of foam is gas, which is eliminated inconspicuously from the vagina. Consequently, foams are less messy, have less leakage and are more pleasant to use. Foams are formulated as oil-in-water emulsions and are stored under gas pressure. They disperse readily to cover vaginal tissue with spermicide immediately after insertion into the vagina.

In all these intravaginal contraceptives, the spermicide is the active ingredient that immobilizes or kills sperm on contact. Some preparations contain two or more spermicides with similar or different mechanisms of action.

Surfactants include the most popular spermicidal compounds in use today. Spermicides such as nonylphenoxypolyethoxyethanol (nonoxynol-9), methoxypolyoxyethylene glycol 550 laurate, p-methanylphenylpolyoxyethylene ether and p-diisobutylphenoxypolyethoxyethanol, break down the sperm wall by attaching to spermatozoa and inhibiting oxygen uptake and fructolysis. Their effect is irreversible loss of motility and permanent disruption of the cell membrane. They affect not only the spermatozoal membrane, but also any bacteria or parasite present in the vagina. These agents vary in the speed with which they immobilize sperm and in the concentration needed to produce their action when combined with various vehicles and seminal fluid. Surfactant spermicides are available in most dosage forms including aerosol foams.

Bactericides used as spermicides include phenylmercuric acetate, quinine compounds and quaternary ammonium compounds, including benzethonium chloride and ricinoleic acid and its compounds. These agents disrupt sperm metabolism by combining with sulfur and hydrogen bonds within the spermatozoa. The mechanisms of action of bactericides and surfactants are often the same and seem to have a synergistic effect when used together.

Acidic agents, such as lactic, boric, tartaric and citric acids and gum acacia, immobilize and in some cases destroy sperm. Small quantities of these acidic agents occasionally may be added to other spermicidal ingredients.

Safety

Two concerns exist about the safety of spermicide preparations. The first concern is the possible effect on the fetus if preparations are used before conception or during an undiagnosed pregnancy. The second is the possible effect on the user. Although one study reported congenital anomalies in infants of women who had obtained a spermicide within 10 months of conception, there was no evidence that the spermicide had been used either before or during pregnancy. Subsequent studies showed no causal association between spermicide use and birth defects. However, a conservative approach is best followed: spermicides should not be used if the woman may already be pregnant. In animal models, some spermicides are absorbed through the vaginal mucosa, but evidence of absorption in humans is lacking. The United States Food and Drug Administration advisory panel on nonprescription contraceptives and other vaginal drug products available in the United States has determined that menfegol, nonoxynol-9 and octoxynol are safe and effective vaginal spermicides; phenylmercuric acetate and phenylmercuric nitrate are categorized as unsafe or ineffective.

Some spermicides rarely cause allergic contact dermatitis reactions in some individuals. Animal testing has been more extensive, but the results cannot be applied to humans. In general, spermicides can promote health by preventing some infections and possibly protecting against cervical neoplasia.

Consumer Counselling

Creams and jellies are formulated for use either alone or with a diaphragm. Products intended for use alone have a higher concentration of spermicide and disperse more readily than products intended for use with a diaphragm. Aerosol foams and foaming tablets are not intended for use with a diaphragm.

The pharmacist should review applicator use and care with the user. A demonstration would be helpful. Proper use of the applicator and proper insertion of the product must be stressed, because the spermicide may be ineffective if not inserted high in the vagina. With aerosol foams, the user must be instructed to return the canister to an upright position before removing the applicator to avoid spraying foam widely. With creams and jellies, the applicator must be screwed onto the tube of spermicide for proper filling. The applicator may be dropped into a glass or cup of water after use to facilitate later cleaning with water and soap.

Many products must be inserted for a minimum time before coitus to enable sufficient dispersion of the spermicide for effective contraception. Generally, intercourse may take place at once with foams, jellies, creams and pastes; however, manufacturers of some jellies, creams and pastes recommend an interval of 5 to 10 minutes following application. With foaming tablets and suppositories, an interval of 10 to 15 minutes is desirable. The package insert should be consulted for specific recommendations.

Spermicidal products usually lose their effectiveness within 1 hour. When using foams, if intercourse has not taken place within 20 minutes, another applicatorful must be inserted. When using contraceptive cream or jelly, another applicatorful must be inserted if intercourse does not take place within 1 hour. Repeated acts of coitus require repeated applications of spermicide. The package insert for each product provides information on times pertaining to that specific product.

Douching after using spermicides is a personal preference but is not necessary. Douching must not be done for 6 to 8 hours after intercourse since it renders the spermicide useless.

The contraceptive effectiveness of both IUDs and condoms increases when used in conjunction with a spermicide. Some birth control clinics recommend using a spermicide for the first 3 months after IUD insertion when the chance of expulsion is greatest, as well as during the fertile days of the menstrual cycle. Use of a spermicidal foam and condoms together at all times results in extremely effective contraception. If a vaginal lubricant is needed during sexual intercourse, a spermicide preparation can be used to good advantage.

Allergic reactions to these products may rarely occur in both men and women. The symptoms may be redness and itching of the genitals, with or without swelling and discharge. The sensitizing agents may be the base, the spermicide or the preservatives used in the product. Suggested treatment is to discontinue use of that specific brand. Often, symptoms do not recur if another product is used. If symptoms are severe, a physician must be consulted.

Other than rare allergic reactions, no adverse reactions to spermicide use have been reported.

Diaphragms

A diaphragm acts as a mechanical barrier to prevent sperm from entering the cervical canal and as a receptacle for a spermicide cream or jelly, which it holds against the cervix. Use of the diaphragm declined significantly with the advent of oral contraceptives and the IUD, but in recent years its popularity has increased.

All diaphragms consist of a vulcanized latex dome and a peripheral steel ring covered with rubber. The main difference between them is the type of steel ring (see Figure 1).

A flat spring diaphragm consists of a flat, narrow steel band that compresses in all planes but is relatively stiff compared to other models. Some women find this type easier to insert than other models.

Coil spring diaphragm rings are made of a rubber-covered, coiled steel wire. They are flexible in all planes and can be easily grasped and folded for insertion. On compression, the rim lies in a flat plane like the flat spring. Since the coil is more flexible and exerts less pressure, some women find it more comfortable than the flat spring.

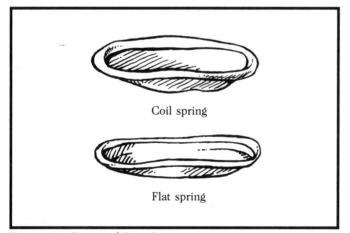

Coil spring

Flat spring

Figure 1 *Types of Diaphragms*

Both the flat spring and the coil spring can be used by women with normal vaginal shape and size and good vaginal muscle tone. Anatomic variations determine the suitability of the fit, hence the contraceptive effectiveness. The two types of diaphragm may not be interchangeable. In cases where the type is not specified by the physician or user, consult the physician or diaphragm fitter.

Failures with contraception while using the diaphragm may be due to incorrect size or incorrect insertion. Counselling can contribute to correct use and optimal contraceptive effectiveness.

Size and Fitting

The size of the vaginal diaphragm is given by the diameter of its rim and is expressed in millimetres (mm). Diaphragms are available in sizes varying from 50 to 105 mm, in increments of 5 mm. The most common fittings are between 65 and 80 mm.

The type and size of the diaphragm must be selected for the individual according to her own specific requirements. Two factors must be considered in selecting the proper size: the depth of the vagina and the tone of the musculature. If the diaphragm is too large or too small, it will not be adequate. If it is too small, it does not fit snugly behind the pubic symphysis and may become dislodged during coitus. It is important to select the largest size tolerated by the user. If it is too large, the diaphragm comes too far forward and may cause discomfort to the user and her sexual partner. A too-large diaphragm may even protrude from the vagina. In either case, the diaphragm is not held securely in place and may sag down, permitting the penis to pass over the front rim, nullifying its contraceptive value.

Effective contraception is possible with correct use of a diaphragm with a spermicide, but most women need instruction and some practice with insertion to feel comfortable with its use. Women's self-help groups and some birth control clinics spend time fitting and teaching women how to use the diaphragm as an effective contraceptive method.

Clinical diaphragm fitting can be accomplished through a four step procedure to manually measure the length of the vaginal canal from the pubic bone to the posterior fornix or by the sequential insertion of differently sized rings or sample diaphragms. The diaphragm fitting must always be checked with the type of diaphragm that will be used.

Safety

Allergic reactions to either the diaphragm or the spermicide may occur in rare cases. Diaphragms have been associated with an increased risk of urinary tract infections. Toxic shock is a more serious potential problem related to the use of the diaphragm.

Toxic shock syndrome is an illness with serious morbidity and mortality. It occurs primarily in healthy menstruating women who use tampons, but it has been reported in other populations. Some nonfatal cases have been associated with the use of a diaphragm. In these cases, the diaphragm was left in place from 24 to 48 hours—long past the time required for contraceptive effectiveness. Women using diaphragms for contraception should be instructed not to leave the diaphragm in place longer than 24 hours nor to use it during menstruation. Symptoms such as fever, diarrhea, vomiting, muscle aches and a sunburn-like rash should be reported to a physician promptly.

Consumer Counselling

Instructions for diaphragm use vary according to the manufacturer. Pharmacists should not assume the user knows the correct use of the diaphragm. Pharmacists should instruct the user to hold the diaphragm with the dome down and to squeeze out 5 to 15 mL of spermicide, spreading it over both sides of the diaphragm and around the rim. In practice, this procedure causes the diaphragm to be slippery and difficult to handle and insert. Frustration arising from difficulty in inserting the diaphragm may lead to poor compliance, and it may be recommended that the spermicide be put around the inside, but not on top, of the rim. It appears to make no difference which side of the diaphragm is in contact with the cervix.

The diaphragm can be inserted while squatting, lying down or standing with one foot propped up. It should be held with the dome down and the rim pinched together between the fingers and thumb. The lips of the vagina are spread with the other hand and the diaphragm inserted into the vagina as far as it will go, making certain the leading rim passes behind the cervix. The front rim is pressed up behind the pubic bone (see Figure 2). The cervix must be completely covered by the diaphragm. (The cervix normally feels like the tip of the nose.)

compliance. Since the diaphragm provides no protection if not used, inserting it up to 12 hours before intercourse is better than not using it at all.

The diaphragm must be left in place 6 to 8 hours after sexual intercourse for maximal contraception. It should not be left in place longer than 24 hours, since this may cause increased incidence of vaginal and other infections.

To remove the diaphragm, the user hooks the index finger behind the edge of the forward rim and pulls gently downward and out (see Figure 3). Sometimes it helps to bear down at this point. Long fingernails can be a hazard and can cause a tear in the diaphragm. The introducer may also be used to remove the diaphragm. It is inserted gently, the hooked end placed behind the edge of the diaphragm and pressure exerted.

Douching is not required, but may be a personal preference. If the

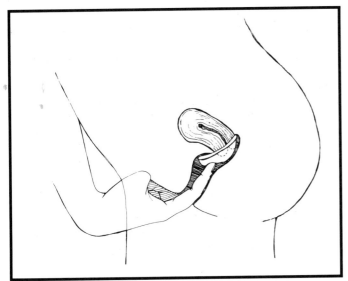

Figure 2 *Inserting a Diaphragm*

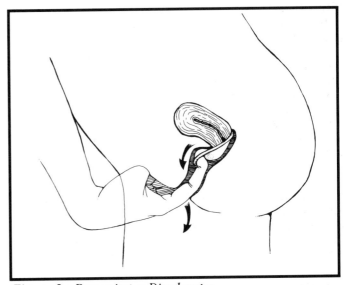

Figure 3 *Removing a Diaphragm*

Some women will find it easier to use an introducer, or inserter, with the diaphragm. The diaphragm is placed on the introducer (over the end and in the notch indicated for that size) and spermicide applied to the diaphragm as usual. It should be applied to the side next to the introducer before its placement there. With the notches facing upward, the introducer is gently pushed into the vagina as far as it will go. A twisting motion of the hand holding the introducer releases the diaphragm. After the introducer is withdrawn, the position of the diaphragm must be checked to ensure proper placement.

Ideally the diaphragm is inserted 30 to 60 minutes before intercourse, eliminating interruption of coitus and allowing time for the spermicide to disperse around the cervical os and onto the vaginal tissues. At one time, it was recommended that if intercourse did not take place within 2 hours, the diaphragm should be removed, rinsed and reinserted with additional spermicide. Also, it was suggested that an additional applicatorful of spermicide be used if coitus was repeated. A recent study shows that spermicide effectiveness persists longer than initially thought. Further studies may prove that the diaphragm may be inserted for periods of up to 12 hours before intercourse and that additional applications of spermicide may not be required for repeated acts of coitus. Both would improve user

user wishes to use a douche, she should not do so for 6 to 8 hours after intercourse. About half the douche solution should be used before removal of the diaphragm and the remainder after removal.

After use, the diaphragm is washed with mild soap and warm water and patted dry. It is then dusted with corn starch and returned to its container. Exposure to detergents, petrolatum (for example, Vaseline) and perfumes hastens deterioration. The diaphragm must be checked for holes before each use by holding it up to the light or by filling it with water and watching for leaks. The light check is better than the water check. The holes tend to occur around the rim. With careful use, the diaphragm may last for years.

The fit of the diaphragm should be checked if there has been a weight loss or gain of 4 kg or more, after pregnancy is terminated by either delivery or abortion, and after pelvic surgery. Otherwise, a check on the fit can be made at the yearly appointment for a Pap test.

If the user complains of pelvic pain, cramps, urinary retention, bladder symptoms or aggravation of recurrent cystitis with the use of the diaphragm, the pharmacist should advise the user to consult a physician. A change in size or rim type may resolve these problems, but diaphragm use may have to be discontinued if symptoms persist.

Cervical Cap

The cervical cap is a soft rubber, thimble shaped cup that fits over the cervix and is held in place by suction between its firm, flexible rim and the surface of the cervix or cervical-vaginal junction. The cervical cap has been shown to have efficacy rates similar to the diaphragm. They have been widely available in Europe for many years, and are approved for use in Canada; however, there are a limited number of physicians here who have been trained to fit the caps. The cap holds a spermicide next to the cervix and exerts its contraceptive effect much like the diaphragm does—as a mechanical barrier to prevent sperm from entering the cervical canal and as a receptacle for the spermicide.

Size and Fitting

Cervical caps may be sized—depending on the type and manufacturer—according to the inner or the outer diameter. Inner diameters may range from 22 to 31 mm, varying by increments of 3 mm. Outer diameters may range from 42 to 54 mm, varying by increments of 6 mm. A cap, determined by trying the various sizes available, which fits snugly enough to maintain suction contact between the cap rim and the cervix or vaginal vault, is chosen.

Safety

Documentation of the safety of the cervical cap is ongoing. As with other latex rubber products, allergic contact dermatitis may rarely occur. A more serious theoretical complication is that of toxic shock syndrome, although this has not yet been reported. A follow-up Pap test is recommended after the first 3 months of cervical cap use, then yearly thereafter.

Consumer Counselling

Instructions vary according to the manufacturer. Most women find the insertion of the cap is more difficult than insertion of a diaphragm, and removal can be tricky.

The cap is filled approximately one-third full with spermicide taking care to avoid applying spermicide to the rim, as this may interfere with the formation of a seal between the cap and the cervix. While the user is in a squatting position, the cap is introduced into the vagina with the index finger of the left hand. The cap is pushed upward in the vagina with the dome facing downward and the rim toward the cervix. The cap is pushed onto the cervix so that the rim attaches to it. The dome of the cap may now be pinched to increase the suction.

To remove the cervical cap, the index finger is placed behind the rim of the cap. A downward motion dislodges the cap from the cervix. The index finger is inserted into the cap (somewhat like a thimble), and the cap is drawn out of the vagina.

Condoms

The condom is the most commonly used contraceptive in the world, for the following reasons: it is available without medical prescription; it is generally free of side effects; it is simple to use and easy to understand; and it helps prevent the spread of STDs. When condoms are used properly and consistently, their effectiveness is better than 97 per cent. If the condom is used with contraceptive jelly or cream and a vaginal barrier, a success rate of 99 per cent can be obtained; if used with a contraceptive foam, a success rate better than 99 per cent is possible. Acceptability of condom use has increased because of the growing need for men to assume their share of birth control responsibility, and because of concern about acquired immune deficiency syndrome (AIDS) and other STDs. The disadvantages of condom use are that it interrupts sexual activity and can reduce sensation for the man.

Although the number of different brands of condoms has increased greatly in the past few years, the basic types remain the same. The many colors and textures do not alter the basic function—preventing sperm from getting into the vagina.

Most condoms on the market are made of latex rubber and are available in plain or teat-end, lubricated or non-lubricated varieties. The teat end provides a reservoir for holding the ejaculate. To prevent painful intercourse, lubrication of the condom is necessary when vaginal secretions are limited. As well, friction may tear the condom on insertion if lubrication is lacking. Condoms lubricated with spermicide are now available. Presumably, the spermicide helps prevent pregnancy if the condom breaks during use. Rubber condoms are less expensive than natural skin condoms.

Animal membrane or skin condoms are made from sheep cecum. They are more expensive than rubber condoms, but are said to be capable of transferring heat and so dull sensation less. Because natural skin condoms do not stretch as rubber condoms do, they are large and may not fit as securely as the latex rubber condoms. Animal membrane condoms are not effective in preventing AIDS.

National standards set for condom manufacture in Canada were implemented in 1978 and include length (greater than or equal to 160 mm), width (45 to 55 mm between rim and 80 mm from closed end, and less than or equal to 70 mm within 80 mm of closed end), a water leakage test for holes (for new condoms and condoms aged in an air oven 12 hours at 68 to 72°C) and a test for strength (bursting volume greater than or equal to 25 L). In general, condoms made by the major manufacturers are of high quality. In Canada, packaging and labelling specifications include a 5 year expiration date.

Consumer Counselling

Instructions for condom use vary with manufacturer. The pharmacist should not assume everyone knows how to use condoms. The condom should be put on before vulvar or vaginal contact. Although there is no confirmation that viable sperm are found in the pre-ejaculatory fluid providing the man has urinated since his last ejaculation, putting on the condom before genital contact is recommended because it causes less interference.

The condom should be unrolled over as much of the erect penis as possible. In the past, it was recommended that air be expelled from both the teat-ended and the plain-ended condoms to avoid rupture of the condom on ejaculation and that an air-free portion be left free at the end of a plain-ended condom to hold the ejaculate. However, no evidence exists that this rupture would occur. Any space left at the tip of the condom is probably flattened against the wall of the vagina during intercourse.

The vagina must be sufficiently lubricated or the condom may cause pain for the woman and may tear on penetration. Lubrication also increases sensitivity. Petrolatum should not be used as a lubricant because it is not easily cleansed from the vagina and it causes latex rubber condoms to deteriorate. A water-soluble jelly can be used if there is inadequate lubrication, but one of the spermicidal jellies, creams or foams is a better choice.

The penis may be removed from the vagina while still erect to prevent spillage. However, as long as the condom is held firmly against the base of the penis during withdrawal, seepage is unlikely. A less abrupt end to coitus may increase user compliance.

If the condom breaks or tears during intercourse, a spermicide should be inserted into the vagina immediately.

Allergic contact dermatitis from condoms may occur in both men and women. The sensitizing agent may be the rubber in the condom or one of the chemicals used in the manufacture of the condom. Symptoms related to condom use in the male may range from itching and penile edema to an eczematous dermatitis that spreads to the scrotum, inguinal area and inner aspects of the thighs. In women, there may be pruritus vulvae or a burning vaginal sensation, with or without accompanying eczematous reactions. A change of brands may be sufficient to eliminate the reaction, but if the condition persists, a physician must be consulted.

A condom should be used whenever a vaginal or other genital infection is present or suspected in either partner. This measure not only helps prevent transmission of the infection to the uninfected partner, but also helps prevent reinfection.

Condoms should be stored in a cool place away from direct sunlight.

Contraceptive Sponge

A disposable contraceptive sponge has recently been introduced to the Canadian market. The sponge is composed of soft polyurethane foam saturated with 1 g of nonoxynol-9. It measures about 5 cm in diameter and 3 cm in thickness. It has a concave dimple in one side designed to fit over the cervix and a woven polyester loop on the other side to facilitate removal. The sponge exerts a contraceptive effect by providing a barrier between sperm and cervix, trapping sperm within the sponge and releasing spermicide contained within the sponge to destroy the sperm.

Although contraceptive effectiveness is less than that achieved with the diaphragm and spermicide, there are some advantages. The sponge provides continuous protection for 24 hours regardless of the frequency of coitus. There is no waiting after insertion. It is easy to use—moistened with water, squeezed gently to remove excess and inserted high in the vagina so it blocks the cervix. There is less messiness than with the diaphragm or spermicides. An important factor in its acceptability is that one size fits all, and it can be purchased in retail outlets without a prescription.

Safety

Side effects of the contraceptive sponge are allergic-type reactions and vaginal irritation. The incidence of both contraceptive failure and side effects is higher that that seen with diaphragm use. Vaginal irritation seems to be a result of excessive absorption of vaginal secretions by the sponge, resulting in vaginal dryness and irritation. The allergic-type reactions have been attributed to the spermicide. As with all vaginal barrier methods of contraception, there is concern about toxic shock syndrome with use of the contraceptive sponge. One study reports 13 confirmed cases of toxic shock syndrome related to use of the contraceptive sponge.

Consumer Counselling

Before use, the sponge should be moistened with clean water and gently squeezed until the spermicide begins to foam. With the loop on the underside, the sponge should be folded in half, and inserted high into the vagina in the same manner as the diaphragm (see Figure 4). Insertion can take place just prior to intercourse, or as long as 24 hours before. The sponge must be left in place for 6 hours after coitus, but total wearing time should not exceed 30 hours. The sponge can be worn while bathing or swimming. Sponges should not be worn

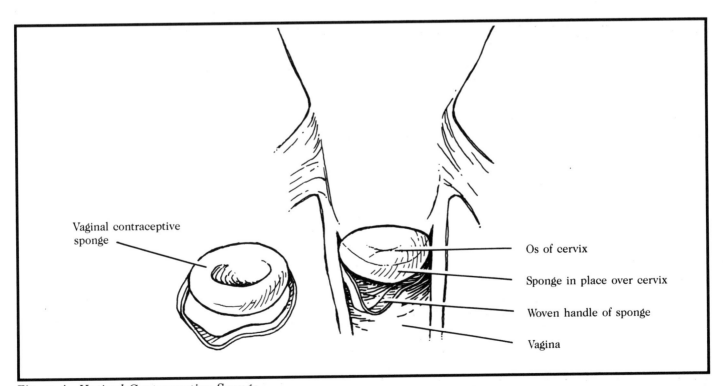

Vaginal contraceptive sponge

Os of cervix

Sponge in place over cervix

Woven handle of sponge

Vagina

Figure 4 *Vaginal Contraceptive Sponge*

while menstruating, for several weeks following pregnancy or if any signs of a vaginal infection are present. If there is an odor or the sponge is discolored upon removal, a physician should be consulted in order to rule out infection. An individual sponge should never be used more than once.

Recent Developments

A condom for women has recently been developed and is undergoing trials in the United States. It consists of two rings connected by a polyurethane sheath. One end is closed and designed to fit high in the vagina, over the cervix, while the other end is open and remains outside the vagina, covering the perineal area (see Figure 5). The device is prelubricated and designed to be discarded after use. It does not need to be fitted by a health care professional. Long-term effectiveness studies have not been completed at this time; however, preliminary studies report the female condom to be less likely to leak or to become dislodged during intercourse than the traditional condom. Theoretically, it provides greater protection from sexually transmitted diseases than traditional condoms, by preventing direct contact with the introitus of the vagina and the base of the penis, both areas which may harbor infective lesions. Vaginal irritation, itching and pain have been reported with the use of the female condom. Further studies are needed to fully assess the safety and efficacy of this barrier device. It is not currently available in Canada.

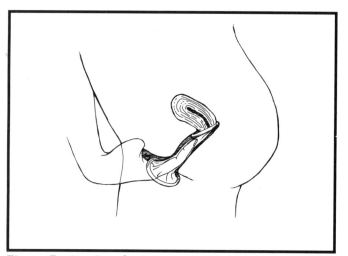

Figure 5 *Condom for Women*

Contraceptives and Sexually Transmitted Diseases

With the advent of serious STDs for which no cure or no adequate treatment exists, preventing disease transmission is extremely important. At present, no cure exists for herpes simplex virus (HSV) or human immunodeficiency virus (HIV), which causes AIDS. Treatment is often inadequate for genital wart infections and occasionally even for uncomplicated gonorrhea that has become resistant to antibiotics. Although there is an effective vaccine for hepatitis B, transmission can occur from an asymptomatic carrier during sexual intercourse.

Many STDs are asymptomatic and carriers cannot be identified readily—a serious medical problem. Abstinence is the only foolproof

preventive measure. For sexually active persons, monogamy carries no risk of acquiring an STD if neither partner is infected. People who have more than one sexual partner can gain some protection against STDs by using barrier methods of contraception.

Condoms play a major role in helping prevent STDs. They protect against the transmission of bacteria and viruses that may be present in the semen, and prevent infection from a penile shaft lesion. In addition, condoms help prevent transmission of infection from the partner to the wearer. Pelvic inflammatory disease occurs less often in women whose partners use condoms.

It has been recognized for many years that condoms help protect the users from STDs, but it is becoming increasingly evident that spermicides and the vaginal barrier devices protect the woman, at least to some extent, from STDs. In vitro studies show that spermicides deactivate many organisms responsible for STDs.

Ask the Consumer

Q. (To a person requesting a douche) Are you using a douche as a method of contraception?

■ Douching is not a contraceptive method, although many women believe it is. If contraception is desired, suggest an effective method.

Q. (To a person requesting a diaphragm) Have you recently been measured for a diaphragm?

■ A number of factors can cause a change in the size of diaphragm required for effective contraception. These factors include a change in weight of 4 kg or more, pregnancy terminated by either abortion or delivery, and pelvic surgery. If any of these events occur, the diaphragm size should be checked.

Q. Have you or your sexual partner ever had itching or irritation of the genital area after you have used this product?

■ Allergic or sensitization reactions that occur with a particular contraceptive product can be avoided by changing to a product with a different formulation. This consideration applies to condoms, diaphragms and spermicides.

Q. Did you know it is recommended condoms be used during sexual intercourse when a vaginal infection is present?

■ When dispensing a prescription for medication intended for treatment of vaginal infections, it is a good idea to suggest condoms be worn by the male partner during sexual intercourse to prevent infection of the man and reinfection of the woman.

Q. Are you using this spermicide cream with or without a diaphragm?

■ Some spermicide creams and jellies intended for use with a diaphragm may not spread as well and have less spermicide than products intended for use alone. It is necessary to determine how the product will be used to provide optimal advice.

Q. Are you using this contraceptive foam alone or with condoms?

■ An extremely high rate of contraceptive effectiveness may be obtained by using these two methods together. Encourage consumers to use this combination rather than either method alone.

Q. Do you understand this contraceptive product must be inserted a period of time before intercourse takes place and, if intercourse does not take place within a certain period of time, another application of spermicide must be inserted for optimal effect?

■ Each spermicide, to exert maximal contraceptive effect, must be allowed sufficient time to spread over vaginal and cervical surfaces. These times vary with the product formulation and must be pointed out to the user.

Q. Are you using this contraceptive method to space your children? Is there any reason why you must not become pregnant?

■ Failures may occur with nonprescription contraceptive methods. If pregnancy is inadvisable—for medical or other reasons—such methods should not be used. Nonprescription methods are probably most useful to individuals wanting to space their children. The use of foam and condoms for a few months after discontinuing oral contraceptives and before pregnancy is a good suggestion.

References

Introduction
Balakrishnan TR, Krotki K, Lapierre-Adamcyk E. Contraceptive use in Canada 1984. Fam Plan Perspect 1985;17(5):209–15.

Edelman DA. Nonprescription vaginal contraception. Int J Gynaecol Obstet 1980;18:340–4.

Grindstaff CF. The pharmacist and family planning: new roles and responsibilities. West Hanover: Chris Mass, 1980.

Hatcher RA, Guest F, Stewart F, et al. Contraceptive technology 1986–87. New York: Irvington Publishers Inc, 1986.

Hatcher RA, Stewart GK, Stewart F, et al. Contraceptive technology 1978–1979. New York: Irvington, 1978.

Sherris JD. Update on condoms—products, protection, production. Popul Rep (H) 1982;10(6):121–56.

Tatum HJ, Connell-Tatum EB. Barrier contraception: a comprehensive overview. Fertil Steril 1981;36(1):1–12.

The Boston Women's Health Book Collective. Our bodies, ourselves. New York: Simon and Schuster, 1976.

Zatuchni GI, Aquiles JS, Speidel JJ, et al, eds. Vaginal contraception: new developments. Hagerstown: Harper-Row, 1979.

Natural Family Planning
Billings E, Westmore A. The Billings method—controlled fertility without drugs or devices. London: Penguin, 1981.

Parenteau-Carreau S. Love and life, fertility and conception prevention. Serena Canada, 1982.

Zatuchni GI, Daly MJ, Sciarra JJ, eds. Gynecology and obstetrics. Philadelphia: Harper-Row, 1983.

Barrier Methods
Jackson M, Berger G, Keith LG. Vaginal contraception. Boston: GK Hall, 1981.
Robins J. Failures of contraceptive practice. NY State J Med 1976;76:361–5.

Spermicides
Abrutyn D, McKenzie BE, Nadaskay N. Teratology study of intravaginally administered nonoxynol-9-containing contraceptive creams in rats. Fertil Steril 1982;37(1):113–7.

Belsky R. Vaginal contraceptives—a time for reappraisal? Popul Rep (H) 1975;3:37–55.

Coleman S, Piotrow PT. Spermicides—simplicity and safety are major assets. Popul Rep (H) 1979;7(5):100.

Fed Reg 1980;45:82014–49.

Fisher AA. Condom dermatitis in either partner. Cutis 1987;39(4):281,284–5.

Hatcher RA, Guest F, Stewart F, et al. Contraceptive technology 1984–1985. New York: Irvington, 1984.

Hendershot GE. Coitus-related cervical cancer risk factors: trends and differentials in racial and religious groups. Am J Public Health 1983; 73(3):299–301.

Jick H, Walker AM, Rothman KJ. Vaginal spermicides and congenital disorders. JAMA 1981;245(13):1329–32.

Schlesinger B, ed. Family planning in Canada: a source book. Toronto: University of Toronto Press, 1977:136.

Shapiro S, Slone D, Heinonon OP. Birth defects and vaginal spermicides. JAMA 1982;247(17):2381–4.

Diaphragms
DeYoung P, Martyn J, Wass H, et al. Toxic shock syndrome associated with a contraceptive diaphragm. Can Med Assoc J 1982;127:611–2.

Finn SD, Latham RH, Roberts P, et al. Association between diaphragm use and urinary tract infection. JAMA 1985;254:240–5.

Hyde L. Toxic shock syndrome associated with diaphragm use. J Fam Pract 1983;16(3):616–20.

Lane ME, Arceo R, Sobrero AJ. Successful use of the diaphragm and jelly by a young population: report of a clinical study. Fam Plan Perspect 1976; 8(2):81–6.

Leitch WS. Longevity of Ortho Cream(R) and Gynol(R) in the contraceptive diaphragm. Contraception 1986;34(4):381–93.

Loomis L, Feder HM Jr. Toxic shock syndrome associated with diaphragm use (Letter). N Engl J Med 1981;305:1585–6.

Sobrero AJ. Vaginal diaphragms. Medical aspects of human sexuality. Toronto: Jay Kay, 1973:23–7.

Strom BL, Collins M, West SL, et al. Sexual activity, contraceptive use, and other risk factors for symptomatic and asymptomatic bacteriuria. Ann Int Med 1987;107:816–23.

Tofte RW, Williams DN. Toxic shock syndrome: clinical and laboratory features in 15 patients. Ann Intern Med 1981;94:149–56.

Wortman J. The diaphragm and other intravaginal barriers—a review. Popul Rep (H) 1976;(4):57–75.

Cervical Cap
Anonymous. The cervical cap. Med Lett Drugs Ther 1988;30:93–4.

Cagen R. The cervical cap as a barrier contraceptive. Contraception 1986; 33(5):487–96.

Weiss BD, Bassford T, Davis T. The cervical cap. Am Fam Physician 1991; 43:517–23.

Condoms
Arnold CB. Proper use of the condom. Medical aspects of human sexuality. New York: Jay Kay, 1975:147–8.

Dalsimer IA, Piotrow PT, Dumm JJ. Condom—an old method meets a new social need. Popul Rep (H) 1974;1:1–19.

Fisher AA. Allergic reactions to contraceptives and douches. Medical aspects of human sexuality. New York: Jay Kay, 1975:110–25.

Free MJ, Skiens EW, Morrow MM. Relationship between condom strength and failure during use. Contraception 1980;22(1):31–7.

Harvey PD. Condoms—a new look. Medical aspects of human sexuality. Toronto: Jay Kay, 1973:70–89.

Contraceptive Sponge
Anonymous. A vaginal contraceptive sponge. Med Lett Drugs Ther 1983; 25:78–80.

Birth control device equal of diaphragm. The Vancouver Province. 1983 Apr 10:B5(col 1).

Falch G, Pearson K, Fleming D, et al. Toxic shock syndrome and the vaginal contraceptive sponge. JAMA 1986;255(2):216–8.

Contraceptives

Kafka D, Gold RB. Food and drug approves vaginal sponge. Fam Plan Perspect 1983;15(3):146–8.

Mills A. Barrier contraception. Clin Obstet Gynecol 1984;11(3):641–78.

Sherris JD, Moore SH, Fox G. New developments in vaginal contraception. Popul Rep (H) 1984;7(1):157–90.

Smith M, Barwin BN. Vaginal mechanical contraceptive devices. Can Med Assoc J 1983;129:699–701,710.

Recent Developments

Leeper MA, Conrardy M. Preliminary evaluation of "Reality", a condom for women. Advances in contraception 1989;5:229–35.

Contraceptives and Sexually Transmitted Diseases

Stone KM, Grimes DA, Magder LS. Primary prevention of sexually transmitted diseases. JAMA 1986;255(13):1763–6.

20
Feminine Care Products

Laura-Lynn Pollock

*An understanding of the physiology of the female repro-
ductive system is necessary for appropriate counselling on
genital hygiene and the choice of feminine care products
such as menstrual pads and tampons. Toxic shock syndrome is a rare but serious problem linked to menstruation and the use of menstrual products. Other menstrual
problems are amenorrhea, dysmenorrhea and premenstrual syndrome. Some nonpharmacologic measures
relieve these problems. Pharmaceutical agents used
include analgesics, nonsteroidal anti-inflammatory drugs,
antihistamines and diuretics. Vaginitis must be correctly
diagnosed and treated with medications specific to each
diagnosis.*

Products promoted for menstrual hygiene and other feminine care
abound on the market. Some are necessary and useful, but others
are more controversial, perhaps even questionable in value.

Pharmacists should understand the conditions that lead a woman
to seek a nonprescription product. They must also be able to counsel
her on the safe use of the product, recommend further medical
follow-up if required, and dispel any myths or misunderstandings that
she may have.

Reproductive Anatomy and Physiology

The visible external genitalia, or the vulva, includes the area of
the mons pubis, the labia minora and majora, and the perineum.
Protected within this region are the clitoris and the vaginal and urethral openings. Situated posterior to the perineum is the anus (see
Figure 1).

The vagina is a tube-like structure at an angle of 45° to the vulva
and extending upward to the uterus. Transverse folds in the vaginal
wall provide the flexibility of shape and size required for intercourse
and childbirth.

Epithelial cells line the vagina. During child-bearing years,
increased estrogen levels cause proliferation of the basal cells in the
epithelium. The glycogen stored by these cells is broken down to
lactic acid by vaginal lactobacilli or Doderlein's bacilli. This action
renders the vaginal environment acidic with a pH of 3.5 to 5.5.

Vaginal Discharge

The vagina has no sweat or sebaceous glands. The normal vaginal
discharge is comprised of components from a variety of other
sources—cervical glands, uterus, fallopian tubes and a transudate
from the capillaries in the vaginal walls.

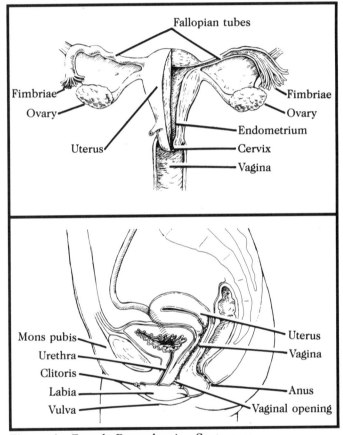

Figure 1   *Female Reproductive System*

This discharge routinely cleanses the vagina and maintains the pH
and bacterial environment essential for normal health. Both the
amount and character of the secretions vary in response to corresponding cyclical fluctuations in estrogen and progesterone levels.
Sometimes the discharge is pasty, whitish in color and scanty. Other
times it is more copious and the consistency of uncooked egg white
(for example, at ovulation). No discharge is apparent on some days.

Vaginal Odor

Vaginal discharge combines with secretions from vulvar, perineal and
urethral glands to produce an odor. The odor is normal and healthy
and should not be unpleasant. A foul or unusual odor may indicate

Feminine Care Products

poor hygiene or the presence of infection. A discolored or purulent discharge may accompany the unpleasant odor in the case of an infection.

Menstrual Cycle

When a female reaches puberty her body undergoes a complex physiological process each month. During this process an ovum is released and the endometrial lining is stimulated to prepare for its implantation. If fertilization and implantation do not occur, the superficial layers of the endometrium are sloughed off and menstrual bleeding occurs.

The age of menarche, when menstruation begins, is commonly around 12 years. On average, menopause occurs at 50 years of age, but menstruation may well continue beyond that age. The average woman experiences about 450 menstrual cycles during her lifetime.

Hormones secreted by the hypothalamus, pituitary gland and ovary are responsible for the ovarian and endometrial changes that occur during the cycle. Figure 2 shows the complex relationship between the various levels of control.

At the time of menses the levels of estrogen and progesterone are at their lowest. The hypothalamus is thus triggered to release a gonadotropin releasing hormone or luteinizing hormone releasing hormone (LHRH).

LHRH stimulates the anterior pituitary to release follicle stimulating hormone (FSH) and luteinizing hormone (LH). These hormones are responsible initially for preparing and developing a primary ovarian follicle.

The developing follicle produces increasing amounts of estrogen, which exerts a negative feedback effect on FSH production. Declining FSH levels inhibit development of additional follicles.

Estrogen levels continue to rise until sufficient to trigger a surge of LH from the anterior pituitary. Ovulation occurs about 30 hours later. The ruptured ovarian follicle then becomes the corpus luteum—a body capable of both estrogen and progesterone production.

During the latter half or luteal phase of the cycle, progesterone and estrogen levels rise until they reach their peak about 18 to 22 days into the 28-day cycle.

If fertilization of the ovum does not occur during the final days of the cycle, the corpus luteum degenerates and estrogen and progesterone levels fall rapidly. Menses occurs and the hormonal cycle begins again.

Although the menstrual cycle is usually discussed in the context of 28 days, there is much individual variability. The normal range can be anywhere from 20 to 40 days, often with minor variations occurring from 1 month to another.

Variations most commonly occur during the preovulatory part of the cycle. The postovulatory phase is usually consistent, lasting 14 days. As an example, in a cycle shorter than 28 days, ovulation occurs before the midpoint of the cycle, sometimes as early as day 7. The converse is true when menstruation occurs at intervals greater than 4 weeks.

The average length of menses is 5 days with the range from 2 to 8 days. During any one menstrual period the characteristics of flow may vary. Sometimes it can be relatively heavy with a red, clotted appearance; at other times the flow may be scanty, with a brownish tinge.

Blood, cervical and uterine secretions, endometrial tissue, mucus and vaginal components make up the material discharged during menstruation. On average, 30 to 50 mL of blood is lost with each menstrual period, although this amount is variable. About 1 per cent of women may lose more than 200 mL.

Genital Hygiene

The perineal region can be adequately cleansed by washing regularly with water and mild soap, including during menstruation.

The vagina is self-cleaning and generally does not require the use of irrigation solutions such as douching products to remain healthy.

Vaginal Douches

Vaginal douching is a process of instilling fluid into the vagina to flush the cavity and remove any discharge or other vaginal contents. It is also used to alter vaginal pH and occasionally to treat infections.

Much controversy surrounds the routine use of douches to cleanse the vagina. Some reports claim douching provides no benefit and may disrupt the vaginal flora or increase the occurrence of irritation. Others claim routine douching causes no harm.

There is some concern that douching may also increase the risk of developing ascending infections of the genital tract, for example, salpingitis. It is difficult to determine if douching is the culprit or if the lifestyles of a large portion of the women who often use douches predispose them to an increased risk of sexually transmitted diseases and their complications.

Overall, occasional douching (2 or 3 times per month, or less) is not harmful if appropriate solutions are used correctly and a vaginal infection is not present. However, douching is not necessary to maintain good personal hygiene.

Douching Technique

Two basic types of douching syringes are the fountain syringe and the bulb syringe. Disposable douching equipment is usually similar to a bulb syringe.

The fountain syringe consists of a rubber bag, tubing and a rounded tip with holes for insertion into the vagina. The bag is filled with douching solution and held about 60 cm above the hips. The force of gravity draws the solution gently into the vagina.

Bulb syringes do not require tubing. The bulb is filled with solution and fitted with a vaginal tip. Squeezing the bulb causes fluid to enter the vagina. Some devices do not require manual pressure on the bulb. The fluid is forced out by the inward pressure exerted by the distended walls of the full bulb. In either case it is important to use only gentle pressure. Excessive force may cause a reflux of the solution and possibly bacteria into the uterus or peritoneal cavity.

The most comfortable position for douching is lying on the back in the bathtub with knees bent. The douche tip is inserted into the vagina with gentle downward pressure as far as it will comfortably go. Fluid is instilled into the vagina either by releasing the valve on the tubing or by gently squeezing the bulb. A feeling of fullness in the abdomen indicates sufficient fluid has been instilled.

To ensure the fluid remains in the vagina long enough to come in contact with all folds of the mucosa, the labia should be held together with one hand. After about 1 minute they can be released and the fluid expelled.

Feminine Care Products

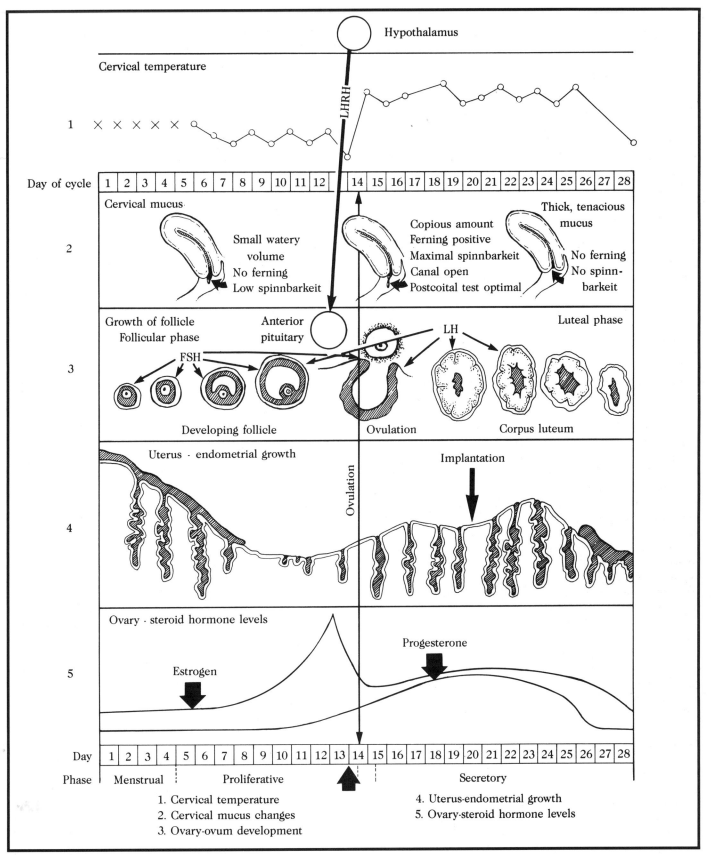

Figure 2 *The Menstrual Cycle*

Feminine Care Products

Consumer Counselling

Several points should be emphasized to ensure proper and safe use of douching products:

- Thoroughly clean reusable douching devices with hot water and soap after each use.
- Do not use douches during pregnancy unless otherwise advised by a physician.
- Douches are not an effective form of contraception.
- If a vaginal spermicide is used for contraception, do not douche for at least 6 hours after intercourse.
- Vulvovaginal irritation may indicate an infection. Although douching may relieve the symptoms, the proper antimicrobial must be used to eradicate the organism.
- Examination by a physician is essential if an infection is suspected.
- Do not douche for at least 24 hours before examination for a suspected vaginal infection, as douching may make the diagnosis difficult and delay treatment.

Pharmacologic Agents

The simplest and perhaps safest douching liquid is warm water. There is no risk of irritation or allergic reactions as with some of the commercial douches.

Vinegar and water provide a mildly acidic solution that may be used for general hygiene or to relieve vaginal irritation. To prepare, mix 15 to 30 mL of vinegar with 1 L of warm water.

Alkaline solutions have also been used and are prepared by mixing 15 to 30 mL of sodium bicarbonate with 1 L of warm water.

Controversy exists regarding the relative efficacy of acidic and alkaline douches. Although both decrease vulvovaginal irritation, some reports claim the alkaline preparation promotes bacterial growth whereas the acidic one does not. This possibility might be considered if a vaginal infection is suspected.

Commercially prepared products contain a variety of ingredients. They are more expensive than home remedies and for hygiene purposes are not superior (see Table I).

When recommending a commercial product, it is important to instruct the consumer on the proper use. Many products come in liquid concentrate or powder, both of which require proper dilution to avoid irritation and toxicities.

Ready-to-use douches with disposable syringes are convenient and eliminate the risk of reinfection from poorly cleaned equipment.

Several commercial products now contain vinegar and water with a minimum number of other ingredients. If a woman does not wish to prepare her own solution at home, a commercial vinegar and water product is an acceptable alternative.

Towelettes and wipes are also available for feminine hygiene. These products are moistened with various astringents, emollients, surfactants, counterirritants, antimicrobials and perfumes. They are convenient to use, but have no proven benefit over regular cleansing with water and mild soap. Irritation and sensitivity reactions are possible due to the ingredients of some products.

Feminine Deodorant Sprays

Aerosol sprays promoted for controlling genital odor are the most questionable of all feminine care products. Normal genital odor does not require the use of such products. Regular gentle washing of the perineal area with soap and water is sufficient.

Infection, poor hygiene or a forgotten vaginal tampon may be responsible for unpleasant odor. These causes must be ruled out

Table I *Ingredients of Vaginal Douching, Cleansing and Deodorant Products*

Class	Compound	Comments
Antimicrobials	Boric acid	Weak bacteriostatic agent; 5% solution may be effective against *Candida albicans;* caution regarding potential toxicities
	Povidone-iodine	Active against candidal and trichomonal infections; use on advice of physician if for infection; may stain clothing—use tampons or pads
	Phenol, thymol, sodium perborate, cetylpyridium chloride	Antiseptic; mild bactericide; fungicide
Astringents	Aluminum, alum, zinc sulfate	May decrease local edema and discharge; irritation may occur—dilute solutions correctly
Counter-irritants	Eucalyptol, methyl salicylate, menthol, phenol, thymol	Anti-inflammatory; antipruritic; mild anesthetic soothing properties; menthol has caused contact dermatitis
Preservatives	Benzalkonium chloride, sorbic acid, paraben	Mild antimicrobial activity at usual concentrations; irritation may occur
Buffers	Sodium citrate, citric acid, boric acid, sodium perborate	pH adjustment to decrease irritation of product
Proteolytics	Papain	Hydrolyses protein component of vaginal discharge; questionable value; allergic reactions are possible
Surfactants	Docusate sodium, nonoxynol–9, sodium lauryl sulfate	Assist in cleansing
pH altering agents	Acetic acid	15 mL in 1 L water decreases microbial growth; may decrease irritation and pruritus
	Sodium bicarbonate	15 mL in 1 L water; antipruritic; may enhance microbial growth

before a woman begins to use genital deodorants. Masking an odor may delay the seeking of necessary medical treatment.

Feminine deodorant sprays contain antimicrobials, emollients, perfumes and propellants. The perfume is probably the major active ingredient in the product.

There is a significant incidence of local, allergic reactions to these products. The use of the product should be discontinued immediately if such a reaction occurs. Corticosteroid therapy may also be indicated for treatment of the reaction.

Feminine Care Products

Potential risks also exist to the respiratory tract if aerosol particles are inhaled. Consumers should be warned to avoid inhaling the product upon application.

In light of the questionable need for genital deodorant sprays and the potential adverse reactions related to their use, it is important that a woman requesting such a product be aware of the limitations to its use and the proper method of application.

Consumer Counselling

Genital deodorant sprays are for external use only. They are not to be applied intravaginally. The spray should not be applied just before sexual intercourse, as it may irritate the vagina or penis. For application, the spray canister is held at least 20 cm from the body. Irritation may occur if the product is applied in excessive amounts or from the chilling effect of the propellant. If irritation or redness occurs, use of the product should be discontinued immediately. If the condition does not improve, the consumer should consult a physician. Deodorant sprays should not be used when wearing a menstrual pad. Pads may increase the contact time of the spray on the body and thus increase the risk of irritation. Tampons should not be inserted immediately after using the spray. The spray should not be applied to broken skin or if lesions are present, such as in the case of herpes.

Local Anesthetic and Antipruritic Creams

Creams with topical anesthetic and/or antipruritic properties are marketed for the treatment of genital irritation. Common ingredients are benzocaine, tripelennamine hydrochloride and resorcinol.

Creams are not recommended for several reasons. When used, they may mask signs of an infection or other condition (for example, sensitivity reaction) and delay treatment. Topical antihistamines are of questionable value both as local anesthetics and in treating allergic conditions. Both topical anesthetics and topical antihistamines can cause local hypersensitivity reactions.

Talcum Powder

Scented and unscented talcum powders are sometimes applied to the perineum for aesthetic purposes. Women using such products should be warned that particles of talc may cause vaginal irritation and infection.

Menstrual Care
Pads and Tampons

Pads are worn against the perineum to absorb menstrual and other vaginal discharge. Disposable pads are made from absorbent cotton, rayon or cellulose while washable, reusable cotton fabric pads are also available. Older style pads were held in place by a light elastic belt. Newer brands are secured to undergarments by adhesive strips, or, in the case of reusable pads, with pins or velcro strips.

Maxi or superabsorbent pads are used during periods of heavier menstrual flow; mini pads and pantyliners are used during times of light flow or between periods to absorb vaginal discharge.

Tampons are wads of cotton, rayon or cellulose worn intravaginally. They absorb menstrual flow and, in the case of superabsorbent products, can also expand and block the vaginal canal. This blockage helps stop unwanted leakage.

Tampons are inserted either by a plunger-style applicator or by pushing the tampon into the vagina with a finger or applicator stick.

The brand of tampon determines the method. Consumers should be aware of the choices of application methods so a suitable product is selected.

The decision to use pads or tampons is a personal choice. Many women prefer tampons because they are more discreet, less bulky, easier to carry in a purse and there is less odor associated with their use.

Although tampons have been worn without any problems by millions of women, there is evidence to link tampon use with three important consequences: vaginal or cervical ulcers, vaginal mucosal changes and toxic shock syndrome.

Drying, layering and microulceration of the vaginal mucosa can occur with a variety of tampon brands. These changes are most prominent with superabsorbent products, but all strengths are implicated. In the early stages these reactions can go undetected as they cause no obvious symptoms. Repetitive use of superabsorbent tampons, especially during periods of light flow, may increase the risk of these transient effects progressing to clinical ulceration.

Both pads and tampons come in scented and unscented versions. Scented or deodorant products are not required, as odor is not a problem if tampons and pads are changed regularly and genitals cleansed normally. As with most scented products, the risk of allergic reaction exists.

Toxic Shock Syndrome

Toxic shock syndrome (TSS) was first described in 1978. It is an acute illness caused by a toxin-producing *Staphylococcus aureus*. Those at risk for TSS include menstruating women using tampons, postpartum women and anyone (male or female) with surgical wound infections or staphylococcal infections.

Symptoms

Affected individuals experience a complex of symptoms that, in combination, are diagnostic of TSS: a sudden high fever (38.8 °C or greater); a diffuse sunburn-like rash and erythema on the palms of the hands and the soles of feet; desquamation of the skin on the palms and soles within 2 weeks of initial symptoms; and low blood pressure (a systolic of less than 90 mm Hg) leading to severe hypotension and shock. In addition, people with TSS present with three or more of the following: nausea, vomiting or diarrhea at the onset of illness; sore throat, or redness of the conjunctiva of the eye; severe myalgias; oliguria and renal impairment with elevated blood urea nitrogen levels; elevated hepatic enzymes and bilirubin indicating hepatic failure; low platelet counts, abnormal bruising and bleeding; confusion, disorientation and loss of consciousness; and cardiac arrhythmias, severe hypotension and shock.

Treatment

A menstruating woman who has any symptoms of TSS should seek medical attention immediately. If she has a vaginal tampon in place it should be removed. TSS is rare, but can be fatal if not recognized early and treated correctly.

Treatment is aimed at reversing the severe hypotension and maintaining circulation and cardiac and renal function. Large volumes of intravenous fluids may be required as well as other supportive care. Antistaphylococcal antibiotics such as beta-lactamase-resistant penicillins, cephalosporins and vancomycin have been used in attempts to eradicate the toxin-producing *Staphylococcus aureus* bacteria implicated in the disease. The beta-lactamase-resistant penicillins seem to decrease the recurrence rate.

Tampons and TSS

Staphylococcus aureus is a common pathogen found on vulvar tissue. The organism may be introduced into the vagina during insertion of the tampon. The vaginal environment and the menstrual exudate provide excellent conditions for bacterial proliferation.

If a toxin is produced it can be absorbed into systemic circulation in a number of ways. It may gain entry through the vaginal wall that has been damaged by the use of the tampon. The microulcerations and other mucosal alterations caused by tampons impair the integrity of the mucosa and decrease its barrier properties.

In the late 1970s, much TSS attention centred around the use of the Rely brand of tampon. This brand has been removed from the market by the manufacturer, but subsequent studies have implicated no one brand more often than any other. Superabsorbent products are considered to present greater risk than regular products.

Current recommendations regarding tampon use and TSS include the following:

- Women who have had TSS should avoid the use of tampons for at least 6 months following the infection.
- Women who have undergone vaginal surgery, childbirth or any other procedure that may have damaged the vaginal epithelium should not use tampons until healing is complete (6 to 8 weeks).
- Women who have no problems with tampon use can continue to use them in their regular fashion. (The risk of TSS is low.)
- Tampons should be changed regularly (about 4 to 6 times daily).
- Avoid use of superabsorbent tampons during days when flow is light. (This may decrease the adverse effects of the tampon on the vaginal tissue.)
- Alternate between pad and tampon use during the menstrual period (for example, use tampons during the day and pads at night).
- Any menstruating woman who develops a high fever, nausea, vomiting, diarrhea, a sunburn-like rash and lightheadedness on rising should immediately remove the tampon and seek medical attention.

Menstrual Problems

Amenorrhea

Amenorrhea is the lack of menstruation. Primary causes are dysfunction of the ovary or pituitary gland or a genetic abnormality. Failure to menstruate at puberty is often the first indication of the problem.

Secondary amenorrhea can be due to a number of factors. Pregnancy, lactation and menopause are normal physiological causes. Other causes can include physical or emotional stress, discontinuation of oral contraceptives, sudden dramatic weight loss or obesity, and thyroid or adrenal dysfunction.

Unexplained failure to menstruate should be assessed by a physician. This evaluation should be based on age, duration of amenorrhea and contributing factors.

Dysmenorrhea

Discomfort or pain while menstruating is called dysmenorrhea. Mild to severe discomfort just before or on the first day of menstruation is common. This cramping and abdominal discomfort usually lasts for 1 to 2 days. Normally it does not interfere with physical or mental

activities. About 10 per cent of women have severe cramping and pain accompanied by nausea, vomiting, headache, backache and diarrhea.

Primary dysmenorrhea is not associated with any underlying medical problem. Secondary dysmenorrhea can be due to such things as intrauterine devices, pelvic inflammatory disease, endometriosis and fibroids.

The exact etiology of primary dysmenorrhea is uncertain. It appears to be associated with increased levels of prostaglandins, which are produced by the endometrium. Prostaglandins and prostaglandin metabolites have been found in above normal levels in menstrual, endometrial and serum samples from women with dysmenorrhea.

High levels of prostaglandins F_{2a} (dinoprost) and E_2 (dinoprostone) may be partly responsible for the increased uterine activity observed with dysmenorrhea. Prostaglandin F_{2a} causes uterine contractions that, if intense, can create pain due to myometrial ischemia. Prostaglandins may also cause the release of intracellular substances, which in turn can contribute to dysmenorrhea. Bradykinins and histamine can promote pain. Heparin, histamine and serotonin may reduce hemostasis and cause longer and heavier periods.

Primary dysmenorrhea occurs only during ovulatory cycles. Estrogen, luteal phase levels of progesterone, and the state of the endometrium all contribute to the ultimate synthesis of prostaglandins.

Treatment

Secondary causes must be ruled out before treating primary dysmenorrhea. Numerous supportive and pharmacologic approaches can control dysmenorrhea. Heating pads, hot water bottles and hot baths may help reduce discomfort. Relaxation activities or exercise have also been useful for some people.

Unless symptoms are unusually severe, nonprescription therapy is the first step in pharmacologic treatment. If nonprescription treatments are not effective, prescription medications are indicated. Most women will respond to nonsteroidal anti-inflammatory agents or oral contraceptives.

Pharmacologic Agents

Ibuprofen, acetaminophen and acetylsalicylic acid (ASA) are the common nonprescription choices.

Ibuprofen is a nonsteroidal anti-inflammatory drug (NSAID) that has been shown to be effective in treating the discomfort of dysmenorrhea. It affects prostaglandin synthesis as well as has analgesic action. Studies show that up to 80 per cent of women with primary dysmenorrhea record improvement with the use of a NSAID, such as ibuprofen, making it a good nonprescription choice for symptomatic treatment of the condition.

Other NSAIDs such as naproxen and mefenamic acid would also be good choices, however, a prescription is required for their use. Due to the wide range of individual variation in response to any one NSAID it would be reasonable to try a prescription NSAID if ibuprofen or other nonprescription analgesics were not successful in controlling the pain.

Depending on the severity of the dysmenorrhea a dose of 200 to 400 mg every 4 to 6 hours could be tried.

Patients should be screened prior to recommending ibuprofen as there are side effects and precautions to consider with its use.

Gastrointestinal problems will necessitate discontinuation of the drug in up to 15 per cent of patients. The majority of this will be due to epigastric pain, abdominal discomfort, nausea and vomiting, abdominal bloating and gas. Rarely, gastrointestinal ulceration and hemorrhage can occur. Caution should be used when recommending ibuprofen for a patient taking an oral anticoagulant such as warfarin. Although ibuprofen appears to have little effect on the hypoprothrombinemic reaction to warfarin, there is a theoretical increased risk of gastric ulcer bleeding when the two drugs are used in combination.

Other adverse effects that can occur are a skin rash, dizziness, headache, fluid retention or visual disturbances.

Ibuprofen should be used with caution in a patient with peptic ulcer disease, a history of gastrointestinal ulceration or with heart failure. It is contraindicated in patients with a known hypersensitivity to ASA or other NSAID or in whom those drugs precipitate asthma-like symptoms, urticaria or rhinitis. Ibuprofen may also increase serum lithium concentrations and thus increase the risk of lithium toxicity for some patients.

ASA is a weak inhibitor of prostaglandin synthesis. Doses of 650 mg every 4 hours relieve dysmenorrhea in up to 30 per cent of individuals. These results have been contradicted by some, but the fact remains that many women with mild to moderate menstrual discomfort use ASA products for relief. Doses of 325 to 1,000 mg every 4 to 6 hours, not exceeding 4 g daily, can be used.

Before an ASA product is recommended to a consumer, potential adverse effects must be assessed. The following individuals should avoid ASA or use it with caution: those who have a history of peptic ulcer disease or gastrointestinal bleeding; people with clotting disorders, vitamin K deficiency or hypoprothrombinemia; people on anticoagulant therapy; people who have asthma or urticarial reactions (they may be more likely to exhibit acute hypersensitivity reactions to ASA); people who have exhibited hypersensitivity reactions to non-steroidal anti-inflammatory agents (there is potential for cross-reactivity with ASA, particularly if the original reaction included asthma-like symptoms); insulin-independent diabetics and those taking an oral hypoglycemic (for example, tolbutamide or chlorpropamide); chronic alcohol abusers (alcohol enhances the ability of ASA to cause gastrointestinal bleeding and irritation); and people taking other potentially ulcerogenic drugs (for example, prednisone and nonsteroidal anti-inflammatory agents).

Intoxication can occur with acute and chronic ingestion. Tinnitus, headache, dizziness, visual changes, confusion, thirst, hyperventilation and gastrointestinal upset are common symptoms. ASA should be discontinued if toxicity is suspected, and a physician should be consulted.

ASA may induce a heavier menstrual flow in some women. If a heavier flow is noticed and is bothersome, ASA use should be discontinued and an alternative product, such as ibuprofen or acetaminophen, substituted.

A variety of ASA products are on the market. The regular, single-entity tablets are the products of choice. Enteric-coated tablets may take longer to reach peak blood levels. This delay decreases their effectiveness during short term, acute use, such as is needed for dysmenorrhea.

Acetaminophen is widely used for dysmenorrhea both alone and in products marketed for this condition. Analgesic doses of 325 to 1,000 mg can be used every 4 to 6 hours, not exceeding 4 g daily.

Acetaminophen is less irritating to the gastrointestinal tract than ibuprofen or ASA, which makes acetaminophen better tolerated by some people. It has not been shown as effective against dysmenorrhea as ibuprofen, however. Significant drug interactions are rare, and hemostasis is not affected. Hypersensitivity reactions have been reported, but cross-reactivity with ibuprofen or ASA is low.

Acute or chronic toxicity is possible. Nausea, vomiting and abdominal pain are usually seen 2 to 3 hours after acute ingestion of a toxic dose (150 mg/kg). Hepatic necrosis may occur, particularly if the overdose is not treated within 16 hours of ingestion. If an overdose of acetaminophen is suspected, the consumer must be referred immediately to an emergency medical facility.

Nonprescription products are available containing ASA or acetaminophen in combination with mild diuretics, antihistamines or both. These products are promoted for use against menstrual discomfort and symptoms of premenstrual syndrome. Diuretics and antihistamines are not recommended for primary dysmenorrhea.

Single-entity products of ibuprofen, ASA or acetaminophen are the logical nonprescription treatments for menstrual cramping and abdominal discomfort. Ibuprofen has been shown to be very effective for symptomatic relief from dysmenorrhea while ASA and acetaminophen are less so. For mild symptoms, however, any of the three drugs could be tried.

Treatment should begin at the first sign of menstrual discomfort and continue until dysmenorrhea stops. As discomfort usually begins at the onset of menses, medication is taken for the first 1 to 3 days of the menstrual period.

A woman who has tried nonprescription options for several cycles and is not getting adequate relief should be referred to a physician for assessment and prescription therapy.

Premenstrual Syndrome

Premenstrual syndrome (PMS) is a complex disorder consisting of the cyclical occurrence of various physical, psychological and behavioral symptoms (see Table II).

Table II *Symptoms of Premenstrual Syndrome*

Psychological	Physical
anxiety, irritability	abdominal bloating
depression, crying	edema
mood swings	weight gain
increased appetite	changes in bowel movements
cravings, binge eating	breast discomfort
lethargy, fatigue	headache, backache
forgetfulness	hot flashes
confusion, clumsiness	acne
sleep disturbances	rhinitis
aggression	palpitations
phobias	

Up to 90 per cent of women experience at least one of the symptoms; with true PMS occurring in about 40 per cent of women. Less than 10 per cent would suffer from a severe form of the syndrome. PMS is distinguished from dysmenorrhea by the difference in symptoms as well as the timing of symptoms in relation to menses. Dysmenorrhea occurs as menstruation begins. PMS symptoms begin at the time of or following ovulation, peak in the days before menses and subside once menstruation has begun. There is a small subset of women whose symptoms will last through menses.

Women in their thirties and forties have a higher incidence and severity of PMS than do younger women. Symptoms may increase after childbirth and after tubal ligation. Dysmenorrhea commonly occurs in younger women and tends to decrease with age and childbirth.

There has been much speculation about the etiology of PMS. Progesterone deficiency has been blamed, because symptoms increase about the time that luteal phase progesterone levels decrease. Estrogen levels may play a role. Other theories implicate fluid retention due to an underlying endocrinological imbalance. Vitamin B_6 and vitamin A deficiencies and changes in glucose tolerance have been suggested. Prostaglandins may play a part in PMS.

Endorphins have been implicated, as well. This theory states that high estrogen and progesterone levels in the luteal phase increase endorphin activity, thus causing fatigue and depression. The sudden drop in endorphins just before menses, paralleling a drop in estrogen and progesterone, may precipitate irritability, anxiety, tension and hostility—symptoms common to acute narcotic withdrawal and also to PMS.

Treatment

It is unlikely PMS has only one cause; until the puzzle is unravelled further, treatments will remain numerous and varied. Each woman should be treated according to her specific needs and symptoms.

Once other medical conditions have been ruled out and a PMS diagnosis made, the first step is to reassure the person that the symptoms are PMS-related and that other women experience similar problems.

General measures can be tried to help eliminate external factors contributing to PMS:

- Decrease salt in the diet when edema and bloating occur to help limit fluid retention.
- Exercise regularly to increase endorphin production.
- Limit intake of sweets and other carbohydrate sources during the period of PMS. Acute increases in carbohydrate intake can cause rapid weight gain in some women. There has also been some evidence to link intake of sweets and high sugar containing food with PMS.
- Reduce stress factors and practice stress management techniques.
- Eliminate intake of stimulants and depressants such as caffeine and alcohol.

Mild analgesics such as ASA, acetaminophen and ibuprofen may relieve minor discomfort and headaches. Prescription and nonprescription diuretics are often used even though they have limited benefit. Contradictory evidence surrounds the efficacy of nonsteroidal anti-inflammatory agents. They may be useful for some women. Nutritional supplements of vitamin B_6, linoleic acid as oil of evening primrose, and high dose multiple vitamin therapy are also used. Progesterone vaginal/rectal suppositories, rectal suspension, and injection have gained widespread popularity. Evidence conflicts on the efficacy of progesterone, but many women claim to find it effective. Bromocriptine can decrease breast tenderness at doses of 2.5 mg twice daily. Other hormone preparations such as oral contraceptives and gonadotropin releasing hormone have limited and unpredictable value. Lithium carbonate, tricyclic antidepressants and benzodiazepines are indicated in cases of severe mood alteration or in individuals suffering from severe anxiety, tension and irritability.

Pharmacologic Agents

The analgesics ASA, acetaminophen and ibuprofen are commonly used to relieve mild pain and headache associated with PMS. They are found as single-entity products. ASA and acetaminophen are also found in combination with mild diuretics and antihistamines. It is best to recommend single-entity products specific for relief of identified symptoms whenever possible.

Doses of 325 to 1,000 mg every 4 to 6 hours, not to exceed 4 g in 24 hours, are recommended for both ASA and acetaminophen. Ibuprofen can be taken in doses of 200 to 400 mg every 4 to 6 hours. (For a more detailed discussion see the section on dysmenorrhea.)

Antihistamines such as pyrilamine maleate are found in some nonprescription products marketed for relief of PMS symptoms. The dose of pyrilamine contained in menstrual products is 12.5 to 25 mg per tablet or capsule. These amounts are well below the recommended oral adult dose of 100 mg.

Women using a product containing an antihistamine should be cautioned about the potential for drowsiness. Use of antihistamines may also increase the lethargy some women experience with PMS.

Pamabrom and caffeine have been included in menstrual products as mild diuretics. These diuretics are of limited benefit in treating PMS, but are safe to use as long as recommended doses are not exceeded.

Pamabrom is a theophylline derivative. The maximum daily dose is 200 mg.

Caffeine is a stimulant and mild diuretic. It is included as a diuretic and to treat the fatigue and lethargy that often occur with PMS. Those individuals who experience PMS symptoms of irritability and anxiety should limit their use of caffeine-containing products.

PMS is sometimes treated with vitamin B_6 (pyridoxine) (50 to 100 mg daily). People using vitamin B_6 should be given proper guidelines on dosage. Some women have exhibited neurotoxicity after consuming high doses, for example, 5 g/day, in attempts to alleviate PMS symptoms. Sensory neuropathy or neuronopathy can occur when excessive pyridoxine is used for several months or more. For these reasons some sources recommend that 100 mg be the daily maximum for vitamin B_6.

Oil of evening primrose contains 9 per cent gamma-linolenic acid (GLA), a fatty acid some believe to be low in women with PMS. GLA is an intermediate in the production of prostaglandin E and, to some degree, prostaglandin E_2.

Doses range from 500 to 1,500 mg twice daily. The benefits of the product have not been widely tested. One study showed some relief of a variety of PMS symptoms when oil of evening primrose was compared with placebo. With the exception of depression, the improvements were not statistically significant.

Vaginitis

A number of microorganisms make up the normal flora of the vagina. Vaginal pH and other environmental factors (such as secretions, glycogen content, and estrogen and progesterone levels) control the balance of bacterial growth and to some degree the organisms found there. When changes in the environment upset the natural balance, or foreign organisms are introduced into the vagina, symptoms of vaginal or cervical infection may result.

Numerous factors, such as certain disease states and medications, seem to predispose some women to vaginitis. Monilial vaginal infections can be associated with the use of broad-spectrum oral antibiotics, oral contraceptives, or with the presence of diabetes mellitus.

Feminine Care Products

Vulvar pruritus and erythema, excessive or unusual vaginal discharge, burning or stinging during intercourse or voiding, or unpleasant odor may indicate infection.

Several organisms commonly cause infection: *Candida albicans, Trichomonas vaginalis, Chlamydia trachomatis* and *Neisseria gonorrhoeae*. Bacterial vaginosis is the current term for what was once known as Gardnerella or nonspecific vaginitis. Although it is generally accepted that Gardnerella vaginalis is implicated in the condition it is believed that there must first be a disruption in the vaginal ecology before this normally occurring bacteria can cause irritation by acting synergistically with other anaerobic organisms in the vagina.

Symptoms vary depending on the organism so it is often difficult to distinguish differences without performing vaginal and cervical cultures. Accurate diagnosis is essential for selecting treatment. Any woman experiencing symptoms that may be due to a vaginal infection must be referred to a physician for assessment (see Table III).

Table III *Common Types of Vaginitis*

Cause	Common symptom(s)	pH	Choice treatment
Candida	Severe pruritus, cottage cheese discharge	4 +	Miconazole, clotrimazole
Trichomonas	Genital wetness or discharge; may be pruritic	6 +	Metronidazole (oral)
Bacterial vaginosis	"Fishy" odor; creamy discharge (gray/yellow)	5–6	Metronidazole (oral), ampicillin
Atrophy	Discharge; genital irritation	7	Estrogen, water-soluble lubricants

Atrophic vaginitis is a problem encountered most often by postmenopausal women. Symptoms result from low estrogen, which causes thinning of the epithelium and increased pH. Lack of vaginal lubrication, discomfort on intercourse and occasional spotting are typical of atrophic vaginitis. Treatment is topical or oral estrogen replacement. Water-soluble lubricant products can also be used for temporary relief during intercourse.

Treatment

Treatment of vaginitis is specific for the organism and usually a prescription medication.

Vaginal douches, anesthetic creams and medicated wipes may provide temporary relief from symptoms, but do not adequately treat the infection.

If vaginal pH alterations are a factor in the infection, a pH-altering douche or gel may be used, but only on the advice of a physician. A common ingredient used to acidify the vagina is acetic acid (vinegar).

Povidone-iodine douches and suppositories have been used to treat *Candida albicans* and Trichomonas infections. More effective prescription therapies are available and are the treatments of choice.

Boric acid has been used to treat vulvovaginal *Candida albicans*.

The most effective dose and regimen have not been conclusively established. Gelatin capsules containing 600 mg boric acid powder inserted into the vagina once daily for 14 days have been found effective in up to 92 per cent of cases. One study claimed a 98 per cent success rate in women with chronic vulvovaginal mycotic infections who were unresponsive to conventional, antifungal therapy. Boric acid vaginal inserts 600 mg were inserted twice daily for 14 to 28 days with several patients requiring 600 mg daily during menses only for an additional 4 months as a prophylactic measure. Treatment caused no untoward effects except a slight watery discharge and a mild burning sensation in some individuals. Toxicity from boric acid appears unlikely when it is used in the recommended manner.

A detailed discussion of douching techniques can be found in the genital hygiene section of this chapter. It is important to reinforce the need to clean the douching apparatus adequately after each use. Cleaning is particularly important when a vaginal infection is involved.

Women who are prone to vaginal infections, particularly monilial or yeast infections, may try some preventive measures to lessen the chance of recurrence. Maintain good genital hygiene. Wearing loose-fitting undergarments and pants and avoiding synthetic underwear or pantyhose may help by allowing adequate ventilation. Some women find that dietary modifications help, such as increasing yogurt in their diets and decreasing yeast products. Some also believe that high dietary sucrose intake is linked to vulvovaginal candidiasis. There is no strong scientific evidence to support this.

Condoms should be worn by the male partner during sexual intercourse whenever an active vaginal infection is present. This will decrease the risk of partners infecting and reinfecting one another.

Ask the Consumer

Genital Hygiene and Vaginitis

Q. Why do you wish to use a douche? Are you experiencing vaginal irritation or unusual discharge?

■ When a woman asks for advice regarding a douching product, it is important to assess the situation before making a recommendation. Vaginal infections are often characterized by vulvovaginal irritation, pruritus and increased or unusual vaginal discharge. Douches should not be used in place of appropriate vaginitis therapy. All suspected cases of vaginitis must be assessed by a physician.

Q. Are you familiar with how to use this douching product?

■ The product must be diluted or mixed correctly to avoid irritation. Douching apparatus may be confusing to someone who has never used it before. Use of the apparatus and proper technique must be explained to the consumer. Only gentle pressure is required when instilling the solution.

Q. Do you have any allergies to soaps, chemicals or perfumes?

■ Some ingredients in douching products can cause hypersensitivity reactions. Always check allergy potential with the consumer before recommending a product.

Chapter 20

Feminine Care Products

Menstrual Care

Q. Have you used this brand of tampons before?

- The method of application varies from brand to brand. Some have plunger-type applicators; others have applicator sticks or are inserted with a finger. The consumer may not realize the difference and accidentally purchase an unsuitable product.

Q. Do you know the symptoms of toxic shock syndrome?

- Although toxic shock syndrome is rare, if the following symptoms occur during menstruation the woman should seek medical attention immediately: sudden high fever, diarrhea, vomiting and sunburn-like rash.

Menstrual Problems

Q. Please describe your menstrual pain.

- Dysmenorrhea is a cramping, labor-like pain centered in the abdomen and lower back. It begins just before or at the onset of menses and lasts for 1 to 3 days. If the pain lasts through menses and increases in severity or is felt at other times in the menstrual cycle, it may be due to an underlying medical disorder and the woman should be assessed by a physician.

Q. Have you tried any medication in the past for menstrual pain? Did it help?

- If nonprescription analgesics have been used for several cycles with no success, prescription therapy is indicated. Refer the consumer to a physician.

Q. Do you have a history of stomach or duodenal ulcers?

- Individuals with any of the above should avoid the use of ASA and ibuprofen if possible. ASA and ibuprofen to a lesser degree can cause gastrointestinal irritation and ulceration. Acetaminophen is the nonprescription drug of choice for such individuals.

Q. Are you taking other medications?

- ASA can interact with a number of medications, including phenytoin, warfarin, probenecid and oral hypoglycemics. Ibuprofen appears to have fewer interactions, but caution should be used when it is in combination with oral anticoagulants, lithium, triamterene and other ulcerogenic agents. Acetaminophen is the drug of choice if a drug interaction is possible with ASA.

Premenstrual Syndrome

Q. What symptoms lead you to believe you have PMS and when did they begin?

- PMS symptoms are many and varied. They usually peak 2 to 3 days before onset of menstruation and resolve rapidly once bleeding begins. They can begin on or any time after ovulation. It is important to rule out any underlying medical condition that may cause the symptoms. Once PMS is suspected, nonprescription treatment can be tried. Women with severe incapacitating symptoms should be referred to a physician.

Q. Are you trying any general measures that help relieve the symptoms?

- A number of lifestyle modifications may help decrease PMS symptoms. They include stress reduction, increased exercise and dietary changes.

Q. What have you used in the past for PMS relief?

- A review of past therapy indicates whether nonprescription options are still available or whether the woman must try prescription therapy next.

Q. Do you have, or have you had, any conditions that preclude you from using ASA, such as peptic ulcer, bleeding disorders or asthma?

- ASA is a common nonprescription product used to treat PMS. As with dysmenorrhea, several factors make ASA an undesirable choice for some people. If the woman has had any of the above conditions or has experienced any adverse reactions to ASA, acetaminophen or in some cases, ibuprofen is the analgesic of choice.

References

Reproductive Anatomy and Physiology

Fritz MA, Speroff L. Current concepts of the endocrine characteristics of normal menstrual function: the key to diagnosis and management of menstrual disorders. Clin Obstet Gynecol 1983;26:647–87.

Huggins GR, Preti G. Vaginal odors and secretions. Clin Obstet Gynecol 1981;24:355–75.

McPherson A, Anderson A, eds. Women's problems in general practice. Oxford: Oxford University Press, 1983.

Sloane E. Biology of women. New York: J Wiley and Sons, 1985.

Spellacy WN. Abnormal bleeding. Clin Obstet Gynecol 1983;26:702–10.

Yarkauskas E. Primary female syndromes—an update. NY State J Med 1990:295–302.

Vaginal Douches

Byers JF. To douche or not to douche. Am Fam Physician 1974;10(3):135–9.

McGowan L. Peritonitis following the vaginal douche and a proposed alternative method for vaginal and vulvar care. Am J Obstet Gynecol 1965; 93:506–9.

Reynolds JEF, ed. Martindale: the extra pharmacopoeia. London: Pharmaceutical Press, 1989.

Rosenberg MJ, Phillips RS, Holmes MD. Vaginal douching. Who and why? J Repro Med 1991;36:753–8.

Sadik F. O-T-C feminine hygiene aids. J Am Pharmacol Assoc 1972;12(11): 565–70.

Zbella EA, Nemec LA, Vermesh M. Vaginal douching: pros, cons, and proper technique. Postgrad Med 1984;76(8):93–5.

Pads and Tampons

Consumer Reports. Menstrual tampons and pads. The medicine show. New York: Pantheon, 1980;214–23.

Freidrich EG. Tampon effects on vaginal health. Clin Obstet Gynecol 1981;24:395–405.

Holt P. The toxic shock syndrome. Maternal and Child Health 1981;July: 268–72.

Todd JK. Therapy of toxic shock syndrome. Curr Ther 1990:45–9.

Dysmenorrhea

Abramowicz M. Drugs for dysmenorrhea. Med Lett Drugs Ther 1979;21:81–3.

Dawood MY. Dysmenorrhea. Clin Obstet Gynecol 1983;26:719–27.

Dawood MY. Dysmenorrhea. J Reprod Med 1985;30:154–65.

Hansten PD, Horn JR. The top 40 drug interactions. Drug Interaction Newsletter 1991;11(1):483-90.

Muse KN. Cyclic pelvic pain. Obstet Gynecol Clin N Amer 1990;17:429–40.

Wenzloff NJ, Shimp L. Therapeutic management of primary dysmenorrhea. Drug Intell Clin Pharm 1984;18:22–6.

Premenstrual Syndrome

Briggs CJ. Evening primrose: la belle de nuit, the king's cureall. Can Pharm J 1986;119:249–54.

Feminine Care Products

Chihal HJ. Premenstrual syndrome: an update for the clinician. Obstet Gynecol Clin N Amer 1990;17:457–77.

Kleijnen J, Ter Piet G, Knipschild P. Vitamin B_6 in the treatment of premenstrual syndrome—a review. Br J Obstet Gynaecol 1990;97:847–52.

Lyon KE, Lyon MA. The premenstrual syndrome, a survey of current treatment practices. J Reprod Med 1984;29:705–11.

Maddocks S, Hahn P, Moller F, Reid RL. A double-blind placebo controlled trial of progesterone vaginal suppositories in the treatment of premenstrual syndrome. Am J Obstet Gynecol 1986;154:573–81.

Nader S. Premenstural syndrome. Tailoring treatment to symptoms. Postgrad Med 1991;90:173–8.

O'Brien PMS. The premenstrual syndrome. J Reprod Med 1985;30:113–23.

Pariser SF, Stern SL, Shank ML, et al. Premenstrual syndrome concerns, controversies, and treatment. Am J Obstet Gynecol 1985;153:599–603.

Puolakka J, Makarainen L, Viinikka L, Ylikorkala O. Biochemical and clinical effects of treating the premenstrual syndrome with prostaglandin synthesis precursors. J Reprod Med 1985;30:149–53.

Reid RL. Premenstrual syndrome: a therapeutic dilemma. Drug Ther 1982;12(4):65–75.

Reid RL, Yen SSC. The premenstrual syndrome. Clin Obstet Gynecol 1983;26:711–7.

Rossignol AM, Bornlander H. Prevalence and severity of premenstrual syndrome—effects of foods and beverages that are sweet or high in sugar content. J Repro Med 1991;36:131–6.

True BL, Goodner SM, Burns EA. Review of the etiology and treatment of premenstrual syndrome. Drug Intell Clin Pharm 1985;19:714–21.

Vaginitis

Doering PL, Santiago TM. Drugs for the treatment of vulvovaginal candidiasis—the comparative efficacy of agents and regimens. Drug Intell Clin Pharm 1990;24:1078–83.

Eschenbach DA. Vaginal infection. Clin Obstet Gynecol 1983;26:186–201.

Fleury FJ. Adult vaginitis. Clin Obstet Gynecol 1981;24:407–35.

Foreman A, Smith CB. Vaginitis. Systematically solving a bothersome problem. Postgrad Med 1990;88:123–33.

Hanna NF, et al. The relation between vaginal pH and the microbiological status in vaginitis. Br J Obstet Gynaecol 1985;92:1267–71.

Henderson JN, Tait IB. The use of povidone iodine (betadine) pessaries in the treatment of candidal and trichomonal vaginitis. Curr Med Res Opin 1975;3(3):157–62.

Jovanovic R, Congema E, Nguyen HT. Antifungal agents vs. boric acid for treating chronic mycotic vulvovaginitis. J Repro Med 1991;36:593–7.

McCue JD. Evaluation and management of vaginitis—an update for primary care practitioners. Arch Int Med 1989;149:565–8.

Sparks JM. Vaginitis. J Repro Med 1991;36:745–52.

Van Slyke KK, Michel VP, Rein MF. Treatment of vulvovaginal candidiasis with boric acid powder. Am J Obstet Gynecol 1981;141:145.

21

Constipation and Laxatives

Revised by Lily Lum. Based on the original chapter by Reina Bendayan

The many causes of constipation necessitate a wide variety of treatments. Nonpharmacologic measures—increasing dietary fibre, fluid intake and physical activity—are recommended in most cases. Bulk-forming agents are relatively safe products for chronic constipation. Osmotic laxatives are used before hospital procedures. Stimulant or contact laxatives such as phenolphthalein are commonly used for self-medication, and are the agents most often involved in cathartic abuse. Emollient and lubricant laxatives may be indicated in some cases. Dosage forms of laxatives may be oral, or packaged for use as suppositories or enemas.

Constipation is a common problem in North America and Europe. Surveys in the United States and England reveal that 17 to 20 per cent of healthy individuals suffer from constipation. This problem is more frequent in females than males and more prevalent among the elderly.

The use of nonprescription laxative preparations is widespread and often irrational. Pharmacists can play an important role in assuring better control and use of these preparations. They also have a responsibility to provide appropriate consumer counselling.

The objectives of this chapter are to define and explain the problem of constipation and its numerous etiologies, to discuss different treatment approaches as well as the efficacy and safety of the major pharmacologic agents in various nonprescription laxative preparations, and to present a comprehensive approach for evaluating and treating constipation.

Defining constipation is difficult. Normal defecation patterns vary significantly: 94 per cent of normal individuals present stool frequencies ranging between 3 per day to 3 per week. One study found the average time between stools in healthy males to be 27 hours. (No similar study has been conducted with women.) Constipation is not a disease, but a symptom that can be defined as an infrequent and generally painful evacuation of feces. It is characterized by flatulence, feelings of malaise, slight anorexia and mild abdominal discomfort or distension. The three types of constipation are spastic, atonic and organic. Spastic constipation is characterized by hard, round, marble-like stools that are difficult to pass. This condition occurs because the sigmoid sphincter allows an insufficient amount of stool to enter the rectum and the defecation urge is not satisfactorily stimulated. Atonic constipation is characterized by large stools that range from hard to soft consistency depending on the laxative used. This condition occurs in elderly, chronically debilitated individuals and in chronic laxative abusers. Organic constipation is induced by diseases, for example, neoplasms and hypothyroidism.

Causes of Constipation

There are many causes of constipation, but the most common are as follows: poor dietary habits, such as a low intake of dietary fibre or an inadequate fluid intake; geriatric condition that leads to decreased tonus of the gut smooth muscle, loss of the gut neuro-muscular reflex activity, loss of awareness of and neglect of the defecation urge; pregnancy; neglect of the defecation urge (certain occupations predispose this problem, for example, truck drivers, waiters and airline personnel); lack of physical activity; immobilization; laxative abuse; psychiatric conditions such as depression; and drug consumption (see Table I). In most cases in the Western world, constipation results from an over-refined, fibre-deficient diet.

Table I *Drugs That Can Induce Constipation*

Analgesics—anti-inflammatory drugs
Antacids (e.g., calcium carbonate, aluminum hydroxide)
Anticholinergics (e.g., dicyclomine, propantheline, benztropine)
Antihypertensive agents (e.g., reserpine, clonidine)
Calcium channel blocker (e.g., verapamil)
Diuretics
Laxatives (if abused)
Iron salts
Narcotics (e.g., codeine)
Phenothiazines (e.g., chlorpromazine)
Tricyclic antidepressants (e.g., amitriptyline)

Treatment

Before recommending a treatment to the constipated individual, pharmacists should check that the consumer has consulted a physician to rule out the presence of an underlying gastrointestinal disease. Pharmacists should also evaluate carefully the person's pharmacotherapeutic profile.

General treatment of constipation includes changes in dietary habits, increasing the intake of whole grain cereals, vegetables and fruits and ensuring a fluid intake of 1.4 to 2.4 L a day. Pharmacists must use caution when counselling consumers suffering from congestive heart failure and renal insufficiency, as these individuals are fluid restricted. Increasing physical activity is also important as it promotes appetite and evacuation. If possible, drugs that decrease intestinal motility should be discontinued. Relief of emotional stress is important if the stress is associated with the constipation problem.

Pharmaceutical Agents

Drug therapy may be required if the general treatment measures do not alleviate the constipation. Laxatives and cathartics are drugs that promote defecation. The terms "laxative" and "cathartic" imply different intensities of drug effect. Laxative effect suggests the elimination of a soft, formed stool whereas cathartic effect implies a more fluid evacuation. Most drugs that promote defecation produce a laxative effect in low dosage, but a cathartic effect in higher dosage. Consequently, when applied to the drugs themselves, the terms are often used interchangeably.

In general, laxatives and cathartics are classified according to their mechanism of action. They include bulk-forming agents, osmotic cathartics, stimulant (contact) cathartics, emollient laxatives and lubricant laxatives.

Dietary Fibre and Bulk-Forming Agents

Dietary fibre and bulk-forming agents are helpful in relieving chronic constipation. Dietary fibre is the portion of plant food that escapes digestion in the small intestine. The related bulk-forming agents are natural and semi-synthetic polysaccharides and cellulose derivatives. Dietary fibre and related agents absorb and retain large amounts of fluids, increasing the bulk of the intestinal contents. The resulting mechanical distention stimulates a reflex peristalsis, while the absorbed water also softens the stools. These effects appear within 24 hours, but if fibre is used repeatedly, the full effect may be delayed for up to several days or longer. When these agents are taken regularly, a soft, formed stool results.

Bran and other bulk-forming agents have been shown to reduce intraluminal rectosigmoid pressure and to relieve symptoms in people with irritable bowel disease and diverticular disease of the colon.

Bran and bulk-forming agents have minimal side effects. The rapid introduction of bran into the diet may cause flatulence, but this effect can be relieved by adjusting the dosage, switching to a different preparation or a different source of fibre, or increasing the fluid intake. Intestinal obstruction has been reported after administering bulk-forming agents, and impaction may result when there is gross intestinal pathology. It is highly recommended to administer at least 250 mL of fluid with each dose of bulk-forming agents and bran.

Bulk-forming agents are relatively safe laxatives and are used in treating people with irritable bowel syndrome, diverticulitis, constipation during pregnancy, or constipation resulting from low residue diets. They may be useful for people who should avoid straining during defecation and for people requiring long-term laxative therapy.

Bran is a by-product of milled wheat. Raw bran contains more than 40 per cent dietary fibre; processed bran contains 25 per cent dietary fibre. To prevent constipation, the usual adult daily dose of crude bran ranges from 6 to 12 g taken orally. Oat bran is inaccurately believed by many to be useful in relieving constipation. Oat bran is rich in soluble fibre; it is the insoluble form of fibre found in wheat bran that is a better constipation reliever.

Methylcellulose and **carboxymethylcellulose sodium** are hydrophilic semi-synthetic derivatives that have similar laxative properties. Cellulose is available in tablets as well as in bulk. The usual adult daily dose ranges from 1 to 6 g.

Psyllium preparations are obtained from plantago seeds, which contain a large amount of natural mucilage that forms a gelatinous mass on contact with water. Several case reports of allergic reactions to psyllium products have been reported in the literature. The reactions range from rhinitis and lacrimation to severe respiratory compromise. Health care workers can become sensitized to the psyllium while handling the product and inhaling the aerosolized psyllium powder.

Psyllium is available in regular and effervescent powder (for example, Metamucil); the effervescent preparation contains 240 mg of sodium per package, which should be considered when treating people on a sodium-restricted diet. The usual adult daily dose ranges from 4 to 10 g, taken one to three times a day. In children more than 6 years old, the daily dose ranges from 1.5 to 15 g.

Polycarbophil is a polyacrylic acid that is cross-linked with divinyl glycol. Polycarbophil is pharmacologically inert and not absorbed from the gut; it is strongly hydrophilic with a high water-binding capacity. Polycarbophil does not interfere significantly with the activity of digestive enzymes. In animal studies, polycarbophil has been shown to be nonabsorbable and free of toxicity.

Polycarbophil calcium (Mitrolan) is available in tablets of 500 mg. The usual daily adult dose is 4 to 6 g in four doses. It is not recommended for people with obstructive bowel disease or for children less than 3 years old.

Plant gums include agar, tragacanth, chondrus, karaya and sterculia. Agar is relatively ineffective as a bulk-forming agent in usual doses (4 to 16 g). Karaya gum in oral doses of 5 to 10 g daily is effective in increasing the bulk of the stool. However, allergic reactions such as urticaria, rhinitis, dermatitis and asthma have been reported. Due to these disadvantages, these agents are not recommended for treating constipation.

Osmotic Laxatives

Saline cathartics and lactulose are effective in emptying the bowel and are used before surgical or radiological bowel procedures. Saline cathartics are magnesium phosphate and sulfate salts. After oral or rectal administration, magnesium, sulfate and phosphate ions are incompletely absorbed from the gastrointestinal tract and retain water in the intestinal lumen through an osmotic effect. The increased intraluminal pressure produces a mechanical stimulus that increases intestinal motility. It has been reported that cholecystokinin secretion, caused by magnesium salts, mediates pancreatic secretion and increases secretion and motility of the small intestine and colon. These effects promote the laxative action.

Full doses of saline cathartics produce a semi-fluid or watery evacuation within 0.5 to 3 hours. Rectal preparations act in about 5 minutes through distention and osmotic activity. Saline laxatives should be accompanied by at least 250 mL of fluid to prevent dehydration and to maximize the laxative effects. However, these laxatives should be administered with great caution to people with impaired renal function, hypertension, congestive heart failure or hypocalcemia. Some absorption of the component ions of the saline cathartics occurs; in certain cases this absorption may produce systemic toxicity. Individuals with renal impairment may experience an accumulation of magnesium, sodium and phosphate ions. Toxic serum concentrations of magnesium may lead to central nervous system depression, muscle weakness, hypotension and electrocardiographic changes. The use of phosphate salts in children under 2 years of age and in people with renal impairment has been reported to produce hyperphosphatemia, hypocalcemia, tetany, hypernatremia and dehydration. These agents should be used with caution; chronic administration must be avoided.

Constipation and Laxatives

Magnesium salts include mainly magnesium sulfate, magnesium hydroxide and magnesium citrate. The oral adult daily recommended doses for magnesium sulfate are 10 to 30 g diluted in 250 mL of water, or magnesium hydroxide 25 to 50 mL as a suspension. Magnesium citrate (15 g/300 mL) is generally used to empty the bowel before radiological examinations of the colon. In adults, the dosage is 300 mL (one bottle) administered with 250 to 300 mL of fluid per hour for 4 to 6 hours before administering the drug and for 3 hours after.

Phosphate salts may be administered orally or by enema. These cathartics include sodium biphosphate and sodium phosphate effervescent. The recommended oral adult daily doses for sodium biphosphate are 3.6 to 7.2 g as a dilute solution, or sodium phosphate 10 g as an effervescent solution. Sodium phosphate enema is used in a dose of 120 mL.

Lactulose is a semi-synthetic disaccharide recommended for preventing and treating portal systemic encephalopathy and chronic constipation. This agent retains water and electrolytes in the lumen because of the osmotic activity of the disaccharide. The osmotic effect of lactulose increases in the distal ileum and colon, where the unabsorbed disaccharide is metabolized by the intestinal microflora to lactate and other organic acids that are only partially absorbed. Lowering the colonic pH stimulates colonic smooth muscle contraction. Onset of the laxative action is 24 to 48 hours. Lactulose may cause flatulence, cramps and abdominal discomfort, especially when therapy is initiated. Nausea and vomiting have also been reported. Excessive dosages can cause diarrhea, loss of fluid and potassium, exacerbation of encephalopathy and hypernatremia. This agent should be used with caution by diabetics, since it contains some digestible sugar.

The usual adult dose of lactulose syrup is 15 mL (10 g of lactulose) to 30 mL daily; this dose can be increased to 60 mL daily if necessary. Osmotic laxatives and lactulose are not good choices to treat constipation, particularly in the elderly, due to the risk of inducing dehydration and electrolyte imbalance. One reference recommends lactulose as a laxative of choice in children less than 1 year of age. The starting dose is 5 to 10 mL daily, to be increased until the formation of soft stools.

Stimulant (Contact) Laxatives

Stimulant (contact) laxatives include different types of compounds, mainly of vegetable origin, for example, anthraquinone derivatives contained in cascara sagrada, aloe, senna and rhubarb; phenolphthalein, other phthaleins and coal tar dyes; ricinoleic acid; resins; and alkaloids of podophyllum, sulfur, and calomel. These agents act on the intestinal mucosa and affect gastrointestinal motility and the absorption of electrolytes and water. The effect of these agents relates to their ability to inhibit intestinal water absorption and increase permeability of the intestinal mucosa. Contact cathartics increase the propulsive peristaltic activity of the intestine by local irritation of the intestinal smooth muscle. The intensity of action is proportional to dosage, but individually effective doses vary. Stimulant laxatives produce severe abdominal cramps frequently, increase mucus secretion and in some individuals, lead to an excessive evacuation of fluids. Dosage of these agents should be adjusted to produce a soft, formed and easily evacuated stool. Contact cathartics are the agents most often involved in cathartic abuse.

Diphenylmethane cathartics include primarily **phenolphthalein** and **bisacodyl**. These agents act on the colon and produce laxative effects in 6 to 12 hours. As phenolphthalein undergoes enterohepatic circulation, its effects last for 3 to 4 days. With bisacodyl rectal suppositories, the laxative effect occurs 15 to 60 minutes after administration.

Phenolphthalein and bisacodyl are usually nontoxic. Major side effects are fluid and electrolyte depletion resulting from an excessive cathartic effect. Allergic reactions, including fixed-drug eruption, Stevens-Johnson syndrome and lupus erythematosus syndrome, have been reported with phenolphthalein. Osteomalacia also has been related to chronic ingestion of phenolphthalein. Phenolphthalein can be secreted into breast milk and may cause diarrhea in the infant. Bisacodyl suppositories may cause a burning sensation; continued administration may cause inflammation of the anus.

The usual daily dose of phenolphthalein in adults is 30 to 100 mg, and in children more than 6 years, 30 to 60 mg. Under the advice of a physician, children 2 to 5 years are given 15 to 20 mg.

For bisacodyl, the usual daily adult dose is 5 to 15 mg orally or 10 mg rectally. For children more than 6 years, the daily dose is 5 mg orally or 10 mg rectally.

Anthraquinone cathartics include senna, cascara sagrada, danthron and casanthranol. The properties of anthraquinone laxatives vary depending on the anthraquinone content and the rate of liberation of the active ingredients from the glycosidic combinations. These agents increase the peristaltic activity of the colon; the laxative effect occurs 6 to 12 hours after ingestion. Adverse effects resulting from this group are mainly excessive cathartic effects, and the urine is dyed red. Prolonged use of anthraquinone laxatives, especially cascara sagrada, can result in a dark pigmentation of the colonic mucosa. This pigmentation is usually reversible 4 to 12 months after the drug is discontinued. The presence of colonic pigmentation helps confirm suspicions of cathartic abuse. Anthraquinone laxatives are secreted into breast milk.

Cascara sagrada (for example, cascara fluid extract and cascara sagrada tablets) is the least potent anthraquinone laxative. United States Pharmacopeia (USP) preparations include the tablets, the fluid extract and the aromatic fluid extract. The recommended dose of the aromatic fluid extract is twice that of plain fluid extract, because about one-half the active cathartic ingredients are destroyed in preparing the aromatic fluid extract. Daily dosages for adults are 300 mg for the tablets, 0.5 to 1.5 mL of fluid extract or 5 mL of aromatic fluid extract. Children 2 to 12 years of age require one-half the adult dose. Children under the age of 6 should only be treated under the advice of a physician.

Casanthranol is a purified mixture of anthranol glycosides extracted from cascara sagrada. It is estimated to be 10 times more potent than whole cascara sagrada. The usual daily dose for adults is 30 mg.

Danthron is a free anthraquinone rather than a glycoside. Its pharmacologic properties and limitations are similar to those of the anthraquinone glycosides. Danthron is partly absorbed from the small intestine and a large part is metabolized and excreted by the kidneys. The urine may become red. Danthron produces a soft or semi-fluid stool 6 to 8 hours after ingestion. The usual dose in adults is 37 to 150 mg; danthron is not recommended for children less than 12 years of age.

In 1987, the U.S. Federal Drug Administration ordered the total recall of nonprescription laxative products containing danthron. It was withdrawn from the U.S. market because studies have shown that danthron can cause liver tumors in rats when given in high doses for an extended period of time. In Canada, many of the danthron-containing laxatives were voluntarily withdrawn or reformulated.

Constipation and Laxatives

Senna preparations are more potent than those of cascara and produce more abdominal pain. Crystalline senna glycosides (sennosides A and B) and standardized concentrations of senna pods form more stable and reliable preparations than those containing senna leaf. The usual daily doses of senna leaf preparations in adults are 0.5 to 2 g as a powder, 2 mL as fluid extract and 8 mL as a syrup. Daily doses of sennosides A and B are 12 to 24 mg. Doses for senna pod preparation are 3 to 6 g twice daily as granules, 10 to 15 mL once or twice daily as syrup and 2 to 4 tablets twice daily. For all senna preparations, the daily dose for children 2 to 5 years (only if under the advice of a physician) is one-quarter the adult dose, and children 6 to 12 years, one-half the adult dose.

Rhubarb, aloe, alloin and **frangula** are the most potent anthraquinone laxatives; their ingestion often results in colic. In view of the availability of similar agents of lesser potency, these agents should not be used.

Castor oil, extracted from the castor plant *Ricinus communis*, is composed primarily of the triglyceride of ricinoleic acid. It produces prompt evacuation of the bowel. The action of castor oil is due to ricinoleic acid, a product of its hydrolysis by intestinal lipases. Ricinoleic acid enhances movement of fecal matter by increasing the contractile activity of the smooth muscle of the small intestine. It may also affect water and electrolyte secretion.

Castor oil is not recommended for managing constipation because regular use may result in excessive loss of fluid and electrolytes. Malabsorption of nutrients may also result because of the erosion of intestinal villi and the disorganization of the microvillus surface. Castor oil should be reserved for use when total evacuation of the colon is desirable, such as before an operation or diagnostic procedure. The usual daily dosages in adults are 15 to 60 mL in a single dose; in children 2 to 12 years, 5 to 15 mL; and in infants less than 2 years, 1 to 5 mL. Children under the age of 6 should be treated only under the advice of a physician.

Emollient Laxatives

Docusate calcium and **docusate sodium** (also known as dioctylcalcium sulfosuccinate and dioctylsodium sulfosuccinate) are emulsifying and dispersing agents. In recommended oral doses, these agents soften fecal matter by facilitating its admixture with aqueous and fatty substances. These laxatives also appear to stimulate secretion of water and electrolytes in the colon. Softening of stools occurs 24 to 72 hours after administration. Stool softeners are indicated for people who are immobilized or infirm, as in orthopedic surgery, the elderly, people with compromised cardiac status, the terminally ill and people with neuromuscular deficits such as muscular sclerosis, muscular dystrophy and Parkinson's disease. Stool softeners may also be administered as adjunctive therapy with drugs that reduce normal peristalsis such as codeine, iron and morphine.

Recommended doses of these agents are well tolerated, although cramping pains may occur. Liquid preparations can sometimes cause nausea. These agents do not interfere with absorption of nutrients from the gastrointestinal tract. They do increase absorption, hepatic intake and toxicity of other drugs administered concurrently. One case of hepatotoxicity has been reported with the concurrent use of docusate and danthron.

Stool softeners are particularly useful in treating constipation caused by hard, dry stools and in conditions in which painful or difficult defecation should be avoided, for example, diseases of the rectum and colon and postpartum constipation. When used in an enema, these agents may facilitate the elimination of impacted fecal matter.

The usual adult daily dosages of docusate sodium are 50 to 300 mg in single or divided doses, and 50 to 100 mg in a solution of 0.1 per cent. For children 6 to 12 years the dosage is 40 to 120 mg; children 3 to 6 years, 20 to 60 mg; and infants less than 3 years, 10 to 40 mg. Children under the age of 6 should be treated only under the advice of a physician. Docusate sodium drops have been administered as a rectal enema in doses of 50 to 100 mg.

Lubricant Laxatives

Mineral oil (liquid petrolatum) and some digestible plant oils (for example, cottonseed oil and olive oil) soften fecal matter and may interfere with colonic absorption of fecal water. Emulsification of mineral oil increases its palatability and wetting properties, but the amount of oil absorbed also may increase. The laxative effect of mineral oil is seen 6 to 8 hours after oral administration. If administered with meals, mineral oil may interfere with absorption of essential fat-soluble substances and may delay gastric emptying. A daily intake of mineral oil for 1 or 2 weeks or longer reduced vitamin K absorption and produced hypoprothrombinemia in 70 per cent of the pregnant women in one study. With prolonged and repeated use, significant absorption of mineral oil may occur. The oil may produce a typical foreign-body reaction characterized by cells of chronic inflammation, including giant cells. This reaction may appear in the intestinal lymph nodes, intestinal mucosa, liver and spleen. To date, one case of hepatic damage has been associated with mineral oil deposits in the liver.

Lipid pneumonia can occur following the oral ingestion of the oil, particularly if it is taken at bedtime. The ingested oil adheres to the pharynx, and small amounts may then be aspirated into the lungs. Pediatric, elderly, debilitated or dysphagic individuals are more prone to develop this type of pneumonia, and the use of mineral oil should be discouraged in this population. If large doses of mineral oil are taken, the oil may leak through the anal sphincter. This leakage may produce anal pruritus, hemorrhoids, cryptitis and other perianal diseases. Leakage can be avoided by reducing or dividing the dose or using a stable emulsion of mineral oil.

Mineral oil is useful in situations where straining at defecation should be avoided (for example, recent myocardial infarction, postpartum constipation, posthemorrhoidectomy or abdominal surgery, hernias, aneurysms and cerebrovascular accidents). The prolonged use of this laxative is not recommended. The usual daily dosage in adults is 15 to 45 mL. Mineral oil should not be used in children under 6 years of age. Heavy mineral oil is specified for internal use as a laxative. Light mineral oil should not be used for internal consumption because of leakage.

Suppositories

Rectal suppositories may be used for evacuating the lower bowel, but they are not effective if the stool is dry and hard.

Glycerin suppositories stimulate the rectal mucosa and may also soften the stool. They promote evacuation 15 to 30 minutes after administration. Some people may experience rectal irritation and discomfort. The usual daily dosage in adults is 3 g (one suppository), and in children less than 6 years, 1 to 1.5 g. Children under the age of 6 should be treated only under the advice of a physician.

Carbon-dioxide-releasing suppositories are of use in evacuating the distal colon. Gentle pressure from the expanding gas stimulates

Table II *Instructions for Consumers*

Laxative agent	Consumer information	Laxative agent	Consumer information
Bulk laxatives	At least 250 mL of liquid should be taken with each dose of bulk laxative; up to 3 days of medication may be necessary to achieve laxative effect.	Emollient laxatives	Do not take with mineral oil. Acts within 24 to 72 hours.
Osmotic laxatives	For occasional use only. Increase fluid intake with the use of saline laxatives. Caution individual patients on low sodium diets and those with renal impairment. Laxative effect occurs in 1/2 to 3 hours.	Lubricants (mineral oil)	For occasional use only. Do not take with meals; do not administer to children less than 6 years of age, pregnant women, bedridden or aged individuals, individuals having difficulty in swallowing, or people who are vomiting; do not administer with stool softeners. Acts within 6 to 8 hours.
• magnesium citrate	Refrigeration retards decomposition of salt solution.		
Stimulant (contact) laxatives	For occasional use only; chronic use may lead to laxative dependency and loss of normal bowel function. Use sparingly in children. Not recommended for use by pregnant women.	Suppositories	Before using suppositories, allow them to stand at room temperature. After removing the wrapper, the suppository should be inserted into the rectum with the tapered end first. Instruct the user to remain reclined for a few minutes after insertion. Best results may be achieved by inserting the suppository after a meal to take advantage of the natural bowel reflexes.
• anthraquinone	May discolor urine and feces; generally administered at bedtime.		
• bisacodyl	Tablets should be swallowed whole, not crushed, chewed or administered within 1 hour of antacids or milk; laxative effect usually occurs in 6 to 12 hours.	Enemas	Temperature of the solution should be warm (35°C–37°C). A reclining posture should be assumed and the container of enema fluid should be positioned slightly above the hips. More thorough cleansing may result if individuals lie on their left side after solution is administered.
• castor oil	Acts within 2 to 6 hours; should not be given at bedtime. Castor oil is not recommended for the treatment of chronic constipation.		

normal activity and defecation reflexes in the lower bowel. The usual adult dosage is one suppository to be retained 15 to 20 minutes.

Suppositories containing bisacodyl are also available.

Enemas

Clinical indications for enemas are surgery, delivery, lower bowel constipation, fecal impaction and barium enema preparation. When administered properly, enemas clean the distal colon by distention. In a crossover study, phosphate enemas were more effective than tap water, soap suds or other saline enemas.

An improperly administered enema can produce fluid and electrolyte imbalances and colonic perforation. Enema fluids that contain substances foreign to the bowel cause mucosal changes or spasms of the intestinal wall. Hydrogen peroxide enemas can cause proctitis and hemorrhaging. Water intoxication results from the use of tap water or soap suds enemas in the presence of megacolon. Refer to the section on drug information for the consumer for the proper method of administering an enema (see Table II).

Drug Interactions

In general, laxatives may decrease absorption of drugs taken concurrently due to their stimulant action on the gastrointestinal tract. Drugs that undergo slow absorption may be particularly affected. For specific drug interactions involving laxatives, refer to Table III.

Combination Products

Many commercially available laxative products contain more than one pharmacologically active ingredient. In general, single-entity products are preferred to those having multiple active agents because of reduced risk of adverse effects, allergic reactions and drug interactions. The laxative dose required by an individual is also more easily titrated when one active principle is involved.

Drug Therapy and Consumer Information

Therapy for spastic constipation requires the combined use of a high-fibre diet, adequate fluid intake, regular exercise, reassurance to overcome emotional factors and, if necessary, appropriate doses of a laxative. The use of bran or one of the bulk laxatives (for example, psyllium) is also recommended. Adequate fluid intake is necessary, and therapy can be pursued for a few months. People who do not respond to bran or bulk laxatives, or who suffer from atonic constipation, require bowel retraining with the periodic administration of enemas and the use of glycerin suppositories just before the bowel movement. Stimulant or saline laxatives can be used for a short period of time. For example, bisacodyl tablets can be administered at bedtime to produce a cathartic effect in the morning. If the constipation is associated with an underlying disease, the pharmacist should refer the person to a physician for further investigation and treatment of the primary disease.

Constipation and Laxatives

Treatment in Different Age Groups

Age is an important factor to consider before recommending a laxative preparation. Constipation in children must be treated with great caution; an excessive cathartic effect can lead rapidly to serum electrolyte disturbances and severe dehydration. It is important to reassure parents of a constipated child, to advise them to avoid the regular use of enemas, saline and contact cathartics, and to consult their pediatrician or family physician. It is difficult to define normal bowel habits for infants and children. Changes in the frequency and the consistency of stools can occur at different periods during the first year of life. Bowel movements generally become less frequent with increasing age of the infant. During the first few months of age, constipation in formula-fed infants can be treated by adding sucrose or dextrose to the formula. Increased fluid intake is highly recommended for children. In older infants, increased bulk in the diet with the administration of bran cereals, fresh vegetables and fruits such as prunes or apricots can be recommended. In cases of fecal impaction, saline enemas can be administered; they should be used only to relieve the impaction.

In elderly people, various psychological changes and factors, such as decreased muscle tone, insufficient fluid intake, poor diet, consumption of medication, presence of disease and laxative abuse, may contribute to the problem of constipation. In this population, implementation of a high residue diet and appropriate fluid intake should be emphasized. Also, the regular administration of a bulk-forming agent (for example, psyllium) can be recommended. If these measures do not effectively relieve constipation, low doses of a stimulant laxative (for example, bisacodyl) can be administered; the long-term use of stimulant laxatives should be avoided. In the case of laxative abuse, it is important to stop administering the drug gradually and to counsel the person on how to re-establish regular bowel habits. Elderly people should avoid saline laxatives as they are more sensitive to serum electrolyte imbalances. Also, the administration of mineral oil should be discouraged as these people are more prone to lipid pneumonia and vitamin deficiencies.

Treatment During Pregnancy and Lactation

Constipation is a common problem during pregnancy; in a survey involving 350 pregnant women, 31 per cent suffered from constipation during the antenatal period. In pregnancy, constipation is usually attributed to a decrease in tone and motility of the nonstriated muscle of the gastrointestinal system. Also, lack of physical exercise and the pressure of the enlarging uterus may delay emptying time of the bowel and contribute to the problem. Treating constipation in pregnant women involves applying the general measures described earlier, particularly an increase in fluid and fibre intake. If these measures are not sufficient, bulk-forming laxatives can be recommended. Mineral oil use should be avoided as it interferes with the absorption of liposoluble vitamins and can lead to hypoprothrombinemia. Chronic use of stimulant and saline laxatives should be avoided because these products may induce a severe electrolyte imbalance. Castor oil should be avoided by pregnant women as the stimulant effect of this agent can cause uterine contractions.

Breast-feeding women should avoid stimulant laxatives, particularly phenolphthalein, cascara and danthron, as they can be secreted into breast milk and can induce diarrhea in the infant.

Figure 1 *Suggested Approach for Treating Constipation*

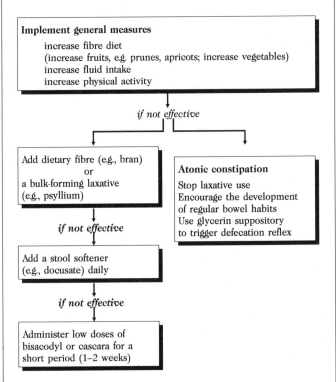

Treatment of Laxative Abuse

Excessive and chronic consumption of laxatives, particularly contact cathartics, may lead to severe diarrhea, abdominal pain, vomiting, weakness, hypokalemia, weight loss, skin pigmentation and steatorrhea.

Long-term use of anthraquinone laxatives can result in atonic constipation. Consumers may find it necessary to use increasingly larger

Table III *Drug Interactions with Laxatives*

Laxative	Drug	Result of interaction
Danthron	Docusate	a case of hepatotoxicity has been reported
Mineral oil	Oral anticoagulants	alterations in anticoagulant effect due to possible decreased absorption of vitamin K
	Vitamins	possible reduction of vitamin A, D, E, K absorption
	Docusate	absorption of mineral oil may be increased
Saline laxatives	Tetracyclines	cations may combine with tetracycline to form complexes that are not readily absorbed
Magnesium salts	Digoxin	pharmacologic effect of digoxin may be decreased due to possible reduced digoxin bioavailability

Constipation and Laxatives

Table IV *Laxative Agents*

Classification and drug	Daily dosage range		Onset of action	Systemic absorption
	Adult	Pediatric (age in years)		
Bulk forming agents				
methylcellulose	1–6 g	1–1.5 g (>6)	24–72 hr	no
psyllium	12–30 g (3 divided doses)	1.5–15 g (>6)	24–72 hr	no
polycarbophil	4–6 g (4 divided doses)	not recommended (<3)	24–72 hr	no
Osmotic agents				
magnesium citrate	15 g (300 mL) (bowel preparation)		0.5–3 hr	yes
magnesium hydroxide	25–50 mL		0.5–3 hr	yes
magnesium sulfate	10–30 g (in 250 mL of water)		0.5–3 hr	yes
sodium phosphate-biphosphate compound	20–45 mL (in half glass cool water)		5–30 min	yes
lactulose	15–60 mL (10 g/15 mL)	5–10 mL (<1)	24–48 hr	no
Stimulant (contact) laxatives				
Anthraquinlone				
cascara sagrada			6–12 hr	yes
tablets	300 mg	150 mg (2–12)		
fluid extract	0.5–1.5 mL			
aromatic fluid extract	5 mL	2.5 mL (2–12)		
danthron	37–150 mg	not recommended (<12)	6–8 hr	yes
sennosides A&B	12–24 mg	3–6 mg (2–5) 6–12 mg (6–12)	8–12 hr	yes
Diphenylmethane				
bisacodyl — oral	5–15 mg	5 mg (>6)	6–12 hr	yes
— rectal	10 mg	10 mg (>6)	15–60 min	
phenolphthalein	30–100 mg	30–60 mg (>6) 15–20 mg (2–5)	6–8 hr	yes
Castor oil	15–60 mL	5–15 mL (2–12) 1–5 mL (<2)	2–6 hr	yes
Emollient laxatives				
docusate calcium	50–500 mg		24–72 hr	yes
docusate sodium	50–300 mg	40–120 mg (6–12) 20–60 mg (3-6) 10–40 mg (<3)	24–72 hr	yes
Lubricants				
mineral oil	15–45 mL		6–8 hr	yes

doses or more potent agents to relieve constipation. Vigorous purgation may produce a paradoxical diarrhea complicated by water and electrolyte depletion.

Pharmacists should be aware that laxatives may be abused for reasons other than a constipation problem. Patients with eating disorders, for example, bulimia, may abuse laxatives for weight control.

The importance of re-establishing regular bowel habits without the use of laxative agents should be stressed to laxative abusers. Bowel retraining takes time, and the person requires constant encouragement and reassurance to refrain from returning to the laxative habit. The following measures are suggested to aid people suspected or known to misuse laxatives:

- Discontinue use of all laxatives.
- Consume larger quantities of fluids and high-fibre foods (for example, vegetables, fruits and cereals).
- If required initially, use a bulk-forming laxative to supplement fibre in the diet.
- Attempt defecation at the same time each day, about 30 minutes after a meal.
- If required, use a glycerin suppository or saline enema to promote initial colonic activity.
- Exercise regularly to promote colonic activity.
- Do not ignore the urge to defecate. Psychiatric support may be necessary in some cases.

Laxative Use in Preparation for Diagnostic Procedures

The colon must be thoroughly cleansed prior to certain gastrointestinal diagnostic procedures such as colonoscopy. To achieve bowel evacuation, various protocols are used. Patients are required to adhere to a clear liquid or low-residue diet 24 hours prior to the procedure. Osmotic or stimulant laxatives are taken by the patients during the preparation period to produce catharsis and consequently, bowel evacuation. Bowel evacuation products are not to be used for routine treatment of constipation.

Several colon electrolyte lavage solutions have been introduced on the Canadian market. They are osmotically balanced electrolyte solutions which contain polyethylene glycol, potassium, bicarbonate, chloride, and sodium sulfate as the predominant salt. The presence of polyethylene glycol in these solutions acts as an osmotic agent to prevent significant water or electrolyte changes when large volumes are ingested. The usual recommended oral adult dose is 240 mL every 10 minutes until approximately 4 L is consumed. The colon is cleansed usually within 4 hours. The most frequent adverse effects include nausea, abdominal fullness and bloating. Colon electrolyte lavage solutions are a safe and effective alternative to other cleansing methods.

Summary

Constipation is a common problem among the Western population. It is important to evaluate the severity of the problem before recommending treatment. In most cases, implementing a diet rich in fibre, increasing fluid intake and increasing physical activity alleviates the condition. If these general measures are not sufficient, and consultation with a physician rules out organic causes such as neoplasms or polyps, drug therapy can be recommended. This recommendation should be based on the type and severity of the constipation, the person's age and the physiopathological conditions present.

Ask the Consumer

Q. What is the usual pattern of your bowel movements? How has it changed and since when? Have you been examined recently by your physician?

- The normal frequency of bowel movements varies from one individual to another. It is important to ask about the consistency of stools and the effort required to pass them to determine whether the person is truly constipated.

Q. Are you experiencing any other symptoms, such as nausea, vomiting, cramps, abdominal pain, weight loss, rectal bleeding or straining during defecation?

- Nausea, vomiting, cramps, abdominal pain and distension may indicate appendicitis or paralytic ileus. Rectal bleeding may indicate the presence of inflammatory bowel diseases. Black stools indicate a blood loss from the upper gastrointestinal tract. If these symptoms are present, refer the person to a physician immediately. In these cases, laxatives are contraindicated. Inappropriate laxative use can mask symptoms and hinder proper medical diagnosis.

Q. Are you currently being treated for any acute or chronic illness? If so, what medication are you taking?

- A person with a history of intestinal disorders or other illnesses associated with constipation should not self-medicate. If the person suffers from certain chronic conditions, such as congestive heart failure, hypertension or chronic renal insufficiency, choosing a laxative requires consideration because of the electrolyte content of some laxative preparations. Drug therapy may also cause constipation, and some people may require the occasional use of a mild laxative.

Q. Have you changed your diet or daily routine recently?

- Constipation can be precipitated by changes in diet, environmental changes, travel and stressful situations. It is important to establish the probable cause of constipation, so a rational approach to management can be recommended. Education regarding prevention of constipation through proper diet, fluid intake and exercise may be required. It is important to stress that laxatives should not normally be used to maintain regular bowel habits.

Q. Have you attempted to relieve your constipation?

- It is important to determine whether appropriate therapeutic measures have been taken.

Q. Have you used a laxative before? If yes, was it effective? How long have you used it?

- It is important to know if the person has already experienced constipation and has used a laxative. The prolonged use of laxatives may produce an atonic colon and severe chronic constipation. If this type of laxative is used, advise the person of the inherent hazards in this practice, as well as suggesting nondrug measures to maintain regular bowel movements.

References

Introduction

Akdamar K, Maumus LT. Management of constipation in the elderly. Geriatrics 1984;39(12):81–3.

Brunton LL. Laxatives. In: Gilman AG, Goodman LS, Rall TW, Murad F. Goodman and Gilman's the pharmacological basis of therapeutics. New York: Macmillan, 1985:994-1003.

Burkitt DP, Trowell HC. Refined carbohydrate foods and disease. London: Academic Press, 1975.

Connell AH, Hilton C, Irvine G, et al. Variation of bowel habits in two population samples. Br Med J 1965;2:1095–9.

Constipation and Laxatives

Deyroede GA. Common sense approach to overcoming constipation. Drug Ther 1978;8:113–7.

Drossman DA, Sandler RS, McKee DC, Lovitz AJ. Bowel patterns among subjects not seeking health care. Use of a questionnaire to identify a population with bowel dysfunction. Gastroenterology 1982;83:529–32.

Erle HR. Constipation. Primary Care 1976;3:301–10.

Klein H. Constipation and fecal impaction. Med Clin North Am 1982; 66:1135–41.

Painter NS. Constipation. Practitioner 1980;224:387–91.

Pietrusko RG. Use and abuse of laxatives. Am J Hosp Pharm 1977;34:291–300.

Rendtorff RC, Kashgarian M. Stool patterns of healthy adult males. Dis Colon Rectum 1967;10:222–8.

Thompson WG. Laxatives: clinical pharmacology and rational use. Drugs 1980; 19:49–58.

Thompson WG, Heaton KW. Functional bowel disorders in apparently healthy people. Gastroenterology 1980;79:283–8.

Bulk-forming Agents

Anonymous. Health News. Toronto: Faculty of Medicine, University of Toronto, 1991;9(2):2.

Anonymous. Calcium polycarbophil (Mitrolan). Med Lett Drugs Ther 1981; 23:52.

Biggs JS, Vesey EJ. Treatment of gastrointestinal disorders of pregnancy. Drugs 1980;19:70–6.

Brodribb AJM. Treatment of symptomatic diverticular disease with a high-fibre diet. Lancet 1977;1:664–6.

Fingl E. Laxatives and cathartics. In: Goodman LS, Gilman A, eds. Goodman and Gilman's the pharmacological basis of therapeutics. New York: Macmillan, 1975:976–86.

Fisher RE. Intestinal obstruction due to psyllium seeds. CA Wes Med 1938;48:190.

Goff S, Grelis ME, Child PG, et al. In vitro effect of a hydrophilic polycarbophil resin on the activity of some digestive enzymes. Fed Proc 1955;14:344.

Ivy AC, Isaacs BL. Karaya gum as a mechanical laxative. An experimental study on animals and man. Am J Dig Dis 1938;5:315–21.

Kallman H. Constipation in the elderly. Am Fam Physician 1983;27(1):179–87.

Maesner JE, Huckendubler-Stephenson S, Johnson MA. Psyllium hydrophilic mucilloid allergic reactions. Drug Intell Clin Pharm 1986;20:548.

Mendeloff AI. Dietary fiber and human health. N Engl J Med 1977;297:811–4.

Parks TG. Diet and diverticular disease. Proc R Soc Med 1974;67:1037–40.

Wand SP. Fecal impaction due to hygroscopic gum laxative. Am J Dig Dis 1940;7:297–8.

Osmotic Laxatives

Abelson WH, Smith RG. Residents handbook of pediatrics—The Hospital for Sick Children, Toronto, Canada. 7th ed. Toronto: BC Decker Inc, 1987:164.

Anonymous. Lactulose (Chronulac) for constipation. Med Lett Drugs Ther 1980;22:2–4.

Bennett A, Eley KG. Intestinal pH and propulsion: an explanation of diarrhoea in lactase deficiency and laxation by lactulose. J Pharm Pharmacol 1976; 28:192–5.

Chesney RW, Haughton PB. Tetany following phosphate enemas in chronic renal disease. Am J Dis Child 1974;127:584–6.

Harvey RF, Read AE. Mode of action of the saline purgatives. Am Heart J 1975;89:810–2.

Kaupeke C, Sprague T, Gitnick GL. Hypernatremia after administration of lactulose (Letter). Ann Intern Med 1977;86:745–6.

Levitt M, Gessert C, Finberg L. Inorganic phosphate poisoning resulting in tetany in an infant. J Pediatr 1973;82:479–81.

McConnel TH. Fatal hypocalcemia from phosphate absorption from laxative preparation (Letter). JAMA 1971;216:147–8.

Mordes JP, Swartz R, Arky RA. Extreme hypermagnesemia as a cause of refractory hypotension. Ann Intern Med 1975;83:657–8.

Stimulant Laxatives

Ammon HV, Thomas PJ, Phillips SF. Effects of oleic and ricinoleic acids on net jejunal water and electrolyte movement. Perfusion studies in man. J Clin Invest 1974;53:374–9.

Anderson PO. Drugs and breast feeding. Semin Perinatol 1979;3:271–8.

Anonymous. Laxative recall. Can Pharm J 1987;120(6):405.

Binder HJ. Pharmacology of laxatives. Ann Rev Pharmacol Toxicol 1977; 17:355–67.

Cass JC, Frederik WS, Montilla E. Phenolphthalein: a review of the medical literature and controlled evaluation of its use as a laxative in the treatment of chronic constipation. Curr Ther Res Clin Exp 1965;7:571–89.

Clain J, Novis BH, Bank S, et al. Cathartic colon with unusual histological features. South Afr Med J 1974;48:216–8.

Drug information for the health care provider. Rockville: United States Pharmacopeial Convention, 1987.

Frame B, Guiang HL, Frost HM, et al. Osteomalacia induced by laxative (phenolphthalein) ingestion. Arch Intern Med 1971;128:794–6.

Gaginella TS, Phillips SF. Ricinoleic acid: current view of an ancient oil. Am J Dig Dis 1975;20:1171–7.

Lewin KJB. Phenolphthalein reaction simulating disseminated (systemic) lupus erythematosus (Letter). Lancet 1962;2:461.

McNeely MD. Drug interference with routine urinalysis. Drug Ther 1974; 4:79–81.

Saunders DR, Sillery J, Rachmilewitz D, et al. Effect of bisacodyl on the structure and function of rodent and human intestine. Gastroenterology 1977;72:849–56.

Savin JA. Current causes of fixed drug eruptions. Br J Dermatol 1970;83:546–8.

Travell J. Pharmacology of stimulant laxatives. Ann Acad Sci 1954;58:416–25.

Wilson JT, Brown RD, Cherek DR, et al. Drug excretion in human breast milk: principles, pharmacokinetics and projected consequences. Clin Pharmacokinet 1980;5:1–66.

Wittoesch JH, Jackman RJ, McDonald JR. Melanosis coli: general review and a study of 887 cases. Dis Colon Rectum 1958;1:172–80.

Emollient Laxatives

Dujovne CA, Shoeman DW. Toxicity of a hepatotoxic laxative preparation in tissue culture and excretion in bile in man. Clin Pharmacol Ther 1972; 13:602–8.

Tolman KG, Hammar S, Sannella JJ. Possible hepatotoxicity of doxidan. Ann Intern Med 1976;84:290–2.

Lubricant Laxatives

Becker GL. The case against mineral oil. Am J Dig Dis 1952;19:344–8.

Blewitt RW, Bradbury K, Greenhall MJ, et al. Hepatic damage associated with mineral oil deposits. Gut 1977;18:476–9.

Freiman DG, Engelberg YH, Merrit WH. Oil aspiration (lipoid) pneumonia in adults; a clinicopathologic study of 47 cases. Arch Intern Med 1940; 66:11–38.

Gennaro AR, ed. Remington's pharmaceutical sciences. Pennsylvania: Mack Publishing Company, 1990:788,1323.

Reynolds JEF, ed. Martindale the extra pharmacopoeia. London: The Pharmaceutical Press, 1989:1322–3.

Suppositories

Bloom A. Suppositories. Practitioner 1971;206:85–90.

Enemas

Kemp R. Enemas. Practitioner 1971;206:81–4.

Page SG Jr, Riley CR, Haag HB. A comparative clinical study of several enemas. JAMA 1955;157:1208–10.

Drug Interactions

Hart LL. Constipation and diarrhea. In: Katcher BS, Young LY, Koda-Kimble MA, eds. Applied therapeutics, the clinical use of drugs. San Francisco: Applied Therapeutics, 1983:101–15.

Kastrup EK, ed. Facts and comparisons. St Louis: JB Lippincott, 1987.

Treatment in Different Age Groups

Feeding babies—a counselling guide on practical solutions to common infant feeding questions. Health and Welfare Canada, 1986.

Constipation and Laxatives

Lamy PP, Krug BH. Review of laxative utilization in a skilled nursing facility. J Am Geriatr Soc 1978;26:544–9.

Olney L. Constipation in childhood. Am Fam Physician 1976;13:85–9.

Treatment During Pregnancy and Lactation

Greenhalf JO. Laxatives in the treatment of constipation in pregnant and breastfeeding mothers. Practitioner 1973;210:259–63.

Treatment of Laxative Abuse

Cooke WT. Laxative abuse. Clin Gastroenterol 1977;6:659–73.

Cummings JH, Slader GE, James OF, et al. Laxative-induced diarrhea: a continuing clinical problem. Br Med J 1974;1:537–41.

Vanin JR, Saylor KE. Laxative abuse: a hazardous habit for weight control. J Am Coll Health 1989;37(5):227–30.

Laxative Use in Preparation for Diagnostic Procedures

Anonymous. Current drug topics. Metrodis, Sunnybrook Medical Centre, Toronto, Ontario, 1986;5(3):4–5.

Gossel TA. The growing market for colonic lavage kits. US Pharmacist 1989;14(4):44,51.

22
Antidiarrheals

Dawn M. Frail

Pathophysiology of the intestinal tract often involves imbalances in fluid absorption and secretion, causing diarrhea. Among the causes of diarrhea are diet, infection, drugs, and psychological and physiological factors. Treatment, which may be specific, supportive or symptomatic, depends on whether the diarrhea is acute or chronic. Supportive therapy—the replacement of lost fluid and electrolytes—is always required. Specific therapy generally involves the use of prescription drugs and is only possible when the cause of the diarrhea is known and is amenable to therapy. Nonprescription products used for symptomatic therapy include adsorbents, absorbents, anticholinergics, antiperistaltics and lactobacillus preparations.

Diarrhea, one of the most common disorders experienced by man, has been studied enough to determine its etiology and most rational treatment. However, the disorder is difficult to define for two major reasons: it is a symptom of a number of completely different conditions and presents in various ways; and normal bowel function varies widely among individuals as frequency of bowel movements can range from 3 times daily to 3 times weekly in normal adults. Diarrhea is clinically defined as an increase in frequency, fluidity and volume of bowel movements for the individual. The significant feature is the change in bowel habit rather than the absolute number of bowel movements, volume or consistency.

Pathophysiology

Diarrhea is a disturbance in the balance between the absorption of water and electrolytes from the lumen of the intestinal tract and the secretion of fluid into the lumen. Under normal conditions about 9 L of fluid enter the gastrointestinal (GI) tract from an individual's diet, saliva, gastric juice, bile, pancreatic juice and small intestinal secretions. All but about 500 mL of this fluid is reabsorbed before it reaches the colon, and a further 350 mL are reabsorbed in the colon. The result of a normal digestive and absorptive process in a healthy adult is a stool weighing 100 to 200 g, of which 60 to 85 per cent is water.

The production of a normal stool depends on the balance between GI fluid secretion and absorption. Fluid secretion and absorption are both regulated by solute movement.

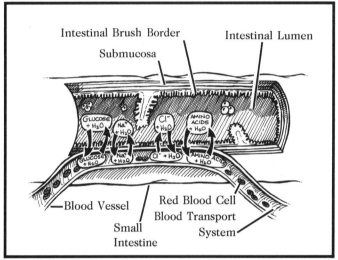

Figure 1 *Fluid Absorption*

Fluid Absorption

Most fluid is absorbed through the villous epithelial cells although some probably passes through the intercellular junctions. Transcellular fluid absorption is linked to solute movement because the passage of solutes across the basolateral membrane causes an increase in the osmotic pressure in the intercellular space. This elevated osmotic pressure pulls fluid from the lumen across the villous epithelial cells and into the submucosa. As solutes such as sodium, chloride, glucose, and amino acids are absorbed, water is absorbed with them. (see Figure 1.) Neutral sodium-chloride absorption is inhibited both by cyclic adenosine monophosphate (c-AMP) and by high intracellular concentrations of calcium. It is thought the constipating side effect of calcium channel blockers is due to the maintenance of low intracellular calcium concentrations secondary to calcium channel blockade. Without calcium inhibition, the absorption of sodium and chloride plus water is enhanced.

Fluid Secretion

Although absorptive processes take place in the villous cells, the crypt cells are thought to be responsible for secretion. The mechanism of chloride secretion from crypt cells is not fully understood, but fluid secretion is linked to it. Compatible with the role of c-AMP and calcium in absorption, chloride secretion is increased both by c-AMP and high intracellular calcium concentrations.

Etiology

Diarrhea results when the balance between fluid absorption and secretion in the GI tract is disrupted. Although an alteration in intestinal motility contributes to the diarrheal state, it is rarely the primary cause. The relationship of smooth muscle activity, propulsion and absorption of GI contents is complex and poorly understood. Reduced fluid absorption or increased fluid secretion can cause large fluid loads in the intestinal lumen. The large fluid load, in turn, causes accelerated transit, thus aggravating an already unbalanced situation.

Since diarrhea is a symptom arising from a number of diverse causes, it is best described by its etiology.

Diet

Diet can be responsible for diarrhea via a number of mechanisms. Spicy foods or chemical irritants such as those found in unripe apples and sour milk may irritate the intestinal mucosa, thereby interfering with its normal functions. Excessive coffee drinking can cause diarrhea and may be the result of the inhibition of phosphodiesterase by methylxanthine, with the consequent elevation of intracellular c-AMP.

Foods often cause an osmotic diarrhea. Osmotic diarrhea occurs with an increase in water-soluble, poorly absorbed solutes in the intestinal lumen. The osmotic pressure created causes an excessive water influx into the duodenum and jejunum. The severity of the diarrhea depends on the ability of the ileum and colon to absorb the excess fluid. A water deficit, rather than electrolyte loss, is the major consequence of osmotic diarrhea. Foods such as vegetables and fruits which contain indigestible fibers may provoke this type of diarrhea.

Osmotic diarrhea can also be the result of a disaccharidase deficiency in the intestinal brush border, particularly a deficiency of the lactose-digesting enzyme lactase. When milk or other lactose-containing products are ingested, lactose hydrolysis is inadequate. The disaccharidase remains in the intestinal lumen, causing retention of water. A lactose deficiency often appears in early adulthood and is most common in Blacks, Asians, Jews and American Indians. A lactose deficiency can also occur temporarily during and following most acute infective diarrheas.

Other sugars that can cause osmotic diarrhea are fructose and sorbitol. Sorbitol is commonly used as a sweetener for sugarless candy. Eating large amounts of such candies has resulted in diarrhea. Apple juice, sometimes recommended as a treatment for diarrhea because of its pectin content, can actually aggravate the condition in the small number of children who suffer from carbohydrate malabsorption. Apple juice contains glucose, fructose, sucrose and sorbitol, which are osmotic diarrheal agents.

Infant diarrhea can accompany weaning from breast to cow's milk due to alterations in the intestinal microbial flora. The new source of milk carries new microorganisms to which the infant has to adjust. This problem can be minimized by using sterilized milk.

Infection

The major cause of acute diarrhea is gastroenteritis, an inflammation of the GI tract caused by bacterial, viral, fungal or parasitic infections. Of these, bacterial pathogens appear to be the major cause of diarrhea in adults and children over 2 years old. The bacterial pathogens can be classified as noninvasive or invasive. (see Table I.)

Noninvasive bacteria, as their name implies, do not damage the gut mucosa directly. They produce enterotoxins that increase the secretion of GI fluid and electrolytes. At a cellular level, this increased

Table I *Bacterial Causes of Acute Diarrhea*

Organism	Onset (hours)	Source
Noninvasive bacteria		
Vibrio cholerae	24–72	Water, shellfish
Escherichia coli	24–72	Direct contact
Clostridium perfringens	8–16	Inadequately cooked meat
Staphylococcus aureus	4–12	Food poisoning
Invasive bacteria		
Shigella	24–72	Direct contact in poor hygienic environment
Salmonella	12–36	Poultry, egg products, raw milk
Vibrio parahaemolyticus	24–72	Raw or cooked fish, shellfish, salad, meat, vegetables
Campylobacter fetus	2–10 days	Poultry, meat, milk, contact with infected animals or people

secretion is probably due to toxin-induced activation of adenylate cyclase in crypt cells, thus causing a secretory diarrhea because of the increased levels of c-AMP. The mechanism by which toxins activate adenylate cyclase is unknown but may involve the stimulation of prostaglandin biosynthesis. Prostaglandins are thought to be mediators of intestinal secretion. The increased c-AMP also inhibits sodium chloride absorption, further compounding the problem. However, the absorptive processes for other solutes, such as glucose and amino acids, remain intact. For this reason, oral glucose rehydration solutions remain effective supportive therapy. Noninvasive bacteria include *Vibrio cholerae*, some strains of *Escherichia coli*, *Clostridium perfringens* and *Staphylococcus aureus*.

Escherichia coli, which is part of the normal flora of the GI tract, is of particular interest because of its role in traveller's diarrhea. It is spread by the fecal-oral route, usually through contaminated food or drinking water. *Clostridium perfringens* and *Staphylococcus aureus* are the major causes of food poisoning. Staphylococcal food poisoning results from eating food contaminated with staphylococci that produce enterotoxin-B. *Clostridium perfringens* food poisoning results from eating meat containing clostridial spores. Clostridial spores can be killed by adequate cooking, but if they enter the GI tract in a viable state, they proliferate and produce enterotoxins.

The bacteria that invade and damage the mucosal tissue account for a small percentage of all acute diarrheal illnesses. Because of the destructive nature of these bacterial infections, there is usually GI inflammation, exudation of serum and blood, impairment of absorption and passive secretion of fluids. Besides direct invasive mechanisms, these bacteria may also produce enterotoxins that contribute in some minor way to the diarrheal state. Most of these organisms have been implicated in the pathogenesis of traveller's diarrhea but generally in conjunction with *Escherichia coli* which remains the major cause. The direct invasive type of infectious diarrhea is more likely to produce fever, abdominal pain and rectal bleeding than is toxin-mediated diarrhea. The presence of these symptoms calls for consultation with a physician. Shigellosis is the most serious of these infections, but is responsive to antibacterial therapy.

Table I lists the bacteria often involved in acute diarrhea, the time of onset of symptoms and the source of infection.

Bacterial pathogens are the major cause of infective diarrheal illness in adults and children over age two, but infections due to the rotavirus are the most common cause of infective diarrhea in younger children.

The mechanism of viral diarrhea is uncertain, but it is believed the absorptive villous epithelium is replaced by secretory crypt epithelium.

Fungal and parasitic infections are generally responsible for only a small percentage of all diarrheal episodes. However, *Cryptosporidium*, a parasite associated with GI and respiratory tract infections in animals, is second only to the rotavirus as a cause of diarrhea at certain times of the year and in certain geographic locations. A Canadian report suggested *Cryptosporidium* be considered a possible cause for summertime diarrhea in children under age six who live in an area where this organism is known to occur.

The dramatically increased incidence of the acquired immune deficiency syndrome (AIDS) has stimulated considerable research. People with AIDS commonly experience diarrhea. Although it is now known that this diarrhea has an infectious etiology, the causative agents are diverse and include *Shigella*, *Campylobacter*, *Giardia lamblia*, *Escherichia histolytica*, *Chlamydia trachomatis*, *Herpes simplex* and *Neisseria gonorrhoeae*.

Drugs

Diarrhea is a common side effect of drugs. In addition to laxatives and magnesium-containing antacids, drugs that induce diarrhea include antibiotics (tetracycline, ampicillin, penicillin, erythromycin, sulfonamides, trimethoprim-sulfamethoxazole, cephalosporins, chloramphenicol, lincomycin and clindamycin), nonsteroidal anti-inflammatory agents, guanethidine, methyldopa, digoxin, quinidine, colchicine and antimetabolites.

Antibiotic-induced diarrhea is common but usually mild. The mechanism is not well understood. Although many antibiotics are mild GI tract irritants, antibiotic-induced diarrhea probably results from suppression of the normal flora, thereby allowing enteropathogenic organisms to proliferate. Withdrawing the antibiotic to allow recolonization of normal gut flora usually eliminates the problem. However, antibiotics may cause a more serious type of diarrhea known as "pseudomembranous colitis." Clindamycin and lincomycin are well known as potential causes of pseudomembranous colitis. The estimated incidence of clindamycin-induced colitis varies widely, from 1 in 10 to 1 in 100,000. Although it occurs more often in females, all age groups may be affected, and an underlying illness or state of debilitation is not a prerequisite. Neither total dose nor duration of therapy can be correlated with onset, duration or severity of colitis. The important point is that onset may not occur until several days or weeks after the therapy is discontinued, and an individual may not associate the diarrhea with the antibiotic.

Almost any antimicrobial can cause pseudomembranous colitis but, next to clindamycin and lincomycin, ampicillin and the cephalosporins (particularly cefotaxime) are implicated most frequently.

Antibiotic-induced pseudomembranous colitis is due to an enterotoxin-producing organism, *Clostridium difficile*. This organism normally forms a minor part of the intestinal flora, but proliferates under certain circumstances during treatment with antibiotics. Metronidazole and oral vancomycin are the drugs of choice to eliminate the organism and improve the condition. However, the condition can recur when metronidazole or vancomycin are discontinued.

Laxatives, by nature of their action, can cause diarrhea. When laxatives are used appropriately, diarrhea does not occur. Laxative abuse by groups such as anorexics and bulimics introduces a whole new problem. (See the chapter on eating disorders.) These individuals use laxatives regularly to accelerate weight loss or counteract binge eating. This use of laxatives is representative of the laxative abuse syndrome (LAS). Because of the self-induced, covert nature of LAS, it is difficult to diagnose and treat. Pharmacists may be in a good position to identify these people through observation of purchasing practices and counselling. These individuals should be referred to a physician, because long-term laxative abuse can cause cathartic colon.

Psychological Factors

Emotional stress, especially anticipation of a disturbing event, is a common cause of mild diarrhea. The emotional stress triggers excessive stimulation of the parasympathetic nerves which results in an increase in GI motility and secretion into the large intestine.

Physiological Conditions

Diarrhea is associated with various physiological conditions such as malabsorption syndromes, pancreatic insufficiency, biliary tract disorders, hypoparathyroidism, diabetes mellitus, ulcerative colitis, carcinoma of the intestinal tract and cirrhosis. After gastric surgery, pyloric dysfunction is common and an osmotic diarrhea occurs because hypertonic stomach contents are rapidly dumped into the duodenum.

Acute versus Chronic Diarrhea

Pharmacists should be able to distinguish between acute and chronic diarrhea, recognizing their causes, symptoms and complications. Any diarrhea lasting more than a few days or occurring intermittently should be investigated by a physician. Likewise, people complaining of blood or mucus in the stool should consult a physician. Chronic diarrhea should never be treated symptomatically. In most cases it can be treated specifically once the cause is determined. Non-prescription antidiarrheals are recommended only for acute, self-limiting cases of diarrhea.

Treatment

Three types of therapy exist for diarrhea: specific, supportive and symptomatic.

Symptomatic therapy is recommended only for acute self-limiting diarrhea, possibly accompanied by loss of appetite, abdominal cramps, nausea and vomiting. Any symptoms suggesting a more serious underlying cause should be referred to a physician. The age and condition of the individual must also be considered. Acute diarrhea is usually only an inconvenience or embarrassment in otherwise healthy adults, but it can be dangerous in elderly or debilitated persons, pregnant women, patients with a medical history of chronic illness and children younger than 3 years of age.

Specific Therapy

Specific therapy is rational only when the cause of the diarrhea is known and amenable to therapy. For example, antibiotics are not generally indicated for acute bacterial diarrhea because they do not shorten the illness; they may even encourage the development of resistant bacterial strains. Antibiotics may also cause diarrhea as a side effect.

Traveller's diarrhea can be treated specifically. The effectiveness of treatment, however, depends on how promptly treatment is started when symptoms occur. The most common regimens recommended are 160 mg of trimethoprim and 800 mg of sulfamethoxazole, 200 mg of trimethoprim alone or 100 mg of doxycycline twice daily for 3 days.

A number of prophylactic regimens have been recommended for traveller's diarrhea. Those requiring antibiotics should be reserved for high-risk travellers for whom the benefit of prophylaxis outweighs the risk of antibiotic resistance and adverse drug reactions. Chemoprophylactic regimens include 160 mg of trimethoprim and 800 mg of sulfamethoxazole, 100 mg of doxycycline, 200 mg of trimethoprim alone, 500 mg of ciprofloxacin or 400 mg of norfloxacin taken daily. A prophylactic regimen using bismuth subsalicylate, a nonprescription drug, is effective for 65 per cent of travellers. However, it requires the traveller to take 60 mL or 2 tablets of the bismuth subsalicylate product (Pepto-Bismol) four times daily. More importantly than drug prophylaxis is the avoidance of foods and liquids that carry the causative bacteria. Conscientious selection of low risk foods and drinks is the best prophylactic measure.

Other causes of diarrhea and their specific treatment include giardiasis and amebiasis, treated with drugs; carcinoma of the colon, with surgery; and ulcerative colitis, with drugs or surgery. For most cases of acute diarrhea, the cause is not determined and the condition cannot be treated specifically.

Supportive Therapy

Supportive therapy is the most important approach to treating diarrhea. The goal is to control the secondary effects, for example, fluid and electrolyte loss. These effects are critical in infants and young children, who are more susceptible to dehydration because they have a greater rate of water turnover in relation to total body water than do adults.

Controversy surrounds the correct procedure for replacing fluid. Starving a child or adult has no rationale. Even during diarrhea the body absorbs about 60 per cent of normal nutrients. A bland diet (for example, toast, crackers, applesauce and bananas) offered in small, frequent amounts does not aggravate the diarrhea. Milk should be withheld for several days because in many cases of acute infectious diarrhea, a temporary lactase deficiency develops. The physician may often prescribe a lactose-free, soy-based formula for infants with diarrhea. For adults, it is probably sufficient to consume water, juice, gelatin products, carbohydrate and electrolyte soft drinks, and clear soups. Decarbonated soft drinks have been recommended as rehydration solutions, but recent evidence does not support this application. For example, cola drinks have an osmolarity that is far too high and an electrolyte content far too low to be suitable for rehydration.

For young children, rehydration is not as simple. In the past, mothers were directed to prepare salt solutions, but this practice is now discouraged because of the possibility of sodium overload from incorrectly prepared solutions. The success of oral rehydration solutions in developing countries has resulted in reevaluating the role of these solutions as a general supportive therapy for diarrhea.

The World Health Organization (WHO) rehydration formula has been used in developing countries since the 1960s (see Table II). Its use was first justified by the finding that sodium absorption through the intestinal mucosa was coupled with glucose and this mechanism remained intact in the presence of cholera. Since water is absorbed along with sodium, rehydration occurs. Still, there was some reluctance to use an oral preparation for infants in developed countries because many physicians wondered whether an infant could drink the volumes of fluid necessary for rehydration therapy, especially if vomiting was present. During the 1970s a number of studies confirmed that most infants can be rehydrated safely by the oral route even if vomiting is present, provided the oral rehydration solution is given in small, frequent feedings. Although most physicians accepted oral rehydration therapy, there were still debates about the composition of the WHO formula. Many American pediatricians feared the sodium content was too high for rehydration of infants suffering from noncholera-induced diarrhea because the sodium loss in these individuals was considerably less than in cholera sufferers. Formulas with a lower sodium content were proposed, but have not been shown to have any benefit over the WHO formula. The WHO formula was revised in 1984 and now contains trisodium citrate instead of sodium bicarbonate (see Table II). The citrate-containing solution is more effective in correcting acidosis and has made the product more stable for storage under conditions of high humidity and temperature.

Table II *Oral Rehydration Solutions for Fluid Replacement in Acute Diarrhea*

	WHO (original)	WHO (revised 1984)
Sodium (mEq/L)	90	90
Chloride (mEq/L)	80	80
Potassium (mEq/L)	20	20
Bicarbonate (mEq/L)	30	–
Citrate (mEq/L)	–	30
Glucose (mEq/L)	111	111

An alternative formula developed and adapted for use by the Center for Disease Control (U.S. Department of Health and Human Services) is easier to prepare in the home and is more suitable for use in developed countries (see Table III). The concentrations of electrolytes are only about half those in the WHO formula and the formula is readily available and inexpensive. A number of dextrose-electrolyte solutions are also available commercially and provide a convenient, consistent source of fluid and electrolyte replacement.

In most cases of acute diarrhea, adults can be rehydrated merely by drinking more fluids or the fluids suggested in Table III. Children less than 3 years of age can also be managed this way if the diarrhea has been present for less than 24 hours and there are no signs of dehydration such as sunken fontanelles, dry mucous membranes, absence of tears, decreased urine output, tachycardia, poor skin turgor and poor responsiveness. If dehydration is suspected, this therapy may be recommended as a stop-gap measure only until a physician can be consulted.

Table III *Home Treatment of Acute Diarrhea*

Glass I	Glass II
240 mL orange, apple or other fruit juice (source of K+)	240 mL tap water (preferably boiled and cooled)
2.5 mL honey or corn syrup (glucose)	1.25 g baking soda (NaHCO₃)
1 pinch salt (NaCl)	

Directions: One glass of each is prepared and taken alternately. Supplement with other fluids.*

*These dextrose-electrolyte solutions may also be obtained commercially.

Symptomatic Therapy

Nonprescription drugs are used for symptomatic therapy. The goal of symptomatic therapy is to stop or reduce the severity of diarrhea by decreasing the frequency, or increasing the consistency, of bowel movements. The therapy merely alleviates the inconvenience of diarrhea; although the stools appear more formed, the fluid and electrolyte loss is not reduced and the underlying pathology remains unchanged. Since fluid and electrolyte losses may be masked and the severity of the condition underestimated, these agents should not be used in pregnant women or in children less than 3 years of age and should only be used with caution in elderly or debilitated persons. It is questionable whether these agents should be used at all, because acute diarrhea is believed to be a normal defense mechanism to rid the body of toxic substances. By trying to stop the diarrhea, the toxic condition may persist.

Nonprescription antidiarrheal preparations contain ingredients classified as adsorbents/absorbents, astringents, anticholinergics, antiperistaltics, lactobacillus preparations and miscellaneous agents. It is important to remember that these preparations provide only symptomatic treatment. Supportive therapy (fluid and electrolyte replacement) must also accompany the treatment of the symptoms.

Pharmaceutical Agents
Adsorbents/Absorbents

Kaolin, a native hydrated aluminum silicate, is classified as an adsorbent and protectant. Although kaolin has been used to treat diarrhea since ancient times, no controlled studies have established its effectiveness. Kaolin is believed to adsorb bacteria, viruses and toxins and thereby reduce the severity of diarrhea. However, early in vitro studies showed it was not an efficient adsorbent. Kaolin may also increase the resistance of intestinal flow by solidifying the colon's contents, although this has not yet been demonstrated. The American Medical Association has stated that if any action is attributable to the adsorbents, it is probably a mild water-binding effect. However, kaolin is considered safe in the usual dose of 12 to 24 g. In Canada, kaolin is found only in combination with pectin.

Pectin, a purified carbohydrate product, is obtained from the dilute acid extract of the inner portion of the rind of citrus fruits and apple pomace. Chemically, it consists of partially methoxylated, polygalacturonic acids. Its exact mechanism as an antidiarrheal is unknown, but it is believed to have adsorbent and protectant properties, to prolong gastric emptying and, perhaps, to have an antibacterial effect by decreasing the pH of the intestine.

The combination of **kaolin and pectin in suspension** is a common antidiarrheal agent. The proportions are usually 20 to 25 per cent kaolin and one per cent pectin. Although the combination has shown some effectiveness in animal studies, it has not been proven effective in humans although it does appear safe. One clinical study evaluated the effectiveness of a kaolin-pectin mixture in treating acute diarrhea. When compared to kaolin alone, pectin alone, diphenoxylate-atropine liquid combination and a placebo, the kaolin-pectin product produced stools that tended to be more formed than those in placebo-treated individuals. However, no difference existed among any of the products in their effect on frequency of bowel movements or water content and weight of the stools. Most cases of diarrhea disappear spontaneously whether treated or not.

Activated attapulgite occurs naturally as magnesium aluminum silicate and is produced by thermal treatment of its hydrous counterpart. Such treatment increases its adsorptive capacity. It is an effective adsorbent. It reduces the number of bowel movements, improves stool consistency and assists (when accompanied by other agents) in relieving cramps. Its usual dose is 6 to 9 g daily.

Hydrophilic agents such as polycarbophil, psyllium and methylcellulose have been used to treat diarrhea. Of these, polycarbophil, a polyacrylic resin, is the most effective hydrophilic agent, absorbing 60 times its weight in water. This agent is believed to absorb water from liquid stools as well as swelling and adding body to the feces. Calcium polycarbophil is used in the only Canadian product (Mitrolan) that contains a hydrophilic agent and is specifically indicated for diarrhea. The calcium salt is used because it can be formulated as a more pharmaceutically acceptable product than polycarbophil. With the calcium salt, calcium ions are replaced by hydrogen in the gastric acid, but this does not make calcium polycarbophil superior to polycarbophil. The effective dose for calcium polycarbophil is 4 to 6 g daily for adults or 1.5 g daily for children 6 to 12 years of age.

Polycarbophil is safe and well tolerated. Intestinal obstruction, which has been reported with most bulk-forming agents, is possible. Consequently, polycarbophil should not be used in people with obstructive bowel disease or in children less than 3 years old.

Recent reports indicate that hydrophilic agents are useful in the symptomatic treatment of chronic diarrhea and for individuals with ileostomies.

Activated charcoal was once thought to bind bacteria, toxins and gas because of its large available surface area. However, these effects have not been demonstrated when treating diarrhea.

Aluminum hydroxide gel is an adsorbent and can cause constipation. It is in fact, used as an antidiarrheal in combination with magnesium-containing antacids to counteract the diarrhea caused by the latter.

Astringents

Bismuth compounds in Canadian products include bismuth subsalicylate and bismuth oxycarbonate. Their exact mechanism of action is not known but they are thought to bind bacterial toxins and/or precipitate protein, thereby decreasing cell permeability in the intestine. Furthermore, in the case of bismuth subsalicylate, the salicylate portion may have an antidiarrheal action since it inhibits prostaglandin synthesis, and prostaglandins may be mediators of intestinal secretion. Evidence to support this theory comes from a study in which acetylsalicylic acid successfully treated diarrhea caused by radiotherapy. However, caution should be exercised in recommending these products to treat children or anyone sensitive to salicylates. Bismuth subsalicylate-containing products can produce

plasma salicylate levels approximating those observed after an analgesic dose of acetylsalicylic acid. Bismuth absorption appears to be
minimal.

As discussed earlier, bismuth subsalicylate is used in the
prophylaxis of traveller's diarrhea. It is also used for the symptomatic
treatment of traveller's diarrhea but has not been shown to be quite
as effective as loperamide for this indication.

Bismuth compounds are converted to bismuth trisulfide in the
intestine and color the stools black. Under certain conditions, this
same reaction can occur in the mouth, producing a disturbing black
discoloration of the oral cavity.

Anticholinergics

Anticholinergics (for example, atropine sulfate, hyoscine hydrobromide and hyoscyamine sulfate) are found in several nonprescription
antidiarrheals. No controlled studies support their effectiveness. Theoretically, they block cholinergic-mediated increases in GI motility.
However, their inclusion in antidiarrheals is questionable because
the relationship between intestinal motility and diarrhea is uncertain. Intestinal motility is decreased only by doses that cause other
adverse effects, so the doses present are too low to be of any value.
Anticholinergics might relieve intestinal spasm and pain, but again,
not in such low doses.

Safety is a major concern with these agents. Children less than
6 years of age are especially susceptible to anticholinergic effects.
People with narrow-angle glaucoma, asthma, chronic obstructive pulmonary disease, heart disease or enlarged prostate are also at risk.

Antiperistaltics

Loperamide is a synthetic opioid that does not penetrate into the
CNS and is therefore devoid of the CNS side effects of the opiates.
Like the opiates, it does inhibit peristaltic activity by acting on the
longitudinal and circular muscles of the intestinal tract. It is an especially effective agent for treating traveller's diarrhea because it provides relief from the cramping. Loperamide should be used cautiously
in patients with infectious diarrhea because slowing intestinal
motility may, in fact, give the organisms more opportunity to invade
and injure the mucosa. The usual adult dose for loperamide is 4 mg
initially followed by 2 mg after each unformed stool to a maximum
of 16 mg per day. Children's doses of loperamide are dependent on
the child's age and weight and should be administered only on the
advice of a physician. The maximum dose in children 2 to 5 years
of age (10 to 20 kg) is 1 mg three times daily; in children 5 to 8 years
of age (20 to 30 kg), 2 mg twice daily; and in children 8 to 12 years
of age (greater than 30 kg), 2 mg three times daily.

Lactobacillus Preparations

Products containing *Lactobacillus acidophilus* or *Lactobacillus bulgaricus* have been promoted as aids for restoring normal intestinal
flora when diarrhea is caused by pathogenic organisms which replace
the normal flora. Most support for the efficacy of these products
comes from case reports or uncontrolled trials. The few controlled
trials show no evidence of efficacy. It has been suggested that yogurt
and buttermilk can be as effective as these lactobacillus preparations.
At this time it is unclear whether lactobacillus preparations are effective or ineffective.

Miscellaneous Agents

A number of other ingredients appear in Canadian nonprescription
antidiarrheal products. Either no scientific or sound theoretical basis
exists for these ingredients or they have never been evaluated as
antidiarrheals. These ingredients are largely obtained from plants.
Tannic acid, rhubarb, wild strawberry leaves and hypericum all have
astringent properties. Rhubarb is also a laxative. Althea is a demulcent and emollient used to treat irritation and inflammation of the
mucous membranes of the mouth and pharynx. Ammonia is used
internally for its restorative action. Aniseed and valerian are carminatives. Ginger is a carminative that is added occasionally to purgatives
in the belief that it prevents abdominal spasms. Blackberry root bark
was used by North American Indians to arrest vomiting and diarrhea.
No evidence exists that any of these agents are useful in treating
diarrhea.

Drug Interactions

Antidiarrheal agents can reduce absorption of other drugs from the
intestine. This effect presumably occurs because of adsorption of the
drug by the antidiarrheal or by an alteration in gut transit time. These
interactions were observed when a kaolin-pectin mixture was given
concurrently with each of lincomycin, clindamycin and digoxin.

The lincomycin-kaolin-pectin interaction is considered clinically
significant. Since there is a high incidence of diarrhea in people
taking lincomycin, they could easily be taking both agents. The GI
absorption of lincomycin is reduced by as much as 90 per cent when
a kaolin-pectin mixture is given concurrently. Kaolin-pectin mixtures
should be avoided during lincomycin therapy or taken at least 2 hours
before or 3 or 4 hours after lincomycin.

Since clindamycin is chemically similar to lincomycin, it was
hypothesized that its absorption might also be reduced by a kaolin-
pectin mixture. However, in one study, the antidiarrheal mixture
reduced the rate but not the extent of clindamycin absorption. This
finding is not surprising since the GI absorption of clindamycin is
not reduced by food as is the absorption of lincomycin.

The concurrent administration of a kaolin-pectin suspension with
a single dose of digoxin resulted in reductions of 41 per cent and
62 per cent in the total amount of digoxin absorbed. When the antidiarrheal mixture was given 2 hours before the digoxin dose there
was no effect on absorption, but when given 2 hours after, absorption was reduced by 20 per cent. This interaction may be avoided
by separating the administration times.

Another possible drug interaction involves absorption of salicylate
from products containing bismuth subsalicylate. People on oral
anticoagulants, sulfinpyrazone, probenecid or any other medications
for which salicylates are contraindicated, should not be given
products containing bismuth subsalicylate.

Although few drug interactions have been reported for nonprescription antidiarrheals, it is wise to avoid giving adsorbent antidiarrheals
concurrently with any other medication.

Summary

If a case of diarrhea is acute and self-limiting and there are no contraindications, an antidiarrheal product may be recommended. It is
best to recommend only rehydration fluids, but if the consumer
insists on a product, the most appropriate choices are calcium polycarbophil, activated attapulgite or loperamide. For traveller's diarrhea,
bismuth subsalicylate preparations can be recommended for
prophylaxis and treatment or loperamide preparations for treatment
only. Special instructions for these products include the following:
• Shake liquid products well before using.

Figure 2 *Suggested Approach for Treating Diarrhea*

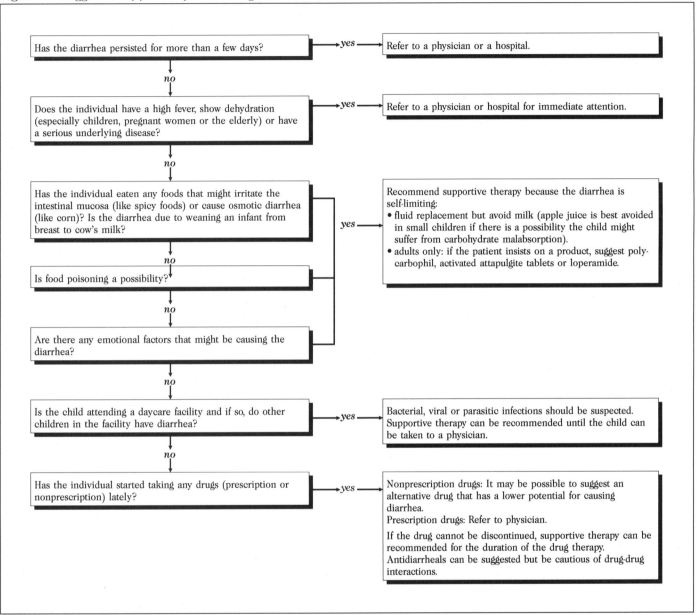

- Do not use products any longer than 2 days without consulting a physician.
- Do not be alarmed if the stools turn black with the bismuth sub-salicylate preparation.
- Continue rehydration fluids while taking medications.
- It is best to avoid cow's milk for a few days.

Additional sources of information:
- *Don't drink the water.* Available from the Canadian Public Health Association, 1565 Carling Avenue, Suite 400, Ottawa, Ontario K1Z 8R1.
- Drinking water purification for travellers. Compendium of Pharmaceuticals and Specialties (CPS) 27 edition (1992), page B91–2.

Ask the Consumer

Q. Is the product for yourself? If not, how old is the person?
- If the person using the product is between 6 and 60 years of age an antidiarrheal may be appropriate, depending on the answers to the other questions. Do not recommend antidiarrheals for children less than 3 years of age. Counsel parents about maintaining adequate hydration. If a child shows signs of dehydration such as tachycardia, poor skin turgor and absence of sweat or tears, a physician should be consulted immediately. The same precautions apply to elderly people. For a child between the ages of 3 and 6 years, it may be appropriate to recommend an antidiarrheal agent, but avoid products containing anticholinergic

ingredients. Anticholinergics should also be avoided by the elderly.

Q. *How long have you had the condition?*
- This question helps determine whether the condition is chronic or acute (and probably self-limiting). Any condition present for more than a few days should not be treated with an antidiarrheal product. It should be investigated by a physician.

Q. *Do the stools contain any blood, pus or mucus, or are they black and tarry?*
- Presence of blood, which may present as a black and tarry stool, usually indicates an inflammatory, infectious or neoplastic disease. It may also indicate the presence of hemorrhoids or an anal fissure. In any event, the person should contact a physician immediately.

Q. *What other symptoms are you experiencing?*
- A person reporting vomiting (which indicates additional fluid loss) or fever should be referred to a physician immediately.

Q. *Have you changed your diet recently?*
- This question is important. In the case of an infant, a formula change may cause diarrhea. Normally the infant adjusts quickly. Likewise, in adults, diarrhea may be associated with certain foods, for example, milk, which may indicate a lactose intolerance.

Q. *Do other people you know have the same symptoms? Did you eat food that might have been contaminated (for example, dairy products, potato salad or warmed-over meat)?*
- Affirmative answers suggest food poisoning, which is usually self-limiting.

Q. *Have you recently travelled to a foreign country?*
- This question helps determine if the condition is traveller's diarrhea.

Q. *Are you currently taking or have you recently taken prescription or nonprescription drugs?*
- A number of nonprescription drugs including laxatives and magnesium-containing antacids may cause diarrhea. Laxatives should be discontinued, and the antacid doses replaced or alternated with a constipating antacid, such as aluminum hydroxide gel. If the consumer is taking a prescription drug, such as a broad-spectrum antibiotic, a nonsteroidal anti-inflammatory agent, guanethidine, methyldopa, digitalis or colchicine, the physician should be consulted immediately. The drug probably will be substituted with another drug or the diarrhea treated symptomatically. Diarrhea and pseudomembranous colitis may appear after such antibiotics as clindamycin and lincomycin are discontinued. A medication history can also determine the presence of any condition or chronic illness, such as diabetes, heart condition or pregnancy, which might make self-medication for diarrhea inadvisable.

References

Introduction
Connell AM, Hilton C, Irvine G, et al. Variation of bowel habit in two population samples. Br Med J 1965;2:1095–9.
Cummings J. Treatment of diarrhea in adults. Prescr J 1977;17:27–39.

Gangarosa EJ. Recent developments in diarrheal diseases. Postgrad Med 1977;62(2):113–7.
Jeejeebhoy KN. Symposium on diarrhea. I. Definition and mechanisms of diarrhea. Can Med Assoc J 1977;116:737–9.
Low-Beer TS, Read AE. Diarrhoea: mechanisms and treatment. Gut 1971; 12:1021–36.
Phillips SF. Diarrhea: a current view of the pathophysiology. Gastroenterology 1972;63(3):495–518.
Phillips SF. Diarrhea: pathogenesis and diagnostic techniques. Postgrad Med 1975;57(1):65–72.

Fluid Absorption
Binder HJ. The pathophysiology of diarrhea. Hosp Pract 1984;19(10):107–18.

Fluid Secretion
Krejs GL, Fordtran JS. Physiology and pathophysiology of ion and water movement in the human intestine. In: Sleisenger MH, Fordtran JS, eds. Gastrointestinal disease: pathophysiology, diagnosis, management. Toronto: WB Saunders, 1977:313–5.

Diet
Babb RR. Coffee, sugars, and chronic diarrhea. Postgrad Med 1984; 75(8):82–7.
Hyams JS, Leichtner AM. Apple juice: an unappreciated cause of chronic diarrhea. Am J Dis Child 1985;139(5):503–5.
Lipin R. Outbreak of diarrhea linked to dietetic candies—New Hampshire. JAMA 1984;252(13):1672.
Morley A, Blenkinsopp J, Nicholls JR, Nicholls JL. Treating diarrhoea. Pharm J 1986;237(6392):164–5.
Pietrusko RG. Drug therapy reviews: pharmacotherapy of diarrhea. Am J Hosp Pharm 1979;36:757–67.
Sadik F. Antidiarrheals. Pharmindex 1985;27(11):8–15.
Turnberg LA. Coffee and the gastrointestinal tract. Gastroenterology 1978; 75(3):529–30.

Infection
Anonymous. The patient with gastroenteritis: module 1. Epidemiology and etiology of acute diarrhea. Am Pharm 1986;26(6):79–82.
Anonymous. Campylobacter enteritis (Editorial). Lancet 1978;2:135–6.
Anonymous. Advice for travelers. Med Lett Drugs Ther 1990;32(815):33–6.
Bissenden JG. Cryptosporidium and diarrhea. Br Med J 1986;293:287–8.
Blaser MJ, Berkowitz ID, LaForce FM, et al. Campylobacter enteritis: clinical and epidemiologic features. Ann Intern Med 1979;91:179–85.
Blaser MJ. Current approach to acute diarrheal illnesses. Drug Ther 1983; 13(2):114–26.
Bradshaw MJ, Harvey RF. Antidiarrhoeal agents: clinical pharmacology and therapeutic use. Drugs 1982;24:440–51.
Carpenter CCJ. Mechanisms of bacterial diarrheas. Am J Med 1980; 68(3):313–6.
Edwards LA. Symposium on diarrhea. 6. Infectious diarrhea. Can Med Assoc J 1977;116:753–5.
Fingl E, Freston JW. Antidiarrhoeal agents and laxatives: changing concepts. Clin Gastroenterol 1979;8:161–85.
Grady GF, Keusch GT. Pathogenesis of bacterial diarrheas (first of two parts). N Engl J Med 1971;285(15):831–41.
Laudano JB, Patton LR. Traveler's diarrhea. Pharm Times 1986;52(7):96–107.
Montessori GA, Bischoff L. Cryptosporidiosis: a cause of summer diarrhea in children. Can Med Assoc J 1985;132(11):1285.
Satterwhite TK, DuPont HL. The patient with acute diarrhea: an algorithm for diagnosis. JAMA 1976;236(23):2662–4.
Skirrow MB. Campylobacter enteritis: a "new" disease. Br Med J 1977;2:9–11.
Tolle SW, Elliot DL. The evaluation and management of acute diarrhea. West J Med 1984;140(2):293–7.

Drugs
Anonymous. Treatment of *Clostridium difficile* diarrhea. Med Lett Drugs Ther 1989;31(803):94–5.

Bartlett JG, Chang TW, Gurwith M, et al. Antibiotic associated pseudo-membranous colitis due to toxin-producing clostridia. N Engl J Med 1978;298:531–4.

Bytzer P, Stokholm M, Anderson I, Klitgaard NA, Schaffalitzky de Muckadell OB. Prevalence of surreptitious laxative abuse in patients with diarrhoea of uncertain origin: a cost benefit analysis of a screening procedure. Gut 1989;30(10):1379–84.

Dhar GJ, Soergel KH. Principles of diarrhea therapy. Am Fam Physician 1979;19(1):164–173.

George WL, Sutter VL, Goldstein EJC, et al. Aetiology of antimicrobial-agent-associated colitis. Lancet 1978;1:802–3.

George RH, Symonds JM, Dimock F, et al. Identification of as a cause of pseudomembranous colitis. Br Med J 1978;1:695.

Hoberman LJ, Eigenbrodt EH, Kilman WJ, et al. Colitis associated with oral clindamycin therapy: a clinical study of 16 patients. Am J Dig Dis 1976;21:1–17.

Keighley MR, Burdon DW, Arabi Y, et al. Randomised controlled trial of vancomycin for pseudomembranous colitis and postoperative diarrhoea. Br Med J 1978;2:1667–9.

Nolan N, Tighe B, Cooney C, O'Briain DS. Cefotaxime and pseudomembranous colitis. Lancet 1985;2(8460):888.

Rifkin GD, Fekety FR, Silva J Jr, et al. Antibiotic-induced colitis implication of a toxin neutralised by Clostridium sordellii antitoxin. Lancet 1977;2:1103–6.

Smith ER, Goulston SJ. Antibiotic-induced diarrhoea. Drugs 1975;10(5):329–32.

Tedesco FJ. Clindamycin-associated colitis. Review of the clinical spectrum of 47 cases. Am J Dig Dis 1976;21:26–32.

Tedesco F, Markham R, Gurwith M, et al. Oral vancomycin for antibiotic-associated pseudomembranous colitis. Lancet 1978;2:226–8.

Vargas J. Sorting out the causes of vomiting and diarrhea. Emerg Med 1988;20(3):138–42,145,148,153,156.

Psychological Factors
Sadik F. Diarrhea therapy. Pharmindex 1989;31(7):7–16.

Treatment
Anonymous. Oral fluids for dehydration. Med Lett Drugs Ther 1987;29(743):63–4.

Anonymous. Nonprescription antidiarrheal drugs. Fed Reg 1986;51:16138.

Anonymous. Water with sugar and salt (Editorial). Lancet 1978;2:300–1.

Bell DR. Diseases of the alimentary system: acute diarrhoea in adults. Br Med J 1976;2:1240–2.

Chatterjee A, Mahalanabis D, Jalan KN, et al. Oral rehydration in infantile diarrhoea. Arch Dis Child 1978;53:284–9.

Chatterjee A, Mahalanabis D, Jalan KN, et al. Evaluation of a sucrose/electrolyte solution for oral rehydration in acute infantile diarrhoea. Lancet 1977;1:1333–5.

Gossel TA, Wuest JR. Antidiarrheals. US Pharmacist 1982;7(7):19–23.

Guay DRP. Traveler's diarrhea. Am Drug 1990;202(2):88,90.

Hatcher G. Diarrhoea. Br Med J 1976;1:571–3.

Hirschhorn N, Kinzie JL, Sachar DB, et al. Decrease in net stool output during intestinal perfusion with glucose-containing solutions. N Engl J Med 1968;279(4):176–81.

Ho G, Grant D. Diarrhea—pathophysiology and treatment. On Cont Pract 1988;15(3):29–38.

Isaacson EL, Delgado JN. Nonprescription antidiarrheal agents. Pharmindex 1979;21:13–5.

Jacknowitz AI. Traveler's diarrhea. US Pharmacist 1986;11(7):10–20.

Lin AYF, Mangione RA. Update on the management of infectious diarrhea. Pharm Times 1988;54(7):138–49.

Mazumder RN, Nath SK, Ashraf H, Patra FC, Alam AN. Oral rehydration solution containing trisodium citrate for treating severe diarrhoea: controlled clinical trial. Br Med J 1991;302(6768):88–9.

Merson MH. Oral rehydration therapy—from theory to practice. WHO Chron 1986;40(3):116–8.

Pierce NF, Hirschhorn N. Oral fluid: a simple weapon against dehydration in diarrhoea. How it works and how to use it. WHO Chron 1977;31(3):87–93.

Randall DL. Therapy of acute diarrheal diseases in children. Drug Ther 1973;3:77–88.

Sack DA, Chowdhury AMAK, Eusof A, et al. Oral hydration in rotavirus diarrhoea: a double blind comparison of sucrose with glucose electrolyte solution. Lancet 1978;2:280–5.

Salazar-Lindo E, Sack RB, Chea-Woo E, et al. Bicarbonate versus citrate in oral rehydration therapy in infants with watery diarrhea: a controlled clinical trial. J Pediatr 1986;108(1):55–60.

Santosham M, Daum RS, Dillman L, et al. Oral rehydration therapy of infantile diarrhea: a controlled study of well-nourished children hospitalized in the United States and Panama. N Engl J Med 1982;306(18):1070–6.

Santosham M, Reid R. Diarrhoea management. World Health 1986;April:8–9.

Stanaszek WF, Campbell G. Case studies in pharmacy practice: pediatric vomiting and diarrhea. US Pharmacist 1978;3:22–4.

Weizman Z. Cola drinks and rehydration in acute diarrhea (Letter). N Engl J Med 1986;315(12):768.

Kaolin
Alestig K, Trollfors B, Stenqvist K. Acute non-specific diarrhoea: studies on the use of charcoal, kaolin-pectin and diphenoxylate. Practitioner 1979;222:859–62.

Gunnison JB, Marshall MS. Adsorption of bacteria by inert particulate reagents. J Bacteriol 1937;33:401–9.

Moss JN, Martin GJ. Adsorption of bacterial toxins by inert particulate materials. Am J Dig Dis 1950;17:18–9.

Pectin
Leeds AR, Ralphs DNL, Ebied F, et al. Pectin in the dumping syndrome: reduction of symptoms and plasma volume changes. Lancet 1981;1:1075–8.

Nalin DR. Treatment of diarrhea (Letter). JAMA 1977;237(19):2035–6.

Portnoy BL, DuPont HL, Pruitt D, et al. Antidiarrheal agents in the treatment of acute diarrhea in children. JAMA 1976;236(7):844–6.

Hydrophilic Agents
Anonymous. Calcium polycarbophil (Mitrolan). Med Lett Drugs Ther 1981;23(11):52.

Rutledge ML, Willner MM, Clayton JM. Clinical comparison of calcium polycarbophil and kaolin-pectin suspensions in the treatment of acute childhood diarrhea. Curr Ther Res 1978;23(4):443–7.

Bismuth Compounds
Anonymous. Salicylate in Pepto-Bismol. Med Lett Drugs Ther 1980;22(15):63.

Feldman S, Chen SL, Pickering LK, et al. Salicylate absorption from a bismuth subsalicylate preparation. Clin Pharmacol Ther 1981;29:788–92.

Johnson PC, Ericsson CD, DuPont HL, et al. Comparison of loperamide with bismuth subsalicylate for the treatment of acute travelers' diarrhea. JAMA 1986;255(6):757–60.

Mennie AT, Dalley VM, Dinneen LC, et al. Treatment of radiation-induced gastrointestinal distress with acetylsalicylate. Lancet 1975;2:942–3.

Pickering LK, Feldman S, Ericsson CD, et al. Absorption of salicylate and bismuth from a bismuth subsalicylate-containing compound (Pepto-Bismol). J Pediatr 1981;99:654–6.

Anticholinergics
Gossel TA. Acute diarrhea. US Pharmacist 1988;13(5):82,84–6,88,90–1.

Miscellaneous Agents
Lewis WH, Elvin-Lewis MPF. Medical botany: plants affecting man's health. New York: J Wiley and Son, 1977.

Drug Interactions
Albert KS, Ayres JW, DiSanto AR, et al. Influence of kaolin-pectin suspension on digoxin bioavailability. J Pharm Sci 1978;67(11):1582–6.

Albert KS, DeSante KA, Welch RD, et al. Pharmacokinetic evaluation of a drug interaction between kaolin-pectin and clindamycin. J Pharm Sci 1978;67(11):1579–82.

Brown DD, Juhl RP. Decreased bioavailability of digoxin due to antacids and kaolin-pectin. N Engl J Med 1976;295(19):1034–7.

Wagner JG. Pharmacokinetics 1. Definitions, modelling and reasons for measuring blood levels and urinary excretion. Drug Intell Clin Pharm 1968; 2:38–42.

Travelling

Anonymous. Don't drink the water. Ottawa: Canadian Public Health Association, 1989.

Lynk AD. Advice for tropical travellers—a guide for the primary care physician. Drugs Ther Maritime Pract 1989;12(1/2):1–8.

23
Hemorrhoids

Revised by Betsy Miller. Based on the original chapter by Oksana I. Andrusiak

A good understanding of the anatomy of the anal canal and the pathogenesis of hemorrhoids is needed to develop a sound rationale for treatment. The four stages of hemorrhoids are distinguishable by their signs and symptoms. Pharmacologic agents to treat hemorrhoids include anesthetics, anti-inflammatory drugs, protectants, counterirritants and keratolytics, astringents, vasoconstrictors, anticholinergics, wound-healing agents and antiseptics in various delivery forms. Some surgical treatments are available under a physician's care.

Hemorrhoids, commonly called piles, have afflicted mankind since ancient times, yet they are poorly understood. Some researchers believe hemorrhoids are a pathological abnormality, but recent work suggests that they are a displacement of normal anorectal structures. Hemorrhoids affect both sexes equally, occurring with greatest frequency in persons between 20 to 50 years of age. More than 50 per cent of the adult population in North America has noticeable symptoms of piles.

Anatomy

The digestive tract terminates with the anal canal, which has a unique appearance. The lower third of the canal is smooth, but in the upper two-thirds, the mucosa is in longitudinal folds called the columns of Morgagni. The two zones meet at the pectinate line, at which point the typical large bowel epithelium abruptly changes to the stratified squamous epithelium of the marginal zone (see Figure 1).

The anal canal is surrounded by two sphincters, which control defecation. The external sphincter, located at the bottom of the anal canal, is under voluntary control. The internal sphincter, a muscle under autonomic control at the top of the anal canal, allows the passage of feces into the anal canal.

Blood to the anal canal is supplied by the superior, middle and inferior rectal arteries, which drain into the portal circulation through the superior rectal veins (see Figures 2 and 3). In the rectum and the anal canal, the veins run close to the arteries. Drainage occurs through two plexuses. The superior venous plexus lies above the pectinate line and is covered by the mucosa of the rectum and the upper anal canal. It drains into the portal system via the inferior mesenteric vein. The inferior venous plexus lies beneath the pectinate line underneath the anal skin and drains into the systemic circulation via the internal iliac veins. Since these two systems interconnect, the portal and systemic circulations are connected in the hemorrhoidal plexuses.

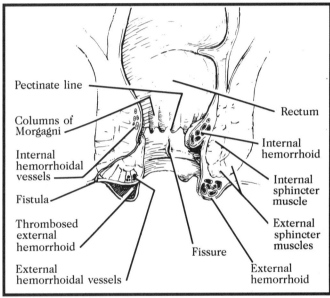

Figure 1 *Anal Canal*

Etiology

Hemorrhoids are often described as varicose veins in the anal canal or clusters of dilated blood vessels. However, neither of these two statements accurately define hemorrhoids. Hemorrhoids are not veins at all. They do not even look like varicose veins. Furthermore, the blood from them is bright red, not dark as one would expect from veins.

The normal anal submucosa consists of veins that have areas of dilatation. The dilated vessels are present at birth and are not a result of disease. Anal cushions are also present in the anal canal. These pads of thickened submucosa contain small arteries and dilated vessels. The anal cushions are found in the right anterior, right posterior and left lateral positions in the anal canal. They assist anal continence by acting "much as a soft washer in a tap." The veins in the cushions are supported by the Treitz muscle and elastic tissue, which also hold the cushions against the internal sphincter in the anal canal.

The attachment of the cushions to the wall of the anal canal is normally quite lax. With increasing age, the anchoring connective tissue fibres start to disintegrate, and the cushions loosen even more. The resulting congestion within the anal canal causes the cushions to

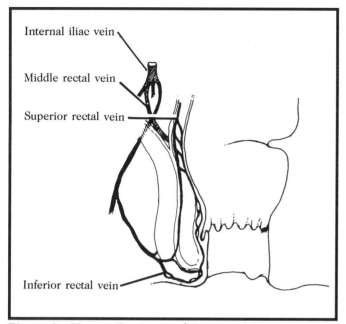

Figure 2 *Venous Drainage of Anorectal Region*

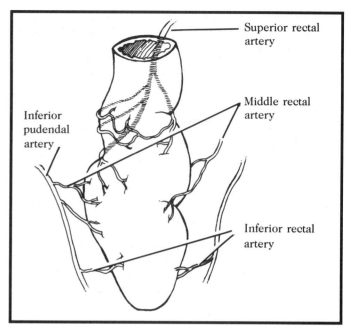

Figure 3 *Anterior View of the Arteries of the Rectum and Anal Canal*

hypertrophy and protrude further down. Thus, hemorrhoids are anal cushions that have been disrupted from their internal attachments.

The main cause of hemorrhoids is straining, usually as a result of constipation. When the individual tries to pass small, firm stools, the intrarectal pressure rises, blocking the venous return from the anal canal and leading to more straining. The shearing action of the fecal mass passing over the area causes a loosening of the underlying connective tissue. Diarrhea can also cause hemorrhoids, due to futile and protracted straining. Regular bowel movements help prevent hemorrhoids.

Other Causes

The suggestion that the human upright position has led to the development of hemorrhoids is unlikely. Hemorrhoids are not a universal problem, but are mainly an affliction of the western world. The condition seldom occurs in the rural populations of Asia and Africa.

Heredity is not an important factor in developing piles. The only connection between heredity and hemorrhoids is the similarity of diet and personal habits in members of the same family.

Hemorrhoids often develop during pregnancy, but pregnancy is not the cause. Pregnancy is now believed to precipitate the onset of hemorrhoids in susceptible women. The woman who experiences piles in the last few months of pregnancy may have become symptomatic due to increased abdominal pressure, allowing already existing piles to present themselves. Other possibilities are that during pregnancy there may be a softening of the elastic tissue that supports the anal cushions or that the woman may be more constipated, especially if she takes an iron supplement. In any case, these hemorrhoids usually resolve after parturition.

Stages of Hemorrhoids

Hemorrhoids may be classified according to their degree of formation. In the first stage, swelling occurs in the anal cushion due to straining. This swelling is seldom noticed by the sufferer, but can be observed by a physician during a rectal examination. First-degree

hemorrhoids are usually painless. However, the passage of hard stools may scrape the swollen cushions and produce slight bleeding, a signal that piles may be developing.

During the second stage, a small part of the anal mucosa or cushion may protrude at the anus during defecation. After the bowel movement, the elastic connective tissue draws the hemorrhoid back into the anal canal.

Third-degree hemorrhoids remain in the prolapsed position after defecation, but may be replaced manually within the anus.

Fourth-degree hemorrhoids cannot be replaced after a bowel movement, and thus create a permanent bulge at the anus. This condition is quite painful, and it is usually at this stage that people see their physician.

Symptoms

Pain, bleeding and protrusion are the major complaints of hemorrhoid sufferers. Other conditions that cause pain and may coincide with hemorrhoids are anal fissures, inflammation and blood clots. Blood clots occur when a vessel within the anal canal expands or bursts. This can occur anywhere along the anal canal or completely outside the anus within a permanently prolapsed pile. The cause is not known, but one possible explanation is that a prolapsed hemorrhoid was pinched by the external sphincter muscle of the anal canal, causing the rupturing of a blood vessel. If no other complications develop, the blood clot usually resolves spontaneously after about one week.

Bleeding is usually noticed as a bright red streak on toilet paper or on the surface of the stool. Blood may also spot the person's underclothing or drip after a bowel movement, especially when the individual is constipated. If the blood is dark in color or present in large amounts, other pathologies may be involved and a physician should be consulted promptly.

Another common complaint of the hemorrhoid sufferer is prolapse, a condition characterized by the protrusion of skin through the anus. Prolapse itself is not a dangerous condition, but may lead to other complaints such as soiling of a mucoid discharge, itching, ulceration, necrotization and false urges. False urges occur when the prolapsed hemorrhoids cause a sense of fullness within the anal canal. Individuals should avoid straining and should not remain on the toilet if they are unsure whether a real need to defecate exists.

Treatment
Nonpharmacological Measures
Hemorrhoids are found primarily in populations consuming the diet of the western world, a diet high in white flour, sugar and fibre-depleted carbohydrate foods. Fibre is the part of fruits, vegetables and whole grains that resists digestion in the gastrointestinal tract. The approximate daily intake of crude fibre in western countries is about 4 g; in some nonindustrialized countries, fibre intake can reach up to 30 g/day.

Fibre's capacity to hold water allows the formation of softer, bulkier stools that can pass through the colon more rapidly. Wheat bran fibre is most effective in relieving constipation; it is better than fibre found in fruits and vegetables because it is more concentrated. Since constipation and straining are major causes of hemorrhoids, increasing the daily intake of fibre by consuming a bran-containing cereal may help to alleviate hemorrhoids. Vegetables and fruits vary in their ability to absorb moisture. Carrots have the greatest absorption capacity of the vegetables, about half that of bran. Other high-absorption vegetables are brussels sprouts, eggplant, spring cabbage and corn. High-absorption fruits include apples, pears and oranges.

Adding fibre to the diet is usually adequate to relieve symptoms of piles in people with first and second degree hemorrhoids. When diet alone is not sufficient to relieve constipation, a stool softener or a bulk-forming laxative may be added.

The second most important preventive measure is good toilet habits. The rectal reflex should not be postponed, or it will weaken. The largest daily meal should be eaten at the same time each day, about 36 hours before a time available for a bowel movement. A healthy meal usually takes 36 hours to digest. One should not remain on the toilet more than 1 to 2 minutes. Straining should be avoided. Any prolapsed hemorrhoids must be replaced with a moistened tissue. After each bowel movement, the anorectal area should be cleaned with soap and water and wiped with a wet toilet tissue.

If these general measures do not relieve hemorrhoidal symptoms, the individual may be advised to use a sitz bath 3 to 4 times daily. A sitz bath consists of a tub of warm water (about 46°C) in which the individual sits for 15 minutes at a time. Plastic sitz baths may be fitted over the toilet seat rim for greater convenience.

Pharmacological Treatment
People are often hesitant or embarrassed to ask for advice about hemorrhoids. The pharmacist should initiate the discussion by asking pertinent questions, such as, "Have you been experiencing constipation?" and "Have you been experiencing any symptoms as a result of the constipation?" These questions will encourage the person to talk about the condition and seek the pharmacist's advice.

Medical treatment is generally symptomatic. A variety of products are available that claim to reduce bleeding and decrease pain and itch. These products may relieve the discomfort, however, the degree of relief attributable to a placebo effect has yet to be determined. Hemorrhoidal products are classified into groups based on the phamacological action of the active ingredients. Available preparations contain local anesthetics, anti-inflammatory agents, protectants,

counterirritants, astringents, vasoconstrictors, anticholinergics, wound-healing agents or antiseptics. The mechanism of action of each of these agents is discussed in the following pages. Available preparations provide only symptomatic relief; none are curative.

The safest compounds are the protectants, vasoconstrictors and some astringents. If not used for prolonged periods, some of the local anesthetics are relatively safe and may relieve pain.

Many of the commercially available hemorrhoidal products contain combinations of 2 or more active ingredients. Generally, there is no fixed limit on the number of ingredients as long as the combination is rational, safe and effective. Obviously, the same is not true for an irrational combination such as one which combines a local anesthetic with a counterirritant.

Local Anesthetics
Local anesthetics block nerve conduction in an effort to relieve itching, irritation and discomfort. Most local anesthetics are classified according to chemical structure into either esters or amides. The esters are usually more sensitizing than the amides. Of the esters, benzocaine and tetracaine are most capable of inducing contact dermatitis.

Local anesthetics may be used internally or externally. The safety of using these compounds intrarectally is not yet fully established. Local anesthetics can be absorbed systemically to a sufficient extent, especially if used intrarectally, to produce systemic toxicity, mainly of the central nervous system and the cardiovascular system. The pharmacist should recommend that products containing local anesthetics be used only in the perianal region or the lower anal canal.

The risk of adverse effects from the absorption of local anesthetics can be decreased by including a vasoconstrictor, for example, epinephrine or phenylephrine. As well as reducing toxicity, the vasoconstrictors increase the duration of action of the anesthetic by slowing down its absorption into the hemorrhoidal tissue.

Local anesthetics temporarily reduce the pain and itch associated with hemorrhoids. They should not be used more than 5 to 7 days at a time because of the danger of masking more serious conditions, such as anal fissures, cryptitis, fistulas, abscesses, and benign or malignant tumors of the lower colon or rectum. Some of the local anesthetics found in commercially available preparations are benzocaine, tetracaine, pramoxine, diperodon, dibucaine and lidocaine.

Benzocaine is an ester-type local anesthetic hydrolyzed in the body to p-aminobenzoic acid. To relieve pain, benzocaine ointment in concentrations of 5 to 10 per cent is used up to 6 times a day. It should not be used more than a few days at a time, because it may mask more serious disorders or result in further itching and irritation due to sensitization.

Benzocaine acts only while in contact with the mucous membrane. Nevertheless, absorption through the rectal mucosa may be rapid resulting in potentially toxic systemic effects. Consequently, application of products containing benzocaine should be restricted to areas below the rectum since drug absorption in the perianal region is poor.

Tetracaine is another ester-type local anesthetic, but it also has vasodilator properties. It is best used with a vasoconstrictor to reduce its rate of absorption and to decrease the risk of adverse effects. It is usually available as a 0.5 per cent ointment or a 1 per cent cream for painful conditions of the anorectal region.

Dibucaine is a local anesthetic of the amide type, suitable for surface or spinal anesthesia. Like tetracaine, it has vasodilator properties and is best used with a vasoconstrictor. The usual strengths found in hemorrhoidal preparations are 0.5 to 1 per cent in ointments and creams, and 2.5 mg in suppositories. Although dibucaine has fewer sensitizing characteristics than benzocaine, the possibility still exists for developing contact allergy in the perianal area.

Pramoxine is a topical anesthetic associated with low degrees of sensitization and toxicity. Structurally unrelated to the esters and amides, it may be useful for people sensitive to these classes of drugs. Pramoxine is applied locally as a 1 per cent cream for the discomfort and pain of hemorrhoids. It acts within 3 to 5 minutes and is applied up to 5 times a day. While less sensitizing than other local anesthetics, it may, as with all local anesthetics, cause allergic reactions.

Diperodon is also used in hemorrhoidal remedies, but some studies have found it ineffective. More research is needed to establish the safety and efficacy of diperodon and other local anesthetics, such as lidocaine, amylocaine and dibucaine, for both internal and external use.

Anti-inflammatory Drugs

Topical corticosteroids are often used in hemorrhoidal preparations to reduce the swelling of inflamed piles. Topical corticosteroids cause vasoconstriction, which reduces the seepage of fluid into interstitial spaces, thereby decreasing intercapillary distention. Corticosteroids also inhibit prostaglandin biosynthesis, which is important because prostaglandins upon release from damaged tissues can initiate an inflammatory response. Hydrocortisone acetate is the corticosteroid used in commercial hemorrhoid products.

Corticosteroids have been associated with several potential problems. First, they may mask signs of infection. Second, systemic absorption may be sufficient to cause adrenal suppression. Third, their antianabolic effects may actually slow the rate of wound healing due to impaired collagen synthesis. Topical application of corticosteroids can produce sensitization in some people.

Protectants

Protectant compounds provide a physical barrier to irritation by forming a protective layer over the mucous membranes lining the anorectal region, thus preventing excessive water loss from the tissues. This is important because drying of the area can intensify any itching, burning or pain already present.

Protectants are quite safe, because, with the exception of bismuth compounds, they are seldom absorbed through intact or broken skin or through mucous membranes. Commonly recommended protectants are aluminum hydroxide gel, kaolin, calamine, cocoa butter, lanolin, mineral oil, white petrolatum and zinc oxide. Cod and shark liver oils are also considered safe protectants.

Counterirritants and Keratolytics

Counterirritants are used to relieve pain and itch by providing a sensation of coolness, which distracts from the sensation of pain. They should not be used intrarectally, as the rectal mucosa does not contain any sensory nerve endings. A recommended counterirritant is menthol in concentrations of 0.25 to 1 per cent. At this strength, menthol may be safely applied externally up to 6 times a day. The main adverse effect of menthol is the potential for sensitivity reactions. Other counterirritants, such as camphor, hydrastis and oil of turpentine, are not recommended since they are considered unsafe or ineffective. Camphor quickly reaches toxic concentrations due to its high lipid solubility. Juniper tar requires further studies into its safety and effectiveness.

Keratolytics appear to have some value in reducing hemorrhoidal itch, but their exact mechanism of action is unknown. Two keratolytics recommended for external use are resorcinol and aluminum chlorhydroxyallantoinate. Allantoin may be applied up to 6 times daily in doses of 0.2 to 2 per cent ointment. Resorcinol as a 1 per cent to 3 per cent ointment may be used with the same frequency.

Astringents

Astringents are used to relieve the irritation and burning sensation of piles by protecting the underlying tissue. They are applied to the skin or mucous membranes. By coagulating proteins in the fluid between epidermal cells, astringents form a superficial protective layer. Their action is almost entirely limited to cell surfaces and the interstitial spaces of the skin and mucous membranes.

The most commonly used astringent is zinc oxide in concentrations of 5 to 25 per cent. It may be applied internally or externally up to 6 times daily after each bowel movement. Witch hazel (hamamelis water) 10 to 50 per cent is recommended for external use only and is available commercially as pads or wipes. These may also be used up to 6 times a day.

Vasoconstrictors

Vasoconstrictors are used temporarily to reduce swelling of hemorrhoidal tissue by constricting blood vessels. However, these products are not effective for itching and should not be used to control bleeding. If bleeding does occur, a physician should be consulted.

Three vasoconstrictors are recommended for external use. These are ephedrine sulfate, epinephrine hydrochloride and phenylephrine hydrochloride aqueous solutions, of which the first and the last mentioned may also be used intrarectally. Only ephedrine sulfate is found in nonprescription hemorrhoidal products. Ephedrine's recommended daily dosage is 2 to 25 mg applied up to 4 times daily. It has a quick onset of action, starting within 1 minute, and the effect lasts 2 to 3 hours.

Unpleasant side effects can occur following absorption of vasoconstrictors. These include increased blood pressure, cardiac arrhythmia, central nervous system disturbances, and aggravation of symptoms of hyperthyroidism. While significant absorption is not very likely when vasoconstrictors are used externally on intact skin, there is a possibility of systemic absorption following application of the drug to abraded and irritated skin.

Anticholinergics

Anticholinergic agents are claimed to act as counterirritants, but no evidence exists that they are effective as such in anorectal conditions. Furthermore, these drugs can be absorbed systemically to produce anticholinergic toxicity. These compounds should not be used in nonprescription hemorrhoidal preparations.

Wound-Healing Agents

No studies have yet found that wound-healing agents relieve hemorrhoidal symptoms. However, these agents claim to accelerate tissue healing and thus relief of symptoms may accompany healing. One substance found in Preparation H, a live yeast cell derivative (LYCD), has been extensively tested in in-vitro and in-vivo wound healing models. LYCD has been shown to stimulate oxygen consumption, increase angiogenesis, and promote collagen synthesis. Preparation H also contains vitamin A in the form of shark liver oil as another agent to promote wound healing. However, no acceptable evidence exists that LYCD or shark liver oil, alone or in combination, can reduce inflammation, cure infection or shrink hemorrhoids.

Antiseptics

The use of antiseptics such as boric acid, benzalkonium chloride, phenol and resorcinol in the anorectal region has been described as scientifically unsound, because an antiseptic's purpose is to inhibit microbial growth in the area where it is used. Although maintaining an aseptic anorectal area should promote healing, it is unlikely that antiseptics make much difference considering the large numbers of microorganisms normally present. It is advisable to keep the perianal area clean with soap and water; antiseptics should be regarded only as possible adjuncts to good personal hygiene. In addition, these agents are considered unsafe (for example, boric acid may produce toxicity) and have not been clearly shown to alleviate hemorrhoidal symptoms.

Delivery Forms

Hemorrhoidal preparations are available in a variety of dosage forms: creams, ointments, suppositories, aerosols and cleansing pads. Ultimately, the choice of delivery form lies with the consumer or physician. Many people prefer suppositories, but these products are often not effective because they tend to slip into the rectum and melt, thus bypassing the anal canal where the medication is needed. Suppositories with a multiple aperture tip may overcome this problem, but the possibility of self-inflicted trauma exists.

In general, creams and ointments are preferable to suppositories. They are easier to apply and usually contain the same or similar ingredients as suppositories. Aerosols may be simplest to use, but delivery tends to be erratic and thus ineffective.

Other Treatment

If drug treatment fails, the individual should be referred to a physician, who may consider one of the following five treatments.

In **sclerotherapy**, the hemorrhoid is injected with a solution of quinine and urea hydrochloride or 5 per cent phenol in almond oil. Sclerotherapy is effective for treating friable bleeding hemorrhoids. The injection results in inflammation and scarring of the pile, which subsequently causes its destruction. This form of treatment is rarely used.

In **rubber band ligation**, two elastic bands are placed over the pedicle of the pile. The aim is to cut off the blood supply and produce necrosis of the hemorrhoid and subsequent sloughing of the lesion. This procedure is indicated for internal hemorrhoids only, because any such procedure below the pectinate line would cause severe pain.

Anal dilatation is the forced dilatation of the anal canal and lower rectum under general anesthesia. It is used primarily for internal hemorrhoids. This procedure should not be used if the individual's main complaints are soiling, prolapse or incontinence, because it would aggravate these conditions while treating the symptoms of hemorrhoids.

Cryotherapy (freezing) may be used for both internal and external hemorrhoids. The pile is frozen using liquid nitrogen or carbon dioxide administered by a probe. The limitations to this method of therapy include foul, copious and prolonged anal discharge and a slow healing process. Cryotherapy is rarely used alone, but may occasionally be combined with rubber band ligation.

Figure 4 *Suggested Approach for Treating Hemorrhoids*

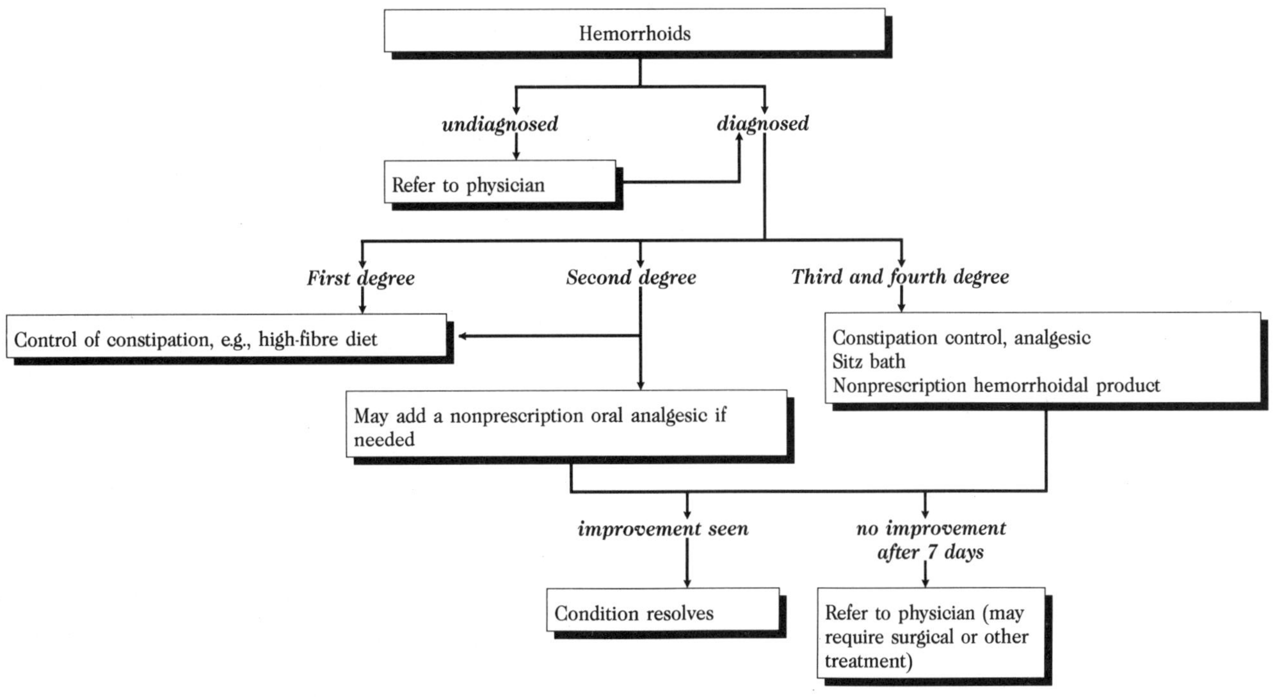

Another less invasive method of cryotherapy is the use of a specially designed device intended to apply controlled cooling to the anorectal tissue. Available without a prescription, Anurex is a reusable medical device that consists of a sealed probe unit slightly smaller than a little finger, filled with a cooling liquid. The probe is stored in the freezer in its vertical position. The patient is instructed to lubricate the probe and the anal area prior to insertion of the probe into the rectum. The probe is inserted and left in position for 6 to 8 minutes before being removed.

Hemorrhoidectomy surgery is generally reserved for treatment of hemorrhoids causing excessive pain and bleeding and resistant to other forms of treatment. A local anesthetic is applied and the hemorrhoid is dissected from the anus. Although the most effective technique, this procedure causes many complications, the worst of which is severe post-operative pain.

Summary

Although many products are available to relieve the symptoms of hemorrhoids, little evidence suggests that the treatment of symptoms has any significant effect on the condition. Since constipation and straining greatly contribute to the development of hemorrhoids, the simplest and cheapest way to prevent hemorrhoids is to add fibre-rich foods to the diet. Eating a daily serving of high-fibre cereal is perhaps the most convenient preventive measure. Fruits and vegetables also contain fibre, but in a less concentrated form; more is needed to achieve the same results as high-fibre cereal.

Laxatives should not be recommended to relieve constipation, as they may produce a state of dependence. Also, diarrhea may occur, which in turn may produce protracted straining and irritation, thereby worsening the condition of the developing hemorrhoids. Symptomatic treatment of hemorrhoids should be as conservative as possible, and precipitating factors such as long visits to the toilet should be avoided. The use of commercial hemorrhoid products should alleviate symptoms of pain, inflammation, burning and itching. If the symptoms persist after more than one week of self-treatment, consumers should see their physician for a more appropriate course of action.

Acknowledgement

Some of the information in this chapter first appeared in *On Continuing Practice*, 14(1):31–36;1987.

Ask the Consumer

Q. What are your symptoms and how long have you experienced them?

■ People with hemorrhoids often complain of pain and the appearance of bright red blood after a bowel movement. Diagnosed, uncomplicated hemorrhoids usually resolve quickly. When symptoms persist for more than one week, a physician should be consulted. If the blood is dark or present in large amounts, refer the individual immediately to a physician for a definitive diagnosis.

Q. Have you been straining at stool?

■ Constipation precipitates the development of hemorrhoids. If the individual has been straining at stool, advise that bowel habits be regulated through a high-fibre diet, adequate fluid intake and good toilet habits.

Q. Have you recently been pregnant?

■ Pregnancy, especially in the third trimester and at parturition, often precipitates hemorrhoids in previously well women. It is believed pregnancy only accentuates an existing problem. Hemorrhoids in these people usually resolve soon after parturition.

Q. Have you tried anything for this condition?

■ Knowing what products have been tried in the past aids in selecting a more appropriate preparation. Also, it may alert the pharmacist to a more serious problem.

References

Introduction

Baeton CGMI. Haemorrhoids, evaluation of methods of treatment. The Netherlands: Van Gorcum and Company, 1985:36–52.
Kaufman HD. The haemorrhoid syndrome. Tunbridge Wells: Abacus Press, 1981:19–33,51–5.

Anatomy

Holt RL. Hemorrhoids: cure and prevention. Tunbridge Wells: Abacus Press, 1980:3–119.
Mallet L. Hemorrhoids. In: Cyr JG, ed. Canadian self-medication. Ottawa: Canadian Pharmaceutical Association, 1984:83–7.
Wood C, ed. Haemorrhoids—current concepts on causation and management. London: Royal Society of Medicine, 1979:3–12.

Etiology and Other Causes

Alexander-Williams J. The nature of piles. Br Med J 1982:285:1064.
Gossel TA. Anorectal disorders. US Pharmacist 1985:10(8):23–4.
Haas PA, et al. The pathogenesis of hemorrhoids. Dis Colon Rectum 1984: 27:442–4.
McCormack TT, et al. Rectal varices are not piles. Br J Surg 1984:71:163.
Thomson H. Rectal disease—nonsurgical treatment of hemorrhoids. Br J Hosp Med 1980:24(4):298.

Treatment—Nonpharmacological Measures

Anonymous. The high fiber diet—its effect on the bowel. Med Lett Drugs Ther 1975:17(23):93.
Burkitt DP, Graham-Stewart CW. Haemorrhoids—postulated pathogenesis and proposed prevention. Postgrad Med J 1975:51:632.

Pharmacological Treatment

AMA drug evaluations. Toronto: WB Saunders, 1983:1337.
Anonymous. Getting to the seat of the problem. FDA Consumer 1980: 14(7):19–23.
Driscoll DF, DeFelice MD, Baptista RJ. Hemorrhoids: etiology and treatment. US Pharmacist 1981:6(5):43–58.
Gossel TA. Hemorrhoidal products. US Pharmacist 1989:14(7):37–42.
Parks J. Hemorrhoids. Can Pharm J 1969:102:67–70.
Thomson H. Piles: their nature and management. Lancet 1975:2:494–5.

Local Anesthetics

Anonymous. Med Lett Drugs Ther 1981:2(23):100.
Benowicz RJ. Non-prescription drugs and their side effects. New York: Grosset and Dunlap, 1977:82–7.
Gossel TA, Stansloski DW, et al. Consumer guide: nonprescription drugs. New York: Publications International, 1981:53–4.
Reynolds JEF, ed. Martindale: the extra pharmacopoeia. London: Pharmaceutical Press, 1982:287,899–902,909–10.
van Ketel WG. Contact allergy to different anti-hemorrhoidal anaesthetics. Contact Dermatitis 1983:9(6):512.

Anti-inflammatory Drugs

Seeman P, Sellers EM, Roschlau WHE, eds. Principles of medical pharmacology. Toronto: University of Toronto Press, 1980:424–5,430.

Stanaszek WF. Case studies in pharmacy practice—hemorrhoids. US Pharmacist 1978:3(3):15–9.

Wound-healing Agents

Anonymous. Med Lett Drugs Ther 1976:18(25):108.

Goodson W, et al. Augmentation of some aspects of wound healing by a "skin respiratory factor." J Surg Res 1976:21:125–9.

Minutes of OTC panel on haemorrhoidal drug products. Fed Reg 1980: 45(103):35653.

Delivery Forms

Carden ABG. Management of haemorrhoids and associated anorectal conditions. Drugs 1972:4:75–80.

Dicaire P, Boucher PC. The treatment of hemorrhoids. Can Pharm J 1985: 118(3):121–2.

Other Treatments

Anonymous Hemorrhoids. Health News (U of Toronto). 1990 Feb: 4.

Anonymous. Med Lett Drugs Ther 1975:17:2.

24
Foot Care

Linda R. Hensman

Self-medication products exist to treat or temporarily relieve many foot conditions. Keratolytics and caustic agents remove corns, calluses and some warts. Protective pads relieve bunions, corns and calluses. Ingrown toenails should not be self-medicated. Athlete's foot is treated with drying and antibacterial agents, followed by antifungal treatment. The diabetic individual needs counselling to prevent the problems of diabetic foot. Good foot hygiene and removal of the cause prevent or relieve many conditions. For permanent relief of most foot conditions, a podiatrist or physician must be consulted.

A wide variety of foot conditions exist, but rarely are they life-threatening. Concern for foot disorders lies in the axiom attributed to Socrates, "To him whose feet hurt, everything hurts." Since aching, tired or painful feet can affect our general sense of well being and often restrict daily activities, it is important to correct these problems.

Foot conditions fall into numerous classifications, including congenital defects, inherent and acquired deformities and disabilities, diseases of the skin, nails, bones, joints and muscles, and circulatory disturbances. This chapter is restricted to a discussion of conditions that may be self-medicated.

An appreciation of the basic structure of the foot helps understand the subsequent discussion on foot disorders (see Figure 1).

Calluses and Corns

Calluses and corns are commonly occurring lesions of the feet that develop at sites of repeated pressure and friction. Often they are asymptomatic, but they may develop into painful lesions for which treatment is commonly sought.

A callus is a localized area of dense hyperkeratosis of the stratum corneum (thickening of the skin). It appears as a raised, slightly yellowish lesion with a normal pattern of skin ridges on the surface. The edges are not well defined and the size may range from a few millimetres (for example, a callus on the top of a toe) to several centimetres (for example, a callus on the ball of the foot). Calluses develop on weight-bearing areas and are most commonly found over the metatarsal heads (on the sole), on the dorsal aspect of the toes and on the heel (see Figure 2).

A callus develops as a protective barrier in response to continuous friction and pressure, often created by improperly fitting or inflexible footwear and backless shoes that allow lateral movement of heels. Orthopedic problems, another common cause, include structural abnormalities causing improper weight distribution, loss of protective fat pads under the skin with aging (for example, over the metatarsal heads) and hammertoes (a flexion deformity of the toe due to contraction of the skin and soft tissue beneath the flexed joint).

Individuals are often unaware of a callus, as it is commonly an asymptomatic lesion. However, as it becomes thicker it may impede circulation and cause a burning sensation. A callus on the heel may build up until it becomes uncomfortable and painful because of complicating fissures.

Corns are also areas of hyperkeratotic tissue. They are usually flat, slightly elevated, well circumscribed lesions, devoid of the normal pattern of skin ridges. In contrast to a callus, a corn usually develops over some bony prominence, such as a bony spur or exostosis. As

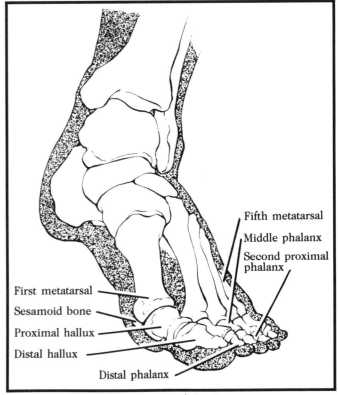

Figure 1 *View of the Bones of the Foot*

Fifth metatarsal
Middle phalanx
Second proximal phalanx
First metatarsal
Sesamoid bone
Proximal hallux
Distal hallux
Distal phalanx

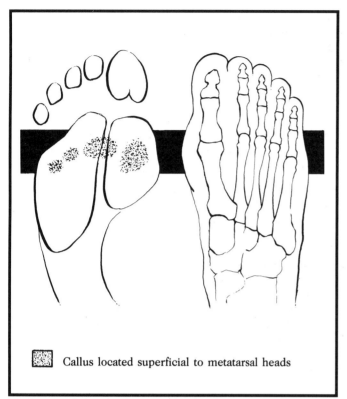

Figure 2 *Sole of a Foot with a Callus*

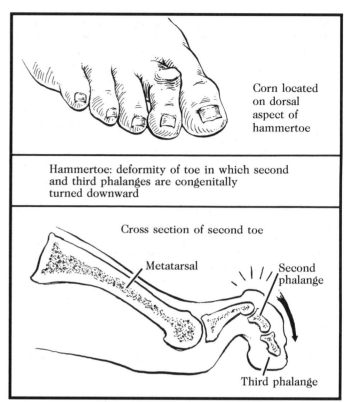

Figure 3 *Corn Located on Dorsal Aspect of Hammertoe*

a result, corns usually have a more compact central core than calluses. The base of the core is at the skin surface, with the apex extending downward and pressing on the nerve endings in the dermal layer. Because of this core, pain results when pressure is applied to the corn.

Both hard and soft corns exist. Hard corns are compact, shiny, hard-surfaced lesions typically occurring on the lateral and superior aspect of the fifth toe, overlying the metatarsophalangeal joints. Soft corns are callused areas usually found in the interdigital webs, particularly between the fourth and fifth toes. Characteristically, soft corns lack a prominent central core and have a whitish color. Accumulated moisture in the web spaces causes maceration of the skin and accounts for the white look of soft corns.

Corns occur because of pressure or friction applied by a bony prominence to the soft tissues and bone of an adjacent toe or metatarsal head. Structural deformities of bones (for example, hammertoes) and compression from improperly fitting shoes increase pressure and friction and initiate or aggravate the development of corns (see Figure 3).

Treatment

Before recommending a treatment, pharmacists must obtain descriptive information about the condition and previous treatment, as well as other medical conditions and current drug therapy. No individual with a history of diabetes mellitus, peripheral vascular disease or serious dermatologic disease should attempt to treat calluses or corns except under the supervision of a physician or podiatrist.

Treatment of corns and calluses with nonprescription products will likely be unsuccessful if the cause is not removed. People who seek advice on products for corn and callus removal must be informed

of the roles played by ill-fitting footwear and foot deformities. Individuals should be advised to wear well fitting, flexible footwear and seek the advice of a physician or podiatrist to correct anatomical foot deformities (for example, hammertoes, bony spurs, flat feet and improper weight distribution). In many cases, a change in footwear or correcting the abnormality resolves the corn or callus. Nonprescription medication may be suggested to individuals seeking more rapid resolution of the condition or who are unwilling to seek the advice of a podiatrist or physician.

Salicylic acid exerts its keratolytic action by increasing endogenous hydration of cells, causing swelling, softening, maceration and ultimately desquamation of the stratum corneum. It is capable of causing this effect in concentrations of 2 per cent or greater on both hyperkeratotic and normal skin. Salicylic acid is useful in treating such hyperkeratotic conditions as corns and calluses. It can also cause superficial tissue damage and necrosis to surrounding normal skin if misapplied or overused.

To treat corns or calluses, salicylic acid preparations of 10 to 40 per cent are used. Salicylic acid is incorporated into dosage forms such as plasters, pastes, collodions and slow release patches. These occlusive dosage forms promote moisture retention, essential for maximum therapeutic benefit with salicylic acid. Without moisture, adequate concentrations of salicylic acid do not soften cornified epithelium.

Because of its destructive effect on normal skin, salicylic acid must be carefully applied to the affected area only. Its use must be discouraged in individuals with diabetes mellitus, peripheral vascular disease or other dermatological conditions in which acute inflammation and ulcer formation is difficult to treat.

Salicylic acid plaster is a uniform mixture of salicylic acid spread on appropriate backing material. It is available at concentrations of 12 to 45 per cent. Since soft corns are highly macerated, moist lesions, products promoted for soft corn removal contain lower concentrations (12 to 20 per cent) of salicylic acid. Applying high concentrations (40 to 45 per cent) may cause excessive tissue destruction and necrosis.

Salicylic acid in collodion is often available in combination with caustic agents such as acetic and lactic acids. Salicylic acid paste is available in concentrations of 15 per cent. Salicylic acid is also available in a karaya gum patch which is designed to permit continuous passive diffusion of dissolved salicylic acid from the patch into the tissue. This vehicle has been designed primarily for the treatment of warts.

Glacial acetic acid and **lactic acid** are included in corn and callus removal products because they possess caustic properties. These agents cause severe destruction when applied to normal tissue; surrounding healthy tissue must be protected when treating lesions with these agents. Most formulations contain less than a 10 per cent concentration of glacial acetic acid or lactic acid. Contraindications to the use of these chemicals are similar to those for salicylic acid.

Product Selection

All available products have effective concentrations of active ingredients. Product selection depends on consumer preference and the condition. No one product has been shown more effective than another in clinical studies.

Plasters and patches are occlusive and adhesive and provide prolonged contact of the drug with the lesion. The backing can be cut to conform to the size and shape of the affected area. Hard corns and calluses are most easily treated with plasters.

Collodion dosage forms are also adherent and occlusive. Their application requires considerable care to avoid spilling the preparation onto surrounding tissues. They may not be the product of choice for individuals who are elderly, "shaky" or have poor eyesight. Collodion products are highly flammable and volatile and must be stored tightly capped and away from heat and sunlight. Where children are present, they may be less desirable than plasters and pastes because of their toxic potential both on ingestion and inhalation. Collodions are more useful for treating corns than calluses.

Pastes are the least adherent and occlusive of the three dosage forms available.

Products containing low concentrations of salicylic acid (12 rather than 40 per cent) are recommended for treating soft corns. Plasters are easier to apply than pastes or collodion products.

Consumer Information

The consumer should always be advised to read and follow the label of the specific product. However, the following instructions are applicable to most corn and callus removal products and should be given to any individual purchasing such a product:
- Soak the affected area in warm water for 10 to 15 minutes to soften the skin. Pat dry.
- If a solution is used, cut a hole in a bandage, and apply it to the area so only the lesion appears through the hole, and then drop on the solution. Apply one drop at a time and allow it to dry or harden. Repeat this procedure until the area is covered. If the solution touches healthy skin, wash it off immediately.
- If a plaster or patch is used, trim it to the shape of the corn or callus.

- If paste is used, apply a sufficient quantity to cover the lesion.
- Cover the lesion with occlusive adhesive tape (for example, Blenderm).
- After 12 to 24 hours, remove the bandage and soak the area in warm water for 10 to 15 minutes.
- Gently remove the soft white tissue by rubbing with a rough towel, pumice stone or callus file, taking care not to rub the adjacent areas.
- Repeat the entire procedure until the corn or callus disappears.

The condition usually resolves in 10 days. Adhering to the treatment regimen is critical to a successful outcome. Selecting a convenient time for treatment (at bedtime, first thing in the morning or both) may be helpful. Individuals should be discouraged from trying to hasten the process by using sharp knives or razor blades to cut dead tissue, as this practice may result in infection.

Protective Pads, Metatarsal Cushions and Arch Supports

Various protective pads are available for use in corn and callus prevention and treatment. Different materials are used, including moleskin, felt and latex foam. The pads are manufactured in a wide variety of shapes and sizes to accommodate the different types and locations of lesions (aperture pads to circle and protect a specific area, crescent pads to protect around and behind an area, and metatarsal cushions). Sheets of moleskin and lambswool are available to construct a pad. When placed over or around the irritated area, the pad reduces friction and pressure, relieves pain and may reduce lesions. These pads may help temporarily, but they do not treat the cause and should not be recommended for continuous use.

If the aim is to protect the area from pressure, pads should be made from material as thick as the area to be protected. In the case of a corn, for example, the pad should not be placed over the lesion, but trimmed to surround the area. Pads to reduce friction should be cut to the shape and size of the area and placed over it. Padding material with adhesive backing (for example, Kurotex) should not be applied over blistered or broken skin. Inserting lambswool between web spaces may be useful therapy for soft corns, as it separates the toes and decreases friction between them.

Also available are commercial arch supports intended to support the foot in the ideal natural position so problems resulting from improper weight distribution (for example, corns and calluses) do not develop. These supports are available in standard sizes and may not suit every foot or foot condition. Those made of sponge rubber and other flexible materials adapt freely to the foot and are of limited benefit. More elaborate arch supports are available in different widths and sizes, but must be adjusted to ensure maximum benefit. To be most effective, arch supports must be custom fitted to the contours of the foot.

Warts (Verrucae)

Warts or verrucae are common skin tumors caused by the human papillomavirus (HPV). Warts begin as smooth-surfaced, skin-colored lesions that enlarge and develop a papillomatous appearance. After attaining a certain size they become stable lesions, although repeated irritation may lead to further enlargements. Warts are usually asymptomatic, but plantar warts may enlarge to the point of producing pain and discomfort.

Warts occur in about 7 to 10 per cent of the population. Children and adolescents are most commonly afflicted except in the case of venereal warts, for which the highest frequency is in the adult population. Warts appear to develop more often in people who perspire excessively on the palms of the hands and soles of the feet and in people who are institutionalized. Also, individuals with depressed cell-mediated immunity (for example, people with Hodgkin's disease or lymphoma and those treated with immunosuppressive agents) have a much greater incidence of progressive and extensive warts than the general population.

The natural history of warts is unpredictable and varies among the different types of warts. Twenty to thirty per cent of all warts resolve spontaneously within 6 months, and 65 per cent involute by 2 years. However, new warts develop more frequently in infected individuals such that the overall prevalence of warts increases in untreated individuals.

Warts are classified according to their location. Verrucae vulgaris or common warts are encountered most often. They are found predominantly on the hands and fingers, but may occur as single or multiple lesions on any part of the body. Common warts are skin-colored to brown lesions that appear initially as smooth-surfaced lesions but enlarge and take a roughened papillomatous texture. They range in size from several millimetres to several centimetres. Verrucae vulgaris are usually easily identified, but on occasion may be confused with deep-seated fungal infections or squamous cell carcinomas.

Periungual verrucae occur at the periphery and base of the nails. Subungual verrucae are located underneath the nail plate and occasionally are found in conjunction with periungual warts. They possess a papillomatous surface similar to common warts.

Flat warts or juvenile warts are asymptomatic lesions occurring primarily on the face, neck and back of hands, although the trunk, legs and arms may be affected. They are smooth, slightly raised, skin-colored to brown lesions approximately 2 to 5 mm in diameter. The lesions are multiple and may coalesce to form linear streaks or small plaques.

Plantar warts occur on the plantar surface of the foot. Several types exist: multiple and tiny, single and large, with or without smaller satellite lesions or grouped to form clusters (mosaic warts). They are well circumscribed, indurated lesions that are usually flat when located on weight bearing surfaces, for example, soles or heels. They appear grayish and friable and often are surrounded by a ring of hyperkeratotic tissue. The surface of the plantar wart may reveal multiple tiny black dots that tend to bleed when the surface is scraped. The presence of these dots may help differentiate plantar warts from similar hyperkeratotic lesions. A definitive diagnosis must be made by a podiatrist or physician.

Condyloma acuminata, or venereal warts, are moist, cauliflower-like lesions that develop on the mucous membranes and at the mucocutaneous junction of the anogenital region. They are sexually transmitted lesions and are not associated with warts elsewhere on the body.

Treatment Measures

A number of factors must be considered when recommending a treatment regimen for warts. The number and type of wart influences the choice of treatment. The size, depth and location will also influence the treatment modality. Therapies that are successful for one type may be inferior or ineffective for other types. Warts that are painful, subject to continual trauma or cosmetically objectionable should be treated. If the wart does not meet these criteria, treatment may not be necessary or at least should proceed cautiously,

as problems associated with treatment are often more bothersome than the primary lesion (for example, painful scar tissue formation, destruction of normal skin surrounding the lesion, secondary infections, and hypopigmentation or hyperpigmentation). Individuals who are naturally or therapeutically immunosuppressed are difficult to treat and treatment may hasten the spread of warts. Finally, people with circulatory disorders or diabetes mellitus should never attempt self-treatment of warts because of the inherent danger of infection. These individuals must be referred to a physician.

Verrucae Vulgaris

Verrucae vulgaris can be managed successfully by a variety of different methods. Dessication and curettage is rapid and painless, but may leave residual scars and alter normal skin pigmentation. Cryotherapy with liquid nitrogen produces discomfort and occasional scarring, but may also cause hypopigmentation or hyperpigmentation. However, these procedures must be performed by a physician or podiatrist.

Nonprescription salicylic acid preparations are promoted for self-treatment of common warts. Researchers found no significant difference between the cure rate of individuals with hand warts treated with cryotherapy and those treated with salicylic acid/lactic acid in flexible collodion. People who self-treated warts with this combination were provided with detailed instructions and followed up at 3 week intervals. Up to 12 weeks of therapy were required to eradicate some warts. Close supervision played a key role in the success of home therapy. Salicylic acid products can be recommended to individuals seeking a home treatment method of common warts.

In general, the therapy of warts other than verrucae vulgaris necessitates the use of prescription products or toxic agents that require physician supervision. Individuals who request advice on treating flat warts, periungual or subungual warts, plantar warts or venereal warts should be referred to a physician or podiatrist. Nonetheless, pharmacists must be aware of the treatments available to these people.

Plantar Warts

A variety of treatments for plantar warts has been used over the years, but no treatment has been found superior to another. Although some nonprescription products are available, most treatments are best undertaken by a physician or podiatrist, because of the unpredictability of therapy, the contagious nature of plantar warts and the potential for toxicity and complications with self-treatment products. Excision or electrodesiccation removes plantar warts, but both procedures may result in scarring, producing more pain and discomfort than the original lesion. Cryotherapy has been used with varying degrees of success to manage plantar warts. More recently, intralesional bleomycin and contact immunotherapy have been used to eradicate plantar warts.

Researchers evaluated several products for plantar wart treatment in a double-blind trial. Over a 12 week period, they compared salicylic acid/lactic acid in flexible collodion (SAL), podophyllum 50 per cent in mineral oil, and flexible collodion in treating simple and mosaic plantar warts. Individuals were given detailed instructions for applying either SAL or flexible collodion at home. People receiving podophyllum were treated at the clinic. The cure rate for SAL (84 per cent) and podophyllum (81 per cent) in simple plantar warts was significantly greater than with collodion alone (66 per cent). The cure rate for mosaic plantar warts was lower than for simple plantar warts (58 per cent versus 75 per cent cured in

12 weeks), illustrating the more resistant nature of mosaic warts to treatment. About one-half the individuals classified as cured at 12 weeks were already cured at 6 weeks. The speed of cure was highest for SAL. Both the SAL and podophyllum treatments were safe and effective in both children and adults; no cases of hypersensitivity or toxicity were reported. Researchers concluded that SAL was a successful home-treatment product for plantar warts. These findings contrast with the failure of previous treatments received by the same individuals. The researchers attributed much of the SAL success to the verbal and written instructions given to the users. Additionally, regular follow-up by a physician ensured the product was used correctly and was not discontinued prematurely.

Nonprescription products can be successful in managing plantar warts when the directions for use are followed consistently. If the warts return or the condition persists after using a product for 12 to 14 weeks, the individual should be referred to a physician or podiatrist.

Flat Warts

Flat warts have been treated most successfully with tretinoin or benzoyl peroxide. The irritant effects of these agents produce erythema and peeling of the warts. Two to three weeks of therapy usually clear the lesions.

Periungual/Subungual Warts

Periungual and subungual warts have been treated by cryotherapy, although this method often produces extreme pain that may last several hours. Application of cantharidin is less painful and more effective for periungual warts. Intralesional bleomycin has been used to treat periungual warts successfully.

Venereal Warts

Cryotherapy, electrocautery and surgical excision can clear venereal warts, but the treatment of choice is podophyllum resin (20 to 25 per cent concentration).

Product Selection

Treatment of warts with **salicylic acid** involves nightly application of the selected product in the same manner as that outlined in corn and callus treatment. However, warts usually require a longer treatment period. Premature discontinuation results in regrowth of the wart. Treatment must continue until all warty tissue is removed. The precautions and product selection guidelines discussed previously apply to managing warts.

Podophyllum and **colchicine** are cytotoxic agents that cause necrosis and sloughing of wart tissue. Podophyllum is usually dispensed as a concentration of 20 to 25 per cent in compound tincture of benzoin or alcohol. Podophyllum is applied sparingly to the wart and washed off in 6 to 8 hours to prevent excess irritation. The low viscosity of the vehicle allows the podophyllum to flow onto the surrounding healthy tissue, which may result in tissue damage. This risk is reduced if the tissue adjacent to the wart is protected with petroleum jelly. A commercially available product (Verban) contains podophyllum 2 per cent and colchicine 0.1 per cent. It should be applied daily to the wart area for 1 to 3 hours and then removed. Its availability as a nonprescription product is due to the low concentrations of colchicine and podophyllum and conservative treatment recommendations. These factors allow its use with minimal supervision.

In addition to topical reactions caused by the irritant effect, podophyllum has caused renal toxicity and peripheral neuropathy, but only when applied to extensive areas, particularly mucous membranes (for example, when venereal warts are treated).

Cantharidin is a potent vesicant that causes exfoliation of the warty tissue. Its lytic action is limited to the epidermal cells and does not extend into deeper tissue; as a result, no scarring occurs with topical application. Cantharidin is applied lightly to the wart area with a stick or swab and allowed to dry. The treated wart is then covered with a nonporous plastic tape. After 24 hours the tape is removed and the wart is covered loosely with a bandage. The cantharidin causes a blister to form. The blister dries within 7 to 10 days and the necrotic tissue peels off. The application may need to be repeated.

Sensitivity to cantharidin varies greatly. Some individuals may complain of a tingling or burning sensation; others experience extreme tenderness. The major disadvantage of cantharidin is that a ring of satellite warts may develop at the periphery of the original lesion. Although cantharidin is classified as a nonprescription drug, it is suggested treatment be performed only by a physician.

Trichloroacetic acid, present in some wart removal products, is a powerful irritant that hydrolyzes protein with resultant acute inflammation. Tissue is destroyed by the corrosion and irritation inherent in its caustic nature. Care must be taken to ensure it does not contact normal tissue.

Bunions

Bunions are deformities of the great toe joint (first metatarsophalangeal joint) that subsequently develop inflammation and swelling of the surrounding bursa and other soft tissues (see Figure 4). Occasionally, bunions develop in the fifth metatarsophalangeal joint. These are referred to as "tailor's bunions" or "bunionettes." Bunions develop when repeated pressure and friction are applied to the joint. Most

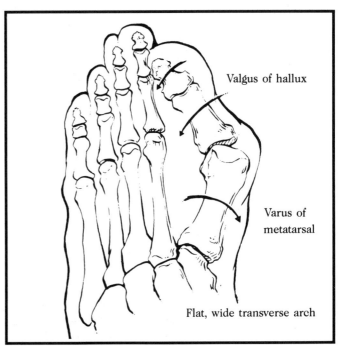

Figure 4 *Bunion Associated with Hallux Valgus*

people who develop bunions have a structural defect of the foot such as a hallux valgus (deviation of the great toe joint toward the medial side of the foot), metatarsus varus (outward deviation of the fifth toe joint) or pronated ("flat") feet.

The symptoms of bunions include pain on the dorsomedial aspect of the first metatarsal head. Often the individual complains of redness and recurrent swelling of the great toe joint and general foot discomfort, sometimes without specific reference to the joint itself. The great majority of people do not have pain in the joint even with gentle movement. This characteristic may help distinguish it from an attack of gout, which often presents in a similar manner. If bunions are left unattended and are continually traumatized, chronic traumatic arthritis and synovitis may develop.

Treatment

Since bunions are commonly aggravated by narrow shoes, wider shoes bring relief to some people. Orthotic devices benefit some people by stabilizing the bones and muscles and retarding joint deviation. Bunion pads and protectors may relieve pain if the padding is thicker than the central prominent area of the bunion. However, all these measures are temporary. People who complain of symptoms suggestive of a bunion are best referred to a physician or podiatrist, so early treatment can be instituted and pain and permanent arthritic damage avoided.

Ingrown Toenails

Toenails that become imbedded into the skin margin surrounding the nail plate are referred to as ingrown toenails. They develop most commonly in the great toe in males (in a 2:1 ratio) and in persons between 10 and 30 years of age. Contrary to popular belief, abnormal convexity of the toenails does not appear to be a predisposing factor. Individuals with thin nails, thick nail folds and medial rotation of the great toe seem most likely to develop the condition. Improper trimming of nails, which allows the nail to grow abnormally into the surrounding tissue may contribute to the condition. This growth causes pressure and pain. If the condition becomes chronic, edematous granulation tissue may develop and the nail edges may appear "heaped up." Bacterial infections may then develop (see Figure 5).

People with ingrown toenails complain of pain, especially when pressure (for example, from tight footwear) is applied to the nail. One or both edges of skin surrounding the nail may be involved, appearing red, swollen and tender. Purulent discharge may be present if an infection develops.

Treatment

At the first sign of an ingrown toenail, clean cotton packing or lambswool may be placed gently under the nail. This procedure lifts the nail up and allows normal growth; if done early in treatment, it may avoid further complications. However, since nails grow very slowly (less than 1 mm per week), this may need to be done for several weeks or months. Other disadvantages are that it may be uncomfortable, irritating or malodorous (since packing attracts moisture). It may be preferable to use more drastic treatment measures particularly in young children. Long-standing cases, especially those associated with an infectious process, must be referred to a podiatrist. No treatment is successful unless the nail plate infiltrating the tissue is removed. Individuals should not attempt this procedure, but should see a podiatrist or physician. Permanent relief from recurrent ingrown toenails often necessitates partial or total removal of the toenail.

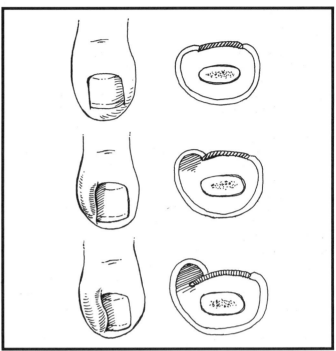

Figure 5 *Development of Ingrown Toenail Showing a Cross Section at Different Stages of Development*

A number of proprietary medications are available to treat ingrown toenails. They contain ingredients such as sodium sulfide and tannic acid and are intended to relieve pressure and pain. No clinical studies have been done to prove their efficacy. The directions accompanying these products suggest inserting cotton packing under the nail, which probably provides the relief.

Ingrown toenails can be avoided if a few rules for nail care are followed:
- Keep nails clean.
- Keep the cuticles free of irritants and the cuticles back by brushing regularly with a nail brush.
- Trim the nails straight across—do not cut down into the corners.
- Do not wear tight shoes and avoid excessive walking.

Athlete's Foot

Athlete's foot is a general term to describe itching, scaling, interdigital lesions of the feet. The clinical spectrum of athlete's foot ranges from mild scaling with periodic pruritus to severe inflammation with exudation, fissuring and denudation. The condition is most commonly characterized by hyperkeratosis, maceration, pruritus, stinging and malodor.

It is widely thought that dermatophyte fungi are wholly responsible for athlete's foot and therefore, it is commonly referred to as tinea pedis. However, clinical studies indicate symptomatic athlete's foot arises from both fungal and bacterial infection. Athlete's foot probably develops in the following manner.

Dermatophytes *(Trichophyton rubrum, Trichophyton mentagrophytes* and *Epidermophyton floccosum)* invade and disrupt the horny layer of the skin, producing drying and scaling that are often asymptomatic lesions. Existence of dermatophyte fungi in these lesions is easily demonstrated by culture or potassium hydroxide examination. Depending upon environmental factors, the condition may or may not progress.

Increased moisture and temperature (for example, hot weather, hyperhidrosis or occlusive footwear) produce maceration of tissue and stimulate overgrowth of bacteria. The bacteria involved are resident aerobic diphtheroids, although in extremely severe cases gram-negative organisms, including Proteus and Pseudomonas species, may be present.

Bacteria and bacterial products invade and easily diffuse through the fungus-damaged horny layer, resulting in hyperkeratotic, pruritic, macerated, symptomatic athlete's foot. Recovery of fungi from these lesions is low.

Although pathogenic fungi are common in the environment, the frequency of fungal infections is relatively low. A number of factors, many not yet defined, influence the susceptibility of individuals to developing a fungal infection. Simple exposure, even to massive quantities of pathogenic fungi, often is not sufficient. Exposure to fungus plus trauma, especially trauma that results in blistering, produces clinical infection. Although males and females appear equally susceptible under experimental conditions, clinically, males develop fungal infections more commonly. Children rarely develop athlete's foot. In shoe-wearing populations of temperate climates, athlete's foot is mainly a seasonal disease, flaring in the summer and quiescent in winter.

People complaining of athlete's foot may present with a variety of lesions and symptoms. Most commonly, the fourth web space is involved, although any web space may be affected. Dry, scaly lesions associated with periodic pruritus appear first. Subsequently, the toe web space may become macerated, whitish and exceedingly pruritic. This condition is often associated with malodor. Small fissures in the areas of toe flexion may develop, and the individual may complain of painful burning or stinging sensations. If untreated, further erosion and erythema and a foul-smelling purulent exudate may develop. Pain may be extensive. The erosion and erythema may spread further over the foot.

Athlete's foot may also present as an off-white, scaling lesion of the soles, particularly along the instep. Inflammation with vesicle formation may also develop. Vesicular eruption is more common on the soles than on the interdigital webs. Initially, vesicles appear yellow, but dry to take on a brown appearance.

With a moderate to severe inflammatory fungal infection of the feet, some people develop a pustular, vesicular inflammatory dermatosis affecting the palm of one hand. This reaction is referred to as an id or dermatophytid reaction.

Interdigital pityriasis, psoriasis, soft corns, dyshidrosis, localized forms of atopic dermatitis and other conditions may be mistaken by the consumer to be athlete's foot. Individuals who fail to respond after a reasonable time (up to 1 month) to such treatment approaches as drying, antibacterial and antifungal therapy must be referred to a physician for further evaluation.

Treatment

Selecting the treatment for athlete's foot depends on the stage of the disease process. In acute, inflammatory athlete's foot, characterized by maceration, erythema, exudation and vesicular eruption, the inflammatory process and bacterial proliferation must be suppressed before antifungal therapy can help. Bacteria can be suppressed in several ways. The simplest is exposure to the air, since drying keeps the resident bacteria at low levels. Individuals should wear sandals or socks that allow good ventilation. Because wearing sandals is not always practical, drying agents such as astringents (for example, aluminum salts) and powders (medicated or nonmedicated) can be recommended. In addition, the use of broad spectrum antibacterial agents, such as antibiotic creams, may be suggested. Severe cases require systemic therapy with antibiotics. Drying and antibacterial agents are not curative, but they make the condition revert to the simple, dry, scaly stage. Antifungal agents can then be used to suppress the fungus that initiated the process. Antifungal treatment alone rarely produces resolution in the acute inflammatory cases. In many cases, the use of antifungal agents during the acute inflammatory stage further sensitizes the skin and worsens the condition.

In the dry, scaly variety of athlete's foot, for which fungi are primarily responsible, antifungal agents alone produce rapid improvement.

Individuals with a history of recurrent episodes of athlete's foot often benefit from maintenance therapy with a drying antifungal powder.

Pharmacologic Agents

The first antifungal agent found clinically effective in dermatophyte infections was sodium propionate. Subsequently, **undecylenic acid** and its salts were found to have the greatest antifungal activity when a large group of fatty acids was tested.

Undecylenic acid is fungistatic and fungicidal as well as possessing antibacterial properties. It is active against a wide variety of pathogenic fungi responsible for superficial mycoses (for example, Epidermophyton, Trichophyton and Microsporum species).

Undecylenic acid may be formulated in combination with zinc undecylenate. Zinc undecylenate exhibits similar antifungal activity to the acid form as well as possessing astringent properties that decrease moisture and its irritation. In clinical trials, undecylenic acid with zinc undecylenate have been shown to be clinically superior to placebo.

Undecylenic acid alone or in combination with zinc undecylenate is available as a powder, cream, ointment, solution, foam or soap. These preparations are usually non-irritating; sensitization is seldom noted. Some individuals may experience a transient, mild, stinging sensation if the preparations are applied to excoriated areas.

Most undecylenic acid products should be applied daily for 2 weeks. If the condition does not improve or if it worsens, a physician should evaluate the condition. The solution may be used full strength and applied directly to the lesions or diluted and used as a soaking solution. If the solution is applied directly to the lesions, it must be allowed to air dry. Otherwise, further maceration and aggravation of the condition may result. The powder may be dusted liberally over the lesions and rubbed gently but thoroughly into the affected area. It may be sprinkled into the socks and shoes daily. The foam may be sprayed between the toes and on other affected areas and allowed to dissipate and dry. The cream or ointment should be rubbed into the lesions well. Excessively thick applications of the ointment should be avoided to prevent moisture retention. Selecting a particular formulation depends on individual preference. None of the products is effective in acutely inflamed, macerated lesions.

Tolnaftate is an effective agent for treating cutaneous fungal infections and interdigital foot lesions due to *Trichophyton rubrum*, *Trichophyton mentagrophytes* and *Epidermophyton floccosum*. It is an antifungal agent only and is ineffective against gram-positive and gram-negative bacteria. Fungal infection of the nails (onychomycosis), which may develop in long-standing cases of athlete's foot, is often unresponsive to topical tolnaftate therapy.

Effective therapy of interdigital lesions requires twice daily applications of tolnaftate for 14 to 28 days. Tolnaftate should be applied sparingly (2 to 3 drops cover the toes and web spaces) to a thoroughly cleansed area. The cream is rubbed thoroughly but gently into the skin. The solution should also be rubbed in well and allowed to dry. Individuals with hyperkeratotic areas may benefit from the use of a keratolytic agent before or during treatment with tolnaftate. Treatment in these cases may have to be extended up to 6 weeks. The concomitant use of wet compresses (for example, Burow's solution) in acute inflammatory cases of athlete's foot does not affect the fungicidal activity of tolnaftate solution. However, tolnaftate treatment alone in these cases is often ineffective owing to the bacterial nature of the infection.

Tolnaftate cream and solution are available in a concentration of 1 per cent. Tolnaftate solution is odorless, greaseless and does not stain clothing or skin.

Tolnaftate is available in a powder formulation that serves a twofold purpose: it acts as a delivery vehicle for tolnaftate and it absorbs moisture, preventing skin maceration. Tolnaftate powder is more effective than the vehicle alone for reducing the incidence of fungal infection in laboratory-confirmed dermatophytosis. The prophylactic use of tolnaftate powder in high-risk individuals may significantly reduce the incidence of fungal infection. Tolnaftate powder should be used only for extremely mild cases or as adjunctive treatment.

Tolnaftate is well tolerated when applied to intact or broken skin. Some people experience a slight stinging sensation on application. Only one report exists of a delayed hypersensitivity reaction to tolnaftate, despite its use by several million people. As with any topical medication, exacerbation of the condition, irritation or sensitization warrants discontinuing use.

In clinical trials when tolnaftate and undecylenic acid were used to treat athlete's foot, the two agents were equally effective, with no agent clinically superior. Both undecylenic acid and tolnaftate are superior to placebo when treating fungal infections. In these studies, individuals applied the products twice daily. Although twice daily application is recommended for tolnaftate, most undecylenic acid products suggest once daily applications. Studies have not been conducted to compare once daily application of undecylenic acid with twice daily applications of tolnaftate.

Haloprogin has a spectrum of activity similar to that of tolnaftate. It is effective against *Trichophyton rubrum, Trichophyton mentagrophytes, Epidermophyton floccosum* and some Candida species. It has been used successfully in managing culture-positive tinea infections.

For fungal infections of the feet, haloprogin should be applied liberally twice daily for 14 to 28 days. Interdigital lesions may require up to 4 weeks of therapy. Haloprogin is available as a cream or solution.

Haloprogin produces local irritation, burning and vesicle formation in some people as well as increased pruritus, maceration and exacerbation of pre-existing lesions. These reactions may occur more often if occlusive footwear is worn.

In a number of clinical studies haloprogin was equal in efficacy to tolnaftate in treating potassium hydroxide-positive and culture-positive fungal infections of the feet. In one study, haloprogin treated patients exhibited lower relapse rates 8 days after treatment was completed. This finding suggests haloprogin may be preferred for individuals who relapse frequently.

Salicylic acid is a keratolytic agent when used in concentrations greater than 2 per cent. It is incorporated into topical antifungal products for two reasons: it aids the removal of hyperkeratotic tissue, thus facilitating the penetration of antifungal agents, and it accelerates exfoliation of the infected tissue.

Salicylic acid alone or combined with benzoic acid may help treat hyperkeratotic areas of athlete's foot, before or during treatment with other antifungal agents. Salicylic acid alone has minimal antifungal activity. Whitfield's Ointment was a widely used proprietary medication containing salicylic acid and benzoic acid. **Benzoic acid** is a fungistatic agent only; eradication of the infection occurs only after the infected skin is shed. Continuous use of the medication for several weeks or months is needed to notice any effect. Because such lengthy therapy is required, agents such as tolnaftate or haloprogin are preferred.

Aluminum salts are recommended for the acute inflammatory stage of athlete's foot because of their astringent action. When applied to damaged skin they act as protein precipitants, causing a superficial protective layer to form. Aluminum salts also harden the skin and reduce exudative secretions. They possess limited antibacterial activity. They help dry the skin surface rather than killing microbial organisms.

Aluminum-containing products are available from which solutions for soaking or applying as wet compresses can be made. When there is extensive involvement of the foot, soaking the foot in a solution is preferred while smaller lesions may have wet compresses applied locally. This procedure should be done 2 to 3 times daily. Excessive use of soaking solutions may result in excessive drying with cracking and fissuring of the skin and worsening of the condition. If inflammatory lesions worsen or do not improve, individuals should discontinue use and seek the advice of a physician. Aluminum-containing powders may be dusted in socks and shoes to assist in reducing moisture.

Product Selection

Selecting a specific product to manage athlete's foot depends on the stage of the disease and the consumer's preference for the type of product (for example, cream or liquid).

All antifungal agents effectively treat culture-positive fungal infection of the feet. The imidazoles such as clotrimazole, miconazole and ketoconazole exhibit a broader spectrum of activity and are more effective than the older antifungal agents. However, unlike tolnaftate, haloprogin and undecylenic acid products are not available without a prescription.

Liquid preparations and creams are useful in moderately involved, dry, scaly lesions of the feet. Powder formulation should be used as adjunctive treatment only. Occlusive based products should be avoided. Hyperkeratotic areas may be treated with keratolytics before or during treatment with antifungals.

Agents useful for the acute stage are limited. Burow's solution (for example, Buro-sol tablets or powder) may be used as soaking solutions or wet compresses. Powders may be useful to assist in drying the lesions. After the initial inflammatory reaction subsides, antifungal therapy may be started. The newer imidazole agents exert an antibacterial effect as well as serving as antifungal agents and may be useful during the acute stage.

Consumer Information

If drug therapy is to be effective in athlete's foot, the individual must comply with the recommended treatment schedules and follow

Table I *Common Foot Care Medications*

Corn, callus and wart treatment
Salicylic acid 40% plaster
Salicylic acid 15% paste
Salicylic acid in flexible collodion
(with or without glacial acetic or lactic acids)

Athlete's foot
Dry, scaly stage
  Tolnaftate
  Haloprogin
  Undecylenic acid, zinc undecylenate
  Salicylic acid/benzoic acid
Acute, macerated, odoriferous stage
  Aluminum salts (direct application or as soaking solutions)
  Dusting powders (medicated or non-medicated)
  Broad spectrum topical antimicrobials

Ingrown toenails, bunions
No drugs of recognized utility

general measures of good hygiene. Pharmacists advising individuals with athlete's foot should provide the following information:

- Clean and dry the feet (especially between the toes) thoroughly every day.
- To avoid excessive irritation and aggravation of the condition, handle the affected area gently.
- Wear sandals or shoes and socks that allow adequate ventilation. Avoid socks made of synthetic fibres as they retain heat and moisture. Light cotton socks are best. Do not wear occlusive footwear, such as rubber boots and athletic shoes.
- Change shoes daily to allow them to dry inside.
- Change socks regularly and wash them thoroughly in hot water.
- Dust the feet, especially between the toes, with a medicated powder to aid drying.

Pharmacists should advise consumers the average time for treatment is 2 to 4 weeks. Extensive involvement, failure to follow the therapeutic program and other variables alter the time required. Relief from symptoms is usually noted within a few days after treatment begins. In more severe cases, relief may be less rapid. The use of antifungal agents alone in acute cases of athlete's foot has limited success; consumers should be informed of treatment to eradicate the bacterial component of the disease.

Consumers who have diabetes mellitus, peripheral vascular disease, or a history of allergies, asthma or dermatological disorders should not self-medicate athlete's foot but should be referred to a physician.

A number of products are available for self-treatment of certain foot conditions (see Table I).

Diabetic Foot Care

Most individuals take their feet for granted. Diabetics cannot afford this luxury, since there is an inclination to a variety of vascular, metabolic and neurological deficiencies that may result in foot problems, more specifically if there is lack of or poor diabetic control. It has been estimated that 20 per cent of all diabetic patient admissions to hospital are for foot lesions.

The diabetic may become afflicted with peripheral neuropathies, such as peripheral neuritis, hyperesthesia and decreased or absent vibratory and temperature sensations. Peripheral neuropathies result in lack of protective sensation, which can lead to soft tissue infections and bone and joint injuries (Charcot's joints) without the diabetic being aware of these changes. Characteristically, minor cuts and scratches go unnoticed. These cuts may serve as a portal of entry for bacteria. As the infection develops, common signs and symptoms of the infectious process (for example, throbbing, increased temperature and pain) may not be noticed, and the minor problem may become an extensive infection.

Ulcers often develop under corns or calluses on the plantar surface of the diabetic foot. When individuals with normal sensory perception develop painful lesions (for example, corns) on the sole of the foot, they unload the area of pressure through limping. The diabetic, lacking normal sensation, continues to apply full pressure on the area. As the lesion grows, it acts as a hard foreign body, eventually causing ulceration. The skin surface may appear normal, but debridement reveals an ulcer in the deeper tissues. If the condition is left unattended, the individual may eventually note a serous exudate or, when secondary infection develops, a purulent discharge.

In addition to lack of sensory perception secondary to neuropathy, many diabetics have impaired circulation, which can be a major limiting factor in maintaining healthy feet. Pathologically, the small vessels in the diabetic have thickened basement membranes. This thickening results in a narrowing of the capillaries, thereby reducing tissue perfusion. A relative hypoxia exists, which, in addition to the high glucose concentrations in the blood, provides an ideal environment for the growth of aerobic and anaerobic bacteria. Some infections may cause thrombosis of the small vessels, leading to gangrene and possibly amputation. Good control of the diabetic condition may limit vascular complications.

Thirty per cent of all diabetics manifest other cutaneous diseases (for example, granuloma annulare, necrobiosis lipoidica, diabeticorum and xanthoma). One major problem is the excessive formation of corns and calluses compared to normal individuals. Although no proven explanation exists, denervated stratum corneum may absorb water to a lesser extent than normal extremities. Additionally, the diabetic foot is frequently characterized by reduced or absent perspiration.

Treatment

Because of the circulatory, neurologic and metabolic deficiencies of the diabetic, minor problems may become severe conditions that are difficult or impossible to treat. It is important the diabetic know and practise preventive foot care. Additionally, the pharmacist should be aware of problems associated with the diabetic foot and should discourage diabetics from self-medicating abnormal foot conditions.

Diabetics are encouraged to follow these recommendations:

- Never attempt self-medication of a foot problem; seek the advice of a physician or podiatrist.
- Inspect feet daily (using a mirror to observe the underside) and seek medical care for any variation from the normal state (for example, cuts, scrapes and ingrown toenails). Early signs of foot trouble may include blisters, changes in skin color, swelling, rashes, increased temperature to touch and slow healing sores.
- Bathe feet daily. Avoid hot water (check temperature first), especially if diminished circulation and sensory perception are a problem. Use a mild soap for cleansing; do not use harsh chemicals. Dry feet thoroughly, especially between the toes. Apply lotion or oil to feet after drying.
- Avoid walking with bare feet as there is always the possibility of

Table II *Common Foot Disorders—Characteristics and Treatment*

Foot condition	Characteristics and treatment	Location	Differential diagnosis	Treatment
Callus	Hyperkeratotic area Raised, yellowish, lesion with normal pattern of skin ridges Poorly defined borders, varying size No central core	On weight-bearing areas such as sole of foot, heel, dorsal aspect of toes	Corn	Remove cause (e.g., friction) Orthotic appliances for weight redistribution if necessary Regular soaking of feet and rubbing or filing away hyperkeratotic tissue Salicylic acid products
Hard corn	Shiny, hard, well-defined lesion Central core Loss of normal pattern of skin ridges	On weight-bearing surface usually over bony prominence such as dorsal aspect of toe joints, side of fifth toe	Callus Plantar wart	Remove cause (e.g., bony prominence and pressure) Soaking and salicylic acid products Temporary use of cushioning pads to relieve pain
Soft corn	Thickening of skin Soft, macerated lesion No central core	Interdigital web space (usually between fourth and fifth toes)	Athlete's foot	Remove cause (bony spur or exostosis) Cushioning (e.g., lambswool between toes) Salicylic acid products
Plantar wart	Varying size and number Well-defined, flat lesion Greyish, friable with black dots in centre Ring of hyperkeratotic tissue	Weight-bearing area (e.g., ball and heel of foot)	Corn Callus	Refer to physician or podiatrist
Bunion	Inflammation of bursa, associated with joint deformity	First to fifth metatarsophalangeal joint	Gouty arthritis	Temporary cushioning to relieve pain Surgical correction
Ingrown toenail	Infiltration of toenail into soft tissue Swollen, red, tender, "heaped-up" tissue margins	Commonly great toe nail		Packing under nail Onychectomy (total or partial)
Athlete's foot	Varying characteristics depending on stage Dry, scaly lesions Macerated, erythematous, hyperkeratotic weeping lesions Fissures Vesicular eruption	Interdigital webs and sole	Psoriasis, soft corn, dermatitis (atopic, contact, etc.), dyshidrosis, etc.	Antifungal agents for dry, scaly variety Drying agents (powders, astringents, open shoes, etc.) for acute macerated stage Antibacterial agents Keratolytic agents for hyperkeratotic lesions

injuring the foot. Minor cuts may serve as an entry for bacteria and infections may develop.

• Have feet measured and shoes fitted professionally. Wear new shoes for short periods of time and visually check the foot for pressure areas.

• Do not wear elastic stockings or socks with tight elastic tops. Do not use hot water bottles or heating pads.

• Have corns or calluses treated periodically by a physician or podiatrist. Do not self-medicate.

• Cut toenails in good light after a bath. Cut by following the shape of the ends of the toes and do not cut too short. Do not cut nails if eyesight is poor; have a physician or podiatrist trim them.

• Have feet checked by physician or nurse at each clinic or office visit.

The pharmacist can play a key role in encouraging diabetic individuals to develop habits that maintain good foot care. (See the chapter on diabetes care.)

Ask the Consumer

Q. Where is the lesion (on top of or between the toes, or on the sole of the foot)? What does it look like (red, white, swollen, soggy or hard)? Is it painful (with or without pressure) or itchy?

■ Since it is often impossible for the pharmacist to observe foot lesions, the consumer must be questioned thoroughly to determine the characteristics of the lesion. This information makes it possible to classify the lesion and leads to the appropriate treatment recommendation. Table II summarizes the characteristics, location, differential diagnosis and treatment of commonly encountered foot problems.

Q. Can you relate the onset of the problem to a particular pair of shoes or boots?

- New or poorly fitting footware can cause some foot disorders. If this may be the reason for the development or aggravation of the lesion, tell the consumer that treatment is ineffective if the cause is not removed. Shoes or boots that are too short, narrow or pointed apply excessive pressure to the feet; loose shoes allow excessive friction and may result in the formation or aggravation of corns, calluses, bunions and ingrown toenails. Occlusive footwear may exacerbate athlete's foot. The individual should discontinue wearing any footwear that seems to worsen the problem.

Q. Have you attempted self-medication? If so, which medication did you use and for how long? How did you apply it? Has it been effective?

- If individuals have not attempted to self-medicate, a treatment plan can be recommended based on classification of the lesion. Therapeutic failures can often be attributed to noncompliance or, less commonly, to misdiagnosis. By asking the above questions, pharmacists can determine if the product has been used appropriately (correct duration of treatment and proper application) and if adjunctive measures have been employed (for example, soaking the lesion and occlusion with salicylic acid products). If the product has been used incorrectly, instruct the individual in correct usage and retreatment. If therapeutic failure does not appear to be due to noncompliance, misdiagnosis is a possibility. At this stage, refer the individual to a physician or podiatrist.

Q. Do you have any other medical problems such as diabetes mellitus or circulatory disorders?

- Individuals with circulatory disorders or diabetes mellitus are highly susceptible to ulceration and infection and have slower healing rates than healthy individuals. These people are particularly prone to complications when keratolytic or caustic agents are applied to the skin or when conditions such as athlete's foot are allowed to progress to the acute stage. They should not attempt to self-medicate any foot disorder until they have consulted a physician or podiatrist.

Q. Do you have a history of asthma, allergies or other skin disorders?

- Atopic dermatitis is a common pruritic skin disease and is associated with asthma and hay fever. When present on the foot, atopic dermatitis may mimic athlete's foot. Individuals with atopic dermatitis have a greater tendency to develop severe exfoliative dermatitis from milder atopic disease when exposed to external irritants, overtreatment, infection and perspiration. People who respond positively to the above questions are best referred to a physician or podiatrist.

References

General

Giannestras NJ. Foot disorders—medical and surgical management. Philadelphia: Lea & Febiger, 1973:351–60.
Gibbs RC. Skin diseases of the feet. St Louis: Warren Green, 1980.
Gilman AG, Goodman LS, Gilman A, eds. Goodman and Gilman's the pharmacological basis of therapeutics. New York: Macmillan, 1980.
Hlavac HF. The foot book: advice for athletes. Mountain View: World Publications, 1977.
Stewart WD, Danto JL, Madden S. Dermatology: diagnosis and treatment of cutaneous disorders. St Louis: CV Mosby, 1974:314–5.

Calluses and Corns

Fritsch WC, Stoughton RB. The effect of temperature and humidity on penetration of C14 acetylsalicylic acid on excised human skin. J Invest Dermatol 1963;41:307–11.
Jahss MH. Disorders of the foot. Philadelphia: WB Saunders, 1982.
Popovich NG. Foot care products. In: Feldmann E, ed. Handbook of nonprescription drugs. Washington: American Pharmaceutical Association, 1977:361–79.
Potter GK. Histopathology of clavi. J Am Podiatry Assoc 1973;63:57–66.
von Weiss JE, Lever WF. Percutaneous salicylic acid intoxication in psoriasis. Arch Dermatol 1964;90:614–9.

Warts

Bart BJ, Biglow J, Vance JC, et al. Salicylic acid in karaya gum patch as a treatment for verucca vulgaris. J Am Acad Dermatol 1989;20:74–6.
Benton C. The management of viral warts. The Practitioner 1988;232:933–8.
Beutner KR, Conant MA, Friedman-Kien AE, et al. Patient applied podofilox for treatment of genital warts. Lancet 1989:831–4.
Bunney MH, Nolan MW, Williams DA. An assessment of methods of treating viral warts by comparative treatment trials based on standard design. Br J Dermatol 1976;94:667–79.
Bunney MH, Hunter JA, Ogilvie MM, et al. The treatment of plantar warts in the home. A critical appraisal of new preparation. Practitioner 1971; 207:194–204.
Edwards A, Atma-Ram A, Thin RN. Podophyltoxin 0.5% vs podophyllin 20% to treat penile warts. Genitourin Med 1988:263–5.
Epstein WL, Kligman AM. Treatment of warts with cantharidin. Arch Dermatol 1958;77:508–11.
Eskelinen A, Mashkilleyson N. Optimum treatment of genital warts. Drugs 1987;34:599–603.
Green D, Jolly HW. Comparative trial of a two dosage schedule of ketoconazole 2% cream for the treatment of tinea pedis. J Am Acad Dermatol 1987; 17(11):53–6.
Massing AM, Epstein WL. Natural history of warts. A two-year study. Arch Dermatol 1963;87:306–10.
Middleton RK, Chan S. Bleomycin treatment of warts. DICP 1990;24:952–3.
Naylor MF, Neldner KH, Yarborough GK, et al. Contact immunotherapy of resistant warts. J Am Acad Dermatol 1988;19(4):679–83.
Rosenberg EW, Amonette RA, Gardner JH. Cantharidin treatment of warts at home (Letter). Arch Dermatol 1977;113:1134.
Sanders BB, Stretcher GS. Warts: diagnosis and treatment. JAMA 1976; 235:2859–61.
Simon S, Brody N. Chronic exuberant verrucae and depressed cellular immunity. Cutis 1981;28:504–6,519.
Soletto RJ, Napoli RC, Gazivoda PL, Hart TJ. A perspective study using bleomycin sulfate in the treatment of plantar veruccae. J Foot Surg 1975; 28(2):141–3.
Spanos NP, Williams V, Gwynn MI. Effects of hypnotic, placebo, and salicylic acid treatments on wart regression. Psychosom Med 1990;52:109–14.
Steele K. Management of cutaneous warts. Aust Fam Phys 1988;17(11):950–2.
Steele K, Irwin WG. Liquid nitrogen and salicylic/lactic acid paint in the treatment of cutaneous warts in general practice. JR Coll Gen Practitioners 1988;38:256–8.
Stoeher GP, Peterson AL, Taylor WJ. Systemic complications of local podophyllin therapy. Ann Intern Med 1978;89:362–4.
Stone KM, Becker TM, Hadgu A, et al. Treatment of external genital warts: a randomized clinical trial comparing podophyllin, cryotherapy and electrodesiccation. Genitourin Med 1990;66:16–9.
Taylor MC. Successful treatment of warts. Postgrad Med 1988;84(8):126–36.
Thivolet J, Viac J, Staquet MJ. Cell-mediated immunity in wart infection. Int J Dermatol 1982;21:94–8.

Ingrown Toenails

Connolly B, Fitzgerald RJ. Pledgets in ingrowing toenails. Arch Dis Child 1988;63:71–2.
Gillette RD. Practical management of ingrown toenails. Postgrad Med 1988;84(8):145–58.

Langford DT, Burke C, Robertson K. Risk factors in onychocryptosis. Br J Surg 1989;76:45–8.

Pearson HK, Bury RN, Wapples J, Watkin DFL. Ingrowing toenails: is there a nail abnormality? J Bone & Joint Surg 1987;69(5):840–2.

Stone OJ. Commonsense advice on treating nail disorders 1989;85(6):279–88.

Athlete's Foot

Amsel LP, Cravitz L, Vanderwyk R, et al. Comparison of in vitro activity of undecylenic acid and tolnaftate against athlete's foot fungi. J Pharm Sci 1979;68:384–5.

Baer RL, Rosenthal SA. The biology of fungus infections of the feet. JAMA 1966;197:1017–20.

Battistini F, Cordero C, Ureuyo FG, et al. The treatment of dermatophytoses of the glabrous skin: a comparison of undecylenic acid and its salt versus tolnaftate. Int J Dermatol 1983;22:388–9.

Carter VH. A controlled study of haloprogin and tolnaftate in tinea pedis. Curr Ther Res 1972;14:307–10.

Chretien JH, Esswein JG, Sharpe LM, et al. Efficacy of undecylenic acid—zinc undecylenate powder in culture positive tinea pedis. Int J Dermatol 1980;19:51–4.

Fuerst JF, Cox GF, Wever SM, et al. Comparison between undecylenic acid and tolnaftate in the treatment of tinea pedis. Cutis 1980;25:544–6.

Gellin GA, Maibach HI, Wachs GN. Contact allergy to tolnaftate. Arch Dermatol 1972;106:715–6.

Green DL, Gutierrez MM. Tinea pedis caused by Hendersonula toryloidea. J Am Acad Dermatol 1987;16(5):1111–4.

Hermann HW. Clinical efficacy studies of haloprogin, a new topical antimicrobial agent. Arch Dermatol 1972;106:839–42.

Jones HE. Therapy of superficial fungal infection. Med Clin North Am 1982;66:873–93.

Katz R, Cahn B. Haloprogin therapy for dermatophyte infections. Arch Dermatol 1972;106:837–8.

Leyden JJ, Kligman AM. Interdigital athlete's foot: new concepts in pathogenesis. Postgrad Med 1977;61:113–6.

Leyden JJ, Kligman AM. Aluminum chloride in the treatment of symptomatic athlete's foot. Arch Dermatol 1975;111:1004–10.

Lyddon FE, et al. Short chain fatty acids in the treatment of dermatophytoses. Int J Dermatol 1980;19(1):24–28.

Pariser DM. Superficial fungal infections: a practical guide for primary care physicians. Postgrad Med 1990;87(5):205–14.

Robinson HM Jr, Raskin J. Tolnaftate, a potent topical antifungal agent. Arch Dermatol 1965;91:372–6.

Smith EB. Topical antifungal agents. In: Dermatologic clinics. Philadelphia: WB Saunders, 1984:109–13.

Smith EB, Dickson JE, Knox JM. Tolnaftate powder in prophylaxis of tinea pedis. South Med J 1974;67:776–8.

Smith EB, Powell RF, Graham JL, Ulrich JA. Topical undecylenic acid in tinea pedis: a new look. Int J Dermatol 1977;16:52–6.

Strauss JS, Kligman AM. An experimental study of tinea pedis and onychomycosis of the foot. Arch Dermatol 1957;76:70–9.

Tschen EH, Becker LE, Ulrich JA, et al. Comparison of over-the-counter agents for tinea pedis. Cutis 1979;23:696–8.

Yoshikawa TT, Chow AW, Guze LB, eds. Infectious disease, diagnosis and management. New York: Wiley, 1980.

Diabetic Foot Care

Boulton AJM. The diabetic foot. Med Clin North Am 1988;72(6):1513–30.

Colwell JA, Halushka PV, Sarji KE, et al. Vascular disease in diabetes-pathophysiological mechanisms and therapy. Arch Intern Med 1979;139:225–30.

Louie TJ, Bartlett JG, Tally FP, et al. Aerobic and anaerobic bacteria in diabetic foot ulcers. Ann Intern Med 1976;85:461–3.

Shenaq SM. Diabetic foot ulcers. Postgrad Med 1989;85(1):323–8.

25
Diabetes Care

William R. Cornish

Diabetes mellitus is classified into five clinical categories, of which the two most common are insulin-dependent (IDDM) and non-insulin-dependent (NIDDM). Long-term complications include macrovascular disease, retinopathy, nephropathy, neuropathy and diabetic foot. Management of diabetes begins with appropriate diet and exercise, but oral hypoglycemic agents and insulin are often necessary. Differing sources, formulations and administration methods of insulin allow consumer-based selection. Monitoring diabetic control with urine glucose, urine ketone and blood glucose testing devices is critical to management.

Several years ago, roadside billboards asked the question, "What do one million Canadians have in common?" The answer, surprisingly, was diabetes mellitus. It has a prevalence in the general population of about 5 per cent. Diabetes has a significant economic impact on society, as shown by United States statistics. In 1980, the overall cost resulting from diabetes was 9.7 billion dollars. This included indirect costs due to loss of productivity, and direct costs reflecting expenditures for medical and related services.

Diabetes is associated with significant morbidity and mortality. Retinopathy is the leading cause of new blindness, nephropathy is the most important cause of adult renal failure, and neuropathy contributes to diabetic foot problems, which may lead to amputation.

Diabetes is a condition that requires the cooperation and continuous commitment of the whole health care team. The nutritionist, physical therapist, pharmacist, social worker, nurse, podiatrist, family physician, endocrinologist and others share a role in diabetes care.

At the centre of this group are the diabetics. These individuals must assume a great degree of responsibility for control of their condition and they require much attention from the health care team to do so successfully. A diet specifying the types and amounts of food and timing of meals must be designed and taught to the patient. An exercise plan should be discussed with the physician. The effects of diet, activity and medication, must be understood before the individual can be responsible for control of blood glucose. The pharmacist can provide information on storage, mixing and injection of many new insulin products, and can monitor medication for drug interactions, particularly with the oral hypoglycemic agents. As well, proper use of blood glucose, urine glucose and ketone monitoring products must be understood to ensure useful feedback to the individual and the team concerning the control of diabetes.

Patients need education, skills training, reinforcement, encouragement and counselling. This is especially true now that sophisticated methods of monitoring and more complicated insulin treatment regimens are utilized in an effort to establish more strict blood glucose control. This is an exciting time for individuals with diabetes and for the health care team. Health care professionals should be knowledgeable and capable of providing answers to the questions asked by consumers. This is the challenge of diabetes care today.

Table I *Classification of Diabetes Mellitus and Other Categories of Glucose Intolerance*

Current terms	Former terms
Clinical categories	
Type I: Insulin-dependent diabetes mellitus (IDDM)	Juvenile diabetes
	Juvenile-onset diabetes
	Ketosis-prone diabetes
	Growth-onset diabetes
	Brittle diabetes
Type II: Non-insulin-dependent diabetes mellitus (NIDDM)	Adult-onset diabetes
Type a: nonobese	Maturity-onset diabetes
Type b: obese	Ketosis-resistant diabetes
	Stable diabetes
	Maturity-onset diabetes of youth
Diabetes mellitus associated with other conditions or syndromes	Secondary diabetes (drug-induced diabetes; impaired glucose tolerance due to other hormonal irregularities)
Impaired glucose tolerance (IGT)	Asymptomatic diabetes
	Chemical diabetes
	Subclinical diabetes
	Borderline diabetes
	Latent diabetes
Gestational diabetes	Gestational diabetes
Statistical risk	
Previous abnormality of glucose tolerance	Latent diabetes
	Prediabetes
Potential abnormality of glucose tolerance	Potential diabetes
	Prediabetes

Adapted from: National Diabetes Data Group. Classification and diagnosis of diabetes mellitus and other categories of glucose intolerance. Diabetes 1979;28(12):1039–57.

Definition and Classification

Diabetes is a metabolic syndrome characterized by glucose intolerance and hyperglycemia. Diabetes is not a single disease entity. Both clinically and genetically, diabetes is a heterogenous group of disorders. Diabetes is currently classified into 5 major clinical categories and 2 classes of statistical risk. This system, introduced in 1979, is shown in Table I along with the terminology used in the former classification system.

In the statistical risk classes, Potential Abnormality of Glucose Tolerance refers to those people considered at risk on a theoretical basis alone. In contrast, Previous Abnormality of Glucose Tolerance includes people who have demonstrated diabetic hyperglycemia or

impaired glucose tolerance in the past, but who now have reverted to normal. Examples include gestational diabetics and formerly obese diabetics who have lost weight.

Gestational diabetes mellitus (GDM) refers only to diabetes that has its onset or recognition during pregnancy. Women who have had GDM are at increased risk for progression to diabetes within 5 to 10 years.

The Impaired Glucose Tolerance category includes people who have mild glucose intolerance of a degree between normal and diabetic, and have a nondiagnostic fasting plasma glucose. Clinically significant renal and retinal complications of diabetes are absent.

Secondary diabetes is that which occurs in association with other conditions that have either caused the diabetes or allowed it to

Figure 1 *Pathogenesis of Insulin Resistance in NIDDM*

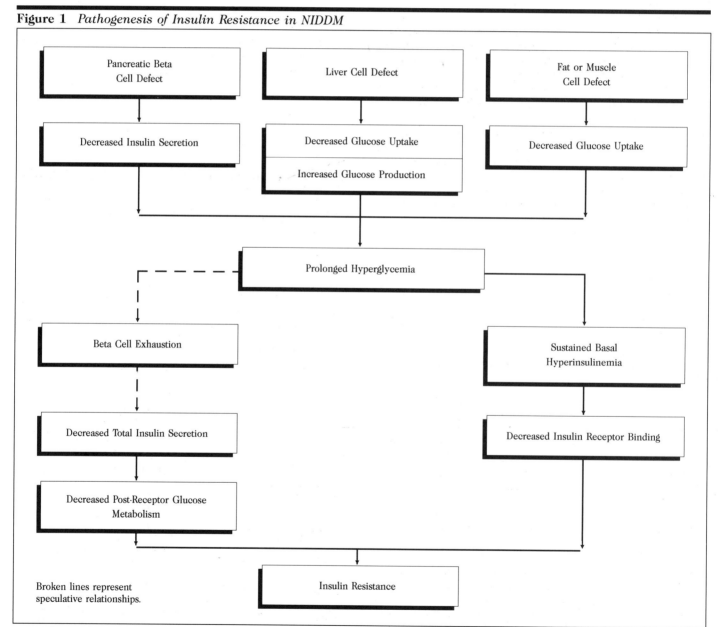

Broken lines represent speculative relationships.

Adapted from: Defronzo RA, Ferrannini E, Koivisto V. New concepts in the pathogenesis and treatment of non-insulin-dependent diabetes mellitus. Am J Med 1983; 74(Suppl 1A):52–81.

develop. Secondary causes include pancreatectomy, cystic fibrosis, chronic pancreatitis, pancreatic carcinoma, hemochromatosis, acromegaly and Cushing's syndrome.

The remaining subclasses, insulin-dependent diabetes mellitus and non-insulin-dependent diabetes mellitus, are discussed in detail below. Together they comprise the vast majority of cases of diabetes.

Insulin-Dependent Diabetes Mellitus (IDDM)

About 5 to 10 per cent of those with diabetes have IDDM or Type I diabetes (formerly called juvenile onset or brittle diabetes). These individuals require injected insulin to prevent ketoacidosis and to sustain life. They are distinct from other diabetics who may require insulin for optimal control of glucose but who are usually resistant to ketosis and can survive without insulin.

IDDM usually appears in youth and has its peak incidence at puberty, or about 14 years of age. A second rise in incidence may occur in later life, after age 40. The onset is commonly abrupt, occurring over several days. Classic signs and symptoms include thirst, increased appetite, excessive urination and weight loss. *fatigue*

The pathogenesis of IDDM is believed to involve the following series of events. First, genetic susceptibility must be present. Second, an environmental event, probably occurring long before diagnosis of diabetes, initiates the process in genetically predisposed individuals. Viral infection is believed to be one common triggering mechanism. Next, the pancreas undergoes an inflammatory response, called insulitis, which is accompanied by infiltration of activated T lymphocytes. The insulin-secreting pancreatic beta cell is transformed so the immune system recognizes it as foreign. Cytotoxic islet cell antibodies are produced and lead to destruction of over 90 per cent of the beta cells in the pancreas. Alpha cells, which secrete glucagon, are spared during this process. *no more insulin produced*

There is a low prevalence of direct inheritance in this type of diabetes. The chance of a child developing IDDM when a first degree relative has the disease is only 5 to 10 per cent. IDDM is strongly associated with the presence of certain histocompatibility antigens (HLA) on the sixth chromosome, the probable site of the IDDM susceptibility genes. *Treatment - insulin, diet*

Non-Insulin-Dependent Diabetes Mellitus (NIDDM)

About 85 to 90 per cent of all diabetics have NIDDM or Type II diabetes (formerly called adult or maturity onset diabetes). It is characterized by a later onset (in middle life or beyond), the presence of endogenous insulin secretion and a resistance to ketosis. The onset of symptoms is much more gradual than in IDDM and diagnosis is often made without classic symptoms, but on routine urinalysis or fasting glucose results. No HLA relationship has been identified, and autoimmune mechanisms are not believed to be involved. The genetic influence is strong, since whenever NIDDM occurs in identical twins, either both or neither of the twins is affected. The risk of developing NIDDM in offspring and siblings is higher than the corresponding risk of inheriting IDDM.

The exact pathogenesis of NIDDM is uncertain. Figure 1 represents one hypothetical sequence of events that combine to produce insulin resistance which is characteristic of NIDDM.

Insulin secretion is impaired in NIDDM. The pancreatic beta cell is less sensitive to glucose stimulation, the response is delayed, the overall secretory capacity is reduced, and there may be excessive late insulin secretion. Hyperglycemia results from impaired insulin

secretion, decreased glucose uptake by muscle, fat and liver cells, and increased glucose production by the liver.

Prolonged hyperglycemia provides a continual stimulus to the pancreas and excessive insulin levels result. This causes an automatic decrease in the number of insulin receptors on target cells, decreases insulin binding and contributes to insulin resistance. Prolonged hyperglycemia in genetically predisposed individuals may cause beta cell exhaustion, a further decrease in insulin secretion and defective postbinding (intracellular) insulin action. Obesity is associated with a reduced number of insulin receptors and contributes to insulin resistance. Weight reduction can improve insulin action in obese patients with NIDDM and improve glucose tolerance.

The distinguishing features of IDDM and NIDDM are summarized in Table II. *Found in a routine blood test*

Carbohydrate Metabolism

Normal homeostatic processes maintain plasma glucose concentrations in the range of 3.3 to 9 mmol/L (60 to 160 mg/dL). Values below 2.2 mmol/L (40 mg/dL) are insufficient to provide adequate fuel for the brain, and those over approximately 10 mmol/L (180 mg/dL) exceed the kidney's capacity for reabsorption of glucose and cause it to spill into the urine.

After consumption of food by a nondiabetic, glucose stimulates the pancreatic beta cells to secrete insulin. This process promotes uptake

Table II *Comparison of Type I and Type II Diabetes*

Feature	Type I (IDDM)	Type II (NIDDM)
Proportion of all diabetics	5–10%	85–90%
Age of onset	usually childhood or adolescence	usually after 40 years
Type of onset	acute, severe	gradual, mild
Signs, symptoms	excessive urination excessive thirst increased appetite	usually no major complaints
Body weight	normal or decreased	obesity in 70–90%
Etiology:		
Autoimmunity	85% have anti-islet antibodies	rarely present
Heredity	25–50% concordance in identical twins	95–100% concordance in identical twins
HLA Association	2.5 times the expected frequency	same frequency as normal population
Physiologic defect	insulin deficiency	resistance to insulin action and impaired insulin secretion
Insulin levels	negligible	variable; often normal or high
Stability	frequent wide blood glucose fluctuations	fairly stable glucose levels
Ketosis	prone to ketosis	ketosis-resistant
Treatment	diet, insulin	reducing diet, oral hypoglycemics, insulin

of glucose from the bloodstream into the tissues for energy or storage. In muscle, glucose may be stored as glycogen, and amino acids converted to protein. In adipose tissues, insulin promotes glucose conversion of fatty acids and their storage as triglycerides. Insulin also promotes the storage of glucose as glycogen in the liver. These processes contribute to an overall anabolic state.

In the fasting state, hypoglycemia is avoided in the nondiabetic as follows. Low glucose levels inhibit insulin release and stimulate release of the counter-regulatory hormones. Glucagon, epinephrine, cortisol and growth hormone promote an increased glucose level, oppose insulin and produce a catabolic state. Glycogen is broken down (by glycogenolysis) in the liver to supply glucose directly. Protein is broken down to provide amino acids that can be used to synthesize glucose in the liver (by gluconeogenesis). In adipose tissue, triglycerides are converted to free fatty acids, which travel to the liver as fuel for gluconeogenesis.

In insulin deficiency, the cells are starved for glucose, which cannot enter from the bloodstream. The above catabolic processes are initiated in a futile attempt to raise intracellular glucose. The results are increased appetite (polyphagia), hyperglycemia, loss of glucose in the urine (glucosuria), a resultant osmotic diuresis (polyuria), dehydration and excessive drinking (polydipsia). Acidic ketone bodies, formed during breakdown of free fatty acids, accumulate in the bloodstream to produce ketoacidosis and are excreted in the urine (ketonuria).

Diabetic ketoacidosis, which may occur in IDDM, is a medical emergency which, if untreated, may result in death. The individual may appear drowsy or unresponsive and have dry skin, possibly rapid, deep breathing, a fruity odor on the breath, and anorexia, vomiting or abdominal pain. Treatment consists of replacing fluid volume using intravenous saline solutions, administering intravenous insulin by infusion and replacing electrolytes lost in the urine.

Patients with NIDDM have adequate insulin activity to avoid ketoacidosis. However, they may develop a hyperglycemic, hyperosmolar, nonketotic coma during periods of stress and loss of control. Prompt attention in the hospital emergency ward is required for this condition as well. The signs and symptoms of hyperglycemia and hypoglycemia are contrasted in Table III.

Hypoglycemia

Hypoglycemia refers to a blood glucose below 2.8 to 3.3 mmol/L (50 to 60 mg/dL). Factors contributing to hypoglycemia in those with diabetes include exercise, excessive dosage of insulin or oral hypoglycemic dosage, insufficient food intake and certain other medications and alcohol. The signs and symptoms usually associated with hypoglycemia are listed in Table III. The severity of symptoms does not directly correlate with the prevailing level of blood glucose. For example, a rapid fall from a high (e.g., 12 mmol/L or 215 mg/dL) to a normal blood glucose level (e.g., 4.4 mmol/L or 80 mg/dL) may induce symptoms in some persons. On the other hand, blood glucose levels of 2.2 mmol/L (40 mg/dL) may occur in others without recognizable symptoms.

The danger of hypoglycemia is that the brain requires normal glucose levels to function properly. Below 2.2 mmol/L (40 mg/dL), the individual often becomes confused, amnesic or somnolent. Loss of consciousness, convulsions, brain damage and even death may occur at glucose levels below 1.1 mmol/L (20 mg/dL).

It is important for those suspected of experiencing hypoglycemia to confirm this by testing blood glucose. The objective of treatment is to restore normal glucose levels without producing hyperglycemia. This goal can be achieved in the conscious individual by oral administration of 10 g of glucose. This amount of glucose is provided by 100 mL of sweetened juice or nondiet soft drink, 2 packets of sugar, 15 mL of jelly, 5 to 6 Life Savers, 4 sugar cubes or 10 mL of honey. The blood glucose should rise by approximately 2.2 to 2.8 mmol/L (40 to 50 mg/dL) within 10 to 15 minutes, and should be confirmed by a repeat blood glucose test. If the response has been inadequate, the treatment should be repeated. If a meal is not scheduled within 30 minutes, small amounts of protein and starch should be eaten.

If the individual is stuporous, a glucose gel preparation (for example, Monoject Insulin Reaction Gel, 40 per cent dextrose, 25 g package) placed in the mouth between the cheek and gums will melt and slide down the esophagus without danger of aspiration.

For severe hypoglycemic reactions in unconscious individuals, glucagon may be injected subcutaneously, to raise blood glucose and restore consciousness, thereby permitting oral carbohydrate ingestion. A response should occur within 5 to 20 minutes after injection of 0.5 to 1 unit of glucagon. It is recommended that those with diabetes keep a supply of glucagon and that a family member or friend be trained to inject it.

Table III *Signs of Hypoglycemia and Hyperglycemia*

Signs	Hypoglycemia (insulin shock)	Hyperglycemia (diabetic coma)
Onset	sudden (hours)	gradual (days)
Overall condition	very weak	extremely ill
Behavior	excited, nervous, irritable, confused (in severe, late stages may be unconscious)	drowsy, may progress to loss of consciousness
Skin	moist, pale (sweating)	dry, flushed
Mouth	moist, numb/tingling tongue	dry
Thirst	absent	intense
Hunger	present	absent
Breath	normal	fruity odor (in IDDM)
Respiration	normal or rapid, shallow	deep, labored (in IDDM)
Blood pressure	normal	low
Pulse	full, bounding	weak, rapid
Pain	headache	abdominal pain
Vomiting	absent	common
Tremor	common	absent
Convulsion	in late stages	absent
Blood glucose	low	high
Urine glucose	absent in second voided specimen	high
Urine ketones	absent	high (in IDDM)

Diagnosis

The diagnosis of diabetes requires only that an individual demonstrate hyperglycemia and signs and symptoms attributable to osmotic diuresis. Individuals with persistently elevated fasting plasma glucose levels (greater than 7.8 mmol/L or 140 mg/dL) on at least 2 occasions have diabetes. Some asymptomatic individuals with normal fasting plasma glucose may be suspected of having diabetes and may warrant investigation. An oral glucose tolerance test requires ingestion of 1.75 g/kg of glucose (maximum 75 g). Plasma glucose is tested at 1, 2 and 3 hours afterward. The criteria for diagnosis are shown in Table IV.

Long-Term Complications

The late complications of diabetes are listed in Table V. The table indicates the increased risk in diabetes for developing each complication relative to the risk in the nondiabetic population, and summarizes the influence of glycemic control on the incidence of complications.

Macrovascular Disease

Ischemic heart disease is involved in about 60 per cent of deaths of adult diabetics. The risk of death from coronary artery disease or stroke is doubled by the presence of diabetes.

This risk rises rapidly with age, but is not strongly correlated with either the duration of diabetes or the severity of hyperglycemia. However, 2 major risk factors for coronary artery disease—increased LDL cholesterol and decreased HDL cholesterol—appear to be related to the severity of hyperglycemia. Better control of blood glucose tends to lower LDL and raise HDL cholesterol, thereby improving the lipid profile in diabetes.

Retinopathy

Diabetic proliferative retinopathy is the leading cause of new cases of blindness in North America. It is present in 50 per cent of cases of blindness diagnosed before age 20, but only 15 per cent of those diagnosed after age 50. Five to 10 per cent of individuals having diabetes for 20 years will become legally blind. In NIDDM, 15 to 25 years after diagnosis, people are 2 to 3 times less likely to have proliferative retinopathy than in IDDM. Minor background changes begin after 5 years, but rarely cause visual loss. Proliferative changes involve growth of new vessels that tend to bleed, causing vitreous hemorrhage. The hemorrhaging can lead to fibrosis and eventual detachment of the retina.

Good glycemic control during the initial 25 years of diabetes is rarely associated with these changes, whereas poor control may lead to 80 per cent proliferative retinopathy and 12 per cent blindness. Intensive treatment is recommended to reduce the frequency and severity of retinal damage. However, once damage is established, an ophthalmologist may use photocoagulation to prevent further proliferation, and vitrectomy to treat hemorrhage. These measures may be successful in avoiding total loss of vision in 60 per cent of advanced cases. These treatments are critical, as blind diabetics often cannot learn braille because of sensory neuropathy.

Cataracts occur in 12 per cent of diabetics by 20 years after diagnosis. However, this incidence has not been shown to be correlated with glycemic control.

Table IV Diagnostic Criteria for Diabetes Mellitus and Gestational Diabetes

NONPREGNANT ADULTS

Diabetes Mellitus. Diagnosis of diabetes mellitus in nonpregnant adults should be restricted to those who have *one* of the following:
- random plasma glucose level of ≥11.1 mmol/L (200 mg/dL) *plus* classic signs and symptoms of diabetes mellitus, e.g., polydipsia, polyuria, polyphagia and weight loss;
- fasting plasma glucose level of ≥7.8 mmol/L (140 mg/dL) on at least 2 occasions; or
- fasting plasma glucose level of <7.8 mmol/L (140 mg/dL) *plus* sustained elevated plasma glucose levels during at least 2 oral glucose tolerance tests. The 2-h sample and at least one other between 0 and 2 h after 75-g glucose dose should be ≥11.1 mmol/L (200 mg/dL). Oral glucose tolerance testing is not necessary if patient has fasting plasma glucose level of ≥7.8 mmol/L (140 mg/dL).

PREGNANT WOMEN

Gestational Diabetes. After an oral glucose load of 100 g, diagnosis of gestational diabetes may be made if 2 plasma glucose values measured in mmol/L (mg/dL) equal or exceed

Fasting	1 h	2 h	3 h
5.8 (105)	10.5 (190)	9.2 (165)	8.1 (145)

Adapted from: Physicians guide to insulin-dependent (Type I) diabetes: diagnosis and treatment. Alexandria: American Diabetes Association, 1988; June.

Table V Long-Term Complications: Relative Risk, Prevalence and Relationship to Control

Complication	Relative risk in diabetes	Prevalence (%) after 25 years of diabetes		
		Overall	Good control	Poor control
Retinopathy	Risk of blindness 25 × normal	60	10	80
Nephropathy	Risk of renal failure 17 × normal	20	<1	20
Neuropathy		50	10	65
Macrovascular disease	Risk of stroke and coronary artery disease 2 × normal	The relationship between glycemic control and macrovascular disease is at present unclear.		

(handwritten: Heart disease)

Nephropathy

Diabetes is the single most important cause of adult renal failure. Before the availability of dialysis and transplantation, nearly 50 per cent of deaths in those diagnosed before age 20 were due to renal failure.

Nephropathy develops as glomerular permeability increases after 5 to 15 years of diabetes. The diagnosis is made upon detecting gross proteinuria. After 15 to 20 years of diabetes, 35 per cent of people with IDDM, but only 13 per cent of those with NIDDM, develop rapidly progressive renal failure. Dialysis or transplantation may be required within another 5 years in these cases.

(handwritten: Treatment - reduce blood pressure)

Good glycemic control over 25 years is rarely associated with proteinuria, whereas poor control contributes to nephropathy in 20 per cent of cases. When proteinuria is established, aggressive treatment of hypertension, not plasma glucose, reduces the risk of developing chronic renal failure and the eventual need for dialysis.

By screening for the presence of albumin in the urine (microalbuminuria), kidney disease can be detected in the early stages. Studies have shown that the use of angiotensin converting enzyme (ACE) inhibitors such as captopril or enalapril can reduce microalbuminuria, improve renal function, and slow or possibly prevent the progression of diabetic nephropathy.

Neuropathy

Neuropathy is perhaps the most frequent complication early in diabetes. The incidence increases rapidly after 15 years to eventually affect 50 per cent of those having diabetes for 30 years. Neuropathy may be present at the diagnosis of NIDDM, since the mild, early course of NIDDM may go undetected. Symptoms of peripheral neuropathy that affect primarily the feet, legs and hands include burning, tingling, pain, numbness, and loss of pain and light touch sensations. This condition is a major contributor to amputations. (See the section on diabetic foot.)

In addition to these sensory defects, the function of the autonomic

Figure 2 *Pathogenesis of the Diabetic Foot Ulcer; peripheral vascular disease and neuropathy may coexist.*

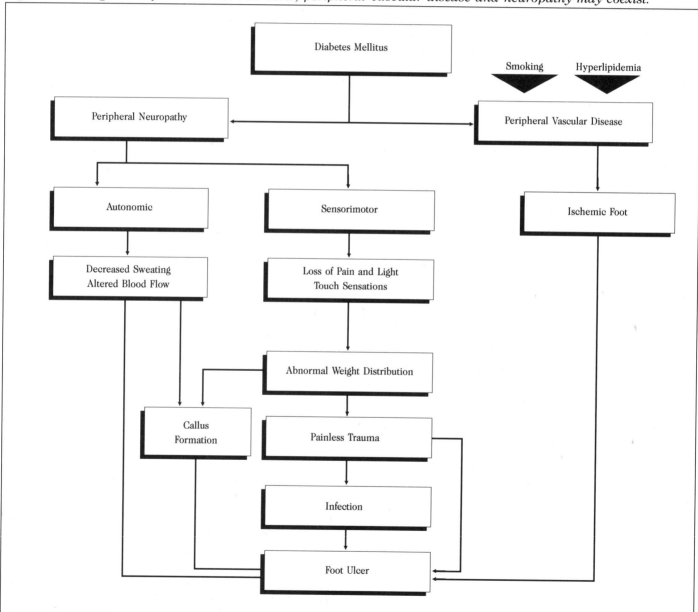

Reprinted from: Boulton AJM, Bowker JH. The diabetic foot. In: Olesfsky JM, Sherwin RS, eds. Diabetes mellitus: management and complications. New York: Churchill Livingstone, 1985:255-75.

nervous system may deteriorate after years of poor metabolic control. Autonomic neuropathy affects many organ systems. Bladder atony and a failure to sense a full bladder may cause urinary hesitancy and may increase the risk of pyelonephritis due to ureteral reflux. Diabetic gastroparesis reduces gastric motility and delays emptying, which can cause anorexia and postprandial vomiting. Metoclopramide, domperidone or cisapride may alleviate these problems. Diabetic diarrhea may cause fecal incontinence. Sexual impotence commonly affects 50 per cent of diabetic males after 10 to 15 years. Postural hypotension without adequate compensatory tachycardia may occur. Deficient sweating and the resulting dry skin may aggravate foot problems. Finally, there may be a loss of awareness of the adrenergic symptoms of hypoglycemia (sweating, tachycardia, nausea and tremulousness). People treated with insulin are thus at increased risk for severe hypoglycemia as falling plasma glucose levels may go unnoticed.

In people with good glycemic control, neuropathy reportedly occurs in only 10 per cent after 25 years; 70 per cent of those poorly controlled have progressive symptoms. Therefore, intensive treatment using multiple daily insulin injections or subcutaneous infusion has been recommended. *good diet, blood sugar testing exercise*

Diabetic Foot

Persons with diabetes are at risk of developing neuropathy and peripheral vascular disease and are 15 times more likely to require amputation of a gangrenous foot than nondiabetic individuals. The (United States) National Diabetes Advisory Board concluded that provision of adequate foot care could reduce the amputation rate by as much as 50 to 75 per cent.

The pathogenesis of diabetic foot ulcer is illustrated in Figure 2. An inadequate blood supply, dryness due to decreased sweating, structural deformities with abnormal weight distribution and loss of sensation all contribute to the potential for developing painless trauma, infection and ulceration.

The costs of amputation in dollar figures and in quality of life can be staggering. Hospital admission, rehabilitation services, loss of income, restriction of physical activities and potential extended care must be considered. Thus, it is extremely important to educate those with diabetes and the health care team in order to prevent foot problems. Experience shows that patients ignore what they cannot feel or see and often fail to seek medical advice until serious ulceration and infection occurs.

Prevention involves daily inspection of the feet and adherence to many other cautions as outlined in Table VI. These points are especially important in the population at greatest risk, those over 40 years of age who have had diabetes for more than 10 years. Avoiding pressure, cold and smoking helps maintain peripheral blood flow. Avoiding cutaneous insults such as hot water, sunburn, keratolytics and ill-fitting footwear are all essential elements of prevention.

Treatment of Diabetes

A theoretical goal of treatment would be to cure diabetes mellitus. One experimental aproach for patients with IDDM involves pancreas transplantation. Over the last 20 years, experience with this approach in 700 patients indicates that success is limited by technical difficulties and immunologic problems such as graft rejection. Some individuals are successful in achieving satisfactory blood glucose levels after surgery, but many are not. It is hoped the availability of

Table VI *Preventing Diabetic Foot Ulcers: Consumer Instructions*

Do
1. Inspect feet daily, using a mirror and with help from a family member. Look at pressure points, and between toes for scratches cuts, blisters.
2. Wash feet daily in tepid water. Avoid extreme temperatures. Dry carefully, especially between toes.
3. Apply lubricant (lotion) after washing.
3. Trim toenails straight across.
5. Always wear stockings properly fitted and change daily.
6. Wear comfortable, roomy shoes. Change often.
7. Inspect inside of shoes daily for foreign objects, sharp protrusions and torn linings.
8. Ensure that physician inspects feet each visit.
9. Consider assessment by a podiatrist; state that you are diabetic.

Don't
1. Don't walk barefoot.
2. Don't use hot water bottles or heating pads. Check bath water temperature before stepping in (85–90°F or 29–30°C is acceptable).
3. Don't wear shoes without stockings.
4. Don't wear sandals with thongs between toes.
5. Don't buy plastic shoes.
6. Don't smoke.
7. Don't use keratolytics (chemicals to remove corns or calluses).
8. Don't cut corns or calluses, except upon advice from physician or podiatrist.
9. Don't wear garters, cross legs or do anything to impair circulation to the feet.

better immunosuppressive regimens may improve results in the future.

Another approach to curing diabetes involves implantation of healthy insulin-secreting islet cells into the pancreas of the diabetic individual. This procedure is still in the experimental stage. The use of cyclosporin very early in the development of IDDM to protect the pancreas from autoimmune destruction has been attempted in some trials. However, such immunosuppression is considered at this time to be a research tool only.

Current management of diabetes includes dietary therapy, exercise, oral hypoglycemic agents and insulin.

Diet

Diet plays a vital role in managing diabetes and is an essential component for optimum results. The 5 goals of dietary therapy as outlined by the American Diabetes Association are listed in Table VII.

Strategies for IDDM and NIDDM

In IDDM, the total daily energy should be consumed consistently throughout the day in 3 regular meals, a bedtime snack and one or more between-meal snacks. Consistent adherence to this meal plan is required to counterbalance the effects of a traditional insulin treatment and exercise program. However, patients controlled by insulin pump or by multiple daily insulin injections (based on blood glucose monitoring results) may be allowed greater flexibility in meal plans.

In obese persons with NIDDM, weight reduction can have beneficial effects on glycemic control, lipid profile, blood pressure and kidney function. Correcting obesity reduces insulin resistance in NIDDM, improves glucose tolerance and can reduce or even eliminate the need for oral hypoglycemic agents or insulin.

To reduce weight, a calorie restriction of 500 to 1,000 kilocalories below the usual daily food intake is recommended. Maintaining reduced body weight requires a lifelong commitment to continued calorie restriction. Unfortunately, experience has shown that few people actually lose much of their excess weight; in those who do, weight loss is often temporary.

Table VII *Goals of Dietary Therapy in Managing Diabetes*

1. To maintain plasma glucose levels as near to physiologic as possible in order to prevent hyperglycemia and hypoglycemia, and to prevent or delay development of long-term complications.

2. To attain and maintain reasonable body weight in adults and normal growth rate in children.

3. To restore optimal plasma lipid levels.

4. To determine an individualized meal plan with consistent timing of meals and snacks to prevent inordinate swings of plasma glucose in insulin-requiring diabetics.

5. To manage weight in obese individuals with NIDDM by alteration of food intake and eating behavior, along with enhancement of activity level.

Adapted from: American Diabetes Association. Nutritional recommendations and principles for individuals with diabetes mellitus:1986. Diabetes Care 1987;10(1):126–32.

Composition of Diet

The diabetic diet is designed to provide the amount of energy required to achieve and maintain the desired body weight. Fat should provide no more than 30 per cent of the total energy. Cholesterol content should not exceed 300 mg per day. Patients with persistently elevated LDL cholesterol have greater risk of cardiovascular disease and should be further restricted to 20 to 25 per cent fat and 100 to 150 mg of cholesterol per day.

The amount of carbohydrates should be liberalized and provide 55 to 60 per cent of calories. Foods containing unrefined carbohydrates are preferred, and simple sugars are best avoided. Most patients should attempt to gradually increase their current daily fibre content to decrease postprandial hyperglycemia and lower cholesterol levels. However, many individuals may consider such high-fibre diets less palatable and may experience gastrointestinal side effects such as abdominal cramping, flatulence or loose stools. In addition, no information is currently available on the long-term effects of fibre on glycemic control.

After ingestion, various carbohydrates elicit different plasma glucose responses. Researchers have compared these responses to that elicited by an equivalent amount of glucose. Based on the degree and duration of hyperglycemia, these responses have been assigned a glycemic index. This data may be used in selecting which types of carbohydrate sources are to be consumed. However, the long-term clinical utility and benefits of a low-index diet have yet to be established.

The North American dietary intake of protein is generally considered excessive. Many persons with diabetes either have, or are at risk of developing, nephropathy. Therefore, the remainder of the diet should contain protein not exceeding about 0.8 g/kg in most cases.

protein not more 50-60g/day

Sodium

Modest restriction of sodium intake is recommended since persons with diabetes frequently become hypertensive. A general maximum daily intake of 3 g of sodium is advised.

Alcohol

Alcohol should be consumed in moderation by persons with diabetes for several reasons. Alcohol can depress the capacity of the liver for gluconeogenesis, thereby impairing the body's ability to recover from hypoglycemia. Since alcohol may potentiate and prolong hypoglycemia, it should be consumed only with a meal. Alcohol yields a high amount of energy and must be considered in overall dietary caloric calculations for weight reduction. Inebriation in a person with diabetes may be mistaken by others for hypoglycemia or insulin shock and is best avoided.

Alcohol ingestion by those taking chlorpropamide may result in an adverse interaction characterized by flushing, headache, dizziness, nausea and vomiting. Excessive alcohol intake is contraindicated in persons taking metformin.

Individuals should not exceed 2 equivalents of alcohol once or twice weekly. One equivalent is represented by 240 mL of beer, 110 mL of wine or 45 mL of distilled beverage. Light beer and dry wine are preferable due to their lower carbohydrate content.

— no more than 2 drinks/wk.

Artificial Sweeteners

The availability of artificial sweeteners is believed to help diabetics adhere to their diets, although recent recommendations now allow for a modest intake of sucrose. Two categories of sweeteners exist. The first category is comprised of fructose, mannitol, sorbitol and xylitol which possess similar energy values to glucose (4 kcal/g) and may interfere with weight reduction if not considered in caloric calculations. There is no evidence of toxicity with these agents. In particular, it is believed that dietary sorbitol does not gain intracellular access and thus does not contribute to developing long-term diabetic complications.

The second category includes the noncaloric sweeteners saccharin, cyclamate and aspartame. Diabetics can avoid excessive intake of any one sweetener by using various agents to distribute any potential risks. The acceptable daily intake of cyclamate is 10 mg/kg. The acceptable daily intake of saccharin in children is 500 mg/day and in adults 1,000 mg/day. The acceptable daily intake of aspartame is 50 mg/kg, equivalent to ingesting 16 cans of soft drink by a 70-kg person. Certain aspartame formulations contain lactose, and it has been recommended that diabetics limit consumption of these products.

Studies show that aspartame is well tolerated in diabetics using dosages in excess of average intake. Two studies found no derangement in diabetic control, no evidence of toxicity and an incidence of adverse reactions no greater than with placebo.

Aspartame is metabolized before absorption to phenylalanine, aspartic acid and methanol. About 10 per cent by weight is converted to methanol. However, these amounts are of no concern. Phenylalanine intake must be restricted in subjects with the rare genetic metabolic disorder phenylketonuria. However, apart from this caution, the American Medical Association concluded in 1985 that use of aspartame in normal humans, including pregnant women, is safe.

See also the section on sugar substitutes in chapter on nutritional products.

Dietetic Products

Special dietetic foods are expensive and generally unnecessary. The nutritional value of such products is believed to be no better than regular foods. Differences are often related only to cost, calories or substitution of sweeteners for sucrose. Several terms are used to describe special food products.

The label "no sugar added" means no sucrose has been added, but the product may contain other simple sugars (fructose or dextrose). "Sugar-free" products contain little or no sugar and are reduced in calories. "Calorie-reduced" products are reduced in calories, but may be inappropriate for diabetics due to simple sugar content. "Carbohydrate-reduced" products may contain large amounts of saturated fats, may be high in calorie content and are to be discouraged in diabetics.

Exercise

Along with diet, exercise is a fundamental component of the diabetes treatment plan. Regular exercise should be encouraged and aerobics are recommended where appropriate. Table VIII outlines the benefits and risks of exercise in diabetics.

People over 40 years of age and those with a previously sedentary lifestyle are advised to undergo a treadmill stress test before initiating an exercise program. Diabetics with foot problems should select appropriate activities such as swimming, rowing or cycling. The poorly controlled diabetic with fasting hyperglycemia (greater than 16.7 mmol/L or 300 mg/dL) is advised to postpone exercise until control is regained.

Non-insulin-dependent diabetics have essentially normal requirements for energy during exercise and supplemental food is not recommended, unless sulfonylurea therapy has been noted to induce hypoglycemia. However, significant adjustments often must be made by insulin-dependent diabetics. The person with IDDM is best advised to avoid strenuous activity within 4 hours of injection of short-acting insulin to avoid its peak action coinciding with the exercise. Since those treated with regular insulin before meals 3 times daily use small doses and adjust according to blood glucose tests, the 4-hour proviso need not contraindicate exercise in these individuals.

The abdomen is the recommended site for injection. Absorption is more predictable and less likely to be enhanced by exercise-induced increase in blood flow, as can occur with leg injections.

If exercise is anticipated and the insulin required for that period has not yet been injected, reductions in dosage of 30 to 35 per cent for intermediate-acting insulins and of 50 to 65 per cent for short-acting types have been recommended. The exact adjustment is highly individual and can be determined only after experience with home blood glucose monitoring (HBGM) and observed responses to various exercises. It is recommended that vigorous exercise be undertaken only if the plasma glucose is in the range of 5.6 to 11.1 mmol/L (100 to 200 mg/dL) and there is no ketosis.

To avoid hypoglycemia from unplanned exercise, depending on results of HBGM, supplemental complex carbohydrate (for example, 25 to 30 g) may be taken before, and possibly during, prolonged activity. Additional food may be required at the next snack or meal.

Postexercise hypoglycemia may result from continued enhancement of insulin sensitivity, repletion of muscle and liver glycogen stores, or the action of intermediate-acting insulin. Food supplements, according to HBGM results, are especially important since the symptoms of hypoglycemia (for example, sweating and palpitations) may not be as readily apparent during exercise.

Table VIII *Exercise in Diabetes*

Benefits

1. Improvement in insulin sensitivity and glucose tolerance, allowing for decreased need for insulin or oral hypoglycemic agent.
2. Facilitation of weight loss in obese non-insulin-dependent diabetics (caloric restriction is a prerequisite).
3. Possible decreased risk of cardiovascular disease.
4. Enriched quality of life through increased work capacity and improved sense of well-being.

Risks

1. Immediate and prolonged hypoglycemia, due to enhanced tissue uptake of glucose, induced either by exercise or by potentiation of the action of insulin or oral hypoglycemic agents.
2. Exacerbation of hyperglycemia and development of ketosis if exercise is undertaken during a state of insulin deficiency.
3. Worsening of diabetic complications (proliferative retinopathy, nephropathy and diabetic foot) is possible with strenuous exercise of certain types.
4. In people with coronary artery disease, exercise can lead to arrhythmias, ischemia or infarction.

Oral Hypoglycemic Agents

Oral hypoglycemic agents play an important role in treating NIDDM. Oral agents are indicated for people failing to achieve adequate control after a 2- to 3-month trial of diet and exercise. Some individuals with NIDDM who have severe fasting hyperglycemia will require treatment with insulin.

Oral hypoglycemic agents currently available in Canada are compared in Table IX with respect to half-life, duration of action, dosage range and frequency, and route of elimination.

Sulfonylureas improve NIDDM by improving insulin secretion by the pancreas and by decreasing insulin resistance in liver, muscle and adipose tissues. Since sulfonylureas directly stimulate pancreatic insulin secretion they may therefore cause hypoglycemia. In contrast, metformin, a biguanide, does not increase insulin secretion and does not cause hypoglycemia. Its beneficial effects appear to result from improved insulin activity which results in increased uptake of glucose into muscle and decreased glucose production by the liver.

Adverse Effects

Hypoglycemia is the most frequent serious adverse effect of sulfonylureas. It can be fatal if not recognized and promptly treated. The patient and the family should be familiar with the signs and symptoms of hypoglycemia and with the methods used to correct it. The incidence of sulfonylurea-induced hypoglycemia is estimated at one to 5 per cent. The agent most often implicated has been chlorpropamide, probably due to its long half-life and enhanced potential for accumulation. Glyburide, despite its shorter apparent half-life, has been increasingly associated with hypoglycemia, perhaps because the drug may accumulate within the beta cells of the pancreas

Table IX *Oral Hypoglycemic Agents*

Sulfonylureas	Other names	Daily dosage		Half-life (hr.)		Duration of action (hr.)	Doses per day	Comments
		Average	Range	Average	Range			
Acetohexamide 0.5g	Dimelor	1.0g	0.25–1.5g	6	4–12	12–18	1–2	• renal excretion of 50% of active metabolite • avoid in renal impairment
Chorpropamide 100mg, 250mg	Apo-Chlorpropamide Diabinese Novo-Propamide	250mg	100–500mg	35	24–60	24–72	1	• renal excretion of 10–60% of active drug • avoid in renal impairment • caution in the elderly
Gliclazide	Diamicron	160mg	80–320mg	10	6–14	16–24	1–2	• inactive metabolites • caution in renal impairment
Glyburide 2.5mg, 5mg	Diabeta Euglucon	7.5mg	2.5–20mg	10	6–16	16–24	1–2	• active metabolites • caution in renal impairment
Tolbutamide 0.5g	Apo-Tolbutamide Mobenol Novo-Butamide Orinase	1.5g	0.5–3	6	4–8	6–12	2–3	• inactive metabolites • preferred agent in renal impairment
Biguanide								
Metformin 0.5g	Glucophage	1.5g	2.5g	2.8	1.5–4.5	8	2–3	• renal excretion of 100% active drug • contraindicated in renal impairment • risk of lactic acidosis

causing excessive insulin secretion in certain circumstances. Factors that increase the risk of hypoglycemia include advanced age, renal impairment, inadequate or irregular nutrition, liver disease, use of a longer acting sulfonylurea and concomitant use of drugs known to potentiate the action of sulfonylureas.

Other adverse effects are generally mild and occur infrequently. About 2 per cent of people experience dose related gastrointestinal upset, which can be minimized by taking the sulfonylurea with meals. Cutaneous reactions occur in 1 to 3 per cent of people and are manifested as mild rashes that are reversible within 2 to 14 days of drug withdrawal. Hematological reactions are rare.

Chlorpropamide causes a unique effect by potentiating the release and action of antidiuretic hormone and in some people this may cause a dilutional hyponatremia which if severe, can cause loss of consciousness. Another reaction seen with chlorpropamide is the disulfiram-like effect which can occur with concomitant ingestion of alcohol. Facial flushing, dizziness, headache, nausea and vomiting may result from this interaction.

The University Group Diabetes Program (UGDP) study from the 1960s reported a 2.5 fold increase in cardiovascular mortality associated with tolbutamide therapy compared with diet alone. These results have been the subject of much debate. In 1979, the American Diabetes Association advised that the present use of sulfonylureas in treating NIDDM should not be restricted nor significantly altered based upon findings from the UGDP study.

Metformin is reported to cause adverse gastrointestinal effects in up to 20 per cent of patients. These include metallic taste, nausea, vomiting, anorexia, abdominal pain and diarrhea. These effects are dose related and can be minimized by administration with meals. Lactic acidosis is a rare but serious complication with a mortality

rate of 40 to 50 per cent. It has developed in individuals treated with another biguanide, phenformin, which was removed from the Canadian market in 1977. However, metformin has not been reported to cause lactic acidosis since its introduction in Canada in 1972. The risk of mortality from lactic acidosis due to metformin is estimated to be no greater than the risk of mortality from hypoglycemia due to glyburide. Therefore, metformin is clearly a safe agent provided that it is not prescribed when contraindicated (see Clinical Use & Efficacy).

Drug Interactions

Other medications may potentiate or diminish the action of oral hypoglycemic agents by one of two mechanisms. The first involves a pharmacokinetic drug interaction with sulfonylureas whereby the protein binding, distribution, metabolism or elimination of the sulfonylurea is altered. The second involves pharmacodynamic interactions whereby another agent alters glucose metabolism through its own intrinsic activity. A list of drugs that interact with the sulfonylureas appears in Table X. The action of metformin can be influenced only by interactants operating through pharmacodynamic mechanisms.

Choice of Drug

The oral hypoglycemic drug of first choice is usually a sulfonylurea. The choice among sulfonylureas is usually based on their kinetic properties, adverse effect profiles, and consideration of individual patient characteristics. For example, the elderly are at increased risk of developing hypoglycemia due to poor eating habits and reduced renal drug elimination. Thus, a short-acting, less potent agent such as tolbutamide may be preferred. Use of acetohexamide and chlorpropamide should be avoided, while gliclazide and glyburide should

Table X *Drug Interactions With Oral Hypoglycemic Agents*

DRUGS THAT MAY POTENTIATE THE HYPOGLYCEMIC EFFECTS OF SULFONYLUREAS

Interacting drugs	Mechanism and comments
* Beta-adrenergic blockers	• decreased gluconeogenesis and glycogenolysis • block most symptoms of hypoglycemia (except sweating) • probably less likely with cardioselective agents (e.g., metoprolol, atenolol)
Chloramphenicol	• decreased hepatic metabolism • decreased renal excretion? • more common in renal insufficiency
Clofibrate	• decreased protein binding • probable decreased metabolism
Coumarin anticoagulants (acenocoumarol, bishydroxycoumarin) (**not** warfarin)	• decreased hepatic metabolism
* Ethanol (acute ingestion)	• decreased gluconeogenesis • especially important in fasting or malnourished individuals
* Monoamine oxidase inhibitors (especially tranylcypromine)	• increased insulin secretion • decreased gluconeogenesis
Pyrazolones (phenylbutazone, sulfinpyrazone)	• decreased protein binding • decreased hepatic metabolism • decreased renal excretion
* Salicylates (includes PAS) (large doses of 4–6 g/day)	• decreased protein binding • increased insulin secretion • decreased gluconeogenesis? • decreased renal excretion?
Some sulfonamides (sulfamethizole, sulfadimethoxine, sulfisoxazole)	• decreased protein binding • decreased hepatic metabolism • decreased renal excretion
* Sympatholytics (clonidine, guanethidine, reserpine, methyldopa?)	• decreased gluconeogenesis • block symptoms of hypoglycemia

DRUGS THAT MAY DIMINISH THE HYPOGLYCEMIC EFFECTS OF SULFONYLUREAS

Interacting drugs	Mechanism and comments
* Beta-adrenoceptor agonists (epinephrine, ephedrine, terbutaline, etc.?)	• alpha-agonists decrease insulin secretion • beta-agonists increase hepatic gluconeogenesis and glycogenolysis
Ethanol (chronic alcoholism)	• increased hepatic metabolism (severe liver disease and acute ethanol can cause hypoglycemia)
* Estrogens (oral contraceptives)	• insulin resistance?
* Glucocorticosteroids	• intrinsic hyperglycemic activity (uncommon with alternate day dosing)
* Nicotinic acid	• insulin resistance
Phenobarbital	• increased hepatic metabolism
* Phenytoin	• decreased insulin secretion
Rifampin	• increased hepatic metabolism • increased hypoglycemia upon withdrawal of rifampin
* Theophylline	• increased gluconeogenesis • increased insulin secretory response to glucose?
* Thiazide diuretics (also ethacrynic acid, furosemide, diazoxide)	• decreased insulin secretion • potassium depletion leading to insulin resistance

*Denotes agents which interact by a pharmacodynamic mechanism. These agents have potential to alter control in metformin treated patients.

be used with caution in these individuals. When compliance may be a concern, a longer-acting agent should be selected for once daily dosing and tolbutamide should not be used.

Chlorpropamide can cause unique adverse effects not shared by the other sulfonylureas, and is reportedly associated with the highest incidence of adverse effects. Considering this and its very long half-life of elimination, chlorpropamide appears to be a less attractive agent. Acetohexamide is not commonly used and has little to offer over other sulfonylureas.

Glyburide is now the most widely used agent. It has an intermediate duration of action, allows fine titration of dosage, and may be given once daily in many individuals. Although glyburide is a newer second generation sulfonylurea, its efficacy is not superior to that of chlorpropamide. It should be noted that glyburide is fast becoming the commonest cause of sulfonylurea-induced severe, prolonged hypoglycemia.

The newest agent, gliclazide, has been marketed in Canada during the past year. Gliclazide appears to possess certain properties not shared by the other sulfonylureas. It is reported to not promote weight gain, it reduces platelet hyperadhesiveness and hyperaggregation, and can restore vascular fibrinolytic activity during therapy in patients with NIDDM. The clinical significance of the latter two observations in relation to the development and progression of the long-term complications of diabetes is unknown.

Metformin is most often used in combination with a sulfonylurea and is prescribed for only 10 per cent of diabetics requiring oral hypoglycemic agents. It is usually added as a second agent for persons who fail to establish adequate control with a sulfonylurea alone. Treatment with metformin is often associated with weight loss, in contrast to sulfonylurea therapy, which promotes weight gain. Metformin may favorably alter serum lipds. Therefore, metformin appears particularly suited for use in grossly obese individuals with NIDDM.

Clinical Use and Efficacy

Oral hypoglycemic agents may be contraindicated in several situations: IDDM; ketoacidosis; hyperosmolar nonketotic coma; lactic acidosis; periods of severe stress; and pregnancy.

Metformin use is contraindicated in people with renal insufficiency, hepatic failure or alcoholism, or cardiovascular disease with severe circulatory impairment and tissue hypoxia.

Diabetes Care

The use of oral hypoglycemic agents is not universally successful. A satisfactory response is more likely to occur in selected individuals with the following characteristics: age at onset of diabetes greater than 40 years; duration of diabetes before treatment less than 5 years; obesity at the time of diagnosis; fasting plasma glucose less than 11 mmol/L (200 mg/dL); no history of previous insulin therapy, or well controlled on less than 20 to 30 units per day; and absence of ketoacidosis, past or present.

A significant proportion of patients (15 to 20 per cent) initially prescribed oral agents may fail to respond adequately. This is termed a primary failure. Of those who achieve satisfactory control, an estimated 5 to 10 per cent per year may subsequently lose control and are termed secondary failures. Common causes of secondary failure include dietary neglect, inadequate drug dosage, metabolic stress (for example, myocardial infarction, trauma, infection, surgery) and deterioration of endogenous insulin secretory capacity. As few as 30 to 50 per cent continue successfully after 10 years on oral hypoglycemic agents.

Treatment is initiated with a minimal dosage and gradually increased as required to achieve control up to the maximal recommended dosage. Elderly, debilitated people and those with hepatic or renal insufficiency require smaller initial and incremental dosages. It is recommended that control be monitored to regulate dosage requirements and to verify continued efficacy. Some authors recommend periodic withdrawal of oral hypoglycemic agents to document the need for continued therapy. It is possible for some individuals with NIDDM to enter a phase of relative remission and to require no medication for varying periods of time.

When control deteriorates, metformin can be added to sulfonylurea therapy. Metformin may convert a secondary failure to success. Alternatively, one can switch to another sulfonylurea. However, there is no rationale for using two different sulfonylureas in one person. Some patients with NIDDM require insulin for adequate control, either continually throughout the course of their diabetes or intermittently during periods of stress to establish blood glucose control and allow for successful maintenance therapy with oral agents.

Insulin
Formulations

Insulins fall into 1 of 4 categories based on their formulation and resultant time course of action. The short-acting insulins include regular and Semilente insulin. The intermediate-acting preparations

Table XI *Canadian Insulin Products*

Type	Source	Product	Dosage Form	Manufacturer
RAPID				
Regular	Beef/Pork	Insulin-Toronto	10 mL vial	Conn-Novo
		Iletin Regular	10 mL vial	Lilly
	Pork	Illetin II Regular	10 mL vial	Lilly
		Velosulin Nordisk	10 mL vial	Nordisk
	SHI	Novolin-Toronto	10 mL vial	Conn-Novo
		Novolin-Toronto Penfill	1.5 mL cartridge	Conn-Novo
		Velosulin Human	10 mL vial	Nordisk
		Velosulin Human	2.5 mL cartridge for Insuject	Nordisk
	BHI	Humulin R	10 mL vial	Lilly
		Humulin R	1.5 mL cartridge for B-D Pen	Lilly
Semilente	Beef/Pork	Semilente Insulin	10 mL vial	Conn-Novo
		Iletin Semilente	10 mL vial	Lilly
INTERMEDIATE				
NPH	Beef/Pork	NPH Insulin	10 mL vial	Conn-Novo
		Iletin NPH	10 mL vial	Lilly
	Pork	Iletin II NPH	10 mL vial	Lilly
		Insulatard Nordisk	10 mL vial	Nordisk
	SHI	Novolin-NPH	10 mL vial	Conn-Novo
		Novolin-NPH Penfill	1.5 mL cartridge	Conn-Novo
		Insulatard Human	10 mL vial	Nordisk
		Insulatard Human	2.5 mL cartridge for Insuject X	Nordisk
	BHI	Humulin N	10 mL vial	Lilly
		Humulin N	1.5 mL cartridge for B-D Pen	Lilly
Lente	Beef/Pork	Lente Insulin	10 mL vial	Conn-Novo
		Iletin Lente	10 mL vial	Lilly
	Pork	Iletin II Lente	10 mL vial	Lilly
	SHI	Novolin-Lente	10 mL vial	Conn-Novo
	BHI	Humulin L	10 mL vial	Lilly

Table XI *(Cont'd) Canadian Insulin Products*

Type	Source	Product	Dosage Form	Manufacturer
LONG ACTING				
PZI	Beef/Pork	Iletin PZI	10 mL vial	Lilly
Ultralente	Beef/Pork	Ultralente Insulin	10 mL vial	Conn-Novo
		Iletin Ultralente	10 mL vial	Lilly
	SHI	Novolin-Ultralente	10 mL vial	Conn-Novo
	BHI	Humulin U	10 mL vial	Lilly
MIXTURES	Pork	Mixtard Nordisk (30% Reg/70% NPH)	10 mL vial	Nordisk
		Initard Nordisk (50% Reg/50% NPH)	10 mL vial	Nordisk
	SHI	Novolin–30/70 (30% Reg/70% NPH)	10 mL vial	Conn-Novo
		Novolin–30/70 Penfill	1.5 mL cartridge	Conn-Novo
		Mixtard 30/70 Human	10 mL vial	Nordisk
		Mixtard 30/70 Human	2.5 mL cartridge for Insuject X	Nordisk
		Mixtard 50/50 Human (50% Reg/50% NPH)	10 mL vial	Nordisk
		Mixtard 15/85 Human (15% Reg/85% NPH)	10 mL vial	Nordisk
	BHI	Humulin 30/70	10 mL vial	Lilly
		Humulin 30/70	1.5 mL cartridge for B-D Pen	Lilly
SPECIAL PRODUCTS				
Concentrated Insulins	Pork	Iletin II Regular** 500 U/mL	20 mL vial	Lilly
	SHI	Actrapid Human** 500 U/mL	10 mL vial	Conn-Novo
Sulphated Insulin	Beef	Sulphated Insulin*	10 mL vial	Conn-Novo
Insulin for S/C Pump	Pork	Velosulin Nordisk	5.7 mL infusor cartridge	Nordisk

*Requires approval for release from Conn-Novo Medical Department
**Emergency Drug Release (Health Protection Branch)
SHI Semi-Synthetic Human Insulin (enzymatically derived from pork)
BHI Biosynthetic Human Insulin (rDNA–recombinant DNA technology)
Conn-Novo Connaught Novo Nordisk (distributor of Connaught Novo and Nordisk products)

are NPH (neutral protamine Hagedorn or isophane) and Lente. PZI (protamine zinc insulin) and Ultralente are long-acting insulin products. Premixed formulations containing various proportions of NPH and regular insulin comprise the fourth category. Canadian insulin products are listed in Table XI.

The accepted standard times for onset, peak and duration of action of the 7 basic insulin formulations are outlined in Table XII. Caution should be used in applying these figures to the individual, since they represent average values from several standard references. Considerable variation in these parameters exists from one person to another and even within one individual from time to time.

Regular insulin is a clear, unmodified solution. It is the only type that may be administered intravenously and is routinely used during treatment of diabetic ketoacidosis, during surgery or during intravenous feeding (parenteral nutrition). Only regular insulin can be injected intramuscularly. This route may be required when the intravenous route is not available and one requires more rapid absorption than that seen after subcutaneous injection.

All other common insulin products are suspensions of insulin modified to extend the action profile and are given only subcutaneously. Two different methods have been used to achieve extended action. First, the protein protamine can be bound with insulin in the presence of zinc to form crystals that delay absorption from the subcutaneous injection site. In NPH insulin, protamine and insulin are present in approximately equal proportions for intermediate action. PZI is formulated with an excess of protamine and thereby becomes a long-acting insulin.

The second method involves modification of insulin in the presence of an acetate buffer and excess zinc. Semilente insulin is comprised of zinc insulin in amorphous form, which produces an activity profile which is slightly delayed compared to that of regular insulin. Ultralente insulin contains zinc insulin in crystalline form, which provides a duration of action of up to 36 hours. Lente insulin is a combination of the former 2 types in a ratio of 3:7, amorphous to crystalline (Semilente to Ultralente) providing an intermediate action.

Table XII *Insulin Formulations: Time Course of Action*

Category	Formulation	Onset (hr)	Peak (hr)	Duration (hr)
Short-Acting	Regular	0.5–1	2.5–5	5–7
	Semilente	1–2	4–10	12–16
Intermediate-Acting	NPH (Isophane)	1–1.5	4–12	18–24
	Lente	1–2.5	7–14	18–24
Long-Acting	PZI (Protamine Zinc)	4–8	14–24	36
	*Ultralente	4–6	18–24	36
Mixtures	Regular/NPH (30/70, etc.)	0.5	2–12	18–24

Notes: 1. These data are averages. The time course of insulin action varies greatly in individuals (see text).
*The values in the table are traditional figures which generally apply to nonhuman insulins. The onset and peak action of some human insulins may occur earlier, and their duration may be shorter (see text).

As shown in Table XI, insulin manufacturers have produced several premixed combination products containing regular and NPH insulin at a fixed ratio of 15:85, 30:70 or 50:50 units/mL of each component. These mixtures produce similar effects to those seen after separate injections of regular and NPH insulin at different sites.

Pharmacokinetics
Absorption

The subcutaneous absorption of insulin is highly irregular. Variability of 25 per cent within the same individual and 50 per cent between two diabetics has been observed. It has been suggested that as much as 80 per cent of the day-to-day fluctuation in blood glucose concentrations can be accounted for by variations in absorption of insulin.

Most of the factors affecting subcutaneous absorption relate to the degree of blood flow present at the injected site. The higher the rate of blood flow, the more rapid the insulin absorption. There are inherent differences in blood flow in different regions of the body. The onset of action of regular insulin is quickest when the injection is in the abdomen, followed by the arm, the buttock and the thigh. In one study, absorption half-lives were 87, 141, 155 and 164 minutes respectively. As well, the depth of injection may increase the rate of absorption if either too deep into the muscle, or too shallow and above the subcutaneous tissue, since these areas are more highly perfused.

Factors increasing the rate of absorption from any one site include exercise of the area, massage and higher ambient temperature. Smoking has been associated with slower insulin absorption due to vasoconstriction of blood vessels.

To decrease the variability of subcutaneous insulin absorption, the following guidelines are recommended. The patient should develop a reproducible injection technique that avoids too shallow or too deep an approach. Routine massage of the injection site is not recommended. Rotation of the site of injection is still considered necessary, but rotation from one anatomical area of the body to another is discouraged. The site rotation should occur within one area, such as the abdomen or thigh. This will prevent the development of lipohypertrophy and promote more reproducible absorption. To avoid an exaggerated hypoglycemic response, the injected area should not be exercised immediately after an injection of regular insulin.

Distribution and Elimination

After absorption, insulin reaches sites of action and elimination via the systemic circulation. In the bloodstream, insulin may be bound to antibodies or may exist in a free state. The degree of binding depends on the antigenicity of the injected insulin and the genetically determined propensity of the individual to respond and produce antibodies. Only free unbound insulin is biologically active and degradable. Therefore, in people with a high degree of insulin binding, the onset of insulin action may be delayed and the duration of effect prolonged. These effects are undesirable, since the diabetic requires a prompt onset of action from preprandial regular insulin injections, and may be at risk for late postprandial hypoglycemia if antibodies prolong insulin action. As well, extensive antibody binding of insulin tends to prolong recovery from hypoglycemia. The major sites of degradation of insulin are the kidney and liver.

Insulin Source

For over 60 years, insulin has been extracted from livestock pancreas. Conventional insulin preparations contain varying amounts of beef and pork insulin in a ratio of about 70:30, depending on species availability.

The structure of the insulin protein derived from 3 sources (beef, pork and human) differs in the amino acid sequences. Pork insulin differs from human insulin by one amino acid, whereas beef insulin differs by having 3 alterations in the amino acid sequence. For this reason, beef insulin is a more foreign protein, more antigenic and more likely to be associated with immunologic complications during therapy. For many years, prior to the availability of human insulins, a pork monospecies insulin product has been available for use by diabetics who do not tolerate the beef/pork combination product.

Insulin identical in structure to human pancreatic insulin has been available since the beginning of the 1980s. Currently, 2 methods are used to produce human insulin. Biosynthetic human insulin (BHI) is produced within *Escherichia coli* bacteria using so-called genetic engineering through recombinant DNA technology. Semisynthetic human insulin (SHI) is produced from pork insulin by enzymatic cleavage of the alanine residue and replacement with threonine.

Table XI lists all insulin products currently available in Canada, indicating the source from which each is derived.

Complications of Insulin Therapy
Antigenicity

Injecting exogenous insulin to treat diabetes can elicit an immune response. Antibodies are produced when the body recognizes the insulin preparation as a foreign substance.

Several factors affect the magnitude of the immune response. The most important of these appears to be the source of the insulin. The amino acid sequence of the beef insulin protein differs from that of the human insulin at 3 places, while that of pork insulin differs at only 1 place. As a result, beef insulin is much more antigenic than pork insulin, which is slightly more antigenic than synthetic human insulin preparations.

The modification of insulins to achieve extended action may contribute to their antigenicity due to the formation of complexes of insulin molecules. Preparations such as NPH and Lente insulin are slightly more antigenic than regular insulin. During storage, slight chemical changes may occur depending on temperature, pH, and insulin and zinc concentration. This process may lead to modification of the insulin molecule and to formation of polymers of insulin in solution. Even the site and mode of injection (by formation of a subcutaneous depot of insulin) may contribute to antigenicity. These points may explain why even human insulin products may be antigenic.

The purity of the insulin product has been an important determinant of antigenicity. The purity of insulin from animal sources has improved gradually over the years. Conventional insulin before 1972 was purified by sequential recrystallization only. This process did not effectively remove contaminants such as proinsulin which was present in a concentration of greater than 10,000 ppm. In 1972, proinsulin concentration was reduced to between 1,000 and 10,000 ppm through the use of gel filtration chromatography, and the resultant level of purity was referred to as "single peak." In 1980, the designation "purified" was introduced to describe insulins purified by ion exchange chromatography and containing less than 10 ppm proinsulin. At present, all Canadian insulin products are highly purified and therefore purity is no longer an important determinant of antigenicity.

Biosynthetic human insulin contains no proinsulin. Its potential contaminants are *Escherichia coli* polypeptides, but the manufacturer states that these are removed during the purification process and are undetectable in the commercial product. The purity of semisynthetic human insulin relates to its content of pork proinsulin, which is invariably less than 10 ppm.

Local Reactions

Local reactions to subcutaneous injection of the older, nonpurified beef/pork insulins were not uncommon, affecting 5 to 10 per cent of users. The incidence with insulin products currently available is believed to be substantially less. Upon initiation of treatment, the local reaction may consist of erythema, swelling, pain or pruritus. In most cases, these effects subside and disappear after a few weeks. If they persist, the severity of the reaction may be decreased by changing to a less antigenic pork or human insulin, or by splitting the injection volume between 2 sites.

Lipoatrophy is a process whereby adipose tissue is lost at the sites of subcutaneous injection of insulin. The exact cause is unknown, but probably relates to the presence of impurities in conventional beef-pork insulins marketed over 20 years ago. The incidence and severity have been progressively declining; from 55 per cent in 1953 to only 10 per cent in 1979, and presumably much lower with the availability of purified, less antigenic insulin preparations. Although it is primarily of cosmetic significance, lipoatrophy may also cause disordered insulin absorption if affected sites are used for subcutaneous injection. When caused by beef/pork insulin, a change to pork or human insulin usually leads to improvement if injections are made into the site of atrophy. In some cases, a mixture of insulin and dexamethasone injected into the site has been of benefit.

Lipohypertrophy—the development of abnormal subcutaneous deposits of adipose tissue or fat pads—may occur as a result of repeated injection of insulin at the same site. This practice must be avoided since insulin absorption from hypertrophied sites can be delayed. Adherence to a plan for rotating injection sites can both prevent and resolve this condition. (See the section on subcutaneous injection of insulin.)

Systemic Reactions

Generalized allergic reactions are rare and occur almost exclusively in diabetics who have had interrupted or intermittent insulin therapy. A large, immediate type of reaction may occur at the injection site and a systemic reaction may involve urticaria, nausea, angioedema, bronchospasm or hypotension. After the acute reaction has been treated, individuals requiring continued treatment with insulin should be hospitalized and desensitized. Desensitization involves giving minute doses (the initial subcutaneous dose is 10^{-5} units) in gradual increments until either the required daily dose is reached or until a large local or mild systemic reaction occurs. At this point, the dose is dropped back to the previously tolerated dose. The process may take a week in hospital. Pork or human insulins are indicated for continued management of individuals allergic to beef/pork insulin.

Immunologic Insulin Resistance

Insulin resistance is a state in which a normal amount of insulin produces a subnormal biologic response. Immunologic insulin resistance is caused by the excessive binding of insulin in the circulation by immunoglobulin G antibodies. Bound insulin is not biologically active and thus dosage increases may be required in order to exceed the binding capacity and produce adequate free insulin concentrations to control blood glucose.

True immunological resistance is present when insulin requirements exceed about 2 units/kg/day. The incidence has been estimated in the past at 0.01 per cent of the insulin-requiring population. Other types of insulin resistance should be ruled out and antibody levels determined to confirm the diagnosis. The availability of more highly purified insulins and the greater use of less antigenic pork and human insulins have made this complication exceedingly rare.

Treatment may involve a switch of insulin type, or corticosteroid therapy. If a beef/pork insulin has been used, pork or human insulin may be of benefit. However, the success rate is less than 100 per cent due to cross-reactivity between species of insulin. Sulfated insulin, available from Connaught Novo Nordisk (upon special request), has been particularly effective in cases with immunological resistance. This chemically modified soluble insulin of beef or pork source has been treated with sulfuric acid, adding 6 sulfate groups to the insulin molecule. This structural change probably leads to a change in configuration of the insulin and a decreased recognition and binding by antibodies. On initiation of treatment, a reduced dosage is required to avoid hypoglycemia, and twice daily injections are usually sufficient.

Corticosteroids may be effective in lowering insulin requirement. Prednisone, 30 mg/day, may be used initially, and may produce a sharp drop in insulin binding. After this response, alternate day dosing is recommended and the prednisone dose may then be tapered and discontinued.

Two preparations of concentrated pork insulin are available in Canada on an emergency use basis, subject to approval by the Health Protection Branch of Health and Welfare Canada. Iletin II Regular (pork) 500 units/mL and Actrapid HM (human) 500 units/mL may be prescribed for those diabetics requiring very large doses of insulin. The concentrated preparation reduces the injection volume, precludes the need for multiple injection sites and may improve insulin absorption due to formation of a smaller subcutaneous depot.

Choice of Insulin by Source

The physician has a choice of 3 types of insulin by source: beef/pork,

pork or human. The 2 types of human insulin, biosynthetic and semi-synthetic, are generally considered interchangeable. Not all formulations of modified insulins are available as pork and/or human insulin. There is currently no pork or human Semilente or protamine zinc insulin. However, the availability of pork and human regular insulin and human Ultralente provides adequate treatment options.

The differences between insulins from various sources are basically the degree of antigenic potential and the cost. The cost of human insulin has fallen to a level which is currently about 20 per cent higher than that of beef/pork insulin. The cost of pork insulin is currently 45 per cent higher than beef/pork and about 20 per cent higher than human insulin.

Many insulin-requiring diabetics in Canada are maintained on beef/pork insulin products. These products have been purified to contain less than 10 ppm proinsulin in all cases. Despite the availability of human insulin, most diabetics have not been switched to the newer products. Either they are adequately tolerating the potentially more antigenic beef/pork variety, and the physician does not wish to introduce a new variable in well controlled individuals, or the cost of switching has been considered prohibitive.

When transferring a patient from beef/pork or pork insulin to human insulin, no initial dosage adjustment is required. However, it is recommended that blood glucose be monitored and insulin dosage be adjusted accordingly. Since antibody levels have been observed to decline in patients transferred from beef/pork to human insulin, insulin dosage reduction may be required during this period.

There is no evidence that better glycemic control can be achieved by using human insulin. The biological response to human insulin (intravenously) is virtually identical to that of pork insulin.

However, subcutaneous absorption of human insulin may occur more rapidly than with beef or pork. This may be due to the greater solubility of human insulin, which has the hydrophilic amino acid threonine in place of the alanine residue found in beef and pork insulin. The duration of action of human NPH may be significantly shorter than beef or pork NPH insulin and a once daily injection of human NPH is less likely to provide a 24 hour duration of action in all patients. Human Ultralente insulin also has a significantly shorter duration of action than the animal source product.

The indications for use of human insulin are as follows. Human insulin should be used to initiate treatment, for intermittent therapy, during pregnancy, and for patients intolerant of animal source insulin. Conversion of all patients from beef/pork or pork insulin to human insulin is neither required nor recommended except in previously noted circumstances.

Clinical Use of Insulin

Indications

Insulin is required to treat all patients with IDDM. Some individuals with NIDDM who cannot be controlled with diet, exercise and oral hypoglycemic agents will require insulin. Women who are sufficiently hyperglycemic during pregnancy to require medication must receive insulin since oral hypoglycemic agents are contraindicated during pregnancy. Patients with NIDDM are commonly treated with insulin during periods of extreme metabolic stress, such as trauma, serious infection or surgery.

Dosing Regimens

Successful replacement of insulin action in diabetes should provide 2 essential components that are present with normal endogenous insulin secretion. First, stable basal insulin concentrations are required between meals and overnight. Second, abrupt increases in insulin levels are required to coincide with absorption of nutrients from meals.

The simplest insulin treatment regimen would consist of a single morning injection of intermediate-acting insulin. However, this is often ineffective in controlling hyperglycemia after breakfast and, therefore, a rapid-acting insulin is usually combined with the intermediate-acting insulin and given as one injection. If the duration of action of the intermediate-acting insulin is not sufficiently long, fasting hyperglycemia before breakfast may require splitting of the daily dose of intermediate-acting insulin into 2 doses, one before breakfast and a second before the evening meal. In some individuals, the peak effect of this dose may occur during sleep at 2 to 4 a.m. and necessitate moving the second dose time to before bedtime to reduce the risk of nocturnal hypoglycemia.

The use of twice daily intermediate-acting insulin is called a *split* regimen. When each injection is combined with short-acting insulin, it is referred to as a *split and mixed regimen*. Figure 3, Panel A depicts this regimen and the usual proportions of the daily insulin dosage given in each component.

The *split and mixed* regimen is an improvement over previous approaches and it facilitates achievement of optimum blood glucose control. The delivery of insulin in 4 components facilitates dosage adjustment in response to blood glucose testing results. The effect of each insulin injection can be determined by testing blood glucose at specific times of the day as follows. The effect of the morning regular insulin dose is tested prior to lunch; the morning intermediate-acting insulin prior to supper; the afternoon regular insulin prior to bedtime; and the afternoon (or evening) intermediate-acting prior to breakfast the following morning. Based upon results of blood glucose monitoring, insulin dosage may be adjusted using a predetermined set of instructions or algorithm prepared by the physician.

Another method for achieving optimum blood glucose control is use of multiple daily injections (MDI) of insulin. This insulin regimen consists of 3 pre-meal injections of regular insulin along with Ultralente insulin injected separately once or twice daily. The long-acting Ultralente insulin provides basal insulin levels throughout a 24 hour period with no appreciable peaks in activity. The regular insulin doses are determined after blood sugar testing prior to meals (see Figure 3, Panel B).

The advantage of this MDI regimen is that mealtimes can be flexible since the insulin designated to cover that food intake has not already been injected earlier in the day. As well, the nature of the meal (amount of carbohydrate, number of calories) is also somewhat flexible since the dosage of pre-meal regular insulin can be adjusted to account for this.

Another method of administering intensive insulin therapy is the continuous subcutaneous insulin infusion (CSII). Briefly, in CSII, insulin is delivered using an electromechanical pump, a length of tubing and a subcutaneous needle implanted usually in the abdomen. The pump can be programmed to deliver insulin at a continuous basal rate and, at the discretion of the user, injects a selected bolus dose of insulin before meals (see Figure 3, Panel C).

The degree of improvement in blood glucose control using CSII and MDI is comparable. It should be noted that CSII is considered an experimental therapeutic procedure. It is usually reserved for patients who fail to achieve adequate blood glucose control using MDI, and those who experience brittle diabetes during pregnancy.

The timing of preprandial doses of regular insulin is crucial for

Figure 3 *Idealized Periods of Insulin Effect with Various Dosing Regimens*

Panel A
Split and mixed regimen (Regular plus NPH or Lente twice daily)

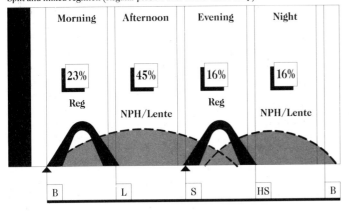

Panel B
MDI regimen (Multiple Daily Injections) (Regular before meals plus Ultralente once daily)

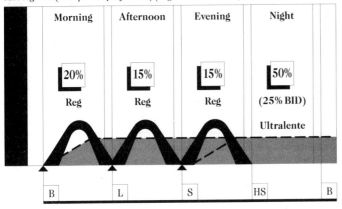

Panel C
CSII (Continuous Subcutaneous Insulin Infusion) (Regular insulin by pump)

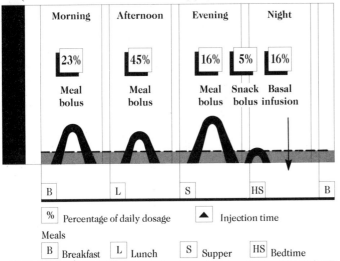

| % | Percentage of daily dosage | ▲ | Injection time |

Meals

| B | Breakfast | L | Lunch | S | Supper | HS | Bedtime |

Adapted from: Skyler JS, Reeves ML. Intensive treatment of Type I diabetes mellitus In: Olefsky JM, Sherwin RS, eds. Diabetes mellitus management and complications. New York: Churchill Livingstone, 1985:31–75.

optimal control of postprandial hyperglycemia. Standard references have recommended an injection 15 to 30 minutes before mealtime. Many people administer regular insulin 15 minutes before eating. However, recent evidence on insulin absorption rates indicates that an earlier injection—30 to 60 minutes before eating—is associated with less exaggerated postprandial hyperglycemia.

Intensive insulin therapy is a demanding treatment program, and many individuals are not able to comply with these demands. It is successful only in certain carefully selected, highly motivated people who can be extensively trained and closely monitored. Even with careful selection, continued success may be difficult to achieve. Individuals themselves must make conscious decisions to begin intensive therapy.

Insulin Administration
Insulin Syringes

Insulin syringes in Canada are calibrated for one strength of insulin, 100 units/mL (U-100). The syringe barrel bears markings that indicate, for a particular volume of U-100 insulin withdrawn, how many units are contained. There are 3 sizes of insulin syringes available. The 1 cc syringe has a 100 unit capacity; the 0.5 cc syringe has a 50 unit capacity; and the 3/10 cc syringe has a 30 unit capacity. The advantage of the 50 and 30 unit syringes is that the narrower barrel allows wider, more easily differentiated graduations to be marked on the syringe. For individuals using lower doses of insulin, these smaller syringes allow greater accuracy in dosing.

Most individuals prefer to use plastic disposable syringes and needles rather than glass syringes intended for reuse. The latter type are heavier, traditionally require sterilization, have a larger dead space volume (see below) and are less convenient, especially for travel. The disadvantages of disposable syringes include greater expense and less durability of the markings on the barrel.

Insulin syringes are made with a permanently attached subcutaneous 28 gauge needle which is commonly 1/2 inch (12.7 mm) long. Extra fine needles, 29 gauge, are now available under the names "Ultra-Fine" and "Ultra Comfort". Syringes with detachable needles have a dead space, that is a volume of insulin remaining in the syringe neck and needle hub when the syringe plunger has been fully depressed. This dead space volume, estimated at 0.04 to 0.09 mL (4 to 9 units) on average, can contribute to inaccuracies in delivery of insulin doses when mixtures are used. The actual volume of the first insulin drawn up will exceed the prescribed amount and the actual volume of the second insulin will be short of the prescribed amount by an equal volume. However, this problem is significant only if the order of mixing is reversed or if a different syringe with a different dead space volume is used. Disposable syringes with permanently attached needles and no dead space volume are the preferred type.

The possibility of reducing treatment expense by reusing disposable syringes and needles has been investigated. Several studies confirm the safety of this practice by reporting no appreciable bacterial contamination of syringe or insulin and no evidence of infection at the injection site. People studied have used the same syringe and needle usually for at least 3 injections, often 6 times and some up to 15 times before changing due to needles becoming blunt, or syringe barrel markings becoming obliterated. Needles were recapped and syringes stored at room temperature or in a refrigerator between injections. Syringes were flushed with air to remove residual insulin.

Withdrawal of One Insulin Type

Using conventional syringes and attached needles, the procedure for withdrawing a dose of one insulin type is outlined below.
- Wash hands thoroughly.
- Do not shake the vial.
- Completely disperse the sediment in insulin suspensions by gently rolling the vial between the palms of the hands. Ensure no clumping occurs and no sediment remains at the bottom of the vial or on the side of the vial. Discard vial if these problems occur.
- Clean the rubber stopper of the vial with alcohol (using a swab, gauze or cotton).
- Using an insulin syringe, draw back the plunger so the leading edge coincides with the required dose.
- Uncap the needle, insert it through the rubber stopper of the upright vial, and push the plunger in completely.
- Turn the vial and the syringe upside down and pull the plunger back slightly past the required dose.
- Inspect the syringe barrel for air bubbles.
- If bubbles are present, flick or tap the barrel until the bubbles rise to the top of the syringe.
- Push in the plunger to the exact dose, thereby expelling the air bubbles back into the vial.
- Return the vial to the upright position and remove the needle and syringe, which are now ready for injection.

Withdrawal and Admixture of Two Insulins

The following is the procedure for preparing a dose of 2 insulin types using the example of 20 units of NPH plus 10 units of regular insulin in one syringe.
- Wash hands thoroughly.
- Do not shake the vial.
- Completely disperse the NPH sediment by gently rolling the vial between the palms of the hands. Ensure no clumping occurs and sediment remains at the bottom of the vial or on the sides of the vial. Discard vial if these problems occur.
- Clean the rubber stoppers of each vial with alcohol.
- Pull back the syringe plunger to the 20-unit mark, insert the needle through the NPH vial stopper, and push the plunger in completely with the vial upright.
- Keeping the thumb on the plunger, remove the needle from the vial, leaving 20 units of air inside.
- Pull back the syringe plunger to the 10-unit mark and insert the needle through the rubber stopper of the upright regular insulin vial.
- Depress the plunger completely, turn the vial and syringe upside down, and withdraw slightly more than 10 units of regular insulin.
- Tap the syringe barrel to send any bubbles to the top, push in the plunger to measure exactly 10 units, and remove the needle from the vial.
- Invert the NPH vial, insert the needle and pull the plunger back from the initial 10-unit mark to the 30-unit mark, thus withdrawing 20 units of NPH.
- Bubbles should not be a problem this time. Do not pull back past the 30-unit mark.
- Remove the needle and syringe from the vial, now ready for injection.

The order of mixing has traditionally involved drawing up short-acting insulin first. This method is designed to maintain the integrity of the regular insulin solution. If modified insulin is drawn up first, inadvertent introduction into the second, soluble insulin vial will cause clouding. More important, repeated contamination of a short-acting preparation with insulin suspensions may lead to a delay in the action profile of the regular insulin. It is essential that soluble insulin retain its prompt onset to remain effective in controlling postprandial hyperglycemia and in supplementing modified insulins during illness.

Insulin Mixtures

Certain types of insulin preparations are physically incompatible and cannot be mixed. The Lente family of insulins are incompatible with PZI and NPH insulins due in part to their buffers and preservatives. Regular insulin by Nordisk (Velosulin) cannot be mixed with Lente-type insulins because its phosphate buffer may precipitate the excess zinc in the Lente products. Other regular insulins are physically compatible with all of the other longer-acting formulations.

Although regular insulin is not physically incompatible when mixed with modified insulins, its activity profile after subcutaneous injection may be altered. The extent of this effect may vary with the type of modified insulin formulation, the ratio of the 2 insulin doses, the duration of mixing and even the species source of insulin.

Both PZI and NPH insulins may contain excess protamine, which can bind with regular insulin in a mixture. In vitro studies of NPH/regular insulin mixtures have detected significant binding of regular insulin, which begins within 5 minutes and equilibrates at about 20 minutes. Despite this finding, clinical studies have not demonstrated a significant blunting of the prompt action of regular insulin in mixture with NPH. This statement is generally applicable regardless of the proportion of the insulin doses mixed, the insulin species, the manufacturer or the duration of mixing. Studies have reported that comparable insulin levels result from regular/NPH mixtures injected promptly after preparation and those stored for 3 weeks or for 3 months. The insulins used in these 2 studies were Velosulin and Insulatard.

There is extensive binding of regular insulin by PZI. After only 15 minutes of mixing, only 25 per cent of the regular insulin dose remains unbound. Therefore, it is recommended that PZI and regular insulin not be mixed.

The Lente family of insulins contain excess zinc, which can bind regular insulin in mixtures. This interaction may convert some of the regular insulin to a Semilente form, which exhibits a more delayed action profile. In vitro, the binding is detectable early as with NPH mixtures, but the Lente types progressively bind regular insulin for up to 24 hours. The extent of binding is greater than that seen with NPH mixtures, and increases as the ratio of Lente to regular insulin increases.

Several studies report that the onset of activity of Lente/regular mixtures is delayed after mixed injection compared with separate injections. Early insulin levels are significantly lower, peak levels are achieved much later, and levels at 8 hours are higher after mixtures. It has been suggested that the complex formed in Lente/regular mixtures is more stable than that formed in NPH/regular mixtures. The latter may dissociate in vivo after injection to liberate regular insulin more readily than Lente/regular mixtures.

The species of Lente/regular insulin combination appears to influence binding. Human mixtures have been shown to bind immediately after mixing, resulting in a significant delay in onset of activity. Nonhuman mixtures of Lente/regular insulin, if injected immediately (within 15 minutes) after preparation, are not similarly affected. One study demonstrated that human Lente and regular insulins injected through one stationary needle, but from consecutive separate syringes, preserved the prompt action of regular insulin. Ultralente insulin has been reported to delay the onset of regular insulin activity in mixtures to a greater extent than does Lente insulin.

The significance of these observations must be kept in perspective. Clinical studies have not demonstrated superior glycemic control in individuals treated with NPH/regular versus Lente/regular mixtures. It must be noted that there is tremendous variability of absorption of any insulin injected subcutaneously. If one considers as well the contribution of diet, exercise, and stress or illness to the difficulties in achieving optimum blood glucose control, the relative impact of insulin binding in mixtures is certainly diminished.

Nevertheless, the following recommendations seem appropriate. First, users should prepare mixtures immediately before injection, and should develop consistency in the length of time the insulins are mixed. It is suggested that NPH be the preferred intermediate-acting insulin for use in mixtures. A commercially available premixed combination of NPH/regular insulin might be recommended for individuals who are unable to prepare admixtures accurately and reproducibly. Individuals maintained on Lente/regular mixtures who must have syringes prepared for them in advance are advised to inject these doses only after 24 hours of storage, to allow equilibration of binding. For example, on the day of the nurse's visit, a syringe prepared on the last visit should be used.

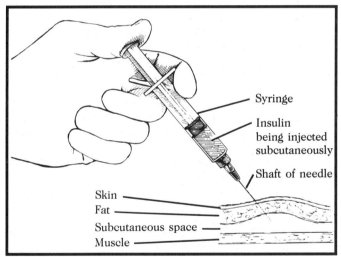

Figure 4 *Subcutaneous Insulin Injection*

Subcutaneous Insulin Injection

Insulin is injected into the subcutaneous tissue, which lies between the fat layer just under the skin and the muscles below (see Figure 4).

Insulin must not be introduced too deeply into muscle or too superficially into the epidermal layers. Absorption rates from these tissues differ significantly, and the standard activity profiles for insulins apply only to subcutaneous injection. The recommended procedure for subcutaneous injection of insulin is described below.

- Clean the injection site with alcohol, using a circular motion from the centre outward. Allow the alcohol to dry. (Some authorities advise aginst the use of alcohol. It is believed by some that alcohol

may disrupt the cutaneous lipid barrier and thereby promote infection. Alcohol may also make injection more painful if not allowed to dry.)

- Remove the needle shield from the syringe. Gently pinch a two-inch fold of skin. Using an angle of between 45 and 90 degrees to the skin, quickly insert the needle with the bevel up. Release the fold of skin. Obese individuals may require a 90 degree angle; thinner people should use a lower angle, nearer 45 degrees, for more shallow penetration.
- Some references recommend that the plunger be pulled back to aspirate for blood. If blood is obtained, the injection is aborted and a new syringe is used to withdraw insulin. Since in practice this tends to be a rare occurrence, many authorities do not insist upon aspiration.
- Slowly depress the plunger to inject insulin over a 3 to 5 second period.
- Pull the needle straight out of the skin. Hold an alcohol swab or cotton ball over the injection site to prevent leakage of insulin.
- After a few seconds, wipe the site, but do not massage the area.
- To prevent abuse of used syringes by others, the needle should be broken off manually or with a device available for this purpose.

Areas recommended for subcutaneous injection of insulin include the upper/outer areas of the arms, the front and sides of the thighs, the buttocks and the abdomen (except around the navel). Each area provides a number of discrete injection sites. A body map such as that depicted in Figure 5 can be used to record the site last used, to avoid frequent re-injection of one site. Traditionally, it was recommended that 21 to 28 days elapse before re-injecting any one site in order to reduce the risk of developing lipoatrophy associated with the use of older, less pure, beef and pork insulins. This required rotating injection sites not only within one anatomical area but also among areas as well. Today, it is still recommended that injection sites be rotated to avoid frequent re-injection of the same site which may lead to development of lipohypertrophy. It is more common now to have the individual rotate sites within only one area of the body, often the abdomen or the thigh. Frequent rotation between areas is not recommended.

Special Devices for Subcutaneous Injection of Insulin

Five **pen-like devices** for subcutaneous injection of insulin are available in Canada. Diabetics might be more likely to accept a MDI regimen if the procedure is more convenient. A separate device is required for each type of insulin used.

Connaught Novo markets 2 devices, Novolin Pen and Novolin Pen II. The Novolin Pen is made of chromium-plated brass and weighs 53 g. A cap can be removed to reveal a detachable needle for subcutaneous injections. The cap is then attached to the other end of the pen to allow dosing of insulin by depressing a button. The barrel accepts a 1.5-mL glass cartridge containing 150 units of insulin called the Novolin Penfill, currently available as Novolin Toronto, Novolin NPH and Novolin 30/70. Cartridges containing insulin suspensions should be carefully shaken up and down 10 times to allow a glass ball to disperse all sediment in the Penfill. They should be stored in a refrigerator until needed or carried as a backup supply. These cartridges can be kept at ambient temperatures up to 37 °C for up to 1 month. The in-use Novolin Pen with cartridge should not be refrigerated. The Novolin Pen is designed primarily for individuals injecting small doses of regular insulin before meals. Depression of

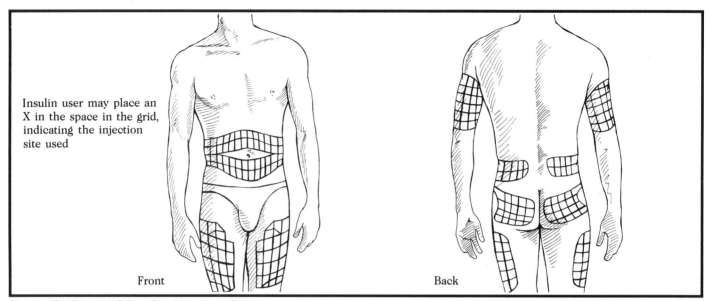

Figure 5 *Potential Insulin Injection Sites*

Adapted from Lilly Diabetes Care

Insulin user may place an X in the space in the grid, indicating the injection site used

Front

Back

the button injects 2 units of insulin, although doses can be delivered in single unit increments.

A second device, the Novolin Pen II, has been marketed for use by those requiring higher doses. The user of this pen can dial to select a dose between 2 and 36 units, in two-unit increments.

The Novolin Pens are safe, efficient, highly reliable and acceptable to most users surveyed. Patients usually find injections with the pen to be quicker and easier than injections using the conventional needle, syringe, and vial.

Two devices, Insuject and Insuject X, are marketed by Nordisk. The components are generally similar to the Novolin Pens except the Insujects deliver insulin by rotating the barrel top in a ratchet manner. The Insuject accepts a 2.5 mL cartridge containing 250 units of Velosulin Human, and the Insuject X takes Insulatard Human NPH or Mixtard 30/70 Human cartridges.

Comparing these 2 devices reveals certain advantages and disadvantages. The Novolin Pen's method of insulin release by plunger is more convenient than the rotation required by the Insuject, especially for injecting hard to reach sites. The Insuject provides a scale by which the remaining insulin may be estimated, even by touch (approximately) for the visually impaired. The Novolin Pen, Insuject and Insuject X allow dosing in increments of one unit rather than the two units of Novolin Pen II. The Insujects and Novolin Pen II provide a dose recall feature that displays the amount injected at the previous dose time. The Insujects allow longer intervals between refill due to the larger cartridge volume. The Novolin Pen II delivers larger doses more conveniently than the others.

Collaboration between Eli Lilly and Becton Dickinson has produced the latest pen-like injector. The B-D Pen accepts newly marketed cartridges containing 1.5 mL (150 units) of Humulin R, Humulin N or Humulin 30/70. The B-D Pen has the capacity to deliver up to 30 units, in single increments.

The **jet injector** was pioneered 40 years ago and has been used for many years to facilitate administration of vaccine during massive immunization campaigns. A high pressure device, it can propel insulin at high velocity through a fine orifice. The shock wave generated pierces the epidermis and causes the insulin to spread into the subcutaneous tissue without using a needle.

Some people, because of pain or psychological aversion to needles, may be more compliant with MDI regimens administered by jet injector. Users experience less immediate pain compared with conventional syringe and needle injection. However, both delayed aching pain and bleeding have been reported with jet injection. The current availability of an adjustable "punch pressure" feature might be expected to diminish somewhat these latter adverse effects.

Insulin absorption following jet injection occurs more rapidly than after conventional injection. Peak insulin concentration is achieved earlier and higher free insulin levels have been reported. The disappearance of insulin may be more rapid after jet injection. The rapid onset of action has been attributed to the wide subcutaneous dispersion of insulin, which avoids formation of a large, slowly absorbed depot as results from conventional injection. Other possible explanations are that the insulin is deposited either too deep into muscle or too shallow nearer the skin. These tissues have greater blood flow than subcutaneous tissue. In theory, more prompt control of postprandial hyperglycemia and a diminished likelihood of late hypoglycemia may be advantages of jet injection. However, better diabetic control has not been demonstrated.

Reported disadvantages of jet injectors include inconvenience and lack of portability of some models, a requirement for regular maintenance, the high cost of the device and the potential for insulin waste due to the dead space inherent in the injector. However, the dead space in a new device, the Preci Jet 50, is reported to be minimal (0.13 to 0.55 units). In the experience of some users, the objective of reduced pain may not be achieved. Few people continue with the device after the first weeks to months of enthusiasm wane.

Currently, 3 types of jet injectors are available in Canada: the Preci-Jet 50, the Medi-jector EZ and the Medi-jector II. A disposable vial adaptor transfers insulin from vial to injector. Mixed injections can be prepared, and the capacity of the device is 50 units (100 units for Medi-jector II). During filling, the device clicks audibly with each unit of insulin drawn and thus can be used by the visually impaired. The power is supplied mechanically, and the devices allow different pressure settings to be selected.

Some diabetics have a strong aversion to penetrating the skin with a needle. A device called **Injectomatic Syringe Injector**, when loaded with a prefilled insulin syringe with a permanently attached needle (Monoject Ultra-Smooth), propels the needle and syringe into the skin. The user must depress the plunger and inject the insulin.

Insulin pumps are portable infusion devices prescribed for Type I diabetics requiring continuous subcutaneous insulin infusion (CSII).

A pump consists of a programmable computer, an electromechanical pump, a reservoir for insulin (syringe or cartridge) and plastic tubing running from the reservoir to a subcutaneous needle. The size and weight of most pumps are comparable and are now considered convenient. The user can attach the pump to a belt or shoulder strap, or carry it in a pocket or purse. The nickel-cadmium rechargeable batteries are usually used for a 24 hour period, replaced with fresh ones and then recharged over at least a 16 hour period. The subcutaneous needle is usually inserted in the abdominal area at a 30 to 45 degree angle to the skin. It is then anchored along with a 10 cm loop of tubing (to minimize traction on the needle) using hypoallergenic tape.

All pumps incorporate several warning alarms. These signals alert the user if the batteries run low, if the insulin reservoir is low, if the pump motor either stops working or "runs away" (delivering excess insulin), if there is significant obstruction to insulin flow to the injection site or if unacceptable programming entries are made.

Individual pumps vary in several ways. The size of insulin reservoir, and hence the required frequency of refilling, varies widely. The rates of basal insulin delivery vary both in the number of individual rates possible and the range of these rates. The range of bolus rates (or doses) and the size of increments permitted is another variable. Each pump may offer certain special features such as memory functions (for example, dose recall) and basal rate programmability that allows for augmented infusion (for example, in the predawn hours).

Several factors should be considered in selecting an insulin pump. These include safety features (alarms), durability, the service record of the manufacturer, the ability of the supplier to provide training, the ease of use and the cosmetic attractiveness to the user. One should look also at clinically desirable special features.

Exposing the pump to extreme temperatures should be avoided. Insulin stability decreases in heat and the insulin may freeze in cold weather. Plastic tubing may become brittle and crack in the cold. Pumps must be removed before exposure to water (showering or swimming).

Storage, Stability and Sterility

Unopened insulin vials should be stored under refrigeration at 2 to 8°C and protected from light. Under these conditions, stability is guaranteed until the expiration date on the box and vial label. Freezing of insulin should be avoided. Vials of frozen insulin should be discarded, since irreversible aggregation and precipitation of insulin usually results.

It is recommended that vials of insulin currently in use be stored at room temperature (maximum 25°C). Injection of cold insulin has been associated with pain and development of lipodystrophy at the site of injection. Also, one study demonstrated that refrigeration impaired the effectiveness of the preservative in sterilizing an insulin vial inoculated with bacteria.

Storage of insulin at room temperature increases the rate of chemical alteration such as deamidation and polymerization of insulin. Insulin suspensions stored for extended periods above 25°C may become difficult to homogenize due to formation of lumps or flakes that resist disintegration. Frequent agitation of insulin, which occurs

when it is carried about by the user, may contribute to the above problem. It has been stated that storage of insulin for several weeks at 25°C is not associated with significant loss of biological potency. One estimate of the rate of loss is 1.5 per cent per month. The general rule of thumb is to allow 1 month only, since ambient room temperature may well exceed 25°C.

Direct sunlight can greatly accelerate the rate of degradation of insulin when compared to storage in the dark at the same temperature. Therefore, the in-use vial is best stored inside the original box if kept at room temperature. Individuals using a low dosage of insulin who will not deplete their vials of insulin within 1 month should refrigerate their in-use vials and remove them well before injection to allow warming.

Any discoloration, turbidity or unusual viscosity in a regular insulin solution indicates deterioration or contamination, and the vial should be discarded. Insulin suspensions should be discarded if the sediment cannot be suspended by rotating the vial, if a clumped, granular precipitate is apparent, or if a deposit of solid particles is seen on the wall of the vial. It has been shown that, if such vials are used to deliver a prescribed volume of intermediate-acting insulin, the user will receive only a fraction of the prescribed dose of insulin.

Insulins contain preservatives such as phenol, metacresol or methylparaben. In one study, these preservatives provided adequate bactericidal protection by sterilizing within 24 hours insulin vials that had been inoculated with bacteria. People who keep in-use insulin vials at room temperature for over 28 days are not at increased risk of infection. Despite poor compliance with handwashing and preparation of vial and skin before injection, bacterial contamination and infection have not been a problem among insulin-requiring diabetics.

On occasion, insulin may have to be drawn up into plastic disposable syringes and stored before use. A recent study reported that biosynthetic human insulins (regular, NPH, commercial and extemporaneous mixtures of regular/NPH) drawn up into plastic syringes retained their stability and sterility for 28 days stored at room temperature or in a refrigerator. These doses should be placed so that the needle end of the syringe points upward. This will prevent sedimentation of insulin suspensions and clogging of the needle. Before use, it is important that the syringe be rolled between the palms for 15 seconds to resuspend the insulin.

Monitoring Diabetic Control

The degree of control achieved by treatment can be assessed by a combination of three methods.

Glycosylated Hemoglobin

The hemoglobin contained in red blood cells reacts with glucose in the blood to form a stable complex called glycosylated hemoglobin. This process occurs slowly over the 3 month life span of the erythrocytes and the extent to which hemoglobin becomes glycosylated depends upon the prevailing blood glucose levels.

Glycosylated hemoglobin values are routinely used to monitor overall glycemic control achieved during the previous 2 to 3 months. Although exact ranges vary among laboratories, a hemoglobin A_{1c} value of 4 to 6 per cent represents slight or infrequent hyperglycemia as seen in very mild diabetes or in intensively treated and very well controlled patients; 8 to 9 per cent indicates a moderate degree of hyperglycemia; and 11 to 13 per cent is reflective of frequent and severe hyperglycemia as seen in very poorly controlled patients.

Urine Glucose Monitoring

Before the introduction of products for home blood glucose monitoring (HBGM) in 1978, glycemic control was monitored by testing the urine for glucose.

Current management of diabetes requires HBGM, particularly for all insulin-treated patients. Nevertheless, some patients are unable or unwilling to perform HBGM and may have to rely upon urine glucose monitoring.

The presence of glucose in the urine signifies that at some point during the collection interval, plasma glucose exceeded the kidneys' capacity to reabsorb glucose. The plasma glucose value at which glucose spills into the urine is termed the patient's renal threshold. One cannot reliably translate the magnitude of glycosuria to the plasma glucose profile in onset, degree, or duration of hyperglycemia. Renal threshold is considered to average 10 mmol/L (180 mg/dL) in most patients. Variations between individuals are common and the threshold, affected by the glomerular filtration rate, may change within the same person due to aging, progression of nephropathy, or pregnancy. The best indication of glycemic control that can be obtained with urine testing is the assurance from consistently negative results that plasma glucose did not exceed the renal threshold value. It is not possible to confirm that lower target levels were achieved, or that hypoglycemia was avoided.

Urine glucose testing measures the percentage of glucose present. This value is dependent on the volume or concentration of urine in the bladder and may not correctly reflect the amount present. A further limitation stems from the potential interference by drugs and other substances. For these reasons, a poor correlation exists between urine glucose and simultaneous plasma glucose values.

Because such wide variability exists, urine glucose testing is not sufficiently reliable to allow monitoring of glycemic control in IDDM, especially when frequent adjustment of insulin dosage is used to achieve control. Urine testing may be sufficient in stable patients in whom control is not urgent, and if HBGM is undesirable to the individual or considered impossible by the physician. It is also indicated in NIDDM individuals whose goal of therapy is to achieve negative urine glucose results after meals.

Urine Collection

There are two techniques for urine collection. The first, termed single-void, is a collection of urine produced since the last void. This test provides a reflection of plasma glucose levels prevailing during the collection interval. The second-void or double-void method involves emptying the bladder 30 minutes before the desired test time, drinking a glass of water, and 30 minutes later voiding again and testing the specimen. The purpose of the double-void is to reflect more accurately plasma glucose levels at the time of testing. However, correlation with plasma glucose has been shown to be similar using single- and double-voided specimens.

A comparison of urine testing results obtained from single- and double-void specimens led the authors of one study to conclude that for routine purposes of monitoring for freedom from glycosuria, the single-void specimen is a better indicator of overall glycemic control. Furthermore, the greater effort required and the inconvenience of the double-void technique may contribute to a decreased compliance with testing.

Timing

In non-insulin-treated patients not testing blood glucose, one goal of treatment might be to achieve freedom from glycosuria. This is best documented by testing a fasting urine glucose upon arising in the morning, and a postprandial sample (for example, 2 hours after supper).

Insulin-treated patients who test only urine glucose may attempt to confirm indirectly the avoidance of hypoglycemia by achieving trace amounts of glucose in the urine. Testing might be done 4 times daily, before meals and at bedtime. In addition, postprandial values may provide some indication of glycemic control.

Testing Systems

Urine testing products currently available in Canada are listed in Table XIII. Only Clinitest tablets use the copper reduction technique for glucose detection. This test is not specific for glucose, and it may give false positive results in the presence of other reducing substances (for example, other sugars, drugs or metabolites). The other products are available as sticks or strips and use a glucose oxidase method for the specific detection of glucose. However, other reducing substances may cause false negative results.

In the **copper reduction reaction**, cupric sulfate (blue to blue-green) is converted to cuprous oxide (yellow to red-orange) by reducing substances. A positive test is evidenced by color changes through this spectrum. Clinitest tablets are used as follows (5-drop method).

- Place 5 drops of urine in a test tube, rinse the dropper and add 10 drops of water.
- Drop 1 tablet into the test tube. Do not shake.
- Watch the tube during the boiling reaction for color changes. Wait 15 seconds after the reaction stops. Shake the tube gently and compare the color with the color chart. Disregard color changes occurring after the 15-second waiting period.

If, during the boiling reaction, the color passes rapidly through orange to dark brown or greenish-brown, interpret the test result as being over 2 per cent. This pass-through phenomenon is seen when heavy glycosuria is detected during the 5-drop method. To avoid this problem, patients expected to have large amounts of glucose in the urine may be instructed to use the 2-drop method (2 drops urine, 10 drops water). This variation detects up to 5 per cent glucose, but requires a special 7-block color chart which is available from the manufacturer upon request. The per cent results given by each method appear in Table XIII.

For many years, Clinitest was the only product capable of detecting urine glucose over 2 per cent. It was considered the most quantitative test and thus was the product most often recommended for individuals requiring more accurate results for achievement of better control. Another advantage of Clinitest was that the presence of ketones in the urine was reported not to interfere with the accuracy of results.

However, Chemstrip uG is capable of detecting up to 5 per cent glucose in urine without interference from ketones and has comparable accuracy.

Other potential advantages reported for Clinitest are the larger color area for reading, colors that are more easily differentiated than strip products and lower expense after initial set-up costs. In addition, spoilage of the tablets, leading to a darker blue mottled appearance, can be more easily detected by the user than with strip products.

The Clinitest system has a number of disadvantages compared with the glucose oxidase systems. The tablets are highly corrosive and poisonous if ingested. They are not recommended for use in homes

Table XIII *Products for Monitoring Urine Glucose and Ketones*

	Product	Manufacturer	Detection range and values	Reading instructions
Glucose	Chemstrip uG	BMC	0　0.1　0.25　0.5　1　2　3　5 g/dL (0　5.5　14　28　56　111　167　280 mmol/L)	1. Read at 120 sec 2. Disregard changes after 180 sec
	Clinitest Tablets	Miles	5–drop method: 0　0.25　0.5　0.75　1　>2 (0　14　28　42　56　>111) 2–drop method: 0　<0.5　0.5　1　2　3　5 (0　<28　28　56　111　167　280)	1. Watch boiling reaction. 2. Observe during 15 sec 3 Read immediately. 4. Beware "pass-through" phenomenon. 5 Disregard changes after 15 sec
	Diastix	Miles	0　0.1　0.25　0.5　1　2 (0　5.5　14　28　56　111)	1. Read at exactly 30 sec 2. Disregard changes after 30 sec
	Tes-Tape	Lilly	0　0.1　0.25　0.5　>2 (0　5.5　14　28　>111)	1. Read at 60 sec 2. If 0.5g/dL or greater, wait 60 sec for final result.
Ketones	Acetest Tablets	Miles	Small　Moderate　Large 20　30–40　80–100 mg/dL (2　3–4　8–10　mmol/dL)	1. Use white paper as background. 2. Read at 30 sec
	Chemstrip K	BMC	Neg　+　++　+++ 0　5–40　40–100　>100 (0　0.5–4　4–10　>10)	1. Read at 120 sec 2. Disregard changes after 180 sec
	Ketostix	Miles	Neg　Trace　Small　Moderate　Large　Larger 0　5　15　40　80　160 (0　0.5　1.5　4　8　16)	1. Read at exactly 15 sec 2. Disregard changes after 15 sec
Glucose and Ketones	Chemstrip uG/K	BMC	(see Chemstrip uG and Chemstrip K)	1. Read glucose and ketones at 120 sec 2. Disregard changes after 180 sec
	Keto-Diastix	Miles	(see Diastix and Ketostix)	1. Read ketones at exactly 15 sec 2. Read glucose at exactly 30 sec 3. Disregard later changes.

BMC=Boehringer Mannheim Canada.

with children. If swallowed, vomiting must not be induced. Large volumes of milk or water must be given immediately. Following accidental external exposure, the area should be flooded with water. Eyeballs must be flushed for at least 20 minutes. Users can receive burns during the boiling reaction, especially those with sensory neuropathy. As noted above, the usual 5-drop method is subject to the pass-through phenomenon, which has been reported to cause error in up to 58 per cent of readings by hospital nurses. Other potential sources of error include adherence of urine or water to the walls of the test tube, or use of an incorrect number of drops. A high incidence of false positive tests has been reported. The timing of the reading is crucial, as the reaction has no endpoint and proceeds past 15 seconds. Performing the test is tedious, time-consuming and inconvenient, requiring equipment that decreases portability. A survey of children with diabetes indicated Clinitest was more difficult to use than strip products such as Diastix or Chemstrip uG.

The **urine glucose testing strips** include Diastix, Chemstrip uG and Tes-Tape. Combination products that also test for ketones in the urine include Keto-Diastix and Chemstrip uG/K. The glucose oxidase enzyme present in the test system catalyzes the reaction of glucose and oxygen to form glucuronic acid and hydrogen peroxide, which, in turn, reacts with a chromogen system to produce color changes.

Instructions for using the various glucose-only products are relatively simple. The strip contains 1 (Diastix) or 2 (Chemstrip) rea-

gent pads, which should not be touched. Instructions are as follows:
- Dip the reagent end of the strip for 1 second in a freshly collected urine specimen or pass it quickly through a stream of urine.
- Gently remove excess urine by tapping or wiping the edge of the strip along the rim of the vessel.
- Compare reagent pad(s) with color blocks on the side of the strip container at designated reading times. (See Table XIII.)

Clinistix is not listed in the table because it is designed to detect the presence, but not the quantity, of glucose in the urine. This product is not indicated for urine glucose monitoring in diabetes.

Tes-Tape is unique since it is not a strip, but a continuous paper tape in a dispenser. It is the most portable of all tests and is inexpensive. However, it has several disadvantages. Tes-Tape may be so sensitive to the presence of low concentrations of glucose that it can register positive results even at levels considered normal for nondiabetic urine. It is reportedly difficult to distinguish between 0.25 per cent and 2 per cent due to colors used. The absence of intermediate color blocks (for example, 0.75 per cent and 1 per cent) between 0.5 per cent and 2 per cent may contribute to this difficulty. In a comparison of urine testing products, correlation of results with laboratory standards indicated Tes-Tape was the least accurate product. Another study reported nonuniform color development along the tape, making interpretation difficult. Minor problems with difficulty in tearing off and tape curling were noted. One paper concluded that

Tes-Tape was too unreliable for quantitative estimation of urine glucose due to poor precision.

Diastix is a product designed to detect 0.1 per cent to 2 per cent glucose in the urine. Within the range of intended use, Diastix has a correlation coefficient with laboratory results greater than the 5-drop Clinitest method. However, there can be some difficulty distinguishing between 1 and 2 per cent due to insufficient color differentiation. Therefore, Diastix is not recommended for people requiring accurate detection of heavy glycosuria. The reading of Diastix at 30 seconds is crucial, since the color reaction continues to progress. Late color changes must be disregarded. High amounts of ketones in the urine may depress glucose results obtained with Diastix.

As with all strips, Diastix should be kept in a cool, dry place (but not refrigerated) with the lid tightly closed on the container. The dessicant in the container can be toxic if ingested. When spoiled, the pale blue test patch becomes greenish or tan-green.

The manufacturer recommends that strips be discarded 4 months after opening the container or by the expiry date printed on the label. To confirm test performance, the company suggests testing a mixture of 5 mL of nondiet Coca-Cola (or 7Up) along with 75 mL of water. The result should read 0.25 to 0.5 per cent, but if a lower result is obtained, the strips should be discarded.

Chemstrip uG has an expanded detection range of up to 5 per cent. Unlike the Diastix products, the Chemstrip uses 2 reagent pads for glucose detection and a corresponding 2-block color chart. The nearest pad is designed for color differentiation from 0.1 to 2 per cent, and the distal pad from 1 to 5 per cent. The strip should be read at 2 minutes and color changes after 3 minutes should be disregarded. Reading time is less crucial than with the Diastix products, which must be read at exactly 30 seconds. There is no interference by urine

ketones with Chemstrip uG, whereas their presence may compromise the accuracy of Diastix test results.

Chemstrip uG is considered by several authors to be the method of choice for urine glucose testing. Its precision, accuracy and sensitivity are considered a significant improvement over other products. Diabetic children expressed preference for Chemstrip uG over Clinitest and Diastix, and may be more likely to comply with their monitoring regimen. A multicentre study reported superiority of Chemstrip uG over Diastix and Clinitest with respect to performance and user preference. Some people consider the reading time of 2 minutes to be a disadvantage. The American Diabetes Association Committee on Therapeutics now recommends patients with IDDM who must rely upon urine glucose monitoring should use either the 2-drop Clinitest method or Chemstrip uG/K. Considering the many disadvantages of Clinitest noted previously, Chemstrip uG/K, for both glucose and ketones, would appear to be the product of choice.

Drug Interference with Urine Glucose Testing

The presence of drugs in the urine may interfere with the accuracy of urine glucose testing. The copper reduction test (Clinitest), because it is not specific for glucose, is subject to false positive results in the presence of other reducing substances. The glucose oxidase tests (all strips) may read false negative in the presence of strong reducing substances, which inhibit the oxidation of the chromogen and diminish the development of the color reaction. False positive results with glucose oxidase tests have been reported only when cleaning substances such as hydrogen peroxide and sodium hypochlorite (bleach) remain in urine collection containers.

The literature on drug interference with urine glucose testing has recently been reviewed and clarified. The results are summarized

Table XIV *Classes of Drugs That Interfere With Urine Glucose Tests*

Group A: drugs that interfere with urine glucose tests	Affected tests	Group B: drugs that may interfere with urine glucose tests	Affected tests	Group C: drugs that do not interfere with urine glucose tests
Ascorbic acid	C, GOT	Chloral hydrate	C	Aminoglycoside antibiotics
ß-Lactam antibiotics*	C	Hyaluronidase	C	Chloramphenicol
Cephalosporins		Nalidixic acid	C	Ciprofloxacin
Penicillins		Nitrofurantoin	C	Ephedrine
Monobactams (aztreonam)		ρ-Aminosalicylic acid	C	Epinephrine
		Phenazopyridine	GOT	Ethacrynic acid
Carbapenems (imipenem)		Probenecid	C	Indomethacin
Levodopa	C, GOT	X-ray contrast media	C, GOT	Isoniazid (INH)
Salicylates	C, GOT			Lincomycin
				Methenamine
				Methyldopa
				Metaproterenol
				Morphine
				Nicotinic acid
				Phenothiazines
				Sulfonamide antibiotics
				Tetracycline antibiotics+
				Thiazide diuretics

In general, drugs cause false positive reactions with Clinitest (C) and false negative reactions with glucose oxidase tests (GOT). GOTs include Diastix, Keto-Diastix, Chemstrip uG 5000, Chemstrip uG 5000 K and Tes-Tape.
*False positive, false negative and uninterpretable results have been reported.
+Some injectable preparations of tetracycline contain large amounts of ascorbic acid.
Adapted from: Rotblatt MD, Koda-Kimble MA. Review of drug interference with urine glucose tests. Diabetes Care 1987;10(1):103–10.

in Table XIV. All potential offending agents have been categorized into 3 classes. Group A includes drugs well documented as causing interference; group B represents those reported to interfere but with poor documentation; and Group C lists those that do not interfere.

Some drugs interfere with only 1 test system. For example, penicillins and cephalosporins may cause false positive results only with Clinitest. Patients receiving these antibiotics should test their urine glucose with a strip product based on the glucose oxidase method. Group B drugs, shown in Table XIV, affect mainly the Clinitest system. However, they should be assumed potentially to interfere with glucose oxidase methods as well. When a drug reportedly affecting both test systems must be taken, home blood glucose monitoring is recommended.

Urine Ketone Monitoring

Normally, the urine is free of ketones. However, in poorly controlled IDDM or during starvation, insulin deficiency and glucagon excess combine to cause the breakdown of fat and the production by the liver of ketones. The 3 ketone compounds formed are beta-hydroxybutyrate, acetoacetate and acetone. When produced in excess, ketones are excreted in the urine and usually reflect loss of control in IDDM which may progress to development of diabetic ketoacidosis and coma.

The basis for ketone testing is that sodium nitroprusside turns a lavender color in the presence of acetoacetate. As the reaction progresses, the color deepens to a darker violet. Acetoacetate is detected by all urine ketone testing products, acetone is detected by Chemstrip K and Chemstrip uG/K, but beta-hydroxybutyrate is not detected by any of these products.

Patients with NIDDM are generally resistant to ketosis and rarely develop ketonuria except during periods of major stress associated with trauma, surgery or severe infection. Therefore, these individuals do not need to test their urine for ketones.

Patients with IDDM should test for ketones when urine glucose exceeds 2 per cent or when blood glucose test results exceed a predefined level (for example, 16.7 mmol/L or 300 mg/dL.) Early detection of significant ketonuria is critical; diabetic ketoacidosis may progress without severe hyperglycemia to warn the patient who tests only blood glucose. Other indications for urine ketone testing include febrile illness, nausea and vomiting, prolonged fasting, stress, and pregnancy.

Products available for urine ketone monitoring are listed in Table XIII. They include products which detect ketones only (Acetest tablets, Chemstrip K, Ketostix) and combination products designed to measure both glucose and ketones (Chemstrip uG/K, Keto-Diastix). Patients with IDDM who monitor blood glucose would use a ketone only test while those who routinely monitor urine glucose would use a combination product.

The table indicates the detection values and reading times for all available products. Acetest tablets require a dropper and a clean, white piece of paper. A drop of urine placed on the tablet is absorbed within 30 seconds (unless the tablet is defective), and color changes are compared with the chart provided. Pink, yellow or tan colors are disregarded. Acetest tablets may be used to detect ketones in serum, plasma or whole blood as well.

Miles Domestic Division recommends the following test to confirm adequate performance of ketone detection. Dilute one-quarter teaspoon of nail polish remover (any brand containing acetone) in 175 mL of water. When tested, this solution should produce results

between "small" and "moderate." If lower readings are obtained, the product should be discarded.

Interference with urine ketone testing may occur. Phenylketonuria, a rare metabolic disorder, may cause a false positive reading with Ketostix, Keto-Diastix and Acetest products. In contrast, although phenylketonuria may produce a color change in Chemstrip products, this is readily distinguishable from all other test results and does not interfere with accurary. Levodopa metabolites may cause false positive results with Ketostix, Keto-Diastix and Acetest.

Blood Glucose Monitoring

Home blood glucose monitoring (HBGM) has become a major adjunct to diabetes care in the past decade. In 1987, the American Diabetes Association estimated this technique was being used by over one million diabetics in the United States. HBGM provides the patient and the health care team with vital clinical information previously unavailable with urine glucose monitoring. Both consumers and care providers should be trained to use the technique accurately, to record results and to respond with changes in therapy designed to achieve better glycemic control.

Indications

HBGM is recommended for all individuals recieving insulin and may also be useful for those not treated with insulin. Use of HBGM is especially important for the following individuals: women who are both pregnant and diabetic; pregnancy complicated by diabetes; patients with a propensity to develop severe ketosis or hypoglycemia (unstable or brittle diabetes); people prone to hypoglycemia who may not experience the usual warning symptoms; people receiving intensive insulin treatment; people with abnormal renal glucose thresholds; color-blind people requiring a digital glucose testing result, or those who require an audible result due to severe visual impairment; and people who have difficulty producing a urine sample (due to neurogenic bladder or severe renal impairment).

Advantages and Disadvantages

As a method of monitoring diabetic control, HBGM has several distinct advantages over urine glucose testing. It allows direct sampling of blood for glucose and provides timely information. Detection and confirmation of hypoglycemia, previously not possible without laboratory testing, allows for early administration of glucose and prevention of serious reactions. Most important, only with HBGM is it possible to attempt tighter glycemic control of diabetes. Patients can now strive to achieve near normal blood glucose values rather than simply shooting for values below the renal threshold. Physicians can instruct patients to adjust insulin dosages based upon results of HBGM to achieve optimum diabetic control.

HBGM benefits the patient in many other ways. It serves as an educational and training tool to improve the understanding of diabetes among patients and their families. The effects of diet, exercise and medication become more apparent through observation of blood glucose results. Many people report increased satisfaction from more active participation in their treatment plan, as well as from enhanced control over their condition. HBGM provides an increased flexibility in lifestyle, because the consequences of varying the time and size of meals and of the type of physical activities may be minimized. Other advantages include greater social acceptability and convenience of HBGM over urine testing, and better rapport between patient and physician.

Table XV *Biochemical Indexes of Metabolic Control in Patients with Diabetes Mellitus.**

Index	Range			
	Good	**Acceptable**	**Fair**	**Poor**
Fasting plasma glucose level—mg/dL (mmol/L)	80–120 (4.4–6.7)	120–140 (6.7–7.8)	140–180 (7.8–10)	>180 (>10)
Postprandial plasma glucose level—mg/dL (mmol/L)[+]	80–140 (4.4–7.8)	140–180 (7.8–10)	180–235 (10–13)	>235 (>13)
Hemoglobin A_{IC} level—percent[‡]	<6.0	6.0–7.5	7.5–9.0	>9.0
Total plasma cholesterol level—mg/dL (mmol/L)	<200 (<5.2)	200–220 (5.2–5.8)	220–240 (5.8–6.3)	>240 (>6.3)
Plasma HDL cholesterol level—mg/dL (mmol/L)	>40 (>1.1)	35–40 (0.9–1.1)	30–35 (0.9–0.8)	<30 (<0.8)
Plasma triglyceride level—mg/dL (mmol/L)	<150 (<1.7)	150–200 (1.7–2.2)	200–240 (2.2–2.7)	>240 (>2.7)

*Based on recommendations of the American Diabetes Association and the European NIDDM Policy Group. HDL denotes high-density liproprotein.
+Measured 2 hours after eating.
‡For total glycosylated hemoglobin, multiply values by 1.2.
Adapted from: Gerich JE. Oral hypoglycemic agents. N Engl J Med 1989;321(8):1231–45.

One disadvantage of HBGM is that it is 10 times more expensive than urine testing. The current annual cost of strips for HBGM (4 tests daily) is approximately $1,200, whereas the cost of strips for urine testing of glucose and ketones would be about $125. One study has looked at the feasibility of splitting a blood glucose test strip lengthwise to allow two tests per strip. The conclusion was that the strip (Chemstrip bG), split with scissors, can be read visually with a reliability comparable to that of the intact strip. The authors recommended splitting as a cost saving measure. The manufacturers do not recommend this procedure due to the reduction in test pad size and readability, and concerns with possible contamination. The added cost of HBGM must be viewed in relation to the staggering costs associated with the complications of diabetes. It is certainly a small price to pay for better monitoring and the potential for achieving tighter control and reduced morbidity. In addition, reimbursement of the costs for HBGM is becoming increasingly available to patients through their health or life insurance plans or through the Canadian Diabetes Association.

Clinical Uses

Patients with IDDM are usually initiated on a frequent regimen of HBGM. Seven samples daily, before and 1 or 2 hours after each meal and at bedtime, are commonly advised. In certain circumstances, a test may be required at 2 to 4 a.m. to check for nocturnal hypoglycemia. The exact regimen varies depending on lifestyle, severity of diabetes, insulin regimen and method of administration, and treatment goals. After initial stabilization, the frequency of monitoring may be decreased. Some individuals may need to test only twice daily, others only 2 or 3 days a week, with more frequent testing again whenever control deteriorates. Extra determinations are recommended before and after exercise and during illness.

Selected individuals on continuous subcutaneous insulin infusion or taking multiple daily injections must perform HBGM and should adjust insulin, diet and exercise to maintain glucose values within a specified target range. This is done through use of a patient specific algorithm devised by the physician. This set of guidelines prescribes dosage adjustments based on observed patterns of testing results. Table XV defines fasting and postprandial target blood glucose ranges associated with good, acceptable, fair and poor degrees of metabolic control. Also listed are similar ranges for glycosylated hemoglobin (Hb A_{1c}) and lipid levels.

Many individuals may not be candidates for intensive insulin therapy and dosage adjustment. In this case, testing results can simply be recorded and reviewed retrospectively by the physician along with glycosylated hemoglobin values to assess control. Adjustments of insulin dosage may be prescribed for a definite period until the next visit. These patients can be instructed to contact the physician when results are outside a predetermined safe range. They are usually expected to be able to recognize emergency situations such as hypoglycemia and ketoacidosis.

HBGM in patients with NIDDM not injecting insulin is less crucial. The pattern of glucose levels is more stable and wide swings with hypoglycemia are unusual. The physician may recommend intermittent testing after a meal to record peak blood glucose levels.

In NIDDM, the primary benefit of HBGM may be as an educational tool to influence behavior. Individuals are encouraged to test blood glucose occasionally in order to learn the body's response to diet, exercise and other factors.

Procedure

Individuals should wash their hands in warm, soapy water and rinse and dry them completely. The warmth, as well as holding the hand below the level of the heart, promotes blood flow to the fingertips. The earlobe, although inconvenient for self-monitoring, may also be used for sample collection. Cleansing with alcohol is optional, since some believe that it disrupts the lipid barrier and may promote skin infection. However, the incidence of infection at blood letting sites is extremely low.

The blood samples are obtained by finger prick using a lancet alone or one incorporated in a special spring loaded device. The depth of penetration of the lancet can be adjusted, by using attachments of variable thickness and by pressing weakly or strongly against the finger, to suit the skin thickness of the individual. It is recommended that the lancet pierce the side of the finger rather than the fleshy tip, since the tip is more highly innervated and, thus, more sensitive to pain. The side of the finger will also have fewer calluses than other areas.

Diabetes Care

Table XVI *Products for Visual Determination of Blood Glucose*

Product Manufacturer	Chemstrip bG (Visual) Boehringer Mannheim	Dextrostix Ames	Glucostix Ames
Detection Range mmol/L (mg/dL)	1.1–44.4 (20–800)	1.4–13.9 (25–250)	1.1–44.4 (20–800)
Reagent pads	two	one	two
Color block values	1.1 (20) 2.2 (40) 4.4 (80) 6.7 (120) 8.9 (160) 11.1 (200) 16.7 (300) 27.8 (500) >44.4 (>800)	0(0) 1.4 (25) 2.5 (45) 5.0 (90) 7.2 (130) 9.7 (175) >13.9 (>250)	1.1 (20) 2.0 (40) 4.0 (70) 6.0 (110) 8.0 (140) 10.0 (180) 14.0 (250) 22.0 (400) >44.0 (>800)
Procedure	• apply blood • wait 60 sec • wipe with cotton wad • wait 60 sec • read if <16.7 • if ≥16.7 wait extra 60 sec	• apply blood • wait 60 sec • wash with 2 sec water stream • gently blot with lint free paper towel • do not wait • read immediately	• apply blood • wait 30 sec • press facial tissue on test pad for 1–2 sec • repeat if necessary • wait 90 sec • read distal pad if <6.0 (110) • if ≥6.0 read proximal pad
Time	120–180 sec	approx 70 sec	120 sec

The user then milks the finger and forms a drop of blood large enough to easily cover the whole reagent pad or pads on the test strip. Care should be taken to avoid spreading or smearing the blood droplet over the pad surface.

Timing begins immediately for a waiting period of 30 to 60 seconds, depending on the product. Then, in most cases, a facial tissue or cotton pledget is used to gently blot the pad and wipe off blood.

One product, Dextrostix, requires that a water bottle be used to direct a 2-second stream of water to wash off the strip before blotting.

Visual Reading

Canadian products for visual determination of blood glucose are listed in Table XVI. The table indicates for each product the detection range, color block values and instructions for use. Two additional products, Accu-Trend and Glucofilm strips incorporate a reference color block system. However, these strips are primarily designed to be read by a blood glucose monitor (Accu-Trend and Glucometer 3 respectively) and are intended to provide only backup visual capacity.

Visual reading of blood glucose strips should be done in good light. The strips have either 1 or 2 reagent pads that develop color during contact with glucose in blood. The inclusion of 2 pads is designed to permit better color differentiation by the reader. One pad reacts to a lower range of glucose values with one color spectrum, and the other pad detects higher values using a different color range. The user should view the lower range first and, if the blood glucose appears to exceed the highest color block, read the higher range (either immediately, or after a further 60 seconds depending on the product).

The color developed in the reagent pad is compared to reference color blocks that appear on the strip container label. Each color block is assigned a glucose value expressed in both mg/dL and mmol/L. When the color of reagent pad falls between 2 color blocks, the result should be estimated at a value between those of the 2 respective blocks. Accurate color comparison and interpolation of the results requires considerable practice.

Certain individuals may not be able to achieve satisfactory testing results through visual reading. Color vision defects develop as retinopathy progresses and are thought to be the result of either diabetic neuropathy of the optic nerve or alteration of normal retinal function. These people perform poorly when reading urine or blood glucose testing products and are usually unaware of their errors. It is recommended that diabetics routinely undergo color vision testing and, upon discovery of deficits, monitor control with the aid of a meter.

Dextrostix was the first avilable blood glucose testing strip. When read visually, the detection range is narrow (1.4 to greater than 13.9 mmol/L or 25 to 250 mg/dL) and the reference color blocks, a series of purple/gray shades, are very difficult to differentiate. One disadvantage is that blood must be removed by washing with a wash bottle for a discrete period. Then, the pad must be blotted and read immediately for an accurate reading. The procedure is complicated and more likely to introduce error than other methods. Visual inspection of Dextrostix has been judged in one study to be too inaccurate to be of practical clinical benefit and it has been recommended that Dextrostix be used only with a meter for best results.

Chemstrip bG was designed for visual determination of blood glucose. The range is broad (1 to 44.4 mmol/L, or 20 to 800 mg/dL) and 2 pads are used throughout the range. When glucose levels are greater than 8.9 mmol/L (150 mg/dL), the distal pad color is given greater weight in estimating the test result; when larger lower than

8.9 mmol/L, the reverse applies. When glucose levels exceed 16.7 mmol/L (300 mg/dL), an additional minute is required before reading. Some people find the need to read the 2 pads simultaneously is difficult and confusing; others achieve accurate results.

Glucostix has the same range of detection as Chemstrip bG, dual reagent pads and a similar procedure for use. However, the 2 reagent pads on the Glucostix strip each detect either a lower or higher range of blood glucose values and do not overlap. The range of colors employed by Glucostix and Chemstrip bG are quite different and may influence patient performance and preference.

Under controlled conditions, visual HBGM can achieve satisfactory accuracy and precision. However, in general use, up to 50 per cent of test values may vary more than 20 per cent from reference values. The quality of results may be diminished by numerous factors related to handling the test strips.

The use of expired or improperly stored strips may invalidate results. All products should be kept in the original container with dessicant and the lid should be tightly closed immediately after opening. Touching the reagent pads with the fingers or other objects is to be avoided. The product should be stored in a cool dry place, but not refrigerated. One manufacturer suggests the container be dated when initially opened and unused strips discarded after 6 months.

Tests carried out at extreme temperatures, below 18°C or above 35°C, may lead to false negative or positive results respectively, due to the temperature dependency of the enzymatic reaction. Since whole blood glucose is being sampled, anemia (hematocrit less than 35 per cent) can falsely elevate test results while polycythemia (hematocrit greater than 55 per cent) can falsely depress test results.

The quality of results in HBGM is also highly dependent on user

Table XVII *Comparison of Blood Glucose Monitors*

Meter Feature	Accu-Chek III (BMC)	Accu-Trend (BMC)	ExacTech (Medisense)	Companion 2 (Medisense)	Glucometer 3 (Ames)	One Touch II (Lifescan)
Warranty	3 years	3 years	4 years	4 years	4 years	3 years
Test strips	Chemstrip BG for AC III	Accu-Trend strips	ExacTech strips	Companion 2 strips	Glucofilm strips	One Touch test strips
Method	wiping method	no wiping	no wiping or blotting	no wiping or blotting	wiping method	no wiping or blotting
Memory Capacity	20 values with date & time	50 values with date & time	1 (most recent value)	10 values no date or time	10 values	250 values with date & time
Battery	6V 1EC/YGI3/A544	3 × 1.5 volt battery	Lithium Lasts 4000 tests	Not replaceable Lasts 2 yrs or 4000 tests	Lithium non-replaceable Lasts 15,000 tests	6VJ size/7K67 lasts 1 yr at 2 tests/day
Time to Read Result	120 sec	20 sec	30 sec	20 sec	60 sec	45 sec
Dimensions (L × W × H)	1.38 m x 6.8 x 2.1 cm	15 × 6.2 × 1.9 cm	pen size/credit card size	9.0 × 5.5 cm credit card size	10.5 × 5.5 cm	12 x 6.5 × 2.5 cm
Weight	135 g	100 g	30 g	40 g	100 g	100 g
Measurement Range	0.5–27.7 mmol/L (9–500 mg/dL)	1.1–33.3 mmol/L (20–600 mg/dL)	2.2–25 mmol/L (40–450 mg/dL)	1.1–33.3 mmol/L (20–600 mg/dL)	1.1–27.8 mmol/L (20–500 mg/dL)	0–33.3 mmol/L (0–600 mg/dL)
Calibration and performance check	–lot specific –program strip with each new vial of test strips –clean meter weekly	–lot specific –program strip with each new vial of test strips	–new vial 2 lot specific strips –test solutions for meter performance	–1 step: lot specific with each new vial of test strips –no cleaning	initial calibration only –check paddle insert –no cleaning	–self calibrated; by manufacturer –check strip: use weekly –clean meter weekly
Computer data systems	Camit EL software program (available in USA)	None	None	Satellite G compatible: in hospital glucose machine with computer capabilities	None	IBM & MAC compatible software program pending
Special Features	–back up visual blood glucose reading –error code: detects user error	–back up visual blood glucose reading –measures plasma glucose instead of whole blood glucose	–works on electrochemical reaction principle instead of photometric	–works on electrochemical reaction instead of photometric	–back up visual blood glucose reading	–readout available in 9 languages –error code: detects user error
Blood letting device	Soft Touch	Soft Touch	ExacTech	ExacTech	Glucolet	Penlet II

Reprinted with permission from: Michael Heffer, B.Sc.Phm., Women's College Hospital, Toronto, Ontario.

skills. Poor technique may diminish the validity of test results. Examples of common errors include the following: excessive time taken to apply blood droplet; use of inadequate volume of blood; uneven application of blood to reagent pad; rubbing or smearing of blood over pad; incomplete, or too vigorous, removal of blood from pad; and inaccurate timing of the blood removal or reading phases of the procedure.

Thorough training of the consumer in all aspects of HBGM is essential to ensure accurate results. User technique should be evaluated at regular intervals and test results compared with those obtained by a laboratory method. The goal is for results to be within 15 per cent of the reference values. Experience has shown that 50 to 70 per cent of people receiving at least some training achieve results within 20 per cent, but that performance may deteriorate with time. Consistently inaccurate results should be investigated and the reasons for the erroneous results corrected.

It is important to remember HBGM measures glucose concentration in capillary whole blood. Measurement of serum or plasma glucose generally gives results (depending upon the hematocrit) 10 to 15 per cent higher than whole blood glucose values.

Meter Reading

Blood glucose monitors currently available in Canada are listed in Table XVII. The table lists many of the features of each device for comparative purposes. Suggested retail prices of the units vary from $80 to $190 and a warranty of 3 to 4 years is common. The size and weight of most devices is similar, with the exception of the 2 much smaller monitors using the newer electrochemical technology rather than the traditional reflectance photometric methods. The memory capacity of these devices varies widely from 1 to 250 results and 3 of the 6 monitors have computer data system compatability. Four devices use strips which require no blotting or wiping of blood from the reagent pad, and these monitors have the shortest reading times. All meters have a broad detection range, with upper limits from 25 to 33.3 mmol/L (450–600 mg/dL). Lower limits of detection include 0, 0.5, 1.1 or 2.2 mmol/L (0, 9, 20, 40 mg/dL). Two monitors use strips with visual capability and therefore offer an alternative to meter determinations.

There are several advantages to blood glucose monitoring with meters. The use of these devices precludes the need to subjectively compare colors and interpolate results. Meters are of obvious benefit to people with color-blindness or other visual impairment. All meters assist the user in accurately timing all steps by providing signals throughout the procedure.

One potential disadvantage of the meters is cost. The current price of most blood glucose meters ranges between $100 and $200. However, financial assistance is available to patients wishing to purchase a meter. Most insurance companies assist their clients by providing a major portion (80 per cent) of the purchase price, and the cost of test strips, subject to consideration of individual circumstances. For people who have no insurance or are denied funding from their insurer, the Canadian Diabetes Association offers financial assistance. In Ontario, for example, the Monitoring for Health Program reimburses 75 per cent of the cost of blood glucose meters (to a maximum of $400 every 5 years); visual or meter blood glucose strips (not urine strips); and blood letting devices and lancets. Consumers should contact their provincial division of the Canadian Diabetes Association.

In choosing a particular meter, the following factors should be considered. The device should be easy to use and have clear, simple instructions. The appearance of the display panel should meet the needs of the user. Calibration must not be difficult for the user, and convenient servicing for the instrument should be available. The meter should be capable of a high degree of accuracy and precision. Special features offered with each device should be considered in relation to the needs of the individual. Portability and cost are 2 additional factors.

Correct handling of the test strip before insertion in the meter is critical to accurate results. Meters yield results within 10 per cent of actual values under controlled conditions.

One unique problem with the validity of HBGM results recorded by users is intentional alteration of test values. In one study, 75 per cent of adults with IDDM reported lower than actual blood glucose values, as determined by use of a meter with memory capability. Overall, 26 per cent of recorded values did not match those stored in the meter. Children have been reported to alter testing technique to register better test results. This was done by altering the timing cycle, scraping the test pad before testing or diluting the blood sample. This deliberate fabrication of results may represent a wish or need to satisfy the physician or parents.

Drug Interference With Blood Glucose Monitoring

One study has examined in vitro the effects of 3 drugs—acetylsalicylic acid, acetaminophen and ascorbic acid—on the accuracy of blood glucose testing. Strong reducing substances can prevent the oxidation of indicator dyes used in glucose oxidase test strips, thereby modifying or impairing color development. The 3 drugs, tested at low to high therapeutic concentrations, were capable of depressing by 20 per cent the test results obtained by Visidex II, Accu-Chek bG and Dextrostix. Interference appeared to depend on drug, concentration and system since each product uses a different dye. Results of HBGM in people on these drugs should be interpreted with caution until further clinical studies evaluate the effect of drug interference in diabetics.

Special Circumstances
Pregnancy

When pregnancy is complicated by diabetes, there is the potential for substantial fetal morbidity and mortality. The rate of congenital malformations can be elevated to 4 to 5 times normal and there can be an increased need for early delivery, usually by caesarean section, due to macrosomatia (birth weight over 4.5 kg). However, meticulous control of maternal glycemia before conception and throughout gestation can greatly diminish these problems for the following reasons. The incidence of congenital malformation relates directly to the lack of control of maternal glycemia during embryogenesis in the first 6 to 8 weeks of gestation. As well, macrosomatia, which results from fetal hyperglycemia associated with fetal hyperinsulinemia, is directly related to maternal glycemic control. For these reasons, any woman with diabetes planning pregnancy should attempt to achieve euglycemia (normal glycosylated hemoglobin results) before conception. Ideally, specialized care should begin 6 months before conception.

During gestation, the goal of therapy is to carefully maintain euglycemia; in nondiabetic pregnant women, plasma glucose levels are lower than in the nonpregnant state. The specific target glucose ranges are 3.3 to 5.8 mmol/L (60 to 105 mg/dL) for preprandial tests and less than 6.7 mmol/L (120 mg/dL) 2 hours after meals. Frequent HBGM is essential, and glycosylated hemoglobin should be measured every 6 weeks.

During pregnancy, regular physical activity is generally encouraged. The use of oral hypoglycemic agents during pregnancy is contra-indicated. If insulin therapy must be initiated, human insulin preparations are recommended since intermittent use of animal source insulin may be more likely to cause immunogenic complications.

Urine glucose testing is not recommended in pregnancy. Any monitoring should involve blood glucose testing to facilitate achievement of normoglycemia.

Travel

Individuals with diabetes must take precautions when travelling. If flying, a request for special meals should be made when making reservations. Snacks such as crackers and cheese, or candies, should be kept on hand to avoid hypoglycemia caused by delayed meals. All diabetes-related supplies should be carried by the individual rather than checked with baggage. This practice prevents damage, delays, losses and harmful exposure of insulin to extreme temperatures.

Individuals should obtain from their physician copies of prescriptions for all medication, needles and syringes. Generic names are more easily understood in foreign countries. A physician's letter explaining the person's condition and needs is recommended. A medical identification bracelet or necklace (for example, Medic Alert) should be worn by all diabetics. If possible, travelling companions should be familiar with diabetes and the recognition and treatment of emergencies.

Ask the Consumer

Q. What type of dietary plan do you follow?

- Type II diabetics are usually overweight and require calorie reduction to achieve ideal body weight and improve diabetic control. Type I diabetics require sufficient food at appropriate frequent intervals to maintain weight and avoid hypoglycemia. Compliance with diet is difficult, but nevertheless essential for overall therapeutic success. All diabetics can benefit from reinforcement and encouragement.

Q. Do you exercise?

- Like diet, exercise is an important part of treatment. In Type II diabetics, adhering to the diet can help reduce weight. In all diabetics, exercise improves the effectiveness of insulin in lowering blood glucose. As well, physical activity can enrich the quality of life, improve the sense of well-being and may decrease the risk of cardiovascular disease. However, caution is required in people with coronary artery disease, those prone to hypoglycemia and diabetics who initiate exercise during significant hyperglycemia. Insulin dosage and food intake may have to be modified for exercise.

Q. Do you take pills for your diabetes?

- Consumers should know the name, strength and dosing frequency of their oral hypoglycemic agents. Oral agents do not lessen the importance of diet and exercise to the successful treatment of NIDDM. If a side effect occurs, the physician may prescribe another agent. Drug interactions between these and other medications may occur. The pharmacist should be aware of any other medications taken by the consumer.

Q. Do you require insulin?

- The consumer should know the brand name, the type of insulin (for example, NPH) and the species source to ensure use of the correct product. The expiry date must be noted, and any preparation of unusual appearance should be discarded. Freezing must be avoided. In-use vials are stored at room temperature and backup supplies refrigerated. Dealing with one pharmacy can help ensure continuous availability of the correct product.

Q. Do you experience hypoglycemia or insulin reactions?

- This unpleasant experience can be potentially dangerous. Consumers must understand the influence of diet, exercise and medication on the blood glucose levels. They should know the time to expect the peak effect from insulin injections. The person and family or friends should be able to recognize the signs and symptoms of low blood glucose and be able to give treatment.

Q. How do you inject your insulin?

- Consumers should be able to demonstrate the accurate withdrawal of insulin (and the preparation of mixtures, if prescribed). Special devices, which bypass insulin withdrawal, deliver insulin from a cartridge through a needle. Jet injectors require insulin withdrawal from the vial, but deliver it subcutaneously without a needle. Insulin pumps are used by a selected few and are prescribed by only a few specialists. Several devices are available to aid insulin withdrawal by the visually impaired.

Q. Do you test your urine?

- Type I diabetics monitor urine for ketones only when blood glucose is very high. Most Type II diabetics monitor urine for glucose. Any one of the convenient strip products is recommended. Available products test for glucose, ketones or both in combination. Product selection should take into account the readability of the color blocks and the timing of the procedure.

Q. Do you monitor your blood sugar?

- Several devices are available for blood letting. Some are pen-like and inconspicuous, and most are adjustable for skin thickness. Proper technique in applying blood to the test strip and in timing the procedure are crucial for accurate results. Considerable practice is required for this and for visual estimation of blood glucose value from color blocks. Periodic assessment of consumer technique is recommended. Many diabetics prefer to use a blood glucose meter to obtain a digital display of the test result, rather than rely on subjective visual assessment. Loss of color vision or acuity may require the consumer to use a meter. Blind diabetics may use a talking meter, which provides an audible test result. Some meters are now capable of storing results in memory.

Q. How do you take care of your feet?

- Daily inspection of the feet by the diabetic or a family member is important. Early detection and correction of minor problems is essential to prevent progression to infection, ulceration, gangrene or amputation. Advice on hygiene, nail clipping, moisturizers, footwear and the avoidance of smoking, sunburn, hot water and keratolytics should be provided to diabetics. Pharmacists can stress the importance of strict adherence to this advice.

Diabetes Care

References

Introduction

Krall LP, Entmacher PS, Drury TF. Life cycle in diabetes: socioeconomic aspects. In: Marble A, Krall LP, Bradley RF, et al, eds. Joslin's diabetes mellitus. Philadelphia: Lea & Febiger, 1985:907–36.

Santiago JV. Overview of the complications of diabetes. Clin Chem 1986; 32(10B):B48–B53.

Definition and Classification

Koda-Kimble MA, Rotblatt MD. Diabetes mellitus. In: Katcher BS, Young LY, Koda-Kimble MA, eds. Applied therapeutics, the clinical use of drugs. Spokane: Applied Therapeutics, 1983:1335–414.

National Diabetes Data Group. Classification and diagnosis of diabetes mellitus and other categories of glucose intolerance. Diabetes 1979;28(12):1039–57.

IDDM

Foster DW. Diabetes mellitus. In: Braunwald E, Isselbacher KJ, Petersdorf RG, Wilson JD, Martin JB, Fauci AS, eds. Harrison's principles of internal medicine. New York: McGraw-Hill, 1987:1778–97.

Krolewski AS, Warram JH, Rand LI, Kalm RC. Epidemiologic approach to the etiology of Type I diabetes mellitus and its complications. N Engl J Med 1987;317(22):1390–8.

Lebovitz HE. Etiology and pathogenesis of diabetes mellitus. Pediatr Clin North Am 1984;31(3):521–30.

NIDDM

DeFronzo RA, Ferrannini E, Koivisto V. New concepts in the pathogenesis and treatment of non-insulin-dependent diabetes mellitus. Am J Med 1983;74(Suppl 1A):52–81.

Skyler JS. Non-insulin-dependent diabetes mellitus: a clinical strategy. Diabetes Care 1984;7(Suppl 1):118–29.

Carbohydrate Metabolism

Zaloga GP, Chernow B. Insulin, glucagon and growth hormone. In: Chernow B, Lake CR, eds. The pharmacologic approach to the critically ill patient. Baltimore: Williams & Wilkins, 1983:562–85.

Hypoglycemia

Anonymous. Miscellaneous antidiabetic agents: glucagon. In: McEvoy GK, ed. American hospital formulary service drug information. Bethesda: American Society of Hospital Pharmacists, 1987:1688–90.

Miles JM, Jensen MD. Complications of insulin-dependent diabetes mellitus: management of insulin reactions and acute illness. Mayo Clin Proc 1986;61:820–4.

Smith RJ. In: Hypoglycemia. Marble A, Krall LP, Bradley RF, et al, eds. Joslin's diabetes mellitus. Philadelphia: Lea & Febiger, 1985:867–81.

Diagnosis

Unger RH, Foster DW. In: Diabetes mellitus. Wilson JD, Foster DW, eds. Williams textbook of endocrinology. Philadelphia: WB Saunders, 1985: 1018–80.

Long-Term Complications

Boulton AJM, Bowker JH. The diabetic foot. In: Olefsky JM, Sherwin RS, eds. Diabetes mellitus: management and complications. New York: Churchill Livingstone, 1985:255–75.

Clements RS, Bell DSH. Complications of diabetes: prevalence, detection, current treatment, and prognosis. Am J Med 1985;79(Suppl 5A):2–7.

Gerich JE. Insulin-dependent diabetes mellitus: pathophysiology. Mayo Clin Proc 1986;61:787–91.

Helfand AE. Preventing diabetic foot problems. Clin Podiatry 1984;1(2): 343–51.

Rosenbloom AL. Long-term complications of Type I (insulin-dependent) diabetes mellitus. Pediatr Ann 1983;12(9):665–84.

Treatment of Diabetes

Feutren G, Assan R, Karsenty G, et al. Cyclosporin increases the rate and length of remissions in insulin-dependent diabetes of recent onset. Lancet 1986;2:119–23.

Lacy PE. Islet transplantation. Clin Chem 1986;32(10B):B76–B82.

Sutherland DER, Goetz FC, Najarian JS. Pancreas transplantation. Clin Chem 1986;32(10B):B83–B96.

Diet

American Diabetes Association. Nutritional recommendations and principles for individuals with diabetes mellitus: 1986. Diabetes Care 1987;10(1): 126–32.

American Medical Association, Council on Scientific Affairs. Aspartame: review of safety issues. JAMA 1985;254(3):400–2.

American Diabetes Association. Glycemic effects of carbohydrates. Diabetes Care 1984;7(6):607–8.

American Diabetes Association. Use of noncaloric sweeteners. Diabetes Care 1987;10(4):526.

Canadian Diabetes Association. Guidelines for the nutritional management of diabetes mellitus in the 1990's. Beta Release 1989;13(3):8–15.

Flood TM, Halford BN, Cooppan R, Marble A. Dietary management of diabetes. In: Marble A, Krall LP, Bradley RF, et al, eds. Joslin's diabetes mellitus. Philadelphia: Lea & Febiger, 1985:357–72.

Gossel TA. A review of asparatame: characteristics, safety and uses. US Pharmacist 1984;9(1):26–30.

Jensen MD, Miles JM. The roles of diet and exercise in the management of patients with insulin-dependent diabetes mellitus. Mayo Clin Proc 1986; 61:813–9.

Morrison AB. Cyclamates in drugs. Information letter 541. Ottawa: Health Protection Branch, 1978:1–2.

Nehrling JK, Kobe P, McLane MP, et al. Aspartame use by persons with diabetes. Diabetes Care 1985;8(5)415–7.

Pagliaro LA, Locock RA. Aspartame. Can Pharm J 1986;119(3):121–3.

Stern SB, Bleicher SJ, Flores A, et al. Administration of aspartame in non-insulin-dependent diabetics. J Toxicol Environ Health 1976;2:429–39.

West KM. Recent trends in dietary management. In: Podolsky S, ed. Clinical diabetes: modern management. New York: Appleton-Century-Crofts, 1980:67–81.

Wood FC, Bierman EL. Is diet the cornerstone in management of diabetes? N Engl J Med 1986;315(19):1224–7.

Exercise

Bergman M, Auerhahn C. Exercise and diabetes. Am Fam Physician 1985;32(4):105–11.

Schiffrin A, Parikh S. Accommodating planned exercise in Type I diabetic patients on intensive treatment. Diabetes Care 1985;8(4):337–42.

Oral Hypoglycemic Agents

American Diabetes Association. The UGDP controversy. Diabetes Care 1979;2(1):1–3.

Asmal AC, Marble A. Oral hypoglycemic agents: an update. Drugs 1984; 28:62–78.

Campbell IW. Metformin and glibenclamide: comparative risks. Br Med J 1984;289:289.

Gerich JE. Oral hypoglycemic agents. N Eng J Med 1989;321(18):1231–45.

Hermann LS. Metformin: a review of its pharmacological properties and therapeutic use. Diabete et Metabolisme 1979;3:233–45.

Jackson RA, Hawa MI, Jaspan JB, et al. Mechanism of metformin action in non-insulin-dependent diabetes. Diabetes 1987;36:632–40.

Jackson JE, Bressler R. Clinical pharmacology of sulfonylurea hypoglycaemic agents. Drugs 1981;22:211–45,295–320.

Kolterman OG, Prince MJ, Olefsky JM. Insulin resistance in non-insulin-dependent diabetes mellitus. Am J Med 1983;74(Suppl 1A)82–101.

Krall LP. Oral hypoglycemic agents. In: Marble A, Frall LP, Bradley RF, et al, eds. Joslin's diabetes mellitus. Philadelphia: Lea & Febiger. 1985:907–36.

Kreisberg RA. The second-generation sulfonylureas: change or progress? Ann Intern Med 1985;102(1):125–6.

Lebovitz HE. Clinical utility of oral hypoglycemic agents in the management of patients with non-insulin-dependent diabetes mellitus. Am J Med 1983;75:94–9.

Diabetes Care

Lucis OJ. The status of metformin in Canada. Can Med Assoc J 1983;128:24–6.

Prendergast BD. Glyburide and glipizide, second generation oral sulfonylurea hypoglycemic agents. Clin Pharm 1984;3:473–85.

Schafer G. Biguanides: a review of history, pharmacodynamics and therapy. Diabete et Metabolisme 1983;9(2):148–63.

Shank WA, Morrison AD. Oral sulfonylureas for the treatment of Type II diabetes: an update. South Med J 1986;79(3):337–43.

Skillman TG, Feldman JM. The pharmacology of sulfonylureas. Am J Med 1981;70:361–72.

Skyler JS. Non-insulin-dependent diabetes mellitus: a clinical strategy. Diabetes Care 1984;7(Suppl 1):118–29.

Vigneri R, Goldfine ID. Role of metformin in treatment of diabetes mellitus. Diabetes Care 1987;10(1):118–22.

Insulin

Anderson JH, Campbell RK. Mixing insulins in 1990. The Diabetes Educator 1990;16(5):380–7.

Anonymous. Antidiabetic agents: insulins. In: McEvoy GK, ed. American hospital formulary service drug information. Bethesda: American Society of Hospital Pharmacists, 1987;1657–68.

Benson EA, et al. Flocculated Humulin-N insulin. N Engl J Med 1987; 316(16):1026–7.

Binder C, Lauritzen TL, Faber O, Pramming S. Insulin pharmacokinetics. Diabetes Care 1984;7(2):188–99.

Bjannes R. Eli Lilly Canada. (Letter to W Cornish, author) 1987;July 7.

Borders LM, Bingham PR, Riddle MC. Traditional insulin-use practices and the incidence of bacterial contamination and infection. Diabetes Care 1984;7(2):121–7.

Brange J. Galenics of insulin: the physico-chemical and pharmaceutical aspects of insulin and insulin preparations. New York: Springer-Verlag, 1987.

Brogard JM, Blickle JF, Paris-Bockel D. Genetically engineered insulin: five years of experience. Drugs Exp Clin Res 1985;11(6):397–406.

Burge C. Connaught Novo. (Letter to W Cornish, author) 1988;April 5.

Cardinale J. Nordisk Gentofte. (Letter to W Cornish, author) 1988;April 5.

Colagiuri S, Villalobos S. Assessing effect of mixing insulins by glucose-clamp technique in subjects with diabetes mellitus. Diabetes Care 1986; 9(6):579–86.

Deckert T. Intermediate-acting insulin preparations: NPH and Lente. Diabetes Care 1980;3(5):623–6.

Deckert T. The immunogenicity of new insulins. Diabetes 1985;34(2):94–6.

Dimitradis GD, Gerich JE. Importance of timing or preprandial subcutaneous insulin administration in the management of diabetes mellitus. Diabetes Care 1983;6(4):374–7.

Forlani G, Santacroce G, Ciavarella A, et al. Effects of mixing short- and intermediate-acting insulins on absorption course and biological effect of short-acting preparation. Diabetes Care 1986;9(6):587–90.

Galloway JA, Spradlin CT, Nelson RL, et al. Factors influencing the absorption, serum insulin concentration and blood glucose responses after injections of regular insulin and various insulin mixtures. Diabetes Care 1981;4(3):366–76.

Gerich JE. Selection of patients for intensive insulin therapy. Arch Intern Med 1985;145:1383–4.

Grammer L. Insulin allergy. Clin Rev Allergy 1986;4:189–200.

Helve E, Pelkonen R, Koivisto VA. Overnight interruption of wearing insulin pump: substitution of dose and injection site of insulin. Diabetes Care 1985;9(6):565–9.

Hunter KR. Change from porcine to human insulin. Br Med J 1986; 293:1099–100.

Klemp P, Staberg B, Madsbad S, Kolendorf K. Smoking reduces insulin absorption from subcutaneous tissue. Br Med J 1982;284:237–8.

Larkins RG. Human insulin. Aust N Z J Med 1983;13:647–51.

Lauritzen T. Pharmacokinetics of subcutaneously administered insulin and its clinical implications. Acta Endocrinol 1985;110(Suppl 272):45–8.

Levandoski LA, White NH, Santiago JV. Localized skin reactions to insulin: insulin lipodystrophies and skin reactions to pumped subcutaneous insulin therapy. Diabetes Care 1982;5(Suppl 1):6–10.

Mecklenburg RS, Guinn TS, Sannar CA, Blumenstein BA. Malfunction of continuous subcutaneous insulin infusion systems: a one-year prospective study of 127 patients. Diabetes Care 1986;9(4):351–5.

Pickup J. Human insulin. Br Med J 1986;292:155–7.

Pietri A, Raskin P. Cutaneous complications of chronic continuous subcutaneous insulin infusion therapy. Diabetes Care 1981;4(6):624–6.

Rathod M, Saravolatz L, Pohlod D, et al. Evaluation of the sterility and stability of insulin from multidose vials used for prolonged periods. Infect Control 1985;6(12):491–4.

Rizza RA. New modes of insulin administration: do they have a role in clinical diabetes? Ann Intern Med 1986;105(1):126–9.

Rizza RA. Treatment options for insulin-dependent diabetes mellitus: a comparison of the artificial endocrine pancreas, continuous subcutaneous insulin infusion and multiple daily insulin injections. Mayo Clin Proc 1986;61:796–805.

Schiffrin A, Mihic M, Leibel BS, Albisser M. Computer-assisted insulin dosage adjustment. Diabetes Care 1985;8(6):545–52.

Skyler JS. Lessons from studies of insulin pharmacokinetics. Diabetes Care 1986;9(6):666–8.

Skyler JS, Skyler DL, Seigler DE, O'Sullivan MJ. Algorithms for adjustment of insulin dosage by patients who monitor blood glucose. Diabetes Care 1981;4(2):311–8.

Skyler JS. Control of diabetes during pregnancy: 1985. JAMA 1986; 255(5):647–8.

Skyler JS, Reeves ML. Intensive treatment of Type I diabetes mellitus. In: Olefsky JM, Sherwin RS, eds. Diabetes mellitus: management and complications. New York: Churchill Livingstone, 1985:31–75.

Tarr, BD, Campbell RK, Workman TM. Stability and sterility of biosynthetic human insulin stored in plastic insulin syringes for 28 days. Am J Hosp Pharm 1991;48:2631–4.

Thorp FK. Insulin pump therapy reconsidered. JAMA 1986;255(5):645–7.

Villeneuve S. Eli Lilly Canada. (Letter to W Cornish, author) 1988;April 15.

White JR, Campbell RK. Guide to mixing insulins. Hosp Pharm 1991; 26:1046–8.

Zell M, Paone RP. Stability of insulin in plastic syringes. Am J Hosp Pharm 1983;40:637–8.

Complications of Insulin Therapy

Chance RE, Root MA, Galloway JA. The immunogenicity of insulin preparations. Acta Endocrinol 1976;83(Suppl 205):185–96.

Cote JR. Single-peak and purified insulins: chemical and clinical evaluation. Hosp Form 1981;16(12):1489–98.

Davidson JK, DeBra DW. Immunological insulin resistance. Diabetes 1978; 27(3):307–18.

Fineberg SE, Galloway JA, Fineberg NS, et al. Immunogenicity of recombinant DNA human insulin. Diabetologia 1983;25:465–9.

Home PD, Alberti KGMM. The new insulins: their characteristics and clinical considerations. Drugs 1982;24:401–13.

Kahn CR. Insulin resistance: a common feature of diabetes mellitus. N Engl J Med 1986;315(4):252–4.

Reeves WG. Immunogenicity of insulin of various origins. Neth J Med 1985;28(Suppl 1):43–6.

Sonnenberg GE, Berger M. Human insulin: much ado about one amino acid? Diabetologia 1983;25:457–9.

Walford S. Insulin antibodies—do they matter? Neth J Med 1985;28(Suppl 1): 47–9.

Young RJ, Hannan WJ, Frier BM, et al. Diabetic lipohypertrophy delays insulin absorption. Diabetes Care 1984;7(5):479–80.

Insulin Administration

American Diabetes Association. Continuous subcutaneous insulin infusion. Diabetes Care 1985;8(5):516–7.

Anonymous. Administering injectable medications. In: Swearington PL, ed. Photo-atlas of nursing procedures. Menlo Park: Addison-Wesley, 1984:103–9.

Anonymous. Drawing and injecting insulin (Pamphlet). Mississauga: Becton Dickinson Canada.

Anonymous. Jet injection of insulin (Editorial). Lancet 1985;1(8438):1140.

Diabetes Care

Anonymous. Let's talk about insulin: a practical guide to insulin therapy (pamphlet). Willowdale: Connaught Nova.

Anonymous. Mixing insulins (Pamphlet). Mississauga: Becton Dickinson Canada.

Anonymous. Syringe reuse. Diabetes Care 1985;8(1):97–8.

Aziz S. Recurrent use of disposable syringe-needle units in diabetic children. Diabetes Care 1984;7(2):118–20.

Berger M. Pharmacokinetics of subcutaneously injected insulin: the miscibility of short- and long-acting insulin preparation. In: Crepaldi G et al, eds. Diabetes, obesity and hyperlipidemias. Elsevier: Science Publishers, 1985:427–31.

Berne C, Eriksson G, Lundgren P. How accurate are insulin mixtures prepared by the patient? Diabetes Care 1986;9(1)23–6.

Bilo JH, Heine RJ, Sikkenk AC, et al. Absorption kinetics and action profiles after sequential subcutaneous administration of human soluble and Lente insulin through one needle. Diabetes Care 1987;10(4):466–9.

Blakeman K. The characteristics and storage requirements of modern insulins. Pharm J 1983;231:711–3.

Bloom A. Syringes for diabetics. Br Med J 1985;290:727–8.

Bosquet F, Grimaldi A, Thervet F. Insulin syringe reuse. Diabetes Care 1986;9(3):310.

Campbell RK. Treating diabetes in the 1980's and beyond. Am Pharm 1984;NS24(12):52–65.

Drug mixtures and compounded prescriptions. In: Fischer JM, Schwinghammer TL, Strauss S, eds. The pharmacist's answer book. Lancaster: Technomic Publishing, 1986:216–21.

Dunn PJ, Jury DR. Multiple dose insulin regimen using the Novo-Pen: initial experience and approximate dose requirements. N Z Med J 1986; 99:226–30.

Fredholm N, Vignati L, Brown S. Insulin pumps: the patients' verdict. Am J Nurs 1984;84(4):36–8.

Halle JP, Lambert J, Lindmayer I, et al. Twice-daily mixed regular and NPH insulin injections with new jet injector versus conventional syringes: pharmacokinetics of insulin absorption. Diabetes Care 1986;9(3):279–82.

Heine RJ, Bilo HJG, Sikkenk AC. Mixing short and intermediate acting insulins in the syringe: effect on postprandial blood glucose concentrations in Type I diabetics. Br Med J 1985;290:204–5.

Heine RJ, Bilo HJG, Fonk J, et al. Absorption kinetics and action profiles of mixtures of short- and intermediate-acting insulins. Diabetologia 1984; 27:558–62.

Jawadi MH, Ho LS. Stability and reproducibility of the biologic activity of premixed short-acting and intermediate-acting insulins. Am J Med 1986; 81:467–71.

Lindmayer I, Menassa K, Lambert J, et al. Development of new jet injector for insulin therapy. Diabetes Care 1986;9(3):294–7.

Malone JI, Lowitt S, Grove P, Shah SC. Comparison of insulin levels after injection by jet stream and disposable insulin syringe. Diabetes Care 1986;9(6):637–40.

Matz R. Syringe reuse. Diabetes Care 1985;9(3):97–8.

Nolte MS, Poon V, Grodsky GM, et al. Reduced solubility of short-acting insulins when mixed with longer-acting insulins. Diabetes 1983;32:1177–81.

Nursing guidelines for managing insulin pumps. In: Swearingen PL, ed. Photo-atlas of nursing procedures. Menlo Park: Addison-Wesley, 1984:117–9.

Olsson P, Hans A, Henning VS. Miscibility of human semisynthetic regular and lente insulin and human biosynthetic regular and NPH insulin. Diabetes Care 1987;10(4):473–7.

Pehling GB, Gerich JE. Comparison of plasma insulin profiles after subcutaneous administration of insulin by jet spray and conventional needle injection in patients with insulin-dependent diabetes mellitus. Mayo Clin Proc 1984;59:751–4.

Peters AL, Davidson MB. Effect of storage on action of NPH and regular insulin mixtures. Diabetes Care 1987;10(6):799–800.

Sugg Welk D. Preventing insulin-induced lipodystrophies. Nursing 1979; 9(12):42–5.

Thatcher G. Insulin injections: the case against random rotation. Am J Nurs 1985;85(6):690–2.

Monitoring Diabetic Control

American Diabetes Association. Concensus statement on self-monitoring of blood glucose. Diabetes Care 1987;10(1):95–9.

American Diabetes Association. On material for testing glucose in the urine. Diabetes Care 1978;1:64–7.

Anonymous. Dextrostix (Product monograph). Etobicoke: Miles Laboratories.

Anonymous. Teaching the diabetic client self-monitoring of blood glucose. In: Swearingen PL, ed. Photo-atlas of nursing procedures. Menlo Park: Addison-Wesley, 1984:152–7.

Anonymous. Chemstrip bG (Product monograph). Dorval: Boehringer Mannheim Canada.

Anonymous. Visidex II (Product monograph). Etobicoke: Miles Laboratories.

Anonymous. Acetest (Product monograph). Etobicoke: Miles Laboratory.

Anonymous. Clinitest (Product monograph). Etobicoke: Miles Laboratories.

Anonymous. Keto-Diastix (Product monograph). Etobicoke: Miles Laboratories.

Anonymous. Chemstrip uG 5000 K (Product monograph). Dorval: Boehringer Mannheim Canada.

Banauch D, Koller PU, Bablock W. Evaluation of Diabur-Test 5000: a cooperative study carried out at 12 diabetes centers. Diabetes Care 1983;6(3):213–8.

Bandi ZL, Myers JL, Bee DE, James GP. Evaluation of determination of glucose in urine with some commercially available dipsticks and tablets. Clin Chem 1982;28(10):2110–5.

Bierman J, Toohey B. Unscientific and opinionated report on meters. Diabetes Educator 1984;9(4):47–50.

Brecher DB, Birrer RB. Home glucose monitoring. Am Fam Physician 1984;29(1):241–4.

Brooks KE, Rawal N, Henderson AR. Laboratory assessment of three new monitors of blood glucose: Accu-Chek II, Glucometer II, and Glucoscan 2000. Clin Chem 1986;3142(12):2195–200.

Chaisson JL, Morrisset R, Hamet P. Precision and cost of techniques for self-monitoring of serum glucose levels. Can Med Assoc J 1984;130:38–43.

Clements RS, Keane NA, Kirk KA, Boshell BR. Comparison of various methods for rapid glucose estimation. Diabetes Care 1981;4(3):392–5.

Feldman JM, Lebovitz FL. Tests for glycosuria: an analysis of factors that cause misleading results. Diabetes 1973;22:115–21.

Gossel TA. Blood glucose self-testing products. US Pharmacist 1986;11(3):91–6.

Gossel TA. Diabetes home testing: urine glucose and ketones. US Pharmacist 1987;12(4):52–62.

Guthrie DW, Hinnen D, Guthrie RA. Single-voided vs double-voided urine testing. Diabetes Care 1979;2(3):269–71.

Hayford JT, Weydert JA, Thompson RG. Validity of urine glucose measurements for estimating plasma glucose concentration. Diabetes Care 1983; 6(1):40–4.

Hilton BA. Diabetic monitoring measures: does practice make perfect? Can Nurse 1982;78(5):26–32.

James RC, Chase GR. Evaluation of some commonly used semiquantitative methods for urinary glucose and ketone determinations. Diabetes 1974; 23(5):474–9.

Ladenson JH, Goldstein D, Greene D, Steffes MW. Panel discussion II: home/hospital monitoring of blood glucose. Clin Chem 1986;32(10B): B71-B75.

Malone JI, Rosenbloom AL, Grgic A, Weber T. The role of urine sugar in diabetic management. Am J Dis Child 1976;130:1324–7.

Marshall SM, Alberti KGMM. Assessment of a new visual test strip for blood glucose monitoring. Diabetes Care 1983;6(6):543–7.

Mazze RS, Shamoon H, Pasmantier R, et al. Reliability of blood glucose monitoring by patients with diabetes mellitus. Am J Med 1984;77:211–7.

McCall AL, Mullin CJ. Home monitoring of diabetes mellitus—a quiet revolution. Clin Lab Med 1986;6(2):215–39.

North DS, Steiner JF, Woodhouse KM, Maddy JA. Home monitors of blood glucose: comparison of precision and accuracy. Diabetes Care 1987; 10(3):360–6.

Podolsky S, Bradley RF. Treatment of diabetes with insulin. In: Podolsky S, ed. Clinical diabetes: modern management. New York: Appleton-Century-Crofts, 1980:91–130.

Rasaiah B. Self-monitoring of the blood glucose level: potential sources of inaccuracy. Can Med Assoc J 1985;132:1357–61.

Rice GK, Galt KA. In vitro drug interference with home blood-glucose-measurement systems. Am J Hosp Pharm 1985;42:2202–7.

Rotblatt MD, Koda-Kimble MA. Review of drug interference with urine glucose tests. Diabetes Care 1987;10(1):103–10.

Schwartz JS, Clancy CM. Glycosylated hemoglobin assays in the management and diagnosis of diabetes mellitus. Ann Intern Med 1984;101(5):710–3.

Shute DT, Oshinskie L. Acquired color vision defects and self-monitoring of blood sugar in diabetics. J Am Optom Assoc 1986;57(11):824–31.

Sobel DO, Balsam M. Comparison of Chemstrip uG, Clinitest and Diastix urine test methods in diabetic children. Diabetes Care 1984;7(3):265–8.

Spraul M, Sonnenberg GE, Berger M. Less expensive, reliable blood glucose self-monitoring. Diabetes Care 1987;10(3):357–9.

Tattersall R, Gale E. Patient self-monitoring of blood glucose and refinements of conventional insulin treatment. Am J Med 1981;70:177–82.

Walford S, Page M, Allison SP. The influence of renal threshold on the interpretation of urine tests for glucose in diabetic patients. Diabetes Care 1980;3(6):672–4.

Wilson DP, Endres RK. Compliance with blood glucose monitoring in children with Type I diabetes mellitus. J Pediatr 1986;108:1022–4.

Pregnancy

American Diabetes Association. Gestational diabetes mellitus. Am Intern Med 1986;105:461.

Anonymous. Summary and recommendations of the second international workshop-conference on gestational diabetes mellitus. Diabetes 1985;34(Suppl 2):123–6.

Coetzee EJ, Jackson WPU. The management of non-insulin-dependent diabetes during pregnancy. Diabetes Res Clin Pract 1986;1:281–7.

Gabbe SG. Management of diabetes mellitus in pregnancy. Am J Obstet Gynecol 1985;153:824–8.

Landon MB, Gabbe SG. Glucose monitoring and insulin adjustment in the pregnant diabetic patient. Clin Obstet Gynecol 1985;28(3):496–506.

Nelson RL. Diabetes and pregnancy: control can make a difference. Mayo Clin Proc 1986;61:825–9.

Skyler JS. Control of diabetes during pregnancy: 1985. JAMA 1986;255(5):647–8.

Travel

Anonymous. Travelling with diabetes (Pamphlet). Toronto: Canadian Diabetes Association, 1986.

26
Ostomy Care and Incontinence

Glenwood H. Schoepp

The colostomy, ileostomy and urostomy are surprisingly common surgical procedures. They create a need for such products as pouches and skin barriers, both of which are available in a variety of forms and sizes. Ostomates need special counselling on peristomal skin care, nutrition and medication use, and on the possible complications of their ostomies. Several support organizations exist. Urinary and fecal incontinence cannot be treated with nonprescription drugs, but pharmacists can provide nonpharmacologic products and counselling. Products include disposable briefs, leg bags, catheters, underpads, urinals and commodes.

Ostomy

An ostomy is an opening into a body cavity or organ or the operation performed to create that opening. When a disease in the gastrointestinal tract becomes life-threatening or difficult to control, ostomy surgery must be performed. More than one million North Americans in all age groups, from newborns to 90-year-olds, have ostomies. Hundreds of thousands of new ostomies are performed here and in the United States every year. Basically, four situations dictate the need for ostomy surgery: the removal of part of the large or small bowel, or the entire large intestine because of disease; to prevent permanent kidney damage from a poorly functioning bladder in children; removal of a urinary bladder because of life-threatening disease; and a temporary ostomy to allow fecal drainage to bypass a diseased or injured organ, permitting that portion to heal (when tissue repair is complete, the surgeon rejoins the intestinal tract).

Types

The most common type of ostomy is the colostomy, followed by the ileostomy. The urostomy is the least common. Colostomies and urostomies are done because of disease, trauma or a birth defect; ileostomies are performed primarily due to disease. Since the success of rehabilitation depends largely on the stoma location, the enterostomal therapist must meticulously select the ostomy site preoperatively.

Enterostomal therapists (ET) are nurses specifically educated in the care of individuals with stomas and draining wounds. Unquestionably, ETs represent the most crucial clinical and counselling resource for ostomates. Other health professionals make use of the expertise of ETs when the need arises.

Colostomy

The sigmoid colostomy usually entails removal of a segment of the descending colon and all the sigmoid colon, rectum and anus. In the descending colostomy, a segment of the sigmoid colon and the rectum and anus are excised. Surgical removal of all the large intestine distal to the ascending colon creates an ascending colostomy. Transverse colostomies (also referred to as double-barrel and loop colostomies), performed to rest a segment of the colon, may be required for as little as several weeks or for more than a year.

Cancer remains one of the most common indications for sigmoid and descending colostomies. Diverticulitis, ulcerative colitis unresponsive to medication, trauma, megacolon, benign tumors and polyps may also necessitate resection of the large bowel. Babies born with imperforate anus or Hirschprung's disease may undergo transverse loop colostomies. Temporary stomas can be performed if the trauma or disease (for example, diverticulitis or cancer) is 10 cm or more away from the rectal sphincter. Sigmoid and descending colostomies may be required at any age, but the typical person is 60 years of age or older.

The nature and consistency of colostomy discharge depends on surgical location. Sigmoid and descending colostomates normally produce one or more firm stools daily. These people may choose irrigation to manage their ostomy and employ closed end pouches or stoma caps between irrigations. In contrast, an ascending colostomy produces frequent, soft, smelly stools with unpredictable timing, and a transverse colostomy produces stools unpredictably, but less frequently. Usually palliative or temporary, transverse colostomies tend to be difficult to manage because they are positioned on the belt line. People with ascending and transverse colostomies can be found in all age groups. They must wear an appliance, a skin barrier, and usually a belt continually.

Ileostomy

An ileostomy results from the surgical removal or bypass of the colon. The distal end of the ileum is brought to the surface of the abdomen to form the stoma. Surgical procedures leading to an ileostomy range from multiple resections of the colon affected by Crohn's disease to total colectomy and proctectomy when ulcerative colitis is involved.

Surgery is generally reserved for patients not responding to medications such as prednisone, salazopyrin or 5-aminosalicylic acid. As ulcerative colitis affects the colon and the rectum only, removal of the large bowel effects a cure. However, Crohn's disease (regional enteritis) can reappear at times in another part of the gastrointestinal tract. People with cancer, congenital defects, trauma and hereditary diseases such as familial polyposis also may require ileostomies. Although relatively new in infants, ileostomy may be performed in cases of necrotizing enterocolitis, a disorder occurring in 3 to 8 per cent of premature infants.

Ileostomates wear drainable pouches and protect their skin with barriers. In 1967, Nils G. Kock created the first ileostomy with an internal ileal reservoir. Since then, a steadily increasing number of these operations have been performed in Canada and the United States, in people with ulcerative colitis or familial polyposis. Significant numbers of complications like malabsorption occur with the ileal Kock pouch (continent ileostomy).

Permanent ileostomies occasionally have troublesome complications necessitating operative revision. Furthermore, in many individuals the psychological impact of a permanent stoma is considerable. Twenty per cent of individuals with permanent stomas experience long-term difficulty in coping. Before surgery, some people express concerns about leakage, odor, noise, sexuality or the presence of an external appliance. In light of these difficulties, other surgical options have been sought for these people.

The ileoanal reservoir was first described as a "restorative procedure" in 1978. Ileoanal reservoir is a generic term for several types of surgical techniques in which an internal pelvic pouch is constructed of ileum and sewn to the anal canal. Three major types of reservoirs are created: the S-shaped, J-shaped and side-to-side. The most popular type in Canada is the J-shaped reservoir. The surgical procedure cures somes diseases, obviates the need for permanent ileostomy and diminishes concern about sexual dysfunction. Since the late 1970s, the ileoanal reservoir has been performed with increasing frequency in specialized hospitals in Canada, the United States and Europe, probably because people like the idea of their own sphincter acting as a natural continence mechanism.

Since both ulcerative colitis and familial polyposis are confined to the mucosa, the function of the sphincter muscle can be preserved by removing just the mucosal lining of the rectum and creating an ileoanal reservoir. Crohn's disease involves not only the mucosa, but also the muscular layers of the bowel; consequently, people with this disease cannot be candidates for the operation.

Considerable time and emotional stamina are needed by people undergoing the operations. (Two or even three operations are usually required.) Moreover, the reservoir does not function like a healthy colon. People typically cite 8 months as the approximate time between the first preoperative visit and the adaptation of the reservoir, the latter signalled by decreased numbers of bowel movements at generally predictable times (for example, transient anal incontinence resolves in 4 to 8 weeks). Mucus discharge increases after the operation, forcing some people to wear protective pads. People with permanent ileostomy or ileoanal reservoir need to empty the appliance or have a bowel movement the same number of times daily (between 5 and 7). An ileoanal reservoir seldom requires irrigation, and the procedure should not be encouraged.

Although ileoanal reservoir appears to be an acceptable alternative to permanent ileostomy, morbidity is significant. The enterostomal therapist plays a key role in minimizing complications (including caustic effluent, anal incontinence, pouchitis, abscesses, and perianal excoriation) and facilitating adaptation. Health professionals will see more people with ileoanal reservoir in future years, as the expertise for the operation spreads from larger centres into smaller communities.

Urostomy

A urostomy involves the genitourinary tract and may be performed on people of any age, including children. To create an ileal conduit, the most common type of urostomy, the bladder is removed and a segment of ileum 10 to 15 cm long is resected from the small intestine to be used as a passage for urine elimination. The surgeon sutures one end closed and uses the other end to create a stoma on the abdominal surface.

Ileal conduits are necessitated sometimes by such afflictions as bladder cancer, chronic cystitis, urinary incontinence, congenital defects and trauma. Youngsters with spina bifida or extrophy of the bladder may also require urostomies. Because the healthy kidney produces 10 to 15 drops of urine per minute, 24 hours a day, a properly fitting pouch must be worn over a urostomy at all times.

Another ostomy surgery likely to be seen more often in the future is the Kock urinary pouch, developed by Dr. Nils Kock and others in Sweden in 1982. The Kock urinary pouch is an internal form of urinary diversion, constructed using about 75 cm of ileum. When the bladder is removed, the pouch acts as a reservoir for urine and at regular intervals, the individual empties the pouch by self-catheterization. The pouch is constructed so that there is a continent nipple between the internal pouch and the stoma on the skin, preventing the outflow of urine while a catheter is inserted into the pouch. There is a second nipple between the pouch and the piece of ileum where the ureters are anastomosed, preventing the reflux of urine up the ureters. The individual catheterizes the pouch every 4 to 6 hours and covers the stoma afterward with a small piece of gauze secured with tape, not unlike a Band-Aid. Highly motivated individuals are preferred for the surgery. People who have undergone several abdominal surgeries or who are obese are less suitable because they are more likely to encounter difficulty with catheterization.

Because small amounts of mucus discharge from the stoma, all people with ostomies wear a small pad over the stoma to prevent spotting of their clothes.

Surgical technique will continue to be modified for a few years because the complication rate is about 20 per cent. Some people heal slowly, bleed or develop infections in the pouch. Revisional surgery may involve straightening the catheterization route, tightening the continence valves or repairing a hernia around the stoma site. In addition, 2 to 3 per cent of people form stones inside the pouch. These problems notwithstanding, the urinary Kock pouch will probably be performed more often because of its capacity of 800 to 1,000 mL (versus 400 to 500 mL for a bladder), and because it offers the individual urinary continence again.

Products and Equipment

Good quality ostomy products are relatively new. Even established companies like Hollister have only been manufacturing for just over 20 years. Individuals with ostomies can choose from disposable (temporary) or reusable (permanent) pouches. When bowel regulation cannot be established and the pouch contents must be emptied frequently throughout the day, drainable pouches work best. Closed-end pouches may be used when regulation is by natural methods or irrigation. For irrigation, a bag of lukewarm water is suspended at

Ostomy Care and Incontinence

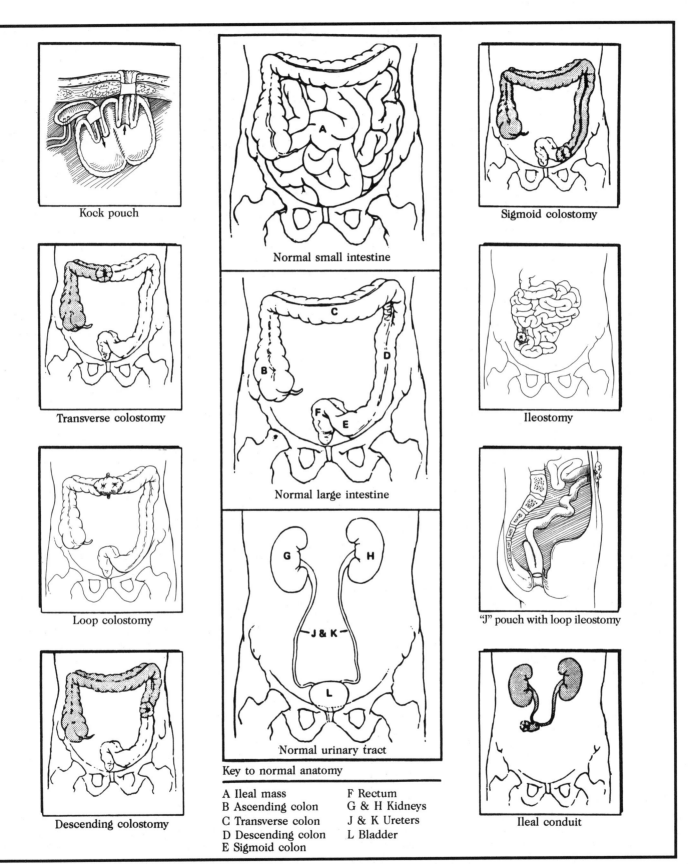

Kock pouch

Normal small intestine

Sigmoid colostomy

Transverse colostomy

Normal large intestine

Ileostomy

Loop colostomy

Normal urinary tract

"J" pouch with loop ileostomy

Descending colostomy

Key to normal anatomy

A Ileal mass   F Rectum
B Ascending colon   G & H Kidneys
C Transverse colon   J & K Ureters
D Descending colon   L Bladder
E Sigmoid colon

Ileal conduit

Figure 1 *Types of Ostomies*

Ostomy Care and Incontinence

shoulder height. The water runs through the stoma into the intestine. The irrigation sets usually feature flexible cones to prevent perforation on insertion and to create a dam against water back-flow.

Most people choose disposable pouches because they are convenient, lightweight, odor-proof and all but invisible under clothing. Drainable disposable pouches last 2 to 7 days, depending on the type of gasket used. Closed-end disposable pouches have to be changed daily or every other day according to the irrigation schedule.

One-piece disposable systems such as Hollister's First Choice line, featuring the skin barrier preattached to the pouch, often have pre-cut stoma openings in numerous sizes. ConvaTec's Active Life products are also popular in the community. They offer a simple peel-and-press application, nonclinging fabric-like pouch backing, and six pre-cut sizes of skin barrier.

In general, two-piece disposable systems consist of a flexible blanket-type skin barrier, mounted with a flange. A drainable or closed-end pouch can then be attached to the flange. Two-piece systems tend to be more popular for institutionalized patients because the pouch can be removed and discarded, while the skin barrier remains intact. Two-piece systems with more flexible flanges (sometimes termed "floating" flanges) will be employed more in future years because they snap more easily onto pouches.

Newer ostomy disposable pouches feature nonclinging fabric backings or pouch covers, both of which make the appliance less noisy, and feel cool and comfortable on the skin. Most pediatric appliances are covered with a diaper or underpants to keep tiny fingers from picking the appliance off.

Reusable appliances also offer the one- and two-piece options.

Figure 2 *Suggested Approach to Skin Care in the Ostomate*

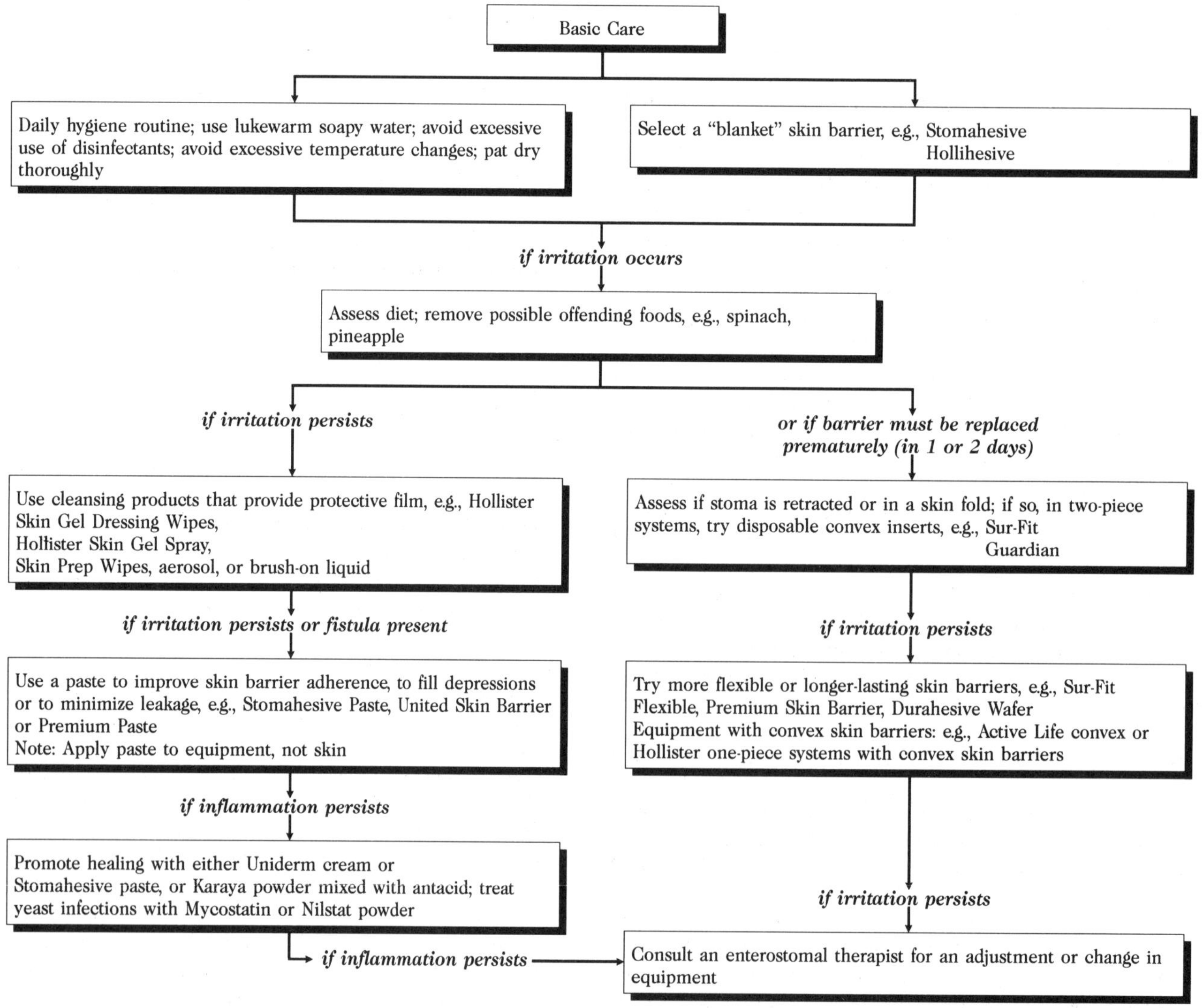

Basic Care

Daily hygiene routine; use lukewarm soapy water; avoid excessive use of disinfectants; avoid excessive temperature changes; pat dry thoroughly

Select a "blanket" skin barrier, e.g., Stomahesive Hollihesive

if irritation occurs

Assess diet; remove possible offending foods, e.g., spinach, pineapple

if irritation persists

or if barrier must be replaced prematurely (in 1 or 2 days)

Use cleansing products that provide protective film, e.g., Hollister Skin Gel Dressing Wipes, Hollister Skin Gel Spray, Skin Prep Wipes, aerosol, or brush-on liquid

Assess if stoma is retracted or in a skin fold; if so, in two-piece systems, try disposable convex inserts, e.g., Sur-Fit Guardian

if irritation persists or fistula present

if irritation persists

Use a paste to improve skin barrier adherence, to fill depressions or to minimize leakage, e.g., Stomahesive Paste, United Skin Barrier or Premium Paste
Note: Apply paste to equipment, not skin

Try more flexible or longer-lasting skin barriers, e.g., Sur-Fit Flexible, Premium Skin Barrier, Durahesive Wafer
Equipment with convex skin barriers: e.g., Active Life convex or Hollister one-piece systems with convex skin barriers

if inflammation persists

Promote healing with either Uniderm cream or Stomahesive paste, or Karaya powder mixed with antacid; treat yeast infections with Mycostatin or Nilstat powder

if irritation persists

if inflammation persists

Consult an enterostomal therapist for an adjustment or change in equipment

Note: The expertise of an enterostomal therapist may be required at any stage in an ostomate's skin care. This algorithm is intended to highlight product selection techniques.

Ostomy Care and Incontinence

Permanent pouches typically can be worn longer than temporary pouches, are more durable and can be custom fitted. Pouches last one or two months and faceplates provide service for 3 to 6 months. Consumers may ask which faceplate is best. Obese individuals with round abdomens require a convex faceplate. Thin people with flat abdomens find a flat faceplate gives the best fit. Manufacturers now produce faceplates with different flexibilities and convexities to meet each individual's needs. Some urostomates or ileostomates prefer reusable, nonadhesive ostomy systems like the VPI appliance, which incorporates a seal ring. Consumers should consult an ET about suitability of VPI before attempting a conversion from disposable equipment.

Most urostomates wear disposable appliances that are either bottom drained through a valve or connected to a bedside urinary collector for overnight drainage.

Ostomates can choose from numerous skin barriers, including wafers, pastes, gels and wipes. The old favorite, karaya gum resin, has fallen out of favor because it melts readily. Manufacturers add karaya gum to some of their pastes to take advantage of the product's natural hypoallergenic and healing properties.

Most individuals prefer a blanket-type barrier like Stomahesive, Hollihesive, Hollister Premium skin barrier or United skin barriers, which can be applied without premoistening. Stomahesive's constituents—gelatin, pectin, sodium carboxymethylcellulose and polyisobutylene—possess a low allergenic potential. United's Soft Guard XL skin barrier does not contain gelatin, and the manufacturer claims this inhibits growth of bacteria or fungi. Hollister Karaya 5 Seal also does not require premoistening, and its high degree of flexibility allows it to mold itself to the skin around the stoma.

The ability of skin barriers to remain in place for several days means they can alleviate the nurse's workload and the user's skin problems, length of stay in hospital and incidence of readmission.

Although most skin barriers give sufficient support to two-piece system components, some people prefer the additional peace of mind offered by an appliance belt, which attaches directly to the flanges on a pouch. Another type of belt—termed a support belt, which is worn over an ostomate's entire equipment, is becoming more popular with active patients. Support belts provide an extra degree of support and confidence during such activities as gardening, golfing, and lifting. Popular models include tbe smaller 3 inch wide belt called Bulgebuster by Nu-Hope and the Cool Comfort larger belt by Nu-Hope, which is available in either 4 or 6 inch widths. These products hold their shape even in a swimming pool or shower.

Popular two-piece ostomy systems—such as ConvaTec's Sur-Fit and Hollister's Guardian S—feature disposable convex inserts that enhance the skin barrier seal around flush or retracted stomas, or stomas situated in skin folds. Convex inserts are manufactured to fit 38-, 45-, or 57-mm flanges.

If the peristomal skin has dips, scars, or creases, Stomahesive, Premium or Karaya paste may be used to fill these depressions, and minimize the potential for leakage. However, pastes should be applied to the equipment, **not** the skin, and allowed to dry 10 to 20 minutes. Where the stoma is flush and the effluent is liquid, allow the paste to dry on the appliance for 4 to 8 hours (that is, overnight). This allows the alcohol in the paste to evaporate, limiting skin breakdown and decreasing the erosion of the skin barrier by the effluent. Pouches last longer as a result.

Several factors affect the selection of ostomy care equipment: the nature of the effluent; anatomic characteristics; skin sensitivities; physical disabilities; method of application and emptying; opaque or transparent pouch option; need to conceal beneath clothing; economics; user preferences; advantages and disadvantages of each appliance system (see Table I); and size of the stoma.

Table I *Comparison of One- and Two-piece Appliances*

One-piece pouch:
Advantages:
• generally better odor barrier
• can empty directly into toilet
• cleaner management for people with poor dexterity and/or poor eyesight

Disadvantages:
• cannot take apart to examine stoma or do procedures like irrigation
• do not have deep convexity, so may require build-up
• larger capacity not available in all product lines

Two-piece pouch:
Advantages:
• can take apart to examine stoma or do daily or twice daily irrigations, installation of medication, etc.

Disadvantages:
• may come apart at the top
• if individual has poor dexterity or eyesight, he/she may find it more difficult to clean and reattach pouch to the flange
• awkward to clean equipment
• generally, poorer odor barrier

Pharmacists should be familiar with the various types of equipment. For someone who wants to conceal the equipment beneath tightly fitting clothing, bulky reusable appliances are less appropriate than disposable ones. Small closed-end pouches are popular for active people involved in sports (for example, swimming) or during sexual intercourse. Each ostomy appliance has unique attachments or matching night drainage bottles. Most equipment cannot be interchanged. For example, the Sur-Fit Urostomy Pouch with Accuseal Tap is designed specifically for use with the Stomahesive Wafer with Sur-Fit Flange or Sur-Fit Flexible.

If the volume of drainage remains consistently high and users are considering the convenience of larger capacity pouches, they can choose between either one- or two-piece systems.

United claims its Soft Guard XL skin barrier lasts twice as long as other barriers, but this seems unlikely for all people, given the unique characteristics of each ostomate. This variation among individuals also applies to other long-lasting skin barriers like Durahesive Wafer.

During the early 1990s, disposable equipment with convex skin barriers were marketed. Examples include Hollister's "148" and "36" numbered series of products, and ConvaTec's "Active Life Convex" group of products which employ Durahesive as the skin barrier, and carry the number prefix "175". These products will grow in popularity because they are one-piece systems which are easy to apply, but even more importantly, they provide improved skin seals and therefore enhance skin protection. These features are particularly beneficial for patients experiencing skin breakdown, or for those patients who find they must change their disposable equipment prematurely (for example, every 1 or 2 days).

Ostomy Care and Incontinence

Products with convex skin barriers are not suitable for everyone. Some patients find the rectangular pouches attached to these unique skin barriers more difficult to empty than traditional bell-shaped pouches. Their comparatively high cost will also limit their popularity.

Complications

Short term ostomy complications including pressure ulcers, rectal/anal skin breakdown and perianal abscesses do occur postsurgically, but relatively infrequently. These problems, largely managed by physicians, are beyond the scope of this chapter. However, practical information from pharmacists can minimize long-term ostomy complications. Some ostomates, particularly those with ileostomies, tend to gain weight because they can eat foods not tolerated before surgery. Ostomates who follow Canada's Food Guide to help plan nutritionally balanced meals and snacks take the first and most important step in reducing dietary problems after ostomy surgery. Prudent dietary considerations can prevent many problems that can occur in varying degrees, such as blockage, constipation, diarrhea, flatus or odor. Eating moderate amounts at regular intervals and chewing foods thoroughly can make a positive difference, too.

Instead of placing severe dietary restrictions on an individual, some authorities advocate trying small quantities of potentially troublesome foods, one at a time, to determine which can be eaten without difficulty. For example, ostomates soon realize spinach can induce explosive diarrhea, red wine causes watery stool and beets color the stool red. Many colostomates control constipation through regular consumption of prune juice or warm lemon juice. On the other end of the scale, naturally laxative foods, such as figs and licorice, can cause diarrhea. If this complication occurs, applesauce, rice or smooth peanut butter thickens the stool. Because of their smaller stoma size, ileostomates are more prone to food blockage; they can reduce the risk by avoiding celery, coconut, popcorn, seeds, pineapple and coleslaw. Fried foods may be particularly difficult to digest. Because of malabsorption, fibre may cause discomfort during the early postoperative period. This information may confuse ostomates, as they are also told they may require bulk-forming agents to normalize their bowel function. People with ostomies should exercise caution in taking laxatives.

Drinking at least 6 cups of fluid each day helps prevent dehydration, particularly in the ileostomate. Ileostomates who require an enhanced salt intake choose foods high in sodium, like ham, corned beef, soya sauce, consommé or soda crackers. Potassium depletion secondary to diarrhea can be ameliorated by eating dried fruits, bananas, oranges, tomatoes, fish or poultry.

Odor from ostomy drainage is imperceptible when the appliance is intact and clamped. To minimize any chance of odor, people with ileostomies typically empty their pouches when one-third to one-half full. Most colostomy pouches have to be emptied once or twice daily. Asparagus makes the urine malodorous, and cheese, eggs, fish, legumes, onions, beer and members of the cabbage family can cause odor in both colostomies and ileostomies. Parsley, yogurt and buttermilk or chewed bismuth subgallate tablets (such as Devrom) or chlorophyll (such as Sudroma) tablets usually help control fecal odor; cranberry juice or vitamin C normally mitigates urinary aroma. Washing the appliance with white vinegar sometimes helps control odor. For severe urinary odor, the physician may order an alkaline-ash diet. Pouch deodorants for instillation into various types of pouches are manufactured as well (for example, Banish II, Uri-Kleen and M-9) and can be recommended as needed.

During the first few weeks postoperatively, the individual may experience much more gas than normal. To avoid episodes of flatus, colostomates and ileostomates restrict their intake of gas-producing foods like beans, broccoli, cabbage, cauliflower, onions, peppers, radishes, sauerkraut, corn and turnips. They also stay away from carbonated beverages, excessively hot or cold beverages, drinking through straws and chewing gum. Other helpful measures include taking a leisurely walk after meals, ensuring dentures fit properly and staying away from foods with air whipped into them such as soufflés, sponge cakes and milk shakes. If gas is a problem, some pouches contain a gas filter lined with charcoal or a small tab located at the top of the flange to release the pressure.

The most common long-term complications of an ostomy involve the skin. Use of a hairdryer on a cool setting for 10 to 15 minutes may help promote healing of many minor skin irritations. Peristomal skin irritation can usually be attributed to a poor skin barrier seal; contact dermatitis can be attributed to equipment components, Candida albicans overgrowth or a too large pouch opening. Stomas flush with the skin or slightly below skin level present management problems because drainage can channel beneath protective skin barriers. Fortunately, most people enjoy excellent equipment fit because of improved surgical technique. Using tincture of benzoin beneath an adhesive vehicle causes blistering of the skin. Similarly, oily preparations (such as Vaseline) prevent adherence of water-tight appliances. In addition, colostomy or ileostomy effluents digest oily vehicles. Since psoriasis may worsen if a skin barrier is placed over a lesion, alternative sites must be selected.

Allergic reactions with a rash may be due to adhesives, pouch materials or product ingredients. How can the consumer differentiate between a yeast infection and mild inflammation around the stoma? Monilial infections usually present as an expanding red rash with some clearing of the redness in the centre. Nystatin powder (for example, Mycostatin or Nilstat) resolves most peristomal monilial infections. (Creams or ointments should not be used, as they prevent appliance adherence.) Mild inflammation leads to superficial redness and mild burning, which can be resolved with UniDerm cream, karaya powder or Stomahesive powder.

A fistula is an abnormal communication between two or more normally disconnected structures or spaces. Fistulae occur for a variety of reasons, including distal obstruction from cancer, Crohn's disease, intra-abdominal abscesses or radiation therapy. Because fistulae are neither well placed nor well constructed, individuals usually cannot pouch themselves. In addition, fistulae drainage often lifts pouches, or "eats" skin barriers, so individuals must look to the enterostomal therapist for assistance. Skin care around a fistula parallels that for an ileostomy. In problem cases, ETs sometimes apply cement between the pouch and skin barrier to reduce the chance of leaks between them. If patients experience chronic, severe skin breakdown, the fistula may have to be flushed (that is, irrigated) by an ET or a physician.

Urinary tract infections often complicate urinary diversions. Alkaline urine may signal the presence of an infection, particularly if accompanied by other symptoms like chills, abdominal cramping or thickened urine. Since the urostomy mucocutaneous junction and stoma are highly colonized with skin flora, taking urine specimens out of the appliance can be highly inaccurate. Accordingly, a deep urine sample is collected from the ileal conduit using a sterile catheter and aseptic technique.

Normally excreted by the ileum, mucus presents in the urine of

Ostomy Care and Incontinence

a urostomate. Some people may mistake the mucus as an indication of a urinary tract infection.

Another complication involves the skin. Epithelial hyperplasia results when alkaline urine bathes the peristomal area. Urine alkalinity also predisposes the urostomate to formation of crystals on or near the pouch opening, which can injure stomal and peristomal tissue. Urinary acidification with vitamin C (but not sodium ascorbate) or adjusting the pouch size sometimes helps alleviate this problem. Cranberry juice may help deodorize the urine, but does not effectively acidify it.

Contrary to common belief, quality of life probably improves rather than worsens after an ostomy operation, especially if consumers receive adequate counselling. Ostomates require a little extra attention from health professionals, particularly if they are new ostomates.

Counselling

Body image is the way people picture their own bodies in their minds, or the way they see themselves. The change in body image as a result of stoma creates anxiety, distortion of self-image, self-depreciation and mourning for a loss. Ostomates' self-perception and their view of how others perceive them are affected. The psychological adjustment during the first year is extensive and is greatly influenced by the cause of the surgery. For a person who has been ill for some time, an ostomy offers resolution of the illness and the opportunity to become well again. On the other hand, someone requiring an emergency operation is totally unprepared and may require more time to accept and adjust to it.

The person who has surgery is not the only one who needs to adjust. Open communication takes down most barriers. For instance, communication can lead to resumption of a sexual relationship. New ostomates often wonder about the quality of their postsurgical sex lives, so detailed counselling is normally required.

The success of counselling centres around empathy for the ostomate's position. The ostomate must be confident the health professional cares and understands. Practical solutions to intimate problems demand frank discussions. For example, during sexual intercourse, the ostomate may wish to fold up the appliance or shift it to one side, so the stoma does not become a barrier between partners.

The physical changes that occur with an ostomy differ according to type of surgery. The male urostomate is typically impotent if the bladder is removed, but the male colostomate may or may not have this problem. If radical excision of the rectum is necessary, such as in cancer, injury to nerves and blood vessels may result in impotence. The male ileostomate is usually able to achieve an erection because rectal excision rarely requires excessive cutting. Anxious people must be counselled that potency may take months or years to return.

Female ostomates are often concerned about pregnancy and delivery. During pregnancy, the base of the stoma enlarges with the abdomen's change of contour, necessitating modification of the appliance and enlargement of the faceplate opening.

Most parents find caring for their child's ostomy challenging at first, but once they master the basic management techniques, they normally cope well with changing a pouch. Children usually become independent in terms of ostomy care by age seven or eight.

The techniques of ostomy management have been updated to alleviate many problems formerly causing people with ostomies to withdraw from society. Because a properly fitted pouch is fundamental to proper management, ostomates must remeasure their

Table II *Drugs which may Discolor Urine*

Drug	Color produced
Aminosalicylic acid	discoloration; red in hypochlorite solution[+]
Amitriptyline	blue-green
Anthraquinone laxatives	reddish in alkaline urine
Chloroquine	rust-yellow to brown
Chlorzoxazone	orange to purplish red
Daunorubicin	red
1, 8-dihydroxy-anthraquinone*	pink to red or red-brown
Dimethylsulfoxide	reddish, due to hemoglobinuria
Heparin sodium	orange
Ibuprofen	red
Indanediones	orange in alkaline urine
Indomethacin	green due to biliverdinemia
Iron sorbitex	black
Levodopa	dark on standing, possibly due to hypochlorite soln[+]
Methocarbamol	dark on standing
Methyldopa	dark on standing, possibly due to hypochlorite soln[+]
Methylene blue	blue or green
Metronidazole	brown or yellow
Nitrofurantoin	rust-yellow to brown
Phenazopyridine	orange to orange-red
Phenolphthalein	pink to purplish red in alkaline urine
Phenolsulfonphthalein (PSP)	pink to red in alkaline urine
Phenothiazines	pink to red or red-brown
Phenylbutazone	brown-green
Phenytoin	pink to red or red-brown
Phosphates	milky
Primaquine	rust-yellow to brown
Quinacrine	rust-yellow to brown
Quinine	black to black
Riboflavin	yellow fluorescence
Rifampin	bright red-orange
Senna	brown
Sulfasalazine	orange-yellow in alkaline urine
Sulfonamides, antibacterial	rust-yellow to brown
Triamterene	pale-blue fluorescence
Warfarin	orange

*Present in many combination products containing docusate sodium.
[+]Hypochlorite solution in toilet bowl from prior use of chlorine bleach cleanser.

Table III *Drugs which may Discolor Feces*

Drug	Color produced*
acetazolamide	black
antacids, aluminum hydroxide types	whitish or speckling
antibiotics, oral	greenish gray
anticoagulants	black
bismuth-containing preparations	greenish-black
charcoal	black
1, 8-dihydroxy-anthraquinone+	brownish staining of rectal mucosa
corticosteroids	black
digitalis	black
ergot preparations	tarry
ferrous salts	black
gold salts	yellow-green
heparin	pink to red or black
hydralazine	black
indomethacin	green due to biliverdinemia
levodopa	black
NSAIDs	pink to red or black
phenazopyridine	orange-red
phenylbutazone	pink to red or black
pyrvinium	red
rifampin	red-orange
salicylates, especially ASA	pink to red or black
senna	yellow

*pink, red or black colors may indicate intestinal bleeding
+present in many combination products containing docusate sodium

stomas periodically, particularly during the first six months after surgery. People who establish a regular routine for changing their appliance probably avoid leakage situations. Urostomates and ileostomates usually change their pouches before a meal since their stomas are generally less active at that time. A commonsense approach to everyday living circumvents many potential pitfalls. For example, heavy lifting may cause herniation around the stoma, and rough contact sports like football may predispose the stoma to laceration or other complications.

Ostomates who travel must take precautions. Most carry their equipment with them in case luggage is lost. Ostomates must consider the climate of the travel location, choice of foods and safety of the drinking water. For example, if the water is not safe to drink, it is equally unsafe to use for irrigation. Three to five drops of tincture of iodine to each litre of water kills all impurities within 15 minutes without making the water unpalatable for drinking. When touring foreign countries, ostomates often avoid salads and fresh fruits because these foods can induce diarrhea. The same risk applies to seafood. If diarrhea continues for more than a few hours, it is wise to seek the services of a physician. Some people ask their physicians to prescribe antidiarrheal medications for prophylaxis before their holiday departure.

Hollister Ltd. publishes a Retailer Directory to assist travellers in times of need. Ostomates can also look in the *Yellow Pages* under "Surgical Supplies," "Hospitals," or "Clinic Pharmacies" if they need appliances or accessories while away from home.

Ostomates who wish to go swimming can make a waterproof equipment seal by using Micropore 5 cm tape around the edges of the faceplate, or by wearing a soft panty girdle under the bathing suit. Covering the stoma is not necessary while bathing or showering because of its natural outward peristaltic contractions. Sur-Fit Flexible need not be removed while bathing, showering or swimming, but after exposure to water, the picture frame support adhesive should be patted dry with a towel.

Medication

Ostomates must choose their pharmacist with as much care as they choose their doctor, although every pharmacist should be able to pass along basic tips about drugs. Ileostomates may not achieve a therapeutic effect from long-acting, enteric-coated or sustained-release drugs, because these products are not adequately absorbed. Liquid formulations are preferred. Similarly, ileostomates must use diuretics with great caution owing to the greater potential for electrolyte imbalance or dehydration. Since cyanocobalamin is normally absorbed in the terminal ileum, vitamin B_{12} must be injected to be effective. Multivitamin products can produce a severe odor in the urine. Ileostomates must avoid laxatives, enemas and rectal thermometers. Although magnesium-containing antacids may induce diarrhea in ileostomates, urostomates must avoid calcium-containing antacids, as a prophylactic measure against calcium stones. Broad-spectrum antibiotics, such as amoxicillin, tetracycline, cotrimoxazole, ciprofloxacin, ofloxacin, cefixime, cefuroxime, ceftriaxone and gentamicin, can cause peristomal fungal infections or diarrhea in intestinal ostomies by altering the normal flora of the gut.

To avoid unnecessary anxiety, people with ostomies must be aware of the effects drugs can exert on urine and fecal color (see Tables II and III).

Ostomates or radiologists may have questions about procedures for bowel preparations such as barium enemas. Barium can be instilled into a colostomy using a foley catheter. The size depends on the size of the bowel lumen. Most ETs recommend colostomates irrigate when they get home, or take milk of magnesia (15 mL three times a day for 3 days). Ileostomates should never take castor oil before a diagnostic test. Irrigations or laxative use afterward are to be avoided. During a postevacuation x-ray, the individual can sit up and rock forward and backward to help move the barium. A Bongort pouch can be used to prevent spillage.

Continuity of care is vital to people with ostomies, beginning pre- and postoperatively with the ET and carried on by pharmacists. To optimize care, knowledge about the particular person must be communicated among members of the team: the doctor, the ET, the family, the pharmacist and the ostomate.

Governments are doing their part, too. Most provincial government health care programs now completely or partially reimburse ostomates for equipment purchases through pharmacies.

Public awareness of gastrointestinal diseases has been enhanced in recent years by efforts like the Cakes for Cures program developed by the Canadian Foundation for Ileitis and Colitis.

Ostomy Care and Incontinence

Support Groups and Organizations

- The Canadian Association for Enterostomal Therapy, 311-167 Lombard Avenue, Winnipeg, Manitoba R3B 0T6.
- The Northwest Society of Intestinal Research, P.O. Box 35567, Station E, Vancouver, British Columbia V6M 4G8.
- The Canadian Foundation for Ileitis and Colitis, 21 St. Clare Avenue E., Suite 301, Toronto, Ontario M4T 1L9.
- United Ostomy Association, 5 Hamilton Avenue, Hamilton, Ontario L8V 2S3.
- The International Association for Medical Assistance to Travellers, 745 Fifth Avenue, New York, New York 10017, USA.
- International Association for Enterostomal Therapy, Inc., P.O. Box 254, New Bedford, Pennsylvania 161400.

Incontinence

Urinary Incontinence

Urination (micturition) does not conform to a uniform pattern, but varies from infancy to old age and between one individual and another. The neurological control of urination is complex. The coordinated reflex activity of the autonomic and somatic nerves maintains a delicate balance between the detrusor muscle and the sphincter mechanisms. Various parasympathetic nerves supply the detrusor muscle, the urethra and the external sphincter, and the pudendal nerves furnish the striated muscles of the pelvic floor. The role of the sympathetic nervous system has recently received more interest. Stimulation of alpha receptors in the proximal urethra leads to contraction; activation of beta receptors relaxes the smooth muscle in the fundus of the bladder. Urination is also centrally controlled. Bladder sensation of fullness and voiding is represented in the spinal thalamic tracts.

Disruption of the voluntary control of urine flow can lead to incontinence. Old terms for urinary incontinence were uninhibited bladder, atonic bladder and spastic bladder. Incontinence is not diagnostic; it is only a symptom reflecting underlying problems. It affects people of all ages. More than one million Canadians suffer from incontinence. Between one-third and one-half of nursing home residents are incontinent, and 5 per cent of those incontinent of urine are also incontinent of feces. The vast majority of adults with bladder problems are women, many of whom live in provinces where seniors comprise a significant percentage of the population (for example, British Columbia).

Types of Urinary Incontinence

Urinary incontinence means different things to different people. To administrators of long-term care facilities, it is defined in terms of financial expenditures. Nursing staffs look at the problem with time-usage in mind. The affected adult most likely defines urinary incontinence with emphasis on the psychological suffering and loss of control over body functions. To avoid such value-laden perceptions, the International Continence Society formulated standard definitions of various types of urinary incontinence.

Stress incontinence is "the involuntary loss of urine when the intravesical pressure exceeds the maximum urethral pressure but in the absence of detrusor activity." Most cases of stress incontinence develop in women who have given birth, due to weakening of the pubococcygeus muscle that supports the bladder.

Urge incontinence is "the involuntary loss of urine associated with a strong desire to void." This type of incontinence often is triggered by intense emotional excitement.

Reflex incontinence is "the involuntary loss of urine caused by abnormal activity in the spinal cord in the absence of sensations, usually associated with the desire to micturate." In such cases, urine escapes without conscious knowledge.

Overflow incontinence is "involuntary loss of urine when the intravesical pressure exceeds the maximum urethral pressure owing to an elevation of intravesical pressure associated with bladder distention, but in the absence of detrusor activity." In other words, pressure within the bladder is greater than pressure in the urethra and the overflow of urine dribbles out.

Established incontinence results primarily from unstable detrusor contractions. Transient urinary incontinence can be attributed to such conditions as confusional states or urinary tract infections.

For the sake of simplicity, urinary incontinence can be grouped under urological/gynecological, neurological, psychosocial and environmental causes. Cases arising from the first category include people experiencing prostatic enlargement, postprostatectomy incontinence, urinary tract infections, vaginitis, fistulae and constipation. Menopause can lead to symptoms of incontinence by weakening the bladder neck support and by rendering hermetic closure of the urethral mucosa less effective. Neurological causes of incontinence include strokes, dementia, cerebral palsy, multiple sclerosis and diabetes mellitus. People with brain lesions or dementia may be unaware of the urge or sensation to defecate or urinate. Strokes render individuals unable to walk to the toilet, or to reach and handle a urinal. A vicious circle then develops. Immobility leads to alterations in bowel tone with the likelihood of constipation, and this process may be a factor in urinary incontinence. Cold air or tight undergarments further complicate the situation.

Unquestionably, psychological causes of incontinence prevail. Depressed people who do not care if they live or die often do not care if they are wet or dry. Emotional breakdown, depression or confusion can precipitate incontinence. Institutionalized people sometimes become incontinent of urine to make a point: they wish to maintain control over all aspects of their lives, including bladder function. The psychosocial impact of urinary or fecal incontinence can be considerable. Venturing out on even the simplest errands and to common social gatherings may become too risky. If a fatalistic attitude prevails, such as "What can you expect at their age?" these people may never regain their self-esteem.

Drugs remain one of the most important environmental causes of urinary incontinence. Diuretics taken in the evening, hypnotics and sedatives that delay the conscious need to void, alcohol and anticholinergics have all been implicated as causes. It is common for an elderly person to be on more than one anticholinergic drug at a time. People may take benztropine, trihexyphenidyl, disopyramide or diphenhydramine concurrently. The antimuscarinic effects of these drugs can so significantly impede urine flow that the bladder's storage capacity is exceeded and overflow incontinence results. Nose drops containing phenylephrine sometimes tighten the bladder neck and result in urinary retention. Methyldopa, prazosin and clonidine can aggravate stress incontinence.

Treatment of Urinary Incontinence

Treating urinary tract incontinence requires an understanding, multifaceted approach. People seek advice on urinary incontinence for three main reasons: they fear the prospect of losing bladder control;

Ostomy Care and Incontinence

they experience an isolated incidence of incontinence (an accident); or they have established incontinence that they attempt to hide. Before starting a particular therapy, the health care team must consider the person's ambulatory ability, degree of manual dexterity, general frailty and motivational level. Individuals must be treated according to biological, not chronological, age. Understanding the pathophysiological mechanisms at work in the elderly lends further rationality to treatment. For instance, mild congestive heart failure may be detected by noting increased urine output during the night and first thing in the morning.

Possible treatments include the following: prescription drugs like oxybutynin; external devices (for example, urinary incontinence garments, catheters, leg bags, night drainage bottles, urinals and underpads); keeping a voiding chart; biofeedback techniques, which sometimes work in cases of urge incontinence; exercises to strengthen the pelvic floor muscles, which can alleviate incontinence in women (examples include walking, running, yoga or even aquacise. Kegel exercises are especially important in cases of stress incontinence. Once voiding starts, the individual contracts and stops the flow of urine, holding for a count of 2 or 3. The process is repeated once or twice per void and is gradually increased to 10 or 20 contractions per set. Women must do these exercises at least 100 times a day to be effective.); consumer education, as correct body position is essential to bladder control (for example, the supine position can inhibit urination); and psychological support (counselling may be necessary to give positive reinforcement and reduce stress).

Prevention

Some cases of urinary incontinence can be prevented. Regularly scheduled toileting time, prevention of fecal impaction and adequate hydration are important physiological components of the prophylaxis and treatment of people afflicted with debilitating illnesses like multi-infarct dementia or Parkinson's disease.

Fecal Incontinence

The rectum, the reservoir for feces, is normally involved in continence and defecation. A valve-like mechanism at the anorectal junction helps prevent the flow of feces into the anal canal until an appropriate time. The competence of this mechanism depends on the tone of the puborectalis muscle in the pelvic floor. This muscle produces the angle at which the rectum forms the anal canal.

If flatus or feces enter the anal canal, stimulation of receptors causes immediate contraction of the external sphincter (of which the puborectalis muscle is a part). Relaxation of the entire sphincter mass occurs with impaction of feces, such as occurs in individuals with idiopathic megacolon, in elderly people and in certain postoperative states. The rectum becomes grossly overloaded, the external sphincters widen and fecal incontinence occurs.

The internal sphincter keeps the anal canal closed in the resting state. In people with Hirschprung's disease, the internal sphincter fails to relax at all, leading to fecal incontinence. Most causes of incontinence can be classified, and their scientific basis is known (see Table IV).

Sudden, explosive diarrhea may well cause an episode of incontinence, even in a normal, healthy person. Some children may become incontinent of feces because they have an impacted stool. Once this problem is corrected, enemas and glycerin suppositories are often used for weeks or months to induce rectal contractions. Impaction can result from neglect to answer the urge to defecate. Incontinence

Table IV Causes of Fecal Incontinence

A. Severe diarrhea
   a. Ulcerative colitis
   b. Crohn's disease
   c. Diverticulitis
   d. Villous papilloma of the rectum
   e. Carcinoma of the rectum
B. Physiological disturbance
   a. Impaction of feces
C. Neurological disease
   a. Cauda equina syndrome
   b. Other central nervous system disorders, including disseminated sclerosis
   c. Neuropathic change in the nerves supplying the pelvic floor muscles
D. Deficiency of the muscle ring
   a. Anorectal agenesis
   b. Traumatic section

Adapted from: Mandelstam D. Incontinence and its management. Dover: Croom Helm, 1986:85.

due to brain damage can be controlled by using laxatives at night to empty the bowel in the morning; drugs known to have constipating effects are given during the day. Trauma causing section of the muscle ring may result during childbirth, surgery for an anal fistula or an automobile accident. Degeneration of the pelvic floor muscles may be due to straining efforts over many years or, in some cases, the result of a difficult labor. Often, postsurgical repair of the traumatized area is protected with a temporary colostomy

Fecal incontinence occurs less often than urinary incontinence. As an isolated symptom, it persists only rarely; almost all cases are treatable. Sometimes people with incontinence forget the obvious. Changes in posture from lying, sitting or standing affect pressure in the alimentary tract. Almost everyone is aware emotional stress plays a significant role in bowel function. Dietary habits of Western civilization over the last hundred years have resulted in a high proportion of people with constipation. The public must be educated to prevent neuropathic changes associated with this trend.

Because fecal incontinence has a multitude of causes, one must carefully assess the person's history before forming an opinion on treatment. Double incontinence can happen, particularly in people like the mentally handicapped or confused elderly.

Products for Urinary and/or Fecal Incontinence

In recent years, a wide variety of products for controlling excretion has been introduced, providing modern solutions to age-old problems. The proper equipment helps ease the financial and psychological impact of incontinence.

Adult disposable undergarments and briefs have gained popularity in the 1980s. Their popularity will undoubtedly grow rapidly in the 1990s because of increasing public awareness of available products, and because of the aging population. These briefs absorb urine or contain fecal material while keeping the skin dry. Many people object to hearing these briefs referred to as diapers, considering the term derogatory.

Several brands are available, so products must be compared to

Ostomy Care and Incontinence

determine which ones best meet an individual's needs and concerns. For instance, some people might need a product at night, but not during the day. People with arthritis or paralysis might require a product that can be applied by rolling from side to side. Similarly, dysphasic people may have difficulty communicating their needs. Before choosing a garment, questions need to be answered. How much urine is expelled during a typical episode? How bulky is the garment and what is its absorbency? Can the garment be used for both fecal and urinary incontinence, or just urinary incontinence? Is it easy to put on?

Depend undergarments by Kimberly-Clark feature a dual-layer absorbent pad of polypropylene fibres, fluff pulp and a superabsorbent material called sodium polyacrylate. A body-side absorbent layer transforms urine into a stable gel. Depend features button-on elastic straps and one-size convenience (fits hip sizes to 135 cm). A thin, form-fitting shape provides freedom of movement and discreet wear under clothes. Depend shields are intended for light to moderate loss of bladder control, while Depend fitted briefs provide security for heavy to complete loss of bladder and/or bowel control.

Procter and Gamble makes the Attends line of incontinence garments, which also incorporates sodium polyacrylate as the absorbent. Although bulkier, the Original Attends brief is more popular in the community; the Trimfit Attends brief line is primarily used in institutions. Trimfit Attends are color-coded by size and can be fitted with waist or hip dimensions. All Attends briefs can be used for bladder or bowel problems. The company also manufactures an Attends undergarment. All three products have a "dry control top sheet," which facilitates the quick transfer of urine away from the body into the absorbent core and inhibits the reverse flow of urine back to the skin. The Serenity line of urinary incontinence products for women was introduced by Johnson & Johnson Inc. in 1991. Serenity Guards, which are very compact, contain a unique corrugated structure which has a superabsorbent powder embedded inside. Serenity offers three levels of absorbency ("light" which is equivalent to shields, "regular" which parallels other regular garments, and "super", which is much like extra absorbency garments).

Knitted, reusable briefs with a disposable pad, such as Dignity by ConvaTec, are less bulky than disposable briefs, but may not be suitable for some people with urinary incontinence, particularly if they are severely debilitated. Looking down to change the pad may cause lightheadedness and increase the chance of falls. Older adults with limited manual dexterity and mobility may encounter difficulty changing the pad, although it can be inserted and placed without removing the pants. If bouts of incontinence are infrequent, one garment or pad change may be needed daily. Knitted briefs are not suitable for adults with fecal incontinence.

People seeking garments for incontinence must consider individual needs, economic factors and expectations of the product. Regardless of the product selected, briefs and pads should never be considered a substitute for physician consultation. Potentially treatable and reversible incontinence might worsen or go undetected and untreated because of indiscriminate use of adult briefs. Moreover, continuous dribbling incontinence can imply a serious pathological or structural abnormality. Incontinence associated with hematuria, or a history of chronic urinary tract infections, necessitates referral to a physician.

Disposable underpads for the bed continue to be widely used in homes and hospitals. The underpad's absorbent layer hugs the skin, and an outer, waterproof absorbent layer protects the bed linens from urine and feces. Family members must avoid overpadding the bed with multiple underpads since this practice is costly and not any more effective.

At one time, the indwelling catheter was considered the only equipment necessary to treat urinary incontinence. However, the high incidence of serious urinary tract infections associated with its usage makes the foley catheter the last form of treatment considered. Adequate hydration, good hygiene at the catheter insertion site and equipment care are essential elements for proper catheter maintenance. In addition, the system should remain closed, with unobstructed urine flow. Besides urinary tract infections, some complications attributed to long-term catheterization include leakage around the catheter due to bladder spasms, blockage of the catheter and fistula formation. Indwelling catheters may be justified temporarily for incontinent individuals who require close fluid monitoring, those who develop nonhealing pressure ulcers and in the terminally ill who otherwise would be uncomfortably wet.

Intermittent catheterization and self-catheterization are possible alternatives to long-term catheter placement for some people. Urethral catheterization may be appropriate for individuals with overflow incontinence resulting from hypotonic bladders secondary to lower motor neuron lesions. Infections occur less often during intermittent catheterization than for catheters in situ.

External urine collection devices like a condom sheath can be fitted over the penis and secured by an adhesive strip. Hollister has developed a convenient, self-adhesive, urinary external catheter that greatly simplifies the penile application procedure. The internal wall of the Hollister Self-Adhesive Urinary External Catheter is coated with an adhesive that holds the catheter securely in place. A tube can be attached to a condom catheter, which can be connected to a leg bag or bedside drainage bag. Moistening the leg bag connector usually eases insertion onto the external or foley catheter. Alternatively, people may wish to try ConvaTec's Accuseal System of urinary drainage, which essentially eliminates any chance of leakage. Since impaired circulation from a tight condom or adhesive strip can lead to serious complications like ulceration, the condom should be checked at least every eight hours.

Male urinals have been around since the nineteenth century. Standing or sitting are the preferred positions for use, especially for men with prostatic hypertrophy or mild urinary obstruction. A woman with limited movement of the hips and thighs may find the typical female urinal uncomfortable to use.

The consumer can choose from fracture style or regular bedpans. Because of their smaller, lower and sloped shape, fracture style bedpans can be slipped under the person, making them particularly useful for those individuals whose physical movement must be restricted. For proper placement of the bedpan to prevent spillage or leaks into the bed, the person flexes at the hips and lowers the buttocks onto the pan, or rolls from a lateral position onto the pan. Extreme care must be taken to protect bony prominences when removing any bedpan.

Mobile or permanent bedside commodes may be necessary for the older adult to regain or retain continence. Mobile commodes can present a safety hazard if a person attempts to sit down or get up while the wheels are unlocked.

Dampness detectors and timing devices sometimes assist in toilet-training retarded adults and in cases of childhood enuresis.

Summary

Incontinence equipment must be selected to best meet the individual's needs. Careful assessment of the disruption and the expectations and capabilities of the person must be performed first. Equipment must never replace an accurate diagnosis.

Sharing information and resources helps health professionals view the incontinent individual in a holistic manner. Because of the universality of incontinence, demands for information from consumers and the numerous new products on the market, health care workers such as pharmacists and nurses will continue to receive frequent demands for counselling. Goals in managing incontinence and ostomies is best summarized by an old proverb: "To cure sometimes. To relieve often. To comfort always."

Suggested Reading
Books
- Broadwell DC, Jackson B. *Principles of Ostomy Care*. CV Mosby Company, 1982 (CV Mosby Co., 11830 Westline Industrial Drive, St. Louis, Missouri 63146, USA)
- Dorr Hullen B, McGinn KA. *The Ostomy Book*. Palo Alto: Bull Publishing, 1980
- Gross L, Bailey Z. *Enterostomal Therapy: Developing Institutional and Community Programs*. Nursing Resources Inc, 1979
- Hutchinson SJ, Shipes E. *The Physical and Psychosocial Care of Children with Stomas*. Charles C Thomas, Publisher, 1981
- Thomson Dr AB. *Idiopathic Inflammatory Bowel Disease*. Ottawa: Canadian Public Health Association, 1982
- Mandelstam D. *Incontinence and Its Management*. Dover: Croom Helm Ltd., 1986
- Palmer MH. *Urinary Incontinence*. Thorofare: Slack Incorporated, 1985
- Smith DB, Johnson DE. *Ostomy Care and the Cancer Patient: Surgical and Clinical Considerations*. Suine and Stratton Inc, 1986

Journals
- *Journal of Enterostomal Therapy*. St. Louis: CV Mosby Company
- *Ostomy Quarterly*. Los Angeles: United Ostomy Association

Manufacturers of Ostomy and Incontinence Products
- ConvaTec, Division of Squibb Canada Inc, 2365 Cote de Liesse Road, Montreal, Quebec H4N 2M7
- Hollister Ltd, 95 Mary Street, Aurora, Ontario L4G 1G3
- Kimberly-Clark of Canada Ltd, 365 Bloor Street East, Toronto, Ontario M4W 3L9
- Pfizer Hospital Products Ltd., United Division, 546 Governors Road, Guelph, Ontario N1H 6K9
- Procter & Gamble Inc., P.O. Box 255, Station A, Toronto, Ontario M5W 1C5
- Canada Care Home Health, Ottawa Ostomy Centre, 1 Raymond Street, Ottawa, Ontario K1R 1A2
- Ontario Ostomy Supply, 60 Shorting Road, Scarborough, Ontario M1S 3S3

Ask the Consumer

Q. What shape is your stoma? Have you noticed a change in size since surgery?
- Pharmacists should be aware that stomas change size postsurgically

so they can confidently answer questions on the subject from ostomates and, more importantly, recognize the need to change inventories to meet the changing equipment needs of the ostomate. Stomas tend to be round, but irregularly shaped stomas are not uncommon. All stomas enlarge somewhat after surgery, but, after a few weeks, postoperative swelling reduces and the stoma assumes its normal shape and size.

Q. Do you bleed from the stoma?
- Stomas are red, mucous membrane tissues containing no sensory nerve endings. Because of their rich blood supply from the intestinal tract, stomas may bleed slightly when rubbed or during routine activities like cleaning. On the other hand, loss of larger amounts of blood from within may signal the return of the disease that necessitated the original surgery. Refer such cases to an enterostomal therapist or physician.

Q. How long do your disposable pouches last?
- Pouches can usually be worn 2 to 7 days, depending on the type of skin barrier used. If the length of equipment life continues to decline, consult an enterostomal therapist to re-evaluate skin barrier and pouch needs.

Q. Should I irrigate my colostomy?
- The decision regarding whether the colostomy should be irrigated is made primarily by the enterostomal therapist. Previous bowel habits, mental ability to learn, physical limitations and the age of the individual all have to be considered. Some people may have questions about the amount of elimination in irrigation and the fact that it seems to vary. Effluent volume is largely determined by food bulk.

Q. How long have you been troubled with urinary incontinence? Did it start gradually, or was it associated with a particular event? Do you have a feeling of urgency, or do you have "accidents"?
- Accidents denote urge incontinence, resulting from emotional excitement. Biofeedback techniques sometimes help treatment.

Q. Do you have a small leakage of urine on slight exertion, such as coughing, sneezing or turning over in bed?
- Stress incontinence results from physical exertion or changes in intra-abdominal pressure. Exercises or medications are useful therapies.

Q. Do you wet yourself without being aware of passing urine? Is the leakage a little or a lot?
- When the pressure in the bladder is greater than that in the urethra, the overflow of urine dribbles out. Anticholinergic drugs commonly cause overflow incontinence.

Q. Do you have a history of constipation? If so, how long has this been a problem?
- Constipation can lead to either urinary or fecal incontinence. The possibility of impaction must be evaluated.

Q. Are you taking any medications such as diuretics, sedatives, antiarthritic medications, antidepressants or sleeping pills?

Ostomy Care and Incontinence

- Many drugs can cause urinary incontinence in the elderly.

Q. Do you have any chronic diseases such as diabetes, multiple sclerosis or diverticulitis?

- Many chronic diseases can lead to urinary and/or fecal incontinence.

References

Ostomy

Broadwell DC, Jackson BS. Principles of ostomy care. St Louis: CV Mosby, 1982:3.

Colostomy

Yen M. Ostomy care. In: Cyr JG, ed. Canadian self-medication. Ottawa: Canadian Pharmaceutical Association, 1984:367.

Ileostomy

Belliveau P, et al. Ileal-anal reservoir: an alternative to permanent ileostomy. J Enterostom Ther 1982;9:44–50.

Broadwell DC, Jackson BS. Principles of ostomy care. St Louis: CV Mosby, 1982:656.

Katcher BS, Young LY, Koda-Kimble MA, eds. Applied therapeutics, the clinical use of drugs. Spokane: Applied Therapeutics, 1983:453–7.

Parks AG, Nicholls RJ. Proctocolectomy without ileostomy for ulcerative colitis. Br Med J 1978;2:85–8.

Roback SA, et al. Necrotizing enterocolitis: an emerging entity in the regional infant intensive care facility. Arch Surg 1974;109:314.

Rolstad BS. Ileoanal reservoir: an overview for patients. Ostomy Quarterly 1986;23(3):81–3.

Rolstad BS, Nemer FD. Management problems associated with ileoanal reservoir. J Enterostom Ther 1985;12:41–8.

Urostomy

Boyd S. Urinary Kock pouch. Ostomy Quarterly 1986;23(2):86–8.

Complications

Broadwell DC, Jackson BS. Principles of ostomy care. St Louis: CV Mosby, 1982:244,253,237.

Counselling

Schilder P. The image and appearance of the human body. New York: Science Editions, 1950.

Medication

Knoben JE, Anderson PO, eds. Handbook of clinical drug data. Hamilton: Drug Intelligence Publications, 1983:59–61.

Meyler L, Herxheimer A. Side effects of drugs. Baltimore: Williams and Wilkins, 1968:237.

Incontinence

Mandelstam D. Incontinence and its management. Dover: Croom Helm, 1986:37,79,85.

McGinnis RH. Understanding incontinence: a urodynamic perspective. Gerontoin 1986;May/June:26–30.

Nesnick N. Medical aspects of urinary incontinence. Paper presented to Attends first invitational symposium on incontinence: rehabilitation and management in the long-term care facility. Dallas, 1985;February 10–2.

Palmer MH. Urinary incontinence. Thorofare: Slack, 1985:12,104,111.

The national nursing home survey. National Center for Health Statistics, Department of Health, Education, and Welfare. 1979;40:79–1794.

27
Diagnostic Aids

Shirley A. Heschuk

Numerous diagnostic aids are used by the self-medicating consumer. Mercury, digital and strip thermometers help assess fever, and basal thermometers help predict ovulation. Urine tests can indicate pregnancy; predict ovulation; measure glucose, ketones, pH and protein; and detect the presence in urine of blood, bacteria, leukocytes and bile pigments. Blood tests measure glucose and ketones. Stool tests check for the presence of fecal occult blood. Airflow meters allow asthmatics to test the efficacy of new medication and blood pressure measuring devices help monitor hypertension.

Nonprescription diagnostic products comprise a rapidly growing area of the home health care market especially with the advent of biotechnology using monoclonal antibodies. Consumers can select products to detect or monitor a wide variety of physiological and pathological conditions. These products allow initial screening and play an important role in the diagnosis of problems that may require further clinical and laboratory examination. Diagnostic aids discussed in this chapter include the following: mercury fever thermometers, digital thermometers, thermometer strips and basal temperature thermometers; urine tests including pregnancy tests and tests for ovulation prediction, glucose, ketones, pH, protein, blood, bacteria (nitrite), leukocytes and bile pigments; blood tests for glucose and ketones (see the chapter on diabetes care for a discussion of glucose and ketone tests); fecal tests for blood; peak expiratory flow meters; and blood pressure measuring devices.

Pharmacists assisting people to select and use diagnostic products and interpret results are advised to understand the following factors: indications for performing the test, including differential diagnosis for positive results and expected user complaints and manifestations; active ingredients and reagent safety; storage instructions and changes in physical properties that indicate a test exceeds its tolerance or no longer meets effective quality standards; instructions for collecting and testing specimens; chemical, physical, physiological or biological principles of the test procedure and its advantages and limitations; normal and abnormal test values and appropriate units of measurement; and test sensitivity and false test results.

Fever as a Diagnostic Aid

Body temperature may provide important information about the presence of illness and about changes in clinical status.

The thermoregulatory centre in the anterior hypothalamus controls body temperature by integrating various physical and chemical processes for heat production (metabolism in liver and muscles) or heat loss (sweating).

Body temperature is subject to individual variation as well as to daily fluctuation due to physiological factors, for example, exercise, digestion, sudden increase or decrease in environmental temperature and excitement. Normal diurnal variation may be as much as 1°C. It is lowest in the early morning and highest about 6 p.m. each day. In women a slight sustained temperature rise follows ovulation during the menstrual cycle.

The average normal oral body temperature is 37°C (range 36 to 37.4°C). (See Table I for a Celsius/Fahrenheit conversion chart.) The normal rectal temperature is 0.5°C higher than the oral temperature and the normal axillary (under the arm) temperature is correspondingly lower.

Fever, or pyrexia, represents regulation of body temperature at an elevated thermoregulatory "set point" above 37°C. The clinical definition of fever is generally accepted to be an oral temperature above the range of 37.5 to 38°C.

Table I *Conversion Chart, Fahrenheit to Celsius and Celsius to Fahrenheit*

°F	°C	°C	°F
95	35.0	0	32.0
96	35.5	35.0	95.0
97	36.1	35.5	95.9
98	36.6	36.0	96.8
99	37.2	36.5	97.7
100	37.7	37.0	98.6
101	38.3	37.5	99.5
102	38.8	38.0	100.4
103	39.4	38.5	101.3
104	40.0	39.0	102.2
105	40.5	39.5	103.1
106	41.1	40.0	104.0
107	41.6	40.5	104.9
108	42.2	41.0	105.8
109	42.7	41.5	106.6
110	43.3	42.0	107.6
$°C = (°F - 32) \times 5/9$		$°F = (°C \times 9/5) + 32$	

Adapted from: Parker WA. In: Cyr JG, ed. Diagnostic aids. Canadian Self-Medication. Ottawa: Canadian Pharmaceutical Association, 1984:374–96.

Diagnostic Aids

The degree of temperature elevation does not necessarily correspond to the severity of the illness, but generally discomfort or malaise appears at about 39.5 to 40°C. The febrile response tends to be greater in children than in adults; some children develop convulsions with relatively mild fevers. These convulsions are thought to have genetic disposition and to be age dependent, occurring in children 9 to 20 months old, and disappearing before they are 5 years old.

Table II Causes of Fever

1. Infections
   • "set point" raised by pyrogen
   • viral, bacterial, rickettsial, fungal, parasitic

2. Heat production exceeds heat loss
   • hyperthyroidism
   • salicylate overdose
   • neuroleptic malignant syndrome
   • malignant hyperthermia

3. Defective heat loss
   • heat stroke
   • anticholinergic drugs

4. Drug-induced
   • amphotericin B or bleomycin therapy
     (via release of pyrogens from white blood cells)
   • hypersensitivity to a drug (unpredictable)
   • idiosyncratic reaction to general anesthetics or
     succinylcholine (malignant hyperthermia)
   • neuroleptic therapy
   • overdose of phenothiazine

Adapted from: Bartle WR. Fever—a diagnostic tool? Can Pharm J 1985; 118(2):54–6.

Rectal temperatures in excess of 41°C are medical emergencies and may result in permanent brain damage; when rectal temperature is more than 43°C, heat stroke occurs and death is common. Data suggests that fevers less than 41°C rarely pose a threat and are better left untreated, to serve as a diagnostic and therapeutic aid.

Table II shows the causes or pathophysiological basis of fever. In some instances the origin of the fever may remain obscure—fever of undetermined origin (FUO)—even after careful diagnostic examination. FUO is defined as fever higher than 39.4°C recorded once daily for at least 3 weeks. Extensive laboratory and physical examination may be required. Most often an infectious disease is the cause but in many cases the diagnosis is never established.

Table III shows the symptomatic treatment of fever.

Measurement of Body Temperature

Temperatures are traditionally measured orally, rectally or axillary using three specific types of mercury-glass thermometers. Table IV describes the three different types of thermometers—oral, rectal, and universal or security—and the difference in bulb construction. The range on mercury fever thermometers is 33 to 44°C. The "normal" mark on all three types of mercury fever thermometers is at 37°C, even though rectal temperatures are usually half a degree higher than oral temperatures.

When the mercury column rises to the maximum temperature

Table III Symptomatic Treatment of Fever

1. Removal of heat
   • remove excessive clothing
   • tepid sponges
     avoid alcohol solutions—toxicity from inhalation or
     absorption through skin

2. Antipyretic drugs
   • ASA—danger of Reye's Syndrome
   • acetaminophen
   • ibuprofen*
     (See chapter on internal analgesics and antipyretics.)

3. Fluid and electrolyte replacements
   • to compensate for that lost through perspiration

*Not for use in children under 12 years of age.
Adapted from: Ryan CF, Vrabel RB. Pediatric antipyretic therapy. US Pharmacist 1978;3:49–64.

mark, it remains there until the mercury is shaken down into the bulb at the bottom of the thermometer.

Rectal temperatures are generally more accurate than oral temperatures. A variety of factors such as recent ingestion of hot or cold food or beverages, mouth breathing and position of the thermometer affect oral temperatures. For oral readings, the thermometer is placed under the rear edge of the tongue and the mouth held firmly closed for 5 to 10 minutes. This type of temperature taking may be difficult for children or for mouth breathers.

Rectal temperatures should be determined only with a rectal or security thermometer—never with an oral thermometer, as the slender glass bulb may break, causing damage to the rectal mucosa.

oral, rectal, axillary + ear thermometers

Table IV Mercury Fever Thermometers

Type	Mercury reservoir	Use
oral	slender bulb	orally, axillary
rectal	blunt pear-shaped bulb	rectally, axillary
universal or security	short stubby bulb	orally, rectally, axillary

Adapted from: Parker WA. Diagnostic aids. In: Cyr JG, ed. Canadian Self-Medication. Ottawa: Canadian Pharmaceutical Association, 1984:379–96.

Lubricating the tip of the rectal thermometer with petroleum jelly facilitates insertion into the rectum and minimizes rectal trauma. The thermometer is inserted to a depth of 2.5 to 5 cm for 3 minutes. This method is recommended for children under age two.

Axillary temperature is easier to determine, safer and less likely to spread infection, but is not as accurate as the rectal or oral method. The lower 2.5 cm of the thermometer is placed in the axillary fold and the arm is held firmly against the side for 3 to 5 minutes.

If the thermometer breaks, the mercury presents little hazard. Only neglible amounts of elemental mercury will be absorbed from the skin, rectum or gastrointestinal tract. Broken glass is of more concern. If a thermometer breaks in the rectum, a physician must be consulted immediately. If a thermometer breaks in the mouth, the individual must spit out all glass fragments and rinse the mouth well

Diagnostic Aids

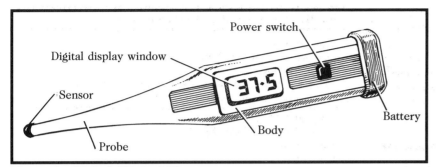

Figure 1 *Digital Clinical Thermometer*

with water. If significant lacerations occur or if glass fragments are swallowed, a physician must be consulted.

Care of Mercury Thermometers

The mercury column must be shaken down after each use. The user grasps the thermometer firmly between the thumb and forefinger at the scale end and shakes vigorously with several snaps of the wrist until the reading is below 37 °C. If the thermometer is dropped or strikes a hard surface, it should be tested before use even if it does not appear broken.

After each use and before re-use, the user cleans the thermometer to avoid contamination. The thermometer is washed carefully with soap and cool (never hot) water, rinsed thoroughly in cool water and stored in a solution of 70 per cent isopropyl alcohol. Before re-use, users should rinse the thermometer in cool water to remove the alcohol.

Digital Clinical Thermometers

Digital clinical thermometers are battery-operated. They are made of hard-to-break materials and are safe for children (see Figure 1).

High-speed response shortens the time necessary to take a temperature reading. Only 1 minute is needed either under the tongue (orally) or rectally and 2 minutes under the arm (axillary). Digital clinical thermometers contain no mercury and therefore require no shaking down as in conventional thermometers. The temperature is read off the digital display window. Body temperatures between 32 and 43 °C are displayed. After use, the user simply wipes the thermometer with an alcohol-dampened cloth.

Subnormal temperature thermometers are available to measure hypothermia in adults, children and infants. The scale range is 25 to 40 °C.

Thermometer Strips

In 1957, researchers evaluating heat losses from the human head found little or no vasoconstriction in the head in response to cold, even when the rest of the body is in a general state of vasoconstriction. The forehead is one of the regions of highest temperature in the head and therefore able to afford thermal transfer to its immediate surroundings. With the identification of a vascular association between the vessels of the forehead and the hypothalamus, a new means has been developed for diagnosing and monitoring fever using forehead temperature.

Forehead temperature is measured with a thin plastic strip coated with encapsulated liquid crystals that change color as a function of temperature. For measurement, the forehead must be clean and dry. The thermometer strip, held by the clear ends, is applied matte side against the skin for 15 to 60 seconds, depending on the product. The thermometer strip is not recommended for children under age 2, as their thermal regulatory system may still be immature.

There are two types of thermometer strips. One measures qualitatively (indicating the existence of a fever) and the other measures quantitatively (indicating the degree of fever). Elevated temperatures should be confirmed with a conventional mercury thermometer.

Thermometer strips are reuseable and should be cleaned with soap and water (not alcohol) and dried thoroughly.

Basal Thermometers

Basal temperature is measured under so-called basal conditions, after a restful night's sleep. It is the normal body temperature taken either rectally or orally (but always by the same method) immediately upon awakening. Any activity may raise the temperature (eating, drinking, smoking or exercising), so take it before getting out of bed. Set electric blankets at the same temperature each night so they are not a factor.

Basal temperature before ovulation usually ranges between 35.8 and 36.7 °C. After ovulation, it rises sharply about 0.3 °C due to the actions of progesterone (the hormone produced by the corpus luteum after ovulation) and stays in that higher range until the next menstrual period begins. To detect accurately this change in temperature, the basal thermometer is extended between each tenth of a degree, making it easy to read. The scale ranges from 35 to 39 °C. (Figure 2 shows the scale of a conventional thermometer versus a basal thermometer.) Digital basal thermometers are now available.

By carefully taking basal temperatures immediately upon waking and recording them on a chart (provided with the basal thermometer), the characteristic rise in temperature after ovulation can be observed. During menses, temperature is not taken; the woman simply marks an "X" on the chart for those days. Any rise in temperature due to illness, emotional upset or a sleepless night is noted on the chart.

The record is kept for at least 3 months to increase the accuracy of ovulation determination (see Figure 3).

An ovum can be fertilized by a sperm 8 to 24 hours after ovulation. Also, sperm can live in the female genital tract for up to 72 hours. For successful fertilization, sexual intercourse must occur

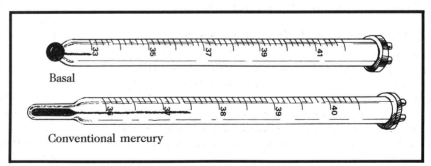

Figure 2 *Basal and Conventional Mercury Thermometers*

either shortly before ovulation—so that sperm are already available when ovulation occurs—or within a few hours after ovulation.

If a woman is using basal temperature charting as a means of contraception (also called the rhythm method), most physiology texts suggest allowing 4 to 5 days on either side of the calculated day of ovulation as the fertile or unsafe phase even when the menstrual cycle is regular. During this time it is advisable for the woman to abstain from sexual activity.

Urine Tests

Urinalysis is a useful method for diagnosing and evaluating many diseases and disease states (see Table V).

The proper collection of urine is one of the most important aspects of urinalysis. It is best to collect the urine at the time specified for a particular test. A diurnal or rhythmic variation in many urinary constituents is noted over the day. About 10 mL of urine is required for most tests. The use of appropriate containers for collection is advisable; if no container is supplied with the test kit, the user may improvise as long as the container is clean (to minimize bacterial contamination) and well rinsed of any detergent residue.

Cleanliness in the collection of the urine specimen allows a more accurate test result. Before collecting a urine sample, women should wash their genital area. The labia are held apart and washed from front to back with a gauze soaked in soap. This procedure is done 2 or 3 times, each time with fresh gauze soaked in soap. To remove any traces of soap, the labia are then wiped again, front to back, with a gauze soaked in water. Specimens from infants and young children can be collected in a disposable collection apparatus consisting of a plastic bag with an adhesive backing around the opening. It fastens to the child to allow voiding directly into the bag.

Most urinalysis tests require a midstream urine sample. A mid-

Table V *Information Obtained by Urinalysis*

Disease of:	Test urine for:
pancreas	glucose, ketones
kidneys (infection)	nitrite, protein
blood	blood
cardiovascular system	blood
respiratory system	pH
electrolyte, acid-base balance	pH
metabolism (CHO, fat, protein)	ketones, pH
pregnancy	HCG (human chorionic gonadotropin)
drug abuse and poisoning	pH, drug itself
liver or biliary disorder	urobilinogen, bilirubin

Adapted from: Gossell TA, Stansloski DW. OTC urine diagnostic products. US Pharmacist 1979;4(5):39–54,72.

stream sample yields a urine specimen with few contaminating bacteria. In collecting the midstream sample, some urine is allowed to pass before catching the specimen. The container must not touch skin or clothing. If the urine is not to be tested immediately, the container is covered so carbon dioxide does not diffuse into the air, making the urine more alkaline. If the specimen is unrefrigerated for more than 1 hour before testing, changes in the constitution of the urine may occur. Bacteria in the urine split the urea, converting it to ammonia and producing an alkaline urine. Marked changes in pH may affect cellular components. For this reason, urine is tested as soon as possible after collection.

Pregnancy Tests

Pregnancy tests are designed to detect the hormone human chori-

Figure 3 *Example of a Basal Temperature Chart*

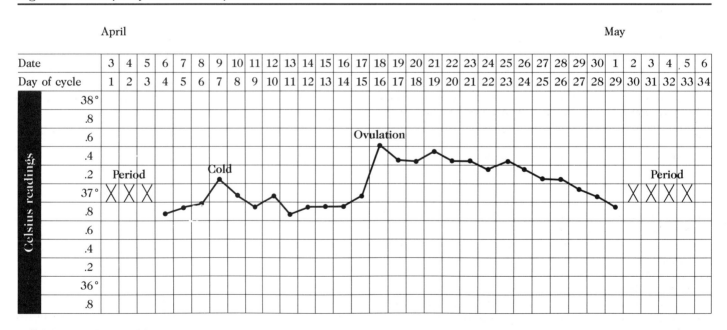

Adapted from: Becton Dickinson basal temperature thermometer (Package insert). Mississauga: Becton Dickinson.

onic gonadotropin (HCG). HCG, a glycoprotein hormone, is not normally present in nonpregnant females as it is produced by the placenta. (See the end of this discussion for other instances where the presence of HCG is not synonymous with conception). From the time the embryo first begins to implant itself in the uterine endometrium (about 5½ to 6 days after ovulation), its trophoblastic cells (developing fetal tissue) release HCG, which signals the corpus luteum that pregnancy has begun. HCG maintains luteal function and prevents its degeneration, thereby forestalling the next menstrual period. In response, the corpus luteum increases in size (several fold) and releases progesterone and estrogen, which in turn stimulate continued development of the endometrium and placenta.

HCG levels begin to rise abruptly within 48 hours of implantation and the hormone appears in the urine 10 to 14 days after conception (concentration range is 100 to 1,000 mIU/mL urine). The HCG level rises rapidly to about 2,500 to 3,000 mIU/mL about 2 weeks past the missed period. HCG levels reach a peak between 8 and 12 weeks of pregnancy (the end of the first trimester) of about 200,000 mIU/mL. Levels drop during the second trimester to reach 2,000 to 4,000 mIU/mL at about 18 weeks. This low level persists until parturition (see Figure 4). The levels of HCG fluctuate during the day and the first morning specimen generally contains the greatest concentration.

Researchers first introduced a test for pregnancy in 1928. The test involved a bioassay for HCG. The woman's urine was injected into an immature female mouse. In 4 to 5 days the mouse was killed and the ovaries examined. The presence of corpus lutea and swelling of the uterus indicated the presence of HCG and a positive test for pregnancy. In 1931, another researcher injected urine from a pregnant woman into a rabbit and the test was completed in 48 hours. Frogs and toads have also been used, but even these bioassays require at least 24 hours. after last period.

In 1960, an immunological method was developed for detecting HCG using hemagglutination-inhibition, which gave confirmation in 2 hours. Immunochemical tests (or immunoassays) for HCG are based on the fact that a potent specific HCG neutralizing antibody may be produced by injecting purified HCG into a rabbit. If antigenic HCG is absorbed into a carrier such as sheep erythrocytes or latex particles, a visible antigen-antibody may be monitored.

The major problem with these early immunochemical tests resulted from the fact that it was difficult to distinguish HCG from other glycoprotein hormones such as luteinizing hormone (LH), follicle-stimulating hormone (FSH) and thyroid stimulating hormone (TSH). All of these hormones are composed of two polypeptide subunits referred to as alpha and beta. The alpha subunits of HCG, LH, FSH and TSH are virtually identical. The beta subunits all differ. The beta subunit of HCG shows a very high degree of homology with that of LH, but has an additional 24 carboxy terminal extension. Antibodies raised against intact HCG (alpha plus beta subunits) rarely distinguish between HCG and LH, but those raised against the free beta subunits showed enhanced specificity for intact HCG plus its free chain. These antibodies formed the essential ingredient in beta-HCG immunoassays. The early home pregnancy tests were hemagglutination or latex agglutination inhibition tube tests using beta-HCG antibodies and turned positive with HCG levels of 750 to 850 mIU/mL urine, 35 days after the last menstrual period.

In the late 1970's, monoclonal antibodies to intact HCG and its free subunits (free alpha and free beta) were raised. This technology

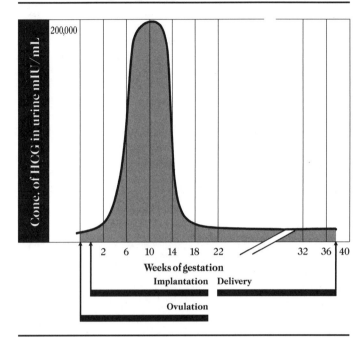

Figure 4   Human Chorionic Gonadotropin Concentration During Pregnancy

Cone. of HCG in urine mIU/mL

200,000

Weeks of gestation

Implantation   Delivery

Ovulation

Adapted from: Goodman HM. Reproduction. In: Mountcastle VB, ed. Medical physiology. St Louis: CV Mosby, 1974:1741–75.

has made available tests which are far more sensitive, with no significant cross-reaction to the LH molecule, and turning positive with HCG levels of 20 to 50 mIU/mL urine, 24 to 27 days after the last menstrual period.

Home pregnancy tests on the market today all involve monoclonal antibody technology.

Monoclonal Antibody Tests for Pregnancy

Monoclonal antibodies are homogeneous immunoglobulins (antibodies) directed at a specific antigen. They are produced by hybridization of myeloma cells (a malignant B-lymphocyte that has the ability of continuous and indefinite reproduction) with sensitized B-lymphocytes (which produces antibodies). The new hybrid cell formed (called a hybridoma) has the desired characteristics of immortality from the myeloma parent and the antibody-producing capability of the normal B-lymphocyte parent. This hybridoma is then isolated and cloned so that each new cell is an exact replica. At this point the monoclonal antibody can be frozen for indefinite storage.

The use of 2 or more monoclonal antibodies in combination, for example antibody to the alpha subunit and to the beta subunit, increases the specificity for HCG. The monoclonal antibody home pregnancy tests incorporate a solid phase monoclonal antibody reaction to the alpha-subunit of HCG and a second monoclonal antibody directed against the beta subunit of HCG. The test includes a reagent consisting of freeze-dried beta-HCG monoclonal antibody conjugated with an enzyme, a color developing solution (substrate), and a plastic indicator which varies according to the product. One area is coated with HCG antibody and the control area is coated with control antibody. Urine is added to the reagent and the plastic indicator with the two areas is placed into this solution and left for varying periods of time according to the product. The beta subunits of HCG in the urine bind to the HCG-antibody coated area. The indicator is rinsed well with water to remove unbound enzyme-label antibody. The color developing solution (substrate) is added and the bound enzyme reacts with the substrate to generate a color. The intensity of this color is proportional to the amount of HCG present in the urine. These tests are also referred to as enzyme-linked immunoassay (ELISA) tests. Advantages of this method include a sensitivity of 50 mIU HCG/mL (therefore it can be used as early as the first day of a missed period), results obtained in 3 to 30 minutes, and increased specificity due to monoclonal antibodies.

A negative test does not necessarily mean the person tested is not pregnant. If menstruation has not begun after 5 days, the test should be repeated. Inaccurate results may be due to poor technique and not following directions. Many tests provide a control—an indicator color or a negative symbol (−)—so that the patient can tell if the test was performed correctly. False negatives are more likely to occur if the menstrual cycle is irregular because it is difficult to judge when to test.

The manufacturers claim the accuracy of the monoclonal antibody pregnancy tests to be 96 to 99 per cent. Even though many of the tests can be performed as early as the first day of the missed period, most manufacturers recommend that to improve accuracy, unless medically imperative, patients should wait at least 6 to 9 days after the missed menstrual period. In early pregnancy HCG concentrations double approximately every 2 days. If earlier detection is medically imperative, serum tests done through the medical practitioner can detect concentrations of 5 mIU/mL HCG within 8 days of ovulation (within/or from 24 to 48 hours of the time of implantation).

The increased sensitivity of assays for HCG has led to several difficulties including false positive results. It has been found that HCG can be produced by nonplacental tissue (for example, the pituitary gland), and has been shown to be present in nonpregnant patients without neoplasms (serum levels of 5 to 25 mIU/mL), in normal males and postmenopausal women (high levels of LH). Some tumors secrete HCG and as a result HCG has become a useful tumor marker in both men and women. These are all detectable at levels less than 25 mIU/mL urine and therefore the levels for a positive pregnancy test has been traditionally set at 25 mIU HCG/mL urine and this level

is usually reached a day or two before the time of a missed period. Technical problems may also cause false positive test results. Table VI lists factors which may influence monoclonal antibody pregnancy test results.

The rapid development of immunochemistry technology, in particular monoclonal antibodies, has greatly increased the sensitivity of pregnancy tests. This allows earlier diagnosis of pregnancy and can contribute to improved prenatal care to minimize potential risks, such as exposure to drugs or irradiation. It can also be an advantage where termination is required.

Table VII lists home pregnancy tests available in Canada.

Urine Testing for Predicting Ovulation

The ovulation predictor tests measure luteinizing hormone (LH), which is always present in female urine but increases dramatically 1 or 2 days before ovulation. This surge in LH levels stimulates ovulation. Once ovulation occurs, the egg can be fertilized for only 8 to 24 hours. This period represents the fertile time.

The use of monoclonal antibody technology allows ovulation predictor tests to be sensitive enough to detect small changes in the amount of urinary LH. Monoclonal antibodies selectively bind to LH in the urine and an enzyme-linked immunoassay (ELISA) indicates the amount of LH bound to the monoclonal antibodies via a change in color intensity on a test stick, test pad or in a test tube, depending on the test. The onset of the LH surge can be detected when there is a significant increase in the intensity of the color over the baseline on a standard chart.

Different ovulation test kits contain supplies for 5 to 9 urine tests to be done on consecutive days. It is important to know the length of the menstrual cycle in order to determine which day testing should begin. To do this, the woman should calculate the average length of her last 3 menstrual cycles. Day 1 is the first day of menses. Each product provides a table in the instruction book to help determine which day she needs to start testing. Generally, if a woman has a 28 day cycle she should begin testing on day 11 or 12 of her cycle. If the menstrual cycle is shorter than 26 days or longer than 32 days, a given method is used to determine the day to begin testing. Some kits offer refills to test for 3 additional days. By increasing the number of days of the month the woman can test, the probability of detecting the LH surge is increased.

This test may be used in conjunction with the basal body temperature method to help estimate the time of ovulation within a few days. Ovulation prediction tests are used by women having trouble conceiving or by those wishing to plan the timing of their pregnancy. They are not meant to be used for contraception. Sperm can survive for up to 72 hours, therefore the optimal days for fertilization include 2 days preceding ovulation, the day of ovulation and the day following.

The accuracy of ovulation prediction tests is influenced by the regularity of the menstrual cycle. Some women do not ovulate every cycle and do not see an increase in LH concentration during these cycles. Certain medications like phenothiazines, medical conditions like ovarian hypofunction or the onset of menopause may cause elevated levels of LH. Decreased levels of LH may be caused by hypopituitarism, psychogenic amenorrhea or anorexia nervosa. Each manufacturer's kit must be read and followed carefully, as there are differences in timing of urine collection and total number of days of testing. Prediction of ovulation is claimed to be anywhere from 85 to 96 per cent accurate, depending on the test. (See Table VIII for ovulation predictor tests available in Canada.)

Table VI *Factors Influencing Accuracy of Monoclonal Antibody Tests for Pregnancy*

False negative	False positive
• Test performed too early	• Hormone fertility drugs containing HCG
• Chilled urine	
• Chilled reagents	• Foreign material—wax from paper cup
• Outdated or deteriorated reagents	• Ectopic production of HCG by nontrophoblastic tumors (e.g. carcinoma of the lungs)
• Test apparatus contamination	• Incomplete or missed abortion
	• Postmenopausal women
• Noncompliance with instructions	• Noncompliance with instructions

Table VII *Home Pregnancy Test Kits Available in Canada*

Product	Manufacturer	mIU HCG/mL urine: Earliest Detection	Reaction Time (minutes)	Endpoint positive	negative	Control	Comments
Advance	Ortho	250: 1 day after m.p.*	30	blue	white	no	stick—1st a.m. urine
Answer Now (1 test or 2)	Carter	25: day of m.p.	3	pink/purple	white	yes—pink in control test area	test key—any urine
Clearblue	Fisons	50: day of m.p.	30	blue	white	no	stick—1st a.m. urine
Clearblue Easy	Fisons	100: day of m.p.	3	blue	white	yes—blue line in control window	1 step—1st a.m. urine
Confidelle	Carter	50: 1 day after m.p.	20–30	blue	yellow	yes—yellow bead	colorbeads
Fact Plus	Ortho	50: 1 day after m.p.	5	(+) symbol	(−) symbol	yes—red color in test window	1 step, any urine
First Response	Carter	50: day of m.p.	1	pink	white	no	test well, any urine

*m.p. = missed period
1–800 numbers—Carter: 1–800–268–3186
　　　　　　　Fisons: 1–800–268–1121
　　　　　　　Ortho: 1–800–567–5667

Urine Glucose Tests

The presence of sugar in the urine (glucosuria or glycosuria) is not necessarily abnormal. For example, sugar (glucose) may appear in the urine after eating a heavy meal or in conjunction with emotional stress. In addition, some people may have a low tubular reabsorption rate for glucose and if the blood glucose level exceeds the reabsorption capacity, glucose spills into the urine. In the majority of cases glucose in the urine is abnormal and is usually due to diabetes mellitus. Urine glucose tests are mainly used for diabetic screening, confirming a diagnosis of diabetes and for monitoring the effectiveness of diabetic control. (See the chapter on diabetes care for more details on these tests).

Normally, urine does not contain enough glucose to react with the nonprescription testing methods. However, when blood glucose levels rise above the usual concentration of 3.3 to 7.8 mmol/L (60 to 140 mg/dL) to exceed the renal threshold of 10 to 11.1 mmol/L (180 to 200 mg/dL), glucosuria appears and can be measured.

Two methods test glucose in the urine: copper reduction tests and glucose oxidase tests. The copper reduction tests are based on reduction of copper by glucose (for example Clinitest tablets). Cupric sulfate (blue) in the presence of glucose yields cuprous oxide (green to orange). The greater the amount of glucose present, the more intense the orange color. This test is nonspecific for glucose and may detect the presence of other reducing substances in the urine (for example, uric acid, ascorbic acid and other sugars such as lactose or fructose). The test tablets are caustic and must be handled with care. The tablets should not be refrigerated, as they may absorb moisture. They should be kept out of light and away from heat. Discolored tablets should be discarded.

Enzyme tests use the enzyme glucose oxidase, which oxidizes glucose to yield gluconic acid and hydrogen peroxide. Hydrogen

Table VIII *Ovulation Predictor Test Kits*

Test	Manufacturer	Reaction Time (minutes)	Endpoint Positive	Negative	Number of Tests/Kit	Comments
Clearplan Easy	Fisons	5	↑blue		5	test urine same time each day
First Response	Carter	10	pink	white	5; 3 refills	1st a.m. urine
Ovukit	Cadna Medical	60	↑blue		6 or 9 sticks	collection of urine between 10 a.m. & 8 p.m.
OvuQuick	Cadna Medical	4	↑blue		6 or 9 pads	collection of urine between 10 a.m. & 8 p.m.

peroxide then reacts with another enzyme, peroxidase, to release oxygen. The amount of oxygen produced, in turn, changes the color of a dye (chromogen).

Manufacturers use different chromogens in their products, therefore, different colors are produced (see Table IX).

Strips of plastic are impregnated with the reagents (enzymes and chromogen). When dipped into urine, the strip changes color according to the amount of glucose in the urine. Each manufacturer has a color chart indicating percentage values of glucose (for example, 0.1 per cent equals 100 mg/dL). The color obtained in the test is matched with this chart.

Large doses of vitamin C (ascorbic acid), which result in urinary concentrations of 40 to 50 mg/dL may decrease the glucose sensitivity of glucose oxidase. Moderate to high urinary ketone levels may depress the color development of tests using glucose oxidase. (See chapter on diabetes care for a complete list of drugs which interfere with urine glucose tests.)

Specimen collection may be of the single-void or double-void type (see the chapter on diabetes care). Changes in the concentration of glycosuria between the first and second voids do not reflect a significant change in plasma glucose. Because the single-void specimen is a good indicator of overall control and the double-void method may be inconvenient, the single-void method is probably more attractive to the consumer.

Impairment of vision or colorblindness may affect the ability of a patient to interpret the results of urine glucose testing.

Despite some inherent problems, urine glucose testing may be beneficial for certain patients. It can be used to supplement blood glucose monitoring or for children or other patients who fear the pain of obtaining a blood sample or those who refuse to test blood. Patients with type II diabetes, which is controlled by diet, may use urine testing 1 to 2 hours after a meal to determine glycemic control.

How often urine testing should be performed depends on the severity of the diabetes and other factors such as illness or stress.

Urine Tests for Ketones

Ketone bodies result from the metabolism of fatty acid and fat. They consist mainly of three substances: acetone, beta-hydroxybutyric acid and acetoacetic acid.

Normally, ketone bodies metabolize completely and only negligible amounts appear in the urine. If fat, instead of carbohydrates, becomes the dominant body fuel (as occurs with starvation, weight-reducing

diets, during pregnancy, after strenuous exercise and with diabetes mellitus), an excessive amount of ketones form and appear in the urine. Beta-hydroxybutyric acid and acetoacetic acid are strong acids; when they accumulate in the blood, the individual becomes acidotic.

Ketonuria (excessive amounts of ketones in the urine) is mainly associated with diabetes mellitus. Diabetics who have too little insulin cannot utilize carbohydrates and proteins and must resort to metabolizing fats. Ketone bodies appear in the urine and can provide early detection of ketoacidosis and diabetic coma.

Tests to detect ketones in the urine are based on a nitroprusside (sodium nitroferricyanide) reaction. A positive result is indicated by a color change from beige to violet or red on reagent strips (see Table X for a product list.) The color is compared to a chart for determining the amount of ketone present. The reagent is sensitive to acetoacetic acid, which can be detected at 5 to 10 mg/dL of urine. It is much less sensitive to acetone (40 to 70 mg/dL) and does not react at all with beta-hydroxybutyric acid, which is the most prevalent. A negative test does not rule out ketoacidosis in a person having suggestive signs and symptoms (polyuria, fatigue, nausea, vomiting and stupor that can progress to coma).

The reagent-impregnated plastic dipstick and tablet products deteriorate on exposure to air, depending on how often the container is opened. To test the sensitivity of the products, a solution of 1.25 mL of acetone (for example, fresh nail polish remover) is added to 500 mL of water. Proper sensitivity of the product is denoted by a small acetone reading on fresh reagent strips. Combination dipstick products test for both glucose and ketones on one reagent strip (see Table XI). However, the presence of ketones may depress the glucose-oxidase reaction, thereby giving a false low-glucose reading. In this case, if ketones are present, it is best to switch to a copper-reduction test for a more accurate quantification of glucose.

False positive results for ketonuria may be caused by the presence of phthaleins, large quantities of phenylketones and levodopa metabolites.

Individuals with Type I insulin-dependent diabetes mellitus (IDDM) should test for ketones if their blood glucose test result exceeds 16.7 mmol/L (300 mg/dL) or if their urine glucose test is 2 per cent (2,000 mg/dL) or more. Type II non-insulin dependent diabetes mellitus (NIDDM) patients rarely develop ketonuria. The appearance of ketone bodies in the urine suggests the diabetes is not adequately controlled, and adjustments to either the medication or the diet can be made promptly.

In the nondiabetic, ketone bodies indicate a small amount of carbohydrate metabolism and excessive fat metabolism.

Urine pH

The normal range of urinary pH is 5 to 7 with a mean of 6.25. Diet,

Table IX *Products to Test for Urinary Glucose*

Product	Manufacturer	Chromogen	Color for positive test
Chemstrip uG	Boehringer-Mannheim	O-tolidine (buff)	green→dark blue
Clinistix	Miles	O-tolidine (buff)	dark purple
Diastix	Miles	iodine complex (blue)	green-brown
Tes-Tape	Lilly	O-tolidine (yellow)	green

Adapted from: Yarborough MC, Campbell RK. Module 2: developing a diabetes program for your pharmacy. Am Pharm 1986;26(2):insert.

Table X *Products to Test for Urinary Ketones*

Name	Manufacturer	Color Negative	Color Positive
Acetest Tablets	Miles	buff	maroon
Chemstrip K	Boehringer-Mannheim	buff	violet
Ketostix	Miles	buff	dark purple

Adapted from: Yarborough MC, Campbell RK. Module 2: developing a diabetes program for your pharmacy. Am Pharm 1986;26(2):insert.

Table XI *Combination Glucose and Ketone Urine Tests*

| | | Color | | | |
| | | Negative | | Positive | |
Name	Manufacturer	Glucose	Ketones	Glucose	Ketones
Chemstrip UG 5000K	Boehringer-Mannheim	buff	buff	blue	violet
Ketodiastix	Miles	buff	buff	blue	violet

drug ingestion, the presence of urinary tract infection and the state of the kidneys influence urinary pH (see Table XII.) The kidney is primarily responsible for maintaining an acid-base balance in the body. Urine pH is an important screening test for diagnosing renal disease, respiratory disease and certain metabolic disorders. Certain medications are more effective if the urine is acid or alkaline. (For example, for greater therapeutic action, methenamine requires an acidic urine.) Urine can be acidified by using ascorbic acid or ammonium chloride or alkalinized with sodium bicarbonate or acetazolamide.

Only a freshly voided urine specimen gives an accurate measure of urinary pH. The urine should be refrigerated if kept for any length of time before analysis. On standing, urine becomes more alkaline due to loss of carbon dioxide and bacterial production of ammonia.

Diagnostic tests for urine pH contain either a double indicator (methyl red and bromphenol blue) or phenaphthazine. The double indicator method gives a quantitative discrimination of color change between pH 5 and pH 9 (orange to green to blue with increasing pH). Phenaphthazine tests have a pH range of 4.5 to 7.5 and color gradations from yellow to deep blue with increasing pH. Color charts are provided with each test. When using a combination dip-and-read product for measuring pH, users must be careful that reagents from another area of strip are not washed into the pH area. This problem can be prevented if the last drop of urine remaining on the strip is removed by touching it to the side of the container before reading.

Protein in Urine

Proteinuria is the excretion of greater than normal amounts of urinary protein. It is usually defined in terms of 24-hour urinary protein excretion. Most healthy persons excrete between 30 and 130 mg of protein a day. The maximum normal level is 150 mg a day or 20 mg/dL of urine. Proteinuria is a classic sign of renal injury or disease (nephritis, nephrotic syndrome, nephrosclerosis and pyelonephritis), but also may be seen in nonrenal diseases (fever, trauma,

Table XII *Factors Which Cause a Change in Urinary pH*

Increase pH (alkaline urine)	Decrease pH (acid urine)
NaHCO$_3$	Salicylates
Antacids	High protein diet
Vegetarian diet	Diarrhea
Milk, dairy products	Citrus fruits
Renal failure	Diabetic ketoacidosis
Urinary tract infection	Hypokalemia
	Large doses of vitamin C

Information from: Fischbach FT, ed. A manual of laboratory diagnostic tests. Philadelphia: JB Lippincott, 1980:103–98.

severe exercise, anemia and cardiac disease). The usual protein excreted is albumin; globulins are excreted to a lesser amount. In severe disease states, up to 4 g/day of protein may be excreted.

Nonprescription qualitative tests for screening are negative at normal protein excretion rates (8 to 10 mg/dL). They use a colorimetric reagent strip test that employs the principle of protein error of a pH indicator: bromphenol blue or tetra-bromphenol blue. Bromphenol blue or tetra-bromphenol blue are yellow at pH 3, but with protein present, the color becomes green-blue. The sensitivity of the test is about 20 to 30 mg albumin per 100 mL of urine. The results are graded as trace and 1 through 4. The test material is more sensitive to albumin than to globulin.

False positive proteinuria may be due to a mixture of pus and red blood cells in urinary tract infections or to menstrual flow. A number of drugs may also cause false positive tests for urine protein (gold, sodium bicarbonate, acetazolamide, penicillin in massive doses, chlorpromazine, sulfisoxazole and others).

Other tests for protein include a turbidimetric test based on the principle that heat or acid causes protein to precipitate. Sulfosalicylic or acetic acid is added to a urine sample, which is heated. The presence of precipitate is noted. False positive tests are caused by several drugs, including phenothiazines, sulfonamides, cephalosporins and large doses of penicillin. A false negative result may be caused by highly alkaline urine. The sensitivity of the turbidimetric method is 5 to 30 mg/dL.

A positive test for protein in the urine may signify a more serious disease, hence, consultation with a physician is warranted.

Blood in Urine

The presence of blood in the urine (hematuria) is relatively common and usually results from renal disease or from bleeding into the urinary tract. The presence of hemoglobin (hemoglobinuria), which results from hemolysis of red blood cells, also implies hematuria. The most frequent causes of hemoglobinuria are infection and immunologic reactions (for example, transfusion reaction).

Only large quantities of blood in the urine can be visually detected (pink, red or brown urine). The presence of various drugs (for example, phenolphthalein, senna, cascara, pyrvinium pamoate and sulfonamide), food (rhubarb and beets) or certain disease states (such as porphyria) may impart a brownish-red color to urine. The detection of occult (hidden) blood in the urine depends upon the peroxidase-like activity of hemoglobin (from lysed red blood cells), which causes a change in the color of a chromogen dye in the presence of oxygen.

Guaiac, O-tolidine and benzidine are the chromogens most often used. The reagent strip is immersed in the urine specimen and after 50 seconds is compared to a color chart. Newer formulations detect 0.05 to 0.3 mg of hemoglobin per 100 mL of urine.

False positive readings may be obtained due to the presence of menstrual blood, myoglobin (resulting from muscle trauma disease) or microbial peroxidase associated with urinary tract infection.

False negative test results occur if the individual is taking large amounts of ascorbic acid.

Using midstream or double-voided urine specimens or use of vaginal tampons during menstruation may help avoid extra-urinary contamination.

Bacteria (Nitrite) in Urine

Bacteriuria (presence of 100,000 or more bacteria per mL of urine) is found in most cases of urinary tract infection (UTI), both symptomatic and asymptomatic.

UTI denotes the presence of a large number of microorganisms, often *Escherichia coli*, in either the lower urinary tract (bladder, cystitis; urethra, urethritis; prostate gland, prostatitis) or upper urinary tract (renal parenchyma, pyelonephritis) or both. The symptoms most commonly associated with cystitis and the acute urethral syndrome are a painful or burning sensation during urination (dysuria), urinary urgency and increased frequency of urination. In addition to these symptoms, people with acute pyelonephritis and acute prostatitis often experience lower back pain, general malaise, nausea, vomiting and fever. Some people can have significant bacteriuria (greater than 100,000 bacteria per mL of urine) and still be asymptomatic. This condition may subsequently develop into overt pyelonephritis.

UTI is 30 times more prevalent in females than in males. The female urethra is relatively short, which allows bacteria easy access to the bladder. Males have greater protection because of the longer urethra and the presence of antimicrobial substances in prostatic secretions. However, in males over 50 years of age, UTI is more common due to prostatic obstruction, urethral catheterization and surgery.

If given enough time, bacteria form nitrites by reducing nitrates normally present in the urine. A specimen taken first thing in the morning is best, as several hours (4 hours minimum) are required for the bladder bacterial population to convert nitrate to nitrite. Nitrite reacts with p-arsanilic acid to produce a diazonium salt, which couples with N-(1-naphthyl) ethylenediamine to form a pink-violet azo dye. This test is specific for nitrite. Sensitivity of this test is about 0.05 mg of nitrite per 100 mL. At least 100,000 bacteria per mL of urine are necessary to form enough nitrite to react with the reagent to produce a pink color.

False positive readings may be produced by medications that color the urine red (for example, phenazopyridine or medication containing methylene blue). False positive test results are unlikely to occur due to nitrite formation by contaminating bacteria introduced during specimen collection, as long as the urine is tested within 4 hours of collection.

False negative test results may be seen if the individuals are taking large doses of ascorbic acid. Significant bacteriuria is not ruled out by a negative test.

Nitrite testing is useful in self-screening for asymptomatic bacteriuria, especially in people with recurrent UTI. A positive test almost always signifies an infection in need of further treatment.

Leukocytes in Urine

The main function of leukocytes (granulocytes and agranulocytes) is to fight infection. Large numbers of leukocytes in the urine usually indicate bacterial infection in the urinary tract. If the infection is in the kidney, the white cells tend to be associated with cellular and granular casts, bacteria, epithelial cells and a few red blood cells.

The determination of leukocytes in the urine is based on a reaction that reveals the presence of esterases in granulocytes. An indoxyl ester is cleaved by these esterases and the liberated indoxyl reacts with a diazonium salt to produce a violet dye.

The color outlined is compared to a color chart with corresponding mean values obtained in a counting chamber. Negative or low leukocyte concentrations correspond to 10 to 25 leukocytes per microlitre. High leukocyte concentration of up to 500 leukocytes per microlitre gives a dark violet color.

This reaction is specific for leukocytes and is not affected by bacteria, trichomonads or erythrocytes in the urine, nor by ascorbic acid or ketones.

Bilirubin and other compounds (for example, nitrofurantoin) that impart a color to the urine may cause a darker reaction color, due to an additive effect.

Urinary proteins in excess of 500 mg/dL or cephalexin in high doses can decrease the intensity of the reaction color.

The leukocyte test is usually marketed in combination or multistick products, and is used mainly for detection of urinary tract infections (for example, Chemstrip or Multistix combination products).

Bile Pigments in Urine

Bilirubin is formed in the reticuloendothelial cells of the spleen and bone marrow from the breakdown of hemoglobin. It is transported via the blood stream to the liver, where it conjugates with glucuronic acid and is excreted with the bile into the duodenum. Here, bacterial action reduces the conjugated bilirubin to urobilinogen. Most of the urobilinogen is excreted in the feces; the rest is reabsorbed into the blood and excreted in the urine.

Normally, urine contains no bilirubin and some urobilinogen. However, in liver damage or hepatic inflammation (for example hepatitis or from hepatotoxic agents) or in biliary obstruction, bilirubin may be found in the blood, which is then excreted into the urine. Also, in hemolytic jaundice, the individual's red blood cells break down faster than normal, producing bilirubin more rapidly than the liver can process it. This excess bilirubin circulates in the blood in both free and conjugated forms. The conjugated forms (monoglucuronide or diglucuronide) are water-soluble and readily excreted by the kidneys.

Urine tests for bilirubin are based on the coupling of bilirubin with a stable diazonium salt (such as 2,6-dichlorobenzenediazonium) in an acidic medium to produce a colored azo dye. The more bilirubin present, the greater the intensity of the dye. Test sensitivity for bilirubin is 0.2 to 0.5 mg/dL.

The quantity of urobilinogen formed in the body depends on the quantity of bilirubin excreted with the bile into the intestine. If large amounts of bilirubin are excreted (as in the instances mentioned above), large amounts of urobilinogen are formed. If the liver's capacity to excrete urobilinogen is limited, a greater amount is excreted in the urine.

Testing for urobilinogen in urine uses the same principle of azocoupling as bilirubin but different diazonium salts (for example, p-dimethylaminobenzaldehyde). Sensitivity is 0.4 mg/dL of urobilinogen. Bilirubin does not react with the same salts, so does not interfere with the test. False readings may be obtained because urobilinogen is extremely unstable in acid urine.

Whether testing for bilirubin or urobilinogen, false low test results

Table XIII *Blood Glucose Monitoring Devices and Accessories*

Blood glucose Monitoring Device	Manufacturer	Strip	Range (mmol/L)	Lancing Device	Blood Removal	Elapsed Time (sec)	Memory	Visual Backup
Accu-Check III	Boehringer-Mannheim	Chemstrip bG	2–22	Autoclix or Soft Touch	wipe	120	20	yes
Accutrend	Boehringer-Mannheim	Accutrend Glucose	1.1–33.3	Soft Touch	no wiping	20	50	yes
Answer*	Horner	Answer	2.2–22.2	Within machine (requires a large drop of blood)	no wiping	60–90	40	no
Companion 2 (credit card size)	Medisense	Medisense	2.2–25	Ultra TLC	no wiping	20	10	no
Diascan	Home Diagnostics	Diascan	0–33		wipe	90	—	no
ExacTech (pen or credit size)	Medisense	ExacTech	2.2–25	Ultra TLC	no wiping	30	1	no
Glucometer GX	Miles	Glucostix	1.4–22	Autolet	blot	50	10	yes
Glucometer 3	Miles	Glucofilm	1:1–27.7	Glucolet	wipe	60	10	yes
Glucosan 3000*	Lifescan	Glucoscan	1.5–2.5	Penlet 2	blot	60	29	no
Hypocount MX (for visually impaired)	Meier Medical Supplies	BM test BG	0–22	none	wipe	60	—	yes
Matchmaker*	Boehringer-Mannheim	Chemstrip bG	2–22	Autoclix or Soft Touch	wipe	60	10	yes
One Touch II	Lifescan	One Touch	0–33	Penlet 2	no wiping	45	250	no
Tracer	Boehringer-Mannheim	Tracer bG	2–22	Autoclix or Soft Touch	wipe	120	7	yes

*Products no longer on market; however, some patients may still be using these meters.

may be seen if individuals take large amounts of vitamin C or if they have elevated concentrations of nitrite (for example, in UTI). Drugs that discolor the urine (such as phenazopyridine) may produce false positive results. Sulfisoxazole and p-aminosalicylic acid may give a false positive reading for urobilinogen.

Blood Tests
Blood Glucose Tests

Normal blood glucose levels range from 3.3 to 7.8 mmol/L (60 to 140 mg/dL). In most cases, any degree of elevated blood sugar (hyperglycemia) indicates diabetes. Other possible causes are as follows: Cushing's disease, acute stress, pheochromocytoma, pituitary adenoma, hyperthyroidism, adenoma of pancreas, pancreatitis, brain trauma and chronic liver disease. Smoking may raise the blood glucose level. Lower blood glucose levels (hypoglycemia) may be the result of an overdose of insulin (the most frequent cause), Addison's disease, bacterial sepsis, islet cell carcinoma, hepatic necrosis, hypothyroidism, glycogen storage disease or psychogenic causes. (See the chapter on diabetes care for more information about blood tests for glucose.)

Blood glucose testing has a few advantages over urine testing. Glucose does not appear in the urine until the renal threshold is reached. Urine tests provide no information about blood glucose fluctuations at concentrations below the renal threshold. They are also unreliable if an individual's renal threshold for glucose is higher or lower than normal clinical values. Blood glucose levels reveal the body's immediate state rather than reflecting its condition several hours earlier. Drinking large amounts of fluid dilutes the urine, making it appear to have less glucose. Conversely, dehydration causes a more concentrated urine with higher glucose concentrations. Urine glucose tests give no warning of impending hypoglycemia (low blood sugar).

The variety of nonprescription blood glucose test products available include strips that are read visually and those that read with the aid of electronic reflectance meters or amperometric meters, like the ExacTech which measures the electric current generated by the glucose oxidase reaction on the strip. All give quantitative readings of blood glucose concentration. Also on the market are various blood collection aids (automatic puncture devices) to obtain blood samples painlessly. (See the chapter on diabetes care for procedure on obtaining blood sample.)

Blood glucose test products use the same glucose oxidase and peroxidase enzyme system as urine glucose tests. Users prick their finger to obtain a blood sample. A drop of capillary blood is placed on the reagent strip and allowed to remain for a specified period of time, after which it is either rinsed, wiped, blotted or left untouched (depending on the meter). The result is read by matching it to the color chart provided by the manufacturer or by placing it into the meter. A quantitative measurement can be made over the range of 1.1 to 44 mmol/L (20 to 800 mg/dL) depending on the meter

memory function capable of storing test results for later analysis vary with each meter. Usually test results can be recalled from the most recent to the oldest and some can be stored together with the date and time of the test. However, it is still advisable for the patient to record the results manually in a log book. Specially designed computer software, when hooked up to a patient's meter will graph and print out the results stored in the meter's memory.

Each meter uses strips designed for that model. Strips are not interchangeable. Some strips can be read visually as well as in the meter. This can be an advantage and may also serve to test the performance of the meter.

Blood glucose monitoring is only as good as the user's techniques and even experienced users make significant errors. Many of the devices are complex and the manuals provided are often difficult to follow, some are geared to a fairly high reading grade level. Inadequate training in the use of meters is one of the main causes of errors. Other causes of error include: inadequate amount and placement of blood on the test strip, failure to calibrate the meter, lack of cleaning and use of outdated strips.

Pharmacists have the unique opportunity to provide the necessary counselling to the patient regarding the myriad of products and devices available for blood glucose monitoring and can serve as a resource to the physician and other health care professionals. (See Table XIII for a product list and see the chapter on diabetes care for more information on blood glucose monitors and reagent strips.)

Blood Tests for Ketones

The measurement of ketones in the blood (ketonemia) does not give as accurate or reliable an estimate of early ketosis as does measurement of ketonuria. The concentration of ketone bodies in the blood is low and cannot be detected until their concentration causes the person to become ketoacidotic. The kidneys are able to concentrate ketones and excrete them in the urine, where they can be detected and measured. (See the section on urine tests for ketones.)

Fecal Occult Blood Testing

Detection of occult (hidden) blood in the stool is useful in detecting disease of the gastrointestinal tract. Numerous factors cause blood to be present in the feces. Ingestion of certain foods or drugs (salicylates, steroids, indomethacin, iron, colchicine and reserpine) is associated with increased gastrointestinal blood loss. Pathologic conditions such as bleeding gums, peptic ulcers, dysentry, ulcerative colitis, hemorrhoids, and fissures or colorectal cancer can cause occult blood in the feces. Cancerous lesions within the colon may bleed even before they are well developed; stool testing for occult blood may help provide early diagnosis. Colorectal cancer is one of the most

prevalent cancers in the western world; the mortality rate is as high as 60 per cent. (See Table XIV for people at high risk.)

A dark red to black tarry appearance in the stool indicates a loss of 0.5 to 0.75 mL of blood from the upper gastrointestinal tract. Chemical testing is required to prevent confusing bloody stool with coloring from diet or drugs.

In the 1960s, the guaiac test for occult blood in the stool was introduced. A positive reaction for hemoglobin is a result of its pseudoperoxidase activity. Guaiac undergoes phenolic oxidation in the presence of hemoglobin in the stool and hydrogen peroxide in the test reagent, turning the stool sample blue.

For tests using the guaiac reaction, false positive results can be caused by any substance with peroxidase activity (certain fresh fruits and uncooked vegetables, such as turnip, horseradish, parsnip, cauliflower, broccoli, cantaloupe, artichoke and mushroom).

Red meat in the diet also causes a false positive test. Drugs such as iron, salicylates and other nonsteroidal anti-inflammatory agents, reserpine and corticosteroids will yield a positive test result (see Table XV). False negative results may occur if the person is taking large amounts of ascorbic acid (an antioxidant). Bleeding in the upper intestinal tract may produce a false negative result due to the fact that hemoglobin may be chemically altered as it passes through the gastrointestinal tract so that it loses its pseudoperoxidase activity. Also, intestinal bacteria may convert hemoglobin to porphyrin, which does not react with guaiac. A negative test for occult blood does not necessarily rule out cancer. Some cancerous lesions do not bleed; others bleed infrequently. Roughage encourages early, small cancerous lesions to bleed and increases the accuracy of the test. Since lesions bleed intermittently, more than one stool specimen must be tested. Testing of 3 consecutive stools is recommended. If the test is intended to detect blood from colorectal cancer, the individual should not begin the procedure if actively bleeding from a known

---

Table XIV Risk Factors for Colorectal Cancer

- Age 40 or over
- Ulcerative colitis (lasting more than 7 years)
- Prior adenoma of colon
- Family history of polyposis syndrome
- Female genital cancer
- Prior cured colorectal cancer

Adapted from: Gossell TA. Fecal occult blood testing products. US Pharmacist 1986;11(4):40–51.

Table XV Occult Fecal Blood Test Interference

False Positive	False Negative
• Foods with peroxidase activity: turnips, horseradish, parsnips, cauliflower broccoli, canteloupe, artichokes, mushrooms (for tests using guaiac reaction) • Red meat or rare meat • Drugs: iron, salicylates, NSAIDs, steroids, reserpine and colchicine • Pathological: bleeding gums, nosebleed, peptic ulcers, dysentry, ulcerative colitis, hemorrhoids, fissures, diverticulitis or proctitis • Menstruation • Toilet bowl cleaners (for tests developed in toilet bowl)	• Failure to ingest high residue diet • Ascorbic Acid (>250 mg daily) • Lesions not bleeding at time of test • Noncompliance with test procedure • Test kit outdated or deteriorated

Adapted from: Home Health Care. Winnipeg: Canadian Council on Continuing Education in Pharmacy, 1988;VIII(4).

source (for example, nosebleed, hemorrhoids, rectal fissures, diarrhea, menstruation, diverticulitis, gastrointestinal ulcers or proctitis).

A person who obtains a positive result for a fecal occult blood test is advised to consult a physician for proper diagnosis. (See Table XVI for available fecal occult blood tests.)

Table XVI *Fecal Occult Blood Tests on Market*

Test	Manufacturer	Comments
Colo Screen Self-Test (CS-T)	Helena Laboratories	Pad contains 4 test areas plus positive and negative controls. 3 pads are included. Patient flushes toilet twice, stools in the toilet, drops a pad in the bowl and looks for a color change (red-orange).
EZ Detect	NMS Pharmaceuticals Ltd	Test pad is dropped in toilet after stool. Appearance of a blue cross indicates positive tests.

Adapted from: Home Health Care. Winnipeg: Canadian Council on Continuing Education in Pharmacy, 1988;VIII(4).

Until the cause for colorectal cancer is discovered, early detection and treatment probably offers the best hope for improving the outcome of this disease. Health and Welfare Canada's Task Force on the Periodic Health Examination has recommended periodic testing of all Canadians over the age of 45 years. This recommendation is under review. Currently, insufficient data exists to indicate that screening for colorectal cancer by fecal occult blood testing reduces mortality from the disease. Controlled clinical trials are now underway, but more time is needed for assessment of survival benefit, risk possibilities and economic feasibility. These trials involve initial screening by fecal occult blood testing and the study of positive occult blood reactions by barium enema, endoscopy or both.

The success of a screening program depends largely on the acceptability of the test to the patients. The collection and handling of a stool sample may inhibit compliance. Newer tests (for example, Coloscreen Self-Test) do not require collection of a stool sample. A test pad is simply dropped into the toilet after a stool has been passed and if there is occult blood present there will be a change in color on an indicator patch. In 1990, Pye, et al, compared the Coloscreen Self-Test with a conventional slide test (Haemoccult). Compliance was higher with the test which did not require collection of a stool sample but it was much less sensitive in detecting colonic and rectal cancers. As a result Pye, et al, did not recommend Coloscreen Self-Test as a suitable test for screening asymptomatic patients. Uchida, et al, have developed a new monoclonal antibody test for fecal occult blood utilizing enzyme-linked immunosorbent (ELISA) of human hemoglobin with much greater specificity for human hemoglobin than previous tests. If and when these tests become available to the home care market, they should improve the rate of detection of colon cancer and eliminate the necessity for dietary and therapeutic restrictions.

Peak Expiratory Flow Rate Measurement Devices

In chronic asthma, resistance to airflow is markedly increased and

this is reflected in expiratory flow rates. Ventilatory function can be determined by measuring how well the individual can blow air out of the lungs. A correlation exists between expiratory flow rates and the forced expiratory volume in 1 second (FEV_1), and forced weight capacity (FVC), or the FEV_1/FVC ratio. Since researchers first defined a test in 1959 to determine the peak expiratory flow rate (PEFR), the test has been widely applied to assess new medications and regimens in the management of asthma. (See Table XVII for indications for use of peak expiratory flow rate meters.)

Table XVII *Indications for the Use of a Home Peak Expiratory Flow Rate Measurement Device*

- diagnosis of precipitants for asthma (cold weather, animal or occupational exposure, exercise)
- assessment of prescribed treatment for asthma
- monitoring the success of aerosolized bronchodilators in the treatment of acute symptoms of asthma
- assessment of acute attacks that require emergency treatment by a physician
- involvement of asthmatic patients in self-management

Adapted from: Home Health Care. Winnipeg: Canadian Council on Continuing Education in Pharmacy, 1988;VIII(4).

The measurement of PEFR requires only that the individual inspire fully and expel the breath forcefully into the peak flow meter. Most peak flow meters consist of a tube with a spring-loaded piston and a longitudinal slot through which air escapes. Air blown into the instrument cannot escape until it has moved and uncovered part of the slot. When the pressure is built up behind the piston to balance the force of the spring, an area of the slot is uncovered and allows escape of the air. The piston comes to rest in a position that depends on the flow rate.

The peak expiratory flow meter is used 10 to 20 minutes after the person inhales a bronchodilator drug to determine the efficacy of prescribed treatment. The meter allows the individual to recognize early changes in airflow resistance and a possible impending asthma attack. Monitoring peak expiratory flow rates, keeping a daily diary of activities and timing the onset of symptoms help determine the specific precipitants of asthma exacerbation and whether the treatment program is beneficial.

Ideally the peak flow rate should be close to a predicted or target value provided on a chart or nomogram with the meter. However, the peak flow rate of normal individuals varies widely. Therefore an ideal or target value for each individual on a particular meter needs to be established. Once the brand of peak flow meter is chosen, it should be used exclusively. Switching between types can result in inconsistent readings. Patients must first identify the normal peak expiratory flow rate readings on awakening and at bedtime, either before using an inhaled bronchodilator, or before and after. Fluctuations from these values should be minimal. Values oscillating within 10 to 50 per cent of the target value signal the need for enhanced therapy. When there is no response to therapy and if the peak flow rate drops below 50 per cent, the patient requires emergency treatment by a physician. (See Table XVIII for a peak expiratory flow rate management plan for treatment of asthma.)

For measurements to be accurate, individuals purchasing these devices must receive proper operating instructions. The elderly or

Table XVIII *Peak Expiratory Flow Rate (PEFR) Management Plan for Treatment of Asthma*

PEFR ,90% of target value	— current management is effective
PEFR = 50 to 89% of target value	— enhanced therapy required
PEFR <50% of target value	— emergency situation contact physician
PEFR <30% of target value (<150–200 L/min)	— go directly to hospital

Adapted from: Schoepp G. Winds of change. Drug Merch 1991;72(11):9–13.

the very young may find it difficult to coordinate a breath with the peak flow meter to register reproducible results.

It is recommended that the devices be cleaned by immersing in soapy water every 2 weeks as it has been reported they can become colonized with fungal growth. (See Table XIX for direction on use of peak flow rate meters. See Table XX for peak expiratory flow rate meters available in Canada.)

Table XIX *Directions for Use of Peak Flow Meter*

1. Attach mouthpiece to peak flow meter.
2. Make sure indicator is at bottom of scale.
3. Do not block the opening with your fingers.
4. Stand up (unless handicapped, in which case, the position should be the same for all maneuvers).
5. Inhale as deeply as possible, then place your mouth firmly around mouthpiece, with lips forming a tight seal (do not block the mouthpiece with the tongue).
6. Blow out as hard and as fast as possible.
7. The indicator will move up the scale. Make note of the final position (peak flow).
8. Slide indicator to bottom of scale and repeat test.
9. Do 3 tests. Record the highest reading.
10. Compare results with predicted average values provided with the peak flow meter.

Adapted from: Chrisman CR, Self TH, Rumback MJ. Use of peak flow meters in asthmatics. Amer Pharm 1991;NS31(5):24–8.

Blood Pressure Measuring Devices

What is hypertension? Criteria for diagnosing hypertension are arbitrary, because arterial pressure rises with age and varies from one occasion of measurement to another. Most authorities consider hypertension to be present when the diastolic blood pressure (DBP) consistently exceeds 90 mm Hg in a person less than 50 years of age and 100 mm Hg in a person more than 60 years of age. (DBP is the minimum pressure during relaxation (diastole) of the ventricles.) The systolic blood pressure (SBP) represents the maximal blood pressure when the ventricles are contracting and its level is considered of less importance in measurement of blood pressure. Systolic hypertension is the term used for blood pressure measurements consistantly greater than 160 mm Hg. In 1984, the Joint National Committee on Detection, Evaluation and Treatment of Blood Pressure (United States National Institute of Health) established the definition of high blood pressure as greater than or equal to 140/90 mm Hg, the numerator refers to the systolic blood pressure and the denominator to the diastolic blood pressure.

Table XX *Peak Expiratory Flow Rate Meters Available in Canada*

Meter	Manufacturer	Range (L/min) Minimum	Maximum
Biotrine Asthma	Biotrine Corporation, Woburn, Mass.	20	480
Assess LR (low range pediatric)	Health Scan Products Inc.	50	375
Assess (adult)	Health Scan Products, Inc.	100	750
Mini-Wright (pediatric)	Clement Clarke International Ltd.	50	350
Mini-Wright (adult)	Clement Clarke International Ltd.	60	800
Pulmo-Graph (low-range pediatric)	Devilbiss Health Care Inc.	0	260
Pulmo-Graph (standard-adult)	Devilbiss Health Care Inc.	50	750

The Canadian Hypertension Society (1990) recommends different levels of blood pressure treatment based on the age of the patient and whether or not the patient has target organ damage. Treatment consists of nonpharmacologic methods, pharmacologic methods or combinations of both. They suggest treating everyone with a DBP consistently at or above 100 mm Hg, and that treatment is also indicated for all hypertensives with a DBP of 90 to 99 mm Hg who have target organ damage (for example, damaged heart or renal problems). One study showed that people with mild hypertension (a DBP of 90 to 104 mm Hg) have double the risk of cardiovascular morbidity than people with normal pressure. Also, if people with a DBP of 90 to 95 mm Hg are left untreated, a significant proportion of this group escalate to higher blood pressure levels within the next decade. People with a DBP between 85 and 89 mm Hg are pre-hypertensives and are advised to adopt lifestyle changes to attempt to lower their blood pressure below 85 mm Hg. If the DBP is 90 to 99 mm Hg, or if SBP is 160 mm Hg or greater, and there is no target organ damage the physician is advised to use clinical judgement in treating patients taking into consideration other risk factors, for example, if there is isolated hypertension or if the patient is less than 18 years old. For patients aged 65 to 74 years of age, therapy is similar to that for people under age 65. The society advises in patients 75 years and older with no target organ damage to treat if DBP is 120 mm Hg or greater or SBP is greater than 180 mm Hg. However, for patients 75 years of age or older with target organ damage, treat if DBP is 100 mm Hg or greater or SBP is 180 mm Hg or greater. This takes into consideration that elderly patients have falsely elevated blood pressure because of calcified arteries. (Table XXI shows risk factors for hypertension and Table XXII shows guidelines on blood pressure treatment.)

Blood pressure readings taken at home or work can provide more valid evaluation of blood pressure status. Quite often patients are apprehensive when they visit the doctor and thus their readings may be falsely elevated (white coat response). Improvement in compliance with drug therapy and hence blood pressure control is

Table XXI *Population Risk Factors for Hypertension*

Factor	Incidence
age	increases porportionally with age
family history	twice as high
race	higher among black
salt intake	higher
obesity	higher
stress	higher
use of oral contraceptives	iatrogenic hypertension
others: cigarette smoking, alcohol consumption, caffeine	contributes to development or aggravation of hypertension

Information from: de Champlain J. The clinical evaluation of hypertension. Can Fam Physician 1985;31:307–12.

Table XXII *Levels of Blood Pressure for Treatment*

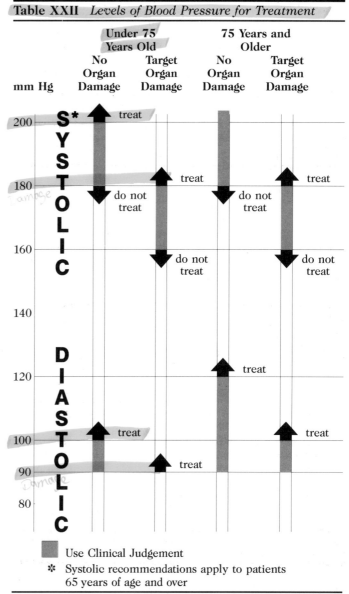

Use Clinical Judgement

* Systolic recommendations apply to patients 65 years of age and over

Reprinted with permission from: The Canadian consensus on hypertension management. Montreal: The Canadian Hypertension Society, 1990.

associated with individuals taking and monitoring their own blood pressure. Use of blood pressure measuring devices is not meant to replace regular visits to the doctor; medication dosages should not be changed except on the advice of a doctor.

Three types of blood pressure measurement devices are a mercury sphygmomanometer, an aneroid sphygmomanometer and an electronic digital readout device. (See Table XXIII for comparison of blood pressure monitoring devices.)

The mercury sphygmomanometer is the most reliable, since the weight of the mercury in this closed system depends upon constant gravitational force. It consists of a hollow glass tube with a mercury reservoir linked to a compression cuff by a piece of rubber tubing. When the cuff is inflated, pressure in the cuff is translated to force on the mercury in the reservoir, causing the mercury to rise in the glass tube. If the mercury column is not exactly at zero when the cuff is deflated, the instrument needs to be recalibrated by the manufacturer. A stethoscope is needed for this method.

The aneroid sphygmomanometer consists of bellows that expand or collapse in response to pressure exerted by the compression cuff. The movement of the bellows rotates a gear, which in turn moves a needle across a calibrated dial. Calibration once a year against a standard mercury manometer is required. The stethoscope is built into the cuff. Most products have an automatic pressure valve to release pressure in the cuff. This type of manometer is easily portable.

The electronic digital display blood pressure monitors are more sophisticated and eliminate the use of a stethoscope. (A microphone is built into the cuff.) The digital monitors offer the advantage of a visual result without the need to listen for the systole and diastole sounds. They feature systolic/diastolic and pulse readings, and a choice of preset inflation pressures with an automatic pressure relief valve for controlled deflation. These devices can be inaccurate, especially if the individual is not familiar with their use. These machines should be calibrated once a year. Some fully automated blood pressure measuring devices are cuffless. The user places a finger through a sleeve, the machine is switched on and readings are shown on a bar graph display. These devices are convenient and easy to use.

When taking blood pressure with manometers requiring a cuff, the user must be relaxed. The arm must be flexed, supported by a firm surface to avoid isometric contraction of the biceps muscle which

will elevate blood pressure readings, and free of restrictive clothing. Taking the reading immediately after eating, smoking or exercising is not advised.

The cuff must have appropriate bladder width (approximately 40 per cent of arm circumference). Some manufacturers make a child-sized cuff. (See Table XXIV for correct cuff size.) Because compression of the aorta on the left side may cause an inaccurate reading, the cuff is applied to the right arm, snugly but not tightly. The lower edge of the cuff should be about 3 cm above the crease of the elbow and the bladder centered over the brachial artery. Some monitors provide a "D-ring" for easy self-application of the cuff. The cuff is inflated to about 30 mm Hg above the pressure at which pulsation disappears. The stethoscope is placed over the brachial artery, and the release valve is used to reduce pressure at a rate of about 2 mm Hg per heartbeat.

Table XXIII *Home Blood Pressure Monitoring Devices*

Device	Advantages	Disadvantages
mercury/gravity sphygmomanometer	• very accurate "gold standard" • rare calibration needed	• bulky • stethoscope required • breakable glass parts
aneroid	• easily portable • relatively inexpensive • built-in stethoscope	• calibration once a year • factory repair
electronic/ automated	• ease of handling • no fine listening judgement required • built-in stethoscope • automatic pressure relief valve • rare calibration needed	• more expensive • less accurate
cuffless/finger monitor	• simple to use • no cuff • very compact, portable	• less accurate

Adapted from: Home Health Care. Winnipeg: Canadian Council on Continuing Education in Pharmacy, 1988;VIII(4).

Table XXIV *Correct Cuff Sizes for Accurate Blood Pressure Measurement*

(Measure arm circumference at the mid point between shoulder and elbow)

Arm Size	Cuff Size	
<33 cm	12 × 33 cm	Regular Cuff
33–41 cm	15 × 33 cm	Large Cuff
>41 cm	18 × 36 cm	Thigh Cuff

Note: Some manufacturers make a child's cuff

Adapted from: Evans CE, Logan AG. The Canadian consensus on hypertension management. Montreal: The Canadian Hypertension Society, 1990:2.

The systolic level (SBP) is equal to 2 mm Hg above the first appearance of a clear tapping sound (phase I Korotkoff). The diastolic level (DBP) is equal to 2 mm Hg above the point at which the sound disappears (phase V Korotkoff). If the sound persists to near 0 mm Hg, the point of muffling of sound (phase IV Korotkoff) indicates diastolic pressure. (See Table XXV for sounds and Korotkoff phases.) With electronic digital display monitors, the diastolic and systolic readings are displayed on the read-out.

The cuff must not be left partially inflated for too long; it may cause venous congestion. At least 1 minute should elapse between readings. The blood pressure in both arms should be taken and the arm with higher pressure used as the reading. The crossing of legs or talking while taking the reading can elevate blood pressure.

Reports on the accuracy of home blood pressure monitors are contradictory. Because of the large number of devices on the market and

Table XXV *Korotkoff Phases*

Phase I	appearance of sound — systolic blood pressure is 2 mm Hg above this
Phase II	sound disappearance
Phase III	sound reappearance
Phase IV	sound muffling
Phase V	sound disappearance — diastolic blood pressure is 2 mm Hg above this

Adapted from: Evans CE, Logan AG. The Canadian consensus on hypertension management. Montreal: The Canadian Hypertension Society, 1990:2.

the confusion of names and model numbers, selection of accurate devices by the consumer or the professional is extremely difficult. There are proposed American Association for the Advancement of Medical Instrumentation (AAMI) standards in the US based on accuracy, reliability and ease of use, but finding data pertaining to a specific device from published studies is very difficult. One study done by Evans, et al, at McMaster University, Hamilton, Ontario compared the accuracy of 23 blood pressure-measuring devices available on the Canadian market. Final selection was based on the accuracy of diastolic pressure readings as this is more critical than systolic readings. Under test conditions, 12 of the 23 devices met all diastolic performance criteria. However, 2 of these failed systolic criteria, 1 of which and 2 others had suboptimal features for home use, for example, either no written instructions on use, no stethoscope provided or no D-ring. They recommended 8 monitors suitable for home use (one is no longer on the market):

Almedic UA241, Almedic UA251 by Almedic
Astropulse 90AC by Marshall Electronics
Lumiscope 100-048 by Lumiscope Co. Inc.
RadioShack 63–661 by Tandy Electronics
Sunbeam 7620 (no D-ring- but rigid cuff) by Hanson Scale Co.
Tycos 7052–11 by Taylor Instrument.

Besides inaccuracy of the device, error can occur in the technique of measurement. Even though instructions may be included with the device, all patients should be given some instruction by professional staff. Patients are best advised to confer with their physician before purchasing a blood pressure monitor. Manufacturers should provide sufficient validation of accuracy.

Elevated blood pressure from any at-home measuring device must be verified by a physician.

Future Tests

As biotechnology knowledge advances, it is expected that non-prescription home diagnostic products, which are more accurate and reliable, easier to use, and less costly, will become available. Some of the areas presently being researched for test kits include: detection of fertility from saliva; sexually transmitted diseases (herpes, chlamydia, gonorrhea, trichomonas and candida); AIDS; strep throat; cancer; monitoring of blood levels of drugs (digoxin, phenytoin, theophylline and carbamazepine); blood levels of cholesterol, alcohol, and certain vitamins/minerals; urine levels for drugs of abuse, calcium or sodium; tests for presence of sulfites in food and beverages; tests for causes of impotence and vision problems. Infra-red light is being investigated to determine blood glucose levels by measuring the amount of light absorbed by the body. This would be a painless alternative for diabetics who regularly prick their finger to obtain a drop of blood to check blood sugar levels.

Summary

Diagnostic aids provide useful monitoring and self-screening tests consumers can perform at home. Consumers' involvement in their own health often enhances compliance with prescribed therapeutic regimens. Many of the tests help consumers identify a medical condition early, providing specific information to be used under the guidance of a physician.

Pharmacists can assist in the proper selection and use of diagnostic test products and the interpretation of results. They can inform consumers of test limitations and recommend any questionable results be referred to a physician. Nonprescription diagnostic aids are not to be used to self-diagnose an illness. The ultimate diagnosis must be made by a physician.

Ask the Consumer

Q. How long has the person appeared feverish? Are there any other signs or symptoms, such as a sore throat? How old is the person?

■ Fever is an important manifestation of illness. For example, it may denote a bacterial or viral infection. It is the most common clinical symptom encountered in children. Markedly elevated or prolonged fevers may result in profound metabolic disturbances as the body tries to maintain a normal body temperature of 37 °C. Discomfort and malaise generally appear about 39.5 to 40 °C. Fever below 41 °C rarely poses a threat; treatment is based primarily on making the individual more comfortable or preventing the occurrence of febrile convulsions in susceptible children. Treatment may involve tepid sponging and use of antipyretic drugs such as acetylsalicylic acid, acetaminophen or ibuprofen. (See the chapter on internal analgesics.) Refer any person with a high fever, especially a child or infant, to a physician before treatment is instituted.

Q. How old is the person for whom the thermometer is being purchased?

■ For children less than 6 years of age, taking temperature orally is not recommended; 5 to 10 minutes are needed to obtain an accurate reading with a mercury fever thermometer, and many children cannot or will not co-operate for this length of time. The rectal route is recommended for children under 2 and the axillary method for children aged 2 to 6 years. The newer digital thermometers, which take only 1 minute to obtain an accurate temperature reading, are safe for any age group and temperatures can be taken orally, rectally or axillary. Rectal temperatures are usually 0.5 °C higher than oral temperatures and axillary temperatures are usually 0.5 °C lower than oral temperatures.

Q. Do you intend to use basal temperature readings as a means of contraception or to increase the probability of conception?

■ Using basal body temperatures (rhythm method) for contraception poses difficulties and risks. Pregnancy can be avoided by abstaining from sexual intercourse for a few days before and after ovulation. However, the exact time of ovulation is difficult to predict; the difficulty is greater if the woman does not have a regular menstrual cycle.

If the rhythm method is used to increase the probability of conception, fertilization may be enhanced if sexual abstinence occurs for a few days before ovulation so the sperm count in the male partner can be increased.

Q. Are your menstrual periods regular? When was your last period? Are you currently taking any medications?

■ Many women have menstrual cycles as short as 18 days or as long as 40 days. Most women (65 per cent) have cycles that average between 25 and 31 days. Once the cycle is established, the variation does not normally exceed 5 days. Irregularity increases the uncertainty of confirming pregnancy. The longer one waits to do a pregnancy test after a missed period, the more likely the urinary human chorionic gonadotropin level is detectable.

Any woman taking medication should consult her physician. Teratogenicity sensitivity is greatest during early organogenesis— from the third week through the third month (first trimester) of pregnancy.

Q. Is the person using the glucose testing products to monitor diabetes? Is the person taking insulin at present? Is the person testing urine or blood for glucose?

■ To control diabetes adequately, glucose levels should be tested, ideally, 4 times daily (before meals and at bedtime). Glucose can be monitored by urinalysis or blood testing. Urine tests depend on a normal renal threshold for glucose. To reflect more accurately the blood glucose concentration at the time of testing, the person is instructed to test a double-voided specimen. This sample reflects blood glucose during the period between voids (30 minutes). Blood glucose testing reveals the body's immediate state and gives warning of impending hypoglycemia. (See the chapter on diabetes care.)

Q. Is the person able to detect different colors?

■ Many diagnostic tests use a color chart to determine results. The person should be able to differentiate colors and shades of one color.

Q. Have you been diagnosed as having high blood pressure? Are you on any medication for this condition? Do you have any auditory problems?

■ Mild hypertension is indicated by a blood pressure reading of over 90 mm Hg diastolic and 140 mm Hg systolic. It should be treated by a physician. Without treatment, mild hypertension greatly increases the risk of cardiovascular disease (cardiac failure, coronary heart disease, stroke and renal failure). Treatment may consist of nondrug therapy, drug therapy or a combination of both. There are 3 types of home blood pressure monitors: mercury sphygmomanometers, aneroid sphygmomanometers and electronic digital monitors. A stethoscope is used with both the mercury and aneroid manometers, so the user must be able to distinguish the heart sounds.

Q. Does the person urinate frequently or have pain or a burning sensation on urination? Is the person catheterized?

■ Urinary tract infection (UTI) denotes the presence of a large number of microorganisms in either the lower urinary tract (bladder, cystitis; urethra, urethritis; prostate gland, prostatitis) or upper urinary tract (renal parenchyma, pyelonephritis) or both. The symptoms most commonly associated with cystitis and acute urethral syndrome are a painful or burning sensation during urination (dysuria), urinary urgency and increased frequency of urination. In addition to these symptoms, people with acute pyelonephritis and acute prostatitis often experience lower back pain, general malaise, nausea, vomiting and fever. In all these circumstances, a significant bacteriuria is present. It can be estimated by chemical tests that rely on the enzymatic activity of viable bacteria, for example, the reduction of nitrate.

Catheterized individuals are more prone to UTI, possibly because bacteria are introduced into the urinary tract when the catheter is inserted.

Q. How old is the person seeking a fecal occult blood testing kit? What symptoms does he or she have?

■ People with high risk of colorectal cancer are age 40 or over. Colorectal cancer may be in an advanced stage of development and still be relatively asymptomatic. A positive fecal occult blood test may detect colorectal cancer even before symptoms occur.

References

Introduction
Gossell TA, Stansloski DW. OTC urine diagnostic products. US Pharmacist 1979;4(5):39–54,72.
Parker WA. Diagnostic aids. In: Cyr JC, ed. Canadian self-medication. Ottawa: Canadian Pharmaceutical Association, 1984:379–96.

Fever as a Diagnostic Aid
Bartle WR. Fever—a diagnostic tool? Can Pharm J 1985;118(2):54–6.
Dinarello CA, Wolff SM. Pathogenesis of fever in man. N Engl J Med 1978; 298:607–12.
Done AK. Treatment of fever in 1982: a review. Am J Med 1983;74 (Suppl 6A):27–35.
Kaufman RE. Fever. In: Shirkey HC, ed. Pediatric therapy. St. Louis: CV Mosby, 1980:287–91.
Kluger MJ. Fever. Pediatrics 1980;66:720–4.
Littlefield LC. General care: fever. In: Katcher BS, Young LY, Koda-Kimble MA, eds. Applied therapeutics, the clinical use of drugs. San Francisco: Applied Therapeutics, 1983:73–83.
McFadden SW, et al. Coma produced by topical application of isopropanol. Pediatrics 1969;43:622.
Orlowski JP. Aspirin and Reye's syndrome: how strong an association? Postgrad Med 1984;75(6):47–54.
Rush JL, Foltz EL. Malignant hyperthermia. J Neurosurg 1977;46:385–90.
Stanaszek WF. Fever of undetermined origin. US Pharmacist 1984;8:10–4.
Stern RC. Pathophysiologic basis for symptomatic treatment of fever. Pediatrics 1977;59:92–8.

Measurement of Body Temperature
Anonymous. Toshiba digital clinical thermometer (Package insert). Montreal: AMG Medical.
Anonymous. Becton, Dickinson basal temperature thermometer (Package insert). Mississauga: Becton, Dickinson.
Benzinger TH. Clinical temperature: new physiological basis. JAMA 1969; 209:1200–6.
Edwards M, Burton AC. Temperature distribution over the human head, especially in the cold. J Appl Physiol 1960;15:209–11.
Froese G, Burton AG. Heat losses from the human head. J Appl Physiol 1957; 10:235–42.
Ryan CF, Vrabel RB. Pediatric antipyretic therapy. US Pharmacist 1978; 3:49–64.

Urine Tests
Fischbach FT, ed. A manual of laboratory diagnostic tests. Philadelphia: JB Lippincott, 1980:103–98.

Pregnancy Tests
Anonymous. Advance (Package insert). Don Mills: Ortho McNeil Inc.
Anonymous. Answer Now (Package insert). Mississauga: Carter Products.
Anonymous. Clearblue Easy (Package insert). Pickering: Fisons Corp Ltd.
Anonymous. Confidelle (Package insert). Mississauga: Carter Products.
Anonymous. Fact Plus (Package insert). Don Mills: Ortho McNeil Inc.
Anonymous. First Response (Package insert). Mississauge: Carter Products.
Anonymous. Pharmacist Letter 1991; March.
Anonymous. The e.p.t. do-it-yourself early pregnancy test. Med Lett Drugs Ther 1978;20:39–40.
Arey LB. Degree of normal menstrual irregularity; analysis of 20,000 calendar records from 1500 individuals. Am J Obstet Gynecol 1939;37:12–29.
Aschheim S, Zondek B. Pregnancy diagnosis with urine by the demonstration of the hormone. Klin Wschr 1928;7:8.
Bucher D, Poulsen F, Rousoe U. More on pregnancy tests (Letter). Clin Chem 1991;37(3):477–8.
Caiola SM. The pharmacist and home-use pregnancy tests. Am Pharmacy 1992;N532(1):57–60.
Emancipator K, Cadoff EM, Burke MD. Analytical versus clinical sensitivity and specificity in pregnancy testing. Am J Obstet Gynecol 1988;158:613–6.
Fields SA, Toffler WL. Pregnancy testing-home and office. The West J Med 1991;154(3):327–8.
Friedman MH, Lapham ME. A simple, rapid procedure for the laboratory diagnosis of early pregnancies. Am J Obstet Gynecol 1931;21:405–10.
Gringauz A. Monoclonal antibodies. US Pharmacist 1985;10(10):38–48.
Gunn DL, Jenkin PM, Gunn AL. Menstrual periodicity: statistical observations on a large sample of normal cases. J Obstet Gynaecol Br Emp 1937;44:839–79.
Hertig AT, Rock J, Adams EC. A description of 34 human ova within the first 17 days of development. Am J Anat 1956;98:435.
Hicks J, Josefsohn M. Reliability of home pregnancy-test kits in the hands of lay persons (Letter). N Engl J Med 1989;320:320.
Horwitz CA. Pregnancy tests 1980: advantages and limitations. Lab Med 1980;11:620.
Horwitz CA, Lee CY. Pregnancy testing. Postgrad Med 1978;63(5):193–6.
Kosasa TS. Measurement of human chorionic gonadotropin. J Reproduct Med 1981;26:201.
Krieg AF. Examination of urine. In: Henry JB, ed. Clinical diagnosis and management by laboratory methods. Philadelphia: WB Saunders, 1979: 559–634.
Lewis C. Human chorionic gonadotropin and its detection by immunochemical methods. Can J Med Technol 1977;39:58–64.
Lind T, Whittaker PG. How positive is a positive pregnancy test? Brit Med J 1988;296:730–1.
Norman RJ, Buck RH, DeMedeiros SF. Measurement of human chorionic gonadotropin (hCG): indications and techniques for the clinical laboratory. Ann Clin Biochem 1990;27:183–94.
Norman RJ. When a positive pregnancy test isn't. Med J Aust 1991;154:718–9.
Porres JM, D'Ambra C, Lord D, Garrity F. Comparison of eight kits for the diagnosis of pregnancy. Am J Clin Pathol 1975;64:452–63.
Ross GT. Clinical relevance of results on the structure of human chorionic gonadotropin. Am J Obstet Gynecol 1977;129:795.
Sheehan C. Current status of pregnancy testing. Am J Med Technol 1983; 49(7):485–8.
Wada HG, Danisch RJ, et al. Enzyme immunoassay of the glycoprotein tropic hormones—choriogonadotropin, lutropin, thyrotropin—with solid phase monoclonal antibody for the alpha-subunit and enzyme-coupled monoclonal antibody specific for the beta-subunit. Clin Chem 1982;28: 1862–6.
Wide L, Gemzell CA. An immunological pregnancy test. Acta Endocrinol 1960;35:261–7.

Urine Testing for Predicting Ovulation
Ferbey B. Home health care. Winnipeg: Canadian Conference on Continuing Education in Pharmacy, 1986:VIII(4).

Diagnostic Aids

Goodman HM. Reproduction. In: Mountcastle VB, ed. Medical physiology. St. Louis: CV Mosby, 1974:1741–75.

Howanitz JH, Howanitz PJ. Immunoassay and related techniques; tumor markers. In: Henry JB, ed. Clinical diagnosis and management by laboratory methods. Philadelphia: WB Saunders, 1984:333–4.

Lum L. Ovulation predictor tests. Pharm Pract 1990;6(8):31–4.

Miyahara RK, Nykamp D. On the shelf and in the future. US Pharmacist 1990;15(3):50–62.

New Drugs volume 5, number 6, Nov/Dec. 1987. (Drug Information Centre Newsletter, Faculty of Pharmacy, University of Toronto.)

Vowles A. Do it yourself. Drug Merch 1990;71(9):21–3.

Urine Glucose Tests

Anonymous. Urinalysis using reagent strip techniques (Pamphlet). Rexdale: Ames.

Malone JI, Rosenbloom AL, Grgic A, Weber T. The role of urine sugar in diabetic management. Am J Dis Child 1976;130:1324–7.

Yarborough MC, Campbell RK. Module 2: developing a diabetes program for your pharmacy. Am Pharm 1986;26(2):insert.

Urine Tests for Ketones

Karam JH. Diabetes mellitus, hypoglycemia and lipoprotein disorders. In: Krupp MA, Chatton MJ, eds. Current medical diagnosis and treatment. Los Altos: Lange, 1982:741–69.

Nelson CJ. A guide to glucose testing urine systems for the pharmacist teaching the diabetic patient. Drug Intell Clin Pharm 1974;8:422–9.

Rosenbloom AL, Malone JI. Recognition of impending ketoacidosis delayed by ketone reagent strip failure. JAMA 1978;240:2462–4.

Protein in Urine

Free AH, Rupe CO, Metzler L. Studies with a new colorimetric test for proteinuria. Clin Chem 1975;3:716.

Abuelo GJ. Proteinuria: diagnostic principles and procedures. Ann Intern Med 1983;98:186–91.

Blood in Urine

Anonymous. Urinalysis with Chemstrip pamphlet. St. Laurent: Boehringer-Mannheim Canada, 1978.

Baran RB, Rowles B. Factors affecting coloration of urine and feces. J Am Pharm Assoc 1973;13:139–42,155.

Bacteria in Urine

Fendler KJ, Elenbaas JK. Urinary tract infections. In: Katcher BS, Young LY, Koda-Kimble MA, eds. Applied therapeutics, the clinical use of drugs. San Francisco: Applied Therapeutics, 1983:749–84.

Kunin CM. New methods for detecting urinary tract infections. Urol Clin North Am 1975;10(2):423.

Rahwan RG. Mechanisms of teratogenesis 1. US Pharmacist 1983;8(2):52,54–7.

Saltmarche A. Bacteriuria, urinary tract infections and the impact of catheters in the elderly. Can Pharm J 1984;6:209–10.

Strommen GL, Barr CE, Tight RR. Urinary tract infections. US Pharmacist 1983;8(10):59–71.

Leukocytes in Urine

Anonymous. Chemstrip 9 (Package insert). Dorval: Boehringer-Mannheim.

Bile Pigments in Urine

Byrne J. Liver function studies part 1: introduction and bilirubin. Nursing 1977;7(7):12–4.

Blood Glucose Tests

Gossel TA. Blood glucose self-testing products. US Pharmacist 1986;11(3):91–6.

Guthrie RA, Karam JH. Self-monitoring of blood glucose. Patient care. 1991;25(5):91–106.

Hernandez C. The answer is at your fingertips: are you trained to respond? Diabetes Dialogue 1985;32(2):33–42.

Home Health Care. Canadian Council on Continuing Education in Pharmacy. Winnipeg 1988; Vol VIII (No. 4).

Schoepp GH. Specialize in diabetes; self-care tips, products to win today's "new diabetic" customer. Drug Merch 1985;11:32–42.

Fecal Occult Blood Testing

Anonymous. Home diagnostic kits for early colorectal cancer detection. Current Trends in Drug Therapy. Rocky Mountain Poison and Drug Foundation 1985;VI(6).

Canadian Task Force on Periodic Health Examination. The periodic health examination. Can Med Assoc J 1979;121:1193–254.

Gilbertsen VA, McHugh RB, Schuman L, et al. The earlier detection of colorectal cancers. A preliminary report of the results of the occult blood study. Cancer 1980;45:2899–901.

Gossel TA. Fecal occult blood testing products. US Pharmacist 1986;11(4):40–51.

Greegor DH. Diagnosis of large-bowel cancer in the asymptomatic patient. JAMA 1967;201(12):123.

Hoogewerf PE, et al. Patient compliance with screening for fecal occult blood in family practice. Can Med Assoc J 1987;137:195–8.

Pye G, Jackson J, Thomas WM, Hardcastle JD. Comparison of Coloscreen Self-Test and Haemoccult fecal occult blood tests in the detection of colorectal cancer in symptomatic patients. Br J Surg 1990;77:630–1.

Simon JB. Occult blood screening for colorectal carcinoma: a critical review. Gastroenterology 1985;88:820–37.

Simon JB. Occult blood screening of Canadians: wise or unwise? Can Med Assoc J 1985;133:647–9.

Uchida K, Matsuse R, et al. Immunochemical detection of human blood in feces. Clin Chim Acta 1990;189:267–74.

Winawer SJ, et al. Current states of fecal occult blood testing in screening for colorectal cancer. CA 1982;32:100

Peak Expiratory Flow Rate Measurement Devices

Beasley R, Cushley M, Holgate ST. A self management plan in the treatment of adult asthma. Thorax 1989;44:200–4

Charlton I, Charlton G, Broomfield J, Mullee MA. Evaluation of peak flow and symptoms, self management plans for control of asthma in general practice. Br Med J 1990;301:1355–9.

Cherniak RM. Chronic and acute asthma: keep to successful management. Postgrad Med 1984;75(2):87–98.

Chiaramonte LT, Prabhu SL. Comparative evaluation of five peak flow devices. J Aller Clin Immunol 1982;69:509–15.

Chrisman CR, Self TH, Rumback MJ. Use of Peak Flow Meters in Asthmatics. Amer Pharm 1991; NS31(5):24–8.

Cross D, Nelson HS. The role of the peak flow meter in the diagnosis and management of asthma. J Allergy Clin Immunol 1991;82(1)(Pt1):120–8.

Leiner GC, Abramowitz S, Small MJ, et al. Expiratory peak flow rate. Standard values for normal subjects. Use as a clinical test of ventilatory function. Am Rev Resp Dis 1963.

Schoepp G. Winds of change. Drug Merch 1991;72(11):9–13.

Wright BM. A miniature Wright peak-flow meter. Br Med J 1978;2:1627–8.

Wright BM, McKerrow CB. Maximum forced expiratory flow rate as a measure of ventilatory capacity. Br Med J 1959;2:1041–7.

Blood Pressure Measuring Devices

Association for the Advancement of Medical Instrumentions: American National Standard for Electronic or Automated Sphygmomanometers. Arlington, Virginia: AAMI, 1987.

de Champlain J. The clinical evaluation of hypertension. Can Fam Physician 1985;31:307–12.

Evans CE, Haynes RB, Goldsmith CH, Hewson SA. Home blood pressure—monitoring: a comparative study of accuracy. J Hypertension 1989;7:133–42.

Evans CE, Logan AG. The Canadian consensus on hypertension management. Montreal: The Canadian Hypertension Society, 1990:1–12.

Fedder DO. Managing the hypertensive patient. US Pharmacist 1986;11(6):54–61.

Fodor JG. Mild hypertension: should it be treated? Can Fam Physician 1985;31:303–4.

Iyriboz Y. Oscillometric finger blood pressure versus brachial auscultative blood pressure recording. J Fam Pract 1990;31(4):376–80.

Johnson AL, Taylor DW, Sackett DL, et al. Self-recording of blood pressure in the management of hypertension. Can Med Assoc J 1978;119:1034–9.

Kannell WB, Gordon T, Schwartz MJ. Systolic vs diastolic blood pressure and risk of coronary heart disease: the Framingham study. Am J Cardiol 1971;27:335–46.

Kirkendall WM, Feinleib M, Freis ED, et al. Recommendation for human blood pressure determination by sphygmomanometers. Circulation 1980;62:1446A-55A.

Larochelle P, Bass MJ, Birkett NJ, et al. Recommendations from the consensus conference on hypertension in the elderly. Can Med Assoc J 1986;135:741–5.

Logan AC. Report of the Canadian hypertension society's consensus conference on the management of mild hypertension. Can Med Assoc J 1984;131:1053–7.

Oed ML. Measuring blood pressure and blood cholesterol: the need for accuracy and precision. US Pharmacist 1990; Cardiovas Dis Suppl:52–6.

Schmidt GR, Hoettels Wenig J. An evaluation of home blood-pressure monitoring devices. Amer Pharm 1989;NS29(91):25–30.

White WB. The assessment of portable, non-invasive blood pressure recorders. J Hypertension 1990;8:591–3.

Future Tests

Anonymous. Etcetera. Can Pharm J 1991;124(8):376.

Bettess S. Home diagnostic agents and testing devices. Winnipeg: Canadian Council on Continuing Education in Pharmacy, 1989:XI(3).

Miyahara RK, Nykamp D. On the shelf and in the future. US Pharmacist 1990;5(3):50–62.

Needham CA. Rapid methods in microbiology for in-office testing. Clin Lab Med 1986;6(2):291–304.

Summary

DiTomasso RA, Colameco S. Patient self-monitoring of behavior. J Fam Pract 1982;15:79.

Gossel TA. Diagnostic products. US Pharmacist 1986;11(2):68–72.

28
Home Health Care

William A. Parker

The growing market of home health care products includes durable medical equipment (ambulatory aids, bathroom safety aids, respiratory therapy equipment), incontinence products (enuresis alarms, catheters and absorbent products), and health supports and appliances (compression products, orthopedic supports and braces). Pharmacists handling these products work closely with other health professionals. Training is available on types, accessories, fitting and use of ambulatory aids—canes, crutches, walkers and wheelchairs. Consumers requesting incontinence products or health supports require special counselling and privacy.

Home health care includes any product or service that allows individuals to remain in their homes instead of in institutions. It is a rapidly growing segment of our health care system, with expected annual growth rates of 20 per cent. Pharmacies have typically enjoyed about 15 per cent of their annual sales from the home health care market, a figure projected to increase. Home health care offers pharmacists a highly clinical, consumer-oriented, health-based practice opportunity coupled with high gross margins, companion sales opportunities and repeat business. It is a team effort involving pharmacists, physicians, allied health practitioners and the consumer, in which the consumer is most often referred to the home health care centre for product selection and training in the proper use and care of the device.

Table I shows the ranges for the consumer mix in American-based home health care centres. As well, some pharmacies do much of their total home health care volume in "industrial sales," such as provision of supplies and equipment to nursing homes and other facilities. Referrals account for about 80 per cent of consumer visits to pharmacies supplying home health care, with actual home health care mix consisting of 40 per cent products and 60 per cent service. Pharmacists can help consumers clarify their perceived needs by having a thorough product knowledge and detailing product advantages, not merely features.

Certain segments of home health care have always been an integral component of pharmacy practice—sick room supplies, first aid needs, dressings and so forth. The aging of our population, consumer preference for in-home versus institutional care, the emphasis on self-care and physical fitness, and government cost containment programs that take people out of hospitals earlier have resulted in a greater need and demand for new home health care products and services not traditionally addressed by pharmacies.

The home health care market is broad, consisting of many possible departments or components (see Table II). Which components are developed depends on many factors, such as pharmacy size and space, costs, expertise and training, consumer mix, support services

Table I *Pharmacy-Based Home Health Care Consumer Mix*

Elderly (chiefly with cancer, arthritis, stroke, ambulatory problems and other ailments)	30–40%
Injured (chiefly with wounds, fractures and burns)	20–30%
Postoperative (chiefly with surgical wounds and related problems)	15–25%
Ostomates	10–20%
Chronic disease (non-elderly, with disease such as diabetes, multiple sclerosis, muscular dystrophy, and cerebral palsy)	5–15%
Sports/Athletic participants	5–10%
Other	5–10%

Adapted from: Home health care marketing manual. Alexandria: National Association of Retail Druggists, 1985.

Table II *Representative Pharmacy Home Health Care Products*

Diagnostic equipment

Apnea monitors
Blood pressure kits
Diabetes products
    Blood glucose monitors & testing materials
    Insulin pumps
    Insulin syringes
    Lancets & holders
    Preci-jects
    Urine testing materials
Ovulation kits & thermometers
Pregnancy testing kits
Pulse meters
Stethoscopes
Stool testing kits
Thermometers

Table II (*Cont'd*) *Representative Pharmacy Home Health Care Products*

Durable medical equipment

Ambulatory aids
  Accessories (e.g., ice-picks, tips)
  Canes (monopod, quad)
  Crutches (axillary, forearm)
  Walkers
  Wheelchairs
  Wheelchair accessories (e.g., cushions, desk arms, leg rests, trays)
Bathroom safety products
  Bathtub lifts
  Bathtub safety rails
  Bathtub safety stools & transfer benches
  Elevated toilet seats
  Grab bars
  Sitz baths
  Toilet safety frames
Patient room
  Beds (hospital) & mattresses (covers, sheets)
  Bed backrests (foam slants)
  Bed boards
  Bed side-rails
  Bed (lap) trays
  Blanket supports
  Commodes
  Geriatric chairs & recliners
  Overbed tables
  Lifts
  Pillows (cervical, wedge)
  Trapeze bars

First aid & skin wound care

Alternating pressure pads
Antichoking devices (airways)
Bandages, gauze, sponges, tapes
Decubitus (bed) pads (e.g., sheepskin)
Detergents & disinfectants
Eye bandages & patches
First aid creams, dressings & kits
Heel & elbow protectors
Surgical dressings (e.g., Duoderm, Opsite)
Swabs, lubricants

Health supports & orthotic appliances

Abdominal supports
Antiembolism stockings
Arm slings
Athletic supports
Auto backrests (e.g., Obus formes)
Braces (ankle, back, elbow, knee, wrist)
Cast covers, shoes
Cervical collars
Compression hosiery, sleeves (Jobst, Sigvaris)
Joint warmers
Lumbosacral supports
Posture aids
Rib belts
Splints & splinting aids
Traction equipment (belts, halters, overbed, overdoor)
Trusses

Table II (*Cont'd*) *Representative Pharmacy Home Health Care Products*

Incontinence & urologic products

Bed pans
Bedwetting alarms
Bladder irrigation trays
Catheters & catheter care trays
Deodorizers
Diapers (disposable, reusable)
Drain & leg bags (disposable, reusable)
External male catheters
Irrigation solutions & syringes
Tubing & connectors
Underpads (disposable)
Underpants (disposable, reusable, liners)
Urinals
Waterproof sheeting

Nutritional therapy

Bags & feeding tubes
Gravity feeding sets
IV equipment & solutions
Liquid nutrition products (e.g., Ensure)
Pumps
Specialty nutrition products (e.g., gluten-free, Lact-Aid)

Ostomy & mastectomy products

Adhesives & adhesive remover
Colostomy pouches
Deodorants
Drains
Karaya powder & rings
Ileostomy pouches
Mastectomy prostheses, bras, clothing, swimsuits
Ostomy skin care, cleansers
Urostomy pouches

Patient aids

Bibs
Breast pumps & shields
Call-bells
Ear syringes
Eating & drinking aids
Finger cots, gloves
Grooming & dressing aids
Hearing aid batteries
Hot water bottles
Invalid rings
Masks
Medical alert (cards, bracelets, necklaces)
Nasal aspirators
Oral hygiene (e.g., swabs)
Patient gowns
Reachers & grippers
Reading & writing aids (e.g., glasses, magnifiers)
Restraints
Shampoo trays
Straws
Telephone aids
Washcloths (disposable)

Table II *(Cont'd) Representative Pharmacy Home Health Care Products*

Rehabilitation & physiotherapy products

- Bathtub whirlpools
- Cold & hot packs
- Elastic bandages
- Foot baths
- Hand exercisers
- Heating pads, lamps
- Ice bags
- Massagers
- Moist heat packs
- Paraffin baths
- Scales
- Stationary bikes
- Treadmills (joggers)
- Weights & weight bags

Respiratory therapy

- Air purifiers
- Aspirators
- Compressors (aerosol)
- Humidifiers
- Mask & tubings
- Nebulizers
- Oxygen concentrators, tanks
- Suction units
- Trach tubes & trach care kits
- Ultrasonic nebulizers
- Vaporizers
- Ventilators

TENS & electrotherapy

- Battery charges, packs
- Electrodes & electrode jelly
- Galvanic stimulators
- Neuromuscle stimulators
- Transepidermal nerve stimulator (TENS) units

Table III *Approximate Share of Total Pharmacy-Based Home Health Care Volume (American)*

Department	Percentage of volume
Supplies: surgical/wound/incontinence	36.5
Durable medical equipment	24.0
Ostomy care	8.0
Respiratory therapy	8.0
Diagnostics	6.0
Health supports and appliances	6.0
Nutritional therapy	5.0
Dialysis home units	4.0
Electromedicals	2.0
Patient aids	0.5
	100.0

Adapted from: Home health care marketing manual. Alexandria: National Association of Retail Druggists, 1985.

such as delivery, repair and on-call arrangements, and so forth. Table III shows an analysis of American pharmacy-based home health care centres and the approximate share of total home health care volume realized per department.

This chapter addresses the role of the pharmacist in providing the following home health care equipment and services: durable medical equipment (such as ambulatory aids and bathroom safety products), respiratory therapy equipment, incontinence and urological products, and health supports and appliances. Discussion of the following home health care components may be found elsewhere in this book: ostomy care; diabetes; diagnostic aids; nutritional therapy; and skin and wound care and dressings (topical first aid).

Durable Medical Equipment

Durable medical equipment (DME) has been defined for the purposes of reimbursement as equipment that can stand repeated use; is primarily and customarily used to serve a medical purpose; is generally not useful to someone in the absence of an illness or injury; and is appropriate for use in the home. Equipment meeting this definition includes ambulatory aids (for example, canes, crutches, walkers, wheelchairs and electric scooters), hospital beds, commodes, bathroom safety equipment (for example, tub rails, grab bars, bath benches and transfer seats) and respiratory therapy equipment.

DME is definitely not a self-service item. Demonstrations, fittings, explanations and training of pharmacy staff are essential, as are the follow-up services of delivery, setup, repairs and maintenance. DME puts great demands on the pharmacy's inventory, selling space and cash flow, especially if rentals accompany sales. Lastly, the pharmacy must be accessible to the handicapped, with wide doors and aisles, ramp access and reserved parking spaces.

Ambulatory Aids

Ambulatory or mobility aids are the most commonly prescribed and requested type of DME. American data reflect the following incidence figures: 2.7 million persons use a cane or walking stick, 88 per cent with chronic problems; 613,000 people are on crutches, 75 per cent with chronic conditions; 700,000 people use walkers, 92 per cent of whom are permanent users; and of 650,000 wheelchair users, 93 per cent are permanent users. If these figures are reduced by a factor of 10 to reflect Canadian demographics, a tremendous need for these products still exists, a need expected to increase with Canada's rapidly aging population. In order of least to most support provided, ambulatory aids include canes, crutches, walkers and wheelchairs.

Canes

Canes are recommended for one of four basic functions: balance; weight transfer; muscle weakness; or regaining confidence in the ability to walk. Individuals should generally carry walking canes on their strong side, that is, on the side opposite the weak limb. This technique provides a greater distance between the cane tip and the weak limb, thus increasing the base of support and balance and decreasing the possibility of falling. For weight transfer, canes are indicated for people who require no greater than 25 to 30 per cent stress-bearing support. Cane users must have good arm, wrist and grip strength on at least one side of the body.

Types: There are many types of canes, handles and accessories, with choice dependent on need, accompanying disorders and personal preference.

Monopod or standard canes, which provide the least support, are available in wood or aluminum. Wooden canes, although the least expensive, must be custom cut to size and should not be rented

Home Health Care

because of wear and tear. Aluminum canes, generally adjustable over the range of 85 to 105 cm, are light in weight, sturdy and hold up well with use. Adjustable aluminum canes are appropriate for either sale or rental. Both wooden and aluminum monopod canes come in a variety of styles and finishes.

Multipod (quad or four-footed) canes provide greater stability than monopod canes due to their widened bases. (Tripod or three-footed canes offer little or no more balance or stability than a monopod cane.) Quad canes also permit greater weight transfer than monopod canes. Quad canes are heavier and require more energy and dexterity on the part of the user. Cane bases range from narrow (about 17.5 by 20 cm; least support) to wide (about 22.5 by 30 cm; most support). Heights are adjustable from about 75 to 97.5 cm. Extra long handles and child sizes are also available. A narrow-based quad cane fits on the standard stair step in the normal cane position. The wide-based quad cane must be turned sideways for use on stairs, which puts the cane handle in an awkward position. To increase stability, the shaft of a multipod cane is not centered on the base plate, but is located closer to one of the sets of legs. Users must be instructed to carry the cane such that the tips closest to the shaft are also the tips closest to their body to increase stability and lessen the likelihood of catching their feet on the cane tip. Users must be cautioned about catching the laterally extended tips of these canes on furniture, walls and other obstructions. Multipod canes of good quality have a hand grip that is rotatable 180° about the shaft to facilitate its use on both sides of the body.

Less commonly used canes include the ortho cane, the forearm or platform cane, and the folding cane. The ortho cane is an adjustable aluminum cane with a curved shaft and a 90° handle. This cane permits the user's weight to be placed directly over the centre of the cane shaft, thus giving maximum support and balance. The forearm cane is indicated for individuals unable to use their hands for weight bearing. With this cane the weight of the body is supported by the forearm. Folding canes, which lack the sturdiness and adjustability of other canes, provide minimal support and balance and are best avoided.

Handles: The "C" or crooked handle is the most common type. It is uncomfortable for some users and may be inappropriate due to its tight curve for individuals with arthritis. Also, the weight of the user's body cannot be placed directly above the cane shaft, thus reducing the cane's stability. The handle may be hooked over the belt or arm when negotiating stairs.

The "T" handle and "D" or shovel handle, which are both more comfortable, allow the full force of the user's weight to be centered over the cane shaft for added stability.

The "J" handle, which is indicated for individuals with weak hands or arthritic involvement of the wrist, has a grip that aligns the fingers and thumb. This grip provides greater comfort and support.

The Ortho Ease Handgrip, manufactured by Lumex, is adjustable from a position parallel to the floor to a 45° angle. This handle is especially indicated for individuals with wrist involvement.

Regardless of style, cane handles should be made of wood or plastic, or covered with a tubular rubber grip. Metal handles are uncomfortable in cold weather, and if the handles become wet through perspiration or other moisture, users may lose their grip. Individuals should be instructed how to rotate handles on quad canes and how to adapt adjustable handgrips like the Ortho Ease.

Accessories: Cane tips are sized by inside diameter or plug size (which corresponds to the outside diameter of the cane shaft) and the base width. Cane and walker tips generally run between American

Standards Association (ASA) sizes 15 (plug size 0.95 cm, base width 2.86 cm) and 19 (2.22 cm, 3.81 cm). The larger rubber crutch tips may be used if greater support is required, but the cane shaft must be built up with tape to accommodate the larger plug size. Cane tips should have a flat or concave base. They must be flexible enough to remain in contact with the ground as the shaft pivots through a step. Users must be instructed to periodically inspect their cane tips for wear and tear, and to see that the tips fit snugly. The tips of all rented canes should be inspected before release. Metal slugs must be placed at the inside base of the tip on metal canes to keep the edge of the shaft from cutting through the tips. For use in winter, ice-gripping tips are available with adjustable metal prongs that can be flipped down and spiked into the ice for added stability.

Cane Fitting: Users stand in a natural position on a hard surface while wearing the same style of shoes they will normally wear while using the cane. The cane tip is placed 10 to 15 cm forward of the foot and 10 to 15 cm lateral to the front of the foot. When the cane is angled back to the hanging arm, the handle of the cane should be at the top of the greater trochanter (the point where the leg can be felt to pivot when lifted) or at the distal crease in the wrist (see Figure 1). This fit results in a bend of 20 to 30° in the user's elbow during normal use, a position that places the muscle groups in the

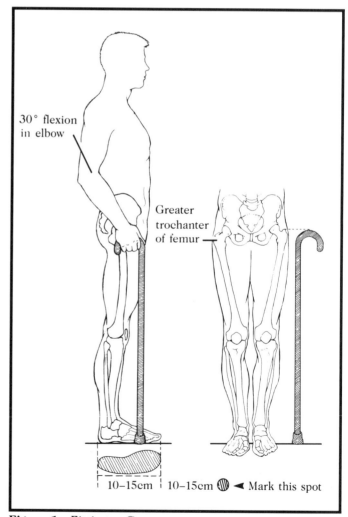

Figure 1 *Fitting a Cane*

Home Health Care

arm in the best position for firm support. (Some people prefer to have elbows at full extension depending on the strength of the muscles and the carrying angle of the hyperextended elbow.) If the individual has scoliosis (an S-shaped curvature of the spine) or other deformity resulting in one shoulder higher than the other, and two canes are indicated, each side must be measured separately.

If the cane is not adjustable and must be cut, it is turned upside down, the hand grip is rested on the floor next to the individual's foot, and a mark is made where the distal crease in the wrist crosses the cane shaft. The cane is cut about 0.6 cm shorter than this mark to allow for the thickness of the cane tip. Wooden canes should be cut with a fine-toothed crosscut saw, and aluminum canes with a tubing cutter. Before cutting, whenever possible, the user should first be given the opportunity to walk with an adjustable aluminum cane adjusted to the measurements taken.

Use: Consumers are instructed to use the cane opposite the weak leg and to step through with the strong leg. A walking gait for an individual with a weak left side is illustrated in Figure 2. If the right side is weak, these directions must be reversed. Walking with two canes is similar to walking with crutches, and the two-point and four-point gaits may be used. Individuals should be cautioned to keep the cane's rubber tip on the floor whenever they move their feet, and to keep the cane (and crutches) below their centre of gravity.

When going up or down stairs, the general rule of "up with the good leg, down with the bad leg" applies. While gripping the handrail with the hand on the strong side, users shift body weight to the weak leg. Then, pulling themselves forward with their hand on the railing, they lift the strong leg up to the next step, followed by the weak leg. The cane is held either in the other hand or hooked over the belt or arm. Quad canes are placed on the step ahead of the user. When travelling down stairs, these steps are reversed, with the weak leg leading followed by the strong leg, one step at a time.

If the handrail is on the weak side, the individual may go up or down the stairs facing backward, leading with the strong leg followed by the weak leg going up, and leading with the weak leg followed by the strong going down, while holding the handrail.

With all ambulatory aids, users must wear nonskid, flat-soled, supportive shoes that can be tied or buckled. If possible, they should remove throw rugs and avoid walking on slippery, waxed or wet floors, and on uneven surfaces. They should always look straight ahead when walking, instead of at their feet, and they should keep their body erect and avoid leaning out over their ambulatory device. If possible, they should walk close to a wall on their stronger or uninjured side for added support. Users should also be instructed not to leave ambulatory aids lying where others may fall over them.

Crutches

Crutches provide greater stability than canes and may be used by individuals having a greater involvement in their lower body. Crutches require greater forearm and upper arm strength than canes, which depend more on hand and wrist strength for their stability and weight-transfer properties. Two primary types are axillary and forearm crutches.

Axillary crutches provide greater support than forearm crutches because they brace both the wrist and elbow. These crutches extend from the ground to the axilla, have a handgrip mounted between two upright supports, have an axillary support and are made of wood or aluminum. Adjustable aluminum axillary crutches are preferred for rental purposes because of their ease of fitting and durability. Wooden crutches are less expensive, but are subject to greater wear and tear. Duralite crutches are similar to regular aluminum crutches except they have a push-button adjustment rather than a wing-nut adjustment, making fitting faster and easier. Another variation, the Ortho crutch, is a single-upright, curved-shafted crutch with a 90° axillary extension. The handgrip is the Ortho Ease Handgrip, a flattened plastic palm surface angled 15° from the horizontal to reduce wrist strain and fatigue. These crutches are versatile—the axillary extension can be removed and replaced by a cuff insert, thus converting the device to a forearm crutch.

There are three steps to fitting an axillary crutch. The first step is to select a crutch from the proper category (see Table IV).

The second step is to determine overall length (see Figure 3). The user stands in a neutral position on a hard surface, wearing the same style of shoes normally worn during everyday activities. A spot is marked on the floor 5 cm laterally from the side of the individual's shoe and 15 cm in front of the toe. From this point, the straight-line distance to the axilla is measured and 5 cm are deducted. This distance is the crutch length from the top of the axillary pad to the bottom of the crutch tip.

The third step is to determine hand grip height (see Figure 3). The hand grip should be at the level of the distal crease in the user's wrist, or level with the greater trochanter. As with canes, this height provides a bend in the user's elbow of 25 to 30° when the hand grip is grasped.

All adjustments must be made with all intended accessories in place (for example, tips, axillary pads and hand-grip cushions). The topmost hole in the lower support of a wooden crutch is never used, otherwise the support may fracture during use. Clearance is essential between the axilla and the top of the axillary pad so the individual's shoulders do not elevate with each swing through the crutch, a practice that can compress the radial nerves, glands and blood vessels, leading to "crutch paralysis."

Forearm crutches (Canadian crutches; Lofstrand crutches, which have open cuffs; and Kenny sticks, which have closed cuffs) provide support to the wrists and elbows. These crutches are indicated for individuals who have good upper body strength. The crutches have a collar or cuff that encircles the forearm and a handgrip that projects forward from the single main shaft. The cuff usually has either a front or side opening. The side opening is often preferred because it allows use of hands for simple tasks (such as opening doors) without having the crutches fall away. Forearm crutches are recommended for amputees and individuals with long-term disabilities who have good elbow and shoulder strength.

In fitting a forearm crutch, users stand with their arms by their side. The length of the extension leg of the crutch is adjusted to a point on the floor 5 cm laterally from the side of the individual's shoe and 15 cm in front of the toe (see Figure 4). Hand grips are adjusted to the level of the greater trochanter or the distal crease in the wrist. Cuff height is then adjusted so it is over the fleshiest part of the forearm, with the top of the cuff about 5 cm below the elbow. If a two-cuffed or Canadian Triceps crutch is used, the top cuff is positioned two-thirds of the way up the humerus. The cuffs can be opened or closed by bending and shaping the band to assure a good fit and to make it easy to change clothing.

Crutch accessories: Axillary pads or crutch tops provide stability and grip to the top of the axillary crutch so it does not slide back and forth during use. The pads are not intended to support weight; during use, weight is transferred through the hands, not the axillae. Hand grip cushions, which may have a lengthwise slit on one side

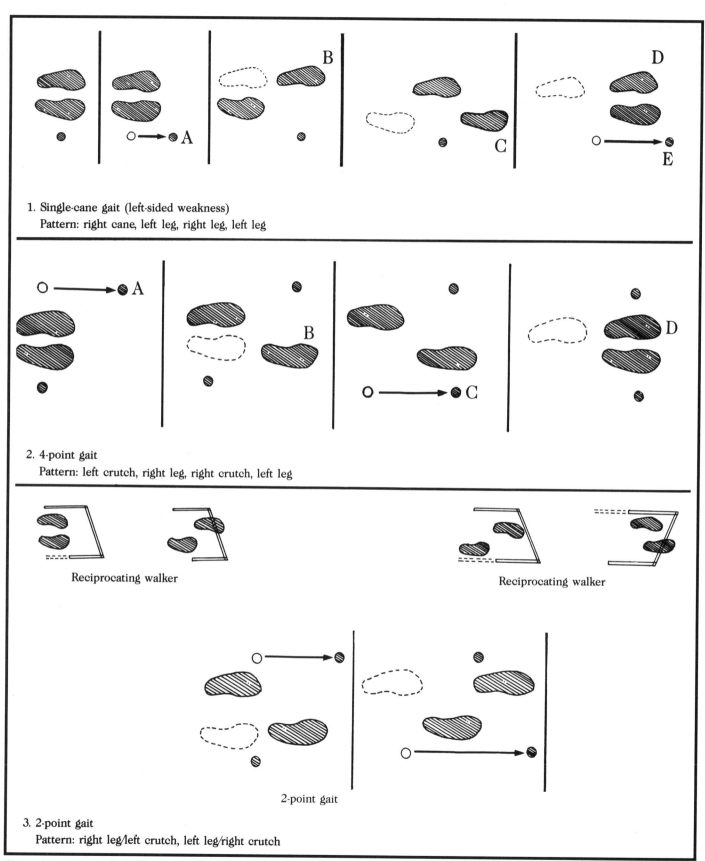

1. Single-cane gait (left-sided weakness)
   Pattern: right cane, left leg, right leg, left leg

2. 4-point gait
   Pattern: left crutch, right leg, right crutch, left leg

   Reciprocating walker

   Reciprocating walker

   2-point gait

3. 2-point gait
   Pattern: right leg/left crutch, left leg/right crutch

Figure 2 *Representative Cane, Crutch and Walker Gaits*

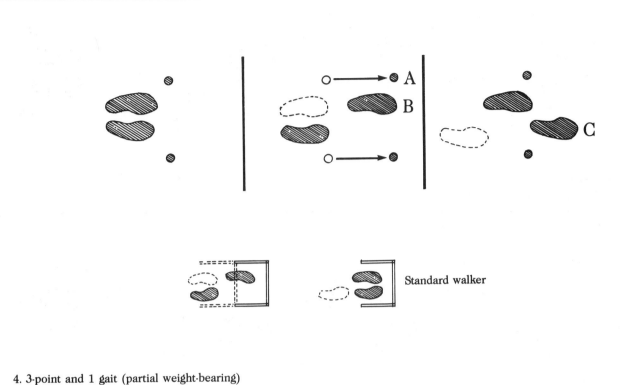

4. 3-point and 1 gait (partial weight-bearing)
   Pattern: both crutches/affected leg, step through with sound leg

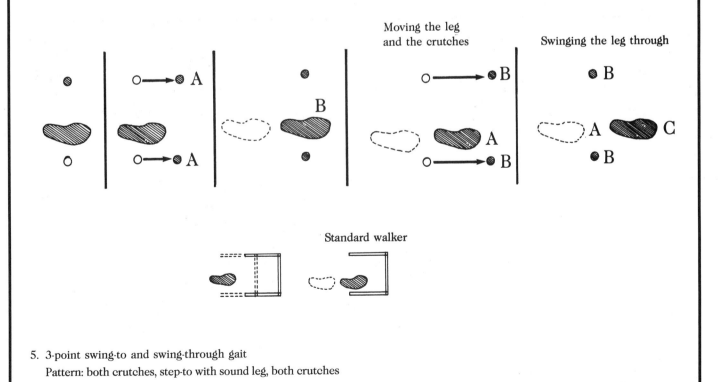

5. 3-point swing-to and swing-through gait
   Pattern: both crutches, step-to with sound leg, both crutches

Figure 2 *(Cont'd) Representative Cane, Crutch and Walker Gaits*

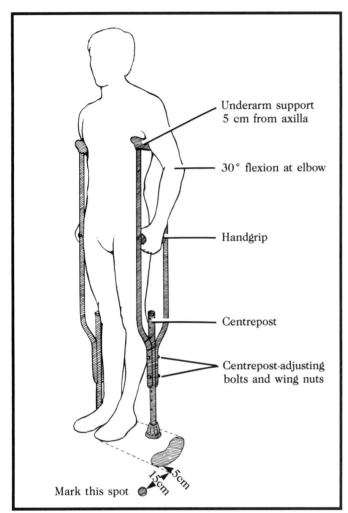

Figure 3 *Fitting an Axillary Crutch*

Underarm support 5 cm from axilla

30° flexion at elbow

Handgrip

Centrepost

Centrepost-adjusting bolts and wing nuts

5cm

15cm

Mark this spot

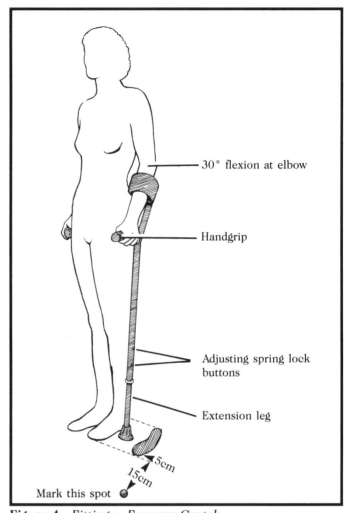

Figure 4 *Fitting a Forearm Crutch*

30° flexion at elbow

Handgrip

Adjusting spring lock buttons

Extension leg

5cm

15cm

Mark this spot

for easy installation, provide comfort and improved hand grip. They may need to be kept in place with strips of adhesive tape to prevent slippage. Axillary pads and hand grip cushions should be provided with all axillary crutches. For hygienic reasons, these accessories should not be rented or resold.

Like cane tips, crutch tips are flat or concave based and the inside diameter can be stated by ASA size number or plug size, ranging from ASA 18 (1.9 cm) to ASA 21 (2.85 cm). For a given diameter of tip, both standard (3.75 cm) and oversized (4.38 cm) base widths are available. Users must inspect their crutch tips periodically for wear and tear and snugness of fit. The tips of all rented crutches should be inspected before release. Tips for aluminum crutches require metal slugs in their bases.

Crutch gaits: Pharmacists should be familiar with the various crutch gaits so they can reinforce instructions given by physicians or therapists, and to aid users who have problems. Any one of five crutch gaits may be used with both axillary and forearm crutches, as well as with walkers (see Figure 2).

The four-point gait is the most common, safest and most stable of the crutch gaits. It is also the slowest. It is best suited to first-time crutch users and those who have poor balance and usually one leg affected, decreased strength or stability, or requiring a wide base of support. The pattern is left crutch, right leg, right crutch, left leg, with

each crutch advanced 20 to 25 cm in front of the user for maximum stability. Three points are always in contact with the ground at any one time.

The two-point gait, which is also used when walking with two canes, is similar to normal walking. It is faster than the four-point gait but requires more balance, since only two points are in contact with the ground at any one time. The pattern is left crutch and right leg moving forward at the same time, followed by the right crutch and left leg at the same time.

The three-point gait, used by individuals with orthopedic conditions requiring nonweight-bearing, such as broken legs or amputations, has two variations. In the swing-to pattern, both crutches move forward together and the unaffected leg steps up even with the crutches. The step-through pattern is similar to the step-to gait, except the legs are brought to a point ahead of the crutches. This variation is the fastest crutch gait, but requires good upper body strength and balance. The user's affected limb does not touch the ground.

The three-point-and-one gait is used when individuals can support their full weight on one leg and 25 to 50 per cent of their weight on the other leg. Both crutches move forward together with the affected leg, the unaffected leg swings through ahead of the crutches, and some weight is placed on the affected limb.

The one-crutch or hemiplegic gait is the same as that for a cane.

Home Health Care

Table IV *Guide to Initial Crutch Size*

User height (cm)	Crutch length (cm)	Crutch type	Length range (cm)
120.0–122.5	80	Child	75–95
125.0–127.5	85		
130.0–132.5	90		
135.0–137.5	95		
140.0–142.5	100	Youth	90–120
145.0–147.5	105		
150.0–152.5	110		
155.0–157.5	115		
160.0–162.5	120	Medium adult	105–137.5
165.0–167.5	125		
170.0–172.5	130		
175.0–177.5	135	Adult	120–150
180.0–182.5	140		
185.0–187.5	145		
190.0–192.5	150	Adult extra	135–165
195.0–197.5	155		

Adapted from: Fassett WE. Ambulatory aids and hospital equipment for the home. In: Catania PN, Rosner M, eds. Home health care practice. Palo Alto: Health Markets Research, 1986:122–55.

The crutch is used opposite the affected leg. The crutch and affected leg move forward at the same time, and the unaffected limb then steps through.

Use: The same usage outlined for canes can be followed by crutch-users. When negotiating stairs, users grasp the crutches in one hand while holding onto the handrail with the other. The swing-through gait is avoided on stairs.

Walkers

Walkers provide greater support than canes or crutches, because they have a wider base and four points in contact with the floor during use. Primary indications for walkers are poor arm strength, fractured hips in older individuals and when stability is of primary concern.

Types: There are two basic frame styles for walkers: the bridge frame and the physical therapy frame. The bridge frame walker has two sides joined by a transverse bar (the bridge) in the front. This bridge is placed fairly high on the frame to allow greater freedom of forward leg movement. Some walkers have the bridge high enough that the user can place it backward over a standard toilet for use as a toilet safety rail. This may be inappropriate for users with significant disability, since the walker is usually higher than a standard toilet safety rail, thus making gripping and transfer more difficult. All folding walkers are of the bridge style. The physical therapy frame is similar in design to the standard bridge frame walker, but the transverse bar is placed lower on the frame. This lower placement results in greater strength and stability since the centre of gravity is lower. It also permits physiotherapists to hang weights on the transverse bar as part of a rehabilitation program. Physical therapy frame walkers are not collapsible.

Besides the choice of frame style, walkers are available as standard (non-folding), folding, reciprocating, side walkers and wheeled walkers. They are also available in different sizes: child (50 to 65 cm high), youth (70 to 80 cm high) and adult (77.5 to 92.5 cm high). All styles have adjustable legs.

Standard walkers are popular in institutions because of their sturdiness and ability to handle heavy use. However, because they do not fold up, they take up extra space in the pharmacy. They are also inconvenient for individuals wishing to travel.

Folding walkers, the most popular, provide flexibility and convenience for travel. They can also fold up one side, enabling their use in small spaces such as a bathroom.

Reciprocating walkers are often used by individuals too weak to use the other models, or for those being retrained in the mechanics of walking. The reciprocating walker has hinges at the ends of the bridge to allow the user to move one side of the walker forward while always keeping two legs of the device in contact with the ground (see Figure 2, the two-point gait). Reciprocating walkers must not be confused with folding walkers. Attempts to use a folding walker as a reciprocating walker can result in injury.

The side walker (hemiplegic or hemi-walker, walkerette and walkane) is indicated for individuals who have lost function of one side of their body or who have lateral instability. Like a cane, this walker is generally carried on the strong side. Side walkers provide greater stability than multipod canes and are less cumbersome than the other walkers.

Wheeled walkers are useful for individuals who cannot lift a regular walker and for older individuals who have poor coordination. However, they are generally considered less stable, and therefore unsafe; if used, they should be equipped with a braking device. Overall, standard adjustable and folding adjustable walkers are the preferred models for pharmacy rentals.

Accessories: Unlike crutch and cane tips, walker tips are generally rounded at the base to minimize their tendency to catch on the floor as the walker is moved. Walker tips range in size from ASA 15 (plug size 0.95 cm) to 21 (2.5 cm). Because of the metal construction of walkers, metal slugs should be inserted in the base of the tips to minimize cutting during use. Frequent inspection for wear and snugness of fit is necessary. Ortho Ease Handgrips (Lumex) may be used on the conventional walker handrail for individuals with wrist involvement. Trays, baskets and other items are available for attaching to the walker's metal frame to permit users to carry small items.

Walker fitting: Walkers are adjusted for height using the same methods as for canes. The legs of the walker are adjusted so the top of the handgrips are level with the greater trochanter or the distal crease in the wrist when standing at the front of the walker. This position results in a bend of 25 to 30° in the elbow during use.

Use: The gaits used by individuals with walkers are the same as the crutch gaits: two-point, three-point (nonweight-bearing), three-point-and-one (partial weight-bearing) and four-point (see Figure 2). Walkers should always be placed about 20 cm in front of the user, and the user walks toward the device while it remains stationary or in full contact with the ground.

Some people tend to lean into the walker while walking up to it, a practice that might result in pushing the walker over. This tendency can be countered by lengthening the two front legs of the walker (with one adjustment), making it tilt back. Handgrip height should then be adjusted at the rear legs.

Reciprocating and side walkers are used differently from standard walkers. With the reciprocating walker, the individual uses the two-point gait as if using two walking canes. The person uses the side of the walker opposite the leg supporting the body weight. The user generally places the side walker off to one side and steps into it with the strong side while dragging the weak side.

Home Health Care

Wheelchairs

Wheelchairs provide the greatest degree of ambulatory support. Hundreds of possible combinations of wheelchair features are available, depending on safety, transfer technique, mode of propulsion, cost and the user's size, body weight, diagnosis, prognosis and style of living (see Figure 5).

Wheelchair fitting: Wheelchairs must be fitted to users, not users to wheelchairs. Ordering and fitting require the same attention given to prescribing drugs (see Figure 6). All measurements are best taken with the user sitting on the wheelchair cushion in a straight-backed chair. User-chair measurements, illustrated in Figure 5, include the following: seat width; seat depth; leg length and seat height; armrest height; and back support height.

Proper **seat width** should provide as wide a space as possible over which to distribute the user's weight. The user measurement should be the width of the hips or thighs, whichever is wider and 5 cm is added to the user measurement to provide at least 2.5 cm clearance on each side of the chair. Excess width prevents the user from reaching the hand rims and propelling the chair with ease. It may also result in a chair that is too wide for typical doorways. If the seat is too narrow, pressure sores may develop over the area of the greater trochanter.

Proper **seat depth** distributes weight evenly over the thighs and buttocks. The user is measured from behind the calf to the back of the buttock. To obtain the chair measurement, 5 to 7.5 cm is subtracted from the user measurement. This figure should result in two fingerbreadths from the back of the knee to the front edge of the seat. Insufficient depth exerts excess weight and pressure on the hips (ischial areas), increasing the risk of pressure sores; excessive depth exerts increased pressure behind the knees (popliteal areas), causing irritation and compromising circulation to the lower limbs.

Proper **seat height** distributes leg weight over the thighs while minimizing pressure on the popliteal areas. The tops of the thighs should be horizontal, parallel to the floor. The user is measured from the heel of the shoe or foot to just under the thigh. The minimum seat height is obtained by adding 5 cm to this leg length (as compression of the seat cushion must be considered). The seat must be high enough that the foot rests are at least 5 cm from the floor. If the seat is too high, the chair will not fit under desks and tables.

Insufficient foot rest height results in the foot rests hitting the ground over uneven surfaces, hitting ramps and increasing popliteal pressure. If the foot rests are too high, the knees rise up, transferring weight and pressure to the buttocks and ischia.

Armrests should support the elbows and forearms while the shoulders are in a relaxed, nonhunched position. With the user's elbows flexed to 90°, the distance is measured between the elbow and the chair seat. For the chair measurement, 2.5 cm are added to the user's measurement. This distance forces the elbows slightly forward, providing a natural brace against forward slumping.

Figure 5 *Fitting a Wheelchair*

	Adult	Junior	Semireclining	Full reclining
1. Seat height (bottom of heel to inner bend of knee plus 7.5 cm clearance)	47.5–50 cm	42.5–50 cm	Same as adult and junior	Same as adult and junior
2. Seat depth (2.5 cm less than length from inner bend of knee to posterior bend of hip	40 cm	40, 35, 32.5 cm	Same as adult and junior	Same as adult and junior
3. Height of backrest (bottom of buttocks to level of shoulders)	40–42.5 cm	40 cm	50–52.5 cm (plus about 25 cm for removable headrest panel)	53.8–56.3 cm (plus about 25 cm for removable headrest panel)
4. Height of armrest (bottom of buttocks to outer bend of elbow)	22.5–23.8 cm	22.5–25 cm	Same as adult and junior	Same as adult and junior
5. Overall height	87.5 cm	80–92.5 cm	97.5 cm (plus about 25 cm for removable headrest panel)	105 cm (plus about 25 cm for removable headrest panel)
6. Overall length	100–105 cm	95–102.5 cm	115–117.5 cm	122.5–125 cm
7. Seat and back width (widest area of hips and shoulders)	45 cm (40 cm for narrow adult; 50 cm for wide adult	40 cm	Same as adult and junior	Same as adult and junior
8. Width open	60–62.5 cm	55–57.5 cm for narrow person; 67.5 cm for wide person	55 cm	55 cm
9. Width closed	25 cm		22.5–25 cm	
10. Weight	20–22.7 kg (10.9–13.6 for lightweight)	18.6–20.5 kg	25–28.2 kg	25.9–29.1 kg

Home Health Care

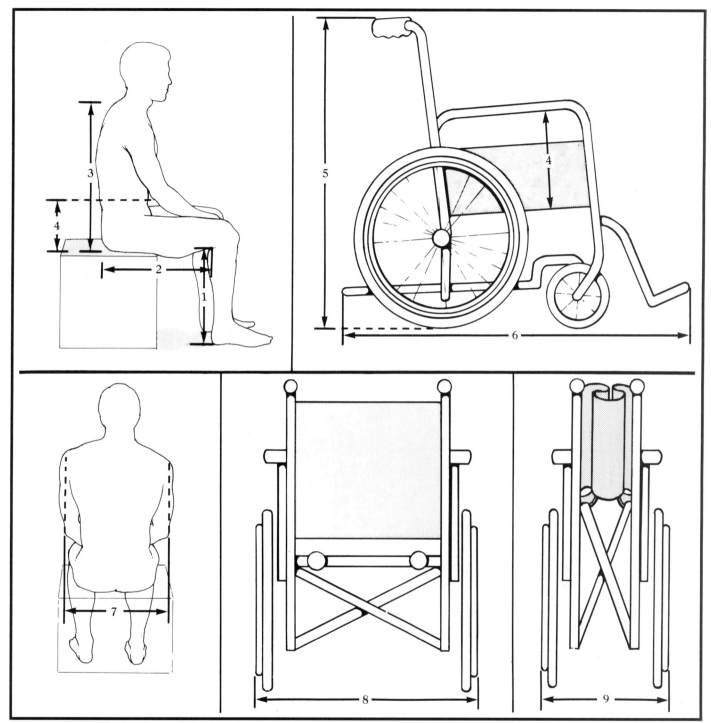

Figure 5 *(Cont'd)   Fitting a Wheelchair*

For **proper back support height**, the distance from the top of the chair seat to just under the user's extended arm is measured. For the chair measurement, 10 cm are subtracted from the user's measurement. There should be support across the scapula because many individuals have weakness of the trunk muscles. It also offers an opportunity for arm excursion. (The back height should be at least 2.5 cm above the inferior angle of the scapula to minimize pressure over these bony prominences.) Inadequate back height provides insufficient support to the upper trunk. Excessive back height in the chairs of users with some ability to propel their chair results in impaired shoulder mobility and decreased chair manoeuverability.

Overall chair width can be estimated by adding 16.25 cm to the seat width when standard armrests are used and 19.38 cm when detachable armrests are used. Wraparound armrests may be used when there is a need to decrease the overall chair width to accomodate narrow doorways.

Figure 6 *Sample Wheelchair Order*

Name _____ Date Ordered_____
Address _____
To whom billed _____ Dealer _____
Brand name _____ Model _____

Size:....................... _____ Adult
_____ Junior
_____ Large child
_____ Small child
_____ Special

Type: .... _____ Fixed back
_____ Added height
_____ Semi-reclining
_____ Full-reclining
_____ Amputee

Brakes: .... _____ Lever
_____ Toggle

Detachable footrests: .... _____ Liftoff
_____ Button
_____ Swinging
_____ Elevating

Footplates: .... _____ Regular
_____ Large

Heel loops:................ _____ Right _____ Left

Armrests: .... _____ Padded
_____ Fixed
_____ Removable
_____ Regular
_____ Adjustable
_____ Desk

Wheels—60 cm: .... _____ 36 spokes
Tires—60 cm: .... _____ Regular
_____ Pneumatic
Axle: .... _____ Regular
_____ Heavy duty
Handrims: .... _____ Regular
_____ Vertical projections
_____ Other
Front casters: .... _____ 20 cm regular
_____ 20 cm semi-pneumatic
Cushion:.................. Seat: _____ 5 cm _____ 7.5 cm _____ 10 cm
_____ Horseshoe
_____ Measurement
_____ Protective covering
_____ Other
Back:..................... _____ 2.5 cm _____ 5 cm
_____ Measurement
_____ Protective covering
Color of
upholstery_____

Additional instructions:

Ordered by _____

Accessories and modifications: The most important wheelchair accessory is the seat-cushion, and every wheelchair should have one. Cushions protect rental units against incontinence. Cushions also help prevent pressure sores, which result from a chair that is too wide or too narrow, or from improperly adjusted foot rests. The most common sites for pressure sores are at the hips, greater trochanters, sacrum and between the knees. The foam rubber or inflatable rubber ring or donut cushion is best for pressure sores between the knees and at the ischial tuberosities (bony prominences of the hip). The inside diameter of a ring cushion should be no greater than 5 cm wider than the ischial tuberosities, which are 10 to 15 cm apart in the adult. For most adults, a cushion of 40 cm with an internal diameter of 11.25 cm is adequate. If an inflatable ring is used, care must be taken not to under- or over-inflate the cushion. The horseshoe cushion (opening to the rear) is best for lesions at the base of the spine. Silicone gel cushions, resin-filled cushions and similar products are also available, but they are expensive and heavy, making them difficult to carry. Pressure sores can result from the inward rotational pressure on the hips caused by the folding chair's hammock seat. In this case a solid insert seat is used beneath the cushion. All cushions should be placed in a removable cloth cover that has ties to secure it to the chair seat back to prevent slipping. All wheelchair cushions can double for use on the user's bed if inserted into a foam mattress designed to accept the cushion and maintain a level surface.

Natural and synthetic sheepskin cushions and pads are also available. Although they permit good drainage and air flow when in direct contact with the skin, they are inadequate when used by themselves and should be used only on top of one of the other cushions.

Gel-filled pads are available to reduce pressure on the elbows and arms. The user can also partly fill two small hot water bottles with water and place them on the armrests.

Elevating leg rests are used by people who have casts on lower extremities, if there are indications of edema in this area, and to prevent contractions because of stiff, contracted or painful joints, as in arthritis. Removable armrests and backrests are useful if lateral or rear transfers must be made. A person with an above-the-knee amputation must have the chair's axle set back to adjust for the change in the centre of gravity. The loss of the weight of the lower extremity shifts the centre of gravity toward the rear of the chair, thus making a conventional chair unsteady and likely to tip over backward. Amputee conversion kits have special adaptors that allow the large rear wheels to be relocated about 6 cm to the rear of the original housing. Weights or sandbags on the footrests help if the chair cannot be modified. A reclining chair back may be indicated for people with respiratory difficulty or for quadriplegics so the lower trunk can be periodically relieved of upper body weight. Safety belts or vests are important accessories for all individuals with decreased trunk or upper body strength. Front wheels are available as solid casters of 12.5 cm or spoked wheels of 20 cm. The solid casters are satisfactory only if the chair is to be used on hard, smooth surfaces; the spoked wheels provide greater manoeuverability and stability, especially on carpeted floors and uneven surfaces. Hard rubber back tires are best for constant indoor use; pneumatic tires are for outside use. Other accessories that may be appropriate include desk attachments for armrests, various types of carrying pouches for attachment to the chair, and commode attachments.

Propulsion techniques: Hemiplegics who propel their chairs with their normal arm and leg need a detachable footrest on their uninvolved side. The seat height must be low enough to permit the user to reach the floor. A one-wheel-drive chair that has both hand rims on the same side may be provided for triplegics having one good upper limb, or for hemiplegics unable to propel themselves as previously described. Brake lever extensions allow the operation of both brakes with one hand. Quadriplegics or people with a poor grasp, such as found in arthritis, may benefit from vertical hand rim projections to aid propulsion.

Users should be cautioned never to lean forward in their chair if they cannot place both feet flat on the floor or if they have poor arm strength or a displaced centre of gravity (for example, leg cast or lower limb amputation).

Transfer Techniques: Brakes are necessary for all transfers. For anterior sliding transfer, swinging detachable footrests permit placement of the chair closer to the surface to or from which the individual is moving. Lateral transfer (with or without the use of a sliding board) requires detachable armrests plus removable footrests. Footrests may not be a problem for standing transfers, but if they are, a single detachable footrest is adequate.

Bathroom Safety Products

Every basic home health care department should have some bathroom safety products. Bathroom safety products form one of the largest home health care markets, for almost every person is a potential customer. As with most home health care items, the greatest demand is among the elderly and disabled. Few homebound people are completely bedridden—most are able to use the bathroom, but not without assistance. Two other important markets are the temporarily disabled (those incapacitated for a relatively short period of time, for example, people with leg fractures) and people who are healthy but seek preventive health care products.

Commodes

Commodes consist of a chair-like frame structure with a toilet seat and a receptacle beneath. Commodes are used whenever a regular toilet is not readily accessible or whenever individuals are unable to move from bed to bathroom.

Several varieties are available: stationary commodes; transport or wheeled commodes; chair commodes, which have upholstered back rests and seats that fit over the toilet seat when the commode is not being used as a toilet (these can double as a chair in the bedroom); folding commodes, which can also serve as shower chairs when the receptacle is removed; and drop-arm commodes, in which either arm can be lowered or removed to facilitate transfer to and from the side of the commode. Backless commodes are also available for this purpose.

Special commode adaptations are also available. The wheelchair commode is a replacement seat insert with a toilet seat and a receptacle. (The wheelchair cushion is placed over the commode insert when the commode is not in use.) In the over-toilet commode, the receptacle is removed, the legs adjusted upward and the entire frame placed over the regular toilet. Over-toilet commodes, which have a splash guard below the toilet seat, provide an elevated toilet seat to facilitate transfers. They also have a safety frame for added security and leverage to assist lowering users to, and raising them from, the toilet seat. Elevated toilet seats fit over the regular toilet seat to raise the seating height for the user. These adaptations also have a splash guard that fits into the toilet bowl. Some devices are like regular toilet seats with elevating supports that clamp onto the toilet; other less expensive models are thick molded-plastic products that sit on top of the regular toilet seat. These have a tendency to stick to the skin and may fall to the floor when the user stands. Most individuals prefer the added stability and security of the clamp-on models.

Special attention should be paid to the splash guard and commode height. Although most people prefer a full splash guard, individuals with poor leg and body control, like paraplegics and quadriplegics, may need elevated toilet seats with partial splash guards (open sides) to attend to personal needs independently (for example, inserting suppositories and cleansing). Standard toilet seats are about 40 cm high. People with stroke, arthritis, hip involvement or similar disability may need to have the rear legs of their commode adjusted higher than the front legs to facilitate use and minimize bending.

Commodes make reasonable rental items, although the receptacle and lid should always be sold separately. Consumers should be told that a receptacle partly filled with water is easier to keep clean than an empty one. Deodorant tablets and drops for use in the receptacle are appropriate companion sales. Commodes must be thoroughly cleansed with detergent and disinfectant between all rentals.

Safety Aids

Safety aids for the bathroom include mats, adhesive strips and spots (for the bottom of the bathtub to prevent slipping), and a variety of tub seats, safety rails and grab bars.

Safety rails and grab bars may be attached around toilets, to the walls of tubs and showers, or clamped over the side of the tub. Wall-mounted bars and rails, which come in a variety of lengths, shapes and angles, generally provide clearance between the bar and the wall of 3.8 cm (resting bar) to 12 cm (arm-hooking bar). Individuals can grab them, rest a limb on them or hook a limb behind the bar. Bathtub safety rails come in different heights (15 to 42 cm) and lengths. Some products incorporate dual height (hi-lo models) to facilitate safe tub entry on the high side and assistance for getting up from the tub on the low side. Bathtub rails should not be used on fibreglass bathtubs. Safety rails and grab bars come in flat boxes, thus taking up little space in the pharmacy. Pharmacists selling these products should be prepared to absorb the cost of installing the devices as part of the purchase price or to refer the consumer to someone who will provide proper and safe installation.

People who cannot sit in or rise from the bottom of the bathtub, or who cannot stand for a shower, may benefit from one of the many bath stools, chairs, benches or lifts. Bath stools are generally made of economical plastic and have drainage holes in the seats. They may have adjustable legs and backrests for people with balance problems. Stools vary in height between 12.5 and 55 cm. Bath chairs, which are more expensive, are available with a U-shaped or cut-out seat to permit the user to remain seated while washing the perineal area. Bath chairs have backs and adjustable legs and may be padded. Bath benches are constructed to have two legs placed inside the tub and two legs outside, thus providing optimal safety. Individuals can be easily transferred from wheelchairs to benches where they can lift their legs into the tub and slide over, thus eliminating the need to stand and reducing chances of slipping. All bath benches have back rests; some models may be padded, some may have cut-out seats,

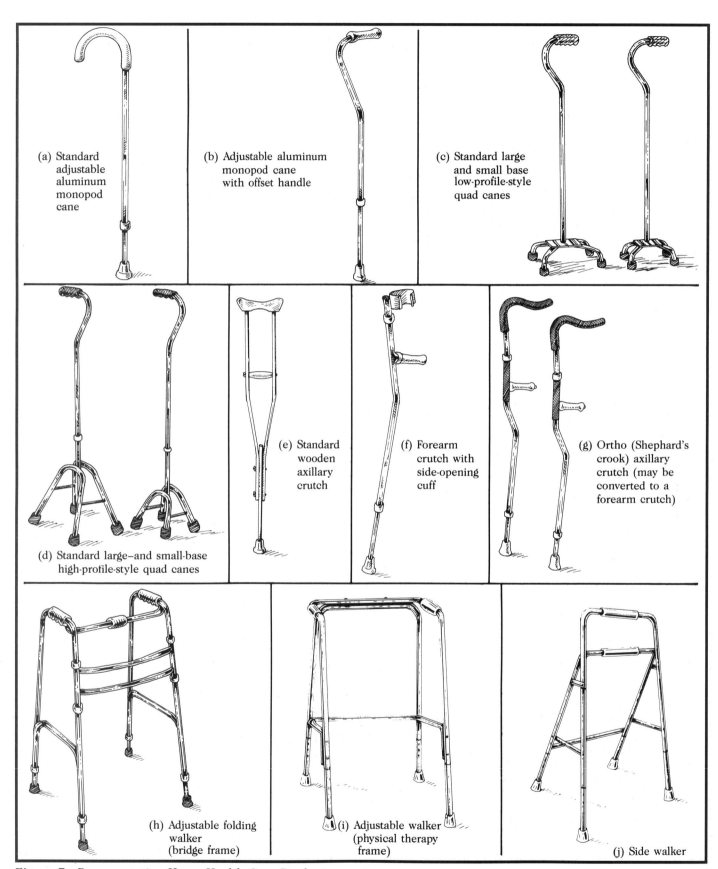

(a) Standard adjustable aluminum monopod cane

(b) Adjustable aluminum monopod cane with offset handle

(c) Standard large and small base low-profile-style quad canes

(d) Standard large–and small-base high-profile-style quad canes

(e) Standard wooden axillary crutch

(f) Forearm crutch with side-opening cuff

(g) Ortho (Shephard's crook) axillary crutch (may be converted to a forearm crutch)

(h) Adjustable folding walker (bridge frame)

(i) Adjustable walker (physical therapy frame)

(j) Side walker

Figure 7 *Representative Home Health Care Products*

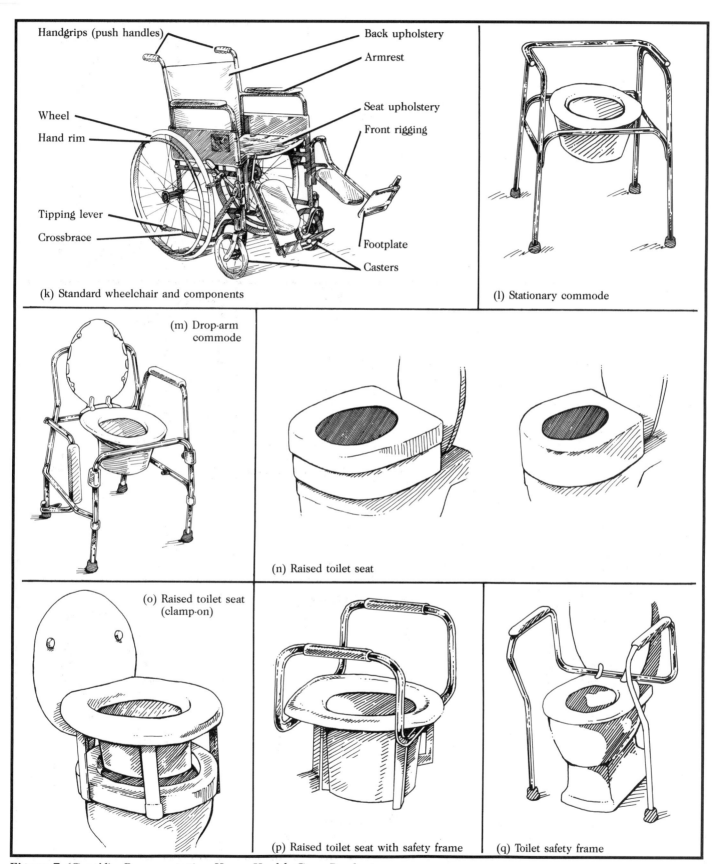

Handgrips (push handles)

Back upholstery

Armrest

Seat upholstery

Front rigging

Wheel

Hand rim

Tipping lever

Crossbrace

Footplate

Casters

(k) Standard wheelchair and components

(l) Stationary commode

(m) Drop-arm commode

(n) Raised toilet seat

(o) Raised toilet seat (clamp-on)

(p) Raised toilet seat with safety frame

(q) Toilet safety frame

Figure 7 *(Cont'd) Representative Home Health Care Products*

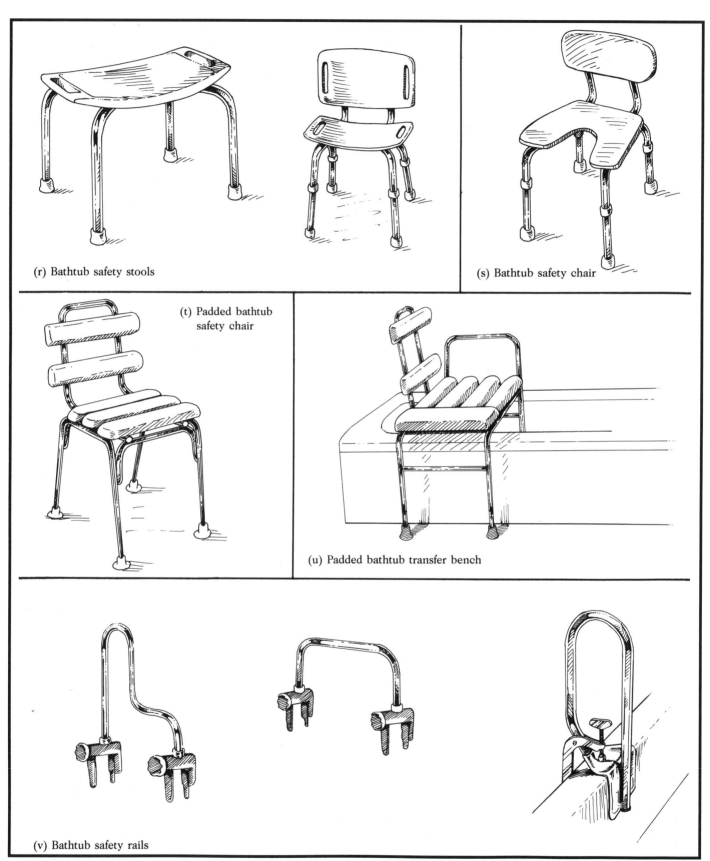

(r) Bathtub safety stools

(s) Bathtub safety chair

(t) Padded bathtub safety chair

(u) Padded bathtub transfer bench

(v) Bathtub safety rails

Figure 7 *(Cont'd) Representative Home Health Care Products*

Home Health Care

and some may have full chair backrests and armrests. All stools, chairs and benches should have slip-resistant leg tips. Water-powered bath lifts are available. They have a swivel seat for easy transfer; water pressure from the bathtub faucet is used to lift a person into and out of the tub.

Auxiliary or companion products may include whirlpool baths, sitz baths for perineal care, hand-held showers, long-handled faucet handles and faucet grippers.

Since many people requiring bath safety products have disorders associated with diminished sensation in the extremities, they are more prone to burns and scalds; water heater temperatures should be reduced to around 45 °C, or a thermostatic mixing valve should be in place.

Respiratory Therapy Equipment

Approximately 3 million Canadians have some degree of chronic respiratory ailment, with 1 million suffering from a clinically significant disease. Fifteen per cent of males and 5 per cent of females over the age of 20 have some significant airflow obstruction. Pharmacy-based home health care may provide products and services to these individuals in the following four areas: environmental conditioning (air cleaners and purifiers, humidifiers, vaporizers); physical therapy (percussors, incentive spirometers); delivery of drug therapy (aerosol compressors, nebulizers, tubings); and delivery of oxygen (oxygen tanks, concentrators, and regulators).

Environmental Conditioning

Air purifiers and humidifiers and vaporizers enjoy two distinct markets and must be so merchandised: as a "demand" (therapeutic) item and as a "lifestyle" (healthy living) item. As well, there is a strong seasonal component associated with their use, with peak demand for air purifiers seen during the dust and pollen-laden summer months while humidifier/vaporizer use peaks during the drier winter months.

Air purifiers differ in size, air moving capability, and effectiveness. Electrostatic or electronic air cleaners are small, portable, inexpensive products that might fit on a desk or table. They electrically charge airborne particles and attract them to a series of oppositely charged plates, releasing ozone in the process. The ozone, which imparts a characteristic odor, may aggravate hyperactive airways. These units are initially about 80 per cent effective in removing harmful airborne particulates, a figure which drops to about 25 per cent over a few days as the plates become dirty. Units should be cleansed with a strong detergent every 3 to 5 days. Dry media air purifiers employ paper or fibre impregnated air cleaning. Although the problem of ozone generation has been removed, these units still fail to move a satisfactory amount of air and require frequent cleaning. While expensive, high efficiency particulate air (HEPA) filtration units are preferred. These units are capable of removing better than 99.9 per cent of airborne particulate matter greater than 0.3 micron in diameter while changing room air 8 to 10 times per hour. These products, which make good rental and sales items, employ a series of progressively smaller outer filters which culminate with an internal, laminar flow hood-type HEPA filter.

Humidifiers and vaporizers both add humidity to the air, but they do so in different ways. Both units can be used to prevent dry throat and skin, loosen up nasal and chest secretions, soothe dry mucous membranes, provide a more comfortable room environment, and eliminate static electricity. Vaporizers account for approximately

50 per cent of the market share while humidifiers and ultrasonic humidifiers account for 30 and 20 per cent, respectively.

Vaporizers heat water to its boiling point and deliver moisture to room air in the form of steam. Tap water should be used (boiling occurs as ionized minerals in the water complete an electrical circuit between the vaporizer's electrodes). Normally, steam will begin to be visible in 2 to 3 minutes, with a steady flow in 15 to 30 minutes. If the water is too hard, boiling water may begin foaming and spilling over, and lights may flicker or household fuses may blow. The tap water should be diluted with distilled water, rain water, or refrigerator defrost water. If the water is too soft, a decrease or absence of steam will be noted. Add one-eighth teaspoon of baking soda to 2 L of water if steam does not appear in 10 minutes. Vaporizers have a medication cup to which vaporizer fluids (volatile oil like camphor and menthol) may be added. Do *not* add medication to the reservoir. Vaporizers should be rinsed with fresh water prior to each filling, and the accumulation of minerals around the edges of the bowl should be removed. Cleaning tablets (for example Solaray Vaporizer Cleaner, Solaray Humidifier Scale Prevention, Hankscraft Vaporizer Cleaning Tablets) should be used approximately every fifth filling to help prevent deposits. The tablets should be placed in the reservoir before operating, and the unit then run until the water becomes cloudy. Rinse well. A nonmetallic object should be used to clean scale build-up around the electrodes. If there are excessive deposits, the electrodes should be soaked overnight in vinegar. Patients must be counselled to use caution to prevent burn injuries due to the hot steam emitted from vaporizers.

Humidifiers and ultrasonic humidifiers add a cool mist to room air. Humidifiers employ a rapidly rotating spindle immersed in water which draws up water and throws it against a screen by centrifugal force. The screen breaks the water into small droplets which are then blown into the room by a high-speed fan. The ultrasonic humidifier, which is quieter but more expensive, employs a transducer rather than a motor. The transducer vibrates over 1.5 million times per second to produce an ultrafine mist. Many ultrasonic humidifiers contain a humidity control and mist output control, and may have a filter for incoming air. If room humidity is higher than what the patient sets on the humidistat, the humidifier will not work. Similarly, if the unit's incoming air filter becomes clogged, the humidifier may produce a bad odor or fail to operate. To prevent calcium deposits and a fine dusting of minerals left behind when water droplets evaporate, patients should use distilled water in their humidifiers. Some ultrasonic units employ an exchangeable demineralizer cartridge that may need periodic changing. Unlike the use of vaporizers, patients should be counselled that medications cannot be added to humidifiers. Patients should clean their humidifiers every 3 days with 4 L of cool tap water and 100 mL of household bleach. The unit should be run for 30 to 90 minutes with this solution, then rinsed clean with warm water and dried. Improperly cleaned humidifiers may present infection hazards. The cool mist provided by humidifiers is not sterile as in the heated steam given off by the vaporizers.

Accessory and companion products for the environmental conditioning department include vaporizer cleaning tablets, demineralizer units for ultrasonic humidifiers, water filters for humidifiers, medication solutions for vaporizers, replacement filters for air purifiers, and pollen and air-warming face masks.

Humidifiers and air purifiers should be kept running in the store to generate interest. Staff should be trained to emphasize product features, such as the therapeutic use of vaporizers and their inexpensive cost versus the better looking, quieter ultrasonic humidifiers, and consumers should be encouraged to trade up units. Lastly, merchandisers should anticipate the primary-use seasons previously discussed.

Physical Therapy

Patients suffering from conditions like chronic bronchitis and cystic fibrosis often produce increased amounts of pulmonary secretions. The mucus, which is often thick and tenacious, may prove difficult for patients to expectorate on their own. One device that may prove helpful to these individuals is a mechanical **percussor**, an electric drill-shaped instrument with an adjustable, vibrating pad that sends shock waves through the chest wall when placed on the back and chest. When preceded by an aerosol inhalation treatment and combined with postural drainage, the percussor is usually effective in loosening mucus found in the lungs and airways.

Monitoring peak expiratory flow rates by means of an **incentive spirometer** or peak flow meter may aid patients assessing the effectiveness of their therapy and/or the early recognition of increasing airflow resistance and an impending asthma attack (see the chapter on Diagnostic Aids.)

Delivery of Drug Therapy

Aerosol nebulizer therapy has become increasingly popular for effective drug treatment of airflow obstruction and related respiratory conditions, like aerosolized pentamidine for AIDS patients with *Pneumocystis carinii* pneumonia. Nebulizers may be effective in treating reversible airflow obstruction where conventional pressurized aerosol or dry powder inhalers have failed. Unlike conventional inhalers, nebulizers require minimal coordination on the part of the patient, thereby ensuring the reliable delivery of an adequate dose. The usual vehicle, normal saline, is itself active in soothing the airways and liquefying secretions. Lastly, nebulizers permit the administration of doses larger than those obtainable from pressurized aerosols.

Although nebulizers may be powered by a gas source such as oxygen, most are powered by an electrically operated air compressor, such as a Medi-mist or Maxi-mist machine. Jet nebulizers found in these types of machines operate on the Venturi principle (see Figure 8). Air forced through a jet placed in a medication nebulizer creates an area of low pressure which draws up the drug solution into the fast moving gas stream, where it is smashed into small droplets. The medication-laden mist is then delivered to the patient by means of a face mask or mouthpiece during normal tidal breathing. Patients must be counselled to keep the jets and tubing cleaned, otherwise they will become plugged and compromise delivery. Aerosol compressors make good rental items while replacement tubings, masks and nebulizers are steady companion sales. Portable compressors are available that will operate off of a car's cigarette lighter for patients requiring therapy while travelling.

Oxygen

The increase in the number of pulmonary disease patients receiving respiratory care, as well as an increase in hospice patients dying at home, has made low flow oxygen therapy a safe, effective and economically viable service for home health care pharmacies.

Medical oxygen may be administered to patients by nasal cannula, by face mask, or via a tracheal or endotracheal tube. Nasal cannulae are often preferred because they tend to remain in place longer, allow the use of the oral cavity while receiving oxygen, and impose less

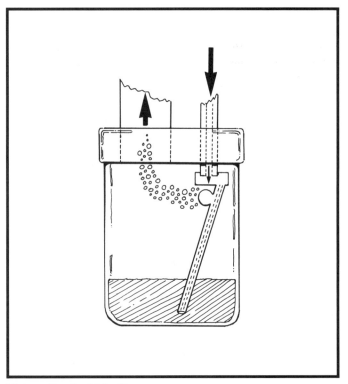

Figure 8 *Jet Nebulizer*

restrictions on the patient with regard to movement and communication. Face masks, on the other hand, permit the delivery of higher concentrations of oxygen and humidity as well as the opportunity to administer certain drugs. Nasal cannulae usually provide from 24 to 50 per cent oxygen with flow rates up to 6 L/minute, while simple oxygen masks deliver approximately 35 to 50 per cent oxygen with flow rates of 5 L/minute or greater. Masks with reservoir bags (disposable nonrebreathing and partial-rebreathing oxygen masks) are capable of delivering much higher concentrations of oxygen with a low flow rate. Jet-mixing "Venturi" masks are also available that will deliver 24, 28 and 35 per cent oxygen dependent on the specific flow rate matched to mask orifice. Both cannula and mask administration require a humidification source to add moisture to the dry oxygen.

Pharmacists may supply oxygen to patients at home in the form of gas (compressed gas system) or by an oxygen concentrator. A compressed gas system is the most costly system for pharmacists to provide. The tanks are heavy, bulky and require frequent replacement. (H or K cylinders last approximately 2½ days at 2 L/minute continuous flow.) They are best indicated for intermittent use at low flow rates. The cylinders are usually rented from the oxygen supplier while pharmacists might rent out the cylinder stand or cart, cylinder wrench, and regulator with gauge. Regulators are used to reduce the cylinder pressure to a level that is safe for patients to use. They also contain a pressure gauge which monitors the volume remaining in the cylinder along with a flow meter that will allow a flow rate between 0.25 and 15 L/minute. A humidifier attachment plus disposable tubings and mask or cannula are sold along with the oxygen. Smaller, portable cylinders and accessories are also available for ambulatory patients. (D cylinders will last 3½ hours at 2 L/minute continuous flow.)

Oxygen concentrators are another means of administering oxygen. Room air is forced into a sieve bed under pressure that traps nitrogen while releasing and storing oxygen. There exists an inverse relationship between flow rates and oxygen concentration. Most concentrators are capable of delivering oxygen flow rates between 0.5 to 6 L/minute with oxygen concentrations between 80 to 98 per cent. Most concentrators are also equipped with a variety of alarms for factors like plugged filters, inadequate pressure, and so forth. Patients should have a backup compressed gas system at home, and pharmacists should have an oximeter or oxygen analyzer for proper monitoring and calibration. While most oxygen concentrators are relatively lightweight, compact, mobile and quiet, they are not intended for ambulatory use like a small oxygen cylinder system.

Pharmacists involved in oxygen services must make the commitment to provide delivery, setup and patient service on a 24-hour basis. Pharmacists should check with local fire departments regarding policies on the storage, transport, and in-home use of gases. While oxygen is not explosive, it is highly combustible in the presence of a flame or spark.

Incontinence Products

Urinary incontinence—the involuntary loss of urine with resultant social and hygienic problems—is a common symptom among the elderly. It is estimated that 500,000 Canadians have a daily need for incontinence products, and another 500,000 are thought to need special absorbent garments occasionally. Between 5 and 10 per cent of people over age 65 living in the community suffer from significant incontinence. In about one-third of these individuals, incontinence is transient and clears either spontaneously or following treatment, such as that for a urinary tract infection. Up to 50 per cent of residents in nursing homes or continuing care facilities suffer from urinary incontinence. Most incontinent individuals are female, and 10 to 25 per cent of those with urinary incontinence also experience fecal incontinence. The frequency and severity of incontinence varies among individuals and may range from occasional dribbling to regular involuntary voiding of large volumes of urine. (See chapter on ostomy and incontinence.)

Overall, incontinent adults exceed the number of babies in diapers by almost 50 per cent. The incontinent elderly purchase 30 per cent of baby diapers and 50 per cent of sanitary pads. Industry figures show the home health care incontinence sales market is growing at an annual rate of 25 per cent; retail pharmacy sales account for 35 per cent of the market, and institutional and catalogue sales account for the rest.

Treatment

Treating urinary incontinence must reflect the underlying cause. Surgical and pharmacotherapeutic treatments are often effective, but various nonsurgical techniques and products are available to a pharmacy-based home health care centre.

Catheterization

Three types of catheter-based treatments exist—indwelling catheters, clean intermittent catheters, and external catheters (males) and collection devices (females). Most catheters are made of soft, flexible rubber and may be opaque or clear. Clear catheters are preferred for self-catheterization, because users can easily see when urine flow begins and when cleaning is ineffective. Indwelling catheters with

silicone and Teflon coatings on the inside and outside, and all-silicone (sialastic) and PVC catheters are also available. These materials reduce friction and discomfort during catheter insertion and removal. They also inhibit catheter encrustations, thus decreasing stones, catheter blockage and infection, and extending the time between catheter changes. Female catheters are generally shorter than male catheters because of the shorter female urethra. Catheter diameter scales, of which the French scale is most commonly used, are shown in Table V.

Table V *Catheter Diameter Scales*

French	10	12	14	16	18	20	22
American	7	8	10	11	12	14	15
English	4	5	6	7	9	11	12
Size (in)	13/100	15/100	18/100	20/100	23/100	26/100	29/10
Size (cm)	0.3302	0.3810	0.4572	0.5080	0.5842	0.6604	0.7366

Adapted from: Eigan BN. Health accessories. In: Gennaro AR, ed. Remington's pharmaceutical sciences. Easton: Mack Publishing, 1985;1824–68.

The **indwelling retention (Foley) catheter** has a balloon (5 or 30 mL) at its insertion end. Two channels run the length of the catheter, one for the passage of urine and one for the injection of sterile water, which inflates the balloon within the bladder, thus securing it. When filling the balloon, it must be remembered that the lumen of the catheter holds approximately 5 mL, a volume that must be added to the total injected. Since this type of catheter results in continuous urine drainage, users must wear a leg-bag collection unit when they are ambulatory and a bedside collection unit when they are recumbent for long periods of time. Collectors should be emptied frequently, rinsed with warm water and cleaned with a solution of white vinegar and water (1:1). Users should have a reserve collector for use while the other is being cleaned and dried. Soft elastic leg-bag straps with Velcro closures add to comfort.

Paraplegics and wheelchair-bound individuals often prefer their leg-bag positioned just above their ankle and fitted with extension tubing to facilitate emptying their bag over a floor drain. Because the use of indwelling catheters is often associated with urinary tract infections, sterile technique is required. This type of incontinence control is generally reserved for people for whom other means of management are unsuitable.

Clean **intermittent catheterization** is a safe and effective means of treating many incontinent people who have bladder hyporeflexia with increased residual urine. This method requires only a clean rather than sterile technique, and is associated with a low incidence of urinary tract infection. Written instructions for catheter insertion and catheter care may be found elsewhere. The straight, clear plastic catheters are intended for brief insertion and removal. They are available in different sizes based on age and sex. Extensions are available for wheelchair-bound individuals.

External devices include the so-called condom catheters for males. Popular and effective, they consist of a penile sheath attached to a drainage catheter. External glue-on collection devices are available for females. These products are satisfactory only in selected cases because of the difficulty of adherence and a good fit. Both products require use of a leg-bag and/or bedside drainage collector with an extension tube as used with the indwelling catheter. Similar external collection devices are available for fecal incontinence.

Home Health Care

Absorbent Products

Adult incontinence garments must fit snugly, be absorbent enough to contain a full void or continuous leakage for several hours, and have elastic gathers at the legs to prevent urine or loose stool from leaking onto outerwear and bedlinens. Children's diapers are a poor substitute for the incontinent adult. Children's diapers fit improperly and have small volume capacity and improper odor control. Feminine hygiene paper products are also inadequate. They are formulated to absorb blood, not urine; urine causes them to bloat, become soggy, leak and release odor. Adult incontinent absorbents have polymers that absorb 50 to 500 times their weight and congeal fluid to prevent leakage. Most products consist of several layers of fabric that permit urine to permeate into underlying absorbent layers, thus maintaining a feeling of being comfortably dry. Many products contain reusable ties, and some contain indicator strips that change color when the undergarment needs changing.

A variety of adult incontinence products are available: disposable or reusable diaper-type garments, briefs and absorbent pant-liners or shields, and absorbent bed underpads. The choice of product depends on the frequency and severity of incontinence. The diaper-type products are recommended for heavy voiders (up to 750 mL in volume with some products). Though effective, these products are relatively expensive, often bulky to wear and require meticulous skin care. (See the chapter on ostomy care and incontinence.) Because of these products' special construction and unique drainage features to keep moisture away from the skin, consumers must be counselled that they do not need to change the garments after each "accident." The undergarment products are loincloth-type absorbent products held in place by elastic straps. These products are good for moderate leakage and occasional dribbling, but are unsatisfactory for bedridden individuals. (Without elastic gathers at the legs and the close fit of diaper-type products, leakage occurs when the user is recumbent.)

Enuresis Alarms

A variety of enuresis alarms (for example, Moses, Palco) are available to help behavior modification, most often in enuretic children. The most successful alarms are those with a wrist alarm and a sensor snap on the underclothing. Success rates may be as high as 85 to 90 per cent, but coaching and instruction of the parents is a prerequisite to success. Wearers often are not awakened by the alarm during initial treatment, so parents must be instructed to arouse the child when the alarm sounds. Criticism has centered on the 15 to 20 per cent relapse rate, but good success rates can be achieved. Success with enuresis alarms has also been demonstrated with institutionalized elderly.

Miscellaneous

Pharmacists should be aware of two other techniques—bladder habit retraining and Kegel exercises—so they can counsel and assist caregivers and incontinent individuals. Bladder habit retraining is time-consuming and labor-intensive, but effective when continually reinforced. Establishing a voiding schedule, and increasing the interval between voidings by consciously delaying urination, have shown significant improvement in 50 to 70 per cent of women under 70 years of age with idiopathic detrusor instability. Exercises to maintain and regain urinary control by strengthening the pelvic floor musculature (Kegel exercises) often help women with stress incontinence. Printed instructions and cassettes are available from Help for Incontinent People (HIP), P.O. Box 544, Union, South Carolina 29379, USA. Another excellent consumer support group is the Simon Foundation of Canada, P.O. Box 3221, Tecumseh, Ontario N8N 2M4, 1–800-265-9595, which publishes a quarterly newsletter and provides patient information and support.

Pharmacy-Consumer Considerations

Pharmacists must allow a consumer's purchase of incontinent supplies to be as discreet as possible. The incontinence department should be well-signed and easy to find to spare the possible embarrassment of asking directions. To encourage people to recognize and seek treatment for voiding dysfunction, the following list of warning signs of bladder control problems developed by HIP should be displayed in the pharmacy: leakage of urine that prevents desired activities; leakage of urine that causes embarrassment; leakage of urine that begins or continues after an operation (hysterectomy, Caesarian section, prostate surgery or rectal surgery); inability to urinate (retention of urine) following an operation; urinating more frequently than usual without a proven bladder infection; needing to rush to the bathroom or losing urine if you do not arrive in time; pain related to filling the bladder or pain related to urination (in the absence of bladder infection); frequent bladder infections; progressive weakness of the urinary stream with or without a feeling of incomplete bladder emptying; and abnormal urination or changes in urination related to a nervous system abnormality (for example, stroke, spinal cord injury or multiple sclerosis).

Displays can be used to show consumers how a garment and pad are worn. Samples of briefs should be available for consumer inspection, along with information explaining how to fit and wear briefs. Absorbent products are bulky and difficult for the elderly to manage, so the pharmacy should have oversized bags for discreet wrapping of purchases, and delivery should be considered. When discussing incontinence supplies with consumers, materials should be referred to as personal protection products rather than diapers. Lastly, the incontinence department should be located near the dispensary, next to the feminine hygiene department as most purchases are made by women. Urinary incontinence is a common symptom among the elderly. People should be made aware that incontinence often can be effectively treated and that measures can be taken to make life as comfortable and dignified as possible.

Health Supports and Appliances

Health supports and appliances serve several purposes: to steady and limit the motions of the joints, ligaments, and muscles in injuries and diseased conditions; to support the pelvic girdle, thereby giving support to the back and abdomen; to support an affected part after the removal of a plaster cast; to rest and support the locomotor structures in general; and, in the case of compression supports, to treat and prevent lower extremity varicosities (varicose veins) and states of impaired lymph flow (for example, post-mastectomy axillary lymphedema).

The health supports department consists of four general types of products: compression therapy (nonprescription—for example, Parke-Davis and Futuro support stockings—and prescription—for example, Sigvaris and Jobst stockings and lymphedema sleeves); nonprescription health supports (for example, Futuro, Tensor, PCP Champion and Camp soft-goods); prescription orthopedic supports (for example, DePuy, Camp and Richards); and orthoses or braces, which give greater motion control than the others.

Home Health Care

More than 40 per cent of Canadians work out daily and 50 per cent of those under 35 years of age participate in a sports activity. It has been estimated that about one million Canadians annually are injured as a result of exercise or sports participation. Pharmacists considering a health supports department in their home health care centre must know what types of injuries and disorders to expect in order to anticipate inventory and product-mix needs. About 10 per cent of hospital emergencies relate to sports injuries. Table VI shows a breakdown of injuries requiring health supports, based on American data. Pharmacists may find these data helpful in planning DME needs and companion-sale products, such as hot and cold packs, slings, cast shoes and cast covers, and similar orthopedic-based products. Compression therapy product needs may be assessed on such factors as percentage of elderly population in the trading area, the

number of vascular surgeons, the number and extent of mastectomies performed, and so forth.

Nonprescription and prescription supports exist for virtually all limbs and body parts from the neck to the ankle. Pharmacists considering involvement with prescription-based health supports require a private fitting room in which to take measurements and fit the appliance. They also require special training in measuring users and fitting appliances. Two, week-long, industry-based fitting schools are run throughout the year, to instruct and certify orthotic fitters. These comparable courses are conducted by Camp International (P.O. Box 495, Trenton, Ontario K8V 5R6) and Airway Surgical Appliances (424 Catherine Street, Ottawa, Ontario K1R 5T8). Pharmacists unable to provide in-pharmacy fitting space may still perform health support fittings in consumers' homes or in nearby hospital or rehabilitation facilities. Performing health support fittings off-premises requires a fitting bag, including tape measure, pliers or stay benders, product reference materials, rubber gloves, sewing kit, business cards, receipt book, insurance forms and three garments—one for the measurements supplied, one a size smaller and one a size larger to account for errors in measurement.

Compression Therapy

Two venous systems exist in the lower extremities—the vein system comprised of deep veins, and the superficial system comprised of the greater and smaller saphenous veins. Interwoven between and around these veins are skeletal muscles that help force blood up the leg when they contract. Since blood flows against gravity to reach the heart, the veins have unidirectional bicuspid valves that direct blood up the legs to the thigh. When the valves fail, reflux of blood occurs at the terminal ends of the veins, leading to distention and varicosities. Valvular incompetence can be irreversible, resulting from thrombosis or disease, and reversible as seen in obesity and pregnancy. Insufficient muscular tone in the legs aggravates incompetent valves. Standing leg pressures consist of approximately 90 mm Hg at the ankle (10 to 15 mm Hg supine pressure), 60 at the knee and 45 at the thigh.

Compression stockings are generally indicated for varicose veins and inactivity of leg muscles (for example, paralysis, bedridden individuals and individuals wearing a cast), when edema of the tissues of the leg results secondary to slowed venous return. In general, support stockings should not be used in the presence of congestive heart failure accompanied by leg or pulmonary edema, infections or lesions of the legs, severe arteriosclerosis or leg deformity.

Nonprescription compression stockings provide about 12 to 18 mm Hg of compression at the ankle and come in stockings and pantyhose. They fit snugly, giving the wearer a sense of mild support while providing a minimal amount of compression. Prescription compression stockings provide four different degrees of compression measured at the ankle—20 to 30 mm Hg, 30 to 40 mm Hg (most commonly prescribed), 40 to 50 mm Hg, and 50 to 60 mm Hg. Most nonprescription supports are closed-toe; the greater pressure stockings usually have an open toe or separate toepiece that does not cause compression. Nonprescription stockings are usually fitted on the basis of user shoe size, height and weight, although some may require measurements at the ankle, calf, knee or thigh depending on the length of the support and the degree of compression.

The lower compressions are indicated for mild venous conditions; the higher compressions are indicated for severe compression needs like lymphedema, post vein stripping and stasis dermatitis. High-compression stockings are used only for ambulatory individuals.

Table VI *Orthopedic Injuries Requiring Health Supports* *

Orthopedic impairments	Incidence
Back & spine	9.3 million
Hip & lower extremity	7.1 million
Shoulder & upper extremity	2.5 million
Brace-wearers	1.4 million

Injuries	
Foot	800,000/year
Toe	300,000/year
Ankle (14% all sports injuries)	800,000/year
Knee (22.5% all sports injuries)	525,000/year → require treatment
Leg (19% all sports injuries)	317,000/year lower leg 182,000/year upper leg
Back (16% all sports injuries)	30 million experience back discomfort/handicapped from back injuries/ailments 6.5 million → confined to bed with back problems at any one time 4.6 million back sprains from physical activities 2.7 million → ruptured discs 2.6 million → chronic intervertebral disc replacements
Fingers	1.7 million/year
Hand	840,000/year
Elbow	238,000/year
Arm (14% all sports injuries)	375,000/year lower arm 84,000/year upper arm
Shoulder	300,000/year
Wrist	475,000/year
Neck	110,000 emergency treatments/year ~6% population → severe neck pain at least once requiring treatment
Head	950,000/year

*Based on American figures.
Adapted from: Selling techniques in the home health care field. Alexandria: National Association of Retail Druggists, 1985.

Non-ambulatory, bedridden individuals may be fitted with so-called anti-embolism stockings (for example, TEDS). Made of white cotton instead of elastomers and having less compression, anti-embolism stockings prevent venous emboli secondary to inactivity. Anti-embolism stockings provide inadequate support for ambulatory individuals.

Besides traditional stockings, there exist a variety of tubular, "stockinette" products like Tubigrip that provide graduated compression with a contoured fit. These products consist of covered elastic threads that, once applied, the elastic moves in the bandage, evening out pressure over varying contours of the body. Shaped support bandages exist for such conditions as varicose veins, gravitational edema (following cast removal), deep vein thrombosis prevention, lymphedema, and post-burn scalding, while straight bandages exist for sprains and strains, soft tissue injuries, joint effusions, general edema, pressure dressings, and so forth. Sizes consist of low, medium and high pressures, with the level of pressure determined by the size of the stockinette used, not the tension with which it is applied. Products should always be applied in a double layer to ensure correct pressure and firm support.

Compression therapy using elastic bandages or wraps should be discouraged. Graduated compression up the leg is essential. An incorrectly applied elastic bandage can result in greater compression in the upper leg than in the lower leg, thereby further impeding circulation. Individuals should be instructed to walk at least 5 minutes out of every half hour to help the calf muscles contract and force blood up the leg. Individuals should also avoid wearing high-heeled shoes, standing in one spot for more than 10 minutes, squatting and crossing their legs, all practices that put added pressure on the veins and reduce circulation. It is also best to avoid using ointments and creams under the stockings, although certain products do permit this. Auxiliary or companion products for individuals with venous insufficiency may include such things as home blood pressure and pulse kits (see chapter on Diagnostic Aids), stethoscopes, leg elevators and various bandage products.

Trusses

A hernia is the protrusion of the intestine and its surrounding membrane (peritoneum) through one of the natural openings in the abdominal wall—the umbilical opening, inguinal openings or the openings for the femoral arteries. Individuals often speak of having a rupture. A rupture is similar to a hernia, except that the protrusion occurs through a previously weakened point in the abdominal musculature, such as a previous surgical incision (incisional hernia). Inguinal hernias are most common, accounting for over 95 per cent of all male hernias (usually manifest as scrotal hernias) and nearly 45 per cent of all female hernias. The incidence of hernias is highest in the infant and elderly populations.

Although hernias may undergo spontaneous resolution, surgery is the usual preferred mode of treatment since strangulation of the intestine is a constant risk. However, some people may require a truss in lieu of surgery, and most individuals require a truss for support during the immediate postoperative period.

Truss Fitting and Consumer Considerations

All trusses must be fitted while the user is lying down so the hernia is reduced (the protruding intestine is returned to the abdominal cavity). If fitting is attempted with the individual in the upright position, the truss itself may cause intestinal strangulation. The choice of truss and location of truss pads depends on the location of the hernia and the individual's weight and general build. Easily protruded hernias require heavier supports. Proper fitting is based on consumer waist size. Once fit, the truss is tested by having the user bend, stoop and squat while observing for protrusion of the intestine past the truss pad. Suspensories consist of a belt with a scrotal pouch that relieves strain and fatigue by reducing the pull on the muscles and cords of the scrotal area. Sizes are determined by the size of the pouch.

Skeletal Supports

The spinal column consists of the cervical spine (7 vertebrae and anterior curve), the thoracic spine (12 vertebrae, posterior curve and attached ribs), the lumbar spine (5 vertebrae and anterior curve), the sacrum (5 tightly joined vertebrae and posterior curve) and the coccyx (3 to 5 vertebrae and posterior curve). The sacrum forms the sacroiliac joint through association with the two innominate bones of the pelvis.

About 3 million Canadians experience back discomfort and disability from back and spinal injuries and ailments, with the back involved in over 15 per cent of all sports injuries. Common anomalies of the spinal column requiring supportive garments and braces include whiplash, trauma to the cervical spine; lordosis (swayback), a hyperextension of the lumbar spine; kyphosis (hunchback), a flexion of the thoracic spine; scoliosis, an S-shaped lateral curve of the thoracolumbar spine; sciatica, extreme pain at the back of the thigh and running down the inside of the leg resulting from rupture or protrusion of an intervertebral disc with subsequent compression on the sciatic nerve; spondylolysis, the breaking down of a vertebral structure; and spondylolisthesis, pain and pelvic deformity resulting from forward subluxation of the lower lumbar vertebrae, usually on the sacrum.

An estimated 6 per cent of the population will, at least once, experience severe neck pain requiring treatment. Common conditions include torticollis (wry neck; a stiff neck caused by spasmodic contraction of neck muscles drawing the head to one side), and whiplash, muscle strain and herniated disc or fracture in the cervical region due to sudden anterior-posterior movement. Neck or **cervical braces** provide support and protection and limit the range of motion, especially flexion and extension. However, with even the most effective cervical orthosis, lateral bending can only be limited to about 50 per cent of normal motion and about 20 per cent of normal rotation.

Soft cervical collars made of foam rubber are indicated for cervical muscle spasm, ligament separation, tendinitis or osteoarthritis, and following cervical laminectomy with fusion, although a hard cervical collar is more often used for this purpose. The collar is usually contoured, being wider at the middle with a depression or cup for the chin, and tapering toward its ends. It provides restriction of motion more through a sensory feedback and a reminder to limit head and neck motion than through actual mechanical restriction of motion. Fitting of soft collars is based on user neck circumference measurement. Collars should be fitted with the neck in a neutral position (head level, eyes straight ahead) unless instructed otherwise. If a slight degree of flexion is ordered, the tapered (closure) end of the collar is placed anteriorly.

Semi-rigid soft collars incorporate a semi-flexible strip of plastic in the collar for added support. Rigid molded plastic collars (for example, the Philadelphia collar) limit anterior-posterior cervical motion to about 30 per cent of normal and provide about 40 per cent of normal rotation and 70 per cent of normal lateral bending. Fitting of rigid collars is based on user neck circumference and the distance from the user's sternal notch on the chest to the point of the mandible (with the head in the desired position). Rigid collars come in different circumference and height categories. Like soft collars, the neck should be in the neutral position unless specified otherwise.

Sacroiliac supports provide support and stabilization for sacral and abdominal muscles and ligaments to aid in relief of lower back discomfort. Lumbosacral supports provide compression to support and stabilize lumbar, sacral and abdominal muscles and ligaments to aid in relief of back discomforts and encourage proper posture. Lumbosacral supports are higher in the front and back than sacroiliac supports, and usually contain posterior boning for additional support. They may also contain posterior casings for insertion of steel stays, but these require a physician's order and the training acquired through one of the fitting schools mentioned earlier. Some sacral supports also accommodate removable and adjustable posterior pockets for insertion of additional padding, rigid supports or thermal pads for reflecting body heat back into the bones and joints of the affected area. Both sacroiliac and lumbosacral supports require a snug hip measurement for proper fitting. Most of these nonprescription supports use hook and pile closures to make the support easy to put on and adjust to desired fit and compression.

Rib belts provide compression to the thorax to minimize chest expansion. They are used to stabilize rib fractures or the thorax after surgery. They may also be used as binders for surgical dressings. Proper fit is based on user chest circumference, just below the nipple line in males and just below the breasts in females. Contoured front panels on women's rib belts reduce the possibility of constriction of breast tissue.

Shoulder braces, either separately or combined with rib belts, support the chest wall, prevent scapular winging and help correct poor posture conditions. Size is determined by under-chest measurement and, in the case of full thorax vests, waist measurement. Some shoulder orthoses also contain side steels for extra back support. Padded clavicle straps for clavicle fractures form a figure eight around the user's shoulder and are fastened in the middle of the upper back with a Velcro closure. The strap, which is padded to provide firm compression in the clavicle area, is fitted on the basis of user chest circumference.

Abdominal binders provide compression to the pendulous abdomen for improving physical appearance and to aid in offsetting the strain on muscles, ligaments and joints. They may also be used for applying compression, when prescribed, after surgery, or as a binder for surgical dressings. Some models feature split-panel design to provide a tailored fit at both the waist and hips. Proper fit is based on user hip measurement, and, like rib belts, women's models have a lower height in the front.

Most **elbow, wrist, thigh, knee** and **ankle braces** consist of either one-way and two-way stretch surgical elastic or neoprene. Neoprene offers several advantages over traditional elasticized supports. It prevents body heat from escaping and therefore helps keep muscles, tendons and ligaments relaxed and helps reduce post-exercise soreness. Neoprene cushions against blows and bumps, and its protection is not diminished when it becomes wet because it does not absorb water. Lastly, it has a multidirectional stretch, thereby giving compression in the joint area. Some products like Coopercare Lastraps contain an insert which allows the product to intercept and neutralize damaging vibrations and shock waves, as well as utilizing natural body heat to keep the muscles warm and stimulate blood flow.

Epicondylitis or so-called "tennis elbow" is a common result of overexertion of the tendon-extensor attachments in the elbow joint (epicondylus medialis and lateralis) by exaggerated, one sided manual activity. The complaints of spontaneous pain and a lack of strength in the forearm extensors making the lifting of objects impossible are precipitated through local pressure and with dorsal extension of the hand against resistance. An effective health support is an epicondylitis clasp. This clasp or tightening strap compresses the forearm musculature at its largest circumference underneath the elbow, without impairing circulation. This produces a change in the trajectory motion of the tendons at their insertion at the epicondylus, thereby changing the local traction and forces on the joint and giving relief. These clasps should only be worn during sporting activities or work known to contribute to the condition.

Various elastic and neoprene elbow supports are also available for wearing over the elbow. They provide little relief for epicondylitis but are of value in providing minor compression on the joint, cushioning and protecting the elbow from bumps, and keeping the muscles, tendons and ligaments warm and relaxed in cases of sprains, strains, inflammation and arthritis. Some of these braces also incorporate an epicondylitis clasp. Fitting of elbow supports is based on consumer elbow circumference measurements.

Wrist braces provide support to the carpal ligaments at the hinge of the wrist in cases of strains and sprains and following cast removal. Use of removable metal splints provides greater support and keeps the wrist in a neutral position to facilitate healing. Fitting of wrist supports is based on user wrist circumference measurements.

The knee, the body's largest polycentric joint, is involved in 23 per cent of all sports injuries. Common injuries include stretched ligaments, torn cartilage, bursitis and patella chondromalacia or "runners knee" (roughening and softening of the posterior surface of the patella due to instability, injury or heredity). A variety of elastic and neoprene wraparound and slip-on knee braces exist to support, rest and cushion the knee. Closed patellar supports aid in the reduction of swelling; open patellar supports provide added stabilization to the knee. Braces with only anterior oval pads provide minimal support, and those with horseshoe-shaped anterior support pads maintain better knee alignment and position, thus offering greater support. Those using flexible stays and hinged side bars with encircling straps provide maximum support for medial-lateral stability. Fitting of knee supports is based on knee circumference measurements of the user.

The ankle is involved in 15 per cent of all sports injuries. Common injuries include sprains, stretched and torn ligaments, tendinitis and arthritis. A variety of elastic, neoprene and canvas wraparound, slip-on and lace-up braces are available to support and cushion the ankle. Some braces incorporate support stays on each side to enhance stability over the ankle joint by splinting the medial and lateral ligaments; some lace-up models also provide an anterior curved stay to minimize dorsiflexion. Aircasts consist of preinflated aircells lining the interior of the brace. These aircells conform to the ankle and gently compress swollen tissue, reducing swelling and edema. They resist inversion and protect sprained ankles against reinjury, often allowing ongoing participation in athletics. Aircells are preinflated and usually do not require further attention. Patients should always wear an absorbent sock for comfort and a laced shoe for maximum support with all ankle braces whenever possible. Fitting ankle supports is based on user ankle circumference measurements.

Companion **sports medicine and health support products** include the following: disposable and reusable hot and cold packs and dry and moist heat heating pads; sacrocushions and back cushions (for example, Obus Forme) for helping maintain correct sitting postures and minimize back fatigue; cervical pillows for supporting the neck and head for more correct sleeping posture and keeping muscles free from pressure, tension and strain; cervical traction kits; arm slings, cast covers and postoperative/cast shoes for fractures, bruises, dislocations or sprains of the foot; foot-care products (for example, blister pads, arch supports, shock-absorbing insoles and foot baths/massagers); and aerobic weights.

A number of points should be kept in mind when fitting health supports. Orthopedic supports and braces should be applied over garments like T-shirts to minimize chafing and appliance-induced discomfort. Weight and pressure are distributed evenly to minimize skin breakdown.

Most health supports fit both males and females. Exceptions include rib belts, abdominal binders, dorsolumbar supports and lumbosacral supports, for which women's garments are cut lower in the front to accommodate breast tissue and minimize tissue breakdown. These women's garments also have a greater hip development (the ratio between hip/waist measurements).

All health supports should be applied in the neutral position—without garment stays, hyperextension or flexion—unless so ordered by the individual's physician. When confronted with in-between sizes, the smaller size is usually chosen to ensure adequate support (but not at the expense of impaired circulation). All straps, stays and closures are marked so users are able to put their garments back on correctly. Consumers should hand wash and air dry all health support garments. Pharmacists should record the individual's name, address, date fitted and measurements, and type, model and size of fitted support for future reference should an adjustment be necessary or a replacement garment required.

Summary

The growing number of elderly, the trend toward self-care, greater subsidization and the increase in services from home health care agencies and hospital outpatient departments assure an increasing number of home health care consumers requiring products and services. Home health care provides all pharmacists with significant opportunity for business and professional growth and development. Although any pharmacy that can free a section of 1.2 to 2.4 metres can handle home health care products, the pharmacist's personal commitment is needed for the expertise to recommend the right equipment and supplies and to instruct consumers in proper use in this highly service-oriented industry. Pharmacists who are serious about developing this specialty need to work closely with medical and paramedical professionals, the industry and suppliers' representatives, and to expand their reading list of journals and publications to include those of allied health and medical specialties. (For example, *Ostomy Quarterly*, occupational therapy and physiotherapy journals and trade magazines, sports medicine publications, and so forth.) Even if the pharmacist chooses not to provide DME services, incontinence products, or health supports and appliances, the information in this chapter should provide the basis for a more intelligent and informed referral to other suppliers.

Suggested Reading
Journals
Home Health Care (Home Health Care Publishing Inc, 26 Dorchester Ave, Toronto, Ontario M8Z 4W3)

Home Health Care Merchandising (Home Health Care Publishing Inc, 26 Dorchester Ave, Toronto, Ontario M8Z 4W3)

Rx Homecare (825 South Barrington Ave, Los Angeles, California 90049)

Homecare Magazine (2048 Cotner Ave, Los Angeles, California 90025)

Homecare Product News (2048 Cotner Ave, Los Angeles, California 90025)

Books
Catania PN, Rosner M, eds. Home Health Care Practice. Palo Alto, California: Health Markets Research, 1986.

Eigan BN. Health accessories. In: Gennaro, AR, ed, Remington's pharmaceutical sciences, 17th ed. Easton, Pennsylvania: Mack Printing, 1985; 1824–68.

Other
Orthotics/Surgical Fitters Programs
Camp International Ltd
P.O. Box 495
Trenton, Ontario K8V 5R6

Airway Surgical Appliances Ltd
424 Catherine Street
Ottawa, Ontario K1R 5T8

Home Health Care Pharmacy Services,
National Association of Retail Druggists
205 Dangerfield Road
Alexandria, Virginia 22314

Courses for the Continuing Education of Pharmacists
Futuro, Cincinnati, Ohio

Ask the Consumer

Q. Why have ambulatory aids been recommended to you?
- The need for ambulatory aids generally falls into one of two groups: short-term rehabilitation following surgery or an accident, and long-term use in conjunction with a debilitating disease or disorder. Knowledge of intended use helps the pharmacist choose the best type of device and appropriate product characteristics (for example, durability and portability).

Q. Is the requested ambulatory aid for yourself or another individual?
- Ambulatory aids must be fitted carefully to an individual to assure safe and effective use. Purchasers who are not the intended users need to provide the desired user measurements. They also require instruction in the proper adjustment, use and maintenance of the device.

Q. Have you been instructed about what ambulatory gait you should use?
- Several different cane, crutch and walker gaits exist. The choice of gait depends on such factors as the type of ambulatory device, the user's strength, balance, mobility and underlying disorder, and

whether weight-bearing is indicated for the affected limb. Most individuals have their gait determined for them by their physician or physiotherapist. However, pharmacists should be familiar with the various gaits so they can reinforce the instructions and assist with the proper use of the ambulatory aid.

Q. Do you have assistance at home?

■ Consumers experiencing ambulatory difficulty and who lack assistance at home may require such devices as a bedside commode or bath bench-transfer seat to maintain their independence. Similarly, handicapped individuals without in-home assistance may require physical changes to their home, such as installation of ramps and lifts, and the purchase of self-help aids to assist eating, dressing and other activities of daily living.

Q. Why do you require a cane?

■ Canes differ in such features as the degree of support and balance they provide (monopod canes least, quad canes most), the amount of strength and dexterity required for use (monopod canes least, quad canes most) and durability (wooden canes least, aluminum canes most). These factors must be matched with consumer needs and limitations.

Q. Have you had a proper home assessment done for your ambulatory aids?

■ Consumers should be instructed in the proper footwear to use and the need to avoid slippery or uneven surfaces, throw rugs, loose cords and wires, and edges of bedspreads and furniture that might catch on ambulatory devices during use. Users may also need instruction on how to properly negotiate stairs with their devices. Such things as narrow doorways, the size of the bathroom, presence of stairs and the need for transfer from one area to another dictates the need for certain product characteristics such as removable wheelchair armrests or seatbacks, walkers, narrow-based quad canes, and folding walkers.

Q. What is the frequency and severity of your incontinence?

■ Incontinence briefs and pant-liners are effective and appropriate for ambulatory individuals with infrequent incontinence and small to moderate volumes of urine. People with more frequent incontinence, those passing moderate to large volumes of urine or stool, or who are recumbent probably require adult, diaper-type absorbent products or other devices, such as external catheters (males) or collection devices.

Q. What medications are you taking and what symptoms accompany your incontinence?

■ Many cases of urinary incontinence in the elderly are associated with and caused by a concurrent urinary tract infection. The presence of such symptoms as urinary frequency, urgency and dysuria necessitate referral to a physician for proper assessment and possible treatment. Poorly controlled diabetes, manifested by such signs and symptoms as polyuria, polydipsia, polyphagia and glucosuria/hyperglycemia, may also aggravate incontinence. The use of certain medications like diuretics and neuroleptics should be reviewed as possible contributors to an incontinent state.

Q. Has your skin started to break down?

■ Bedridden, wheelchair-bound and incontinent individuals are prone to pressure sores. Pharmacists can help prevent this complication by stressing the importance of keeping the skin dry, keeping sheets dry, smooth and unwrinkled, avoiding dragging individuals across bedding, and relieving pressure by frequent turning and the use of auxiliary devices like bed and seat cushions, sheepskin pads, and elbow and heel protectors. Wheelchair adjustment and seat inserts may be required.

Q. Why have compression stockings been recommended to you?

■ The choice of stocking (below-the-knee, above-the-knee or full-thigh) and degree of ankle compression depend on the type and severity of lower limb edema and varicosity and the mobility of the individual. Antiembolism stockings are indicated for the bedridden person; compression supports are reserved for the ambulatory individual.

Q. What are the user's measurements and how many days has it been since the operation or injury?

■ Health supports and garments must be individually sized and fitted to ensure proper support and immobility without compromising circulation or comfort or promoting skin breakdown. Common measurements include snug ankle, calf, knee, thigh, hip, chest and elbow sizings and looser waist and neck sizings. Fitting supports and appliances soon after surgery or injury may be associated with significant swelling, a factor that compromises fit and may necessitate a readjustment or refitting at a later time.

References

Introduction

Home health care marketing manual. Alexandria: National Association of Retail Druggists, 1985.

Kyriakos T. Homing in on a moving target. Drug Merch 1987;68(3):33–45.

Selling techniques in the home health care field. Alexandria: National Association of Retail Druggists, 1985.

Durable Medical Equipment

Cassak DJ. Competitors in home health care. In: Catania, PN; Rosner M, eds. Home health care practice. Palo Alto: Health Markets Research 1986;15–28.

Ambulatory Aids

Eigan BN. Health accessories. In: Gennaro AR, ed. Remington's pharmaceutical sciences. Easton: Mack Publishing, 1985:1824–68.

Fassett WE. Ambulatory aids and hospital equipment for the home. Catania, PN; Rosner M, eds. Home health care practice. Palo Alto: Health Markets Research, 1986:122–55.

Miller RY. Home health care. Ambulatory aids: crutches and walkers. US Pharmacist 1987;12(2):119–26.

Miller RY. Home health care. How to recommend the right cane for your patrons. US Pharmacist 1987;12(1):109–14.

Principles of home care for the convalescent. Patient aids. (A course for the continuing education of pharmacists.) Cincinnati: Futuro, 1984.

Incontinence Products

Gregory JG, Purcell MH. Urinary incontinence in the elderly: ways to relieve it without surgery. Postgrad Med 1986;80:253–62.

Help for incontinent people (Pamphlet). Union, SC.

Hogan DB, Parker WA, Sitland P. Urinary incontinence in the elderly. Drugs Ther Maritime Practitioners 1985;8:11–5.

Incontinence: the new dynamic category (Pamphlet). Montreal: Med-I-Pant, 1986.

Jeter KF. The patient with urinary incontinence. In: Catania, PN, Rosner M, eds. Home health care practice. Palo Alto: Health Markets Research, 1986:168–79.

Williams ME, Panill FC. Urinary incontinence in the elderly: physiology, pathophysiology, diagnosis, and treatment. Ann Intern Med 1982; 97:895–907.

Zoritto ML. The management of urinary incontinence in the elderly. Can Pharm J 1986;119:184–7.

Health Supports and Appliances

Kyriakos T. Cash in on fitness. Drug Merch 1986;67(3):24–8.

Principles and applications of health supports. (A course for the continuing education of pharmacists). Cincinnati: Futuro, 1987.

Compression Therapy

Miller RY. Home health care. Support stockings. US Pharmacist 1987; 12(3):128–34.

Principles and applications of elastic support hosiery. (A course for the continuing education of pharmacists.) Cincinnati: Futuro, 1987.

Skeletal Supports

Harris JD. Cervical orthoses. In: Redford JB, ed. Orthotics etcetera. Baltimore: Williams and Wilkins, 1986:100–21.

29
Baby Care

Revised by Michel Quesnel.
Based on the original chapter by Michel Quesnel and Pierre Dicaire

Pharmacists are often asked for advice on how to feed and care for infants. Breast-feeding has a number of advantages over commercial formulas. Parents choosing commercial formulas must consider a number of nutritional and individual factors. Babies also have special hygiene needs. Other concerns include diaper dermatitis, colic, teething, cradle cap, colds, fever, Reye's syndrome, diarrhea and providing a safe environment.

Feeding

Milk, used whole or as a mixture, is the most important source of nutrition for babies. Mother's milk is unanimously recognized as the best food for the newborn and young infant. The immunological protection and sense of security it provides cannot be copied even by the best modern technology (see Table I).

A comparison of the major nutritional components of breast milk and Canadian commercial infant formulas helps the pharmacist understand the basic chemistry behind each formula and the major differences to better advise parents on their choice of preparations and uses.

The majority of commercial formulas are milk-based. They are modified and transformed with the help of today's technology to try to equal, in quality and quantity, the components of human milk (proteins, lipids, carbohydrates, vitamins and minerals). Milk-based infant formulas are made in one of two ways. One method involves adding lactose and vegetable oil to fat-free milk solids to reach levels recommended for infant formulas. The second method involves adding lactoserum (whey) to nonfat cow's milk (see Table II).

Protein

Proteins provide the infant with all the amino acids essential to normal growth. Government regulations require a minimum quantity of protein, therefore the quantity is comparable in all commercial formulas. Differences are apparent in the quality of protein used (see Table III).

Commercial milk formulas are composed of two types of proteins—casein and lactoserum—that are found in a 40:60 ratio in most regular commercial formulas. In contrast, the ratio of casein to lactoserum in cow's milk is 80:20.

The claimed advantage of the higher ratio of lactoserum is that it produces a softer curd, which is more easily digested and absorbed

by the newborn than the casein-dominant formulas. The protein ratio is even more important to pre-term infants, because the protein profile influences the acid-base balance. Problems of metabolic acidosis and hyperazotemia are more common in pre-term infants fed cow's milk.

Table I	*Advantages of Mother's Milk*	
Immunological	**Nutritional**	**Psychological**
No allergy to human proteins	Less protein, therefore less excretion of nitrogen	Promotes sensory stimulation
Less contamination		Promotes confidence in infant and mother
Immunoglobulin A protects intestinal mucosa	Less casein, therefore more digestible	
*Bifidogenous factor	Fewer minerals, therefore renal load is better	Promotes emotional stability
Presence of lysozymes, which are bactericidal	Calcium: Phophorous ratio=2:1, therefore increased absorption of calcium	Promotes mother-child relationship
Presence of lactoferrins, which prevent bacterial development	Saturated fatty acid digestion	
Presence of macrophages for phagocytosis	Cholesterol •myelinization of nerves •synthesis of steroid hormones •promotes production of bile acids	
Presence of interferons, which are antiviral and antibacterial		
Antistaphylococcal factor	No preparation, inexpensive, fresh, always ideal temperature	
	No additives or adjuvants	

*Lactose is responsible for the bifidogenous factor, that is, the digestion of lactose created in an acid environment not favorable to the proliferation of microorganisms responsible for gastroenteritis.

Table II *Commercial Formulas*

Types of milk (Manufacturer)	Proteins g/dL	Ratio casein: lactoserum	Lipids g/dL	Carbohydrates g/dL	CAL/mL	Osmolarity (mOsm/L)	Renal solute load (mOsm/L)	Elemental iron mg/dL	Forms	Dilutions	Shelf-life if prepared	Particulars	Advantages (see legend)
Human	Human 1.1	40:60	4.5	Lactose 6.8	0.72±	273	77	0.15	—	—	May be frozen but freezing does not preserve immunological properties of human milk	—	See Table I
Cow's	Bovine	82:18	Bovine 3.8	Lactose 5.0	0.63	290	228	0.05	—	—	—	Homogenized not recommended before 6 months; 2% not before 1 year	—
Similac with Whey Ross	Bovine 1.5	40:60	LCT 3.6 Soy-coconut	Lactose 7.2	0.67	260	108	0.15 or 1.2	Ready-to-serve Concentrated powder	1:1 1:60	48 hours 24 hours	• with or without iron • vegetable lipid source • whey protein source: 60% or 18%	1, 2, 7
Regular Similac Ross		82:18											
S-M-A Wyeth	Bovine 1.5	40:60	LCT 3.6 Soy-coconut Sesame	Lactose 7.2	0.67	270	90	0.15 or 1.3	Ready-to-serve 385 mL Concentrated powder	1:1 1:60	48 hours 24 hours	• with or without iron • vegetable lipid source • whey protein source: 60%	1, 2, 7
Enfalac Mead Johnson	Bovine 1.5	40:60	LCT 3.8 Soy-coconut Corn Soy oil 60% Copra 40%	Lactose 7.0	0.67	260	102	0.15 or 1.2	Ready-to-serve Concentrated powder	1:1 1:30	48 hours 24 hours	• with or without iron • vegetable lipid source therefore more digestible • whey protein source	1, 2
Isomil Ross	Soy (isolate) 2.0	—	LCT 3.6 Soy-coconut	Sucrose Maltose 6.8	0.67	228	126	1.2	Ready-to-serve Concentrated powder	1:1 1:60	24 hours	• no lactose • vegetable protein source	3, 6
Meat-base Gerber	Beef heart 2.7	—	Bovine and sesame 3.5	Sucrose Maltose 6.8	0.67	—	—	1.37	Concentrated	1:1	24 hours	• no lactose • protein source can be other than beef	3, 6
Nursoy Wyeth	Soy (isolate) 2.3	—	LCT 3.6 Soy-coconut	Sucrose Maltose 6.8	0.67	185	130	1.3	Powder	1:30	24 hours	• improved homogeneity when mixing • vegetable protein source	4, 6

Baby Care

Table II (Cont'd) Commercial Formulas

Types of milk (Manufacturer)	Proteins g/dL	Ratio casein: lactoserum	Lipids g/dL	Carbohydrates g/dL	CAL/mL	Osmolarity (mOsm/L)	Renal solute load (mOsm/L)	Elemental iron mg/dL	Forms	Dilutions	Shelf-life if prepared	Particulars	Advantages (see legend)
Nutramigen Mead Johnson	Hydrolyzed casein 2.2	—	LCT 3.6 Corn	Sucrose Dextrin Starch 8.8	0.67	400	160	1.3	Powder	1:62	48 hours	•no lactose •vegetable protein source •higher molarity	3, 4, 6
Prosobee Mead Johnson	Soy (isolate) 2.5	—	LCT 3.4 Soy-coconut	Maltose Dextrose Glucose polymer	0.67	180	130	1.3	Ready-to-serve Concentrated powder	1:1 1:30	24 hours	•liquid form without lactose •powder without lactose and sucrose •formula to be used during diagnosis if allergy is suspected	3, 6
Portagen Mead Johnson	Bovine 2.0	—	LCT (13%) corn MCT (87%) 3.4	Sucrose Dextrin Maltose 8.1	0.67	237	150	1.3	—	—	—	•no lactose •lipid source: MCT	5, 6
Pregestimil Mead Johnson	Hydrolyzed casein 1.9	—	LCT (60%) MCT (40%) Corn and coconut 2.7	Starch Dextrin Maltose 9.2	0.67	297	125	1.3	Powder	1 cup: 29oz. give 1 quart	24 hours	•no lactose •no bovine proteins	3, 4, 5
RCF Ross	Soy 2.0	—	LCT 3.6 Soy-coconut	Add: 5.2 g	0.68	Depending on CHO added	—	0.15	Concentrated	1:1 + 52 g of CHO	24 hours	•no carbohydrates •no bovine proteins •deficient in iron	5
Similac-24 LBW Ross	Bovine 2.2	—	LCT (50%) MCT (50%) 4.5 Corn-coconut	Lactose 8.5	0.81	260	147	1.2	Powder	1:60	48 hours	•rich source of MCT •high in calories	8
Enfamil-24 LBW Mead Johnson	Bovine 2.4	—	LCT (60%) MCT (40%) 4.1 Corn-coconut	Lactose 8.9	0.80	264	147	1.2	Powder	—	24 hours	•high in calories •lipid (MCT and LCT)	8

Table II *(Cont'd) Commercial Formulas*

Types of milk (Manufacturer)	Proteins g/dL	Ratio casein: lactoserum	Lipids g/dL	Carbohydrates g/dL	CAL/mL	Osmolarity (mOsm/L)	Renal solute load (mOsm/L)	Elemental iron mg/dL	Forms	Dilutions	Shelf-life if prepared	Particulars	Advantages (see legend)
Similac PM 60/40 Ross	Bovine 1.58	—	LCT 3.7 Corn-coconut	Lactose Maltose 6.88	0.68	239	92	0.15	Ready-to-serve powder	1:60	24 hours	• vegetable lipid source • low protein and mineral content • for infants weighing less than 1,500 g	—
Similac Special-care 20 Ross	Bovine 1.8	—	MCT 3.7 Corn-coconut	Lactose Maltose 7.17	0.68	260	—	0.24	Ready-to-serve	—	24 hours	• vegetable lipid source rich in MCT • for infants weighing less than 2,000 g	8
Similac Special-care Ross	Bovine 2.2	—	LCT 4.4	Lactose 8.6	0.81	260	—	0.3	Ready-to-serve	—	24 hours	• for infants weighing less than 2,000 g	8
Lofenalac Mead Johnson	Hydrolyzed casein 2.3	—	LCT 2.7 Corn	Starch Dextrin Maltose 8.8	0.68	454	140	1.3	Powder	9.5 g in 2oz. of water	—	• no lactose • hydrolyzed casein protein • low phenylalanine content	—
Milumil Milupa	1.8	82:18	LCT 3.1 Coconut-soy	Lactose Maltose Starch 8.2	0.68	380 to 410	—	1.1	Granulated	1:30	24 hours 1 month	• high casein content • high starch content	—
Alactamil Mead Johnson	1.5	—	3.7	6.9	—	—	—	1.2	—	—	—	• no lactose • protein is soy based	3
Alimentum Ross	1.86	—	3.75	6.89	—	—	—	1.2	—	—	—	• casein hydrolysate	4

LCT=long chain triglycerides (vegetable origin, unsaturated)
MCT=medium-chain triglycerides (vegetable origin, unsaturated)
Osmolarity must be less than 400 Osm/L. If the formula is too concentrated, it can cause such problems as enterocolitis, diarrhea and dehydration.
Osmolarity connected with carbohydrate and mineral content varies according to the amount of kcal/L.
Soy-based formulas have a low osmolarity;
Powders have a high osmolarity for the same product.
Renal load in aqueous solution: The relation of proteins and minerals contained in the formula is expressed as the amount of
mEq of NA-K-CL+4 mOsm/urea/g of protein per litre of formula,
for example: human milk=99 mEq; cow's milk=314 mEq; infant feeding
formulas=125 to 150 mEq
Iron content of Regular formulas is currently 0.11 to 0.15 mg/mL,
but this could increase depending on future recommendations of pediatricians.

Advantages
1. Supplement; alternative to nursing; substitute in full term infant with intolerance to bovine lipids
2. Infant requiring more iron between 3 to 4 months (use formulas enriched with iron); prevention of iron-deficiency anemias
3. Newborn allergic to milk; intolerance to bovine proteins and lactose
4. Newborn sensitive to intact proteins
5. Newborn with lipid restriction such as cystic fibrosis (lipase enzyme), heart disease and steatorrhea: formulas with MCT have an advantage
6. Newborn intolerance to lactose, newborn with galactosemia, disaccharidase deficiency
7. Newborn with heart disease (congenital)
8. Newborn weighing less than 2 kg and pre-term less than 37 weeks

Table III *Types of Proteins*

Sources	P.E.R.[a]	Comments
Animal (casein)	100	increased allergenicity, decreased digestibility
Human (whey)	100	nonallergenic, increased digestibility
Beef hearts	80	
Vegetables (soya)	70	less allergenic, increased digestibility
Hydrolyzed casein	100	less allergenic, increased digestibility

[a] P.E.R.: Protein Efficiency Ratio—reflects the weight gain per g of protein fed (casein being the standard). If a formula has a P.E.R. less than 100 per cent of casein, the amount of protein (g/100 kcal) should be increased to compensate for the lower P.E.R.

Although breast-feeding should always be encouraged, health care workers should assure parents that commercial formulas are nutritionally sound and promote normal growth and development when used properly. Commercial formulas usually supply all an infant's nutritional needs until 4 to 6 months of age, when solids may be introduced.

Depending on the population studied, the estimate of cow's milk allergies vary (0.3 to 7 per cent). This low percentage explains why most commercial formulas are cow-milk based. The industry has developed soy-based formulas for the 1 in 13 infants allergic to regular formulas (see Table II). However, studies show that 40 per cent of newborns allergic to regular formulas may become allergic to soy-based formulas.

Recent studies show that the ratio of casein to lactoserum, which was thought to be 40:60 in breast milk, is really 20:80. Therefore, qualitatively, no commercial formula on the market today can claim to closely resemble mother's milk (a claim often made in the past for lactoserum-enriched formulas). Also, those enriched with lactoserum contain not human, but bovine (cow) lactoserum, which contains the molecule beta-lactoglobulin. This molecule, responsible for allergy problems, is absent from human milk (see Table IV). Human lactoserum is more easily digested than bovine lactoserum, but the digestibility of bovine lactoserum compared to casein is about the same.

The casein to lactoserum ratio is important, because it directly affects amino acid metabolism. Recent studies show that the plasma concentration of amino acids in babies fed with formulas enriched with lactoserum is not similar to the concentration of amino acids in breast-fed babies. Formulas enriched with lactoserum have an advantage for pre-term infants because a high-ratio casein formula can produce acidosis. Some practitioners consider enriched formulas unnecessary to produce a pattern and plasma concentration of amino

Table IV *Differences Among Types of Milk*

Factor	Cow's milk	Mother's milk	Infant feeding formulas
Allergenicity	More frequent	Less frequent	Less frequent, varies according to type of protein or carbohydrates used
Aqueous solution	Increased density in aqueous solution	Ideal aqueous solution density 270 to 300 mOsm/L	
Digestion (curds)	Forms large, hard and indigestible curds. Slows gastric evacuation	Forms small curds, easy to digest which do not slow gastric evacuation	Forms small curds, easy to digest which do not slow gastric evacuation
Fats	More difficult to absorb, infant gets 2/3 of the quantity required		
Iron	Deficient in iron, increased risk of anemia or aggravating existing anemia	Has enough iron first 4 months if mother's intake is adequate	Meets daily standard requirement
Proteins	Protein content more than 3 times higher than mother's milk	Ideal protein content: 1.5 g/100 kcal and more	
Protein content and aqueous solution density	Increased protein content and aqueous solution density: 321 mOsm/L. Promotes and predisposes to edema, hypernatremic dehydration	Ideal protein content and aqueous solution density: mother's milk 99 mOsm/L	Infant feeding formulas: 135 to 140 mOsm/L
Vitamins and minerals	Deficient in vitamin C, zinc and copper	Has essential vitamins and minerals if mother's intake is adequate	Has daily requirement in vitamins and minerals recommended for newborn
Comments	2%: not before 1 year old. Homogenized: not before 6 months old. Skim milk: not before 2 years old.		Check fluoride according to formula type and region.

Adapted from: Anonymous. Current issues in feeding the normal infant. Pediatrics 1985;75(1):000.

Table V *Carbohydrates in Commercial Formulas*

Carbohyrate	Comments
Lactose (polysaccharide)	• Predominant carbohydrate in breast milk and commercial standard formulas • Hydrolyzed by enzyme lactase to glucose and galactose • Indirectly improves calcium absorption • Creates an acidic environment which discourages the growth of pathogenic bacteria • It is the least sweet tasting, ideal for supplementing breast milk (one sixth as sweet as sucrose) • Avoid if lactose intolerant and in premature infants (born during the seventh and eighth months). Premature infants may be able to hydrolyze only one third the amount of lactose hydrolyzed by term infants
Sucrose (polysaccharide)	• Sweeter taste (avoid if looking for formula supplement when breast-feeding) • Avoid if infant suffers from diarrhea • Avoid in feeding, because sucrose readily splits into fructose which is not dealt with well by neonate liver and may lead to acidosis and hypoglycemia
Maltose (polysacchride)	• Sweeter taste (one third as sweet as sucrose) • Well tolerated
Galactose (monosaccharide)	• Easily digested
Fructose (monosaccharide)	• Easily digested
Glucose (monosaccharide)	• Easily digested

acids similar to the ones found in the breast-fed baby. Until further studies show the contrary, formulas enriched with lactoserum are unnecessary for a normal-term infant.

Lipids

Fat, a concentrated source of energy, provides anywhere from 40 to 50 per cent of total food energy. The major roles of this component are to act as carrier of fat-soluble vitamins, to help with the absorption of calcium, and to supply essential fatty acids not synthesized by the human body (linoleic-arachidonic) and that are important for myelination and nervous system development.

Any deficiency in these essential fatty acids can lead to such problems as growth retardation, skin changes, hair loss and increase in metabolic rate. The Committee on Nutrition of the American Academy of Pediatrics recommends a minimum of 3.3 g of fat per 100 kcal to a maximum of 6 g/100 kcal. An intake of linoleic acid of 300 mg/100 kcal or about 2.4 per cent of total calories is also necessary. Although linoleic acid is 4 per cent of the total energy of human milk, the minimum amount required in commercial formulas is still controversial.

Chemically, fats may be classified as saturated or unsaturated. Saturated fats are harder to digest and more poorly absorbed than

unsaturated fats such as vegetable oils, especially in the first 6 months of life. Most commercial formulas have replaced butterfat with vegetable oil to attain this higher digestibility. Vegetable oil digestibility is decreased with large amounts of long-chain fatty acids, so the shorter the chains, the better the absorption. Soy and corn oils are easier to digest than coconut oil, which contains a higher number of long-chain saturated fatty acids.

Finally, some formulas are free of, or low in, fats. These formulas are regarded as therapeutic and should be used under medical supervision (see Table II).

Carbohydrates

No well defined, absolute requirements exist for carbohydrates in infancy. However, carbohydrates provide 40 per cent or more of the infant's energy requirements. Some authorities claim that more than 50 per cent of calories derived from carbohydrates are contraindicated, because the infant's ability to hydrolyse disaccharides is compromised, resulting in loose, acidic, watery stools.

The sources of carbohydrates used in infant formulas are disaccharides (lactose, sucrose, maltose) and monosaccharides (galactose, fructose, glucose). Some formulas contain polysaccharides (starch) (see Table V).

In human milk, the content of carbohydrates is about 7 g/mL of which 30 per cent is lactose and the remainder is oligosaccharides. Human milk does not contain fructose or sucrose. Lactose is hydrolyzed by the enzyme lactase and is absorbed as glucose and galactose. Lactose is the predominant carbohydrate in both breast milk and commercial formulas and is important for growth and other functions (see Table V). Infants who lack the enzyme lactase, needed to digest the carbohydrate, are lactose-intolerant. These babies can benefit from soy-based formulas, because the carbohydrates used are a combination of 2 or more of glucose, corn syrup, saccharose and sucrose, which are tolerated by lactose-intolerant infants (see Table II).

Electrolytes (Renal Solute Load)

Other important considerations when choosing or making recommendations on a formula are the renal solute load, osmolarity and osmolality of the formula.

Renal solute load is the excess dietary proteins and electrolytes that must be excreted by the kidney. It can be calculated by the sum of mEq of sodium, potassium and chloride plus 4 mOsm of urea per g of protein in a litre of formula. The renal solute loads of human milk and cow's milk are 79 and 228 mOsm /L, respectively.

Osmolarity refers to the concentration of solute in a solution per unit of total volume of solution and is expressed as mOsm/L of formula. Human milk has an osmolarity of 273 mOsm/L. Commercial formulas with an osmolarity greater than 400 mOsm/L must have a warning statement on the label, because hyperosmolar formulas can contribute to necrotizing enterocolitis, especially during the early neonatal period.

Osmolality relates to the carbohydrate and mineral content of the formula and refers to the concentration of solute in a solution per unit of solvent. It is expressed as mOsm/kg. The osmolality of human milk is 300 mOsm/kg of water.

To avoid an excess of protein-electrolytes, commercially prepared formulas must contain levels of protein and electrolytes in amounts that prevent excess water loss and do not overburden immature kidneys. At present, all commercial formulas, with few exceptions, meet the proper requirements. However, an additional step—dilution—is required in preparing concentrated and powder formulas. The pharmacist can ensure the mixing (dilution) instructions are well understood by the parents. Errors in dilution during preparation increase the renal solute load, osmolarity, osmolality and produce an hyperosmolal state that brings on diarrhea and dehydration which can be fatal to the child.

Finally, the pharmacist should discourage the use of whole, unmodified cow's milk during the first 6 months of life and 2 per cent or skim milk during the first 12 months because of the high protein and mineral content of unmodified cow's milk (see Table IV).

Vitamin and Mineral Requirements

The Food and Drug Act has established the minimum dosage of vitamins and minerals for commercial preparations. These preparations are complete and contain all the essential elements necessary for the infant. It is therefore unnecessary to add any vitamin-mineral supplements, except fluoride when needed (see Table VI). However, supplements may be recommended for special needs depending on whether the infant is breast-fed or formula-fed, and pre-term or term (see Table VI).

A child nourished by breast milk may need a daily supplement of vitamin D (400 IU) during the first 6 months (especially if the child is born in winter). An iron requirement of 0.7 mg/day of **elemental**

Table VI *Vitamin and Mineral Supplements for Pre-term and Full-term Infants When Receiving Mother's Milk or Commercial Formulas*

	Supplement	Comment
Breast-fed infants		
Term	Vit. D	Because of its antirachitic properties a supplement of 400 IU/day may be required (first 6 months)
	Vit. B$_{12}$	If the mother is a strict vegetarian (to prevent megaloblastic anemia)
	Iron	The neonatal stores may be depleted after 6 months or more, iron in a prophylactic dosage of 1 mg/kg/day is suggested until 12 months, but not necessary if solid foods and iron fortified cereals are introduced
	Fluoride	Before recommending a fluoride supplement, the fluoride content of the area water supply must be considered

Age	Conc. of Fluoride in Drinking Water (ppm)		
	<0.3	0.3–0.7	>0.7
<2 years	0.25mg/day	—	—
2–3 years	0.50mg/day	0.25mg/day	—
>3 years	1.00mg/day	0.50mg/day	—

Pre-term	Phosphate	Prior to reaching a body weight of 2.5 kg or calorie intake of 300 kcal/day, a multivitamin supplement plus folate is needed, 0.1 mg/day
		Iron supplements may start sooner (2 months but not before) and need higher doses (2 mg/kg/day). A supplement of phosphate might be required: breast (150 mg/L), formula (450 mg/L)
Formula-fed infants		
Full-terms	None, except iron at 4 to 6 months	Iron fortified formula must be used for all formula-fed infants. Level of iron in fortified formula: 7 to 13 mg/day of iron. Level of 7 mg/day: recommendation of Health and Welfare
		The consumption of adequate amounts of formulas exclude the first 6 months and introduction of solid foods negates the need for supplements
		N.B. Pediatricians recommend an iron-fortified formula after 4 to 6 months
	Fluoride depending on the region	Also when using formulas, either ready-to-serve, concentrated or powdered, fluoride should be administered if the water contains less than 0.3 ppm or if using spring water containing adequate fluoride levels
Pre-terms	Vit. E	They require special formulas with modified contents
	Iron	Because of a more rapid growth rate, a greater nutrient need and reduced intestinal absorption, the pre-term infant requires more vitamin and mineral supplements. However, amounts have not been established for low birth weight infants and the American Academy of Pediatrics recommends the same amounts as the normal formulas except for vit. E. Low birth weight infants consume smaller quantities of formula, so to fulfill the needs of the infant, certain special formulas exist (for example, Similac special care) which have added vitamins, but respect the guidelines set by the Food and Drug Act.
		A daily supplement of iron in the form of ferrous sulfate is recommended when iron-fortified formula is not used.

Table VII *Feeding and Supplement Guidelines For Infants*

Age (months)	Feeding	Liquids*			Supplements			Solids
		Mother's milk	Infant feeding formulas	Juice	Vit. D	Iron	Fluoride	
1–4	Liquids only, no solid foods	590 mL/day (1 to 3 months) 920 mL/day (4 months)	590 mL/day (1 to 3 months) 920 mL/day (4 months)	No	400 IU	7 mg	0.25 mg	None
5	Liquids and cereals on medical advice	1 010 mL/day	1 010 mL/day	Yes	400 IU	7 mg	0.25 mg	Baby cereal enriched with iron, do not add cereal to bottle
6	Liquids and cereals on medical advice	1 010 mL/day*	100 mL/day	Yes	400 IU	7 mg	0.25 mg	3 to 5 tbsp. (cereal) 2 to 5 tbsp. (fruit) 2 to 5 tbsp. (vegetable puree)

*The liquid volumes are calculated on the basis of 110 to 120 kcal/kg/day and most formulas contain 67 kcal/100 mL.

iron for the first year is needed, to meet the iron needs for hemoglobin synthesis (see Table VII). An iron supplement can be avoided if the infant has been introduced to cereal or meat or if the child takes an iron-fortified formula. Cow's milk does not meet the child's needs for vitamin C, vitamin E and iron (see Table VIII).

Product Selection

The pharmacist can help parents determine whether breast-feeding or commercial formulas best meet their needs by discussing advantages and disadvantages of both (see Table IV). If commercial formulas are chosen, the pharmacist can reassure the parents that these formulas offer a good substitute for breast milk and promote normal growth and development.

Once the type of formula (standard versus physician-advised therapeutic) has been determined to meet the needs of the infant, a number of points must be considered before making a recommendation on type or form (ready-to-serve, concentrated or powder): attitude and preference of the parents; need and use of the formula (occasional feeding, supplement to breast-feeding or for travelling); parents' ability to follow directions; sanitary conditions; water supply (innocuity of the water); available storage facilities for the prepared formulas; cost; and convenience.

Concentrated formulas are the most economical and easiest to prepare of the commercial formulas. Mothers who breast-feed and only partly bottle-feed may find the powder form more economical, but it requires additional manipulation and adequate mixing. If in doubt about water supply, the ready-to-use form is safest, but most expensive.

Formula Preparation

Parents feeding their infant with commercial formula for the first time often feel overwhelmed by the complexity of the operation. These parents would surely appreciate receiving brochures on formula preparation from their pharmacist. Recommendations for the preparation of bottle feeding depend on sanitary conditions in the home, water supply, type of equipment used and formula base.

There are three methods of sterilization: the aseptic method, the terminal heating method, and the single-bottle method. Although all methods are acceptable and are generally described in brochures furnished by the manufacturers, certain details should be pointed out. In our environment the aseptic method is acceptable, although it represents a higher risk of contamination. It has the least effect on the thermolabile component of the formula and is the only method recommended for bottles with inner disposable plastic bags (see Table IX). The terminal method is safer and recommended especially

Table VIII *Vitamin Content of Different Types of Milk*

Content per L	Human milk	Commercial formulas	Unmodified cow's milk	2%	Skim milk
Vitamin A (IU)	2,500	2,500	1,500	1,500	1,500
Vitamin D (IU)	22	400	360	360	360
Vitamin E (IU)	1.8	15	0.8	–	–
Thiamine (mg)	0.14	0.65	0.4	0.4	0.4
Riboflavin (mg)	0.37	1.0	1.7	1.7	1.4
Niacin (mg)	1.8	7.0	8.7	8.9	9.1
Vitamin B$_6$ (mg)	0.11	0.4	0.4	0.4	0.4
Folic acid	52	50	50	50	50
Vitamin C (mg)	52	55	15	10	10

Table IX *Bottle and Formula Preparation*

Aseptic method	Terminal heat method	Single-bottle
After feeding, rinse bottle-nipple with cool water.	Same as aseptic method.	Same as aseptic method.
Wash day supply of bottles, nipples and caps in hot water and rinse thoroughly.	Same as aseptic method.	Same as aseptic method.
Boil all utensils required for mixing and preparing of formula as well as bottles, nipples and caps for 5 min. Remove items and place on clean towel. Boil amount of water necessary for formula dilution for 5 min. Remove and let cool to room temperature.	Wash all utensils required for mixing and preparing of formula. Prepare formula with tap water (watch for over or underdilution) and pour into clean nursing bottles, attach the nipples and cover them loosely with caps.	Same as terminal heat method.
Rinse top of formula can with soap and hot water. Open and add the required amount, dilute with boiled water and mix.	Place in sterilizer or in deep cooking utensil. Add water to mid point of bottles. Cover and boil gently for 25 min.	Same as terminal heat method.
Pour the formula into pre-sterilized bottles and attach the nipples and cap with aseptic care.	Remove from heat, cool slightly and tighten.	Same as terminal heat method.
Store in refrigerator until feeding (24 to 48 hours).	Same as aseptic method.	Feed the infant when formula is at room temperature.

when the hygiene condition of the household and environment is not satisfactory. The drawback to this method is that it destroys the thermolabile components such as vitamin C present in the formula. The single-bottle method is good when breast-feeding is supplemented with occasional bottles of formula.

Recommendations

Infants 4 months and over should receive a formula enriched with iron (depending if cereal or solid foods are given). The nutrition recommendations of Health and Welfare state that formula-fed infants should receive iron-fortified formula. Solid food should be introduced around 5 to 6 months and rarely before 4 months. Breast-feeding mothers who want to use formula occasionally should wait at least 3 to 4 weeks after starting breast-feeding before giving the baby formula to allow time for lactation to stabilize. No vitamins are required for full-term formula-fed infants. Some vitamins are required for breast-fed infants.

If using a microwave oven to heat a bottle, parents should remove the cap and nipple first, as these should not be put in the microwave.

They should be sure the heat is distributed evenly before giving the bottle to the infant (shaking the bottle before checking the temperature). Parents should check the expiry date of the formula and read the manufacturer's preparation instructions carefully. Prepared formula should be refrigerated and not kept beyond the manufacturer's recommendation (24 to 48 hours). Parents should discard unused portions after feeding. They should not use whole unmodified cow's milk during the baby's first 6 months, nor 2 per cent or skim milk during the first 12 months. Before using a fluoride supplement, parents should consider the fluoride content of area water and the age of the infant.

Hygiene

The first form of communication for the baby is through body contact with parents. Bathing should be a source of pleasure, relaxation, communication and freedom with your baby. Tactile manipulations necessary for bathing and frolicking in the water provide the infant with a source of intense pleasure and allow new experiences in discovering the world. Optimal communication occurs when the infant feels safe in an atmosphere of calm. Parents promote such an atmosphere when they feel the same calm and satisfaction.

The aims and benefits of bathing a baby are numerous. Daily bathing (unless the baby is sick) stimulates circulation and offers the baby an opportunity to exercise. In hot weather, bathing is a source of refreshment. Bath time reassures the parents by allowing them to examine their babies and assess their general state. Bathing promotes the infant/parent relationship through touching, speaking and seeing. It is a good time for parents and infants to get to know each other.

Bathing Materials

The following materials are useful for the baby's bathtime care: bath towel; soft washcloth; mild soap; brush and/or comb; personal clothing; cotton wads; mild shampoo; water basin; sink or large bath; ethyl alcohol; cotton swabs; moisturizing lotion; and vegetable oil. The newborn can be bathed in the bathroom, kitchen or any other room with suitable conditions. The room should be comfortable (22 to 23°C) and without drafts. The working area should be large enough to arrange the required material before the bath. By arranging materials before the bath, the parents respect the basic rule of never leaving infants alone in the bath and constantly monitoring them to avoid falls. The height of the work table should enable parents to be comfortable, that is, to avoid inappropriate stretching and crouching for long periods of time, both of which cause fatigue.

If possible, the child should be bathed before being fed, since increased activity during the bath increases the possibility of regurgitation after a meal.

The folds in a child's skin easily conserve moisture and become a preferred place for irritations. The areas behind the auricle, between the fingers and toes, the armpits, the groin and the area between the buttocks should be rinsed carefully and dried well.

Care of the Umbilical Cord

The umbilicus usually heals within 8 to 10 days. The cord falls off easily by itself and should never be rushed. To allow rapid healing, the umbilical cord should be kept dry by exposing it to air if possible and by applying alcohol with a cotton swab 3 to 4 times a day.

Baby Care

(Alcohol dries the cord and prevents growth of fungus and bacteria in the navel.) At each daily bath, parents should clean the navel region with water and mild soap, then rinse it well and dry it to prevent infection. Cream, lotion or oil should not be applied as these substances slow the drying process and can lead to infection. Dressings on the navel also slow drying and should not be used. Other suggestions include lowering the diaper to below the cord; using nonclinging, loose clothing; and placing the baby on a side rather than on the stomach when sleeping. A physician should be notified immediately if a discharge or foul odor comes from the navel or if the skin becomes extremely red.

Sponge Bathing

The child is reassured by gentle, firm gestures and by being held tightly. Talking to the baby during the bath also increases the pleasure.

Parents and caregivers should wash the baby's eyes first with clean, moist cotton wads, one for each eye. Washing should be from the inside corner of the eye outward. If the tear duct is blocked, the parents should gently massage along the eyelid below the eye, starting from the middle of the eye and going toward the corner near the nose, 2 or 3 times a day. If the infant's eyes run a great deal and if the secretions are substantial enough to cause the eyelids to stick together, the parents should consult a health professional.

Parents can wash the face and outer parts of the ears with a moist, clean face cloth, without using soap. They should never use oil as it can damage the inside of the ears and the respiratory tract. Cotton swabs should never be used to clean the ears and nose because one move by the child can injure the fragile mucous membranes. Also, a cotton swab used in the inner part of the ear can push the cerumen against the tympanic wall and prevent the normal drying process and expulsion of the cerumen.

Parents can rinse the baby's scalp with a face cloth. They can wash the head with a mild shampoo 2 or 3 times a week, rubbing the scalp gently with the palm of the hand. The head should be rinsed and well dried to prevent a soap residue forming a film on the scalp (see cradle cap below).

The preferred position for holding the baby is the "football" position. The head and nape of the neck are supported by the hand while the hips are supported by the upper arm. In this position it is easy to wash behind the ears and neck.

Parents should undress the baby in stages and remember that the infant gets cold quickly. After applying a mild soap on the face cloth, they should wash the arms, torso, legs, feet and back and finish with the genitals. They should rinse well and dry gently.

Occasional dry skin is normal for the newborn. Only in cases of dry skin should moisturizing lotion (without perfume) or lanolin be applied to soften the skin and make it supple. The use of oil or powder on the body is not recommended except in the diaper area, as it blocks the pores of the skin and retains secretions, causing irritation. The particles of powder can be inhaled by the child, irritating the respiratory tract.

Care of the Genitals

For a girl, parents should delicately clean the vulva with water and mild soap, from the front (urinary meatus) to the back (anus) to avoid contaminating the vagina and urethra with fecal matter. The area should be rinsed well.

For a boy, if the foreskin sticks too much to the glans, parents should not manipulate it excessively to loosen it, but should consult a physician. If the baby is circumcised, parents should follow the doctor's instructions. Prepuce adhesion to the glans is a normal phenomenon up to the age of 3. It is not necessary to maintain a meticulous hygiene of the penis before then. At about age 3, retraction of the penis will be normal and complete. At this age, while the child is bathing the parent should completely retract the prepuce and wash the penis with soap and water.

Care of the Nails

To improve general appearance and prevent scratches, especially to the face, it is important to cut a child's fingernails and toenails regularly. Nail scissors are preferable. Trimming is easiest when the child is sleeping, minimizing accidents caused when the baby moves. The nails should be cut straight across and slightly rounded at the corners.

Diaper Dermatitis*

Diaper dermatitis (diaper rash) is an irritation of babies' skin characterized by redness, itching and burning. The condition, which is limited to the diaper area, causes the baby to be irritable and may lead to difficulty sleeping. Other skin conditions may also affect the diaper area: fungus infections that develop as a result of thrush or taking broad spectrum oral antibiotics; bacterial infections; intertrigo; or erosion of the urinary meatus dermatitis. Such conditions should not be confused with diaper dermatitis. Babies with these complications should be seen by a physician.

Various factors can cause or contribute to diaper dermatitis: an occluded area promoting dampness; mechanical irritation caused by the diaper rubbing against the skin; irritation caused by stools or their breakdown products; and chemical irritation caused by the diaper itself or various health products (soaps, perfumes, softeners, creams). The breakdown of urine into ammonia explains only certain cases of diaper dermatitis.

Prevention

Two general rules can be followed to prevent diaper dermatitis. The first is to avoid using irritants; the second, to ensure the baby is clean and dry.

Diapers

Diapers should be changed frequently, at least every 2 hours during the day and twice at night. Parents should not "double" diapers nor wrap them too tightly. They should avoid plastic pants (air-tight environment).

With cloth diapers, parents should use disposable inner linings. The diapers should be washed properly: rinsed, soaked, disinfected (bleached), washed with mild detergent, rinsed in water and vinegar and dried.

With disposable diapers, parents should avoid using perfumed products and plastics that fit too tightly. The edges should be rolled to prevent the baby's skin from touching plastic.

Washing the Baby

If the baby is soiled, the diaper area should be washed with a mild

---

*This section is reprinted from The Canadian Pharmaceutical Journal, November, 1986.

soap each time the diaper is changed. Parents should dry the skin thoroughly, wiping softly rather than rubbing. Afterward, the baby should be left without a diaper for several minutes to let the skin dry completely. A fresh diaper is put on and clothing avoided that is too warm or too tight.

Health Products

Among baby products, powders are the only agents considered useful in preventing diaper dermatitis. They exert a drying action and protect against rubbing. Products containing zinc oxide or silicone are protectors used to treat diaper dermatitis. Petrolatum and baby lotions are considered ineffective.

Treatment

Most cases of diaper dermatitis can be treated with protecting agents that form a barrier between the skin and the irritating products. By talking with the baby's parents, pharmacists may be able to detect infections or other conditions that require medical attention. The pharmacist should not promote the sale of antifungal agents or anti-inflammatory agents unless a physician has seen the baby.

Diaper dermatitis tends to heal itself when its causes are eliminated. Treated properly, it is usually cured in less than a week. If it persists beyond one week, the baby should be seen by a physician.

Colic

A baby's first cry plays a major role in adapting the cardiovascular and respiratory systems to the extrauterine world. During the first few months after birth, the baby's cries communicate various sensations and emotions such as hunger, thirst, pain, temperature change, discomfort caused by a dirty diaper and social needs. Most babies also cry without apparent reason, which leads to the question of what are the limits of normal crying.

One study shows that duration of crying increases progressively from birth to 6 weeks, attaining an average maximum of 2 hours and 45 minutes per day. After that, the maximum decreases to about 1 hour a day by the age of 12 weeks. Some babies cry much more than average. This situation has been given a number of names, but colic is the most common. It is also referred to as infantile colic, evening colic, 3 month colic and infantile hypertonia.

Colic is defined as a condition in a young infant "who, otherwise healthy and well fed, has paroxysms of irritability, fussing or crying lasting for a total of more than 3 hours a day and occurring on more than 3 days in any one week. The formulation becomes clearer if the word 'paroxysm' is interpreted as crying at full force, not just any degree of fussing."

Etiology

The baby with colic cries uncontrollably, this behavior originating from no known stimulus. The crying tends to occur cyclically, especially at the end of the afternoon and the beginning of the evening, when stress and tension within the family are usually at their peak. The baby has cramps and spasms, most often at set times, especially during the first 3 to 4 months of life; the infant screams, cries, and becomes red, the stomach hardens, hands are often moist, fists are clenched, knees are drawn up to the chest and much intestinal gas is emitted. The baby is irritable and inconsolable. Problems in sleeping are often noted. The attack ends only when the infant is completely exhausted, but apparently is visibly relieved with a bowel movement or the elimination of intestinal gas.

The exact incidence of colic is not well known, because it has not been precisely defined. Studies have given figures ranging from 7 to 40 per cent.

Some studies give a smaller incidence of 10 to 15 per cent. The incidence in premature babies is higher but the onset is delayed until 39 to 44 weeks of gestational age. The incidence is independent of the baby's sex and is highest at 2 to 6 weeks of age. It usually ceases at 2 to 3 months and occasionally at 4 months. Attacks often occur in the evening after feeding; sudden attacks of pain are produced at regular intervals, most often between 6 p.m. and 10 p.m.

It is not known if intestinal gas causes colic. Most mothers believe their colicky babies suffer from pain located in the abdomen. This belief is not based on any objective evidence and probably will never be confirmed nor refuted.

Colic is a normal phenomenon of infancy. When medical history and examination do not show any peculiar characteristics, parents can be reassured that the baby is not suffering from any serious problem. If there is a risk of child abuse or the family is exhausted, hospitalization for a few days may be necessary.

Causes

Leading causes of colic appear to be emotional. Nervous infants have a marked tendency toward colic. This anxiety in the newborn can be caused by an insecure environment, nervous parents, the mother's postpartum anxiety and the parents' inexperience in holding the child in an appropriate way. Certain authors share the view that some colicky babies do not have stomach aches, but simply a difficult temperament. According to them it is a variation of the normal. Other possible explanations include immaturity of the baby's central nervous system and not holding the baby often enough.

Aerophagia (an unconscious and involuntary ingestion of air) can occur—for example, after using a feeding bottle with a too rigid nipple or with an opening that is too small or too large. The infant swallows air with each suck. Air in the stomach prevents babies from eating as much as they want. Also, swallowed air creates abdominal distension and spasms. The more the baby cries the more air is swallowed, resulting in increasing discomfort.

The amount of milk swallowed by the newborn (too much or not enough), speed of drinking (for example, too fast), the temperature of the milk (for example, too cold) and the introduction of new foods are all factors that can bring on colic. Air in the stomach prevents some babies from eating as much as they want. If a breast-feeding mother observes colic after a change in her diet, she should eliminate the offending food (for example, caffeine-containing foods or foods that produce gas such as cabbage, turnip, beans or corn). Introducing solid food to the infant before 3 months can also cause problems as can intolerance to lactose taken by the baby, or taken by the mother if the baby is breast-fed. Immaturity of the gastrointestinal tract can also cause cramps.

According to some authors, colic results from insufficient stimulation through movement. This hypothesis is still unconfirmed, but might explain the increasing popularity of the baby-carrier. Several clinicians attribute colic to spasms or other vague dysfunctions of the smooth musculature of the intestine. Intestinal immaturity may cause a physiological deficiency in lactase. Non-hydrolysed lactase fermentation in the intestine results in formation of excessive

Baby Care

amounts of intestinal gas and painful distension. Passive inhalation of tobacco can also cause colic.

Factors that do not affect colic include mother's age, social class, type of birth (natural or caesarean), prematurity, birth weight, loss or gain of weight, vomiting, diarrhea, constipation, number of bowel movements per day, infant's sex, medication taken by the mother before, during or after the birth and progesterone deficiency.

Treatment

Parents and caregivers should help the infant burp during and after feeding to expel air swallowed during feeding. They should also evaluate the infant's diet according to needs so the baby does not get too hungry or eat too much. A baby under 3 months of age should not be fed more often than 2½ hours after a previous bottle. Some colicky babies tend to increase the amount of milk to compensate. Parents should avoid giving in to this false surge of appetite. They should always let the infant drink slowly in a calm, relaxed atmosphere.

Solid food should not be introduced before 5 months (see Table VII). The child should not be given whole cow's milk before 6 months or 2 per cent or skim milk before 12 months.

If the baby is bottle-fed, parents should examine the nipple of the feeding bottle to prevent excessive swallowing of air (the liquid should drip at the rate of 1 drop per second). They should avoid glass feeding bottles, which promote swallowing of air. Plastic feeding bottles or plastic bags should be used. The pharmacist can advise a preparation of hydrolysate of casein for 2 weeks (for example, Alimentum, Nutramigen or Progestimil). If no change is noted after 2 weeks, parents should return to the original formula and make no other change in food. An intolerance for bovine proteins generally produces an intolerance for soya proteins during colic attacks. Parents should avoid multiple changes in the milk formula.

A breast-feeding mother can try avoiding milk products for a week. If no change is noted, the mother can reintroduce milk products into her diet, since they are essential to good nutrition. However, if a change is noticed, the mother should stay off milk products and consult a pharmacist to select appropriate calcium supplements. She should avoid gas-producing foods and medication (for example, brewer's yeast), foods often implicated in allergies (for example, peanut butter, tomatoes and shell-fish), milk products and citrus fruits, and discontinue use of spices, chocolate, alcohol and coffee.

The health care worker can suggest ways to prevent the infant from taking in too much air while feeding. The infant should be well supported during feeding. Parents can promote sucking between meals by giving the baby an unsugared soother.

After 5 months (see Table VII), if the baby's physician advises starting solid food, parents should not give the baby vegetables that cause gas such as green peas, turnips, cabbage, corn or dry beans.

Parents can provide auditory stimulation, preferably gentle music. They should avoid overstimulation, which can cause anxiety. A baby under 4 months should not be left crying. At this age babies cannot be spoiled. A response by the parent or caregiver within 90 seconds of when the infant starts to cry consoles the baby quickly.

Parents can try more contact with the infant through gentle stroking and heat on the stomach. Placing a parent's warm hand on the abdomen is soothing. Warmth can also be applied using a hot-water bottle wrapped in cloth, pressing the infant against an adult in a baby carrier (preferably carried in front rather than behind), or

placing the infant on the stomach of the mother, father or another adult (to hear the heart beat).

Parents can rock the baby, or reproduce a rhythmic movement with a regular beat (for example, a car ride, turning on a vacuum cleaner or hair dryer, or holding the baby in a seat on an electric dryer or washer.)

Parents should be patient and try to keep calm. They should not feel guilty; colic is rarely the parents' fault. The caregiver can try to hold the baby about 3 hours a day when the baby is not crying. This holding reduces crying by 50 per cent.

The baby should not be allowed to sleep more than 3 consecutive hours during the day. The baby is more tired and sleeps longer at night; if the colic attacks occurred during the night, they will now occur during the day.

Parents can prevent excessive fatigue by using a diaper service or disposable diapers; if the baby is not breast-fed, by using a ready-to-serve formula; sharing the daily home routine with the spouse and other family members; employing a housecleaner, if possible; and hiring a babysitter to care for the baby a few hours a day, if possible.

Sedatives

As a last resort and with medical supervision, sedatives can be administered for a short period of treatment.

Antispasmodics

Because of their antimuscarinic effect on the gastrointestinal tract, anticholinergics can alleviate the intensity of the spasm by causing a decrease of tone and intestinal motility. The decrease in motility can increase the accumulation of gas in the intestine. More than an effective spasmolytic dose can have secondary effects such as constipation, dryness of the mouth and blurred vision. Treatment with drugs such as dicyclomine in a dosage of 5 mg 3 to 4 times daily is effective.

Carminatives

Carminatives are volatile oils (peppermint oil and anise), once used in gripe water to promote elimination of gas. No study has ever demonstrated their effectiveness. Their clinical use has been abandoned. The content of gripe water by 5 mL of volume is as follows: baking soda 50 mg; anise water, 0.180 mL; ginger tincture 0.062 mL; and alcohol 0.246 mL. Bicarbonate reacts with gastric acidity to form carbon dioxide and water. The gas formed increases the infant's flatulence. The ginger tincture in gripe water produces negligible antispasmodic effect in this concentration. Alcohol is contraindicated for infants.

Antiflatulents

The only nonprescription antiflatulent available is simethicone, also known as dimethicone and dimethylpolysiloxane. It is sold under the name of Ovol pediatric drops (1 mL equals 40 mg). Even though no convincing clinical studies prove the effectiveness of silicone polymer for colic caused by flatulence, silicone polymer has been shown to modify the surface tension of air bubbles trapped in the mucus of the intestinal wall. This modification allows their coalescence and dispersion, also facilitating the expulsion of gas. Since simethicone is not absorbed into the blood stream and excretion is solely through the bowels, no secondary effects of toxicity are observed. According to some authors, 125 to 250 mg 4 to 6 times a day are necessary—a much greater quantity than the recommended doses. If the parents still insist on a medicinal treatment after the pharmacist recommends the nonmedicinal approach, the pharmacist can suggest antiflatulents.

Others

Other treatment possibilities include laxatives (glycerin suppositories) and analgesics (acetaminophen). These products should be used only on the advice of a physician.

Parents should discuss colic with their physician at the infant's regular 2 month, 4 month and 6 month visits. They should also consult a physician if fever, vomiting and constipation accompany inconsolable crying; non-medicinal therapeutic measures appear to have no effect within one week; no improvement is seen after 7 days of medicinal treatment advised by a pharmacist; the parent is exhausted and unable to continue with close supervision of the infant; the infant cries more than 4 consecutive hours without being consoled; or growth is slow.

Teething

Even before birth, the gums contain the roots of the teeth. First, the child acquires the 20 temporary or milk teeth, and later the permanent dentition. Generally, babies begin teething at about 5 to 10 months, but they are all different and some can wait one year before the first tooth appears.

Most dentists suggest an early start to cleaning baby teeth. Cleaning should begin from the first showing of the first tooth to develop good oral hygiene habits early. A soft toothbrush is used.

Cutting a tooth is sometimes painful, but does not last more than a few days. Symptoms of teething include excessive salivation; red, swollen, sensitive gums; loss of appetite; frequent crying; moderate diarrhea; fever; and problems sleeping.

Treatment

Chewing and biting are good exercises as the pressure helps push the tooth through the gums. The child can also be given dry bread, teething biscuits or ice rolled in a piece of cloth.

Some teething devices contain gel-like substances that are cooled in the refrigerator. Some of these objects can be pierced by an aggressive biter and the contents, not necessarily sterile, can be swallowed. Parents should give babies special teething objects that are safe, secure, unbreakable and large enough to prevent ingestion (information is available from Consumer and Corporate Affairs Canada).

If the baby starts to chew on the bars of the crib, the bars should be covered with a protective soft shield. Parents must be vigilant to prevent their child from putting pointed objects or objects covered with lead paint in the mouth.

Sucking can irritate inflamed gums. Parents should check the nipple hole of the feeding bottle for adequate flow, to avoid unnecessary sucking. If possible, the child should drink from a glass or cup during this period. The child should not be given biscuits with a high sugar content. Overnight bottles should be avoided.

Certain medications recommended by health professionals reduce swollen gums and give temporary relief. However, pharmacists should avoid recommending medication without properly explaining the uses and dangers of these products.

In general, pharmaceutical agents responsible for temporary relief are called topical anesthetics. These products are considered effective at concentrations of benzocaine above 5 per cent. However, the safety of the product must be evaluated for use with children and teething. The soothing effect provided by these agents must be balanced against such dangers as choking (difficulty in swallowing), burns (food too hot) and tongue biting.

Consumers should avoid applying topical anesthetics less than 1 hour before meals. A Q-Tip can apply the right amount to the defined area of the mouth when using anesthetic gels. Parents should avoid excessive amounts and watch for unnecessary products that have no therapeutic value and can provoke allergic reactions.

Promethazine (for example, Phenergan) has been criticized due to its effect on the cardiorespiratory system and the potential danger of causing apnea, which can be life-threatening. The manufacturer has issued a warning not to use the product with children less than 2 years old.

Cradle Cap

Cradle cap is a term often used to describe yellowish, greasy scales on the scalp. It can begin at birth and ceases spontaneously at 5 to 6 months. It comes from "vernix caseosa," the greasy film covering the skin at birth. It may appear as dry scales on the scalp. Certain authors attribute an antigenic cause to cradle cap, which coincides with the antigenic stimulation of the sebaceous gland during the passage of the maternal androgene through the placenta. To prevent cradle cap, parents should wash the baby's hair and scalp thoroughly 2 to 3 times per week with a mild shampoo. They should always rinse with clean water and dry.

Treatment

Cotton soaked in oil (mineral or vegetable) can be applied in the evening. After about 12 hours, parents can brush the child's scalp with a fine soft brush to remove loose scales. They should gently clean off residual oil with a soft shampoo and dry. The treatment can be repeated if results are not satisfactory.

Other measures to remove scales are as follows:
- Warm the oil slightly (testing for comfortable temperature before application).
- Make compresses about 1 to 3 hours before applying the shampoo.
- Use a keratolytic agent in low concentration under a doctor's supervision (for example, Sebutone which contains sulfur 2 per cent, acetylsalicylic acid 2 per cent, coal tar 0.5 per cent or a mild corticosteroid at 1 per cent.)

If symptoms persist more than a few weeks and treatment does not improve the condition, parents should consult a physician. The problem might be seborrheic or atopic dermatitis.

Colds, Fever and Influenza

Infants are afflicted with 6 to 12 colds and cases of influenza a year, and many of these develop into otitis media infections. Colds are caused by viruses for which there are no pharmacologic cures. (See the chapter on the common cold.) Although several agents are available to relieve symptoms, emphasis must be placed on nonpharmacologic measures, some of which are described below. Medication should be used only as a last resort, as infants are sensitive to adverse

Table X *Treatment for Colds, Fever and Influenza*

Choice of products

•Fever or pain
| Acetaminophen (maximum 5 doses/day) | 10 to 15 mg/kg every 4 hours |

•Congestion and/or rhinorrhea
Pseudoephedrine	1.0 mg/kg every 8 hours
Phenylpropanolamine	0.5 mg/kg every 6 hours
Chlorpheniramine	0.1 mg/kg every 6 hours
Terfenadine	1.0 mg/kg every 12 hours
Triprolidine	0.16 mg/kg every 8 hours

•Irritating dry cough
| Dextromethorphan | 0.3 mg/kg every 6 hours |
| Chlophedianol | 0.4 mg/kg every 8 hours |

Adapted from: Kastrup EK, ed. Facts and comparisons. St. Louis: JB Lippincott, 1983.

effects from it. (See Table X for a discussion of products available to treat colds, fever and influenza.)

General Treatment

Parents should ensure plentiful hydration. The surrounding relative humidity should be increased to a minimum level of 50 per cent (preferably with humidifiers). The caregiver can encourage the infant to rest. A physician should be consulted if there is difficulty breathing or if the cough is hollow and persistent.

Congestion

Increasing the surrounding humidity helps ease congestion. The child's nose should be wiped as often as possible. If the secretions are viscous and difficult to remove, they can be diluted with a saline solution in drops or in a nasal spray. Under the advice of a physician, a nasal pump can be used as a suction device to drain the child's nose and sinuses.

The use of all these measures can greatly improve the child's comfort during the 7 to 10 day duration of the infection.

In some cases, pharmacologic treatment may be required. When medication is used, the indications and contraindications are the same as for the adult. The adverse effects are also the same. The dosage must be adjusted according to the weight of the child, never according to age.

Pharmacists can use some general rules to decide which product to recommend:

• Avoid suppositories; they are poorly absorbed and contain ingredients of doubtful effectiveness.

• Avoid liniments; in addition to irritating the respiratory tract, their absorption through the soft skin of the infant may cause toxic systemic effects.

• Promote buying single products that treat only one symptom at a time. Several products should be used if many symptoms are present simultaneously.

• Parents should use the medication as little as possible and for the shortest time possible.

• Avoid expectorants; they are not effective at the manufacturer's recommended dosage.

• It is not necessary to use products specially formulated for children; they are generally more expensive. Syrups for adults can be used if doses are calculated with precision in terms of the weight of the child.

Fever

Before the temperature of a child is evaluated, it should be known that temperature normally varies by 0.5 to 1°C between morning and evening. These variations are normal and do not indicate the presence of a fever.

The fever itself is useful. It increases production of interferon, stimulates the motility of T-lymphocytes and leucocytes and decreases viral reproduction. Thus, it is a useful defence mechanism and a good diagnostic tool.

Fever frightens people because it can cause convulsions (although rarely) if it reaches 41°C or if the temperature rises quickly. These convulsions occur in 4 per cent of children under 7 years of age, generally less than 24 hours after the beginning of the fever and often even before the parents are aware of the presence of the fever.

When temperature rises more than 0.5°C (depending on the site), the child is considered to have a fever. Medication should be used only when temperature rises at least more than 1°C in the presence of other symptoms. Caregivers should consider the general health of the child, the behavior, whether the child is eating and drinking, and any other accompanying symptoms. (See the chapter on diagnostic aids for information on taking temperature.)

Treatment

Treatment of fever is controversial, since fever does not cause damage, always resolves by itself and may trigger immune defences. Moreover, it has never been shown that treatment lessens the attacks of convulsions. Treatment is popular for three reasons: it increases the child's comfort; it has low toxicity; and it reassures the parents and health professionals.

Parents should uncover or undress the child and lower the surrounding temperature. They should ensure good hydration. The child should be washed, rubbed or bathed in lukewarm water (not cold water or alcohol).

If these measures are not sufficient, a medicinal treatment can be considered. Acetaminophen 10 to 15 mg/kg every 4 hours (maximum 5 doses per day) can be given. (Giving it 20 minutes before bathing the child increases effectiveness.) The Canadian Pediatric Society recommends avoiding the use of acetylsalicylic acid (ASA) for children unless the child is prescribed ASA by a physician for a specific medical condition. (See the section on Reye's syndrome.) Acetaminophen in suppositories should be avoided, because absorption is erratic and unpredictable.

Pharmacists should refer the child to a doctor if the fever persists for more than 24 hours despite treatment; the temperature rises to 40°C or more; or the child's condition seems to require it.

Reye's Syndrome

Reye's syndrome is a disease that affects children, usually under 16 years of age, when they are recovering from a viral infection (influenza, varicella, etc.). This disease is relatively rare: 600 to 1,200 cases per year in the United States. Research and improvements in medical treatment have resulted in the mortality rate dropping to about 30 per cent at present. Survivors often suffer such problems as cerebral disorders, epilepsy, and hemiplegia.

Table XI *Reye's Syndrome*	
Clinical presentation	
Phase I:	Persistent vomiting and lethargy; in very young children vomiting is rare; instead there is hyperventilation. Sometimes there is an apparent remission between phases I and II. Medical examination is mandatory.
Phase II:	Disorientation; apathy or irritability; aggressiveness; hyperventilation; delirium; hyperreflexia. At this stage, the child still responds to external stimuli.
Phase III:	Corporeal rigidity; insensitivity to external stimuli; coma.
Phase IV:	Rigidity; deepening coma; decerebration; dilated pupils not responding to light.
Phase V:	Convulsions; fixed and dilated pupils; absence of tendon reflex; flaccid paralysis; cardiorespiratory insufficiency. Death in 3 to 5 days if treatment is not successful.

Adapted from: Berkow R, ed. The merck manual of diagnosis and therapy. Rahway: Merck, Sharpe and Dohme, 1982:5–7.

Table XII *Infantile Diarrhea*	
Acute diarrhea	**Chronic diarrhea**
•has more than 50 different origins of which some are still unknown. The most frequent cause is infection	•results generally from multiple factors and underlying problems such as major pathologies of one or more organs, food intolerances, malabsorption syndrome, malnutrition
•characterized by the sudden increase in the frequency and liquidity of stools in ordinarily healthy subjects	•characterized by episodes of recurrent or persistent liquid stools which bring on anorexia, weight loss and weakness due to water and electrolyte losses
•usually accompanied by vomiting and low grade fever; the latter usually resolves quickly but diarrhea may persist 3 to 4 days and improve over another 3 to 4 days	•the prognosis is uncertain and self-medication should be avoided
•can disappear without treatment or with certain nonprescription medications if the manifestations are not severe	•does not present the same concern for rapid electrolyte changes but it may be accompanied by signs of failure to thrive

Reye's syndrome almost always develops in children who have taken ASA less than 3 months after an influenza viral infection. A causal link has not been clearly established between the consumption of ASA and the syndrome, but the correlation is sufficiently conclusive for the American Academy of Pediatrics to recommend that children under 16 years of age avoid ASA if they have had an influenza viral infection less than 3 months earlier. In Great Britain, all products for children that contain ASA were taken off the market in the spring of 1986. In 1986, the Canadian Pediatric Society's Committee on Drugs and Hazardous Substances recommended to Health and Welfare Canada that serious consideration should be given to the removal of nonprescription children's ASA products. Health and Welfare Canada now require all products containing ASA for internal use be labelled with a caution that children and teenagers should not use this medication for chickenpox or flu symptoms before a doctor is consulted about Reye's syndrome, a rare but serious condition.

The pathogenesis of the syndrome is said to come from hepatic impairment, which prevents normal metabolism, causing hypoglycemia, an increase in the blood's concentration of ammonia and inhibition of the normal metabolism of fatty acids. Cerebral edema follows, with an increase in intercranial pressure and neuronal damage caused by inhibition of the sodium pump of these cells. (See Table XI for the stages of the syndrome.)

Infantile Diarrhea

Infantile diarrhea, acute or chronic, is a commonly encountered problem. Diarrhea is a condition in which the frequency and liquidity of stools increase abnormally. Some physicians put more emphasis on liquidity than frequency. (See the chapter on antidiarrheals.) However, children who are breast-fed have 4 to 6 liquid bowel movements compared to babies fed with commercial formulas. It is important for health care workers to reassure anxious parents. Although the condition is self-limiting, lasting from a few to several days with

conservative management including administration of fluids, it is potentially life threatening if dehydration and electrolyte imbalance occur. In such cases, a physician should be consulted for proper assessment.

A number of products are labelled for treatment of diarrhea and for rehydration. For the purpose of the chapter, the emphasis of discussion will be on acute diarrhea rather than chronic diarrhea (see Table XII).

Causes

Four documented causes of infant diarrhea are bacterial-viral infections, food intolerance (diet), irritable bowel syndrome and drugs.

Bacterial and Viral Infections

Hospitals have reported that more than 50 per cent of cases of diarrhea in children in winter have a proven viral origin (rotavirus or adenovirus). The incubation period is 12 to 48 hours. In general, bacterial infection is present in more than 10 per cent of stools examined. The stools have shown positive for Salmonella (most frequent, incubation period from 12 to 72 hours); *Yersinia enterocolitica* (incubation period from 12 to 72 hours); Shigella (incubation period from 12 to 72 hours); and *Camphylobacter fetus* (this organism is increasing in frequency; incubation period 2 to 10 days).

Viral infections often cause some destruction of the mucosa in the upper intestinal tract. The intestinal epithelial cells, regenerated from intestinal mucosa damaged by viral infection, temporarily secrete sodium, leading to accumulation of fluid in the lumen and hence vomiting and diarrhea. The mechanism of acute infection with bacteria is different. The bacteria secrete toxins that go into the crypt cells and produce a malfunction of these cells. The cells look normal, but don't function normally.

Table XIII *Needs for Electrolytes and Glucose/24 Hours*

Sodium	Potassium	Calcium	Magnesium	Phosphorus	Glucose
2–4 mEq/kg	1.5–2.5 mEq/kg	50–100 mg/kg	0.5–1 mEq/kg	15–50 mg/kg	2.5–5.0 g/kg
25 mEq/L	20 mEq/L	5–9 mEq/L	3 mEq/L	3 mEq/L	5%

Adapted from: Pereira VL. L'enfant déshydraté. Actualité médicale 1983;30–1,38–9.

Food Intolerance

Acute diarrhea can occur in children as a result of food hypersensitivity (for example, to raisins, fresh fruits such as peaches and strawberries, or lactose). Abuse of juice, especially apple juice, is another cause of subacute or chronic diarrhea.

Irritable Bowel Syndrome

Irritable bowel syndrome is rarely seen in young infants; it is more common in children over 1 year old and adolescents. Recent studies suggest that 15 per cent of children under the age of 2 years have chronic diarrhea. Some may have an early onset of irritable bowel syndrome. Many cases of diarrhea seem to be related to dietary imbalance or excesses in the diet (for example, juice).

Drugs

Another noninfectious cause of acute diarrhea may include administration of drugs such as antibiotics, iron supplements, laxatives and others. Post-antibiotic diarrhea is often seen, especially with wide-spectrum antibiotics (such as ampicillin). Post-antibiotic diarrhea is one of the common causes of diarrhea in children because of frequent use of antibiotics. All antibiotics can cause diarrhea or softer stools.

Treatment

Many people with diarrhea or whose children have diarrhea never see a doctor. They go to their pharmacist to seek advice. (See the chapter on antidiarrheals for risks of antidiarrheal agents and a discussion of the pharmacist's role.)

The available products deal with three specific aspects of diarrhea: treatment of the symptoms; treatment of the cause; and treatment of the effects of diarrhea (water loss and electrolyte imbalance).

The general conclusion regarding nonprescription antidiarrheal agents is that most are not effective, although most are safe to use if they do not delay the diagnosis of a serious infection or medical condition. Nonprescription drug intervention is not indicated for infantile diarrhea. The major disadvantage is possibly delaying medical assessment of the severity of the diarrhea. For example, absorbents (kaolin-pectin) may make stools look better, but they do not alter measured water loss and these agents can cause vomiting.

What is the role of oral fluid and electrolyte therapy? Rehydration (fluid and electrolyte replacement) is the major objective. The concentration of electrolytes, mostly sodium, chloride and potassium, must be adequate to ensure the right needs (see Table XIII).

Today, a number of solutions on the market satisfy the needs of oral fluid and electrolyte replacement. These solutions are better than some home recipes, which can cause hypernatremic dehydration if prepared incorrectly.

Soft drinks and glucose water, widely used in oral rehydration, are largely deficient in sodium, chloride and potassium. Juices (orange and apple) are largely deficient in sodium and chloride, and their use is not advisable because of the possibility of producing hyponatremia. However, soft drinks and diluted juices can be used for short periods of time for children over age 2 with mild non-pathological losses (no serious symptoms such as flushed skin, acute weight loss, dry mucous membranes, tachycardia, low blood pressure and delirium).

Another factor to consider is osmolality. If osmolality is too high, juices can increase the severity of the diarrhea. For this reason, juices must be diluted before they are administered.

Finally, solutions employed in oral rehydration should consist of monosaccharides rather than disaccharides. Monosaccharides have better intestinal absorption. The concentration of monosaccharides must be about 2 to 5 per cent. Soft drinks contain 8 to 10 per cent disaccharides and only a trace of electrolytes. Children, particularly under age 2, should be given a commercial solution (see Table XIV).

Authorities suggest the proportion of glucose should be about 2 to 3 per cent. The sodium level should be about 40 to 60 mmol/L. The solution should contain less chloride than sodium and about 20 to 30 mmol/L of potassium.

The rehydration solution recommended by the World Health Organization (WHO) is higher in sodium and chloride than most commercial solutions sold in Canada. The WHO based its recommendations on studies with cholera, in which much more electrolyte is lost than with the acute diarrhea seen in North American children, for whom much less sodium is therefore needed. All solutions containing glucose-sucrose to stimulate the sodium pump and to prevent ketosis should be between 2 and 3 per cent. (Some authorities prefer 5 per cent.) The quantity of sodium should be between 40 and 60 mmol/L. (The exact amount is controversial.)

The dosages of commercial oral electrolyte and carbohydrate solutions are 100 to 150 mL/kg/day depending on the severity of the diarrhea.

It is important to stop giving the child milk (especially if the child is young) for 24 hours and in some cases longer. A child who is more than 6 months of age can be given yogurt and cheese because these foods contain more lactase and are digested more easily than whole milk or commercial formulas containing lactose as the soul source

Table XIV *Rehydration Solutions*

	Ingredients	WHO formula	Pedialyte	Lytren	Gastrolyte
mmol/L	Sodium	90	45	50	50
	Potassium	20	20	25	20
	Chloride	80	35	45	52
	Citrate	30	10	30	–
	Bicarbonate	–	–	–	18
	Dextrose	111	139	111	101

of carbohydrate. Parents should give the child clear fluids and introduce diluted milk after a 24 hour period. For older children not dependent on milk as their only source of nutrition, diluted milk is introduced later, after giving fruits and vegetables.

Clear fluids should be given only for a short period. It is important to give the child something nutritious. Children under 1 year of age have a transient lactase deficiency for 2 to 3 weeks. Children over 1 year can often tolerate the reintroduction of milk products as soon as the acute diarrhea is over. If not, they can try a half-strength soya-based formula within 24 to 48 hours; if this is tolerated they can progress to full strength and finally to their usual source of milk.

Providing a Safe Environment

Accidents, trauma and poisoning are responsible for more than half the deaths and infirmities in children under age 15. More deaths are caused by these three means than by infections, malformations and cancer put together. The following are responsible for most accidents: objects (for example, fire, medications, household products, toys, car seats, walkers, playpens and strollers); environment (lack of surveillance, playground, cigarettes, matches, tools left unstored and electrical appliances); and the children themselves (curiosity and ignorance of danger).

Poisoning is the eighth most common source of accidental death in children. Medications are responsible for 50 per cent of the poisonings. Pharmacists can advise the following general guidelines to help eliminate this cause:

- Keep all necessary medication in a safe place. Discard unnecessary medication. If possible, keep medication in a locked cabinet.
- Make sure all medication and dangerous products are well identified.
- When buying medication, make sure the product is in a childproof container.
- A child learns through example; avoid taking medication in front of children.
- Do not try to convince children to take medication by telling them it is candy.
- Know what to do in an emergency, for example, if the child chokes.
- Place the telephone number of the nearest poison control centre on or near your phone. Familiarize yourself with procedures to take in case of poisoning (for example, if vomiting should be stimulated or the victim taken to a hospital emergency). In case vomiting may be required, know how and when to use ipecac syrup (or call your pharmacist).
- Avoid storing toxic substances in bottles generally used for food.
- Domestic plants often attract children; when buying a plant for the household, get proper information concerning its toxicity (for example, what happens if the child touches it or bites it). Examples of toxic plants include begonias, poinsettias, diffenbachias, philodendrons, rhubarb leaves and caladium.
- Keep all electrical cords out of reach of children. Cover electrical plugs with special safety caps.
- Avoid leaving cigarettes unattended even for a few seconds.
- Always tie a few knots in plastic bags before storing or discarding them.
- Make sure the cord on the telephone receiver does not hang freely and within the child's reach.
- Do not leave anything heavy, hot or sharp on table mats.

- Make sure all staircases are properly sealed off with the right equipment.
- Toys are an immense source of pleasure for the child, but they can also be a source of danger. Select toys with great care. Pamphlets and guidelines are available from Consumer and Corporate Affairs Canada to instruct parents on selecting and maintaining toys, mobiles, automobile seats, cribs, playpens and other items.

Ask the Consumer

Feeding (Commercial Formulas)

Q. What is the child's age and weight?
- Age dictates the use of a specific kind of formula over use of whole cow's milk. Whole cow's milk should not be given to a child under 6 months of age.

Q. Is the child receiving formula or breast milk?
- If the baby is breast-fed, powder is a good choice for occasional feeding, as it is less expensive than other available preparations such as ready-to-serve or concentrated form.

Q. Are there any dietary restrictions?
- Infants with lactase deficiencies need special formulas.

Q. Are there any problems such as spitting up, vomiting, colic or diarrhea?
- All these symptoms may indicate milk protein allergies or possible disaccharidase deficiency.

Q. Is your child receiving any supplements (vitamins, minerals or fluoride)?
- Depending on the type of milk and local water supply, there may be overconsumption or deficiencies.

Diaper Dermatitis

Q. Is the rash mainly in the diaper area? Are the folds of the diaper area affected?
- Diaper rash is confined mainly to the diaper area, whereas heat rash occurs in areas of sweating and friction. A general rash often relates to an allergy susceptibility.

Q. How long has the rash been present?
- If it has persisted for more than 1 week, refer the consumer to a physician.

Q. Has there been a change in diet recently?
- Foods rich in protein can cause irritation. Introduction of allergenic foods such as cereal, fruit and vegetables can also cause a rash. A change in milk formula can be a cause, as can a change in the mother's diet if she is breast-feeding.

Q. What type of diapers do you use? If cloth, what detergent, rinsing solution and fabric softener do you use to launder them?
- For cloth diapers, wash them properly (rinse, soak, disinfect, wash with a mild detergent (for example, Ivory Snow), rinse in water and

vinegar and dry.) Use disposable inner diapers. If using disposable diapers, avoid perfumed products and plastics that fit too tightly.

Q. How frequently do you change the diapers? Do you use plastic pants or a system of double diapering?

■ Diapers should be changed at least every 2 hours during the day and twice at night. Avoid plastic pants and double diapering as they produce a damp airtight environment.

Q. What soap do you use to wash the baby?

■ Recommend a mild soap (for example, White Dove or Ivory).

Q. Ask the mother if she has recently observed vaginal itching or discharge. Has the baby had white spots in the mouth or on the tongue recently? Has the baby recently been treated with oral antibiotics for an infection (impetigo, otitis or strep throat) or antifungal agents for thrush?

■ Other conditions such as fungal infections resulting from thrush can be mistaken for diaper dermatitis. If suspected, the infant should be referred to a physician.

Q. Are you using prescription or nonprescription medication at present to treat the diaper rash? If so, what products and how? Who recommended them?

■ Most cases of diaper dermatitis can be treated with protecting agents that form a barrier between the skin and the irritating agents. Pharmacists should not recommend antifungal or anti-inflammatory agents unless a physician has seen the baby.

Colic

Q. What age is your child?

■ Colic is rare after 4 months of age.

Q. How much does the child weigh?

■ If medicinal treatment is necessary, the dosage in mg/kg is recommended.

Q. Describe the infant's symptoms. Is the child inconsolable? How often does he/she cry, and when? Is the stomach hard and is the infant drawing the knees up to the chest? Is the child constipated? How long have you observed these symptoms?

Q. Has the diet of the infant changed recently (change in formula, change from breast-feeding to formula, use of whole milk or 2 per cent, introduction of food, food causing flatulence such as cabbage, turnips, beans and corn, underfeeding or overfeeding)? If the infant is breast-fed, has the diet of the mother changed? Does the mother use tobacco or eat foods that produce gas or contain caffeine (for example, tea, coffee or cola drinks)? Is she taking medication?

Q. Describe in a few sentences one of your normal days.

■ Check the mother's emotional state, the home environment and the attitude toward the baby crying. If the mother appears to be exhausted and unable to cope, refer her to a physician.

Q. Show how you bottle-feed your infant.

■ Check the technique of holding the baby during feeding. Check the nipples, the type of bottle, the temperature of the milk, the speed at which the baby feeds and the burping method.

Q. Do you currently use nonprescription medication to treat colic? If yes, who advised it? What product are you using and how long have you used it? What dosage? How do you administer it? Has there been any improvement in the baby's condition?

Q. Are you currently using medication specifically prescribed by a doctor to treat colic? If yes, what are you using and how long have you used it? Do you know what the side effects are? What type of physician (general practitioner or specialist) prescribed it? What dosage and when? How do you administer it? Have you observed an improvement since beginning treatment? Do you have a follow-up appointment with the physician?

Cradle Cap

Q. How old is the child? When did the condition start? Can you describe the problem?

■ These questions help to establish whether the condition is cradle cap or dermatitis.

Q. Are other parts of the body affected?

■ If the answer is yes, the condition is probably seborrheic or atopic dermatitis.

Q. Are there other related symptoms?

■ Scratching can indicate atopic dermatitis or a secondary infection.

Q. Are you using any treatment at present?

Infantile Diarrhea

Q. How old is the child?

■ If the child is less than 3 years of age, an antidiarrheal should not be recommended and the parents should be advised about maintaining adequate hydration.

Q. How much does the child weigh?

■ The child's weight is important in determining the degree of hydration.

Q. How long has the child had diarrhea (number of days)?

■ Neither chronic or acute diarrhea present for more than a few days should be treated with antidiarrheal products, but should be referred to a physician.

Q. Is the child suffering from other symptoms (for example, fever or vomiting)?

- The pharmacist should be looking for the presence of fever and vomiting, which indicate additional fluid loss and referral to a physician.

Q. Is the child taking any medication (antibiotic, laxative)?
- The use of broad spectrum antibiotics such as ampicillin, erythromycin and others can cause diarrhea in infants.

Q. Has there been any change in the child's diet?
- A formula change may cause diarrhea or soften liquid stools. Diarrhea may be associated with certain foods (for example, milk products if the child has a lactose intolerance).

References

Feeding
Anderson SA, Chinn HI, Fisher KD. History and current status of infant formulas. Am J Clin Nutr 1982;35:381–97.

Anonymous. Oral nutrition supplement. In: Kastrup EK, ed. Facts and comparisons. St Louis: JB Lippincott, 1986:58–60.

Anonymous. The promotion of breast feeding. Pediatrics 1982;69:654–61.

Anonymous. Current issues in feeding the normal infant. Pediatrics 1985; 75(1).

Bahna SL. Control of milk allergy: a challenge for physicians, mothers and industry. Ann Allergy 1978;41:1–2.

Canadian Paediatric Society Nutrition Committee. Infant feeding. Can J Public Health 1979;70:376–85.

Committee on Nutrition, American Academy of Pediatrics. Commentary on breast feeding and infant formulas, including proposed standards for formulas. Pediatrics 1976;57:278–85.

Daglish S. Breastfeeding and allergy. Can Pharm J 1983;116:334–6.

Fomon SJ. Infant nutrition. Philadelphia: WB Saunders, 1974:16,158–62,362.

Handbook of infant formulas. Downsview: Wyeth, 1969:86–8.

Hendricks S. Les preparations pour nourrissons. Le Pharmacien 1982; Nov:22–6.

Janas LM, Picciano MF, Hatch TF. Indices of protein metabolism in term infants fed human milk, whey-predominant formula or cow's milk formula. Pediatrics 1985;75(4):775–84.

Maser JE. Nutritional composition of commercial infant formulas. Can Pharm J 1983;116:337–40.

McDonald N. Baby care. In: Cyr JG, ed. Canadian self-medication. Ottawa: Canadian Pharmaceutical Association, 1984.

McKenzie MW, Bender KJ, Seals AJ. Infant formula products. In: Handbook of nonprescription drugs. Washington: American Pharmaceutical Association, 1986:316–41.

Myres AW. Recent developments in nutrition and infant feeding. Can Pharm J 1980;113:11–5.

Product specifications, label declarations, instructions and data provided by the manufacturers. Mead Johnson, Ross, and Wyeth; 1986.

Standard de nutrition au Canada (Pamphlet). Ottawa: Health and Welfare Canada, 1975.

Vaughan VC, McKay RJ. Textbook of pediatrics. Philadelphia: WB Saunders, 1983:190–205.

Yip CMK. Pediatric nutritional products. In Chiles VK, ed.: Canadian self-medication. Ottawa: Canadian Pharmaceutical Association, 1981:241–54.

Hygiene
Doren N, Le Henaff D, eds. Mieux vivre avec son enfant: alimentation et soins du nourrisson de la naissance à deux ans. Québec: Hôpital de l'Enfant-Jésus, Département de santé communautaire, 1983.

St Onge E. C'est pour quand, le bain de bébé. Revue Prénatale 1984;7(2):66–9.

Diaper Dermatitis
Chevalier R, Dicaire P. Diaper dermatitis. Can Pharm J 1986;119:628–9.

Colic
Behrman RE, Vaughan VC, Nelson WE, eds. Nelson textbook of pediatrics. Philadelphia: WB Saunders, 1983:163.

Blais D, et al. Les médicaments: votre santé et vous. Ma Caisse 1986;23(3).

Br Med J 1984;288:901,1230.

Cosluj W. Colic: primary excessive crying as an infant-environment interaction. Pediatr Clin North Am 1984;31(5):993-1006.

Feeding babies (Pamphlet). Ottawa: Health and Welfare Canada, 1986.

Illingworth RS. Infantile colic revisited. Arch Dis Child 1985;60:981–5.

Julien G. Au jour le jour. Départements de santé communautaire du centre hospitalier régional de la Beauce, 1985.

Schmitt BD. The prevention of sleep problems and colic. Pediatr Clin North Am 1986;33(4):763–74.

Weber ML, Chicoine L, et al. Guide thérapeutique pédiatrique. Montréal: Presses de l'université de Montréal, 1986.

Weber M. Le nourisson qui pleure ou les coliques infantile. Medical du Canada 1985;juin:114.

Weissbluth M, Christoffel KK, Davis AT. Treatment of infantile colic with dicyclomine hydrochloride. J Pediatrics 1984;104:951–5.

Teething
Anonymous. Les soins dentaires. Actualités pharmaceutiques 1979;avril:58–61.

Information letter. Montreal: Rhone-Poulenc Pharma, 1986.

Lemay H. La cavite buccale. Quebec Pharmacie 1983;Oct:38–40.

Savard J-G. Des dents saines pour toute la famille. Quebec: Promotion Mondiales, 1979.

Cradle Cap
Bear JM, Rook A. The newborn. Rook A, Wilkinson DS, Ebling FJG, eds. Textbook of dermatology. Oxford: Blackwell Scientific, 1979;185–212.

Bystun AM, Shulack JI. Pediatric dermatology therapy. In: Weinberg S, Hoekelman RA, eds. Pediatric dermatology for the primary care practitioner. Toronto: McGraw-Hill, 1978;14–22.

Doren N, Le Henaff D, eds. Mieux vivre avec son enfant: alimentation et soins du nourrisson de la naissance a deux ans. Québec: Hôpital de l'Enfant-Jésus, Département de santé communautaire, 1983.

Robert P, et al. Dermopharmacologie clinique. St-Hyacinthe: Edisem, 1985:58.

Stephenson MJ. Fever management in pediatric care. Cont Pediatr 1986; Sep-Oct:23–9.

Colds, Fever & Influenza
Anonymous. Over-the-counter cough remedies. Med Lett Drugs Ther 1979; 21:103–4.

Anonymous. The right solution: oral rehydration therapy for the management of acute diarrhea. Mississauga: Medical Education Services, 1985.

Berkow R, ed. The Merck manual of diagnosis and therapy. Rahway: Merck, Sharpe and Dohme, 1982:5–7,1886.

Bernheim HA, Block LH, Atkins E. Fever: pathogenesis and pathophysiology. Ann Intern Med 1979;91:261.

Boisjoly L. La fièvre. Québec Pharmacie 1985;Feb:32,75–6.

Donaldson JF. Therapy of acute fever: a comparative approach. Hosp Pract 1981;16:125.

Kastrup EK, ed. Facts and comparisons. St Louis: JB Lippincott, 1983.

Knoben JE, Anderson PO, Watanabe AS, eds. Handbook of clinical drug data. Hamilton: Drug Intelligence Publications, 1978;533–4.

Paisley J. Acute gastroenteritis syndrome in children. Primary Care 1984; 11(3):513–26.

Waldman RJ, et al. Aspirin as a risk factor in Reye's syndrome. JAMA, 1982;247:3089.

Infantile Diarrhea
Behrman RE, Vaughan VC, Nelson WE, eds. Nelson textbook of pediatrics. Toronto: WB Saunders, 1983:610–2,920–1.

Ferrier PE. Préecis de pediatrie. St-Hyacinthe: Edisem, 1984:202–7.

Hirschhorn N. The treatment of acute diarrhea in children, an historical and physiological perspective. Am J Clin Nutr 1980;33:637–63.

Pereira VL. L'enfant deshydraté. Actualité Médicale 1983;30–1,38–9.

Portnoy BL, DuPont HL, Pruitt D, et al. Antidiarrheal agents in the treatment of acute diarrhea in children. JAMA 1976;236:844–6.

Rees L, Brook CGD. Gradual reintroduction of full-strength milk after acute gastroenteritis in children. Lancet 1979;1:770–1.

Santosham M, Daum RS, Dillman L, et al. Oral rehydration therapy, of infantile diarrhea. N Engl J Med 1982;306:1070–6.

Providing a Safe Environment

Baker D. Toy safety. Cont Pediatr 1986;Nov-Dec:36–42.

Dossier securitaire (bébé Butler);328-6444:5–7,11–12,15,18,22–25,27.

Is your child safe (Pamphlet)? Ottawa: Consumer and Corporate Affairs.

30
Nutritional Products

Robert A. Locock and Louis A. Pagliaro

Many consumers supplement their daily diet with vitamin and mineral products, including multiple-vitamin products, single-entity vitamins, calcium and iron. The value of such nutritional supplements must be weighed against the risks of inappropriate use, such as hypervitaminosis or drug interactions. Consumers may need dietary counselling on low-cholesterol foods, natural fibre and vitamin-rich foods. Consumers may also request information on the sugar substitutes—saccharin, cyclamate and aspartame.

Canadians commonly self-medicate with various nutritional products. In so doing, they often seek the advice of pharmacists. This chapter discusses nutritional products from a pharmaceutical and therapeutic perspective, with particular emphasis on the major vitamins and minerals found in Canadian self-medication products. Special diets and sugar substitutes are also discussed as they relate to self-medication.

Vitamins

Vitamins are components of natural food distinct from minerals and the three major sources of food energy (carbohydrates, fat and protein). They are generally present in normal foods in extremely small concentrations, but are essential for normal growth and health. Often vitamins act as coenzymes in the body's metabolic processes. When vitamins are absent from the diet or not properly absorbed from food, a specific deficiency condition associated with each vitamin can occur (see Table I). Single deficiency diseases are rare in North America. Poor nutritional status usually involves a host of nonspecific symptoms caused by borderline intake of a number of nutrients, including vitamins.

Vitamins can be divided into two groups according to solubility. Those easily soluble in water are referred to collectively as water-soluble vitamins and include the B complex of vitamins and vitamin C. Those easily soluble in fat are referred to collectively as fat-soluble vitamins and include vitamins A, D, E and K. This classification has some therapeutic relevance: water-soluble vitamins are generally considered safer, because an overdose usually does not accumulate in the body, but spills over into the urine. However, noted exceptions to this rule are listed in the section on hypervitaminosis.

The active forms of some vitamins are produced within the body itself; for example, vitamin D is changed to its active form when ultraviolet light from the sun acts on a precursor of the vitamin in exposed skin. The body can convert carotenoids, such as beta-carotene, into vitamin A. Fruits, green and orange vegetables, and juices are good sources of vitamin A from carotenoids. Intestinal bacteria can synthesize vitamin K and some B vitamins. Thus, the intestinal bacteria contribute to meeting human daily requirements

Table I *Major Vitamins*

Vitamin	Major functions in body	Possible result of deficiency
Ascorbic acid (Vitamin C)	Maintenance of intercellular matrix of cartilage, bone, and dentine, collagen synthesis, enhancement of iron absorption, metabolism of carbohydrates	Degeneration of skin, teeth, blood vessels, epithelial hemorrhages, scurvy
Biotin (Vitamin H)	Coenzyme for fat synthesis, amino acid metabolism glycogen formation, involved in carboxylation reactions	Fatigue, lethargy, depression, anorexia, nausea, seborrheic dermatitis, muscular pains
Choline	Constituent of phospholipids, precursor of acetylcholine, metabolism of fat	Not yet clearly established
Cyanocobalamin (Vitamin B$_{12}$)	Coenzyme in transfer of single-carbon units in nucleic acid metabolism, synthesis of red blood cells and protein including myelin formation	Pernicious anemia, growth retardation, neurologic disorders (degeneration of myelin sheaths), confusion, psychosis
Folic acid (Folacin) (Vitamin M) (Vitamin B$_c$)	Coenzyme (reduced form) involved in transfer of one carbon unit in nucleic and amino acid (protein) metabolism (this involved in blood cell, heme, DNA and RNA formation)	Megaloblastic anemia, growth deficiency, gastrointestinal disturbances, diarrhea, glossitis

Table I (Cont'd) Major Vitamins

Vitamin	Major functions in body	Possible result of deficiency
Niacin (Nicotinic acid) (Vitamin B₃)	Constituents of coenzymes NAD and NADP; metabolism of carbohydrate, fat and protein, used therapeutically to lower serum triglycerides; niacin is interconvertible with niacinamide in the body	Pellagra, skin and gastrointestinal lesions, diarrhea, nervous or mental disorders, hyperpigmentation
Pantothenic acid (Vitamin B₅)	Constituent of coenzyme A, synthesis of porphyrins and acetylcholine; metabolism of carbohydrate, fat and protein	Fatigue, sleep disturbances, impaired coordination, nausea, burning sensation in feet
Pyridoxine (Vitamin B₆)	Coenzyme involved in amino acid (protein) metabolism (pyridoxal phosphate), facilitates conversion of tryptophan to niacin; helps prevent hypochromic anemia; necessary for the formation of myelin sheath surrounding nerve tissue	Peripheral neuropathy, irritability, convulsions, muscular twitching, dermatitis near eyes, cheilosis, kidney stones, glossitis
Riboflavin (Vitamin B₂)	Constituents of coenzymes FAD and FMN, metabolism of carbohydrate and protein; involved in the formation of red blood cells and the production of corticosteroids	Lesions of eye, cheilosis, glossitis, photophobia; normochromic, normocytic anemia
Thiamine (Vitamin B₁)	Coenzyme in reactions involving removal of carbon dioxide; metabolism of carboydrate, fat, and protein	Beriberi; peripheral nerve changes, polyneuritis, fatigue, edema, tachycardia, heart failure; Wernicke-Korsakoff syndrome
Vitamin A (Retinol)	Synthesis of rhodopsin (photosensitive pigment in the eye); normal development of epithelium, bones and teeth; steroid hormonal synthesis	Night blindness, xerophthalmia, dry skin, peripheral neuropathy
Vitamin D (Cholecalciferol) (Ergocalciferol)	Regulation of calcium absorption and metabolism necessary for the formation and mineralization of bones and teeth	Osteomalacia (adults), rickets and growth failure (children), muscle spasms
Vitamin E (Tocopherol)	Not yet clearly established; antioxidant effect appears to protect cell membranes from deterioration	Hemolysis of red blood cells (infants); not yet clearly established (adults)

Table I (Cont'd) Major Vitamins

Vitamin	Major functions in body	Possible result of deficiency
Vitamin K	Synthesis of prothrombin in the liver	Hemorrhage, delayed wound healing

for these nutrients. NAD, the coenzyme form of niacin, can be produced in the body from the essential amino acid tryptophan.

The amount of a particular vitamin needed to maintain normal good health and growth varies according to such factors as age, sex and stage of life (see Table II).

Recommended nutrient intakes (RNIs) of vitamins are amounts suggested by a panel of scientific experts to prevent development of symptoms of deficiency disease and to help maintain long-term health in the average individual. RNIs are established at levels that meet or exceed the actual requirements of nearly all healthy people (about 97.5 per cent). Some people have requirements greater than the RNI. A well balanced diet following Canada's food guide provides sufficient vitamins for healthy adults maintaining their normal body weight (see Figure 1). Vitamin supplements may be required for individuals on restricted diets; individuals who cannot tolerate certain foods (for example, milk) because of allergies or other conditions; growing children; pregnant or nursing women; people under stress (psychological or physical); people receiving drugs that interact with vitamins to cause a deficiency (see Table III); and the elderly.

When choosing a vitamin preparation, one is often confronted with the choice between natural and synthetic products. For example, vitamin C derived from rose hips or oranges is a natural vitamin, whereas vitamin C produced in a chemical plant is a synthetic vitamin. However, the chemical structure of the vitamin in each case is exactly the same. Thus, the body cannot differentiate between natural and synthetic vitamins. Indeed, many "natural" vitamin preparations have some of the same vitamin in synthetic form added to them to decrease the cost and bulk of the product.

Hypervitaminosis

When taking vitamins, one can get "too much of a good thing." Megadosing, generally defined as consuming 10 times the RNI of a specific vitamin, is associated with some risk. This problem is of particular clinical concern for the fat-soluble vitamins A and D, and the water-soluble vitamins niacin and ascorbic acid.

Chronic use of 40,000 IU or more of vitamin A per day in adults may result in increased central nervous system pressure and resultant pseudotumor cerebri or related disorders (for example, headaches and irritability); hepatosplenomegaly; hyperostosis; stomatitis; alopecia; anorexia; dry skin; and hemorrhagic papilledema, which may cause blindness. In addition, large doses of vitamin A may cause fetal malformations. Women planning to become pregnant in the immediate future should not consume supplements containing more than 10,000 IU of vitamin A.

Use of 75,000 IU or more of vitamin D per day in adults for several weeks may result in such symptoms of toxicity as osteoporosis associated with bone resorption; hypercalcemia, causing anorexia; hypercalciuria and associated urinary stones; polyuria; weakness; nephrocalcinosis; nausea; and diarrhea.

Use of 3 to 10 g/day of niacin can result in liver failure (for example, hyperbilirubinemia, hepatic cell injury, portal fibrosis, cholestasis),

Nutritional Products

Table II *Recommended Nutrient Intake of Canadians*[a]

Age	Sex	Weight kg	Protein (g/day)	Vit. A (RE[b] /day)	Vit. D (µg/ day)	Vit. E (mg /day)	Vit. C (mg /day)	Folate (µg /day)	Thiamin (mg /day)	Riboflavin (mg /day)	Niacin (NE[c] /day)	Vit. B$_{12}$ (µg /day)	Calcium (mg /day)	Phosphorus (mg /day	Magnesium (mg /day)	Iron (mg /day)	Iodine (µg /day)	Zinc (mg /day)
Months																		
0–4	Both	6.0	12[d]	400	10	3	20	50	0.3	0.3	4	0.3	250[e]	150	20	0.3[f]	30	2[f]
5-12	Both	9.0	12	400	10	3	20	50	0.4	0.5	7	0.3	400	200	32	7	40	3
Years																		
1	Both	11	19	400	10	3	20	65	0.5	0.6	8	0.3	500	300	40	6	55	4
2–3	Both	14	22	400	5	4	20	80	0.6	0.7	9	0.4	550	350	50	6	65	4
4–6	Both	18	26	500	5	5	25	90	0.7	0.9	13	0.5	600	400	65	8	85	5
7–9	M	25	30	700	2.5	7	25	125	0.9	1.1	16	0.8	700	500	100	8	110	7
	F	25	30	700	2.5	6	25	125	0.8	1.0	14	0.8	700	500	100	8	95	7
10–12	M	34	38	800	2.5	8	25	170	1.0	1.3	18	1.0	900	700	130	8	125	9
	F	36	40	800	5	7	25	180	0.9	1.1	16	1.0	1100	800	135	8	110	9
13–15	M	50	50	900	5	9	30	150	1.1	1.4	20	1.5	1100	900	185	10	160	12
	F	48	42	800	5	7	30	145	0.9	1.1	16	1.5	1000	850	180	13	160	9
16–18	M	62	55	1000	5	10	40[g]	185	1.3	1.6	23	1.9	900	1000	230	10	160	12
	F	53	43	800	2.5	7	30[g]	160	0.8	1.1	15	1.9	700	850	200	12	160	9
19–24	M	71	58	1000	2.5	10	40[g]	210	1.2	1.5	22	2.0	800	1000	240	9	160	12
	F	58	43	800	2.5	7	30[g]	175	0.8	1.1	15	2.0	700	850	200	13	160	9
25–49	M	74	61	1000	2.5	9	40[g]	220	1.1	1.4	19	2.0	800	1000	250	9	160	12
	F	59	44	800	2.5	6	30[g]	175	0.8	1.0	14	2.0	700	850	200	13	160	9
50–74	M	73	60	1000	5	7	40[g]	220	0.9	1.3	16	2.0	800	1000	250	9	160	12
	F	63	47	800	5	6	30[g]	190	0.8[h]	1.0[h]	14[h]	2.0	800	850	210	8	160	9
75 +	M	69	57	1000	5	6	40[g]	205	0.8	1.0	14	2.0	800	1000	230	9	160	12
	F	64	47	800	5	5	30[g]	190	0.8[h]	1.0[h]	14[h]	2.0	800	850	210	8	160	9
Pregnancy (additional)																		
1st Trimester			5	100	2.5	2	0	300	0.1	0.1	0.1	1.0	500	200	15	0	25	6
2nd Trimester			20	100	2.5	2	10	300	0.1	0.3	0.2	1.0	500	200	45	5	25	6
3rd Trimester			24	100	2.5	2	10	300	0.1	0.3	0.2	1.0	500	200	45	10	25	6
Lactation (additional)			20	400	2.5	3	25	100	0.2	0.4	0.3	0.5	500	200	65	0	50	6

[a]Recommended Nutrient Intakes (RNIs) are expressed on a daily basis, but should be regarded as the average recommended intake over a period of time, such as a week.

[b]Retinol Equivalents. 1 RE = 1µg or 3.33 I.U. retinol. 1 RE = 6g or 10 I.U. beta-carotene.

[c]Niacin Equivalents. 1 NE = 1 mg niacin or 60 mg tryptophan. About 3% of ingested tryptophan is oxidized to niacin.

[d]Protein is assumed to be from breast milk and must be adjusted for infant formula.

[e]Infant formula with high phosphorus should contain 375 mg calcium.

[f]Breast milk is assumed to be the source of the mineral.

[g]Smokers should increase vitamin C by 50%.

[h]Level below which intake should not fall.

Adapted from: Health and Welfare Canada. Nutrition Recommendations. The Report of the Scientific Review Committee. 1990.

hyperglycemia, lactic acidosis, hyperuricemia, peptic ulceration, diarrhea, flushing of the face, itching, abdominal cramps, headache, dry skin, skin rash or pigmentation of the skin. Niacinamide, another form of the same vitamin, is unlikely to cause these symptoms at similar doses. Niacin may be used to lower blood triglycerides. It is reported to be as effective as lovastatin in lowering serum levels of very low density lipoproteins and low density lipoproteins and in raising the serum level of high density lipoproteins. Niacin is not as beneficial as lovastatin in its cholesterol-lowering effect. It should be noted that slow-release formulations of niacin are much more toxic to the liver than plain preparations.

Consumption of 1 g/day or more of ascorbic acid can result in nausea; abdominal cramps; urinary stone formation due to oxaluria (usually greater than 4 g/day); increased uric acid clearance; rebound scurvy following the sudden cessation of high dose supplements of ascorbic acid; and diarrhea due to the osmotic effect of large amounts

Figure 1 *Canada's Food Guide Recommendations*

Milk and milk products	Meat, fish, poultry and alternates
Children up to 11 years 2–3 servings Adolescents 3–4 servings Pregnant and nursing women 3–4 servings Adults 2 servings Skim, 2%, whole, buttermilk, reconstituted dry or evaporated milk may be used as a beverage or as the main ingredient in other foods. Cheese may also be chosen. **Some examples of one serving** 250mL (1 cup) milk 175mL (¾ cup) yoghurt 45g (1½ ounces) cheddar or process cheese In addition, a supplement of vitamin D is recommended when milk is consumed which does not contain added vitamin D.	2 servings **Some examples of one serving** 60 to 90g (2–3 ounces) cooked lean meat, fish, poultry or liver 60mL (4 tablespoons) peanut butter 250mL (1 cup) cooked dried peas, beans or lentils 125mL (½ cup) nuts or seeds 60g (2 ounces) cheddar cheese 125mL (½ cup) cottage cheese 2 eggs

Breads and cereals	Fruits and vegetables
3–5 servings Whole grain or enriched. Whole grain products are recommended. **Some examples of one serving** 1 slice bread 125mL (½ cup) cooked cereal 175mL (¾ cup) ready-to-eat cereal 1 roll or muffin 125 to 175mL (½ –¾ cup) cooked rice, macaroni, spaghetti or noodles ½ hamburger or wiener bun	4–5 servings Include at least two vegetables. Choose a variety of both vegetables and fruits—cooked, raw or their juices. Include yellow, green or green leafy vegetables. **Some examples of one serving** 125mL (½ cup) vegetables or fruits—fresh, frozen or canned 125mL (½ cup) juice—fresh, frozen or canned 1 medium-sized potato, carrot, tomato, peach, apple, orange or banana

of ascorbic acid in the gastrointestinal tract. Long-term use may interfere with cyanocobalamin absorption. Large doses may also cause hemolysis in individuals with G-6-PD deficiency.

These examples give ample indication that vitamins are not harmless. Inappropriate use can result in much more harm than simply wasting one's money.

Vitamin E (The Vitamin in Search of a Disease)

Vitamin E has been promoted vigorously. Its use for various conditions is highly controversial. It has been claimed to increase virility and sexual endurance, to overcome sterility and to promote a successful pregnancy. Large doses of vitamin E have been claimed useful in treating disorders such as coronary heart disease, muscular weakness, arthritis, diabetes and skin disorders (particularly the elimination of scars with topical application). This vitamin is also said to improve athletic ability, retard aging, increase lung resistance to air pollution and prevent cataracts associated with aging. Many claims for vitamin E are the result of either isolated case reports or extrapolation to humans of tests carried out in animals. Although promoted for many therapeutic effects, current evidence is insufficient to support these claims.

A deficiency disease associated with vitamin E occurs almost exclusively in premature infants, in whom a shortage can cause hemolytic anemia. A primary vitamin E deficiency has never been recognized in otherwise healthy children or adults. However, vitamin E deficiency has been reported in people with long-standing fat malabsorption.

Diets containing large amounts of polyunsaturated fatty acids may increase the requirement for vitamin E. Such diets are often prescribed to individuals at risk for coronary heart disease. However, most dietary sources of polyunsaturates also contain large amounts of vitamin E, making supplementation generally unnecessary. Vitamin E is commonly found as an ingredient in food supplements. Promoters of these diet supplements emphasize its role as an antioxidant.

Vitamin E appears to act primarily as an antioxidant that inhibits oxidation of essential cellular constituents and prevents the formation of toxic oxidation products. Vitamin E may protect fatty acids in cell membranes from oxidative attack. Vitamin E may also function specifically to minimize the negative effects of increased oxygen consumption during aerobic exercise.

Vitamin E, like other fat-soluble vitamins, is stored in adipose tissues, which serve as storage sites protecting against vitamin deficiency for longer periods of time than with the water-soluble vitamins. Individuals have taken doses of up to 300 mg/day or more of vitamin E for extended periods without causing any apparent harm. In others, large doses of vitamin E may cause fatigue, gastrointestinal complaints, headache, blurred vision and dermatitis. Large doses of vitamin E can reportedly antagonize vitamin K and prolong prothrombin time. This reported drug interaction may result in a marked potentiation of oral anticoagulants. Thus, people requiring anticoagulant therapy with warfarin or related drugs generally should avoid supplemental vitamin E and drastic changes in vitamin E consumption once stabilized on an anticoagulant dosage schedule.

Table III *Nutrient-Drug Interactions*

Vitamin/ Mineral	Interacting Drugs	Mechanism/Effect on nutrient
Calcium	anticonvulsants	Accelerated catabolism related to vitamin D depletion
	corticosteroids	Reduced absorption
	diuretics (except thiazides), gentamicin	Increased renal excretion
	laxatives	Increased fecal excretion
	tetracyclines	Reduced absorption (usually of more concern clinically for the reduced absorption of tetracycline)
	thiazide diuretics	Decreased renal excretion
Cyanocobalamin	aminosalicylic acid	Decreased cyanocobalamin absorption
	chloramphenicol	Reticulocytosis associated with cyanocobalamin therapy of pernicious anemia may be decreased or delayed
	cholestyramine	Depletion of intrinsic factor
	colchicine	Malabsorption of cyanocobalamin
	potassium chloride	Lowers ileal pH, inhibiting cyanocobalamin absorption
Folic acid	aminosalicylic acid	Decreased gastrointestinal absorption of folic acid
	methotrexate, pyrimethamine, triamterene, trimethoprim	Conversion of folate to tetrahydrofolate is inhibited (note that this is the intended therapeutic mechanism)
	oral contraceptives (estrogen containing), phenytoin, phenobarbital, primidone	Interference with intestinal absorption of folate and increased catabolism
Iron	antacids, cimetidine	Decreased gastrointestinal absorption of iron salts
	bicarbonate, cholestyramine	Blockage of absorption
	acetylsalicylic acid, coumarin, heparin	Increased iron loss
	oral contraceptives	Increased iron absorption and decreased menstrual iron loss
	isoniazid	Impaired iron incorporation into red blood cells
	chloramphenicol	Suppressed hemoglobin synthesis

Table III *(Cont'd) Nutrient-Drug Interactions*

Vitamin/ Mineral	Interacting Drugs	Mechanism/Effect on nutrient
Magnesium	alcohol, amphotericin B, diuretics, digitalis, gentamicin	Increased renal excretion
Niacin	corticosteroids, estrogens	Increased production of niacin
	isoniazid	Interference with conversion of tryptophan to niacin
	fluorouracil, mercaptopurine	Blockage of intracellular synthesis of pyridine nucleotides
Phosphate	antacids	Binding of phosphate in the gastrointestinal tract preventing its absorption
Potassium	amphotericin B, carbenicillin, diuretics, laxatives, mineralocorticoids ticarcillin	Increased renal or gastrointestinal excretion
	amiloride, captopril, enalapril, lisinopril, spironolactone, triamterene	Decreased renal excretion of potassium
Pyridoxine	cycloserine, isoniazid	Impaired conversion of pyridoxine into pyridoxal and pyridoxamine
	hydralazine, isoniazid, levodopa	Increased excretion of pyridoxine
	penicillamine	Direct competitor for apoenzyme, causing decreased pyridoxine availability; increased excretion
Riboflavin	Antacids containing magnesium, metoclopramide, oral contraceptives, thyroxine	Decreased absorption
Sodium	Amitriptyline, carbamazepine, chlorpropamide, cyclophosphamide, tolbutamide, vincristine	Induction of inappropriate antidiuretic hormone syndrome secretion
	Clofibrate, ethacrynic acid, furosemide, oxytocin, thiazide diuretics	Increased renal excretion
	Laxatives (abuse)	Increased intestinal excretion

Nutritional Products

Table III (Cont'd) Nutrient-Drug Interactions

Vitamin/ Mineral	Interacting Drugs	Mechanism/Effect on nutrient
Thiamine	alcohol, digitalis	Increased thiamine requirement due to diuretic effect
Vitamin A	cholestyramine, clofibrate, mineral oil, neomycin	Impaired intestinal absorption of vitamin
Vitamin D	antacids, cholestryamine, clofibrate, laxatives, mineral oil, neomycin	Impaired intestinal absorption of vitamin
	anticonvulsants, glutethimide	Induction of hepatic microsomal enzymes
	corticosteroids	Interference with hepatic metabolism
	thiazide diuretics	Increased effects of vitamin D
Vitamin E	clofibrate, cholestyramine	Impaired gastrointestinal absorption
	oral contraceptives	Decreased serum concentration
Vitamin K	cholestyramine, mineral oil	Impaired gastrointestinal absorption
	acetylsalicylic acid, coumarin anticoagulants, salicylates	Blockage of synthesis of coagulation factors from vitamin K

Table IV Essential Minerals

Mineral	Major function(s) in body	Possible results of deficiency
Major Minerals		
Calcium (Ca)	Development of bones and teeth; blood clotting, normal nerve and muscle function	Stunted growth, rickets, osteomalacia, osteoporosis, confusion, cramps, tetany
Chlorine (Cl)	Formation of gastric juice, acid-base balance, activation of salivary amylase	Muscle cramps, mental apathy, reduced appetite, alkalosis
Iron (Fe)	Constituent of hemoglobin and enzymes of energy metabolism, cellular respiration	Iron deficiency anemia, oral lesions, koilonychia, anorexia
Magnesium (Mg)	Activates enzymes of protein synthesis, relaxation of skeletal muscles, nerve function	Growth failure, behavioral disturbances (e.g., confusion, disorientation), carphologia, vasodilation, weakness, spasms, loss of muscle control, tetany

Table IV (Cont'd) Essential Minerals

Mineral	Major function(s) in body	Possible results of deficiency
Phosphorous (P)	Bone and tooth formation, acid-base balance, storage and release of energy (ADP, ATP)	Weakness, demineralization of bone, anorexia, fatigue
Potassium (K)	Acid-base and body water (fluid) balance, normal nerve and muscle function, metabolism of carbohydrate and protein	Muscular weakness, constipation, polyuria, paralysis, apnea
Sodium (Na)	Body water (fluid) balance, nerve transmission	Thirst, apathy, confusion, dizziness, nausea, muscle weakness, abdominal cramps, diarrhea, dehydration, shock
Sulfur (S)	Maintenance of protein structure, collagen synthesis (cartilage and tendon), consitituent of nucleic acids and vitamins	Related to lack of sulfur amino acids and resultant poor growth and development
Trace Minerals		
Chromium (Cr)	Involved in glucose and energy metabolism	Not yet clearly established (reportedly associated with increased blood sugar and weight loss)
Cobalt (Co)	Constituent of cyanocobalamin	Not yet clearly established (except as related to cyanocobalamin deficiency and resultant pernicious anemia)
Copper (Cu)	Constituent of enzymes associated with iron metabolism, oxygen transport, melanin formation, and mitochondrial function	Anemia, bone and growth changes, impaired cellular metabolism, mental deterioration
Fluorine (F)	Maintenance of bone structure	Increased tooth decay, defective bone growth
Iodine (I)	Constituent of thyroid hormones, regulation of metabolic rate	Goiter (adults), cretinism (children) anorexia, dry skin
Manganese (Mn)	Constituent of enzymes involved in fat synthesis, protein synthesis, and carbohydrate metabolism	Poor growth, disturbances of nervous system, reproductive abnormalities, increased prothrombin time
Molybdenum (Mo)	Constituent of some enzymes (e.g., xanthine oxidase)	Not yet clearly established (deficiency noted in individuals receiving long-term parenteral nutrition; may be associated with esophageal cancer)

Table IV *(Cont'd) Essential Minerals*

Mineral	Major function(s) in body	Possible results of deficiency
Selenium (Se)	Functions in close association with vitamin E, metabolism of fat	Keshan disease, congestive heart failure, macrocytosis and pseudoalbinism in children
Zinc (Zn)	Constituent of enzymes of digestion; metabolism of carbohydrates, fats, and protein	Growth failure, small sex glands, delayed wound healing and growth, acrodermatitis enteropathica, alopecia

Table V *Osteoporosis Risk Factors*

Endogenous risk factors	Exogenous risk factors
Female gender Postmenopausal Caucasian or Oriental race Small body frame Low body weight Increasing age Positive family history	Low calcium intake High protein supplemental diet Immobilization Sedentary life style Drugs that decrease serum calcium (not yet clearly demonstrated, but a theoretical concern) (see Table III). Endocrine disorders (for example, Cushing's disease, hyperthyroidism)

Minerals

A mineral is an inorganic element or compound occurring in nature. Minerals are essential constituents of all living cells. Major minerals commonly found in Canadian self-medication products (including some important trace minerals) are listed in Table IV along with their major functions and the physiologic results associated with body deficiencies. Two minerals, calcium and iron, because of their importance to the body and prominence in self-medication products and advertising, are also discussed separately below.

Calcium

Calcium is the major component of bones and teeth and is essential for blood clotting and for normal neuromuscular function. Approximately 99 per cent of the body's calcium is stored in the skeleton (bones and teeth) as a reservoir; the remaining 1 per cent is distributed throughout the body. Calcium in the blood is found in approximately equal percentages either in unionized or ionized forms. The unionized form is bound to serum proteins (primarily albumin). The ionized or free form is physiologically active.

Physiologically, vitamin D is responsible for stimulating calcium absorption from the small intestine and for mobilizing bone calcium.

The recommended nutrient intake of calcium is 375 to 1,100 mg in infants and children up to 12 years of age and 700 to 1,100 mg for children over 12 and adults. Higher dosages (for example, 1,500 mg/day) may be required for postmenopausal women who are not receiving supplemental estrogen therapy. Individuals with malabsorption syndromes or uremia may suffer from hypocalcemia even when dietary or supplemental intake matches the RNI. Symptoms of hypocalcemia include rickets or growth impairment in children, osteomalacia, muscle pain, poor development of teeth, tetany and bleeding tendencies. Too much calcium consumed and absorbed by the body results in hypercalcemia, although excess calcium is not usually absorbed unless there is also excess vitamin D. Symptoms of hypercalcemia include anorexia, confusion, delirium, constipation, nausea, vomiting, polyuria, muscle weakness, renal stones, stupor and coma.

Osteoporosis

Because osteoporosis affects so many elderly women (about 25 to 40 per cent) much attention has been directed in the medical literature and lay press toward the benefits of prevention. Osteoporosis is a condition of decreased bone density and mass usually resulting from a negative calcium balance in the body, during which calcium is mobilized or resorbed from bone storage sites to meet the body's calcium requirements. Hip, wrist and vertebral fractures are the major morbidities associated with this loss of calcium from the bone. Risk factors for developing osteoporosis have been identified and can be divided into two categories, endogenous and exogenous (see Table V). These factors contribute to decreased bone calcium levels primarily by decreasing absorption and increasing elimination.

Various drugs (for example, estrogens, fluoride and vitamin D) are currently used to treat osteoporosis. However, the best form of treatment is prevention, and calcium is the mainstay of prevention. Calcium can be obtained readily from natural sources (for example, about 300 mg of elemental calcium are in 240 mL of milk), but many people find a calcium supplement more convenient. Individuals at risk for osteoporosis should usually consume 1,000 to 1,500 mg of elemental calcium daily if they can tolerate the calcium and have no contraindications to its use. In choosing a supplement, one should pay particular attention not only to dosage, but also to the salt form. Of the available salt forms, calcium carbonate is fairly well absorbed and contains the highest percentage of elemental calcium (about 40 per cent); it is generally the preferred form (see Table VI). Vitamin D facilitates calcium absorption and utilization in the body.

Drug Interactions

Calcium can be involved in several potentially significant drug interactions. For example, calcium and digitalis have similar effects on the heart muscle; therefore, digitalis administered to a hypercalcemic person may result in heart block. Calcium (as a divalent cation) can bind to tetracycline and decrease its gastrointestinal absorption if the two are concomitantly administered by the oral route. Dosing

Table VI *Available Calcium Salt Forms*

Calcium salt	% elemental calcium
Calcium carbonate	40
Tricalcium phosphate	39
Calcium chloride	36
Dibasic calcium phosphate	29.5
Calcium lactate	18.3
Calcium gluconate	9
Calcium glubionate	6.5

of these two products should be spaced 2 or more hours apart to avoid this interaction.

Iron

Iron is essential to hemoglobin formation and function and as such is essential to life. About 10 per cent of oral elemental iron is absorbed from the gastrointestinal tract. Vitamin C increases the gastrointestinal absorption of orally administered iron preparations. The trace minerals cobalt, copper and manganese are necessary for proper physiologic utilization of iron. The RNI for iron is only 8 to 13 mg for adults. The reason the requirement is so small is that the body conserves iron quite well. The major source of loss of iron from the body is bleeding. Often gastrointestinal bleeds can result in significant iron loss and resultant anemia. If menstrual flow is significant, it, too, can contribute to or cause clinically significant iron deficiency. For this last reason, iron supplements are often recommended as relatively inexpensive insurance for women between the ages of menarche and menopause. Most of the popular one-a-day vitamin/mineral supplements contain sufficient amounts of iron to meet this prophylactic requirement.

Iron deficiency anemia is a widespread problem in Canada. It occurs particularly in young children, teenaged boys and girls, women of childbearing age and the elderly. Although it causes few deaths, it contributes to poor health and suboptimal performance in many people. Various tests can be performed to measure directly for iron deficiency (for example, total iron binding capacity). An indirect measure of hemoglobin, which contains about 0.34 per cent iron, is more commonly available and used. Normal hemoglobin values range from 12 to 14 g/dL in females and from 14 to 17 g/dL in males. Signs and symptoms of iron deficiency include decreased hemoglobin; decreased energy and vitality; pale complexion; and slowed growth and development in children.

Individuals taking iron supplements should be advised of possible adverse effects. All iron products tend to irritate the gastrointestinal mucosal lining and may cause nausea, cramping or diarrhea. If the diarrhea is severe it can be accompanied by black and tarry stools. (Black and tarry stools may also be a symptom of significant bleeding within the gastrointestinal tract.) These symptoms can often be decreased by administering other salt forms (for example, ferrous gluconate and ferrous fumarate) or by taking the iron preparation with meals. Conversely, constipation is a frequently observed side effect of iron therapy. Individuals troubled by constipation with iron preparations may try one that combines iron with a stool softener (for example, docusate sodium).

Iron preparations can be extremely toxic if overdosed. Symptoms of iron poisoning include vomiting, restlessness, decreased blood pressure, increased respiration, cyanosis and coma. Each year many children are inadvertently poisoned by iron preparations (partly because many of the tablet formulations look like candy such as M&M's or Smarties). Consumers should be particularly careful to educate their children properly to the danger of inappropriate use of medications (be they prescription or nonprescription), never to treat or refer to medication as "candy" and to store iron preparations and all medications safely out of the reach of children.

Drug Interactions

Iron preparations can be involved in several clinically significant drug interactions. For example, iron, like calcium and other divalent and trivalent cations, can significantly decrease the gastrointestinal absorption of tetracycline if the two products are administered concomitantly by the oral route. Therefore, oral iron preparations should be administered 2 hours before or after tetracyclines to decrease the formation of chelates (insoluble drug-metal binding products) that in turn decrease gastrointestinal absorption. Concomitant administration of antacids and oral iron preparations may decrease the absorption of iron. These two preparations should also be dosed 2 or more hours apart.

Drug-Nutrient Interactions

Drug therapy may significantly affect nutritional status by changing absorption, transport mechanisms, metabolism and rates of excretion of various vitamins and minerals. The importance of these effects has been recognized only recently; however, the effects vitamins and minerals can have on drug therapy have been well documented for some time (for example, the interaction of milk products that contain calcium and the tetracyline antibiotics discussed earlier). The most common drug-induced vitamin deficiencies affect folic acid, pyridoxine and vitamin A (see Table III).

Folic acid is absorbed by active transport in the small intestine. Therefore, drugs such as phenobarbital, phenytoin and primidone, which affect folate absorption in the small intestine, may induce a folic acid deficiency. In addition, high doses of folic acid may antagonize the anticonvulsant effect of these drugs. Methotrexate, pyrimethamine, trimethoprim and triamterene, which inhibit the conversion of folate to tetrahydrofolate (the active metabolite) by blocking the enzyme dihydrofolate reductase, can also induce a folic acid deficiency. This is also the mechanism behind the antineoplastic and antibacterial effects of methotrexate, pyrimethamine and trimethoprim.

Several drugs are pyridoxine antagonists. These include isoniazid, cycloserine and other antituberculous drugs that inhibit the enzyme pyridoxal kinase and result in impaired synthesis of pyridoxal phosphate; hydralazine, isoniazid and levodopa, which form hydrazones with pyridoxal phosphate, causing increased excretion of this coenzyme; and penicillamine, a direct competitor for the apoenzyme, which diminishes pyridoxal coenzyme activity. In addition, use of oral contraceptives has been associated with pyridoxine depletion. Clinically, pyridoxine reduces the efficacy and increases the toxicity of levodopa because it is a cofactor in levodopa metabolism. Pyridoxine should not be supplemented in individuals treated with levodopa alone without the concurrent use of a decarboxylase inhibitor (such as carbidopa).

Drugs that impair absorption of vitamin A include mineral oil and retinol, which solubilize beta-carotene and cause vitamin A passage into the feces, and neomycin, which inhibits pancreatic lipase, inactivates bile salts and causes mucosal damage. Cholestyramine, a bile acid sequestrant, may also interfere with absorption of vitamin A and all other fat-soluble vitamins, as may clofibrate, by precipitating bile salts in the common bile duct.

Minerals derived from foods may be affected by several factors, including concurrently used drugs; the volume of free water used to administer a drug; and the minerals (salts) that are an inherent part of the drug (for example, sodium and potassium salts of drugs). Some important minerals affected include sodium, potassium, calcium, iron and magnesium.

Although diuretics primarily promote sodium excretion, renal homeostatic mechanisms generally protect against excessive sodium loss. However, if diuretics are overused or if sodium intake is insufficient, hyponatremia can occur. Potassium depletion can likewise occur with diuretic use (except potassium-sparing diuretics), as well as with the use of many other drugs (for example, acetazolamide, amphotericin B, carbenicillin, mineralocorticoids and ticarcillin). Chronic laxative use can cause excessive fecal loss of both potassium and calcium. Many drugs influence serum levels of calcium. Anticonvulsants accelerate calcium metabolism; glucocorticoids antagonize vitamin D activity in the gastrointestinal tract, thus reducing calcium absorption; diuretics such as furosemide, ethacrynic acid and triamterene, as well as digitoxin and gentamicin, can cause increased renal excretion of calcium. Drugs that decrease iron absorption include bicarbonate and cholestyramine. Several drugs (for example, acetylsalicylic acid, coumarin and heparin) cause iron loss by promoting gastrointestinal blood loss. Oral contraceptives and drugs that induce hemolysis increase iron absorption. Hypomagnesemia may result in people with any drug-induced malabsorption syndrome, as well as in people who chronically abuse alcohol, or use drugs such as diuretics and amphotericin B, which increase the renal excretion of magnesium.

Special Diets

Dietary standards, published by governmental agencies concerned with the prevention of deficiency diseases and the body's requirement for nutrients, have been available for many years. Recently dietary guidelines have focused on the prevention of chronic degenerative diseases and the risks of overconsumption of fats and sugars. The United Kingdom Government Committee on Medical Aspects of Food Policy has published guidelines for meeting the body's physiological need for nutrients and also for reducing the risk of several diet-related diseases. The National Academy of Science in the United States has published an interdisciplinary report "Diet and Health: Implications for Reducing Chronic Disease Risk". The nine guidelines reported in this publication are reproduced in Table VII. As indicated above, the first guideline is important since a major preventive treatment of heart disease is nutritive. The primary dietary substance implicated as a factor in developing atherosclerosis, coronary heart disease and stroke is dietary fat, including cholesterol and saturated fatty acids. High blood cholesterol levels increase the chance of having a heart attack; according to the National Heart, Lung, and Blood Institute of the United States, individuals with a blood cholesterol above 260 mg have four times the risk of developing heart disease as those with a level of 190 mg.

Cholesterol and saturated triglycerides (fats) are found in significant amounts in foods such as beef, pork, milk products and eggs, and in many oils (for example, palm oil and coconut oil). Cholesterol is transported in the blood in spherical particles, or complexes, composed of triglycerides, phospholipids and proteins. These particles are known as lipoproteins. The major cholesterol-containing lipoproteins are referred to as either low density lipoproteins (containing about 75 per cent lipids, including 40 to 45 per cent cholesterol) or high density lipoproteins (containing about 50 per cent lipids, including 20 to 25 per cent cholesterol).

Low density lipoproteins may promote heart disease by penetrating the coronary artery wall where they are broken down enzymatically to cholesterol, cholesterol ester and protein. Then, the cholesterol and cholesterol ester may be deposited in the artery wall, becoming

Table VII *Dietary Guidelines for Reducing Chronic Disease Risk*

1. Reduce total fat intake to 30 per cent or less calories. Reduce saturated fat intake to less than 10 per cent of calories and the intake of cholesterol to less than 300 mg daily.
2. Every day eat 5 or more servings (250 g) of a combination of vegetables and fruits, especially green and yellow vegetables and citrus fruits.
3. Maintain protein intake at moderate levels (less than 1.6 g/kg body weight for adults).
4. Balance food intake and physical activity to maintain appropriate weight.
5. Limit consumption of alcohol to less than 30 mL of pure alcohol in a single day.
6. Limit total daily intake of sodium chloride to 6 g or less.
7. Maintain adequate calcium intake.
8. Avoid taking dietary supplements in excess of the recommended daily allowance in any one day.
9. Maintain an optimal intake of fluoride.

Adapted from: Committee on Diet and Health, Food and Nutrition Board, Commission on Life Sciences, National Research Council. Diet and Health: Implications for reducing chronic disease risk. Washington: National Academy Press, 1989.

major constituents of atherosclerotic plaque. High density lipoproteins may reduce the individual's risk of coronary heart disease by transporting cholesterol out of the cells. Thus, lipoproteins can be considered good or bad depending on type. When high density lipoprotein levels are expressed in proportion to low density lipoprotein levels, a ratio of at least 1:3 is desirable. Women tend to have better lipoprotein ratios than men, contributing to significantly lower incidence of heart disease in women.

Ways to increase blood levels of high density lipoproteins include endurance exercise and losing weight. Although cholesterol and triglyceride levels can be controlled by drug therapy, a report from the American Medical Association recommends diet therapy be tried first, since it is generally safer than drug therapy and if successful may preclude the need for drug therapy.

The "Greenland diet" (fish oil capsules taken up to a maximum of 3 g/day) has been promoted to prevent heart disease. In 1970, Danish researchers observed that Greenland Inuit had a low rate of heart disease despite a diet high in fat and cholesterol. Blood samples from these Inuit were low in fats (particularly triglycerides), low in cholesterol and high in high density lipoprotein cholesterol. It was also noted that the blood samples had a longer than normal coagulation time with decreased platelet aggregation. These effects were ascribed to fish oil components called omega-3 fatty acids.

It has been known for some time that polyunsaturated fatty acids such as linoleic acid, an omega-6 fatty acid from seed and vegetable oils, may lower low density lipoprotein cholesterol levels in blood. The long-chain, highly unsaturated omega-3 fatty acids also competitively inhibit the synthesis of thromboxane A, a vasoconstrictive substance that promotes platelet aggregation. This activity of the omega-3 fatty acids may result in a decreased tendency toward forming atherosclerotic plaques. Hence, fish oil capsules are promoted to prevent heart disease. Several general reviews on the biological effects of fish oils on lipid and lipoprotein metabolism and cardiovascular disease have been published recently.

Nutritional Products

Table VIII *Attributes of Some Alternative Sweeteners*

Sweetener	Source	Sweetness Relative to Sucrose	Toxicity	Use/Comments
Saccharin	Synthetic	300	Carcinogen?	Restricted in Canada and U.S.
Cyclamate	Synthetic	30	Carcinogen?	Restricted in Canada and U.S.
Acesulfame-K	Synthetic	200	None	Approved 1988 in U.S. for use in food and soft drinks
Thaumatin	Plant	3,000	None	Used as a partial sweetener
Stevioside	Plant	300	None	Menthol-like bitter aftertaste
Xylitol	Plant	1	None	Slowly absorbed,
Sorbitol	Plant	0.6	None	excessive amounts can
Mannitol	Plant	0.5	None	cause diarrhea
Dihydrochalcones	Plant	2,000	Testicular atrophy in dogs	Licorice-like aftertaste
Aspartame	Synthetic	200	None	Taste closet to sucrose

Adapted from: Sanyude S. Alternative sweeteners. Can Pharm J 1990;123(10):456.

However, fish oil capsules are not without potential hazard. Diarrhea has occurred after taking 4 to 6 capsules per day. Longer blood coagulation times can be a complication in the event of an accident or emergency surgery and can be particularly dangerous for people taking anticoagulants or large doses of ASA. In addition, if cod liver oil is taken, it is advisable not to exceed the recommended dosage based on its vitamin A and D content, as hypervitaminosis A or D can occur.

Diets low in natural fibre have been associated with increased incidence of atherosclerosis, colon cancer, diverticulosis, gallstones, hiatus hernia, rectal hemorrhoids and other disorders. However, the effectiveness of a high-fibre diet in directly decreasing the incidence of these conditions has not been substantiated. It has been clearly substantiated that increased intake of dietary fibre helps prevent and treat constipation and can reduce both the constipation and diarrhea associated with irritable bowel syndrome. (See the chapter on laxatives.) More research is needed on the nutritional requirements and potential therapeutic benefit of the various forms of dietary fibre.

Vitamin-rich foods, particularly those containing vitamin C and beta-carotene (which is convertible to vitamin A in the body), have been associated with decreased cancer risk. However, it has not been demonstrated whether the effects are related to the vitamin content of these foods or to other factors such as increased dietary fibre content of these foods and decreased fat intake.

Sugar Substitutes

Low-nutrient sweeteners are used commonly by individuals who need or want to reduce their intake of carbohydrates (for example, diabetics and dieters) and by those seeking to avoid or reduce dental caries. Consumers and food manufacturers may add these sweeteners to foods to enhance flavors and acceptability or to manage nutrient value and shelf-life. The separate table-top sweeteners (for example, Equal) are available in aqueous solution with small amounts of preservatives or in powdered or granulated preparations with agents such as dextrose or lactose that provide bulk and add calories (energy) to the preparation (see Table VIII).

Saccharin

Saccharin was first synthesized over 100 years ago and has been used commercially for over 80 years to sweeten foods and beverages. When saccharin is combined with aspartame or cyclamates the sweetness is greater than that provided by the individual sweeteners. Sucaryl was marketed in Canada as a combination of saccharin and cyclamate but now contains only cyclamate.

Saccharin is stable. It is 300 times sweeter than sucrose and is excreted in unchanged form in the urine. A slight metallic aftertaste is often observed by some saccharin users, but saccharin is generally found to have an acceptable taste. It has been used in soft drinks, table-top sweeteners and a wide variety of other beverages, foods and pharmaceuticals.

Saccharin has been investigated, reviewed and debated more than any other food additive in North America. Several early studies found bladder tumors in male rats exposed to extremely high doses of saccharin in utero, during the post-natal period and in two-generation studies. Other single-generation feeding studies in which animals were fed saccharin for a lifetime failed to demonstrate an association between saccharin intake and bladder cancer. In reviewing all available animal and human data, the National Cancer Institute has concluded there is no overall association between saccharin intake and human bladder cancer. However, it remains banned in Canada.

Cyclamate

Cyclamate is an artificial, non-caloric sweetener approximately 30 times sweeter than sucrose on a mg per mg basis. In the past, it has been widely used in low-calorie foods and beverages. Like saccharin, it is not metabolized in the liver, but is variably metabolized in the gastrointestinal tract. Cyclamate is excreted primarily in unchanged form in the urine.

Cyclamate was banned in the United States in 1970; however, a petition to the Food and Drug Administration currently seeks to reapprove cyclamate. The United States National Academy of Sciences has stated that "the totality of evidence from studies in animals does not indicate that cyclamate or its major metabolite, cyclohexylamine, is carcinogenic by itself."

Cyclamate is used world-wide. The Joint Expert Committee on Food Additives of the World Health Organization has established the generally acceptable daily intake of cyclamate to be 10 mg/kg of body weight. Cyclamates are permitted for use as table-top sweeteners in Canada, but must have a warning on the label.

Aspartame

Aspartame, a noncarbohydrate sweetener, was originally approved by the Food and Drug Administration in the United States for use in 1974. However, objections raised on the grounds of safety and questions about test data delayed final approval until 1981. Aspartame was then approved for use with the label to read "contains phenylalanine" as a caution to those individuals with phenylketonuria. The FDA approved the use of aspartame in soft drinks in 1983. In 1984 the Center for Disease Control, after a review of consumer complaints, concluded that the complaints "do not provide evidence of the existence of serious, widespread adverse health consequences attendant to the use of aspartame."

Aspartame is a simple peptide made up of 2 amino acids, L-aspartic acid and L-phenylalanine. It has been suggested that aspartame is no more hazardous than protein in the diet. The highest estimate of daily aspartame use ranges from 22 to 34 mg/kg of body weight (that is, if aspartame replaced all the sugar in the diet) and the quantities of phenylalanine and aspartic acid provided by dietary protein range from 52 to 229 mg/kg of body weight and 80 to 395 mg/kg of body weight respectively. Thus, intake of aspartame appears to have an insignificant effect, compared to normal dietary intake, on the levels of these amino acids.

Aspartame is about 180 times as sweet as sucrose on a mg per mg basis. The energy provided by the normal use of aspartame is minimal. Aspartame may be hydrolyzed in the gastrointestinal tract to aspartate, phenylalanine and methanol by proteolytic and hydrolytic enzymes. Aspartame may also be absorbed directly into mucosal cells by peptide transport mechanisms and subsequently broken down within the cell to aspartate, phenylalanine and methanol. Thus, in either case, the safety of aspartame relates not to aspartame itself, but to the potential harmful effects of these hydrolysis products.

The peak plasma level of phenylalanine in normal subjects and in phenylketonuric heterozygotes indicates a potential risk for this subset of the population. Thus, the Food and Drug Administration requires cautionary labelling of aspartame. Phenylketonuria occurs in about one person in every 50 to 75 as a heterozygous state. It has been shown that the phenylketonuria heterozygotes metabolize the phenylalanine portion of aspartame more slowly than normal subjects. However, peak phenylalanine values in these subjects were still well below those associated with toxic effects. Individuals who are homozygotic for the autosomal recessive trait of phenylketonuria are at risk for potential toxicity and should avoid aspartame-containing products.

The hydrolysis product methanol has been measured in human subjects given aspartame up to 200 mg/kg of body weight. No significant changes in blood formate (a toxic methanol metabolite) were found; however, urinary formate excretion increased over preloading levels. This increase suggests some risk from the methanol content of aspartame. This potential risk appears to be even greater for people receiving large doses of disulfiram, which prevents the further metabolism of formate. However, risk for the normal individual appears to be minimal.

The overall conclusion from all available data on aspartame is that, despite some potential (and perhaps primarily theoretical) concerns, this alternative sweetener is safe for use.

Acesulfame Potassium

Acesulfame potassium is a sweetener 200 times sweeter than sucrose. Acesulfame has some structural resemblance to saccharin and this has raised the question of its carcinogenicity. However acesulfame has not been shown to be teratogenic or mutagenic in various test systems and in animal studies acesulfame has not caused any dose-related malignancies, even after prolonged exposure to very large doses. Acesulfame potassium is soluble in water and heat stable in the temperature range required for food storage and processing. Acesulfame potassium (Sunette–Hoechst) was recently approved in the United States for use as a noncaloric table-top sweetener and as an ingredient in chewing gum, powdered beverages, gelatins, and puddings. Acesulfame in high doses can induce insulin secretion in vivo.

Consumer Counselling

Consumers often ask pharmacists for advice when choosing vitamin and mineral supplements. The following are some general helpful comments. House brands are usually as good as and often much less expensive than nationally advertised brands. Synthetic vitamins are as good as and generally much less expensive than natural vitamins. Pharmacists should advise consumers to check the expiration date on vitamin packages. The product should be good for at least 6 to 12 months from the date of purchase. Consumers should protect vitamins from excessive heat, light and moisture. Generally, vitamins are best stored in a room other than the washroom. Liquid vitamin or mineral preparations may be best for infants and elderly individuals who have difficulty swallowing tablets or capsules. Consumers should follow the label instructions exactly unless otherwise directed by their physician. All vitamins and minerals should be stored safely out of the reach of children.

Ask the Consumer

Q. Is the vitamin/mineral preparation for you or someone else?
- Vitamin and mineral requirements differ according to several parameters, including age and gender. The individual making the purchase is not necessarily the intended consumer.

Q. Do you have any chronic diseases or conditions that may affect your diet (for example, diabetes mellitus)?
- This question provides information about nutrient requirements over and above those normal for the healthy individual. In addition,

Nutritional Products

if the condition is particularly complex or severe, discussion with, or referral to, the consumer's physician may be appropriate.

Q. Are you currently taking any prescription or nonprescription medications?

- Assess possible vitamin/nutrient interactions to avoid or minimize them. Inquire also about "social" drug use. For example, excessive alcohol consumption relates to deficiencies in the water-soluble vitamins, particularly the B-complex, and tobacco smoking has been related to increased requirements for vitamin C.

Q. Do you eat meats, vegetables, dairy products and grains every day? What is your typical daily diet?

- This information gives an initial impression of whether a vitamin or mineral deficiency is likely, and, if it is, which vitamins or minerals are probably required.

Q. Are you currently using any vitamins or mineral supplements? If you are, which specific product(s) do you use and how do you generally use them (for example, 1 tablet daily)?

- This information is necessary to establish an adequate baseline regarding current vitamin or mineral supplementation and to properly determine what changes, if any, should be recommended. This information will also be useful in detecting actual and potential abuse (overuse) of the vitamin/mineral supplements.

Q. Why are you requesting a vitamin/mineral supplement? What related symptoms have you had? Have the symptoms appeared suddenly or gradually?

- The person may have a related (for example, endocrine) or other severe underlying disorder and should be referred for appropriate diagnosis and treatment. The consumer also may have serious misconceptions about the need for and benefits of vitamin therapy that should be addressed and corrected before making any recommendations.

Other appropriate questions may come from these initial questions or from the consumer's clinical presentation. Questions should be tailored to the individual and fully answered before the pharmacist recommends vitamin or mineral supplements, thus providing the consumer with optimal benefits of this therapy and minimizing potential adverse effects.

References

General
Hui YH. Human nutrition and diet therapy. Monterey: Wadsworth, 1983.
McCarthy-Rice C. Nutritional supplements. Pharm Pract 1986;2:6–8,10,12.
Sanders HJ. Nutrition and health. Chem Eng News 1979;57(13):27–46.

Vitamins
Covington TL. Vitamins: part I—common myths. Facts and Comp Drug Newsletter 1987;6:54–5.
DiPalma JR, Thayer WS. Use of niacin as a drug. Ann Rev Nutr 1991;11:153.
Earthman TP, Odom L, Mullens CA. Lactic acidosis associated with high dose niacin therapy. S Med J 1991;84:496–7.
Henkin Y, Johnson KC, Segrest JP. Rechallenge with crystalline niacin after drug-induced hepatitis from sustained release niacin. J Am Med Assoc 1990;264:241–3.

Krogh CME, ed. Compendium of pharmaceuticals and specialities. Ottawa: Canadian Pharmaceutical Association, 1992.
Lewis JG. Adverse reactions to vitamins. Reactions 1980;Jul11:1–2.
Mullen GE, Greenson JK, Mitchell MC. Fulminant hepatic failure after ingestion of sustained-release nicotinic acid. Ann Intern Med 1989; 111:253–5.
Yamanaka WK. Vitamins and cancer prevention: how much do we know? Postgrad Med 1987;82(3):149–51,153.

Vitamin E
Bieri JG, Corash L, Hubbard VS. Medical uses of vitamin E. N Engl J Med 1983;308:1063–71.

Calcium
Anonymous. Food and drug interactions. Health and Welfare Canada Dispatch 1982;50:1–3.
Bauwens SF, Drinka PJ, Boh LE. Pathogenesis and management of primary osteoporosis. Clin Pharm 1986;5:639–59.
Covington TL. Calcium: the miracle mineral? Facts and Comp Drug Newsletter 1986;5:33–4.
Covington TL. Osteoporosis. Am Pharm 1986;NS26(11):47–50.
Nordin BEC, Morris HA. The calcium deficiency model for osteoporosis. Nutri Rev 1989;47:65–72.
Sagraves R, Van Tyle JH. Osteoporosis in women: the importance of calcium. Pharm Times 1986;52:104–13.
Steinberg SK, Cornish P. An overview of calcium and the use of oral calcium supplements. Can Pharm J 1987;120:168–73.
Stevenson JC. Pathophysiology of osteoporosis. Triangle 1988;27:47–52.

Selenium
Anonymous. Newly recognized signs of selenium deficiency in humans. Nutri Rev 1989;47:117–9.
Coombs GF. Selenium in foods. Adv Food Res 1988;32:85–113.

Drug-Nutrient Interactions
Roe DA. Drug-induced nutritional deficiencies. Westport: AVI Publishers, 1985.

Special Diets
Committee on Diet and Health, Food and Nutrition Board, Commission on Life Sciences, National Research Council. Diet and Health: Implications for Reducing Chronic Disease Risk. Washington: National Academy Press, 1989.
Connor WE. Effects of omega-3 fatty acids in hypertriglyceridemic states. Semin Thromb Hemost 1988;14:271–84.
Leaf A, Weber PC. Cardiovascular effects of omega-3 fatty acids. N Engl J Med 1988;318:549–57.
Li Wan Po A. Dietary Supplements (7) Fish Oils. Pharm J 1991; (Jan 19):83–5.
Mason PM. A better prescription for the British diet. Pharm J 1991; (Aug 17):204–5.
Miller RW. The fight against heart disease. Part 1: diet, exercise and other keys to a healthy heart. FDA Consumer 1986;20(1):8–13.
Mueller BA, Talbert RL. Biological mechanisms and cardiovascular effects of omega-3 fatty acids. Clin Pharm 1988;7:795–807.
Yetiv JZ. Clinical applications of fish oils. J Am Med Assoc 1988;260:665–70.
Zanula E. The Greenland diet: can fish oils prevent heart disease? FDA Consumer 1986;20(8):6–8.

Sugar Substitutes
Anonymous. Med Lett 1988;30:116.
Baines CJ. Table top artificial sweeteners: current use in Canada. Can Dent Assoc J 1985;51:427–8.
Liang Y, Steinbach G, Maier V, Pfeiffer EF. The effect of artificial sweetener on insulin secretion. 1. The effect of acesulfame K on insulin secretion in the rat (studies in vivo). Horm Metabol Res 1987;19:233–38.
Mackay DAM. Factors associated with the acceptance of sugar and sugar substitutes by the public. Int Dent J 1985;35:201–9.
Pagliaro LA, Locock RA. Aspartame. Can Pharm J 1986;119:121–3.
Sanyude S. Artificial Sweeteners. Can Pharm J 1990;123:455–60.

31
Eating Disorders

Revised by Jane Blouin and Arthur G. Blouin.
Based on original chapter by Jane Blouin, Arthur G. Blouin and Peter Aubin

Obesity, anorexia nervosa and bulimia present numerous medical risks. The causes of these eating disorders are both biological and psychosocial. Treatment is primarily psychoeducational, although research continues on pharmacologic agents. Nonprescription products used and abused by people with eating disorders include purgatives, emetics, appetite suppressants, diet aids and dietary supplements. Individuals with eating disorders are also more likely than the general population to abuse other drugs such as sleeping pills, analgesics and alcohol.

Self-medication is extremely common in individuals suffering from eating disorders. Ample evidence exists that this group uses nonprescription medication more often than the normal population, and that there are grave risks in abusing these products. Further, one hallmark of eating disorders is the tendency for individuals to feel ashamed of their symptoms, and thus remain undiagnosed and untreated. For these reasons, pharmacists must be familiar with eating disorders and the attendant patterns of nonprescription drug consumption and abuse.

Diagnosis

The definition of obesity varies from a diagnosis based on normal data on body mass index (BMI), measured as kg/m², to one based on data relating BMI to mortality and morbidity rates. The optimal BMI is 22.5 ±2.5 for men, and 21.5 ±2.5 for women. A BMI of 30 kg/m² or over is in the range of obesity, and is associated with elevated morbidity and mortality rates. Obesity is considered a medical condition, rather than a psychiatric disorder. The eating disorders bulimia and anorexia nervosa, on the other hand, have been defined in standard psychiatric diagnostic manuals.

To be given a diagnosis of anorexia nervosa, an individual must satisfy the following criteria: refusal to maintain body weight over a minimal normal weight for age and height, leading to a body weight 15 per cent or more below expected; intense fear of becoming obese, even when underweight; disturbance in the self-perception of body size, shape or weight (for example, feeling fat when emaciated); and, in females, absence of at least 3 consecutive menstrual cycles.

The requirements for the diagnosis of bulimia are as follows: recurrent episodes of binge-eating unusually large quantities of food in

Figure 1   *Body Mass Index (BMI)*

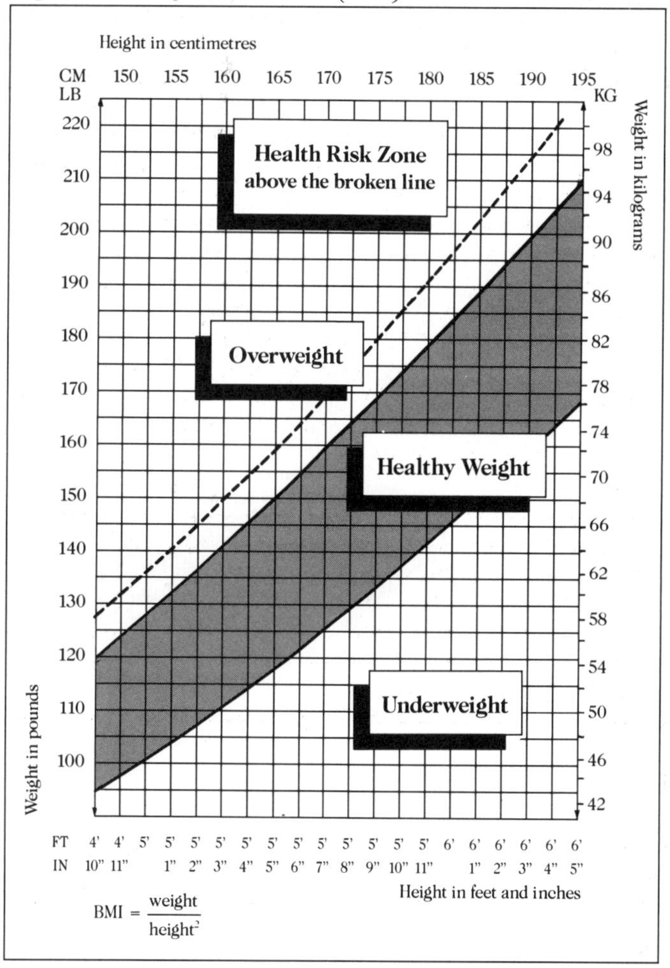

$$BMI = \frac{weight}{height^2}$$

discrete periods of time (that is, 2 hours or less) at least twice a week for at least 3 months; the sense that the binging is out of the individual's control; persistent overconcern with body shape and weight; and attempts to prevent weight gain through self-induced vomiting, use of laxatives, strict dieting, fasting or vigorous exercise.

Prevalence

Recent data suggest that 80 per cent of American men and 70 per cent of American women over age 40 are above the optimal weight range. It is estimated that 45 per cent of Canadians are over the optimal BMI, and less than 12 per cent have a BMI in excess of 30 kg/m².

Anorexia occurs in roughly one per cent of the female college-aged population. Epidemiological research indicates a lifetime North American population prevalence of 0.1 per cent for anorexia nervosa. The incidence of anorexia appears to have doubled in the last two decades.

Bulimia occurs in roughly 4.5 to 18 per cent of college-aged women. Bulimia is believed to be at least 10 times more prevalent than anorexia. The number of people presenting with bulimic symptoms and the number of journal articles concerning bulimia has increased dramatically in the last decade. This may represent an actual increase in prevalence, but is also because the disorder has only been defined in standard psychiatric diagnostic manuals in this decade.

Obesity is more common in women than men, but the over-representation of women in anorectic and bulimic populations is far more extreme—about 95 per cent.

Medical Risks

The medical risks involved in eating disorders are manifold; their presence and severity depend on the intensity and duration of various specific symptoms, rather than the actual eating disorder diagnosis. Binge-eating, which may occur in all three eating disorders, may lead to heart failure, edema, or gastric dilation or rupture. Chronic obesity is linked to increased risk of many diseases, such as diabetes, gout, hypertension and coronary atherosclerosis. Other medical risks include skin excoriation (especially in skin folds), immobility, knee problems such as torn meniscus, and respiratory difficulties. Malnourishment, common in both bulimia and anorexia nervosa, often results in amenorrhea, heart failure, renal dysfunction, various electrolyte disorders, anemia and constipation. Self-induced vomiting, again most common in anorexia and bulimia, often results in hypokalemia, metabolic alkalosis, oral cavity trauma and aspiration pneumonitis. Laxative abuse, common in all eating disorders, can cause hypocalcemia, hypokalemia, hypokalemic cardiomyopathy, hypokalemic ileus and cathartic colon. Diuretic abuse is also a cause of hypokalemia and hyponatremia in these people.

Prognosis

Obesity is universally acknowledged as a condition relatively resistant to treatment. Although initial weight loss is often achieved in people seeking treatment, long-term maintenance of weight loss occurs for only 10 to 15 per cent of individuals.

The prognosis for people with anorexia or bulimia generally depends on the extent to which the person also suffers from other psychiatric disorders, such as depression or personality disorders. The prognosis for anorexia or bulimia alone, or in combination with depression, is usually good when treated with medication and/or psychotherapy. If the eating disorder coexists with a severe personality or character disorder, treatment success is usually extremely limited.

Pathogenesis

The isolation of a single definitive cause of any of the eating disorders has eluded vigorous research. It is increasingly accepted that obesity, bulimia and anorexia are determined by some combination (which may vary for each affected individual) of biological and psychosocial factors.

Biological Factors

Abundant evidence exists that obesity runs in families, although, clearly, either genetic or environmental factors may account for this finding. The obese may have inherited a higher set point weight than the nonobese. This theory suggests that the genetically determined set-point weight is vigorously defended by the functioning of the ventrolateral hypothalamus, the "feeding centre" of the brain, and the ventromedial hypothalamus, the "satiety centre." The activity of these cerebral nuclei promotes the initiation and termination of eating at a given caloric level or set point. If less food is ingested, the individual's basal metabolic rate (BMR) slows down and energy, in the form of adipose tissue, is conserved. Alternatively, increases in caloric intake result in increases in BMR, again stabilizing weight.

The ability of individuals suffering from anorexia nervosa to achieve a weight below their inherited set point appears to argue against the set point theory. However, closer examination reveals evidence to support the theory. Many individuals suffering from anorexia or bulimia manage to achieve stable though suboptimal weights ingesting less than 500 calories per day. These people may survive solely because of drastically reduced BMR. Binge-eating, the major symptom of bulimia and a frequent symptom of anorexia, may be the hypothalamic response to a diet that is hypocaloric for the inherited set-point weight, though the individual may not appear drastically underweight.

A classic experiment demonstrating the deleterious effects of restrictive dieting was done 30 years ago. The results indicate that prolonged dietary restriction not only causes weight loss, but also depression, inability to concentrate and preoccupation with food. After normal diets are resumed, these symptoms, as well as binge-eating, persist for several weeks to months after the individual regains the original weight.

Abnormally high endogenous opioid activity is a factor of etiological significance in obesity. This abnormality may underlie the reduced energy expenditure, higher pain threshold and susceptibility to depression after losing weight observed in obese individuals.

In eating disorders, carbohydrate craving and the impaired satiety response to food may be mediated by functional deficiencies of the neurochemical serotonin. One study found weight-recovered bulimic anorectics had deficient cerebrospinal fluid levels of a serotonergic metabolite, compared to nonbulimic or restricting (that is, nonbinging) anorectics. Serotonergic deficiencies may underlie the urge to binge-eat in obesity, as well as in bulimia and anorexia. Carbohydrate ingestion is known to facilitate central serotonin activity; binge eating may therefore be an attempt to elevate deficient levels of serotonin. Levels of brain serotonin are known to fluctuate seasonally, and may underlie the disruptions in mood and food intake observed in Seasonal Affective Disorder. Blouin et al have also found that bulimic symptoms are markedly exacerbated in the winter months, compared to summer months. Restricting anorectics may suffer from an excess of serotonin, which may promote a chronic sense of satiety.

Other research implicates other neurochemical abnormalities, such as noradrenergic dysfunction.

Although vulnerability to serotonergic dysfunction may be genetically determined, binge-eating is almost invariably associated with a history of prolonged restrictive dieting. The hypocaloric diet impairs the normal insulin response to ingested carbohydrates, which, in turn, limits the rate at which peripheral tryptophan (the serotonin precursor) gains access to the brain. This process results in reduced synthesis of serotonin centrally. At least 90 per cent of women with bulimia report that binge-eating is preceded by a prolonged period of restrictive dieting. Thus, dieting may be regarded as the trigger of the urge to binge-eat in the eating disorders.

Psychosocial Factors

Moderately obese and overweight individuals have repeatedly been found to have no greater degree of any type of psychopathology than nonobese control groups. Nonetheless, many obese individuals come to regard their bodies as grotesque, which, in turn, may lead to social and emotional withdrawal. On the other hand, individuals seeking treatment for eating disorders typically present with symptoms of low self-esteem; more than half the people with anorexia or bulimia suffer clinical depression. Generally, they tend also to be perfectionist, distrustful and unable to identify their own emotions accurately.

Perhaps this cluster of psychological symptoms renders people with anorexia or bulimia more vulnerable to our culture's intense emphasis on thinness as the physical ideal, especially for women. Few North Americans are able to achieve the almost impossible ideal of thinness promoted by the media and the fashion and entertainment industries; for perfectionist people with low self-esteem, this failure is devastating and results in obsessive preoccupation with thinness. It must be more than coincidence that as the female physical role models of Miss America contestants and *Playboy* centrefolds have become increasingly thin over the last two decades, the incidence of anorexia and bulimia has dramatically increased.

Treatment

Treatment of eating disorders has been geared to the increasing, if still limited, understanding of their pathogenesis.

Psychoeducational Approaches

Success has been achieved with cognitive-behavioral treatment approaches in group and individual settings. Often a simple psychoeducational approach is effective, warning of the medical risks of binge-eating, purging and dieting and outlining alternative methods of weight control focused on regular diet and exercise. For people with anorexia nervosa or bulimia, this treatment should be conducted in a hospital setting, although community self-help groups can be a useful adjunct to professional treatment. Most major Canadian cities have an eating disorders clinic in a general hospital, where people are treated on an outpatient basis. Further information on such clinics can be obtained through the National Eating Disorders Information Centre in Toronto (416–483-5213). Obese people who are not binge-eating or purging may benefit from organizations such as Weight Watchers or Overeaters Anonymous, but not from diet centres prescribing hypocaloric diets (for example, less than 1,500 calories per day). Nonobese individuals who are preoccupied with their shape or weight, but who are not binge-eating, purging or underweight, can get help from Anti-diet programs available through many community health organizations. These programs educate people about our culture's unrealistic emphasis on thinness. They are designed to assist people toward a healthier perception of their bodies.

Pharmacologic Approaches

Psychopharmacologic treatment of eating disorders has recently been the focus of intensive research. Tricyclic antidepressant medication has been used with some success in treating bulimia in both depressed and nondepressed individuals. Antidepressant trials have met limited success in treating anorexia nervosa. For example, the serotonergic antagonist cyproheptadine has been used with variable success in treating anorexia. Compared to placebo, cyproheptadine appears helpful in stimulating weight gain and alleviating depression in restricting anorectics, but is not superior to placebo in treating bulimic anorectics. The effectiveness of these agents may be mediated not so much through their pharmacologic antidepressant properties, but through their effects on central or peripheral appetite mechanisms.

Binge-eating has been reduced substantially when treated with the anorexiant fenfluramine, a specific serotonergic agonist, in both obese and bulimic people. Fenfluramine may also reduce binge-eating in bulimic anorexics, but has not been tried due to the risk of weight loss in dangerously underweight individuals. Laboratory studies indicate underweight rats gain weight when administered fenfluramine; overweight animals lose weight.

Other anorexiant agents have been used to treat obesity, notably amphetamine congeners. Pharmacists and physicians are well aware these agents must be prescribed cautiously due to the side effects, abuse potential, tolerance and addiction dangers associated with amphetamines. Although fenfluramine is also an amphetamine derivative, it does not possess the same type and degree of amphetamine-like dangers as the other anorexiants.

Both fenfluramine and fluoxetine, a serotonergic reuptake blocker antidepressant, effectively promote weight loss in obese individuals. Tricyclic antidepressants reduce the depressive symptoms that often accompany weight loss in people being treated for obesity through dietary manipulation. Finally, opiate antagonists such as naltrexone and naloxone have met with some success in the treatment of obesity. It is important to note, however, that weight loss achieved through pharmacologic treatment may not be maintained on discontinuation of medication, and may compromise the long-term success of behavioral psychotherapy when the two treatments are combined.

Self-medication

Nonprescription products used by individuals with eating disorders fall into several categories: laxatives, emetics, appetite suppressants, diet aids, dietary supplements and agents geared to relief of concomitant symptoms of eating disorders. A major psychological characteristic of individuals with eating disorders, especially those with anorexia and bulimia, is the tendency to think and act impulsively and in extremes. It is this characteristic, commonly referred to as black-and-white thinking, which renders nonprescription medication dangerous in the hands of these people. They are more apt to abuse the product than are other people, ignoring manufacturers' recommendations for moderate use.

Another point of interest is the finding that 67 per cent of women with bulimia have reported stealing, compared to only 14 per cent

Eating Disorders

of control subjects. Items most often stolen include food for binges, as well as nonprescription medication products.

Laxatives

The most commonly abused purgative in patients with eating disorders (especially bulimic patients) is laxatives. Laxative abuse has been found to occur in approximately 52 to 62 per cent of women with eating disorders. This is obviously far greater than the incidence of 2.5 per cent of a normal sample of Canadian adults who regularly use laxatives. Of note is the fact that, of the 3 to 4 per cent of high school students who use laxatives, 55 per cent have symptoms of an eating disorder. Laxative users of high school age are clearly at risk for having or developing an eating disorder. Amongst eating disordered patients using laxatives, 55 per cent use laxatives several times per week, 30 per cent use laxatives daily, and 15 per cent use laxatives several times per day. Furthermore, 27.5 per cent use 11 to 20 times the recommended dose per occasion, while another 15 per cent use more than 20 times the recommended dose. The most commonly used brands of laxatives are the stimulant types (for example, Ex-Lax and Correctol).

What most of these women are unaware of, however, is that laxative use has been found to be totally ineffective as a means of weight loss. Although the stimulant type of laxatives promptly produces a watery diarrhea with an accompanying sense of weight loss, this is actually simply the result of temporary fluid loss, as the caloric absorption prevented by the laxative is minimal. Further, they are generally unaware that laxative abuse can severely impair the functioning of the gastrointestinal tract, leading to chronic problems with diarrhea, constipation, gastrointestinal bleeding, abdominal pain, cathartic colon and electrolyte abnormalities, especially hypokalemia. Several researchers have noted that pseudo-Bartter's syndrome, characterized by hypokalemia, systemic alkalosis, elevated angiotensin and normal blood pressure, is a common consequence of laxative abuse. Hypocalcemia and concomitant metabolic alkalosis are frequent sequelae of severe laxative abuse, and can lead to carpopedal spasm and tetany. Dehydration typically follows from chronic laxative abuse, and can ultimately result in reflex peripheral edema, especially during withdrawal from the laxatives.

Education of these clients, regarding the ineffectiveness, medical dangers, and withdrawal from laxative abuse is obviously essential. Most laxative abusers experience a resolution of the fluid retention, and return to normal bowel functions in 10 days of cessation of laxative use. They should be advised to discontinue use of the stimulant type of laxatives, while increasing their fluid intake, engaging in regular physical exercise, and ensuring their diet is high in fibre. It is crucial that they understand the futility of increasing their use of laxatives in response to fluid retention. However, monitoring their bowel functions is important as, in more severe cases, the temporary use of lactulose may be necessary to prevent fecal impaction.

Diuretics

Diuretic abuse is less frequent, but occurs in 16 per cent (British sample) to 34 per cent (US sample) of bulimic women. Again, this is higher than the incidence of 1.2 per cent seen in a normal control population. In the US sample, 10.2 per cent of eating disordered women were found to use diuretics on a daily basis. Diuretic use in general is considered a risk factor for eating disorders, as 50 per cent of a recent study sample who reported diuretic use were also found

to have significant symptoms of an eating disorder. In nonprescription preparations, diuretic agents are most commonly found in products promoted to relieve premenstrual symptoms. Of these, the most popular in Canada is Midol-PMS, containing the diuretic agent pamabrom, and Diurex, which contains caffeine. These agents are far less harmful than prescription diuretics containing furosemide, which are commonly abused by eating disordered individuals. Frequently, patients will obtain large doses of prescription diuretics by surreptitiously obtaining prescriptions from several physicians.

The main complication seen with prescription diuretic abuse is hypokalemia, but hyponatremia, hyperuricemia, hyperglycemia, hypomagnesemia, hypertiglyceridemia, hypercholesterolemia and dehydration are also common metabolic complications of diuretic abuse.

These effects may be reversible with discontinuation of diuretic use, but withdrawal often results in rebound fluid retention. Clients are well advised to reduce their salt intake during this period.

Insulin Manipulation

There are several reports in the literature of diabetics who also suffer from eating disorders deliberately manipulating or abusing their insulin dosages, to avoid the "fattening" effects of insulin. Obviously, this can lead to potentially fatal ketoacidosis.

Emetics

Individuals with eating disorders also frequently consume emetics to assist them in vomiting. Most often, ipecac is used, although there are reports of patients ingesting nicotine or laundry detergent for emetic purposes. Of patients with eating disorders, 28 per cent have used ipecac at some point in the course of their disorder, while roughly 5 per cent report using it currently. Of those who have used ipecac, almost 40 per cent report its use more than 10 times.

Large doses of ipecac may be absorbed, and the emetine hydrochloride base may cause widespread progressive myopathy, characterized by severe disruption of the sarcomeres and sarcotubular system. In addition to general muscle weakness. The toxic effects may include lethal heart complications including dysrhythmias, conduction disturbances, and myocarditis. Emetine-induced myopathy is clinically reversible with discontinuation of ipecac consumption, but educating those who use ipecac for emetic purposes is obviously of crucial importance.

Appetite Suppressants

Diet pills have been reported to be used by 50 per cent of American women with bulimia and anorexia nervosa, while 26 per cent of American women with bulimia use them currently. Of bulimic women taking diet pills, 31 per cent use pills several times per day, 38 per cent several times per week, and the remainder once or more per month. The use of diet pills is probably greater in the US than in Canada, however, as the most popular nonprescription anorexiant, phenylpropanolamine (PPA) is only available in Canada in cough and cold combination products for relief of nasal congestion. The reason for this is that the effectiveness of PPA as an appetite suppressant has not been well established. Further, reported problems associated with frequent use of PPA include elevated blood pressure, renal failure, seizures, agitation, and transient neurological deficits. Canadian diet pills, such as Dexatrim, contain benzocaine, bulk agents,

Eating Disorders

and vitamins. Benzocaine is thought to suppress appetite by decreasing the peripheral sensory desire for food in the mouth, or by decreasing taste sensitivity. Possible complications with abuse of benzocaine include methemoglobinemia, and lowered threshold for asthmatic attacks in sensitive individuals. Glucose-containing preparations are believed to exert anorectic effects through elevating blood glucose levels and consequently inhibiting the appetite centre. Their effectiveness is, at best, controversial. Finally, bulk-producing agents include various natural and semi-synthetic polysaccharides and cellulose derivatives, which create a feeling of fullness through distending the stomach and or intestines when hydrated. While safe when used according to manufacturer's recommendations, these products can lead to flatulence, intestinal obstruction, and diarrhea with attendant fluid, electrolyte and nutrient loss, if abused.

Another American study found that prescription amphetamines were used regularly by 60 per cent of women with bulimia, compared to 20 per cent of normal control subjects. Anorectic doses of this medication can result in adverse cardiovascular and CNS effects common to amphetaminergic agents.

Diet Aids

Another frequent strategy designed to assist eating disordered individuals in restricting their food intake is to chew large quantities of "sugar-free" gums and mints. Despite the intoduction of aspartame as an artificial sweetener, many of these gums and mints contain fairly large amounts of the polyalcohol sugar sorbitol (0.55 to 2.2 g). The ingestion of 10 to 20 g (approximately 10 pieces of gum or mints) per day of sorbitol can cause fairly severe abdominal distress, including gas, bloating, cramping, and diarrhea. While some individuals may ingest large quantities of sorbitol deliberately for its laxative effects, many may be unaware of the link between their abdominal distress and the gums or mints they consume to ward off the urge to binge. In providing education to affected individuals, it is important to distinguish between these two groups of sorbitol abusers, and counsel them accordingly.

The intentional abuse of sodium bicarbonate, through ingesting several tablespoons of baking soda, in order to deaden appetite, has been observed in some anorexic patients. Sodium bicarbonate abuse can be a potentially fatal cause of hypokalemic metabolic alkalosis, and while not a common practice amongst eating disordered individuals, certainly warrants a vigilant awareness of its potential occurrence in patients with repeated unexplained electrolyte imbalance.

Formula diets using liquid, powder or solid formulations are often popular with individuals who distrust their ability to control food intake less rigidly. However, the rigidity and monotony of the recommended regimens result in poor compliance. These diets are generally hypocaloric for prolonged use and promote rebound binge-eating. Thus, these diets are often counterproductive for people with eating disorders. Prolonged use can lead to constipation due to lack of bulk.

Dietary Supplements

In a misguided attempt to ward off vitamin and electrolyte disturbances secondary to restrictive dieting or purging, people with eating disorders often self-medicate with massive quantities of vitamin and mineral pills, potassium, calcium or zinc supplements, and so forth. Overuse may lead to the toxicity associated with vitamin and mineral overdose. (See the chapter on nutritional products.)

Other Forms of Self-medication

Individuals with eating disorders are attracted to a number of other nonprescription medications for relief of symptoms indirectly related to the eating disorder. First among these are sleeping pills. Sleep difficulties, common in this population, may be associated with disruptions in serotonergic functioning, known to play a critical role in maintaining normal sleep-wake patterns. (See the chapter on sleep disorders and nonprescription sleep aids.)

Pain-killers are used less often by obese people than by nonobese control people. This may be attributable to chronically elevated levels of endogenous opioids in the obese. Therefore, anorectics may also overuse analgesic medication, as suboptimal levels of opioid activity are believed to characterize that group.

Believing the pill causes them to look fat, women with eating disorders often seek alternative methods of birth control, or use no contraception at all.

In a recent survey of women with bulimia, 34.4 per cent indicated having a problem with alcohol or other drugs; 23 per cent acknowledged a history of alcohol abuse; and 17.7 per cent indicated

Figure 2 *Suggested Approach to Consumers Seeking Information On Weight Control Products*

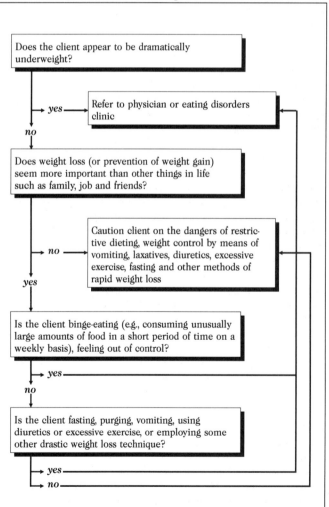

a history of treatment for chemical dependence. A recent survey of cocaine abusers revealed that 22 per cent met the criteria for bulimia, 2 per cent met criteria for anorexia nervosa and an additional 7 per cent had both eating disorders. Individuals with eating disorders appear to be vulnerable to a variety of substance abuse disorders. This observation underlines the need for care in discussing the use of nonprescription medication with this group.

Summary

Pharmacists, physicians and other health professionals are becoming acutely aware of the potentially dangerous use of nonprescription medication by individuals with eating disorders. Some nonprescription weight control products may assist obese individuals in weight reduction, and are reasonably safe if used strictly according to directions. However, if the pharmacist suspects the individual suffers from bulimia or anorexia nervosa, or possesses symptoms of these disorders (for example, binge-eating, hypocaloric dieting or purging), the pharmacist should discourage use of weight control products and purgatives and suggest sources of treatment in the community.

Ask the Consumer

Q. Is this weight control product for you?
■ If a product is for an individual who is normal weight or underweight, advise the consumer that weight loss below the body's set-point weight may precipitate food preoccupation, concentration difficulties and binge-eating.

Q. How much weight do you want to lose?
■ Those who plan to lose more than 2 to 4 kg are more at risk for weight rebound, especially if the loss occurs quickly.

Q. Do you plan to use this medication in conjunction with a low-calorie diet?
■ If the individual's proposed diet is hypocaloric (for example, less than 1,500 calories per day), there is risk of food preoccupation, binge-eating, concentration difficulties, vitamin and mineral deficiencies and later weight rebound.

Q. Do you exercise regularly?
■ Advise the individual that exercise is a far more effective, long-lasting and healthier means of weight control than restrictive dieting.

Q. Do you use any other methods to achieve weight control?
■ If the individual admits to laxative use, self-induced vomiting, fasting or other methods of purging, referral to a physician or an eating disorders clinic may be appropriate.

Q. Have you previously tried any nonprescription weight control products?
■ If a product was tried unsuccessfully, another product may be suggested. Alternatively, if there have been prolonged and unsuccessful attempts at self-medication, referral to a physician may be most appropriate.

Q. Describe your typical daily diet.
■ Intake below 1,500 calories daily should be discouraged. Evidence of binge-eating or severely restrictive intake may indicate that referral for assessment of an eating disorder may be appropriate.

Q. Do you often find yourself eating when you are not physically hungry?
■ A positive response may indicate that eating is used as a means of coping with psychological stress, and thus may not be helped by medication alone.

References

Eating Disorders

Anonymous. Diagnostic and statistical manual of mental disorders (Third Edition—Revised): DSM-111-R. Washington: American Psychiatric Association, 1987.

Barlow J, Blouin J, Blouin A, Perez E. Treatment of bulimia with desipramine: a double-blind crossover study. Can J Psychiat 1988;33:129–33.

Blouin A, Blouin J, Perez E, et al. Treatment of bulimia with fenfluramine and desipramine. J Clin Psychopharmacol, 1988;8: 261–9.

Blouin AG, Blouin JH, Aubin P, Carter J, Goldstein C, Boyer H, Perez E. Seasonal patterns of bulimia nervosa. Am J Psychiatry 1992;149:73–81.

Blundell JE. Is there a role for serotonin (5-hydroxytryptamine) in feeding? Int J Obesity 1977;1:15–42.

Bray GA. Overweight is risking fate: definition, classification, prevalence and risks. Wurtman RJ, Wurtman JJ, eds. Human obesity. Ann NY Acad Sci 1987;499:14–28.

Carlsson A, Svennerholm L, Winblad B. Seasonal and circadian monoamine variations in human brains examined post-mortem. Acta Psychiatr Scand 1980;61(Suppl 280):75–85.

Fairburn C. Cognitive-behavioural treatment for bulimia. In: Garner DM, Garfinkel PE, eds. Handbook of psychotherapy for anorexia nervosa and bulimia. New York: Guilford Press, 1985:160–91.

Foch TT, McClearn GE. Genetics, body weight and obesity. In: Stunkard AJ, ed. Obesity. Philadelphia: WB Saunders, 1980:48–71.

Garner DM, Rockert W, Olmsted MP, Johnson C, Coscina DV. Psycho-educational principles in the treatment of anorexia nervosa and bulimia. In: Garner DM, Garfinkel PE, eds. Handbook of psychotherapy for anorexia nervosa and bulimia. New York: Guilford Press, 1985:513–70.

Garner DM, Garfinkel PE, Schwartz D, Thompson M. Cultural expectations of thinness in women. Psychol Reports 1980;47:483–91.

Garner DM, Olmsted MP, Polivy J. Development and validation of a multidimensional eating disorder inventory for anorexia nervosa and bulimia. Int J Eat Dis 1983;2:15–34.

Gold MS, Sternbach HA. Endorphins in obesity and in the regulation of appetite and weight. Int Psychiat 1984;2(6):203–7.

Goldberg SC, Halmi KA, Eckert ED, et al. Cyproheptadine in anorexia nervosa. Br J Psychiat 1979;134:67–70.

Gross HA, Lake CR, Ebert MH, et al. Catecholemine metabolism in primary anorexia nervosa. J Clin Endocrinol Metab 1979;49:805–9.

Guy-Grand BJ. A new approach to the treatment of obesity. Wurtman RJ, Wurtman JJ, eds. Human obesity. Ann NY Acad Sci 1987;499:313–7.

Healy K, Conroy RM, Walsh N. The prevalence of binge-eating and bulimia in 1063 college students. J Psychiatr Res 1985;19(2/3):161–6.

Herzog DB, Copeland PM. Eating disorders. N Engl J Med 1985;313:295–303.

Hughes PL, Wells LA, Cunningham CJ, Ilstrup DM. Treating bulimia with desipramine: a double-blind placebo-controlled study. Arch Gen Psychiatry 1986;43:182–6.

Johnson C. Initial consultation for patients with bulimia and anorexia nervosa. In: Garner DM, Garfinkel PE, eds. Handbook of psychotherapy for anorexia nervosa and bulimia. New York: Guilford Press, 1985:19–53.

Jonas JM, Gold MS, Sweeney D, Pottash ALC. Eating disorders and cocaine abuse: a survey of 259 cocaine abusers. J Clin Psychiatry 1987;48(2):47–50.

Eating Disorders

Jones DJ, Fox MM, Babigian HM, Hutton HE. Epidemiology of anorexia nervosa in Monroe County, New York: 1960–1976. Psychosom Med 1980; 42:551–8.

Kaye WH, Ebert MH, Gwirtsman HE, Weiss SR. Differences in brain serotonergic metabolism between bulimic and nonbulimic patients with anorexia nervosa. Am J Psychiatr 1984;141(12):1598–601.

Keesey RE. A set point analysis of the regulation of body weight. In: Stunkard AJ, ed. Obesity. Philadelphia: WB Saunders, 1980:144–65.

Keys A, Brozek J, Henschel A, et al. The biology of human starvation. Minneapolis: University of Minnesota Press, 1950.

Needleman HL, Waber D. The use of amitryptiline in anorexia nervosa. In: Vigersky RA, ed. Anorexia nervosa. New York: Raven Press, 1977.

O'Rourke D, Wurtman JJ, Brzesinski A. Treatment of seasonal affective disorder with d-fenfluramine. Ann NY Acad Sci 1987;499:329–30.

Polivy J, Herman CP. Dieting and binging: a causal analysis. Am Psychol 1985;40(2):193–201.

Rand CS, Kuldau JM, Yost RL. Obesity and postoperative pain. J Psychosom Res 1985;29(1):43–8.

Robins LN, Helzer JE, Weissman MM, et al. Lifetime prevalence of psychiatric disorders in three sites. Arch Gen Psychiatry 1984;41:949–58.

Sabry ZI. Nutrition: a national priority. A report by nutrition Canada to the Department of National Health and Welfare. Ottawa: Information Canada, 1973.

Simopoulos AP. Characteristics of obesity. Wurtman RJ, Wurtman JJ, eds. Human obesity. Ann NY Acad Sci 1987;499:4–13.

Stangler RS, Printz AM. DSM III: psychiatric diagnosis in a university population. Am J Psychiatr 1980;137:937–40.

Vigersky RA, Andersen AE, Thompson RH, Loriaux DL. Hypothalamic dysfunction in amenorrhea associated with simple weight loss. N Engl J Med 1977;297:1141–5.

Wadden TA, Stunkard AJ. Psychopathology and obesity. Wurtman RJ, Wurtman JJ, eds. Human obesity. Ann NY Acad Sci 1987;499:55–65.

Walsh BT, Gladis M, Roose SP. Food intake and mood in anorexia nervosa and bulimia. Wurtman RJ, Wurtman JJ, eds. Human obesity. Ann NY Acad Sci 1987;499:231–8.

Weiss SR, Ebert MH. Psychological and behavioural characteristics of normal-weight bulimics and normal-weight controls. Psychosom Med 1983;45(4):293–303.

Willi J, Grossman S. Epidemiology of anorexia nervosa in a defined region of Switzerland. Am J Psychiatr 1983;140:564–7.

Wurtman JJ, Wurtman RJ. Studies on the appetite for carbohydrates in rats and humans. J Psychiatr Res 1983;17:213–21.

Wurtman JJ, Wurtman RJ, Growdon J, et al. Carbohydrate craving in obese people: suppression by treatments affecting serotonergic transmission. Int J Eat Dis 1981;1:2–15.

Treatment

Cohen RY, Stunkard AJ. Behaviour therapy and pharmacotherapy of obesity: a review of the literature. Behav Med Update 1983;4(3):7–12.

Ferguson JM. Fluoxetine-induced weight loss in overweight, nondepressed subjects. Am J Psychiatr 1986;143(11):1496–9.

Halmi KA, Eckert E, LaDu TJ, Cohen J. Anorexia nervosa: treatment efficacy of cyproheptadine and amitryptyline. Arch Gen Psychiatry 1986;43:177–81.

Levitsky DA, Strupp BJ, Lupoli J. Tolerance to anorectic drugs: pharmacological or artifactual. Pharmacol Biochem Beh 1981;14(5):661–7.

Nutzinger DO, Cayiroglu S, Sachs G, Zapotoczky HG. Emotional problems during weight reduction: advantages of combined behaviour therapy and antidepressive drug therapy for obesity. J Behav Ther Exper Psychiatry 1985;16(3):217–21.

Pinder RM, Brogden R, Sawyer PR, et al. Fenfluramine: a review of its pharmacological properties and therapeutic efficacy in obesity. Drugs 1975;10:241–323.

Vigersky RA, Loriaux DL. The effect of cyproheptadine in anorexia nervosa: a double-blind trial. In: Vigersky RA, ed. Anorexia nervosa. New York: Raven Press, 1977:349–56.

Wurtman RJ, Wurtman JJ. Nutrients, neurotransmitter synthesis and control of food intake. In: Stunkard AJ, Stellar E, eds. Eating and its disorders. New York: Raven Press, 1984.

Laxatives and Diuretic Abuse

Adam O, Goebel FD: Secondary gout and pseudo-Bartter syndrome in females with laxative abuse. Klinische Wochenschrift 1987;65:833–9.

Aubin P. Self medication in bulimics and normal controls. [Thesis]. Ottawa: Carleton University, 1987.

Bo-Linn G, Santa Ana A, Morawski SG, Fordtran JS. Purging and calorie-absorption in bulimic patients and normal women. Ann Intern Med 1983;99:14–7.

Fairburn CG, Cooper PJ. The clinical features of bulimia nervosa. Br J Psychiat 1984;144:238–46.

Johnson CL, Stuckey MK, Lewis LD, Schwartz DM. Bulimia: a descriptive survey of 316 cases. Int J Eat Dis 1983;2(1):3–16.

Karpinski K. Summary report: national nonprescription drug survey. Ottawa: Food Statistics and Operational Planning Division, Health and Welfare, 1987.

Lachenmyer JR, Muni-Brander P, Belford S. Laxative abuse for weight control in adolescents. Int J Eat Dis 1988;7:849–52.

Mitchell JE, Pomeroy C, Huber M. A clinicians guide to the eating disorder's medicine cabinet. Int J Eat Dis 1988;7:211–23.

Mitchell JE, Hatsukami D, Eckert ED, Pyle RL. Characteristics of 275 patients with bulimia. Am J Psychiatr 1985;142(4):482–5.

Mitchell JE, Pomeroy C, Seppala M, Huber M. Diuretic use as a marker for eating problems and affective disorders among women. J Clin Psychiatry 1988;49:267–70.

Promeroy C, Mitchell JE, Seim H, Seppala M. Prescription diuretic abuse in patients with bulimia nervosa. J Fam Pract 1988;27:493–6.

Insulin Manipulation

Featherstone HJ, Beitman BD. Diabetic hyperglycemia and glycosuria as a manifestation of bulimia. South Med J 1984;77(7):936–7.

Rodin GM, Daneman D, Johnson LE, et al. Anorexia nervosa and bulimia in female adolescents with insulin dependent diabetes mellitus: a systematic study. J Psychiatr Res 1985;19(2/3):381–4.

Emetics

Halbig L, Gutmann L, Goebel H, Brick J, Schochet S. Ultrastructural pathology in emetine-induced myopathy. Acta Neuropathol 1988;75:577–82.

Rich CL. Self-induced vomiting: psychiatric considerations. JAMA 1978; 239:2688–9.

Short DD, Blinder BB. Nicotine used as emetic by a patient with bulimia. Am J Psychiatr 1985;142(2):272.

Tolstoi LG. Ipecac-induced toxicity in eating disorders. Int J Eat Dis 1990;9:371–5.

Diet Aids and Dietary Supplements

Bennett W. Dietary treatments of obesity. Wurtman RJ, Wurtman JJ, eds. Human obesity. Ann NY Acad Sci 1987;499:250–63.

Kennedy S. Sodium bicarbonate abuse in anorexia nervosa. J Clin Psychiatry 1988;49:168.

Ohlrich ES, Aughey DR, Dixon RM. Sorbitol abuse among eating-disordered patients. Psychosom 1989;30:541–3.

32

Sleep Disorders and Nonprescription Sleep Aids

Revised by Irene Worthington. Based on the original chapter by Susan E. MacKenzie

Numerous factors can alter the normal pattern of the sleep-wake cycle: stress, travel, drugs, alcohol, foods, medical conditions, biological conditions or changes in daily schedule. Consumers with insomnia should be counselled on its causes. Nondrug treatment is recommended, but nonprescription sleep aids that may be used include diphenhydramine and other ethanolamine antihistamines, mephenesin and salicylamide. Pharmacists should also be aware of the symptoms of narcolepsy and sleep apnea, two important sleep disorders for which consumers should be referred to a physician.

In the last two decades, with the advent of sleep laboratory studies, an increasing amount of information about sleep disorders has been accumulated. The pharmacist should be aware of the general treatment measures for the more common sleep disorders—insomnia, narcolepsy and sleep apnea—and what drug treatments are contraindicated in these disorders.

Many people self-medicate at one time or another for the treatment of insomnia. Thus, the pharmacist plays an important role in dealing with these individuals. In managing narcolepsy and sleep apnea, two sleep disorders that until recently were considered rare, nonprescription sleep aids and prescription sedative-hypnotics are contraindicated. In particular, sedative-hypnotics may prove fatal to people with sleep apnea.

Sleep Architecture

The human body operates under the guidance of a 24-hour biologic clock known as circadian rhythm. This rhythm tells the body how much time to spend in sleep, when to sleep and what changes in biologic parameters are associated with sleeping and waking. Circadian rhythm varies with age and between sexes. Two principles are useful in the evaluation and treatment of sleep disorders: the longer a person is awake before bedtime, the greater the likelihood of sleep; and the best sleep occurs at the optimal time, as determined by the biologic circadian clock. The two optimal times are: nocturnal bedtime and mid-afternoon. Exposure to bright light in the evening (6 to 9 p.m.) or early morning (5 to 7 a.m.) can alter this circadian pattern.

The regulation of sleep, wakefulness and level of arousal as well as the coordination of eye movements is under control of the reticular activating system. Central nervous system neurotransmitters, such as serotonin, catecholamines, acetylcholine and amino acids, as well as peptides and humoral sleep factors, help regulate the sleep-wake cycle.

Frequent sampling of blood during the 24-hour sleep-wake cycle demonstrates alterations in the pattern of pituitary hormones during the night's sleep. Sleep synchronizes several hormonal rhythms. A major surge of growth hormone is secreted after sleep onset, associated with the stages of deepest sleep. Adrenocorticotrophic hormone-cortisol (ACTH-cortisol) is not secreted just before and for several hours after sleep onset. During the latter half of the night's sleep, ACTH-cortisol secretion occurs as a series of individual episodes, the accumulation of which produces the characteristic high concentrations on awakening. Prolactin secretion in men and women increases during the night, with the highest concentrations just after sleep onset. The prolactin concentration falls rapidly to normal daytime levels after awakening. Thyrotropin is secreted only minimally during the waking day, but has a secretory surge just before sleep onset in the evening. Sleep also appears to inhibit secretion of thyroid-stimulating hormone (TSH) throughout the night.

Two stages of sleep have been identified in the normal adult in sleep laboratory studies (polysomnography) using electroencephalographic (EEG), electro-oculographic (EOG) and electromyographic

Table I	*Stages of Sleep in the Adult*	
	Characteristics	**% Sleep time**
NREM		
Stage one:	Transition between sleep and wakefulness	5%–10%
Stage two:	Light sleep, subject is easily awakened	50%
Stage three:	Slow-wave or delta-wave sleep (as seen on EEG)	15%
Stage four:	Slow-wave sleep (deepest sleep)	10% (decreases with age)
REM	Dream sleep	20%–25%

Sleep Disorders and Nonprescription Sleep Aids

(EMG) studies: rapid eye movement (REM) sleep and non-REM (NREM) sleep. NREM sleep is divided into four stages (see Table I). Stage one is a transient phase, usually occurring at the onset of sleep. If awakened from stage one, people may claim they were not really asleep but only dozing, so this stage is generally regarded as a transition stage between wakefulness and sleep. Stage two is unequivocal sleep, although a person can be aroused easily. Stages three and four are the phases of deepest sleep and together are often described as delta-wave or slow wave sleep (as seen on an EEG).

During NREM sleep, muscle tone is retained but an EEG records little mental or physical activity. Generally, NREM sleep is associated with a decrease in heart rate, blood pressure, respiration rate and body temperature. During REM sleep, these parameters increase or become more variable, or both. There is negligible muscle tone except for the eye muscles, performing scanning movements. Most dreaming occurs in REM sleep and is most consistently recalled if the person is awakened at this time.

The normal adult sleep pattern consists of REM sleep alternating with NREM sleep about every 90 to 100 minutes, with the first REM period occurring about 90 to 100 minutes after the onset of sleep. The sequence of stages one, two, three and four typically occurs at sleep onset. The sequence is then reversed (stages four, three and two) and REM sleep ensues (see Figure 1).

The normal sleep pattern of the night consists of 3 to 5 such sleep cycles, with an increasing duration and percentage of the REM sleep during the latter half of the sleep period. Stages three and four occur predominantly during the first third of the sleep period. Stage one sleep occupies about 5 to 10 per cent, stage two about 50 per cent, stage three about 15 per cent, stage four about 10 per cent and REM sleep about 20 per cent of the average 450 minutes of total sleep (see Table I).

In the elderly, sleep patterns change dramatically. By age 60, the deeper levels (stages three and four) of NREM sleep have decreased. REM sleep remains proportional throughout adulthood, but declines sharply after age 69. Sleep latency and sleep fragmentation increase. By age 75, sleep is composed primarily of the lighter sleep stages interrupted by frequent night awakenings (see Figure 1).

The elderly are less efficient in fulfilling their 24-hour sleep requirement. They spend more hours in bed but experience fragmented sleep, awaken earlier and nap during the day. As well, there are many medical, psychiatric and situational causes for insomnia in the elderly. In the elderly, the incidence of sleep apnea and nocturnal myoclonus may be as high as 40 per cent. Sedative-hypnotic agents should not be indiscriminately prescribed until the reasons have been fully investigated.

Researchers have found a number of similarities in the sleep studies of chronic insomniacs. Typically, these people have a shorter sleep time and smaller amounts of REM and stages three and four sleep than normal people. The chronic insomniac often exhibits greater concentrations of stages three and four sleep in the first half of the night, in contrast to normal sleepers (see Figure 1).

Insomnia

Because the amount of sleep required varies between individuals, insomnia should be defined as the inability to obtain the amount of sleep a person needs for optimal functioning and well-being. The average time spent in sleep decreases from 16 to 18 hours at birth

Figure 1 *Cycles of Sleep Stages in an 8-Hour Sleep*

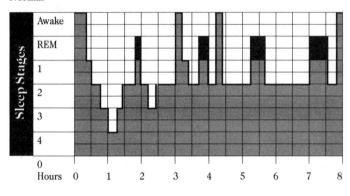

Normal

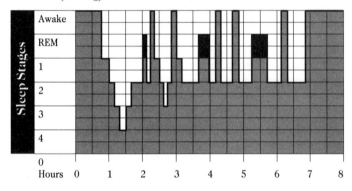

Insomniac (no drug)

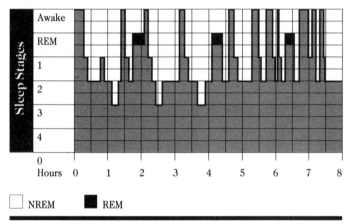

Elderly

☐ NREM   ■ REM

to nine hours at 12 to 18 years. Young adults average 8 to 10 hours of sleep daily. Documented cases exist of people who regularly function on a few hours of sleep per night. On the other hand, some individuals require 9, 10 or more hours of sleep each night; if restricted to 8 hours, they feel sleepy and cannot effectively accomplish their daily work. Insomnia is therefore a relatively subjective complaint.

Insomnia is the most frequently encountered sleep disorder. It may be transient or chronic (more than 3 weeks). Studies have shown that poor sleep is associated with increased mortality and a variety

Sleep Disorders and Nonprescription Sleep Aids

Table II *Some Conditions Which Disrupt Normal Sleep Patterns*

Medical

Pain, e.g. rheumatoid arthritis, cancer, headaches
Sleep apnea
Hyperthyroidism
Chronic obstructive pulmonary disease, asthma
Nocturnal cramps or myoclonus
Hypoglycemia
Narcolepsy
Parkinson's disease
Multiple sclerosis
Hypertension
Cardiovascular insufficiency
Esophageal reflux

Psychiatric

Depression
Schizophrenia
Anxiety and panic disorders
Mania
Dementia
Obsessive-compulsive disorder
Anorexia nervosa
Post-traumatic stress

Other

Pregnancy

Adapted from: Gillin JC, Byerley WF. The diagnosis and management of insomnia. N Engl J Med 1990;322:239–48.

of cognitive deficits. Although data on the prevalence of sleep disorders are fragmentary, a significant percentage of the adult population has frequent and chronic complaints about the quality and amount of sleep. Numerous surveys have tried to determine the nature and prevalence of sleep complaints in various large populations (in the United States, Great Britain, Scotland and Italy) using different techniques (telephone interviews, medical record examinations and questionnaires) on different subgroups (institution and community dwellers). A summary of the results shows the following trends:

- In the general population, about one-third of people surveyed have some difficulty related to sleep. Most people with chronic insomnia report difficulty falling asleep.
- This difficulty may occur in combination with staying asleep or early final awakening. In most people, sleep difficulty starts before age 40.
- Twenty per cent of the adult population surveyed seeks some form of medication for insomnia.
- Insomnia occurs more often among women and elderly people.
- The number of sedative-hypnotics used for sleep increases in those over age 60.

Causes

Transient or short-term sleep disturbances may occur in response to various stresses such as work-related difficulties, interpersonal conflicts, financial problems or major life changes such as marriage, birth of a child or bereavement. Transient insomnia can also be part of

the jet-lag syndrome, resulting from rapid travel through various time zones. Insomnia is often present when work shifts change. In some people, especially the elderly, insomnia may be more chronic and may be caused by an irregular schedule of activity and rest.

Medical conditions that cause pain, discomfort, anxiety or depression are often accompanied by insomnia. These conditions include: cardiovascular and pulmonary disorders (for example, asthma), gastrointestinal disease, renal insufficiency, endocrine disorders, neurological disorders and eating disorders (see Table II). Drugs prescribed for the treatment of certain medical or psychiatric conditions, including amphetamines or other stimulants, energizing antidepressants, steroids, central adrenergic blockers and bronchodilators, can contribute to disturbed sleep (see Table III).

People taking benzodiazepine hypnotic agents with short elimination half-lives (for example, triazolam), may awaken frequently, especially during the second half of the night. They may also have sleep difficulties after abrupt termination of the drug (rebound insomnia).

Caffeinated beverages, such as colas and coffee, and cigarette smoking can also cause sleep disruption, particularly difficulty falling asleep. Alcohol is a short-acting drug that may help an individual fall asleep, but after several hours, sleep becomes disturbed and fragmented.

Drug-Induced Insomnia

The effects of drugs on the sleep stages have been studied extensively, although primarily in normal volunteer subjects rather than people with sleep disorders. The effects of sedative-hypnotics on sleep depend on the specific drug, the dose and the frequency of administration. The effects of sedative-hypnotics on patterns of normal sleep are:

- decreased sleep latency (time to fall asleep)
- increased duration of stage two NREM sleep
- decreased duration of REM sleep
- decreased duration of slow-wave sleep.

The sleep pattern is further disrupted after abrupt withdrawal from chronic use of sedative-hypnotic agents, such as the benzodiazepines. After withdrawal of the hypnotic agent, the frequency of occurrence and duration of REM activity markedly increases, or rebounds, which may lead to such symptoms as nightmares. In addition, daytime symptoms appear, including restlessness, nervousness, generalized muscle aches and, in severe cases, drug withdrawal symptoms such as confusion, hallucinations and grand mal seizures. The withdrawal

Table III *Some Drugs Which May Disrupt Normal Sleep Patterns*

Alcohol	Levodopa
Amphetamines	Meprobamate
Barbiturates	MAO inhibitors
Benzodiazepines	Neuroleptics
Beta blockers	Nicotine
Caffeine	Selegiline
Clozapine	Sympathomimetics
Corticosteroids	Theophylline preparations
Ethchlorvynol	Tricyclic antidepressants

Adapted from: Hill LA. Drug induced sleep changes. Hosp Pharm 1990; 25:1120.

Sleep Disorders and Nonprescription Sleep Aids

syndrome tends to occur more quickly (1 to 3 days) and more acutely with the shorter-acting benzodiazepines such as triazolam. It is important in chronic hypnotic drug users that withdrawal be gradual with close clinical supervision.

Caffeine-Induced Insomnia

Caffeine-containing beverages occupy a significant position in North American consumption patterns. Eight of 10 adults consume coffee, ingesting an average of 3½ cups per day; 17 per cent of these people drink more than 5 cups per day. Caffeine is also present in regular and herbal teas, many soft drinks and chocolate (see Table IV). As well, nearly 200 American and 100 Canadian nonprescription and prescription drug products contain caffeine for its central nervous system stimulating effects, for vascular headache relief or to enhance analgesia (see Table V). Nonprescription stimulant products containing caffeine are available in Canada as single-entity products such as Wake-Ups or as combination products such as Alert (see Table VI).

Caffeine has long been known to have stimulant properties. Oral caffeine in doses of 100 to 400 mg every 3 to 4 hours is an effective stimulant and will restore mental alertness in adults. Since one cup of percolated coffee can contain up to 175 mg of caffeine, drinking one or more cups of coffee leads to increased alertness. Caffeine intake 30 to 60 minutes before bedtime significantly delays sleep onset, decreases total sleep time, alters normal sleep patterns and decreases the subjective quality of sleep. It increases stage two sleep and decreases stages three and four sleep; REM sleep may be altered and the number of awakenings may be increased. These effects on sleep appear to be dose-dependent. Wide variation in individual sensitivity to the sleep-altering effects of caffeine exists. More nondrinkers of coffee than habitual heavy coffee drinkers (greater than 4 cups per day) report an increase in sleep latency and a decrease in sleep quality after drinking coffee prior to bedtime.

Table IV Caffeine Content of Foods and Beverages

Product	Caffeine (mg)
Coffees (per 150 mL)	
Automatic percolated	75–140
Instant	60–90
Decaffeinated	2–6
Filter drip	110–180
Teas (per 150 mL)	
Herbal	24–130
Weak (bag)	20–45
Medium (bag)	48–70
Strong (bag)	70–110
Iced	30–80
Medium-brewed (loose)	70–80
Soft Drinks (per 360 mL)	
Mountain Dew	54
Pepsi-Cola	38
Coca-Cola	33
Tab	32
7Up	0
Ginger Ale	0
Cocoa Products	
Hot cocoa (240 mL)	50
Bittersweet baking chocolate (30 g)	25–35
Milk chocolate bar (30 g)	3–6
Chocolate milk (225 mL)	2–7

Table V Nonprescription Medications Containing Less than 50 mg of Caffeine

A&C preparations	15–30
Anacin	32.4
Anacin with Codeine	32
Ancasal 8	16
Antidol tablets	32.4
Arco pain tablets	30
Atasol-8	30
Calmine tablets	32.4
Casse Grippe Cunard Cap Adult	16.2
Codaminophen tab 1/8 gr	30
Corytab	16
Cotabs	15
Cunard Casse Grippe Cap Enfant	8.1
C2 preparations	15
Dolomine 37 tablets	32.4
Dristan AF preparations	16–32
Emercidin D tablets	30
Emertabs	16.2
Exdol-8	30
Kalmex tablets	4
Lenoltec No 1	15
Medacidin-D tablets	30
Midol	32.4
Neo-Tigol	15
Nervine	30
Novo AC&C 8 mg tablets	15
Novogesic C8	15
Oradrine	32.4
Oradrine-2	32.4
Paradol	15
Rawleigh Cold tablets	16
Sinugex 38 tablets	16
Triaminicin tablets	30
217 preparations	30
222 preparations	30
Tylenol No 1 preparations	15

Table VI Medications Containing More than 50 mg of Caffeine

Alert	100
Astone capsules	55
Cafergot preparations	100
Caffedrine tablets	100
Chase Caffeine tablets	100
Ergodryl capsules	100
Excedrin preparations	65
Gravergol capsules	100
Instantine preparations	64.8
Megral tablets	100
Norgesic Forte	60
Wake-ups	100
Wigraine tablets	100

The clearance of caffeine from the body is significantly influenced by disease, concurrent drug use, smoking, pregnancy and duration of use. People with alcoholic liver disease metabolize caffeine more slowly. Caffeine clearance from the body is enhanced by smoking but is decreased in pregnancy. Caffeine clearance is inhibited by ingesting cimetidine or some quinolone antibiotics (for example, ciprofloxacin). Caffeine does not reverse the effects of ethanol on the central nervous system.

High doses of caffeine (more than 1 g a day or 10 cups of coffee), or caffeinism, can produce pharmacologic effects including irritability, agitation, anxiety, reflex hyperexcitability, tremulousness, dizziness, vertigo, insomnia, occasional muscle twitchings and toxic sensory disturbances such as ringing in the ears and visual flashes of light. Noncentral nervous system symptoms of caffeinism include palpitations, extrasystoles, tachycardia, arrhythmias, flushing, nausea, vomiting, diarrhea, epigastric pain, dehydration, fever and edema.

Consumers should be advised that overuse of caffeine-containing medications, foods or beverages can be a cause of insomnia, although a certain degree of tolerance does occur.

Pregnant women and nursing mothers should be advised against the use of nonprescription stimulants containing caffeine. They should limit the amount of caffeine they otherwise consume. Children are more susceptible than adults to excitation by caffeine and related compounds. Tea, coffee and other caffeine-containing products should be excluded from children's diets.

Alcohol-Induced Insomnia

Alcohol exerts one of the most disrupting influences on sleep quality. Light alcohol consumption may disturb the lower levels of sleep; sustained drinking leads to disrupted and shortened REM sleep, with insomnia and daytime sleepiness. Even drinkers who are not chronic alcoholics exhibit disrupted REM and deep sleep if alcohol is taken too close to bedtime. When the chronic alcoholic withdraws from alcohol, REM sleep occurs more frequently in the sleep cycle and lasts for longer periods of time, causing a REM rebound effect.

Nonpharmacologic Management of Insomnia

When consumers complain of insomnia, it is important to question them for possible causes. (A list of suitable questions can be found in the Ask the Consumer section of this chapter.)

A number of general measures to manage the insomnia without medication may be recommended (see Tables VII and VIII). Following the same routine each night before going to bed and not postponing bedtime is beneficial. However, the bedtime schedule should remain flexible; a person should not go to bed if wide awake. Rather, the person should try to relax, perhaps by reading. A hot milk drink at bedtime may help the person to fall asleep. The bedroom should be as dark and quiet as possible. Daytime naps should be avoided. Beverages containing caffeine should not be consumed for several hours before bedtime.

A gradual increase in daily activity and exercise is helpful, with the exception of exercise near bedtime, which may have an arousing effect. Some people are helped by ensuring they awake at a specific hour each morning; again, some degree of flexibility should be exercised. Education and reassurance are especially useful in alleviating the fear of sleeplessness. Behavioral approaches, including relaxation techniques and biofeedback may combat difficulty falling asleep.

Table VII *General Recommendations for the Treatment of Insomnia*

Recommendation	Comment
Plan daytime activities and exercise	Exercise regularly but not too close to bedtime.
Maintain sleep-wake routine	Develop schedule for retiring (but maintain flexibility); "wind down" before going to bed; go to bed when sleepy. Wake up at same time each morning, including weekends. Do not nap during daytime.
Use bed only for sleeping (or sexual activities)	Do not read, watch television or eat in bed. If unable to sleep, get up and move to another room; stay up until sleepy and return to bed; repeat this as often as necessary throughout the night.
Improve sleep environment	Minimize disruptive stimuli such as noise and light; expect an "adaptation effect" in new environment. Avoid extreme hot or cold temperatures.
Avoid drug-induced sleep disturbances	Minimize use of caffeine and cigarettes; avoid caffeine after lunch. Recognize that alcohol may cause fragmentation of sleep. Be aware that stimulants and other drugs may disturb sleep; recognize sleep disturbances after withdrawal of drug treatment.
Other	Be tolerant of occasional sleeplessness; avoid rumination over sleep difficulty; try relaxation exercises; a hot bath; eat a light snack at bedtime (for example, milk and crackers).

Table VIII *Recommendations for the Treatment of Insomnia in Elderly Persons*

Provide education about changes in sleep patterns with increased age.
Discourage multiple daytime naps.
Include naps, if taken, in 24-hour sleep totals.
Suggest activities, hobbies and special interests to pursue and quiet, relaxing activities prior to bedtime.
Daily exercise.
Delay onset of sleep to a regular time, slightly after sleepiness occurs.
Avoid caffeine, alcohol, nicotine or large meals several hours before bedtime.
Rule out presence of depression or medical disorder.
Rule out drug-induced insomnia.

Behavioral techniques are based on the concept that insomniacs have excessive rumination and high levels of anxiety and arousal before sleep.

Nonprescription Sleep Aids

Sedative-hypnotic agents should only be used when the nonpharmacologic measures fail and when other causes for insomnia have been ruled out. They should only be used in combination with the nonpharmacologic measures to improve the person's sleep. Both nonprescription sleep aids and prescription sedative-hypnotic agents are available. Nonprescription sleep aids are generally used to reduce the time taken to fall asleep.

A nonprescription sleep aid is defined by the United States Food and Drug Administration (FDA) as a substance that helps an individual fall asleep or a substance used for relief of occasional sleeplessness. Current literature agrees that available sleep aids or nonprescription sedatives are of little value in treating insomnia.

Antihistamines

Although not as potent as the benzodiazepines, diphenhydramine in a dose of 50 to 100 mg may be effective as a nonprescription sleep aid. When reviewing the existing evidence in the literature regarding sedative and sleep-inducing properties of diphenhydramine, the FDA found conflicting data.

A double-blind crossover study tested diphenhydramine 50 mg versus placebo in 111 people (aged 18 to 70 years) with mild to moderate insomnia. Researchers found that diphenhydramine was significantly more effective than placebo in decreasing sleep latency and nighttime awakenings and in improving depth, quality and duration of sleep. Although drowsiness, dizziness, grogginess and tiredness were reported more often on the drug than on placebo, subjects still claimed to feel more rested in the morning after taking diphenhydramine. A treatment preference rating showed more than twice as many subjects preferred treatment with diphenhydramine than placebo, and 18 subjects had no preference. Best results were seen in younger subjects with low levels of anxiety and those with significant difficulties in falling asleep.

While this study supports the hypnotic effects of 50 mg of diphenhydramine in treating mild to moderate insomnia of the type most likely self-treated with nonprescription sleep aids, the drug-placebo differences were only moderate.

Diphenhydramine is a potent antihistamine of the ethanolamine group with a high incidence of sedation and anticholinergic effects. Other side effects include dizziness, disturbed coordination and muscle weakness. Paradoxically, children may experience central nervous system stimulation. Diphenhydramine should be administered with caution to patients with convulsive disorders. Individuals may become tolerant to the sedation after 2 to 3 days, but should be cautioned against any activity that is potentially hazardous and requires mental alertness, such as operating machinery or driving.

Diphenhydramine exhibits such anticholinergic side effects as dryness of mouth, urinary retention, constipation, dizziness and blurred vision. Because of these side effects, diphenhydramine should be given with caution to people with narrow-angle glaucoma, prostatic hypertrophy or cardiovascular disease. Anticholinergic side effects can be particularly troublesome to the elderly. As well, patients taking any other medication with a high degree of anticholinergic side effects (that is, antidepressants, antipsychotics, benztropine, oxybutynin) may experience an additive effect.

The central nervous system depressant effects of diphenhydramine are enhanced by other central nervous system depressants, including barbiturates, antipsychotics, antidepressants, anxiolytics and alcohol.

Although diphenhydramine appears to be relatively safe for use in pregnancy, it should probably not be recommended as a sleep aid for pregnant women. There are relatively few studies of antihistamine use during lactation. Diphenhydramine is excreted in breast milk but probably in small amounts. Occasional use of bedtime doses, after the last feeding of the day, may minimize the amount of drug the infant receives. However, frequent use of high doses should be avoided.

Diphenhydramine has not been linked to many serious accidental overdoses. When diphenhydramine is ingested in large doses, the sedative and anticholinergic properties predominate. The syndrome of poisoning in children and young adults includes hallucinations, excitement, ataxia, incoordination, athetosis (slow, involuntary, purposeless movement) and convulsions. These symptoms are the result of centrally-mediated anticholinergic effects. Fixed, dilated pupils with a flushed face and fever are common peripheral anticholinergic effects. Coma may develop and the individual may die of cardiopulmonary arrest. Adults usually present with central nervous system depression leading to coma. Seizures, fever and flushing are not common in adults. Symptoms of overdose occur within 0.5 to 2 hours after ingestion. Treatment consists of supportive and symptomatic therapy including emesis and saline cathartics (if the person is conscious, has not lost the gag reflex and is not convulsing), gastric lavage and administration of activated charcoal as well as artificial respiration and management of anticholinergic effects, including convulsions.

Because the ethanolamine antihistamines are the most sedating of the antihistamines, they are often used as nighttime sleep aids. For example, products containing doxylamine succinate are marketed for individuals experiencing mild to moderate insomnia. Methapyrilene was withdrawn from these formulations due to potential carcinogenicity.

Other Nonprescription Sleep Aids

Mephenesin, a centrally-acting skeletal muscle relaxant, is a compound in some nonprescription sleep aids. Because of its sedative side effects, it has been included in nonprescription sleep aids. However, its efficacy as a sedative has not been established.

Salicylamide is also a compound found in some nonprescription sleep aids. Salicylamide has analgesic, anti-inflammatory and antipyretic properties. It is included in some sleep aids due to its side effect of drowsiness. However, salicylamide is not recommended for use because its effects are unreliable. Although it has sedative properties, the doses contained in nonprescription preparations may be ineffective. Salicylamide is an amide of salicylic acid, but is not converted to salicylate in the body. Individuals who are sensitive to acetylsalicylic acid (ASA) apparently are not sensitive to salicylamide. There is some evidence showing that ASA, used occasionally, may be effective for inducing sleep.

L-tryptophan is an essential amino acid ingested daily in amounts of 1 to 2 g in a normal diet. L-tryptophan is also a precursor of serotonin, a neurotransmitter, which plays a role in regulating sleep. Tryptophan has been advocated as a "natural" sedative-hypnotic as it is a natural substance to the body and is relatively free of toxicity. Unlike the benzodiazepines, it does not appear to distort the usual sleep architecture.

Numerous studies have investigated the hypnotic properties of L-tryptophan. These studies have yielded conflicting results. A number of trials have shown that in some patients, L-tryptophan may

Sleep Disorders and Nonprescription Sleep Aids

reduce sleep onset latency without significantly altering the quality of sleep. Suggested starting doses are 1 to 2 g at bedtime, increasing up to 5 g if necessary.

L-tryptophan is relatively non-toxic in low doses. In animal studies, L-tryptophan has caused renal damage, increased incidence of bladder tumors, pulmonary edema, glycosuria and decreased survival of the animal embryo and neonate. Tryptophan has been claimed to be both a carcinogen and a protective agent against carcinogens.

In man, high doses of L-tryptophan (5 to 12 g) can produce nausea and vomiting, headache, dizziness, drowsiness, hyperglycemia, worsening of chorea (involuntary movements) in Huntington's disease, temporal lobe epilepsy and encephalopathy. Anticholinergic side effects (for example dry mouth, blurred vision, urinary hesitancy, constipation) may also occur. Recently, an epidemic of eosinophilia-myalgia syndrome (EMS) was associated with ingestion of a contaminant or by-product of L-tryptophan manufactured by a single Japanese company. The majority of cases have occurred in the United States with more than 75 per cent of cases reported in women. Doses of L-tryptophan have ranged from less than 100 mg to more than 1.5 g per day. EMS is characterized by rapid onset (usually 1 to 2 weeks) of intense myalgias and a total eosinophil count exceeding 10^9 cells per litre of blood. Various skin lesions (edema, induration, maculopapular or urticarial rashes, alopecia, pruritus) may develop, especially during the early phase of the illness. Life-threatening complications such as ascending polyneuropathy resulting in respiratory failure (the most common cause of death in EMS) have been reported. No reports of EMS have been attributed to the commercially available L-tryptophan in Canada.

L-tryptophan should not be combined with MAO inhibitors or fluoxetine due to potentiation of serotonergic effects resulting in delirium, myoclonus, hypomania, shivering and hyper-reflexia. L-tryptophan should be avoided by pregnant women, patients with liver problems or a history of epilepsy.

In summary, although L-tryptophan may be an effective hypnotic in some patients, long-term safety and efficacy have not been established. L-tryptophan was previously available in Canada as a nonprescription sleep aid. It is currently a prescription drug, indicated for use as an adjunct to antidepressant drug treatment.

Consumer Counselling

Individuals should be advised that insomnia is usually a temporary, self-limiting condition caused by changes in location, daily schedule or stress. Medical, psychiatric or drug-related causes should be ruled out. Anyone using a nonprescription sleep aid containing any sedative agent (such as diphenhydramine) should be cautioned about the potential daytime problems of drowsiness, for example when driving a car and when operating dangerous machinery. They should also be advised to avoid the concurrent use of alcohol and other drugs that potentiate central nervous system depression.

Pregnant women should be advised against the use of diphenhydramine until the expected merits and possible risks are discussed with their physicians. Nursing mothers should be advised that occasional use of diphenhydramine at bedtime may be permissible but frequent use of high doses should be avoided.

An occasional sleeping pill may be of some benefit, but consumers should be advised that chronic use is ineffective in most people with insomnia. Persistent insomnia can be an indication of an underlying disease; such people should be referred to a physician.

Narcolepsy

Narcolepsy is a syndrome of excessive daytime sleepiness associated with abnormal manifestations of REM sleep that may include cataplexy, sleep paralysis and hypnagogic hallucinations. Excessive daytime sleepiness occurs every day, regardless of the amount of sleep obtained at night. Sleepiness occurs mainly in boring, sedentary situations and is partially alleviated by motor activity and mental stimulation.

Cataplexy is a brief, sudden loss of skeletal muscle tone, often following an emotional stimulus such as laughter, anger or excitement. The decrease in muscle tone may be as subtle as a slight drop of the jaw or as profound as a complete loss of tone in most peripheral skeletal muscles. During the cataplectic episode, the person remains aware of the surroundings, which helps to differentiate an episode of cataplexy from a seizure. About 60 per cent of narcoleptic people manifest this symptom. Tricyclic antidepressants such as imipramine or clomipramine may reduce the frequency and severity of cataplectic episodes.

About 60 per cent of patients with narcolepsy experience sleep paralysis and hallucinations. Sleep paralysis is the total inability to move any muscles when falling asleep or waking up. Normal people may have occasional sleep paralysis when awakening. Hypnagogic hallucinations are vivid, dream-like experiences that occur as the individual is falling asleep. The hallucinations may be visual, auditory or tactile. Cataplexy, hypnagogic hallucinations and sleep paralysis improve or disappear with age in about one-third of patients but the degree of sleepiness rarely decreases.

The incidence of narcolepsy is estimated to be between 1 in 1,000 and 1 in 10,000 in the United States, with an equal distribution amongst males and females. It occurs more often than other well known neurological conditions such as multiple sclerosis. There is a familial tendency for narcolepsy. Narcolepsy usually develops in the teens and continues throughout adulthood. Sleep laboratory studies have eliminated much of the ambiguity from the diagnostic procedures for this disease. The cause of narcolepsy is unknown, although neurotransmitters involved in the regulation of sleep-waking states are implicated (for example, serotonin, norepinephrine and acetylcholine).

The usual treatment of narcolepsy includes symptomatic treatment of excessive daytime drowsiness with central nervous system stimulants such as dextroamphetamine, methylphenidate or pemoline. The auxiliary symptoms (cataplexy, sleep paralysis and hypnagogic hallucinations) are treated with tricyclic antidepressants (for example, protriptyline, imipramine). Treatment of narcolepsy is often unsatisfactory. Stimulants can cause insomnia, hypertension, palpitations and at higher doses may mimic symptoms of schizophrenia. Tolerance occurs with these agents; to prevent escalation of dosage requirements, drug holidays may be recommended or use may be restricted to times when the individual must remain awake. Tricyclic antidepressants can also cause such undesirable side effects as dry mouth, tachycardia, constipation and urinary retention.

Other drugs which have been tried in the treatment of narcolepsy include selegiline (a MAO-type B inhibitor), mazindol (an imidazole derivative), propranolol, L-tyrosine (an amino acid) and codeine.

Consumer Counselling

Nonprescription sleep aids are generally contraindicated for people with narcolepsy as daytime sleepiness increases and the altered sleep-wake cycle is further disrupted. However, patients with disturbed nocturnal sleep as the primary complaint may benefit from short-activity hypnotics once or twice a week. Consumers complaining of the symptoms of narcolepsy should be referred to a physician.

Sleep Apnea

Sleep apnea is now considered an important sleep disorder because of its deleterious effects on the cardiovascular system and possibly increased risk of death. Sleep apnea is a cessation of breathing lasting 10 seconds or more and occurring 30 or more times during a 7 hour period of sleep. Daytime symptoms such as excessive sleepiness; impairment of intellectual performance, personality changes, psychiatric disturbances and morning headache may occur. Nocturnal symptoms of snoring, gasping or snorting sounds, excessive body movements, diaphoresis (profuse sweating) and enuresis also occur. Systemic hypertension is a common consequence of obstructive sleep apnea. The hypoxia and carbon dioxide retention associated with the nocturnal apneic events may contribute to the development of polycythemia (increase in total red cell mass of the blood) and the cardiovascular complications of pulmonary hypertension, cardiomegaly, right-sided heart failure and persistent cardiac arrhythmias. These symptoms are progressive unless the sleep apnea is treated.

Sleep apnea is more prevalent in men and is often associated with obesity and hypertension. Onset of sleep apnea generally occurs in adulthood, usually over age 30. Diagnosis and treatment of sleep apnea are crucial because of its serious medical consequences.

Apneas are characterized as central, obstructive or mixed. In central apnea, thoracic and abdominal respiratory effort is absent, whereas in obstructive apnea respiratory efforts persist but are ineffective due to upper airway blockage. Obstructive sleep apnea should be suspected if patients experience both hypersomnia and snoring. In mixed apnea, the episode begins with the absence of respiratory effort followed by upper airway obstruction. Often all three types of sleep apneic episodes are noted in the same person. Most people, however, are categorized as having either central or obstructive sleep apnea depending on the predominant type of apnea during a sleep recording. Of these two types, obstructive sleep apnea is by far the most common, occurring in 1 to 4 per cent of the adult population.

Typically, people with obstructive sleep apnea fall asleep easily but their nocturnal sleep is disrupted. Near the end of each of their repetitive respiratory pauses, there is a short arousal (probably related to hypercapnea) and resumption of breathing. Despite these repetitive brief arousals, the person does not usually awaken fully. The repetitive breath cessations cause marked disruption of sleep stage patterns; deep sleep (stages three and four) is significantly reduced or entirely absent and the amount of lighter sleep (stages one and two) is increased. The sleep cycle may be so disrupted that periods of REM sleep occur at sleep-onset rather than after 70 to 90 minutes of NREM sleep, which is the normal pattern. The percentage of REM sleep usually approximates normal levels, but its distribution is more fragmented. Usually the longest and severest periods of apnea occur during REM sleep.

Causes

There is much speculation about the exact pathogenesis of sleep apnea but it appears to be multifactorial. People with this disorder may have anatomically smaller pharyngeal areas. Occasionally, gross anatomic factors such as mandibular malformation, micrognathia (small jaw), tonsillar and adenoidal hypertrophy, nasal septal deviation, acromegaly, vocal cord paralysis or glottal web play major contributory roles. Nasal obstruction, often of an allergic origin, is associated with a considerable increase in sleep apneic episodes. Hypothyroidism has also been linked with obstructive sleep apnea. Alcohol ingestion and sleep deprivation have been shown to increase the number and severity of sleep apneic events. Genetic factors may play a role as well.

Treatment

Underlying medical illnesses such as congestive heart failure, chronic and reversible respiratory disorders and metabolic abnormalities that may impair upper airway functioning should be improved, if possible. Weight reduction in obese individuals is recommended.

In cases of severe obstructive sleep apnea, a tracheostomy may be required to relieve the symptoms and alleviate the long-term cardiovascular effects of this disorder. Another surgical procedure for obstructive sleep apnea is the uvulopalatopharyngoplasty which yields a response rate of only 40 to 50 per cent and is not currently recommended as first-line therapy. With this procedure the pharyngeal airspace is enlarged surgically. Other nonsurgical treatments used for obstructive sleep apnea include a tongue-retaining device and continuous positive airway pressure applied through the nares. Continuous positive airway pressure is associated with the greatest overall effectiveness and acceptability.

The use of medication is indicated primarily for milder cases of sleep apnea. No single agent has been found to be universally effective in the treatment of sleep apnea. Protriptyline may be useful in some patients but the drug causes a high incidence of anticholinergic side effects and there is a risk of arrhythmias. Medroxyprogesterone acetate has limited success but may improve right-sided heart failure due to sleep apnea. Acetazolamide is the most effective treatment of central sleep apnea, but side effects may limit long-term treatment. Some patients with mixed apneas may worsen on acetazolamide. Other drugs have been tried but are not recommended, because they are either impractical to administer (for example, naloxone, strychnine, nicotine gum) or further studies are required to establish efficacy (for example, tryptophan). Oral theophylline is not recommended due to lack of studies. Drugs which have been found to be ineffective in the treatment of sleep apnea include almitrine, atropine, baclofen, bromocriptine), doxapram and prochlorperazine.

In people with sleep apnea, drugs that depress the central ventilatory drive, such as sedative-hypnotics (for example, benzodiazepines, barbiturates), narcotics, sedating analgesics, beta-blockers and alcohol, should be avoided.

Consumer Counselling

Although people with sleep apnea complain of poor sleep at night, hypnotics are strictly contraindicated. Hypnotics depress respiratory function and thus further aggravate sleep apnea. Consumers complaining of the symptoms of sleep apnea (that is, hypersomnia, snoring) should be referred to a physician.

Additional Information

Emotional support and information for people with sleep disorders and their families may be provided by contacting the national office

Sleep Disorders and Nonprescription Sleep Aids

of Sleep/Wake Disorders Canada, Box 223, Postal Station S, Toronto, Ontario M5M 4L7; (416) 398-1627 or regional offices at: Vancouver/ Burnaby, BC (604) 433-8467; Calgary, Alta (403) 282-4263; Edmonton, Alta, (403) 467-2411; Montreal (Fr) (514) 486-1030; (Eng) (514) 697-2041; Saint John, NB (506) 633-4636.

Ask the Consumer

Q. How long have you experienced insomnia? Do you have difficulty sleeping on a regular basis or only occasionally? What is the pattern of your sleep? Do you have difficulty falling asleep or do you awaken in the early hours of the morning?

■ Nonprescription sleep aids are recommended to treat occasional sleeplessness. Anyone with persistent insomnia problems should be referred to a physician as the insomnia may be a symptom of an underlying medical or psychiatric disorder. Nonprescription sleep aids may decrease the time taken to fall asleep.

Q. Can you associate the insomnia with a specific occurrence, such as change in work shifts, worry, grief or pain?

■ Often events or symptoms such as these may cause secondary insomnia. If people recognize the underlying reason for their sleeplessness, they may be able to minimize the cause themselves.

Q. Do you now take or have you recently been taking medication for anxiety, depression, insomnia or any other illness?

■ Many drugs, during treatment or upon withdrawal, can induce changes in normal sleep patterns that can result in insomnia (see Table III).

Q. Do you drink cola beverages, coffee or tea? Are you taking any medication that may contain caffeine?

■ Cola beverages, coffee, tea and certain medications may contain significant amounts of caffeine, especially if consumed in large amounts. Caffeine is a powerful central nervous system stimulant that can produce insomnia. Caffeine-containing products should be avoided for several hours before bedtime.

Q. Do you use alcohol to help you sleep?

■ Alcohol may help some people fall asleep but it interferes with sleep stage organization, leading to frequent awakenings during the night and early morning awakening. Alcohol is not recommended as a sleep aid.

Q. Do you snore? Do you suffer from daytime sleepiness? Do you nap during the day? Do you experience a restless sleep?

■ Before trying a nonprescription sleep aid, consumers should be encouraged to discuss their symptoms with their physician. A sleep aid may only aggravate symptoms.

Q. Have you used sleep aid products before? Were they helpful?

■ A consumer's experience with sleep aids indicates what might be effective, and helps in choosing a product to recommend.

References

Introduction
Kales A, Kales JD. Sleep disorders. Recent findings in the diagnosis and treatment of disturbed sleep. N Engl J Med 1974;290:487–99.

Sleep Architecture
Bloom FE. Neurohumoral transmission and the central nervous system. In: Gilman AG, Goodman LS, Rall TW, Murad F, eds. Goodman and Gilman's the pharmacological basis of therapeutics. New York: Macmillan, 1985:237.
Goldson RL. Management of sleep disorders in the elderly. Drugs 1981;21: 390–6.
Gottlieb GL. Sleep disorders and their management—special considerations in the elderly. Am J Med 1990;88(Suppl 3A):29s–33s.
Martin JB. The sleep-wake cycle and disorders of sleep. In: Petersdorf RG, Adams RD, Braunwald E, et al, eds. Harrison's principles of internal medicine. New York: McGraw-Hill, 1983:118–24.
Prinz PN, Raskind M. Aging and sleep disorders. In: Williams RL, Karacan I, eds. Sleep disorders: diagnosis and treatment. New York: Wiley Medical, 1978:303–21.
Salamy JG. Sleep: some concepts and constructs. In: Williams RL, Karacan I, eds. Pharmacology of sleep. New York: Wiley Med, 1976:53–82.
Warnes H. Psychophysiology of sleep. Mod Med Can 1977;32(1):40–7.
Wincor MZ. Sleep disorders. US Pharmacist 1990;15(1):26–44.
Zorzitto ML. Sleep in the elderly. Mod Med Can 1983;38(1):77–82.

Insomnia
Balter MB, Bauer ML. Patterns of prescribing and use of hypnotics in the United States. In: Clift AD, ed. Sleep disturbance and hypnotic drug dependence. Amsterdam: Excerpta Medica, 1975.
Chen CN. Sleep, depression and antidepressants. Br J Psychiat 1979;135: 385–402.
Cox TC, Jacobs MR, Leblanc AE, Marshman JA. Drugs and drug abuse. Toronto: Addiction Research Foundation, 1983:205–11.
Gillin JC, Byerley WF. The diagnosis and management of insomnia. N Engl J Med 1990;322(4):239–48.
Guttman D. A survey of drug-taking behavior of the elderly. Research report. National Institute of Drug Abuse Services, 1977.
Hauri PJ, Esther MS. Insomnia. Mayo Clin Proc 1990;65:869–82.
Johns MW. Sleep and hypnotic drugs. Drugs 1975;9:448–78.
Kales A, Kales JD. Evaluation and treatment of insomnia. New York: Oxford University Press, 1984.
Kales A, Kales JD, Bixler EO. Insomnia: an approach to management and treatment. Psychiatr Ann 1974;4:28–44.
Kales A, Soldatos CR, Kales JD. Sleep disorders: insomnia, sleepwalking, night terrors, nightmares, and enuresis. Ann Intern Med 1987;106:582–92.
Kales A, Kales JD. Sleep laboratory studies of hypnotic drugs: efficacy and withdrawal effects. J Clin Psychopharmacol 1983;3(2):140–50.

Drug-induced Insomnia
Hill LA. Drug-induced sleep changes. Hosp Pharm 1990;25:1119–20.
Johnstone GJ, Parker WA. Practical management of benzodiazepine withdrawal. Can Pharm J 1983;116:459–63.
Nuotto E, Mattila MJ, Seppala T, et al. Coffee and caffeine and alcohol effects on psychomotor function. Clin Pharmacol Ther 1982;31:68–76.
Trevor AJ, Way WL. Sedative-hypnotics. In: Katzung BG, ed. Basic and clinical pharmacology. Norwalk: Appleton and Lange, 1987:248.

Caffeine-Induced Insomnia
Caffeine: how much is too much? Faculty of Medicine Health News. Toronto: University of Toronto, 1985;3(3):1–4.
Canadian drug identification code. Ottawa: Health and Welfare Canada, 1991.
Cole JO, Pope HG, LaBrie R, et al. Assessing the subjective stimulants in casual users. Clin Pharmacol Ther 1987;24:243–52.

Sleep Disorders and Nonprescription Sleep Aids

Curatolo PW, Robertson D. The health consequences of caffeine. Ann Intern Med 1983;98:641–53.

Greden JF. Anxiety or caffeinism: a diagnostic dilemma. Am J Psychiatr 1974; 131:1089–92.

Karacan I, Thornby JI, Anch AM, et al. Dose-related sleep disturbances induced by coffee and caffeine. Clin Pharmacol Ther 1976;20:682–9.

Macaulay T, Gallant CJ, Hooper SH, et al. Caffeine content of herbal and fast-food beverages. J Can Diet Assoc 1984;45:150–6.

Over-the-counter nighttime sleep-aid and stimulant products. Fed Reg 1978; 42:25544.

Parker WA. Caffeine-induced psychosis. Can J Hosp Pharm 1986;39(1):13–5.

Parsons WD, Neims AH. Effect of smoking on caffeine clearance. Clin Pharmacol Ther 1978;24:40–5.

Raebel MA, Black J. The caffeine controversy: what are the facts? Hosp Pharm 1984;19:257–67.

Nonpharmacologic Management of Insomnia

Coates TJ, Thorsen CE. What to use instead of sleeping pills. JAMA 1978; 240:2311–2.

Antihistamines

Anderson PO. Drug use during breast feeding. Clin Pharm 1991;10:604.

Anonymous. Antihistamines. The United States pharmacopeia. Kingsport: United States Pharmacopeial Convention, 1982:117.

Briggs GG, Freeman RK, Yaffe SJ, eds. Drugs in pregnancy and lactation. Baltimore: Williams and Wilkins, 1990:213–5.

Garnett WR. Diphenhydramine. Am Pharm 1986;NS26(2):35–40.

Marketing status of ingredients recommended for over-the-counter use: amendment to enforcement policy and diphenhydramine; marketing status as a nighttime sleep aid drug product for over-the-counter human use. Fed Reg 1982;April 23.

McEvoy GK, ed. American hospital formulary service. Bethesda: American Society of Hospital Pharmacists, 1983.

Rickels K, Morris RJ, Newman H, et al. Diphenhydramine in insomniac family practice patients: a double-blind study. J Clin Pharmacol 1983;23:234–42.

Sunshine A, Zighelboim I, Laska E. Hypnotic activity of diphenhydramine, methapyrilene and placebo. J Clin Pharmacol 1978;18:425–31.

Mephenesin

Bianchine JR. Drugs for Parkinson's disease, spasticity and acute muscle spasms. In: Gilman AG, Goodman LS, Rall TW, Murad F, eds. Goodman and Gilman's the pharmacological basis of therapeutics. New York: Macmillan, 1985:473–90.

Salicylamide

Flower RJ, Moncada S, Vane JR. Analgesic-antipyretics and anti-inflammatory agents: drugs employed in the treatment of gout. In: Gilman AG, Goodman LS, Rall TW, Murad F, eds. Goodman and Gilman's the pharmacological basis of therapeutics. New York: Macmillan, 1985:686.

L-tryptophan

Fitten LJ, Profita J, Bidder TG. L-tryptophan as a hypnotic in special patients. J Am Geriatr Soc 1985;33:294–7.

Hartmann E, Spinweber CL. Sleep induced by L-tryptophan: effect of dosages within the normal dietary intake. J Nerv Ment Dis 1979;167:497–9.

Hartmann E, Lindsley JG, Spinweber C. Chronic insomnia: effects of tryptophan, flurazepam, secobarbital and placebo. Psychopharmacology 1983; 80:138–42.

Hartmann E, Chung R. Sleep-inducing effects of L-tryptophan. J Pharm Pharmacol 1972;24:242.

Kazura JW. Eosinophilia-myalgia syndrome. Cleve Clin J Med 1991;58:267–70.

Li Wan Po A, Maguire T. Tryptophan: useful dietary supplement or a health hazard? The Pharmaceutical Journal 1990;244:484–5.

Lindsley JG, Hartmann EL, Mitchell W. Selectivity in response to L-tryptophan among insomniac subjects: a preliminary report. Sleep 1983;6(3):247–56.

Linnoila M, Viukari M, Numminen A, et al. Efficacy and side effects of chloral hydrate and tryptophan as sleeping aids in psychogeriatric patients. Int Pharmacopsychiatry 1980;15:124.

Nickel A. Tryptan: no association with eosinophilia-myalgia syndrome. Can Med Assoc J 1990;143(11):1155–6.

Ostrom J. Tryptophan: a review of its use for depression and sleep. Hosp Form 1981:1164–75.

Pervan Z. Eosinophilia-myalgia syndrome associated with L-tryptophan use. Med J Aust 1991;154:565–6.

Rubin T. Urinary hesitancy with therapeutic doses of L-tryptophan. Drug Intell Clin Pharm 1981;15:996–8.

Schneider-Helmert D, Spinweber CL. Evaluation of L-tryptophan for treatment of insomnia: a review. Psychopharmacology 1986;89:1–7.

Slutsker L, Hoesley FC, Miller L, et al. Eosinophilia-myalgia syndrome associated with exposure to tryptophan from a single manufacturer. JAMA 1990;264:213–7.

Narcolepsy

Aldrich MS. Narcolepsy. N Engl J Med 1990;323:389–93.

Campbell KR. The treatment of narcolepsy and cataplexy. Drug Intell Clin Pharm 1981;15:257–62.

Dement WC, Carskadon WA, Guilleminault C, et al. Narcolepsy, diagnosis and treatment. Primary Care 1976;3:609–23.

Kales A, Vela-Bueno A, Kales JD. Sleep disorders: sleep apnea and narcolepsy. Ann Intern Med 1987;106:434–43.

Zarcone V. Narcolepsy. N Engl J Med 1973;288:1156–66.

Sleep Apnea

Guilleminault C, Dement WC. Sleep apnea syndromes and related sleep disorders. In: Williams RL, Karacan I, eds. Sleep disorders: diagnosis and treatment. New York: J Wiley and Sons, 1978:9–28.

Kimoff RJ, Cosio MG, McGregor M. Clinical features and treatment of obstructive sleep apnea. Can Med Assoc J 1991;144:689–95.

Schott WJ, Middleton RK, Mart LL. Drug treatment for sleep apnea. Drug Intell Clin Pharm 1989;23:308–11.

Schroeder JS, Motta J, Guilleminault C. Hemodynamic studies in sleep apnea. In: Guilleminault C, Dement WC, eds. Sleep apnea syndromes. New York: AR Liss, 1978:177.

Simmons FB, Guilleminault C, Silvestri R. Snoring, and some obstructive sleep apnea, can be cured by oropharyngeal surgery: palatopharyngoplasty. Arch Otolaryngol 1983;109:503–7.

33

Herbal Medicines

R. Frank Chandler

Drugs are derived from many sources, including herbs. Concurrent with man's evolution, drugs have evolved from the use of whole herbs and their simple extracts to highly refined chemical entities. Within the last two decades, the use of herbs as medicine has undergone a dramatic revitalization. Herbs are now widely available commercially. Unfortunately, regulations to ensure quality products and their safe and effective use are largely nonexistent and ineffective. Traditional herbal medicines are widely regarded as safe. While this may be true for intermittent short-term usage, little is known regarding the possible toxicities from chronic use. It is known that, in a few instances, chronic use of traditional herbal medicines will lead to severe and even fatal outcomes. Therefore, herbal medicines—like conventional or allopathic medicines— must be used cautiously. Pharmacists should be aware of the safety and efficacy issues.

Man has depended on plants for shelter, clothing, food and medicine throughout history. Through trial and error man has learned which plants are safe to eat, which are poisonous and which are effective medicines. In some cases, as stated by Paracelsus over 500 years ago, *"Dosis sola facit venenum"*, that is, the dose alone makes the difference. Even the common potato can be fatal!

Neanderthal man appears to have valued and revered a number of herbs as medicinal agents. Today, 60,000 years later, about two-thirds of the world's population still depends almost exclusively on herbs for its medications. Furthermore, about 25 per cent of all prescription drugs in developed countries contain active constituents obtained from flowering plants and trees. Nonprescription drugs and herbal preparations are also used extensively in developed countries as adjuvants or alternatives to conventional or allopathic medicine. The use of herbs for these indications has increased substantially in recent years. In 1984 it was estimated they represented a $750 million market in Canada.

The major reasons cited for this trend are concern over the side effects and cost of allopathic medicines, lack of faith in these medicines, hope that a cure will emerge to treat their chronic or terminal illness and/or the belief that herbal preparations, used in their natural state, are not harmful to humans. This belief in harmlessness defies common knowledge and is contrary to a substantial body of scientific evidence.

The unlimited and unquestioned use of herbal preparations, especially in the light of existing scientific knowledge, contributes to the concerns regarding the safety of their use.

The misidentification of self-collected plant material can result in serious and even fatal poisoning. The most dramatic examples of this type of accidental poisoning are cases in which teas were prepared from mistakenly collected foxglove (Digitalis).

Inadequate quality control of herbal drugs, which permits inferior products to reach the market, is also a significant concern. Indeed, many of the concerns that follow are the consequence of this lack of control. The literature contains many examples of herbal preparations which were of poor quality and where the characteristic constituents were present only in negligible amounts or absent altogether.

Undeclared ingredients of herbal remedies can lead to unforeseen reactions. Intentional adulteration of herbal preparations with toxic components or allopathic medications continues to be a major concern. Agents such as heavy metals, atropine-like alkaloids, cocaine, synthetic corticosteroids and/or nonsteroidal anti-inflammatory drugs, estrogen-like substances, and other drugs have all been found in herbal preparations. Deaths from products containing some of these contaminants have been recorded.

Herbal products in a number of developed countries are not controlled by the respective drug regulations and can, therefore, escape pre-marketing surveillance of their toxic potential by posing as dietary supplements. As a consequence, numerous patients may be exposed to unnecessary risk before the results of independent risk-assessments are available.

Another potential risk arises when uninformed individuals consume doses of herbal remedies larger than tradition provides. This situation usually occurs when the consumer believes natural products are safe—even at excessive doses.

Literature advocating the benefits of herbal preparations abounds. A significant portion of this literature presents only the alleged beneficial aspects of the herbs in question, even if that entails reiterating outdated and uncritical information. Known or potential adverse effects are frequently missing or minimized, either purposely or out of ignorance. The persistent promotion of these products and the revived interest in herbal remedies can bring about the reintroduction of herbal products that have been previously abandoned because of their ineffectiveness and/or their adverse reaction profile.

Adverse outcomes may arise when disorders, which modern therapy can treat and for which life-threatening complications (for

Herbal Medicines

example, hypertension) can be prevented, are treated with an ineffective remedy. Death can be a consequence.

Acute toxic reactions to an herbal product, such as dermatological reactions, are quite likely to be recognized by herbal healers and the consumer. However, they are equally unlikely to recognize the subtle, chronic effects of some compounds. Thus, it is unlikely that the chronic toxicities of pyrrolizidine alkaloids, safrole, aristolchic acids, hydrogen cyanide, or other toxic compounds would be associated with the long term use of the associated herbs.

There is no doubt, however, that some of the botanicals that have been used traditionally as foods or medicines can produce dangerous and sometimes even lethal poisoning. Calls to American Poison Control Centers concerning plants constitute about 10 per cent of all inquiries. Most of these calls concern children under 3 years of age and only a small number report symptoms. Vulto and de Smet have recently summarized the unwanted effects of some 120 botanical medicines or their purified constituents. These effects range from mild irritations to death.

An area of increasing concern, and one for which there is little information, is the effect of herbal medicines on the developing fetus or nursing infant. A recent report serves to document the hazards associated with two commonly used herbs. A Swiss woman consumed an herbal tea, purchased from her pharmacy, daily throughout her pregnancy. Her infant died 11 days after birth from severe jaundice, massive hepatomegaly and ascites. The tea has been found to contain *Tussilago farfara* (coltsfoot) and *Petasites officinalis* (butterbur), both members of the Compositae family and both known to contain hepatotoxic pyrrolizidine alkaloids.

There is also convincing evidence that drugs of abuse can affect neuroendocrine and gonadal function resulting in infertility and sexual dysfunction. Caffeine, in the form of commonly consumed beverages, has been associated with late spontaneous abortion. Furthermore, the deleterious outcome in animals clearly demonstrates that herbs are not always benign to the unborn. Yet pregnant women frequently use herbal beverages during pregnancy as substitutes for caffeine-containing beverages or for their medicinal effects. Additionally, herbs (including some potentially dangerous ones) are employed by some in the practice of midwifery.

Before a patient consumes an herbal beverage or herbal remedy, the risk-benefit ratio must be considered. Products that have laxative, diuretic or gastrointestinal stimulating properties should be used with great caution, if at all. Furthermore, plants containing known toxins and their close relatives should not be consumed during pregnancy.

There is also an alarming lack of scientific data about the possibility of drug interactions between herbal remedies and allopathic medicines. Herbal products have the potential to enhance the activity of allopathic medications when their bioactivities are of a similar nature. Similarly, they may reduce the absorption of allopathic medicines due to the presence of tannins or phytates. There is a similar lack of knowledge about their kinetic behavior.

With such a list of problems associated with herbal remedies, the question "Can they be consumed safely?" naturally arises. If the consumer follows some simple steps, as with allopathic medicines, herbal remedies can be both safe and effective.

Considering the above information, a number of factors should concern all those who use, sell or counsel on the use and properties of herbs. To assist with the selection of herbal remedies, the consumer has been recently provided with a set of guidelines for the appropriate use of herbal products (see Table I).

Some additional questions should also be foremost in the mind of anyone selling or counselling on the use of herbal remedies or teas:

- Is the use of the herb based on known effectiveness or only on traditional use?
- Is it safe or is its safety one of historical use only?
- Is it closely related to plants with known toxicities?
- Are the identity and quality of the herb or preparation guaranteed?
- Are there known or possible interactions with allopathic medicines?

For many herbs, the answers to one or more of these questions are unknown. For others, the answers are known or, at least, considerable information is available.

Plants Regarded as Poisons

A poison is any substance that, in relatively small amounts, produces injury to the body by its chemical action. Most of us can probably relate an incident or story involving a plant or plant product in an untoward event. Many poisons are highly active substances, and since ancient times have served the purposes of murder and suicide. In suitable doses they may also be important as medicines. The occurrence of other, pharmacologically less active substances make a plant poisonous because they are present in high concentration or because they accumulate with chronic use. Often, the only difference between medicinal and poisonous plants is the dose. The poisonous nature of a plant (its active constituents) can be and often is subject to the plant part, the degree of maturity of the plant and environmental conditions.

Some plants are generally regarded as poisonous rather than medicinal. The following are examples, although most also have medicinal applications: the jequerity bean (*Abrus precatorius*), water

---

Table I *Guidelines for Appropriate Use of Herbal Products*

- Buy herbal remedies from reliable and trusted sources.
- Purchase an herbal remedy only if the package clearly states which herb(s) it contains.
- Always ask for the exact directions for use.
- Do not collect herbs in the wild, unless you are well-able to distinguish poisonous and innocuous herbs from one another.
- Store herbal remedies as you would allopathic medicines.
- Do not use herbal remedies that you have kept for years.
- Do not use herbal remedies for serious illnesses.
- Stop using an herbal remedy if you start experiencing side effects.
- Do not exceed the dose range stated in the directions for use.
- To avoid possible chronic effects, do not use herbal remedies for prolonged periods.
- If you are pregnant or breast-feeding and want to use an herbal remedy, do so only after consulting your physician or pharmacist.
- Your physician or pharmacist must be informed if you are using an herbal remedy simultaneously with other medicines.

Adapted from: de Smet PGAM. Drugs used in nonorthodox medicine. In: Dukes MNG, Beeley L, eds. Side effects of drugs Annual 14. Amsterdam: Elsevier, 1990:429–51.

hemlock (*Cicuta maculata*), poison hemlock (*Conium maculatum*), bittersweet (*Solanum dulcamara*), deadly nightshade (*Atropa belladonna*), lily-of-the-valley (*Convallaria majalis*), daffodil (*Narcissus* species), castor bean (*Ricinus communis*), nux-vomica (*Strychnos nux-vomica*) and mistletoe (*Viscum album*).

Plants Generally Regarded as Foods

On the other extreme of the scale are the plants generally regarded as safe to consume as foods. Few would challenge the safety of asparagus, lettuce, broccoli, cucumber, carrots, peas, kidney beans, apricots and potatoes. However, in spite of their general safety, the last three can cause severe toxicity. Fatalities caused by apricots and potatoes have been recorded. The toxins (lectins) in kidney beans (*Phaseolus vulgaris*), which cause severe stomach upset, are destroyed by boiling. The kernels of apricots (*Prunus armeniaca*)—indeed the seeds of most plants of the rose family (Rosaceae)—contain hydrogen cyanide and can be fatal if consumed in sufficient quantity. Potato (*Solanum tuberosum*) sprouts, fruit, vines and green tubers contain the poisonous alkaloid solanine, which may cause stomach upset, vomiting, headaches and death. Only the tuber, free of green portions, should be consumed.

Plants Used as Medicines

Between those plants generally regarded as foods and those regarded as poisons are many plants used for their medicinal value. Most of these uses have evolved over the centuries from their original traditional uses.

Allopathic Medicines Derived from Herbs

Some herbs or their products have become entrenched in current allopathic medicine. No viable alternatives exist for some of these medicines. As such, they play a major role not only in medicine, but also in commerce. Between 1959 and 1980, drugs obtained from flowering plants and trees were present in about 25 per cent of all prescriptions dispensed in the United States. This use represented an estimated $3 billion in sales in 1973 and $8 billion in 1980. Following are a few examples of familiar medicines included in this category.

Foxglove (*Digitalis purpurea*), used in domestic medicine in the United Kingdom as far back as the tenth century, was introduced into medical practice by Dr. William Withering in 1775. He obtained knowledge of its value in dropsy (edema) from an old woman herbalist. Its mechanism of action in congestive heart failure and the nature of its active ingredients were determined later. Digoxin, the major constituent of *Digitalis lanata*, has largely replaced foxglove and its major constituent, digitoxin, in current medical practice.

Quinine, still one of the most important antimalarial drugs, was first isolated from cinchona bark (*Cinchona* species) in 1820. However, the value of this medicine had been known to the Europeans since 1739, when it was revealed that a Peruvian Indian medicine man had "cured" a Jesuit missionary of malaria by administering a cinchona bark preparation. Several synthetic antimalarial drugs have been introduced to the market, but quinine is regaining importance in treating chloroquine resistant organisms.

Before the advent of cimetidine, **carbenoxolone** was the only effective therapeutic agent available that stimulated the healing of gastric and duodenal ulcers. Carbenoxolone is derived from glycyrrhetinic acid, the major sapogenin of licorice (*Glycyrrhiza glabra*)—a plant long used to alleviate gastric pain and oral ulcers.

For centuries, **snakeroot** (*Rauwolfia serpentina*) was used in India to treat a variety of illnesses ranging from snakebite to insanity. Not until 1952 was the value of this plant and its alkaloids recognized. Reserpine was the first drug available to effectively control some forms of anxiety and psychosis. It is also useful in essential hypertension. Rauwolfia and reserpine are still the basis of several preparations used for their antihypertensive and antipsychotic effects.

Tubocurarine, isolated from *Chondodendron tomentosum*, is one of the major alkaloids of curare, a South American arrow poison. Its skeletal muscle relaxant action (paralyzing effect on voluntary muscles) has been successfully transferred to the operating theatre. It allows for muscle relaxation without deep anesthesia.

Although beneficial, and in some cases without an alternative choice, each of these drugs has its own list of adverse effects. These drugs demand judicious use by qualified medical practitioners.

Food-Herbs with Medicinal Applications

A number of herbs are known primarily as foods, although they may also be used for a variety of medicinal purposes and may even be toxic.

One of the best examples is probably **parsley** (*Petroselinum crispum*). The leaves of parsley have been used for centuries as a garnish and nutrient. Parsley seeds were traditionally used as a carminative and the root as a diuretic. The plant has been used to treat arthritis, and the plant and its oil have been used as emmenagogues (drugs that promote menstrual flow). Adverse effects from ingesting the oil have included headache, giddiness, loss of balance, convulsions and renal damage. The oil comprises about 0.1 per cent of the root and about 5 per cent of the seeds and contains at least two biologically active compounds, apiol and myristicin. Apiol is an antipyretic and, like myristicin, a uterine stimulant. Apiol was once available in capsules for use as an abortifacient. The Russians have an apiol product used to stimulate uterine contractions during labor. These constituents are likely responsible for the observed diuretic effect of parsley. Because these compounds may stimulate the uterine muscles, the seeds, juice and oil of parsley should not be administered to pregnant women. Oil of apiol is a prescription drug in Canada.

Another widely used plant is **cassava**. Cassava (*Manihot esculenta* or *Manihot utilissima*) is a small shrub native to Brazil and widely cultivated throughout the tropics. The rhizomes are used in many parts of the world as a starchy food similar to potatoes or rice. Cassava has also been employed as a medicinal herb, primarily for dermatological ailments and as a counterirritant.

Traditional methods of preparation as a food consist of carefully washing and cooking the rhizomes to remove the hydrogen cyanide (HCN) present throughout cassava. The skin of sweet cassava (*Manihot dulcis*) and possibly the flesh may also contain HCN, therefore the cassava must be peeled before eating. The HCN is present as the water-soluble glucoside linamarin.

Commercially, the fleshy rhizomes of cassava and sweet cassava are washed, sliced and pulped. The pulp is placed on a strainer and the starch washed out by a powerful stream of water. The starch is allowed to settle; it is then removed and dried. The starch thus prepared is known as Brazilian-, Bahai-, Rio-, or Para-arrowroot or manioca starch and may be used as a nutrient, a thickening agent or in preparing tapioca.

Herbal Medicines

The HCN in cassava has been the cause of both acute and chronic toxicity, the latter especially in some African populations where it is consumed regularly.

Poke, pokeberry, pokeweed or **pokeroot** (*Phytolacca americana*) has long been a favorite spring potherb in the southern United States. The young leaves and shoots are boiled, usually twice, and eaten as greens, like spinach. Occasionally, a few young leaves are added to salads to provide a tang. Commercial preparations are also available. As an herbal remedy, pokeroot has been promoted primarily as an emetic, cathartic and remedy for chronic rheumatism. Overdoses have sometimes been fatal.

Pokeroot is a common weed of southeastern Canada and the eastern United States, growing to a height of 2 metres. The white flowers develop into juicy, dark purple berries. All parts of pokeweed are toxic, with the poison in highest concentration in the rootstalks, less in the mature leaves and stems, and least in the berries. Leaves collected in the spring before acquiring a red color are edible if boiled for 5 minutes, rinsed and reboiled. Similarly, the berries are edible when cooked. Poisoning often results when pokeroot is collected in error for parsnips, Jerusalem artichoke or horseradish.

Ingestion of the poisonous parts of pokeroot causes severe stomach cramping, nausea with persistent diarrhea and vomiting, slow and difficult breathing, weakness, spasms, hypotension, severe convulsions and death. Several investigations have reported deaths in children following the ingestion of uncooked berries or pokeberry juice. The toxic principle is thought to be a triterpoid saponin, phytolaccigenin, of undetermined structure.

Poke presents a much more insidious risk to health than acute poisoning. It contains a proteinaceous mitogen that may produce blood abnormalities when absorbed. The Food and Drug Administration of the United States (FDA) classifies this herb as one of undefined safety, adding that it "contains an acidic steroid saponin. Emetic action is slow but of long duration. Narcotic effects have been observed."

The Herb Trade Association (a former consumer education organization) issued a policy statement declaring pokeroot must not be sold as an herbal beverage or food. It further recommended all packages containing pokeroot carry an appropriate statement warning of the product's toxicity and its potential danger when taken internally. However, one author states, "With or without a warning label, pokeroot is definitely not recommended for either internal or external use by human beings."

Thus, many plants are used primarily as foods, even in the presence of known and severe side effects. Still others depend on proper preparation to render them safe, or at least free of obvious side effects.

Flavors and Spices as Medicines

Most flavors and spices used as medicines are also employed in low amounts for their familiar flavor or the zest they add to foods. Some are used to flavor medicines. In higher doses, most exhibit a medicinal action. Most flavors are volatile oils. As a group, they are noted for their carminative and stomachic activities. When employed as a food they are subject to the standards for preparation and adulteration found in Part B of the Canadian Food and Drug Regulations. When used as herbal remedies, they do not always comply with these regulations. Other herbs (for example, hibiscus and passion flower) are not subject to these controls. The following examples illustrate how some herbs are used as flavors or spices and medicines.

Aniseed, or anise, is the dried ripe fruit of *Pimpinella anisum*. The fruit ("seeds") contains 1 to 3 per cent volatile oil (anise oil). Anethole (80 to 90 per cent) is the primary ingredient. Anise oil is also obtained from Chinese star anise (*Illicium verum*). This oil also contains 80 to 90 per cent anethole, but, unlike *Pimpinella anisum*, contains traces of safrole, a known carcinogen. The safety of anethole has been questioned, but it was concluded that it does "not seem to be potent enough or persistent enough to be of serious practical concern at this time." The FDA lists both herbs as safe. The Food and Drug Regulations state that *Pimpinella anisum* is the spice, and both *Pimpinella anisum* and Chinese star anise may be used in obtaining anise oil.

Apart from its extensive use as a licorice flavor in foods, beverages, drugs, cosmetics and confectionaries, anise oil is a well established folk remedy for treating flatulence, colic, dyspepsia and hard, dry coughs. The carminative and expectorant activities of the oil have been established, and anise oil is the active ingredient in a number of proprietary cough remedies. It is also present in a number of stimulant laxative preparations to diminish the griping (cramping of the bowels). The oil should be used with caution; as little as 1 mL can result in nausea, vomiting, pulmonary edema and seizures.

Although anise exhibits many biological activities, it is used primarily as a condiment and flavor. Anise may cause sensitization in some individuals. However, it is safe and effective when employed in the traditional manner.

Fenugreek is one of the most versatile seed spices and one of the oldest recorded medicinal plants. Fenugreek (*Trigonella foenumgraecum*) consists of the dried, ripe seeds of a small, southern European herb. The taste of the seed accounts for its use as a spice and flavor, especially in imitation maple syrup and curry.

Fenugreek seeds contain a hydrophilic mucilage that has a soothing effect on the skin and mucous membranes. This effect accounts for its external use in various ointments and poultices. Internally, the mucilage has a soothing effect on the gastrointestinal tract and may be of benefit in coughs and minor mouth and stomach disorders. Fenugreek also displays a laxative action due to the indigestible nature of the hydrophilic mucilage. Its reported hypoglycemic activity is equivocal. The plant appears to produce no serious toxic effects.

Due to its content of sapogenins, particularly diosgenin, fenugreek seed is a potential future source of sapogenins for the manufacture of steroid hormones. Because it is an annual herb, the time required for its planting-to-harvesting is much shorter than that for *Dioscorea* species, the current source of diosgenin, and fenugreek may eventually prove to have a distinct advantage.

The Canadian Food and Drug Regulations state that *oregano*, as a spice, is the dried leaves of *Origanum vulgare* or other Origanum species. However, oregano is known to be derived from several genera of plants, mainly from two families, Labiatae and Verbenaceae. The two most commonly encountered genera are Origanum and Lippia. Over two dozen species yield leaves or flowering tops that have the flavor recognized as oregano. The most commonly used plants are *Origanum vulgare*, *Lippia graveolens* and *Lippia palmeri*. The latter two are referred to as Mexican oregano.

The botanical distinction between oregano and marjoram is not well defined. Carvacrol is the main constituent of the volatile oils of oregano, marjoram, thyme and summer savory.

Oregano is not a significant medicinal herb. The literature lists it as useful in toothache, oral inflammations, rheumatism and nervous headaches. It is also recommended as a carminative, a diaphoretic,

Herbal Medicines

a tonic and an emmenagogue. Because of its fragrance, it was also used as a strewing herb.

Noting that oregano had been used as an emmenagogue, the Expert Advisory Committee on Herbs and Botanical Preparations of Health and Welfare Canada suggested oregano be labelled to indicate its contraindication in pregnancy. However, even allowing for liberal usage in cooking, it is inconceivable that anyone might ingest enough (one quarter of the average kitchen spice bottle) oregano in one meal to induce toxicity. Of greater concern is the purchase of oil of oregano, thyme or marjoram, as toxic doses could then be easily consumed.

Oil of wintergreen (*Gaultheria procumbens*) is used as a flavoring agent in candies, chewing gum, soft drinks (for example, root beer) and dental preparations. The leaves and berries, which persist through the winter, have been used by the Indians as survival food. The berries have been used in pies and the leaves to make an herbal tea. Both are used as a condiment and as a refreshing nibble, especially on a hot day in the woods.

All parts of the plant yield oil of wintergreen, which contains about 95 per cent methyl salicylate. It is primarily a counterirritant, analgesic and antipyretic, but is also used as a carminative, antiseptic, anti-inflammatory agent, diuretic and stimulant, and for many other uses. Small doses stimulate the stomach, but large doses cause vomiting.

Toxicity is unlikely to occur from ingesting the plant. However, as little as 10 mL of the oil (representing about 1 kg of the leaves) can be fatal to a child.

The major use of **hops** (*Humulus lupulus*) is flavoring and preserving beer. Since the Middle Ages, when it was observed that hop pickers tired easily, this herb has been reputed to have sedative and hypnotic effects. The active ingredients are thought to be the bitter, acidic compounds humulone and lupulone, but their action is erratic owing to instability in light and air. Different varieties of hops seem to vary considerably in their sedative effects. Despite lack of scientific proof for the central nervous system depressant effects of hops in humans, the herb and its extracts are widely used in herbal sedative preparations. Hops are generally regarded as safe although they have been known to cause contact dermatitis.

Medicinal Teas

Many herbs are consumed as teas, whether for beverage or medicinal purposes. To use the volatile oils or delicate plant parts such as flowers and soft leaves, the herbs are steeped in water that has been brought to a boil, usually in a tightly covered container. The herbs are allowed to steep for 10 to 20 minutes. To extract the essences from coarser leaves, stems, barks and roots, the herbs are simmered uncovered until the volume of water decreases by about half through evaporation. The beverage teas are made using 1 to 5 g of herb per 500 mL of water; medicinal teas are usually made using about 30 g of herb. Thus, medicinal teas range from about 6 to 60 times stronger than beverage teas. If fresh herbs are used, the quantity of plant material is doubled. The usual dose of medicinal teas is one half to one cup (125 to 250 mL) taken 3 times daily.

Consumption of more than 3 cups a day of any herbal beverage, including regular tea and coffee, is considered by some to be immoderate. Herbs used in herbal beverages cover the full range of safety; from those offering only flavoring and coloring to those that are quite toxic, including chronic toxicity.

The red flowers of **hibiscus** (*Hibiscus sabdariffa*) are popular ingredients in jams, jellies, sauces, acidic beverages and teas. Hibiscus contains various pigments plus relatively large amounts of citric acid (12 to 17 per cent), hibisic acid (23 per cent, the lactone of hydroxycitric acid) and lesser amounts of malic, tartaric and other acids. The pigments impart a red color to the preparation. The acids are responsible for the tart, refreshing taste of various hibiscus beverages. In medicinal preparations they probably account for the mild laxative and diuretic effects attributed to the plant. Other medicinal claims for this plant need to be verified. Hibiscus is free from known or suspected side effects.

Two plants, closely related botanically, chemically and pharmacologically, have long enjoyed popularity as beverages and folk remedies for digestive disorders, cramps and various skin conditions. The plants are known as German or wild **chamomile** and Roman or garden chamomile (*Matricaria chamomilla* and *Anthemis nobilis*, respectively). The active ingredients of these plants are found in the volatile oil, which is particularly abundant in the mature flower heads.

Although numerous claims are made for chamomile, most are without adequate support. Scientific evidence supports three major medical claims made for these plants. In common with many other aromatic plants, chamomile possesses carminative activity and therefore aids digestion. The terpenes, chamazulen and alpha-bisabolol, are major components of the volatile oil and are primarily responsible for the anti-inflammatory activity used for various afflictions of the skin and mucous membranes. The terpenes and other constituents also exhibit a smooth muscle spasmolytic activity, useful in treating various cramps, especially menstrual cramps. The flavonoids (for example, apigenin, luteolin, and quercetin) and coumarins (for example, scopoletin-7-beta-glucoside) enhance this activity. It is therefore apparent the therapeutic value of chamomile does not rest on a single constituent, but on a complex mixture of chemically different compounds.

Since much of the value of this plant lies in its volatile oil, it is unfortunate that even a strong tea contains only about 10 to 15 per cent of the volatile oil originally present in the plant material.

Because these "drugs" include the flower heads, and therefore pollen, tea made from them may cause contact dermatitis or other hypersensitivity reactions in allergic individuals. The contact dermatitis is thought to be due to the presence of the alpha-methylene-gamma-lactone group of the sesquiterpene lactones present. Although these reactions are not common, individuals allergic to ragweed, asters, chrysanthemums or other members of the Compositae family should be cautious about using chamomile. In non-allergic individuals, no serious undesirable effects have been reported with moderate use of chamomile. Chamomile is generally regarded as safe.

Another popular herbal tea, formerly also generally regarded as safe, is now known to be a serious chronic poison and is responsible for a number of deaths. The hepatotoxicity of the pyrrolizidine alkaloids found in **Gordolobos** tea has been widely publicized. The tea is used extensively in the southwest for many common ailments, such as sore throats. It is used daily by some. The symptoms may occur rapidly, especially in young people, but more commonly take decades to appear. Symptoms may progress even after withdrawal of the herb. At least in part, the use of this tea accounts for the high death rate from cirrhosis in Arizona, which consistently runs up to 25 per cent above the national average, even when corrected for deaths known to be due to alcoholism.

Gordolobos is not a consistent preparation, but commonly contains plants rich in pyrrolizidine alkaloids, such as *Senecio longilobos*. The plants from which the teas are derived grow throughout southwestern and western United States. Some, or close relatives, are found in northern United States and parts of Canada. The teas are widely available through commercial distribution. Various species of Crotalaria are also responsible for much of the liver disease in Jamaica, where the plant is used as a bush tea.

Traditional Herbal Medicine

The list of herbs used as traditional drugs is virtually endless. A few examples demonstrate how some of these are, or have been, useful medicines. Other examples touch on the problems encountered and questions that need to be answered. A summary of some data on a number of popular herbs is presented in Table II.

Valerian (*Valeriana officinalis*) is a popular plant used as a sedative/hypnotic, especially in parts of Europe. It is a common constituent in herbal preparations intended for tranquilization or sedation. A group of constituents known as the valepotriates has been shown to possess definite central nervous system depressant effects in humans and is marketed as a sedative in Germany. Other constituents augment this activity. This depressant activity is not synergistic with alcohol and the incidence of undesirable side effects is less than with diazepam. The valepotriates exhibit cytotoxic and antitumor activities. The valepotriate content of valerian can vary widely; this variation depends mainly on conditions of preparation and storage. No toxicities for valerian or the valepotriates have been reported in humans and no adverse effects could be attributed to valerian in controlled clinical trials. Although there is little evidence that the valepotriates are effective cytotoxic agents in vivo, there is concern about the safety of valerian preparations, particularly following long-term use.

Valerian appears to be a safe and effective drug. Stabilization and standardization of the constituents should produce products of considerable importance to the layman and medical practitioners.

Traditionally, **feverfew** (*Tanacetum parthenium*, synonym: *Chrysanthemum parthenium*) has been used as an antipyretic, an antispasmodic, an emmenagogue, a carminative and an anthelmintic. More recently it has become popular in Europe as a prophylactic treatment for migraine headaches. Its extracts have been claimed to relieve menstrual pain, asthma and arthritis.

The chemistry of feverfew is poorly defined. The plant is rich in sesquiterpene lactones, principally parthenolide. The sesquiterpene lactones have been cited as the active and toxic ingredients of feverfew. Members of this class of compounds possess spasmolytic activity. An aqueous solution dramatically suppresses prostaglandin synthesis. The mechansim of action is not known, but appears to differ from that of the salicylates. Feverfew extracts are also potent inhibitors of serotonin-release from platelets and polymorphonuclear leucocyte granules, providing a possible connection between the claimed benefits of feverfew in migraines and arthritis.

Several clinical studies have clearly established the beneficial effects of feverfew as a prophylactic against migraines, decreasing both the incidence and severity of symptoms. The abrupt withdrawal of feverfew in one study led to incapacitating headaches in some people. Most subjects experienced anxiety, poor sleep and muscle and joint stiffness. This effect has been referred to as "postfeverfew syndrome."

Side effects are noted by about 20 per cent of feverfew users, the most troublesome (11 per cent) being mouth ulcerations. Other side effects include widespread inflammation of the oral mucosa and tongue, often with swelling of the lips and loss of taste. Dermatitis and increased heart rate were reported by some users.

The herb has been used to promote menstruation and therefore should be regarded as an abortifacient.

Feverfew, with its established beneficial effects and its relatively low incidence of adverse effects, represents a solid prospect for effective prophylactic therapy for migraine headaches. At the very least, studies with this herb should help elucidate the nature of migraines.

Coltsfoot (*Tussilago farfara*) is one of several plants recently identified as potentially hazardous when consumed chronically. *Tussilago* is derived from the Latin *tussis*, meaning cough, and the plant has a long history of use as an antitussive. Either the leaves or the flower heads are used. The active ingredient in the plant is a mucilage that acts as a demulcent and expectorant.

Although coltsfoot is effective for the purposes claimed, the leaves and flowers contain pyrrolizidine alkaloids. Some of these alkaloids are hepatotoxic and carcinogenic. Senkirkine is present in young flowers and senecionine is found with it in the leaves. Both are known hepatotoxins and carcinogens.

No cases of confirmed coltsfoot poisoning have been reported, but this is not surprising as the pyrrolizidine alkaloids are chronic, cumulative poisons. The argument that the plant has buffers or neutralizers to prevent the toxic effects is not supported by one study in which rats were fed coltsfoot in their diet. Two-thirds of those receiving greater than 4 per cent coltsfoot in their diet developed hemangioendothelial sarcoma of the liver. This demonstrates that coltsfoot can no longer be considered safe therapy. The recent death from hepatotoxicity of an infant whose mother consumed an herbal tea which contained coltsfoot reinforces this. This situation raises the question of long-term safety of all herbal preparations.

Comfrey (*Symphytum officinale*) is one of the most common herbs sold in North America and one for which modern herbalists display a high degree of enthusiasm. The leaves or roots have been widely promoted and used as poultices to heal wounds, burns, sprains, swellings and bruises. Comfrey has been claimed to heal gastric ulcers and hemorrhoids, and to suppress bronchial congestion and inflammation.

The healing properties of comfrey are probably due to its content of allantoin, an agent that promotes cell proliferation. Ointments containing comfrey have been found to possess an anti-inflammatory activity, which appears to be related to the presence of allatoin, rosmarinic acid or a hydrocolloid polysaccharide. The roots contain 0.6 to 0.8 per cent allantoin and 4 to 6.5 per cent tannin; the leaves contain 1.3 per cent allantoin and 8 to 9 per cent tannins. Large amounts of mucilage are present in both roots and leaves.

Despite its common use, the long-term ingestion of comfrey may pose a health hazard. Like Gordolobos tea and coltsfoot, comfrey contains several pyrrolizidine alkaloids known to be hepatotoxic and carcinogenic. The type and amount of alkaloids present vary with plant part and species of Symphytum. Echimidine is the most toxic of the alkaloids found in Symphytum, but does not appear in *Symphytum officinale*. The roots and leaves of this plant are hepatotoxic and carcinogenic (liver and urinary bladder) in rats fed in concentrations as low as 0.5 and 8 per cent of their diet, respectively. Numerous human toxicities also appear in the literature.

Pyrrolizidine alkaloids are recognized as compounds of toxicological significance. A detailed report of human pyrrolizidine toxicity described an outbreak of hepatic disease among Afghani villagers who ate wheat contaminated with Heliotropium seeds, which contain hepatotoxic alkaloids. Within two years, 23 per cent of the 7,200 inhabitants observed had severe liver impairment.

Oral ingestion of pyrrolizidine-containing plants, such as comfrey, poses the greatest risk. The alkaloids are converted to pyrrole-like derivatives, which are responsible for toxicity following ingestion. Additionally, the alkaloids of comfrey applied to the skin of rats were detected in the urine. Lactating rats in the experiment excreted pyrrolizidine alkaloids into breast milk.

The Henry Doubleday Research Association (growers and marketers of comfrey in the United Kingdom) stated publicly that until further research clarifies the long-term health hazard of comfrey ingestion, "no human being or animal should eat, drink, or take comfrey in any form." Based on lack of scientific evidence of a therapeutic effect, the consumption of comfrey and its teas cannot be recommended until further evidence demonstrates comfrey's safety and efficacy.

Drug-Herb Interactions

Only a few cases of drug-herb interactions are reported in the literature. However, since many herbs contain biologically active substances, the possibility of interactions should always be kept in mind. Significant reactions are more likely if herbs possess cardiac, diuretic, sedative, hypotensive, hypertensive, hypoglycemic or anticoagulant effects.

Licorice has salt-retaining effects and may upset the control of hypertension, as may other diuretic herbal remedies. Licorice can also decrease serum potassium and may induce arrhythmias and heart failure. This effect can be compounded by drugs that similarly cause potassium loss. Licorice also exhibits a pronounced anti-inflammatory effect, which may be accompanied by side effects similar to those brought on by excessive secretion of aldosterone (pseudoaldosteronism). This effect has possible serious implications for people receiving steroid therapy and those with hypertension. Since chewing tobacco contains a high proportion of licorice extract, the incidence of pseudoaldosteronism may be expected to increase.

Many herbal preparations contain cardiac glycosides (for example, lily-of-the-valley, *Convallaria majalis*; false hellebore, *Adonis vernalis*; and strophanthus, *Strophanthus kombe*) or agents with similar activity (for example, hawthorn, *Crataegus oxyacantha*) that may potentiate the actions and toxicity of digoxin or other prescribed cardiac glycosides.

One common class of herbal remedies consists of numerous plants reputed to have diuretic activity (for example, bearberry, *Arctostaphylos uva-ursi*; buchu, *Barosma betulina*; juniper, Juniperus species; and St. John's wort, *Hypericum perforatum*). These herbs can induce adverse effects if taken concurrently with prescribed diuretics, cardiac glycosides, antihypertensive drugs or muscle relaxants.

Horse chestnut (*Aesculus hippocastanum*) contains esculoside, a coumarin-like substance that may potentiate the anticoagulant effect of coumarins.

Plants with reputed hypoglycemic activity (for example, burdock, *Arctium lappa*, and karela, *Momordica charantia*) may upset the control of diabetes mellitus.

Plants known or reputed to have sedative activity (for example, hops, *Humulus lupulus*; passion flower, *Passiflora incarnata*; skullcap, *Scuttelaria laterifolia*; and valerian, *Valeriana officinalis*) are often found in herbal preparations. Potential interactions with alcohol, antihistamines, hypnotics and other drugs are similar to those for any central nervous system depressant.

Preparations containing ephedra (ma-huang, Ephedra species) may exhibit the pressor effect of ephedrine, the main alkaloid present. Such preparations should not be used in the presence of hypertension, coronary thrombosis or MAO inhibitors.

Other plants (hawthorn, *Crataegus oxyacantha*; and mistletoe, *Viscum album*) are reputed to reduce blood pressure. Hypotension may result, especially when taken concomitantly with antihypertensive or diuretic drugs.

Adverse Reactions to Herbs

The recent trend toward greater use of herbs has been accompanied by a growing list of adverse effects. The problem is significant enough to warrant coverage in *Iatrogenic Diseases* and *Meyler's Side Effects of Drugs*.

The most common adverse reaction to plants is an allergic response. Usually, this response is seen as hayfever or dermatological conditions. Only rarely is it of a serious nature.

Pyrrolizidine alkaloid poisoning, as discussed earlier, is presented as a major concern in both the above texts. Case studies from Africa, Asia, South and Central America, Britain and the United States are presented. Human exposure to pyrrolizidine alkaloids usually results from accidental contamination of foodstuffs or the deliberate use of plants containing the alkaloids in herbal preparations. These alkaloids cause a characteristic progressive liver disease, ranging from an acute stage, especially in children under 7 years of age, with hepatomegaly and ascites; through a subacute, persistent and often symptomless hepatomegaly; to a chronic, cirrhotic stage. Death may occur at either the acute or chronic stage. Potentially dangerous herbs in this context are comfrey (*Symphytum* species), coltsfoot (*Tussilago farfara*), the ragworts and groundsels (*Senecio* species) and butterbur (*Petasites officinalis*).

Plants containing atropine and related alkaloids (for example, thorn apple, *Datura stramonium*; mandrake, *Mandragora officanarum*; belladonna, *Atropa belladonna*; and henbane, *Hyoscyamus niger*) can cause acute toxicities. Herbs containing these alkaloids have been used for centuries in folk medicine and mystical rites, primarily because of their anticholinergic properties and the consequent hallucinogenic potential. Poisoning has occurred from eating or smoking the leaves or drinking a tea. Fatalities have occurred. Adulteration of other herbs with ones containing atropine and related alkaloids is also a problem.

Many other plants containing psychoactive substances are not only used as medicines, but often for recreational purposes, sometimes with serious adverse effects. Still others have oxytocic effects (for example, devil's claw, *Harpagophytum procumbens*; broom, *Sarothamnus scoparius*) and should not be used by pregnant women.

Since herbs contain biologically active substances, their use can be expected to give rise to adverse reactions. Acute reactions are often identified, and often are extensions of their effects (for example, diarrhea, hypotension, hypoglycemia, hypokalemia and paralysis). The more subtle chronic toxicities such as carcinogenicity, mutagenicity and hepatotoxicity almost certainly will continue to be difficult to correlate to use of a given herb.

Adulteration of herbal preparations in commercial products gives rise to further toxic consequences.

Herbal Medicines

Table II *Commonly Available Herbs Used for Beverages and Medicines[a,b]*

Common name	Botanical name	Part used	Major uses	Main ingredients[c]	Side effects[d]	Apparent efficacy[e]	Probable safety[f]	Comments
Aloe	*Aloe barbadensis*	fresh juice	wound healing, burns	gel (mucilage)		+	+, 3	loses its healing activity if dried; aloe gel prudent to avoid in pregnancy
		dried latex	cathartic	anthraquinones	diarrhea; cramping	+	+, 3	habitual use may cause excessive irritation to the colon; aloe latex contraindicated in pregnancy; aloe gel prudent to avoid during pregnancy
Angelica	*Angelica archangelica*	root, fruit, leaves	diuretic, carminative, emmenagogue, etc. flavor	volatile oil		–	–, 2	contraindicated in pregnancy
Anise (Star anise)	*Pimpinella anisum* (*Illicium verum*)	fruit (seed)	carminative, coughs, dyspepsia; flavor	volatile oil (anethole)	oil may cause nausea, vomiting, seizures and pulmonary edema	NA	NA, 2 (NA, 1)	licorice flavor
Arnica	*Arnica montana*	flower heads	anti-inflammatory, analgesic	unidentified	ingestion can cause severe gastrointestinal and CNS disturbances and can result in death	+	+, 1	plant should not be ingested
Bearberry	see: Uva ursi							
Black cohosh	*Cimicifuga racemosa*	rhizomes and roots	antirheumatic, uterine stimulant, etc.	actein, cimicifugin	nausea and vomiting	–	±, 1	may potentiate hypotensive drugs; contraindicated in pregnancy
Borage	*Borago officinalis*	leaves and tops	diuretic, astringent (diarrhea)	tannins, mucilage	–	– to ±	±, 3	contains traces of pyrrolizidine alkaloids; prudent to avoid during pregnancy
Broom	*Cytisus scoparius*	flowering tops	diuretic, cathartic, emetic, sedative	sparteine, hydroxytyramine	–	+	–, 1	mind-altering properties when smoked; contraindicated in pregnancy

Table II (Cont'd) *Commonly Available Herbs Used for Beverages and Medicines*[a,b]

Common name	Botanical name	Part used	Major uses	Main ingredients[c]	Side effects[d]	Apparent efficacy[e]	Probable safety[f]	Comments
Buchu	*Barosma* spp.	leaves	urinary antiseptic, diuretic	diosphenol	-	± to +	+, 2	prudent to avoid during pregnancy
Burdock	*Arctium* spp.	roots	skin disorders, diuretic	polyhenolic acids	-	-	+, 2	
Calamus	*Acorus calamus*	rhizomes	digestive aid, coughs, flavor	volatile oil	-	±	- or +, 1	some varieties contain the carcinogen, ß-asrone; prudent to avoid during pregnancy
Capsicum	*Capsicum* spp.	fruit	counterirritant, digestive aid	capsaicin	burning sensation, rarely blisters	+	+, 2	affects nerve endings but not capillaries
Catnip	*Nepeta cataria*	leaves and tops	carminative, sedative, etc.	volatile oil (nepetalactone)	oil may cause CNS toxicity	±	+, 3	possible psychotropic when smoked
Cayenne	see Capsicum							
Chamomile	*Matricaria chamomilla* *Anthemis nobilis*	flower heads	carminative, anti-inflammatory, antispasmodic	volatile oil, (chamazulene, alpha-bisabolol)	contact dermatitis	+	+, 3	
Chaparral	*Larrea tridentata*	leaves and twigs	diuretic, antiseptic, anticancer	nordihydro-guaiaretic acid	lesions in the mesenteric lymph nodes and kidneys	-	-, 2	prudent to avoid during pregnancy
Coltsfoot	*Tussilago farfara*	leaves and/or flower heads	antitussive, demulcent	mucilage		+	-, 2	low levels of pyrrolizidine alkaloids; prudent to avoid during pregnancy
Comfrey	*Symphytum officinale*	roots and leaves	wound healing agent	allantoin, mucilage, tannin	hepatotoxic, carcinogenic	+	-, 2	contains high levels of pyrrolizidine alkaloids. Canadian laws recently amended to permit only the leaves of *S. officinale* eligible for DINs. Prudent to avoid during pregnancy

Herbal Medicines

Table II (*Cont'd*) *Commonly Available Herbs Used for Beverages and Medicines*[a,b]

Common name	Botanical name	Part used	Major uses	Main ingredients[c]	Side effects[d]	Apparent efficacy[e]	Probable safety[f]	Comments
Dandelion	*Taraxacum officinale*	roots and leave	diuretic, laxative, digestive aid	inulin, bitter resins	–	±	+, 3	leaves weaker in action
Devil's claw	*Harpagophytum procumbens*	tubers	antirheumatic, anti-inflammatory	harpagoside	–	–	+, 2	activity is still controversial; contraindicated in pregnancy
Dioscorea	*Dioscorea* spp.	tubers	none	diosgenin	–	NA	NA, 1	source of most steroid drugs
Fennel	*Foeniculum vulgare*	fruit (seeds)	carminative, coughs, digestive	volatile oil (anethole)	oil may cause nausea, vomiting, seizures and pulmonary edema	+	+, 3	
Fenugreek	*Trigonella foenumgraecum*	seeds	demulcent, laxative, digestive aid, flavor	mucilage	–	±	+, 2	also contains diosgenin and others
Feverfew	*Tanacetum parthenium* (syn = *Chrysanthemum parthenium*	leaves	migraine prevention; carminative, antipyretic, emmenagogue	parthenolide	oral ulcers	+	+, 3	contraindicated in pregnancy
Garlic	*Allium sativum*	bulbs	hypertension, atherosclerosis; antibacterial, diuretic, antihyperlipemic, antitumor, etc.	allicin	contact dermatitis	+ +	+, NA	
Gentian	*Gentiana lutea*	rhizomes and roots	appetite stimulant, digestive aid	gentiopicrin and amarogentin	nausea and vomiting	+	+, 2	
Ginger	*Zingiber officinale*	rhizomes	motion sickness prevention; carminative	volatile oil, resin	–	+	+, NA	
Ginseng	*Panax* spp.	roots	tonic, adaptogen (anti-stress)	triterpene glycosides	"corticosteroid poisoning"	±	±, 3	
Goldenseal	*Hydrastis canadensis*	rhizomes and roots	dyspepsia, stop post-partum bleeding	hydrastine, berberine	dangerous in high doses	± to +	+, 1	contraindicated in pregnancy

Table II (Cont'd) *Commonly Available Herbs Used for Beverages and Medicines*[a,b]

Common name	Botanical name	Part used	Major uses	Main ingredients[c]	Side effects[d]	Apparent efficacy[e]	Probable safety[f]	Comments
Hawthorn	Crataegus oxyacantha	fruit, leaves, flowers	vasodilation, hypotensive	flavonoids and triterpene glycosides	−	+	+, 1	may enhance digitalis toxicity
Hibiscus	Hibiscus sabdariffa	flowers	diuretic, laxative, coloring agent	citric and hibiscic acid, pigments	−	± to +	+, 3	
Hops	Humulus lupulus	fruit (strobiles)	sedative; flavoring and preserving beer	polyphenolics	dermatitis	+ to + +	+, 2	occasionally smoked to obtain a mild euphoria
Horsetail	Equisetum spp.	aerial parts	diuretic, astringent, antihemorrhagic	saponin, flavones, alkaloids	−	− to ±	+, 1	prudent to avoid during pregnancy; contains thiaminase
Hydrangea	Hydrangea arborescens Hydrangea paniculata	rhizomes and roots, leaves	diuretic, lithotriptic; mild euphoric	flavonoids, resins, mucilage, phenolic and cyanogenic glycosides	vertigo in large doses, vomiting, nausea	− +	±, 2 −, 2	leaves are smoked; narrow margin between pleasure and toxicity
Juniper	Juniper communis	fruit (berries)	diuretic, antiseptic, carminative, flavor	volatile oil, resin, flavonoids	kidney irritation, contact dermatitis	+	±, 1	the berries and oil are contraindicated in pregnancy and kidney disease. Related species should not be used
Licorice	Glycyrrhiza glabra	rhizomes and roots	expectorant, demulcent, flavor, etc.	glycyrrhizin	sodium retention, hypokalemia, "pseudo-aldosteronism"	+	±, 1	may be of use in Herpes infections
Life root	Senecio aureus	entire plant	emmenagogue	pyrrolizidine alkaloids	hepatotoxic	±	−, 1	contraindicated in pregnancy
Linden flowers	Tilia spp.	flowers	diaphoretic, beverage	flavonoids, volatile oil	−	+	+, 2	contraindicated in heart disease
Lobelia	Lobelia inflata	leaves and tops	nauseant expectorant; psychotropic; antiasthmatic	lobeline	vomiting, paralysis, convulsions	+ NA	±, 1 −, 1 NA	nicotine-like action; death can result; prudent to avoid during pregnancy

Table II (Cont'd) *Commonly Available Herbs Used for Beverages and Medicines*[a,b]

Common name	Botanical name	Part used	Major uses	Main ingredients[c]	Side effects[d]	Apparent efficacy[e]	Probable safety[f]	Comments
Mistletoe	*Phoradendron tomentosum*	leaves	hypertensive, smooth muscle stimulant;	phoratoxins, tyramine	gastric irritation, bradycardia, hemagglutination	±	−, 1	cytotoxicity of lectins being studied for anticancer activity; contraindicated in presence of MAO inhibitor; prudent to avoid during pregnancy
	Viscum alba	leaves	hypotensive, antispasmodic	viscotoxins		±	−, 1	
Mormon tea	*Ephedra nevadensis*	stems	diuretic, astringent (diarrhea); tonic	tannin, volatile oil	constipation	+ −	±g, 1 ±g, 1	N.Am. *Ephedra* devoid of alkaloids
Nettle	*Urtica dioica*	aerial parts	diuretic, astringent; antiasthmatic, antirheumatic	unidentified	local irritation to the stinging hairs	+ −	+, 3 +, 3	
Parsley	*Petroselinum crispum*	leaves and stems; fruit (seeds), roots	digestive aid, diuretic; digestive aid, diuretic, emmenagogue	volatile oil (apiole and myristicin), furanocoumarins	nausea, vomiting, dizziness, swollen liver, polyneuritis, phototoxicity	± +	+, 2 ± to +, 2	roots and oil are contraindicated in pregnancy
Passion flower	*Passiflora incarnata*	flowering and fruiting tops	sedative, antispasmodic	alkaloids, flavonoids, maltol	hypotension	± to +	+, 2	
Pau d'Arco	*Tabebuia* spp.	bark	anticancer, antimicrobial	naphthaquinones (lapachol)	nausea, vomiting, anemia, hemorrhage	−	±, 1	therapeutic index is low
Pennyroyal	*Hedeoma pulegioides*	leaves, oil	carminative, diaphoretic,	volatile oil (pulegone)	nausea, vomiting, diarrhea, CNS depression, kidney irritant	± + to ±	±, 2 −, 2	contraindicated in pregnancy
	Mentha pulegium		emmenagogue, abortifacient	volatile oil (pulegone)				
Poke root	*Phytolacca americana*	roots, leaves	antirheumatic, laxative, inflammatory conditions of the upper respiratory tract, anticancer	phytolaccigein, mitogens	severe cramping, vomiting, weakness, hypotension, spasms, death	−	−, 0	should not be consumed

Table II (Cont'd) *Commonly Available Herbs Used for Beverages and Medicines*[a,b]

Common name	Botanical name	Part used	Major uses	Main ingredients[c]	Side effects[d]	Apparent efficacy[e]	Probable safety[f]	Comments
Red clover	*Trifolium pratense*	flowers	expectorant, anticancer	phenolic glycosides	–	–	+, 3	
St. John's wart	*Hypericum perforatum*	leaves and tops	tranquilizer, anti-inflammatory	volatile oil, tannins, hypericin	photosensitizer	+	+, 1	
Sarsaparilla	*Smilax* spp.	roots	diuretic, flavor	volatile oil, sapogenins	none recorded	+	+, 2	
Sassafras	*Sassafras albidum*	root bark	antirheumatic, tonic, diuretic, diaphoretic	volatile oil (safrole)	hepatotoxic, carcinogenic	–	–, 2	*Sassafras* and safrole are listed as food adulterants in Food and Drug Regulations B.01.046; contraindicated in pregnancy
			flavor	safrole		–	–, NA	
Skullcap	*Scutellaria lateriflora*	aerial parts	sedative, antispasmodic	volatile oil, flavonoids	–	–	+, 2	considered to be essentially inactive
Senega	*Polygala senega*	roots	expectorant, emetic, diaphoretic	saponins	nausea, vomiting, diarrhea	+	+, NA	low therapeutic index; prudent to avoid during pregnancy
Senna	*Cassia acutifolia* *Cassia angustifolia*	leaflets, pods	cathartic	anthraquinones (sennosides)	griping	+	+, 1	habitual use may cause excessive irritation to the colon; prudent to avoid during pregnancy
Shavegrass	*Equisetum hyemale*	aerial parts	diuretic, hemostatic, astringent	tannin, alkaloids (nicotine, equisetine)	lassitude, diarrhea	NA	NA, 1	confusion exists regarding safety; prudent to avoid during pregnancy
Snakeroot	see Senega							
Taheebo	see Pau d'Arco							
Tansy	*Tanacetum vulgare*	leaves and flowers	anthelmintic, emmenagogue, tonic	volatile oil (thujone)	nausea, vomiting, convulsions, death	±	– to ±, 2	contraindicated in pregnancy; oil is quite toxic
Tubocurarine	*Chondodendron tomentosum*	bark and stems	skeletal muscle relaxant	alkaloids	hypotension, cardiovascular collapse, respiratory failure	NA	NA, NA	a constituent of curare

Table II (Cont'd) *Commonly Available Herbs Used for Beverages and Medicines*[a,b]

Common name	Botanical name	Part used	Major uses	Main ingredients[c]	Side effects[d]	Apparent efficacy[e]	Probable safety[f]	Comments
Uva ursi	*Arctostaphylos uva-ursi*	leaves	diuretic, astringent, urinary antiseptic	arbutin (prodrug of hydroquinolone), ursolic acid, isoquercetin	mild CNS depression	+	+, 2	urine is often green
Valerian	*Valerianna officinalis*	rhizomes and roots	tranquilizer	valepotriates	-	+	+, 2	disagreeable odor; commercial products available in Europe
Wintergreen	*Gaultheria procumbens*	leaves and stems	counterirritant, analgesic, flavor	volatile oil (methylsalicylate)	oil is toxic (salicylism)	NA	NA, 1	
Wormwood	*Artemesia absinthium*	leaves and tops	anthelmintic, flavor, tonic, mind-altering effects	volatile oil (thujone), sesquiterpene lactones (absinthin)	absinthism (trembling, convulsions, dementia, death)	+	−, 1	contraindicated in pregnancy. Thujone is thought to be the toxic ingredient. It is nearly water-insoluble (teas); therefore teas may not be as toxic as alcoholic extracts
Yellow dock	*Rumex crispus*	rhizomes and roots	astringent, laxative	tannins, anthraquinones	diarrhea, nausea, polyuria	+	+[g], 1	prudent to avoid during pregnancy

a. This table was adapted primarily from Tyler VE. The new honest herbal. Philadelphia: GF Stickley, 1987. This table first appeared in *Drugs and Therapeutics for Maritime Practitioners* 1987;10(5). Brian Tuttle, editor, has kindly given permission to reprint it here.

b. The table does not comment on the desirability or feasibility of using any of the herbal remedies listed, even those indicated as being apparently efficacious and probably safe. Appropriate references should be consulted for detailed explanations of the many complex factors regarding the use of these drugs which could not be included in this brief summary.

c. This column indicates the major ingredient(s) or class(es) of compounds identified. This may not be the active ingredient as often these have not been identified.

d. This column lists the symptoms most commonly seen following doses generally considered to be excessive.

e. Efficacy as scored by Tyler: + =effective; ± =efficacy inconclusive; − =ineffective; NA=not listed.

f. Safety, in normal individuals when used appropriately, as scored in the first column by Tyler: + =safe; ± =safety inconclusive; − =not safe; and in the second column by Duke: 0=very dangerous, Duke wouldn't drink a cup of it; 1=more dangerous than coffee, Duke wouldn't be afraid to drink 1 cup containing 10 g of herb steeped; 2=as dangerous as coffee, Duke wouldn't be afraid to drink 2 cups a day; 3=Duke considers it safer than coffee and wouldn't hesitate, for health reasons, to drink 3 cups a day; NA=not listed.

g. All tannin-rich drugs may have carcinogenic potential in long-term usage.

Products on the Market

The array of herbal products on the market probably exceeds that of prescription medications. Many preparations are designed to stimulate an obvious body function. For example, they exhibit diuretic, laxative, diaphoretic, sialogogue or emmenagogue activity. Many others are formulated to aid digestion or to act as sedatives. Still others may be promoted for specific applications. There are preparations designed to affect virtually every body system. In short, herbal products represent another form of nonprescription self-medication. However, a major difference exists between nonprescription herbals and nonprescription pharmaceuticals. Currently, in Canada and elsewhere, there are few controls over herbal remedies. The herbs are usually traded by common name only. This practice may result in ambiguity, with the potential for therapeutic failure or hazardous results. What does a package labelled "ginseng" really contain? Is it roots or leaves? Is it *Panax ginseng, Panax quinquefolium, Eleutherococcus senticosus* or a hazardous substitute? Although each of these three plants is claimed to exhibit similar activity, the latter, known as Russian or Siberian ginseng, is much less expensive at the wholesale level.

Is the comfrey on the shelf *Symphytum officinale* or *Symphytum x uplandium*? Evidence is growing that the latter, known as Russian comfrey, contains the more toxic pyrrolizidine alkaloid echimidine. Several herbs are sold under the name Gordolobos Tea. Some, such as *Senecio longilobos*, Crotalaria species and Heliotropium species, contain high concentrations of the toxic pyrrolizidine alkaloids; others like *Verbascum thapsus* do not.

Quality assurance is another problem. Since most herbs and their preparations are classified as foods, they are not regulated by monographs to contain delineated amounts of active constituents. The quality of herbs varies widely, as has been shown for feverfew and for the ginsenoside content of commercial ginseng preparations. In some cases the herbal medicines have not even contained the correct herbal ingredient.

Adulteration is also not unheard of, and often the adulterant is potentially more harmful than the original herb. One example involved a woman admitted to hospital with signs of atropine poisoning. She had consumed an herbal tea claimed to be burdock root, but analysis revealed the dried tea contained 30 mg/g of atropine-like alkaloids. Some herbal remedies have been adulterated with allopathic medicines. An antirheumatic preparation from Hong Kong contained aminopyrine, phenylbutazone, indomethacin, phenacetin and dexamethasone. Other preparations are adulterated with inorganic substances such as arsenic, mercury, tin, zinc and lead.

Quality assurance of herbal remedies relies solely on good manufacturing practice, with adequate authentication of individual herbs. The above examples make it painfully obvious that such procedures are not necessarily performed.

Herbal products should meet the same high standards as prescription and nonprescription medicines. Lack of knowledge of the active constituents makes this goal difficult; lack of vigorous monographs ensures continuing chaos.

Regulation of Herbal Remedies

In 1984, Health and Welfare Canada initiated steps to modify the regulatory concepts and procedures for herbal products to ensure better service to the Canadian consumer. An Expert Advisory Committee was established to review safety and regulatory control mechanisms for herbs and botanicals sold as foods.

The committee identified four basic classifications of herbs: herbs and botanical preparations unacceptable for use in or as food; herbs and botanical preparations generally acceptable as food; herbs and botanical preparations acceptable as food under specified conditions; and herbs and botanical preparations generally used for medicinal purposes.

In reviewing the safety of herbs and botanical preparations, the committee concluded that a small number of substances should be prohibited for use in or as foods. It recommended that these substances be added to the list of food adulterants found in the Food and Drug Regulations.

The committee focused on the need for improved standards for identity and quality of herbs and botanical preparations and improvements in advertising and marketing practices. Recognizing the important role of the industry that imports, manufactures and distributes these products, the committee recommended the industry develop appropriate standards as well as a voluntary Code of Ethics and Advertising Practice.

The committee also recognized that although certain herbs and botanical preparations are sold as foods, they are intended primarily for medicinal purposes. The report recommends a new drug subcategory be considered to permit registration of folkloric remedies under specified conditions.

Role of the Pharmacist

Substantive evidence of efficacy must be available to permit a labelling claim of therapeutic utility. This requirement has led to the current, curious situation in which essentially all traditional herbal drugs have been removed from the shelves of pharmacies and from the supervision of knowledgeable pharmacists. But such plant drugs have not ceased to be sold and used. Instead, they have found their way into the stocks of the retail or mail-order stores where, under the guise of herbs, teas, health foods, food supplements, nutritional products and the like, they are labelled only with the name (usually just a common name) of the product. No claim of effectiveness for any condition appears on the label of these containers, nor does it appear in any leaflet or advertisement that directly accompanies the drug, because that technically qualifies as part of the labelling.

Sales staff generally avoid specific recommendations on use of a product to preclude potential charges of unlicensed practice of medicine. If customers wish to know the use of a particular drug, clerks usually refer them to a selection of books, pamphlets and other materials that list the drugs and provide information. This encourages the consuming public to become its own medical counsel, a practice of questionable wisdom and acknowledged risk.

Associated with this situation is the resurgence of quackery. Useless and sometimes even dangerous drugs are sold by nonprofessionals to people who hope their conditions, not alleviated by recognized drugs, will yield to folkloric treatments of unproven value.

The above is not meant to imply that all herbalists lack knowledge or that all herbal products are of no value. Some herbalists are knowledgeable about plant drugs and some of the remedies are also useful. However, a number of individuals take advantage of the relative lack of regulatory controls and make a mockery of the whole practice of traditional medicine.

The resurgence of interest in herbal medicine that originated during the last 2 decades shows every promise of continuing its rapid development. The knowledgeable pharmacist of today must have a working knowledge of herbal remedies. Pharmacists must be able to provide accurate, objective answers to such questions as: Do herbal remedies work? Are they safe? Are they of good quality? Pharmacists must be educated about herbal remedies to become more involved in the supply of accurate information and herbal remedies of good quality.

Summary

Are plants (herbs) food or medicine? Are they safe? Effective? Clearly, the answers depend on the herb under consideration. Most herbs used in sufficient quantities elicit a pharmacologic effect. Natural is not synonymous with safe. Many herbs are extremely poisonous. Five thousand years of folklore do not guarantee absolute safety.

Most herbal remedies appear to do no harm, some may help the consumer, some occasionally cause adverse effects and others are outright hazardous. They may interact with conventional medicines taken concurrently. They may carry hazards for certain people such as pregnant women or people with chronic ailments like heart disease, diabetes or severe allergies. Individuals should inform their physician and pharmacist if they are taking herbal medicines. Above all, people should not abandon conventional treatment without their doctor's knowledge.

Ask the Consumer

Q. Are you aware your herbal medicine may cause adverse effects?

■ The same side effects that occur with prescription and nonprescription medicines can also occur with herbal remedies, as they represent nearly every class of pharmacologic agents.

Q. Are you taking any herbal beverages or medicines concurrently with your prescribed medication?

■ Interactions between herbal remedies and prescription or nonprescription medicines may be expected to occur as readily as those between the latter two classes. Potentiation of prescription or nonprescription medicines by herbal remedies is likely to be the most common type of interaction.

Q. Are you aware there is no legislated guarantee of the quality of any herbal medicine, even those generally regarded as safe and effective?

■ Identification, adulteration and quality control are the three major problems. Herbs should be traded only by their Latin names, as common names often refer to more than one plant, especially in different geographic areas. Herbs have been deliberately adulterated for economy (supplier provides cheaper herb, charges for more expensive one) or for the "benefit" of the consumer (adulterant is often a potent chemical that provides an effect quickly). Without employing adequate analytical or animal assays, neither the purveyor nor the purchaser knows the strength of the preparation supplied.

Q. In spite of its long-standing use, are you aware that the ingestion of comfrey is associated with chronic toxicity?

■ Comfrey (*Symphytum officinale*) has been shown to contain sizable quantities of pyrrolizidine alkaloids known to be hepatotoxic and carcinogenic. Animal studies have confirmed the toxicity, and human toxicities have recently been reported. Other species of Symphytum, often sold as comfrey, are known to contain even more toxic alkaloids. The major problem here is that the toxicities are usually chronic, sometimes taking 30 to 40 years to become obvious.

Q. Are you fully aware of the potential hazards of this herb when it is used as an emmenagogue?

■ An emmenagogue is an agent that induces menstrual flow. An abortion may result if a pregnant woman uses a preparation of this nature. Emmenagogues are commonly used to induce abortions, but the hazards are considerable, as many emmenagogues do not always produce a complete abortion.

Q. Do you know how to prepare this herb as a medicinal tea?

■ Medicinal teas are usually prepared by simmering about 30 g of herb in about 500 mL of water. When the volume has been reduced to about one-half, the tea is filtered from the extracted herb. Medicinal teas are usually 6 to 60 times stronger than beverage teas.

References

Introduction

Anderson LA, Phillipson JD. Herbal medicine, education and the pharmacist. Pharm J 1986;236:303–5:311.

Bain RJI. Accidental digitalis poisoning due to drinking herbal tea. Br Med J 1985;290:1624.

Bender GA, ed. Great moments in medicine. Detroit: Parke-Davis, 1961.

Blackwell WH. Poisonous and medicinal plants. Englewood Cliffs: Prentice-Hall, 1990.

Bunce KL. The use of herbs in midwifery. J Nurse-Midwifery 1987;32:255–9.

Carrera G, Mitjavila S, Derache R. Effet de l'acide tannique sur l'absorption de la vitamine B_{12} chez le rat. CR Acad Sci Paris Ser D 1973;27:239–42.

Corrigan D. Phytotherapy. Int Pharm J 1987;1:96–101.

de Smet PAGM. Kruidenmiddelen en volksgezondheid. Pharm Weekbl 1987;122:1069.

de Smet PAGM. 'Chien Pu Wan' pillen. Pharm Weekbl 1986;121:437–42.

de Smet PAGM. Drugs used in non-orthodox medicine. In: Dukes MNG, Beeley L, eds. Side effects of drugs annual 14. Amsterdam: Elsevier, 1990:429–51.

de Smet PAGM, Keller K, Hansel R, Chandler RF, eds. Adverse effects of herbal drugs 1. Heidelberg: Springer-Verlag, 1992.

Der Marderosian A, Liberti L. Natural product medicine. Philadelphia: GF Stickley, 1988.

Dobbs RJ, Baird IMCL. Effect of a wholemeal and white bread on iron absorption in normal people. Br Med J 1977;1:1641–2.

Dubick MA. Historical perspectives on the use of herbal preparations to promote health. J Nutr 1986;116:1348–54.

Ehudin-Pagano E, Paluzzi PA, Ivory LC, McCartney M. The use of herbs in nurse-midwifery practice. J Nurse-Midwifery 1987;32:260–2.

Farnsworth NR. The role of medicinal plants in drug development. In: Krogsgaard-Larsen P, Christensen SB, Kofod H, eds. Natural products and drug development. Copenhagen: Munksgaard, 1983:17–30.

Farnsworth NR. The role of ethnopharmacology in drug development. Ciba Foundation Symposium 154. Bioactive compounds from plants. Toronto: John Wiley and Sons, 1990:2–21.

Herbal Medicines

Frohne D, Pfander HJ. A colour atlas of poisonous plants. London: Wolfe Publishing, 1984:13–29,63–4. Translated by NG Bisset.

Groenewegen WA, Heptinstall S. Amounts of feverfew in commercial preparations of the herb (Letter). Lancet 1986;1:44–5.

Harrison P. Herbal remedies. Protect Yourself 1984;April:11–14.

James LF. Plant-induced congenital malformations in animals. World Rev Nutr Diet 1977;26:208–24.

Keeler RF. Teratogens in plants. J Anim Sci 1984;58:1029–39.

Kingsbury JM. Poisonous plants of the US and Canada. Englewood Cliffs: Prentice-Hall, 1964.

Lampe KF, McCann MA. AMA handbook of poisonous and injurious plants. Chicago: American Medical Association, 1985.

Lewis WH. Reporting adverse reactions to herbal ingestants. J Am Med Assoc 1978;240:109–10.

Liberti LE, Der Marderosian A. Evaluation of commercial ginseng products. J Pharm Sci 1978;67:1487–9.

Montgomery B. First US report connecting death to popular Chicano, Indian herbal tea. JAMA 1977;238:1233–4.

Morton JF. Atlas of medicinal plants of Middle America. Springfield: CC Thomas, 1981.

Rhoads PM, Tong TG, Banner Jr W, Anderson R. Anticholinergic poisonings associated with commercial burdock root tea. Clin Toxicol 1985;22:581–4.

Roulet M, Laurini R, Rivier L, Calame A. Hepatic venoocclusive disease in newborn infant of a woman drinking herbal tea. J Pediatr 1988;112:433–6.

Siegel RK, Elsohly MA, Plowman T, et al. Cocaine in herbal tea. J Am Med Assoc 1986;255:40.

Smith CG, Asch RH. Drug abuse and reproduction. Fertil Steril 1987; 48:355–73.

Solecki RS, Shanidar IV. A Neanderthal flower burial in northern Iraq. Science 1975;190:880–1.

Sprang R. Toxicity of tea containing pyrrolizidine alkaloids. J Pediatr 1989; 115:1025.

Srisuphan W, Bracken MB. Caffeine consumption during pregnancy and association with late spontaneous abortion. Am J Obstet Gynecol 1986; 154:14–20.

Swanson AB, Chambliss DD, Blomquist JC, et al. The mutagenicities of safrole, estragole, eugenol, trans-anethole, and some of their known or possible metabolites for Salmonella typhimurium mutants. Mutat Res 1979;60: 143–5.

Talalaj S, Czechowicz A. Hazardous herbal remedies are still on the market. Med J Aust 1990;153:302.

Tyler VE. The new honest herbal. Philadelphia: GF Stickley, 1987.

Vulto AG, de Smet PAGM. Drugs used in nonorthodox medicine. In: Dukes MNG, ed. Meyler's side effects of drugs. Amsterdam: Elsevier, 1988:999–1032.

Vulto AG, Buurma H. Drugs used in nonorthodox medicine. In: Dukes MNG, ed. Meyler's side effects of drugs. Amsterdam: Elsevier, 1984:886–907.

Westbrooks RG, Preacher JW. Poisonous plants of eastern North America. Columbia: University of South Carolina Press, 1986.

Yamanaka H, Nagao M, Sugimura T. Mutagenicity of pyrrolizidine alkaloids in the Salmonella/mammalian-microsome test. Mutat Res 1979;68:211–6.

Plants Regarded as Poisons

Dorland's pocket medical dictionary. London: WB Saunders, 1959.

Frohne D, Pfander HJ. A colour atlas of poisonous plants. London: Wolfe Publishing, 1984:13–29,63–4. Translated by NG Bisset.

Plants Generally Regarded as Foods

Chandler RF, Anderson LA, Phillipson JD. Laetrile in perspective. Can Pharm J 1984;117:517–20.

Dreisbach RH. Handbook of poisoning: prevention, diagnosis and treatment. Los Altos: Lange Medical Publications, 1980:246–50.

Duke JA. Handbook of medicinal herbs. Boca Raton: CRC Press, 1985.

Frohne D, Pfander HJ. A colour atlas of poisonous plants. London: Wolfe Publishing, 1984:13–29,63–4. Translated by NG Bisset.

Allopathic Medicines Derived from Herbs

Canadian drug identification code. Ottawa: Health and Welfare Canada, 1990.

Chandler RF. Licorice, more than just a flavor. Can Pharm J 1985;118:421–4.

Der Marderosian A, Liberti L. Natural product medicine. Philadelphia: GF Stickley, 1988.

Farnsworth NR. The role of medicinal plants in drug development. In: Krogsgaard-Larsen P, Christensen SB, Kofod H, eds. Natural products and drug development. Copenhagen: Munksgaard, 1983:17–30.

Farnsworth NR. The role of ethnopharmacology in drug development. Ciba Foundation Symposium 154. Bioactive compounds from plants. Toronto: John Wiley and Sons, 1990;2–21.

Farnsworth NR, Bingel AS. Problems and prospects of discovering new drugs from higher plants by pharmacological screening. In: Wagner H, Wolff P, eds. New natural products and plant drugs with pharmacological, biological or therapeutic activity. New York: Springer-Verlag, 1977:1–22.

Gibson MR. Glycyrrhiza in old and new perspectives. Lloydia 1978;41:348–54.

Grieve M. A modern herbal. New York: Hafner Publishing, 1967:487–93,520–1.

Krogh CME, ed. Compendium of pharmaceuticals and specialties. Ottawa: Canadian Pharmaceutical Association, 1991.

Leung AY. Encyclopedia of common natural ingredients used in food, drugs, and cosmetics. New York: John Wiley and Sons, 1980.

Tyler VE, Brady LR, Robbers JE. Pharmacognosy. Philadelphia: Lea & Febiger, 1988:176,203–25,482–5.

Youngken HW. Textbook of pharmacognosy. Toronto: Blakiston, 1948: 520–1,785–96,812–22.

Food-Herbs with Medicinal Applications

Anonymous. In: Liberti LE, ed. The Lawrence review of natural products. Collegeville: Pharmaceutical Information Associates, 1986; Sept.

Departmental consolidation of the food and drugs act and of the food and drug regulations. Ottawa: Health and Welfare, 1985.

Duke JA. Handbook of medicinal herbs. Boca Raton: CRC Press, 1985.

Hardin JW, Arena JM. Human poisoning from native and cultivated plants. Durham: Duke University Press, 1974:69–73,118–9.

Lewis WH, Elvin-Lewis MPF. Medical botany: plants affecting man's health. New York: John Wiley and Sons, 1977:5, 32,90–91,97–100,213–9.

Trease GE, Evans WC. Pharmacognosy. London: Bailliere Tindall, 1989:535–7.

Tyler VE, Brady LR, Robbers JE. Pharmacognosy. Philadelphia: Lea & Febiger, 1988:176,203–25,482–5.

Tyler VE. The new honest herbal. Philadelphia: GF Stickley, 1987.

Youngken HW. Textbook of pharmacognosy. Toronto: Blakiston, 1948: 520–1,785–96,812–22.

Flavors & Spices as Medicines

Anonymous. In: Liberti LE, ed. The Lawrence review of natural products. Collegeville: Pharmaceutical Information Associates, 1986; Sept.

Canadian drug identification code. Ottawa: Health and Welfare Canada, 1990.

Chandler RF. Juniper, an inconspicuous but insidious drug. Can Pharm J 1986;119:562–6.

Departmental consolidation of the food and drugs act and of the food and drug regulations. Ottawa: Health and Welfare, 1985.

Duke JA. Handbook of medicinal herbs. Boca Raton: CRC Press, 1985.

Grieve M. A modern herbal. New York: Hafner Publishing, 1967:487–93,520–1.

Hawkes D, Chandler RF. Aniseed—a spice, a flavour, a drug. Can Pharm J 1984;117:28–9.

Leung AY. Encyclopedia of common natural ingredients used in food, drugs, and cosmetics. New York: John Wiley and Sons, 1980.

Marcus C, Lichtenstein EP. Interactions of naturally occurring food plant components with insecticides and pentobarbital in rats and mice. J Agric Food Chem 1982;30:563–8.

Miller EC, Swanson AB, Phillips DH, et al. Structure-activity studies of the carcinogenicities in the mouse and rat of some naturally occurring and synthetic alkenylbenzenes related to safrole and estragole. Cancer Res 1983;43:1124–34.

Morton JF. Atlas of medicinal plants of Middle America. Springfield: CC Thomas, 1981.

Osol A, Hoover JE, eds. Remington's pharmaceutical sciences. Easton: Mack Publishing, 1975:1228.

Report of the expert advisory committee on herbs and botanical preparations. Ottawa: Health Protection Branch, Health and Welfare Canada, 1986.

Herbal Medicines

Review of 171 herbs used in brewing teas. FDA Special Publication, 1975;1–32.

Spoerke DG Jr. Herbal medication: use and misuse. Hosp Formul 1980; 15:941–2,945,949–51.

Tierra M. The way of herbs. Santa Cruz: Unity Press, 1980;29–30,69,89–90.

Tyler VE, Brady LR, Robbers JE. Pharmacognosy. Philadelphia: Lea & Febiger, 1988:176,203–25,482–5.

Tyler VE. The new honest herbal. Philadelphia: GF Stickley, 1987.

Windholz M, ed. The Merck index. Rahway: Merck Sharpe and Dohme 1983. Report of the expert advisory committee on herbs and botanical preparations. Ottawa: Health Protection Branch, Health and Welfare Canada, 1986.

Medicinal Teas

Chandler RF, Hooper SN, Harvey MJ. Ethnobotany and phytochemistry of yarrow, Achillea millefolium compositae. Econ Bot 1982;36:203–23.

Der Marderosian A. Medicinal teas—boon or bane? Drug Ther 1977; 7(2):178–81,184–5,188.

Duke JA. Handbook of medicinal herbs. Boca Raton: CRC Press, 1985.

Leung AY. Encyclopedia of common natural ingredients used in food, drugs, and cosmetics. New York: John Wiley and Sons, 1980.

Mitchell J, Rook A. Botanical dermatology. Vancouver: Greengrass, 1979; 186–7,212.

Montgomery B. First US report connecting death to popular Chicano, Indian herbal tea. JAMA 1977;238:1233–4.

Rodriguez E, Towers GHN, Mitchell JC. Biological activities of sesquiterpene lactones. Phytochemistry 1976;15:1573–80.

Roland AE, Smith EC. The flora of Nova Scotia. Halifax: The Nova Scotia Museum, 1969:697–701.

Tierra M. The way of herbs. Santa Cruz: Unity Press, 1980;29–30,69,89–90.

Tyler, VE. The new honest herbal. Philadelphia: GF Stickley, 1987.

Traditional Herbal Medicine

Anonymous. Comfrey. In: Olin BR, ed. The Lawrence review of natural products. St. Louis: Facts and Comparisons, 1990;Oct.

Anonymous. Valerian. In: Olin BR, ed. The Lawrence review of natural products. St. Louis: Facts and Comparisons, 1991;Oct.

Awang DVC. Comfrey. Can Pharm J 1987;120:100–4.

Awang DVC. Feverfew. Can Pharm J 1989;122:266–70.

Beliveau J. Valeriana officinalis. Can Pharm J 1986;119:24–7.

Bounthanh C, Bergmann C, Beck JP, et al. Valepotriates, a new class of cytotoxic and antitumor agents. Planta Med 1981;41:21–8.

British Herbal Medicine Association. British herbal pharmacopeia. Bournemouth: Megaron Press, 1983.

Chandler RF. Juniper, an inconspicuous but insidious drug. Can Pharm J 1986;119:562–6.

Chandler RF. Herbal Medicines. In: Clarke C, ed. Self-Medication. Ottawa: Can Pharm Assoc 1985;517–32.

Cooper CR, ed. Herbal remedies. Hosp Formul 1982;17:1387,1391–2.

Der Marderosian A, Liberti L. National product medicine. Philadelphia: GF Stickley, 1988.

Duke JA. Handbook of medicinal herbs. Boca Raton: CRC Press, 1985.

Frohne D, Pfander HJ. A colour atlas of poisonous plants. London: Wolfe Publishing, 1984:13–29,63–4. Translated by NG Bisset.

Hamon NW. Garlic and the genus Allium. Can Pharm J 1987;120:492–7.

Johnson ES, Kadam NP, Hylands DM, Hylands PJ. Efficacy of feverfew as prophylactic treatment of migraine. Br Med J 1985;291:569–73.

Leung AY. Encyclopedia of common natural ingredients used in food, drugs, and cosmetics. New York: John Wiley and Sons, 1980.

Locock RA. Acorus calamus. Can Pharm J 1987;120:340–2,344.

Locock RA. Mistletoe. Can Pharm J 1986;119:124–7.

Montgomery B. First US report connecting death to popular Chicano, Indian herbal tea. JAMA 1977;238:1233–4.

Pharmaceutical Society of Great Britain. The British pharmaceutical codex. London: Pharmaceutical Press, 1934:569–70,689–90,695,712–3,738,914–5.

Roulet M, Laurini R, Rivier L, Calame A. Hepatic venoocclusive disease in newborn infant of a woman drinking herbal tea. J Pediatr 1988;112:433–6.

Schedule No. 670. Canada Gazette Part II:2530.

Spoerke DG Jr. Herbal medications. Santa Barbara: Woodbridge Press, 1990.

Tyler VE. The new honest herbal. Philadelphia: GF Stickley, 1987.

Warren RG. The anti-migraine activity of feverfew (Tanacetum parthenium). Aust J Pharm 1986;67:475–7.

Drug—Herb Interactions

Anonymous. Herbal medicines—safe and effective? Drug Ther Bull 1986; 24:97–100.

Anonymous. In: Liberti LE, ed. The Lawrence review of natural products. Collegeville: Pharmaceutical Information Associates, 1986; Sept.

Aslam M, Stockley IH. Interaction between curry ingredient (karela) and drug (chlorpropamide) (Letter). Lancet 1979;1:607.

Blachley JD, Knochel JP. Tobacco chewer's hypokalemia: licorice revisited. N Engl J Med 1980;302:784–5.

British Herbal Medicine Association. British herbal pharmacopeia. Bournemouth: Megaron Press, 1983.

Capasso F, Mascolo N, et al. Glycyrrhetinic acid, leucocytes and prostaglandins. J Pharm Pharmacol 1983;35:332–5.

Chandler RF. Licorice, more than just a flavor. Can Pharm J 1985;118:421–4.

Gibson MR. Glycyrrhiza in old and new perspectives. Lloydia 1978;41:348–54.

Penn RG. Adverse reactions to herbal preparations. In: D'Arcy PF, Griffin JP, eds. Iatrogenic diseases. Oxford: Oxford University Press, 1981:205–17.

Tyler VE. The new honest herbal. Philadelphia: GF Stickley, 1987.

Vulto AG, Buurma H. Drugs used in nonorthodox medicine. In: Dukes MNG, ed. Meyler's side effects of drugs. Amsterdam: Elsevier, 1984:886–907.

Adverse Reactions to Herbs

Anonymous. Herbal medicines—safe and effective? Drug Ther Bull 1986; 24:97–100.

Anonymous. Toxic reactions to plant products sold in health food stores. Med Lett Drugs Ther 1979;21:29–31.

Mitchell J, Rook A. Botanical dermatology. Vancouver: Greengrass, 1979: 186–7,212.

Montgomery B. First US report connecting death to popular Chicao, Indian herbal tea. JAMA 1977;238:1233–4.

Penn RG. Adverse reactions to herbal preparations. In: D'Arcy PF, Griffin JP, eds. Iatrogenic diseases. Oxford: Oxford University Press, 1981;205–17.

Roulet M, Laurini R, Rivier L, Calame A. Hepatic venoocclusive disease in newborn infant of a woman drinking herbal tea. J Pediatr 1988;112:433–6.

Siegel RK. Herbal intoxication: psychoactive effects from herbal cigarettes, tea and capsules. JAMA 1976;236:473–7.

Talalaj S, Czechowicz A. Hazardous herbal remedies are still on the market. Med J Aust 1990;153:302.

Vulto AG, Buurma H. Drugs used in nonorthodox medicine. In: Dukes MNG, ed. Meyler's side effects of drugs. Amsterdam: Elsevier, 1984:886–907.

Vulto AG, de Smet PAGM. Drugs used in nonorthodox medicine. Dukes MNG, ed. Meyler's side effects of drugs, 11th ed. Amsterdam: Elsevier, 1988: 999–1032.

Products on the Market

Anderson LA, Phillipson JD. Herbal medicine, education and the pharmacist. Pharm J 1986;236:303–5:311.

Awang DVC. Comfrey Can Pharm J 1987;120:100–4.

Bryson PD, Watanabe AS, Rumack BH, Murphy RC. Burdock root tea poisoning. JAMA 1978;239:2157.

Dukes MNG. Drugs used in non-orthodox medicine. In: Dukes MNG, ed. Meyler's side effects of drugs. Amsterdam: Excerpta Medica, 1980:786.

Groenewegen WA, Heptinstall S. Amounts of feverfew in commercial preparations of the herb (Letter). Lancet 1986;1:44–5.

Montgomery B. First US report connecting death to popular Chicao, Indian herbal tea. JAMA 1977;238:1233–4.

Penn RG. Adverse reactions to herbal preparations. In: D'Arcy PF, Griffin JP, eds. Iatrogenic diseases. Oxford: Oxford University Press, 1981:205–17.

Phillipson JD, Anderson LA. Ginseng—quality, safety and efficacy? Pharm J 1984;232:161–5.

Vulto AG, Buurma H. Drugs used in nonorthodox medicine. In: Dukes MNG, ed. Meyler's side effects of drugs. Amsterdam: Elsevier, 1984:886–907.

Regulation of Herbal Remedies

Chandler RF, Hooper SN, Harvey MJ. Ethnobotany and phytochemistry of

Herbal Medicines

yarrow, Achillea millefolium compositae. Econ Bot 1982;36:203–23.

Morrison AB. Herbs and botanical preparations. Information letter no. 666. Ottawa: Health Protection Branch, Health and Welfare Canada, 1984; Aug 15.

Report of the expert advisory committee on herbs and botanical preparations.

Ottawa: Health Protection Branch, Health and Welfare Canada, 1986.

Role of the Pharmacist

Tyler VE, Brady LR, Robbers JE. Pharmacognosy. Philadelphia: Lea & Febiger, 1988:176,203–25,482–5.

34

Poisoning and Overdose

Revised by Debra A. Kent. Based on the original chapter by Ingrid S. Sketris

The general management of poisoning or overdose begins with basic first aid to support the person's vital functions. Emesis or gastric lavage may be indicated in some cases to rid the body of the poison. Activated charcoal adsorbs poison in the intestinal tract, and cathartics are sometimes used to speed the transit of the charcoal-poison mixture through the tract. Pharmacists can educate consumers on how to prevent poisonings in the home. Treating poisonings requires knowledge, training and experience; pharmacists should keep the number of the local poison control centre or emergency facility convenient for prompt referral.

Poisoning remains a problem in Canada, with approximately 96,000 poisoning exposures resulting in 450 deaths reported in 1987. Children under 5 years of age account for about 65 per cent of poisonings. About 39,000 poisonings (41 per cent) involved drugs. Of all poisonings due to drugs, prescription drugs were involved in 35 per cent, narcotic and controlled drugs in 8 per cent and either nonprescription or unknown drugs in 58 per cent of cases. Nonprescription drugs most often implicated (expressed as a percentage of all poisonings involving drugs) are acetaminophen (13.2 per cent), acetylsalicylic acid (8.7 per cent), antihistamines (7.5 per cent), vitamins (4.7 per cent), cough preparations (2.8 per cent), camphor (1.5 per cent) and iron (0.13 per cent).

Since nonprescription drugs are often involved in poisonings, the pharmacist should advise consumers, especially parents, about proper storage of these products. Pharmacists should know and remind parents of the telephone number of the local poison control centre and first aid measures if accidental or intentional poisoning occurs.

General Management

Treating poisonings usually consists of providing basic first aid, supporting the person's vital functions, preventing the poison not yet absorbed from entering the bloodstream, hastening the removal of the poison from the blood and using an antidote if applicable.

Initially, the person is assessed and treated according to the signs and symptoms present. The basic principle to follow is to treat the person, not the poison.

If exposure is via inhalation, the person is removed from the site and an airway established. The first aider must open doors and windows and avoid breathing fumes. Oxygen and artificial respiration are given as needed.

If exposure is topical, the skin is flooded with water for 10 minutes. Contaminated clothing is removed and placed in a plastic bag. The exposed area may be washed gently with mild soap and rinsed well with water. The first aider must avoid exposure to the poison, as skin absorption is possible. People in contact with the exposed person should wear protective clothing, preferably gloves, mask and gown. These items are disposed of in a plastic bag if the exposure is deemed dangerous.

If the exposure is ocular, the first aider irrigates the eyes using a gentle stream of lukewarm tap water from a pitcher, 5 to 7.5 cm from the eye, for 5 minutes. If exposure involves alkali substances or soluble zinc salts the eyes should be irrigated for at least 15 minutes. The eyelid must not be forced open. The exposed person blinks as much as possible while the eye is flooded. If exposure is significant, if symptoms persist or if damage is apparent, an ophthalmologist should be consulted.

If a caustic or irritating chemical, household product or plant has been ingested, the poison is diluted unless contraindications exist. The affected person is given small amounts of water (30 to 60 mL for children, and 90 to 120 mL for adults) to dilute the substance. Diluents may decrease tissue damage if they are given promptly after ingestion. They may irrigate any residual caustic from the mucous membranes of the oropharynx. Diluents must not be given to people with severe respiratory distress or who have signs of gastric or esophageal perforation, shock or upper airway obstruction. Diluents must not be used if the person cannot swallow, is unconscious or is having seizures. Diluents must not be used if drugs in tablet or capsule form are ingested, as diluents may increase absorption. The first aider avoids dilution with large amounts of fluid, as this action may increase absorption of the poison or cause unnecessary vomiting. Swallowed milk can make esophagoscopy more difficult. All cases of ingestion of alkaline or acid substances should be referred by telephone to the poison control centre for evaluation, regardless of symptomatology, to determine if medical assessment is necessary.

Acids should never be neutralized with sodium bicarbonate or bases with vinegar. Neutralization can increase tissue damage because the reaction liberates heat.

Pharmacists and first aiders, after performing first aid, should consult their local poison control centres for information on all poisons and treatments with which they are not familiar and for all potentially serious poisonings.

If the person requires medical attention, the airway and breathing are established first and then the blood pressure and pulse are stabilized. Temperature, blood pressure and pulse are monitored closely. In addition, depending on the history and physical findings, some comatose people may require oxygen, naloxone and 50 per cent dextrose in water. Assisted ventilation, intravenous fluid and electrolytes, and catecholamines may be needed. Analeptic agents (for example, caffeine, methylphenidate and doxapram) are contraindicated as they can predispose the person to seizures and uncontrolled agitation.

Emesis and Gastric Lavage

The indications for inducing emesis and employing gastric lavage have recently been revised. (A discussion of indications, contraindications and agents to induce emesis is in the chapter on emetics and antiemetics.) Activated charcoal is becoming the usual first method of gastrointestinal decontamination in many acutely poisoned people presenting to the emergency room. Ipecac syrup may still be useful in treating poisoned children at home or those people who have ingested poisons not adsorbed by activated charcoal. If emesis is induced at home, it is essential for the health practitioner to follow up treatment with telephone calls to check on the person's status, as persistent vomiting and diarrhea may occur with the use of ipecac syrup. If emesis is contraindicated, gastric lavage may be performed in the hospital emergency department to remove the poison.

Emesis and gastric lavage have limited value once the drug passes the pylorus of the stomach. They may even waste valuable time, which could be used to place activated charcoal in the gastrointestinal tract. Substances usually pass through the pylorus within one hour of ingestion; transit may be delayed if gastric motility is reduced (for example, by anticholinergic or narcotic drugs) or if the drug has formed concretions.

Activated Charcoal

Activated charcoal is commonly used as initial therapy in poisoned individuals presenting to the emergency room. It also may be used after emesis or gastric lavage. Activated charcoal adsorbs the poison in the intestinal tract and allows it to pass with the stool, thus preventing its absorption. Activated charcoal is the residue of burnt organic matter (for example, wood), which is activated by treatment at high temperatures with various gases and acids to increase its surface area. Charcoal tablets, charcoal briquets, burnt toast and universal antidote (50 per cent burnt toast, 25 per cent tannic acid or strong tea, and 25 per cent magnesium oxide or milk of magnesia) are all ineffective and should not be used. Activated charcoal is not effective for adsorbing cyanide, lithium, acids or alkalis, iron, fluoride, boric acid, lead, ethyl alcohol, methyl alcohol, or petroleum distillates. It may impair endoscopic visualization of the esophagus if used with acid or alkali ingestion. Activated charcoal will bind with ipecac syrup and cause it to lose its efficacy. Activated charcoal may be required in mixed overdoses that include acetaminophen, but it should not be administered concurrently with oral N-acetylcysteine as binding may occur.

Relative efficacies of gastrointestinal decontamination procedures have been compared in human volunteers with varying results. Caution needs to be used in extrapolating data from studies using non-toxic doses in healthy human volunteers to the poisoning situation involving massive doses in uncontrolled environments.

The dose of activated charcoal is 50 to 100 g in adults and 10 to 25 g in children (1 g/kg). It is administered as an aqueous slurry (that is, having a soup-like consistency), using at least 30 to 60 mL of water for each 10 g of activated charcoal, or in combination with a cathartic such as sorbitol. It is given over 15 minutes to avoid gastric distention and emesis.

The administration of multiple doses, such as 25 to 50 g every 4 to 6 hours, may increase clearance, decrease the half-life and prevent desorption of some poisons from the charcoal. Multiple doses of activated charcoal should not be used in people with intestinal obstruction or peritonitis. It should be used with extreme caution in people with adynamic ileus or absent bowel sounds. Activated charcoal is administered until the person improves and drug concentration decreases. Activated charcoal has been shown to increase the elimination of amitriptyline, carbamazepine, dapsone, dextropropoxyphene, digitoxin, digoxin, phenobarbital, phenylbutazone, sotalol and theophylline. It has been suggested that activated charcoal, by adsorbing drugs in the gastrointestinal fluids, creates a concentration gradient between blood and the gastrointestinal fluid. This gradient causes the drug to diffuse back into the gastrointestinal fluid. Activated charcoal must be replaced as it is excreted.

Activated charcoal does not appear to have many side effects. Constipation may occur, but can be alleviated by using a cathartic. Pulmonary aspiration causing airway obstruction has also been reported. The user should be warned that the stool probably will be black.

It has been suggested that activated charcoal be kept in homes as an alternative to ipecac syrup. This practice has not been well evaluated and is not currently recommended by the American or Canadian Associations of Poison Control Centres.

Cathartics

Cathartics may speed the transit of the charcoal-poison complex through the gastrointestinal tract and may prevent desorption of the poison. Studies in normal volunteers have raised doubts about the effectiveness of cathartics in managing poisonings. Nonetheless, they continue to be widely used. Oil-based cathartics are not used as they may increase absorption of lipophilic drugs or may cause lipid aspiration pneumonia if the individual vomits. Saline cathartics (magnesium sulfate, sodium sulfate, magnesium citrate) or sorbitol are usually recommended.

The dose of sodium or magnesium sulfate is 250 mg/kg of a 10 to 25 per cent solution up to 30 g per dose. The dose of magnesium citrate is 4 mL/kg up to 300 mL for adults and 0.5 mL/kg for children. The recommended dose of sorbitol is 1–2 g/kg. Many premixed activated charcoal preparations contain 70 per cent sorbitol solutions. To prevent excessive catharsis in children the 70 per cent sorbitol solution should be diluted with equal parts of water to produce a 35 per cent solution or a commercial 20 per cent solution should be used.

Fluid and electrolyte status must be monitored carefully in very young and very old individuals. Cathartics should be used with extreme caution in people with adynamic ileus or absent bowel sounds. Cathartics should not be used in people with abdominal trauma, intestinal obstruction or severe diarrhea. Sodium-containing cathartics should be avoided by individuals with hypertension or congestive heart failure; magnesium-containing cathartics should be avoided by people with renal failure. When using multiple doses of activated charcoal, cathartics should not be given with each dose;

Poisoning and Overdose

Table I *Poisoning with Nonprescription Drugs*

Substance	Toxic dose[1]	Toxic symptoms[2]	General management[3]	Special therapy[4]
Acetaminophen	ingestions of ≥140mg/kg need serum acetaminophen level and liver enzyme determination; 5.5 g has caused toxicity in an adult; 5 g over 24 hours has been fatal in a child	nausea, anorexia, vomiting, abdominal discomfort, diaphoresis, 1–24 hr; symptoms decrease, 24–48 hr; hepatic toxicity, 3–5 days	consider gastrointestinal decontamination	N–acetylcysteine: I.V. protocol: 150 mg/kg over 15 min, then 50 mg/kg over 4 hr, then 100 mg/kg over 16 hr. Oral protocol: 140 mg/kg initially, then 70 mg/kg every 4 hr for 17 doses
Anesthetics (topical)	variable; usually >5–10 mg/kg in adults; 300–600 mg lidocaine orally in a child; excessive topical application has been reported; death has resulted from aspiration following topical administration to the oral mucosa	gastrointestinal irritation, hypotension, arrhythmias, convulsions, bradycardia, methemoglobinemia, aspiration	consider gastrointestinal decontamination; ipecac should not be used due to the potential for aspiration or development of seizures	oxygen if cyanotic; methylene blue 1–2 mg/kg I.V. of a 1% solution over 5–10 min
Antacids	toxicity unlikely	calcium carbonate may cause hypercalcemia; sodium bicarbonate may cause hypernatremia and metabolic alkalosis; a concretion may occur during concomitant ranitidine therapy	gastrointestinal decontamination usually not necessary	
Antihistamines	variable; 3–4 times recommended total daily dose may cause symptoms in children; symptoms may occur from topical administration	children: hyperexcitability, tremors, ataxia, hallucinations; adults: CNS depression, convulsions, anticholinergic effects, arrhythmias, shock	consider gastrointestinal decontamination	do not use salicylates to reduce fever
Ascorbic acid	not usually toxic; may cause precipitation of cysteine or oxalate stones in predisposed individuals when used in high doses	gastrointestinal irritation, diarrhea	gastrointestinal decontamination not usually necessary.	
Atropine	variable; adults 100 mg; children 10 mg may be lethal; toxicity reported following administration of eye drops	dilation of pupils, hyperpyrexia, hallucinations, convulsions, tachycardia	consider gastrointestinal decontamination	physostigmine only for life threatening symptoms unresponsive to other therapies
Benzalkonium chloride	1–3 g in adults may be lethal	gastrointestinal irritation, shock, convulsions, paralysis	consider dilution; do not use ipecac syrup or activated charcoal if concentrated solution (>10%) ingested	oxygen if cyanotic

Table I *(Cont'd) Poisoning with Nonprescription Drugs*

Substance	Toxic dose[1]	Toxic symptoms[2]	General management[3]	Special therapy[4]
Benzyl benzoate	low order of toxicity; adults 1 g/kg; children 18 g; may be lethal	gastrointestinal irritation, CNS stimulation, incoordination, convulsions	gastrointestinal decontamination not usually necessary	
Boric acid	variable; toxicity from single acute ingestion is rare; 200 mg/kg may produce toxicity; symptoms may occur following chronic or multiple exposures; fatalities seen with repeated application to raw skin	gastrointestinal irritation, convulsions, renal failure, skin eruptions, CNS depression	consider gastrointestinal decontamination; activated charcoal not very effective	
Bromides	adults 20–30 g may be lethal	gastrointestinal irritation, apathy, hallucination, delirium, paralysis, skin eruptions, coma	consider gastrointestinal decontamination; activated charcoal is effective for organic but not inorganic poisonings	sodium chloride or ammonium chloride to promote excretion
Caffeine	adults 150–200 mg/kg may be lethal; toxic effect in adults at 15 mg/kg	gastrointestinal irritation, CNS stimulation, paralysis, convulsions, coma, hypotension, cardiac arrhythmias, hyperglycemia, metabolic acidosis	consider gastrointestinal decontamination	
Camphor	children 1 g may be lethal; 30 mg/kg may see major toxic symptoms	gastrointestinal irritation, CNS stimulation, convulsions, coma, hepatotoxicity	ipecac is contraindicated since convulsions may occur suddenly and without warning; consider dilution, nasogastric aspiration and activated charcoal	
Chlorates (sodium or potassium)	adults 15 g; children 2 g may be lethal	gastrointestinal irritation, hemolysis, convulsions, methemoglobinemia, coma	dilution; consider gastrointestinal decontamination	sodium thiosulfate 2–5 g in 200 mL of 5% sodium bicarbonate, orally
Dextromethorphan	10–30 mg/kg may be toxic; as little as 90 mg in a 3 month child over 24 hr has resulted in toxic symptoms	neasea, vomiting, constipation, lethargy, ataxia, hallucinations, excitation, respiratory depression	consider gastrointestinal decontamination	naloxone 0.01–0.1 mg/kg (child); 0.4–2.0 mg (adult) I.V. push: repeat as needed to a maximum 10 mg

Chapter 34

Poisoning and Overdose

Table I (Cont'd) Poisoning with Nonprescription Drugs

Substance	Toxic dose[1]	Toxic symptoms[2]	General management[3]	Special therapy[4]
Ephedrine/ Pseudoephedrine	severe toxicity from these agents alone is rare; 2–3 times therapeutic dose of ephedrine may be toxic; 4–5 times therapeutic dose of pseudo-ephedrine may be toxic	gastrointestinal irritation, agitation, convulsions, hyperpyrexia, dilated pupils, tachycardia, arrhythmias hypertension	consider gastrointestinal decontamination	
Fluorides	32–64 mg/kg fluoride ion may be lethal; children may be symptomatic at 3–8 mg/kg; >10 mg/kg fluoride ion may be toxic	gastrointestinal irritation, hypocalcemia, tetany, convulsions, arrhythmias, hyperkalemia	give milk; consider ipecac syrup if greater than 8 mg/kg fluoride ion ingested; activated charcoal not very effective	calcium salts orally to bind fluoride; calcium gluconate 10% IV. may be needed in severe ingestion causing hypocalcemia
Hydrogen peroxide	low toxicity with 3–6% solution; severe burns with concentrated solutions	gastrointestinal irritation, abdominal distension, rupture secondary to gaseous expansion	dilution; gastrointestinal decontamination is usually not necessary and may complicate burns from concentrated solution (>10%); activated charcoal not very effective	gastric distention may require decompression via a nasogastric tube
Iodine	2–4 g of free iodine may be lethal in adults	gastrointestinal irritation, renal failure, shock, metabolic acidosis, esophageal stricture	consider dilution; do not induce vomiting if concentrated solution ingested; activated charcoal not likely effective	if concentrated solution ingested give milk, flour or starch
Iron	children 300–600 mg may be lethal; symptoms at 20–60 mg/kg	gastrointestinal irritation 1–6 hr; asymptomatic 6–24 hr; metabolic acidosis, hypotension, convulsions, fever, coma 12–24 hr; liver and renal failure 2–4 days	consider ipecac syrup; activated charcoal not very effective; whole bowel irrigation may be useful	deferoxamine 15 mg/kg/hr I.V. infusion (up to 90 mg/kg every 8 hr) or 90 mg/kg to a maximum of 1 g administered I.M. q8h (I.M. administration only if I.V. route unavailable)
Isopropanol	adult 90 mL has produced toxicity; 2–4 mL/kg may be lethal; in children coma and respiratory depression have followed sponge bathing	gastrointestinal irritation, CNS depression, respiratory depression, hypotension, hyperglycemia, hypoglycemia (rare), renal damage	consider gastrointestinal decontamination; activated charcoal not very effective	give glucose containing substances if hypoglycemia occurs
Magnesium sulfate	low toxicity in acute exposure; 30 g lethal in adult with renal damage	gastrointestinal irritation, CNS depression, dehydration, respiratory depression, cardiac arrest	dilute if concentrated solution; consider ipecac syrup; activated charcoal not very effective	calcium gluconate 1 mL/kg of a 10% solution IV. slowly up to a total of 10 mL
Merbromin	not readily absorbed; low toxicity from acute exposure	gastrointestinal irritation, renal damage	consider gastrointestinal decontamination	
Mineral Oil	low toxicity unless aspirated	nausea, diarrhea; respiratory distress on aspiration	gastrointestinal decontamination not usually necessary	

517

Poisoning and Overdose

Table I (Cont'd) *Poisoning with Nonprescription Drugs*

Substance	Toxic dose[1]	Toxic symptoms[2]	General management[3]	Special therapy[4]
Narcotics	highly variable; codeine: 5 mg/kg in children and 7–14 mg/kg in adults; symptoms at 1 mg/kg	pinpoint pupils, respiratory depression, hypotension, pulmonary edema, bradycardia, convulsions, renal damage	consider gastrointestinal decontamination	naloxone 0.01–0.1 mg/kg (child) 0.4–2.0 mg (adult) I.V. push, repeat as needed to a maximum of 10 mg; continuous naloxone infusion may be used
Nitrites/Nitrates	nitroglycerin 200 mg may be lethal	gastrointestinal irritation, hypotension, cyanosis, methemoglobinemia	consider gastrointestinal decontamination	oxygen if cyanotic; methylene blue 1–2 mg/kg I.V. of a 1% solution over 5–10 min
Phenolphthalein	rarely causes toxicity; child 600 mg; adult 2 g	gastrointestinal irritation, fluid and electrolyte disturbances, hypersensitivity	consider gastrointestinal decontamination; do not give a cathartic	
Phenols	adults 1–15 g; topical exposure can cause burns (if conc >5%) and systemic toxicity	gastrointestinal irritation, CNS stimulation, coma, arrhythmias, renal damage, esophageal stricture, anion gap metabolic acidosis	consider dilution; do not use ipecac syrup or activated charcoal if a concentrated solution (>5%) ingested	
Phenylpropanolamine	50–75 mg may cause symptoms; death following 400 mg in an adult	hypertension, headache, intracranial hemorrhage, arrhythmias, renal failure	consider gastrointestinal decontamination	
Piperonyl butoxide	rarely toxic	gastrointestinal irritation, mild CNS depression	dilute; gastrointestinal decontamination not usually necessary	
Podophyllin	topical application of 1 g; oral, 325 mg may be lethal	confusion, dizziness lethargy, hypotension, renal failure, arrhythmias	consider gastrointestinal decontamination	
Salicylate	mild to moderate toxicity 100–300 mg/kg; severe 300–500 mg/kg; chronic 100 mg/kg/24 hr over 2 days; caution needed with very young or old, chronic ingestion or with enteric-coated tablets; methyl salicylate: 4 mL fatal in child	gastrointestinal irritation, hyperthermia, hyperpnea, CNS stimulation, coma, convulsions, hypoglycemia, hyperglycemia, metabolic acidosis, hypokalemia, respiratory alkalosis, tinnitus, pulmonary edema, arrhythmias	consider gastrointestinal decontamination	glucose, vitamin K, sodium bicarbonate, potassium
Silver nitrate	2 g may be lethal	gastrointestinal irritation, hypotension, convulsions, methemoglobinemia	consider dilution; do not induce vomiting or use activated charcoal due to corrosive nature of silver nitrate	oxygen if cyanotic; methylene blue 1–2 mg/kg I.V. of a 1% solution over 5–10 min for methemoglobinemia
Sodium bicarbonate	30 g baking soda can cause convulsions in a child; 10 g/kg in adult will produce hypernatremia	gastrointestinal irritation, hypernatremia, convulsions, shock	consider gastrointestinal decontamination; activated charcoal not very effective	

Poisoning and Overdose

Table I (Cont'd) *Poisoning with Nonprescription Drugs*

Substance	Toxic dose[1]	Toxic symptoms[2]	General management[3]	Special therapy[4]
Sodium chloride	adults: oral lethal dose 3 g/kg; children: 15–30 g can cause hypernatremia	gastrointestinal irritation, hypernatremia, convulsions, shock	consider gastrointestinal decontamination; activated charcoal not very effective	
Sodium hydroxide (e.g., Clinitest)	one Clinitest tablet has caused esophageal stricture following ingestion	gastrointestinal irritation, respiratory distress, esophageal injuries	consider dilution; do not use ipecac syrup or activated charcoal due to corrosive nature of sodium hydroxide	
Talc	systemic toxicity unlikely	respiratory distress if inhaled		
Vitamin A	acute: >100,000 IU in infants and 300,000 IU in children may cause toxicity; chronic: adults 25,000–75,000 IU daily for 3 weeks; children 25,000 IU daily for 3 weeks	headache, irritability, benign intracranial hypertension, diplopia, papilledema, skin ulcerations, nausea, vomiting, hepatosplenomegaly, teratogenesis	consider gastrointestinal decontamination	
Vitamin C	see Ascorbic acid			
Vitamin D	not acutely toxic; children 5,000 IU daily; adults 75,000 IU daily over several weeks	gastrointestinal irritation, renal damage, hypercalcemia, arrhythmias	consider gastrointestinal decontamination	diuresis, prednisone, calcitonin, sodium edetate, mithramycin to treat hypercalcemia
Vitamin E	not usually toxic acutely; chronic ingestion may produce symptoms	gastrointestinal upset, lethargy, headache	gastrointestinal decontamination not usually necessary	
Zinc chloride, sulfate, acetate	adults 3.5 g zinc chloride, 10 g zinc sulfate may be lethal	gastrointestinal irritation, liver and renal damage, hyperglycemia	consider dilution; do not induce vomiting or use activated charcoal due to corrosive nature of zinc	chelation with calcium disodium edetate if large body burden of zinc
Zinc oxide	adults 10 g may cause toxicity	gastrointestinal irritation	gastrointestinal decontamination not usually necessary	chelation with calcium disodium edetate is effective, but not usually necessary[3]

[1]Toxic or lethal dose reported where known. Such levels have been reported in as few as one person per billion exposures, perhaps giving a misleading impression of the normal toxicity. Toxic symptoms may occur below this dose. Each person should be assessed individually.

[2]Some of the more common toxic symptoms are reported. Symptoms may be delayed many hours in some cases.

[3]If severity of ingestion warrants treatment and no contraindications exist. Diluents should not be administered in people with severe respiratory distress or who have signs of gastric or esophageal perforation, shock or upper airway obstruction, or those who are unable to swallow, are convulsing or comatose. Ipecac syrup should be administered only if recent ingestion of potential severity where activated charcoal is

not being considered as ipecac administration delays the administration of activated charcoal. Do not use ipecac syrup in children under 6 months of age, if the individual is without a gag reflex, obtunded, convulsing or comatose or likely to rapidly become obtunded, comatose or convulsing or in an individual who has vomited profusely. Activated charcoal should not be administered if there is an intestinal obstruction; it should be used extremely cautiously in people with decreased intestinal peristalsis.

[4]Only drug therapy is listed. Protocols should be consulted for indication of antidotes. Forced diuresis, hemodialysis or charcoal hemoperfusion may benefit in some cases. If unfamiliar with administration of antidotes call the Poison Control Centre for monitoring protocols.

Poisoning and Overdose

Figure 1 *Suggested Approach for Treating a Poisoning*

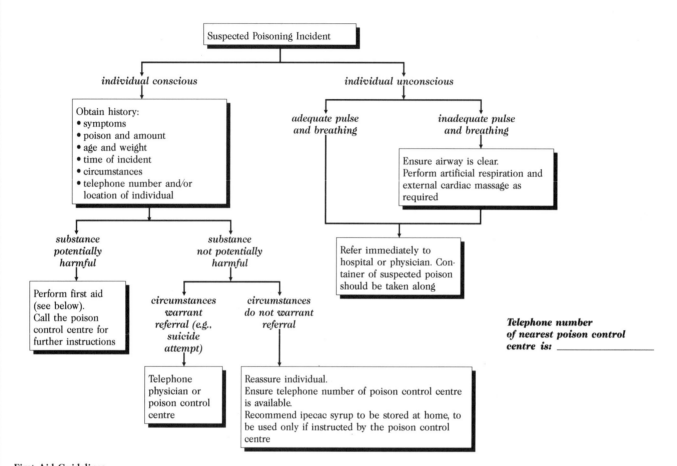

First Aid Guidelines

Poison Route

Skin: Flush skin with water for 10 minutes. Remove contaminated clothing. Wash area with mild soap and water. Avoid further exposure to poison.

Eyes: Irrigate eyes with gentle stream of water from a pitcher 5–7.5 cm from the eye for 5 minutes. Have the individual blink as much as possible. Do not force eyelid open.

Inhalation: Ensure breathing is adequate. Artificial respiration may be necessary. Doors and windows may have to be opened wide and individual removed from site.

Oral: For irritating substances (e.g., cosmetics, chemicals), unless the individual has severe respiratory distress or great difficulty swallowing, dilute with water. Give 30-60 mL in children and 90–120 mL in adults. Do not give fluids in the case of tablets or capsules until toxicity has been assessed.

excessive diarrhea may occur with resultant fluid and electrolyte disturbances.

Poisoning with Nonprescription Drugs

A list has been compiled of some ingredients of nonprescription drugs that may be potentially toxic (see Table I). The lethal or toxic dose (if known) and symptoms that may occur are also provided. Available data are poor and incomplete for some agents due to the small number of cases reported. Symptoms may occur at lower doses or may be delayed, especially with enteric-coated preparations. Each person must be assessed individually, based on age, weight, time since ingestion, amount ingested and symptoms. All suicide attempts and potential cases of child neglect should be referred to a health care

facility. If the person is coming into an emergency department, the pharmacist should give instructions to bring the original container and a sample of the emesis (if any) in a clean jar.

Treating poisonings requires knowledge, training and experience. Poison control centres have been established to provide comprehensive poison information services. Pharmacists should refer all calls to the poison control centre after they have provided first aid instructions. *The Compendium of Pharmaceuticals and Specialties* lists poison control centres in Canada. Adequate follow-up is essential for all potentially toxic ingestions and poison control centres are staffed with trained personnel to do this.

Preventing Poisonings

Pharmacists have a role to play in educating consumers on how to

Poisoning and Overdose

prevent poisonings. The following recommendations apply to pharmacists advising consumers.

- Instruct parents to have ipecac syrup at home to be used only on the advice of the poison control centre, pharmacist or physician.
- Tell the consumer to have the telephone number of the poison control centre readily accessible.
- Assist parents and grandparents in selecting nonprescription drug products with the best closures and recommend reasonable quantities
- Avoid recommending products that look like candy.
- Prescription drugs should be dispensed in containers with safety closures.
- Tell consumers to store all drugs in original containers with labels intact; keep them out of reach of children; and replace them for safe storage immediately after use with lids securely fastened.
- Remind consumers to read all labels on containers and follow directions accurately. Be aware that some directions for first aid may be outdated and even be harmful.
- Tell consumers to discard outdated or unused medications by flushing them down the toilet or taking them to the pharmacy for disposal.

Suggested Readings

Pharmacists may find the following references on poisoning useful additions to their library:

- Freeman Kent DA, Willis GA, eds. *Poison management manual.* Ottawa: Canadian Pharmaceutical Association, 1989.
- Dreisbach RH, ed. *Handbook of poisoning: prevention, diagnosis and treatment.* Los Altos: Lange, 1987.
- Goldfrank LR, Flomenbaum NE, Lewin A, et al, eds. *Toxicologic emergencies.* Norwalk: Appleton-Century-Crofts, 1990.
- Haddad LM, Winchester JF, eds. *Clinical management of poisoning and drug overdose.* Philadelphia: WB Saunders, 1990.

Ask the Consumer

Q. How old is the person?

- Ipecac syrup should not be administered at home to a child less than 6 months of age or an adult over 65 years of age. The age of the person may affect assessment and treatment; for example, age affects the person's metabolism and hence distribution of the drug. Cathartics must be used cautiously in both the very young and very old due to potential fluid and electrolyte imbalance.

Q. How much does the person weigh?

- This information is needed to calculate the toxic or lethal dose on a basis of mg/kg (for solids, such as acetylsalicylic acid) or mL/kg (for liquids, such as isopropanol).

Q. What has been ingested? Was alcohol also ingested?

- Ask about the type of product, the specific brand, ingredients, manufacturer, identification markings on the capsules or tablets, and information about treatment of poisoning on the label. Treatment information on the label may be outdated. Determine if inducing vomiting is contraindicated such as in the case of ingesting a corrosive product. Determine if alcohol was also

consumed; it may potentiate the central nervous system depressant effect of some drugs.

Q. What is the container size? When was it purchased?

- Information on container size, purchase date of the product and how often it was used helps in estimating container fullness. The size of the container opening can provide information on how much a child may have ingested. Pharmacy client records may be useful for estimating the amount ingested.

Q. When was the substance ingested?

- Peak serum drug concentration may be delayed up to 24 hours with enteric-coated tablets and products such as chloral hydrate that form conglomerates.

Q. How does the person feel?

- Refer symptomatic people to the emergency department. Many asymptomatic people may also need a referral.

Q. Does the person have any chronic diseases or take any chronic medications?

- Certain disease states and drugs predispose a person to toxicity.

Q. Were other children involved?

- Often the toxic substance is shared among several children.

Q. Have you tried any remedies?

- Although the ingestant may be nontoxic, the home remedy may be toxic. For example, salt water used to induce emesis in children has been fatal.

Q. How did the poisoning happen?

- All suicide attempts and suspected cases of child abuse must be referred.

Q. Do you know about the poison control centre?

- If the situation is dangerous, the caller must be told to call the poison control centre for immediate instructions, information about product ingredients and any additional information.

  If the situation is not dangerous, the caller should be reassured and provided with information on the poison control centre, first aid and poison prevention.

References

Introduction

Poison control statistics, 1987. Ottawa: Health and Welfare Canada, 1987.

General Management

Dean BL, Peterson R, Garrettson LK, et al. American association of poison control centers policy statement. Gastrointestinal dilution with water as a first aid procedure in poisoning. Vet Hum Toxicol 1983;25:55–6.

Henderson ML, Picchioni AL, Chin L. Evaluation of oral dilution as a first aid measure in poisoning. J Pharm Sci 1966;55:1311–3.

Knopp R. Caustic ingestions. JACEP 1979;8:329–36.

Rumack BH, Burrington JD. Caustic ingestions: a rational look at diluents. Clin Toxicol 1977;11:27–34.

Emesis and Gastric Lavage

Kulig K, Bar-Or D, Cantrill SV, et al. Management of acutely poisoned patients

Poisoning and Overdose

without gastric emptying. Ann Emerg Med 1985;14:562–7.

Mowry JB, Sketris IS, Czajka PA. Ipecac syrup for poisonings at home: availability, compliance, and response monitored by telephone. Am J Hosp Pharm 1981;38:1028–30.

Vale JA, Meredith TJ, Proudfoot AT. Syrup of ipecacuanha: is it really useful? Br Med J 1986;293:1321.

Activated Charcoal

Comstock EG, Boisaubain EV, Comstock BS, et al. Assessment of the efficacy of activated charcoal following gastric lavage in acute drug emergencies. J Toxicol Clin Toxicol 1982;19:149–63.

Cooney DO. In vitro evidence for ipecac inactivation by activated charcoal. J Pharm Sci 1978;67:426–7.

Curtis RA, Barone J, Giacona N. Efficacy of ipecac and activated charcoal/cathartic: prevention of salicylate absorption in a simulated overdose. Arch Intern Med 1984;144:48–52.

Greensher J, Mofenson HC, Picchioni AL, et al. Activated charcoal updated. JACEP 1979;8:261–3.

Jackson JE, Picchioni AL, Chin L. Contraindications for activated charcoal use (Letter). Ann Emerg Med 1980;9:599.

Katona BG, Siegel EG, Cluxton RJ. The new black magic: activated charcoal and new therapeutic uses. J Emerg Med 1987;5:9–18.

Klein-Schwartz W, Oderda GM. Adsorption of oral antidotes for acetaminophen poisoning (methionine and N-acetylcysteine) by activated charcoal. Clin Toxicol 1981;18:283–90.

Levy G. Gastrointestinal clearance of drugs with activated charcoal (Editorial). N Engl J Med 1982;307:676–8.

Neuvonen PJ. Clinical pharmacokinetics of oral activated charcoal in acute intoxications. Clin Pharmacokinetic 1982;7:465–89.

Pollack MM, Dunbar BS, Holbrook PR, et al. Aspiration of activated charcoal and gastric contents. Ann Emerg Med 1981;10:528–9.

Sketris IS, Mowry JB, Czajka PA, et al. Saline catharsis: effect on aspirin bioavailability in combination with activated charcoal. J Clin Pharmacol 1982;22:59–64.

Tenebein M, Cohen S, Sitar DS. Efficacy of ipecac induced emesis, orogastric lavage, and activated charcoal for acute drug overdose. Ann Emerg Med 1987;16:838–41.

Tenebein M. Pediatric toxicology: current controversies and recent advances. Curr Probl Pediatr 1986;16:183–233.

Cathartics

Dreisbach RH, ed. Handbook of poisoning: prevention, diagnosis and treatment. Los Altos: Lange Medical Publications, 1987.

Easom JM, Caracio TR, Lovejoy FH. Evaluation of activated charcoal and magnesium citrate in the prevention of aspirin absorption in humans. Clin Pharm 1982;1:154–6.

Farley TA. Severe hypernatremic dehydration after use of an activated charcoal-sorbitol suspension. J Pediatr 1986;109:716–22.

McNamara RM, Aaron CK, Gemborys M, Daviheiser S. Sorbitol catharsis does not enhance efficacy of charcoal in a simulated acetaminophen overdose. Ann Emerg Med 1988;17:243–6.

Minocha A, Herold DA, Burns DE, et al. Effect of activated charcoal sorbitol mixture in healthy individuals. J Toxicol Clin Toxicol 1985;22:529–36.

Riegel JM, Becker CE. Use of cathartics in toxic ingestions. Ann Emerg Med 1981;10:254–8.

Rumack BH, ed. Poisindex. Denver: Micromedex, 1991.

Poisoning with Nonprescription Drugs

Ackland FM. Hallucinations in a child drinking triprolidine/pseudoephedrine linctus. Lancet 1984;1(8387):1180.

Alexander CB, McBay AJ, Hudson RP. Isopranolol and isopropanol deaths—ten years' experience. J Forensic Sci 1982;27:541–8.

Amitai Y, Whitesell L, Lovejoy FH. Death following accidental lidocaine overdose in a child (Letter). N Engl J Med 1986;314:182–3.

Anonymous. Phenylpropanolamine over the counter (Editorial). Lancet 1982;1:839.

Aronow R, Spiegel RW. Implications of camphor poisoning. Drug Intell Clin Pharm 1976;10:631–4.

Banner W, Tong TG. Iron poisoning. Pediatr Clin North Am 1986;33:393–409.

Bayless JM, Tinanoff N. Diagnosis and treatment of acute fluoride toxicity. J Am Dent Assoc 1985;110:209–11.

Buchanan N, Cane RD, Glantz R, et al. Phenolphthalein poisoning: a case report. S Afr Med J 1976;50:1060–1.

Burruss GL, Van Voorst SJ, Crawford AJ, et al. Small bowel obstruction from an antacid bezoar: a ranitidine-antacid interaction? South Med J 1986;79:917–8.

Cotton WH, Davidson PJ. Aspiration of baby powder (Letter). N Engl J Med 1985;313:1662.

Dietz AJ Jr. Amphetamine-like reactions to phenylpropanolamine. JAMA 1981;245:601–2.

Dipalma JR. Vitamin toxicity. Am Fam Physician 1978;18:106–9.

Done AK. Aspirin overdosage: incidence, diagnosis, and management. Pediatr 1978;62:890–7.

Down PF, Polak A, Regan RJ. A family with massive acute vitamin D intoxication. Postgrad Med J 1979;55:897–902.

Duffy WB, Senekjian HO, Knight TF, et al. Acute renal failure due to phenylpropanolamine. South Med J 1981;74:1548–9.

Dyck RF, Bear RA, Goldstein MB, et al. Iodine/iodide toxic reaction: case report with emphasis on nature of metabolic acidosis. Can Med Assoc J 1979;120:704–6.

Farris WA, Erdman JW Jr. Protracted hypervitaminosis A following long-term, low-level intake. JAMA 1982;247:1217–8.

Feldman MD, Behar M. A case of massive diphenhydramine abuse and withdrawal from use of the drug (Letter). JAMA 1986;255:3119–20.

Filley CM, Graff-Radford NR, Lacy JR, et al. Neurologic manifestations of podophyllin toxicity. Neurol 1982;32:308–11.

Filloux F. Toxic encephalopathy caused by topically applied diphenhydramine. J Pediatr 1986;108:1018–20.

Fischman RA, Fairclough GF, Cheigh JS. Iodide and negative anion gap (Letter). N Engl J Med 1978;298:1035–6.

Freeman Kent DA, Willis GA, eds. Poison management manual. Ottawa: Canadian Pharmaceutical Association, 1989.

Fruncillo RJ, Gibbons W, Bowman SM. CNS toxicity after ingestion of topical lidocaine (Letter). N Engl J Med 1982;306:426–7.

Garriott JC, Simmons LM, Poklis A, et al. Five cases of fatal overdose from caffeine-containing "look-alike" drugs. J Analyt Toxicol 1985;9:141–3.

Goldfrank LR, Bresnitz EA, Howland MA. Antiseptics. In: Goldfrank LR, Flomenbaum NE, Lewin A, et al, eds. Toxicologic emergencies. Norwalk: Appleton-Century-Crofts, 1990:249–56.

Hall AH, Rumack BH. Management of acute acetaminophen overdose. Am Fam Physician 1986;33:107–14.

Hays DP, Johnson BF, Perry R. Prolonged hallucinations following a modest overdose of tripelennamine. Clin Toxicol 1980;16:331–3.

Heifetz SB, Horowitz HS. Amounts of fluoride in self-administered dental products: safety considerations for children. Pediatr 1986;77:876–82.

Helliwell M, Nunn J. Mortality in sodium chlorate poisoning. Br Med J 1979;1:1119.

Hestand HE, Teske DW. Diphenhydramine hydrochloride intoxication. J Pediatr 1977;90:1017–8.

Hooper RG, Conner CS, Rumack BH. Acute poisoning from over-the-counter sleep preparations. JACEP 1979;8:98–100.

Horne MK, Waterman MR, Simon LM, et al. Methemoglobinemia from sniffing butyl nitrite. Ann Intern Med 1979;91:417–8.

Howell JM. Alkaline ingestions. Ann Emerg Med 1986;15:820–5.

Howrie DL, Wolfson JH. Phenylpropanolamine induced hypertensive seizures. J Pediatr 1983;102:143–5.

Inkeles SB, Connor WE, Illingworth DR. Hepatic and dermatologic manifestations of chronic hypervitaminosis A in adults. Am J Med 1986;80:491–6.

Josephson GW, Stine RJ. Caffeine intoxication: a case of paroxysmal atrial tachycardia. JACEP 1976;5:776–8.

Kingswood JC, Routledge PA, Lazarus JH. A report of overdose with astemizole. Human Toxicol 1986;5:43–4.

Koeppel C, Tenczer J, Schirop Th, Ibe K. Camphor poisoning: abuse of camphor as a stimulant. Arch Toxicol 1982;51:101–6.

Krenzelok EP, Anderson GM, Mirick M. Massive diphenhydramine overdose resulting in death. Ann Emerg Med 1982;11:212–3.

Poisoning and Overdose

Lacouture PG, Wason S, Temple AR, et al. Emergency assessment of severity in iron overdose by clinical and laboratory methods. J Pediatr 1981; 99:89–91.

LaMantia RS, Andrews CE. Acute vitamin A intoxication. South Med J 1981;74:1012–4.

Larson WL, Rogers A. Overdosage from phenylpropranolamine: experience of the Hennepin regional poison center. Vet Hum Toxicol 1986;28:546–8.

Leslie PJ, Dyson EH, Proudfoot AT. Opiate toxicity after self poisoning with aspirin and codeine. Br Med J 1986;292:96.

Lewis JM, Klein-Schwartz W, Benson BE, et al. Continuous naloxone infusion in pediatric narcotic overdose. Am J Dis Child 1984;138:944–6.

Lewis JG. Adverse reactions to vitamins. Adverse Drug Reactions Bull 1980; 82:296–9.

Logie AW, Scott CM. Fatal overdosage of phenylpropanolamine. Br Med J 1984;289:591.

Lombaert A, Carton H. Benign intracranial hypertension due to A-hypervitaminosis in adults and adolescents. Eur Neurol 1976;14:340–50.

Mallory A, Schaefer JW. Clinitest ingestion. Br Med J 1977;2:105–7.

Manoguerra AS. Iron. In: Skoutakis VA, ed. Clinical toxicology of drugs: principles and practice. Philadelphia: Lea & Febiger, 1982:271–8.

Martinez TT, Jaeger RW, deCastro FJ, et al. A comparison of the absorption and metabolism of isopropyl alcohol by oral, dermal and inhalation routes. Vet Hum Toxicol 1986;28:233–6.

McCormick MA, Lacouture PG, Gaudreault P, et al. Hazards associated with diaper changing. JAMA 1982;248:2159–60.

McFarland MF, McFarland J. Accidental ingestion of podophyllum. Clin Toxicol 1981;8:973–7.

McGuigan MA. Benzocaine-induced methemoglobinemia (Letter). Can Med Assoc J 1981;125:816.

McGuigan MA. Death due to salicylate poisoning in Ontario. Can Med Assoc J 1986;135:891–4.

Mesnard B, Ginn DR. Excessive phenylpropanolamine ingestion followed by subarachnoid hemorrhage (Letter). South Med J 1984;77(7):939.

Mofenson HC, Caraccio TR, Miller H, et al. Lidocaine toxicity from topical mucosal application. Clin Pediatr 1983;22:190–2.

Monsour PA, Kruger BJ, Petrie AF, et al. Acute fluoride poisoning after ingestion of sodium fluoride tablets. Med J Aust 1984;141:503–5.

Moriarity RW. Guide to managing narcotic overdose. Drug Ther 1982;12: 153,157,160–1.

Nogen AG, Bremner JE. Fatal acetaminophen overdosage in a young child. J Pediatr 1978;92:832–3.

Normann SA, Manoguerra AS. Prospective review of cough/cold preparation ingestion guidelines (Abstract). Vet Hum Toxicol 1986;28:493.

Noseda A, Adler M, Ketelbant P, et al. Massive vitamin A intoxication with ascites and pleural effusion. J Clin Gastroenterol 1985;7:344–9.

Olson ML, McEvoy GK. Methemoglobinemia induced by local anesthetics. Am J Hosp Pharm 1981;38:89–93.

Paterson CR. Vitamin D poisoning: survey of causes in 21 patients with hypercalcaemia. Lancet 1980;1:1164–5.

Pentel P. Toxicity of over-the-counter stimulants. JAMA 1984;252:1898–903.

Potter JL. Acute zinc chloride ingestion in a young child. Ann Emerg Med 1981;10:267–9.

Prescott LF. Treatment of severe acetaminophen poisoning with intravenous acetylcysteine. Arch Intern Med 1981;141:386–9.

Puczynski MS, Phillip E, Rust C. Cardiopulmonary arrest due to misuse of viscous lidocaine. Arch Otolaryngol 1985;111:768–9.

Roberts HJ. Perspective on vitamin E as therapy. JAMA 1981;246:129–33.

Rothstein P, Dornbusch J, Shaywitz BA. Prolonged seizures associated with the use of viscous lidocaine. J Pediatr 1982;101:461–3.

Rumack BH, Peterson RC, Koch GG, et al. Acetaminophen overdose: 662 cases with evaluation of oral acetylcysteine treatment. Arch Intern Med 1981; 141:380–5.

Sawyer DR, Conner CS, Rumack BH. Managing acute toxicity from nonprescription stimulants. Clin Pharm 1982;1:529–33.

Siegel E, Wason S. Camphor toxicity. Pediatr Clin North Am 1986;33:375–9.

Spector R. Activated charcoal for gastrointestinal decontamination of the poisoned patient. Iowa Med 1986;76:231–8.

Swetnam SM, Florman AL. Probable acetaminophen toxicity in an 18-month-old infant due to repeated overdosing. Clin Pediatr 1984;23:104–5.

Taylor CD, Cowart CO, Ryan NT. Isopropanol intoxication: managing the coma. Hosp Pract 1985;20:173–5.

Temple AR. Acute and chronic effects of aspirin toxicity and their treatment. Arch Intern Med 1981;141:364–9.

Thornton WE. Sleep aids and sedatives. JACEP 1977;6:408–12.

Troutman WG. The pharmacist and poisoning (Editorial). Am J Hosp Pharm 1978;35:1351.

Veltri JC. Regional poison control services. Hosp Formul, 1982; 1469–72,1479–81,1484–6.

Winek CL, Wahba W, Williams K, et al. Caffeine fatality: a case report. Forensic Sci Int 1985;29:207–11.

Yolken R, Konecny P, McCarthy P. Acute fluoride poisoning. Pediatr 1976; 58:90–3.

Appendix A

Nonprescription Chemicals

Dawn M. Frail

The purpose of this appendix is to provide the pharmacist with a concise list of chemical products which are largely and, in some cases, exclusively sold in pharmacies as nonprescription items. Table I lists these substances alphabetically, gives their uses, directions for use, and specific information on storage, toxicity, etc.

It should be noted the indications and doses stated on many product packages do not agree with those recommended in the literature. For example, the indications for use on one bottle of camphorated oil state the product can be used to treat symptoms of bronchitis and chest colds. This might lead the consumer to use such a product for inhalation or even use it orally. Similarly, while references do state that camphor spirit can be taken internally as a stimulant and carminative, the oral dose which appears on the label of this product is unconfirmed (see Table I).

This appendix will not address the treatment of toxicity or overdose with these substances (see the chapter on poisoning and overdose); however, it is important to remember that many of these substances are potentially toxic. For example, menthol, camphor, and eucalyptol are often regarded as inactive ingredients but have, in fact,

been responsible for a number of adverse effects and deaths when these substances were inhaled in high concentrations.

In addition to the information given in Table I, certain chemicals warrant special mention. Potassium nitrate (known as saltpeter) and sulfur are used in the production of fireworks and gunpowder. The purchase of these items by children should be supervised. Historically, potassium nitrate has been known as an anti-aphrodisiac; however, there is no information in the literature to support this indication. (Since potassium nitrate does have a mild diuretic effect, this could be the physiological basis for an anti-aphrodisiac effect in males). Presumably, the internal doses given on the packages of potassium nitrate represent diuretic doses, but most packages do not state indications for the product and several companies differ in their recommended doses.

Salts of lemon are commonly referred to as oxalic acid. However, salts of lemon actually contain both oxalic acid and cream of tartar.

At one time sodium borate (borax) was recommended as a mouthwash or gargle in the treatment of aphthous ulcers. In view of its proven toxicity, it has been limited to external use only.

Table I *Chemicals with Pharmaceutical Applications*

Substance	Other Names	Uses	Directions for Use	Comments
Acetone		Solvent for fats, oils, waxes, resins, rubber, plastics, lacquers, varnishes, and rubber cements		Store away from heat in an airtight container. Protect from light. One of the solvents abused in glue sniffing
		Vehicle for drying skin		
		Nail polish remover		
Aluminum potassium sulfate	Alum, aluminum ammonium sulfate	Precipitates proteins and is a powerful astringer	Apply directly to canker sores	Store in airtight containers, available as a powder or as a solid (styptic pencil)
		Hemostatic	Apply directly to the wound	
		Hyperhidrosis	Bathe in a 2% w/v solution twice daily	
		Softens corns and soothes sore feet	Soak feet in a 5–10% w/v solution once daily	
		Throat gargle or douche	5 mL dissolved in 300 mL water 3 to 4 times daily	
		Making pickles	Use a pinch in each bottle of pickles	

Table I *(Cont'd)* *Chemicals with Pharmaceutical Applications*

Substance	Other Names	Uses	Directions for Use	Comments
Ammonium bicarbonate or ammonium carbonate	Smelling salts, Baker's ammonia	Reflex expectorant	200–600 mg orally or by inhalation once daily	Store in a cool place and keep tightly closed
		Carminative		
		As a leavening agent in place of sodium bicarbonate		
Aromatic ammonia spirit		Rubefacient, counterirritant		Store in a cool place and keep tightly closed
Ascorbic acid	Vitamin C	Vitamin and antioxidant (prevents darkening and flavor changes in fruit; restores the original color of sliced meat)	For freezing, canning, and preserving; mix 1.25–2.5 mL with each 250 mL of sugar syrup	Store in airtight, nonmetallic containers, protect from light
Boric acid	Boracic acid	Weak bacteriostatic and fungistatic		Do not use internally
Camphor (solid)		Plasticizer, anti-infective	External use only, store in airtight containers in a cool place	
Camphorated oil (camphor 20%)	Camphor liniment	Counterirritant, antipruritic		As for camphor
Camphor spirit (camphor 10%)		Counterirritant, antipruritic		As for camphor
		Stimulant and carminative	Orally: 30 drops on 5 mL of sugar	
Citric acid		Acidulant (in making lemonade, lemon pie and pharmaceuticals)		Store in a cool place in airtight containers
Compound benzoin tincture	Friar's Balsam	Inhalation in bronchitis and acute laryngitis	5 mL added to 500 mL hot water	Store in a cool place, protect from light
		Internally as a reflex expectorant	4 mL on sugar	
		Antiseptic and styptic	Apply directly to the wound	
		Vehicle for podophyllin		
Copper sulfate		Ophthalmic astringent	Apply a 0.25–5% w/v solution to the eye	
		Treatment of eczema, impetigo, and intertrigo	Copper and Zinc Sulphates Lotion (BPC 1973) is applied as a wet dressing once or twice a day	
		Prevent the growth of algae in swimming pools	Add to pool water to make a concentration of 0.5–1 ppm	
Dextrose monohydrate	Dextrose, glucose, grape sugar	Nutrient replenisher	See chapter on antidiarrheals	The sweetening power is less than that of ordinary sugar

Table I *(Cont'd)* *Chemicals with Pharmaceutical Applications*

Substance	Other Names	Uses	Directions for Use	Comments
Eucalyptus oil		Inhalation in bronchitis and asthma	1.7 mL added to 500 mL hot water once daily	Store in a cool place. Protect from light.
		Internally for catarrh	1–4 drops on sugar	Can have adverse effects if inhaled in high concentrations
		Rubefacient	25% solution with olive oil	
		Aromatic in sauna	Place a few drops near the heat source	
Glycerin	Glycerol	Laxative		
		Externally for its humectant properties		
		To levigate powders and prepare ointments		
Halazone	Water purifying tablets 4-(dichlorosulphamoyl) benzoic acid	Drinking water purification	Dissolve five 4 mg tablets in 1 L of water. Allow to stand 30 minutes, then shake well prior to use	Protect tablets from light and humidity. Do not swallow tablets whole
Hamamelis water	Distilled witch hazel, witch hazel	Astringent, hemostatic	Apply directly to area	
Lemon, salts of	Rust and stain remover, oxalic acid	For removing ink, iron rust and fruit stains, cleaning leather and metals, and for removing the color from calico printing (removes potassium permanganate stains from enamel tubs)	Sprinkle powder over stains and pour hot water through it; repeat if necessary; rinse thoroughly with clear water	All traces of powder must be washed away before ironing. Corrosive; avoid contact with eyes or skin; do not keep near food or beverages; store in airtight containers
Magnesium sulfate	Epsom salts	Purgative	Adult dose: 5–15 mL in 250 mL of water before breakfast	Keep tightly closed; should not be used in persons with kidney ailments or when abdominal pain nausea, or vomiting is present.
		Laxative	Adult dose: 2.5–5 mL in 250 mL of water before breakfast	Note that there is a dried magnesium sulfate available. The dried form can be used instead of the crystalline form. The dried form tends to produce cloudy solutions whereas the crystalline form gives a clear solution
		Enema	A 50% w/v solution	
		A soak for its osmotic action	A 3% w/v solution once or twice a day	
Menthol		Carminative		
		Inhalation in bronchitis and sinusitis		Can have adverse effects if inhaled in high concentrations
		Antipruritic	1.25–16% w/v topically	
Methylsalicylate	Wintergreen oil	Counterirritant	10–60% w/v topically	External use only; store in a cool place in airtight containers; protect from light
		Solvent to clean coal tar from glassware		

Table I *(Cont'd) Chemicals with Pharmaceutical Applications*

Substance	Other Names	Uses	Directions for Use	Comments
Nitrous ether spirit	Sweet nitre spirit, sweet spirits of nitre	Diaphoretic		Store in a cool place in airtight containers; protect from light; not for internal use
Olive oil		Laxative	When given as a rectal injection: 100 to 500 mL warmed to 32°C	Store in airtight containers
		Emollient		
		For cooking and salads		
Peppermint spirit (peppermint oil 10%)	Peppermint essence, essence of peppermint	Carminative	Adults: 5–30 drops on sugar or in sweetened water Children: 2–5 drops according to age	Store in airtight containers, protect from light
		Flavoring agent		
		Perfumery		
Potassium nitrate	Saltpeter	In making fireworks		Store in airtight containers. Historically used as an anti-aphrodisiac but no evidence supports this indication
		Preservative		
		Diuretic	Adults: 300–1 000 mg daily	
Pumice		To remove stains from skin or nails	Make a thin paste with water or hydrogen peroxide and rub lightly	
		To remove tartar from teeth	Make a paste as above and apply using a toothbrush with an up and down movement	
Rose water		In the preparation of Indian foods		
		Perfumery		
Sodium borate	Borax, sodium tetraborate	To soften bath water	30 mL in bath	Store in cool place in airtight containers; poison
		To whiten clothes and remove stains and add brilliance to glassware	30 mL in wash water	
		At one time used as mouthwash or gargle in treating aphthous ulcers but due to toxicity, it is now limited to external use only		
Sublimed sulfur	Flowers of sulfur	Antiseptic and parasiticide	Use as a 10% ointment in soft paraffin. Apply 2–3 times daily	
		Acne therapy		
		Laxative	2.5–5 g 2–3 times daily in honey or molasses	
Tartaric acid	Cream of tartar	Acidulant (in making lemonade, lemon pies, etc.)		
Turpentine spirit		Rubefacient		Protect from light, store in airtight containers; not to be taken internally, avoid inhaling fumes
		To remove stains of paints, varnishes, waxes and resins		

References

Anonymous. Aerosols for colds. Med Lett Drugs Ther 1973;15:86–8.

Aronow R, Spigiel RW. Implications of camphor poisoning. Drug Intell Clin Pharm 1976;10:631–4.

Budavari S, ed. The Merck index: an encyclopedia of chemicals, drugs and biologicals. Rahway: Merck, 1989.

Chilcote RR, Williams B, Wolff LJ, et al. Sudden death in an infant from methemoglobinemia after administration of "sweet spirits of nitre". Pediatrics 1977;59(2):280–2.

Duhan SPS, Garg SN, Roy SK. Effect of age of plant on the quality of essential oil of peppermint. Indian J Pharm 1975;37:41–2.

Feig SA. Methemoglobinemia. In: Nathan DG, Oski FA, eds. Hematology of infancy and childhood. Philadelphia: Saunders, 1974:378.

Jass HE. Description and commentary on the OTC panel reviews: external analgesic products. Cosmet Toilet 1980;95:44–6.

Koppel C, Tenczer J, Schirop T, et al. Camphor poisoning; abuse of camphor as a stimulant. Arch Toxicol 1982;51:101–6.

Mercer FL. Trees and shrubs constitute the sources for important medicinals. Pharm Times 1977;43:103–10.

Phelan WJ. Camphor poisoning; over-the-counter dangers. Pediatrics 1976; 57(3):428–31.

Trestrail JH, Spartz ME. Camphorated and castor oil confusion and its toxic results. Clin Toxicol 1977;11(2):151–8.

Plakogiannis FM, Yaakob M. Influence of ointment bases on the in vitro release of methyl salicylate. Pharm Acta Helv 1977;52(10)236–8.

Reynolds JEF, ed. Martindale: the extra pharmacopoeia, London: Pharmaceutical Press, 1989.

Roberts MS, Favretto WA, Meyer A, et al. Topical bioavailability of methyl salicylate. Aust NZ J Med 1982;12:303–5.

Skoglund RR, Ware LL Jr, Schanberger JE. Prolonged seizures due to contact and inhalation exposure to camphor. A case report. Clin Pediatr 1977; 16(10):901–2.

Skoutakis VA, Koumbourlis TC. Camphor intoxication: diagnosis and management. Clin Toxicol Consult 1981;3(4):131–6.

Watson HR, Hems R, Rowsell DG, et al. New compounds with the menthol cooling effect. J Soc Cosmet Chem 1978;29:185–200.

Wilson JW. A substitute for chloroform in prescriptions (Corresp). Arch Dermatol 1977;113:982.